Frontiers in Reproduction
and Fertility Control

Frontiers in Reproduction and Fertility Control

A Review of the Reproductive Sciences and Contraceptive Development

Roy O. Greep
Project Director

Marjorie A. Koblinsky
Assistant Project Director

Sponsored by the Ford Foundation

The MIT Press
Cambridge, Massachusetts, and London, England

This book was set in V-I-P Times Roman by The MIT Press Computer Composition Group and printed on R & E Book and bound by The Alpine Press Inc. in the United States of America

Library of Congress Cataloging in Publication Data

Main entry under title:

Frontiers in reproduction and fertility control.
 Includes indexes.
 1. Human reproduction. 2. Contraception. I. Greep, Roy Orval, 1905– II. Koblinsky, Marjorie A. III. Ford Foundation.
QP251.F76   612'.6   77–24454
ISBN 0–262–07068–5

Contents

Contributors   ix

Preface   xiii

1   The Gonadotropic Hormones, LH (ICSH)   Harold Papkoff, Robert J. Ryan,
    and FSH   1   and Darrell N. Ward

2   The Chemistry and Biology of Human   Om P. Bahl
    Chorionic Gonadotropin and Its
    Subunits   11

3   Prolactin   25   Henry G. Friesen

4   Steroid Hormone Secretions   33   Seymour Lieberman, Erlio Gurpide,
                                                Mortimer Lipsett, and Hilton Salhanick

5   Hormonal Regulation of the Development,   J. M. Bahr, G. T. Ross, and
    Maturation, and Ovulation of the   A. V. Nalbandov
    Ovarian Follicle   40

6   The Endocrinology of Ovulation and   D. T. Baird and R. V. Short
    Corpus Luteum Formation, Function,
    and Luteolysis in Women   44

7   Induction of Ovulation   49   Carl Gemzell

8   Feedback Regulation of Reproductive   Neena B. Schwartz, Donald J. Dierschke,
    Cycles in Rats, Sheep, Monkeys, and   Charles E. McCormack, and Paul W. Waltz
    Humans, with Particular Attention to
    Computer Modeling   55

9   Secretion of Gonadotropins   90   Roger Guillemin, S. M. McCann,
                                                C. H. Sawyer, and J. M. Davidson

10 Brain Neurotransmitters and the Hypothalamic Control of Pituitary Gonadotropin Secretion 103

Richard J. Wurtman

11 Hypothalamic Influences on Pituitary Function in Humans 108

S. S. C. Yen, F. Naftolin, A. Lein, D. Krieger, and R. Utiger

12 Reproductive Immunology 128

K. A. Laurence

13 The Oviduct 132

R. J. Blandau, B. Brackett, R. M. Brenner, J. L. Boling, S. H. Broderson, C. Hamner, and L. Mastroianni, Jr.

14 The Biology of the Uterus 146

D. G. Porter and C. A. Finn

15 Embryogenesis 157

Anne McLaren

16 Clinical and Epidemiological Aspects of Induced Abortion 167

Christopher Tietze

17 Systemic Contragestational Agents 170

Sheldon J. Segal

18 Female Sterilization 178

Ralph M. Richart and Katherine F. Darabi

19 Intrauterine Contraception 188

Howard J. Tatum

20 The Morning-After Pill: A Report on Postcoital Contraception and Interception 203

John McLean Morris

21 Injectable Contraceptive Preparations 209

Daniel R. Mishell, Jr.

22 Bioengineering Aspects of Reproduction and Contraceptive Development 214

Thomas J. Lardner

23 The Role of Prostaglandins in Reproduction 219

Vivian J. Goldberg and Peter W. Ramwell

24   **Hormonal Control of Gene Expression in Reproductive Tissues**   236   Bert W. O'Malley

25   **Hormone-Receptor Interaction in the Mechanism of Reproductive Hormone Action**   245   E. V. Jensen, K. J. Catt, J. Gorski, and H. G. Williams-Ashman

26   **The Control of Testicular Function**   264   Emil Steinberger, Ronald S. Swerdloff, and Richard Horton

27   **Spermatogenesis**   293   Yves Clermont

28   **The Ultrastructure and Functions of the Sertoli Cell**   302   Don W. Fawcett

29   **Leydig Cells**   321   William B. Neaves

30   **The Blood-Testis Barrier**   338   B. P. Setchell

31   **The Structure of the Spermatozoon**   353   Don W. Fawcett

32   **The Metabolism of Mammalian Spermatozoa**   379   R. A. P. Harrison

33   **The Mammalian Accessory Sex Glands: A Morphological and Functional Analysis**   402   L. F. Cavazos

34   **The Epididymis**   411   David W. Hamilton

35   **Semen: Metabolism, Antigenicity, Storage, and Artificial Insemination**   427   Thaddeus Mann

36   **Capacitation of Spermatozoa and Fertilization in Mammals**   434   M. C. Chang, C. R. Austin, J. M. Bedford, B. G. Brackett, R. H. F. Hunter, and R. Yanagimachi

37   **Sperm Motility**   452   I. R. Gibbons

38 **Regulation of Male Fertility** **458**   C. Alvin Paulsen

39 **Assessment of Clinical Testing Methodology** **466**   Aníbal Faúndes and Ellen Hardy

40 **Historical Charts** **479**

Name Index **565**

Subject Index **571**

Contributors

C. R. Austin
Physiological Laboratory
Cambridge University
Cambridge, England

Om P. Bahl
Division of Cell and Molecular Biology
State University of New York at Buffalo
Buffalo, NY 14620

J. M. Bahr
Department of Animal Science
University of Illinois
Urbana, IL 61801

D. T. Baird
M.R.C. Unit of Reproductive Biology
Edinburgh, Scotland

J. M. Bedford
Department of Anatomy
Cornell University Medical College
1300 York Ave.
New York, NY 10021

R. J. Blandau
Department of Anatomy
University of Washington School of Medicine
Seattle, WA 98195

J. L. Boling
Department of Anatomy
University of Washington School of Medicine
Seattle, WA 98195

B. G. Brackett
Department of Obstetrics and Gynecology
University of Pennsylvania School of Medicine
Philadelphia, PA 19174

R. M. Brenner
Department of Anatomy
University of Oregon Health Science Center
School of Medicine
3181 S. W. Sam Jackson Park Road
Portland, OR 97201

S. H. Broderson
Department of Anatomy
University of Washington School of Medicine
Seattle, WA 98195

K. J. Catt
National Institute of Child Health and Human Development
National Institutes of Health
Bethesda, MD 20014

L. F. Cavazos
Department of Anatomy
Tufts University School of Medicine
Boston, MA 12111

M. C. Chang
Worcester Foundation for Experimental Biology
222 Maple Avenue
Shrewsbury, MA 01545

Yves Clermont
Department of Anatomy
McGill University
Montreal, Canada

Katherine F. Darabi
International Institute for the Study of Human Reproduction
College of Physicians and Surgeons
Columbia University
New York, NY 10032

J. M. Davidson
Department of Physiology
Stanford University
Stanford, CA 94305

Donald J. Dierschke
Department of Meat and Animal Science
University of Wisconsin
1223 Capitol Court
Madison, WI 53706

Aníbal Faúndes
Department of Obstetrics and Gynecology
State University of Campinas
Campinas, São Paulo, Brazil

Don W. Fawcett
Department of Anatomy
Harvard Medical School
Boston, MA 02115

C. A. Finn
Department of Physiology
The Royal Veterinary College
London NW10TU England

Henry G. Friesen
Department of Physiology
University of Manitoba
770 Bannatyne Ave.
Winnipeg, Manitoba R3E OW3
Canada

Carl Gemzell
Department of Obstetrics and Gynecology
Downstate Medical Center
Brooklyn, NY 11203

I. R. Gibbons
Pacific Biomedical Research Center
University of Hawaii
Honolulu, HI 96822

Vivian J. Goldberg
Department of Physiology and Biophysics
Georgetown Medical Center
Washington, D.C. 20007

J. Gorski
Department of Biochemistry
University of Wisconsin
Madison, WI 53706

Roger Guillemin
Neuroendocrinology Laboratory
The Salk Institute for Biological Studies
La Jolla, CA 92037

Erlio Gurpide
Department of Biochemistry and Obstetrics
Mt. Sinai School of Medicine
1176 Fifth Ave.
New York, NY 10029

David W. Hamilton
Department of Anatomy
Harvard Medical School
Boston, MA 02115

C. Hamner
Department of Obstetrics and Gynecology
University of Virginia School of Medicine
Charlottesville, VA 22901

Ellen Hardy
Department of Obstetrics and Gynecology
State University of Campinas
Campinas, São Paulo, Brazil

R. A. P. Harrison
A.R.C. Unit of Reproductive Physiology and
Biochemistry
307 Huntingdon Road
Cambridge, CB3 0JQ, England

Richard Horton
Department of Medicine
University of Southern California/Los Angeles County
Medical Center
Los Angeles, CA 90033

R. H. F. Hunter
University of Edinburgh
Edinburgh, Scotland

Elwood V. Jensen
Department of Biophysics
Ben May Laboratory for Cancer Research
University of Chicago
950 E. 59th St.
Chicago, IL 60637

D. Krieger
Division of Endocrinology
Mt. Sinai Medical Center
1 E. 100th St.
New York, NY 10029

Thomas J. Lardner
Department of Theoretical and Applied Mechanics
Talbot Laboratory
University of Illinois
Urbana, IL 61801

K. A. Laurence
The Population Council
Rockefeller University
New York, NY 10021

A. Lein
Department of Reproductive Medicine
University of California
San Diego School of Medicine
La Jolla, CA 92037

Seymour Lieberman
Department of Biochemistry
College of Physicians and Surgeons
Columbia University
New York, NY 10032

Mortimer Lipsett
Clinical Research Center
National Institutes of Health
Bethesda, MD 20014

Thaddeus Mann
Reproductive Research Branch
National Institute of Child Health and
Human Development
National Institutes of Health
Bethesda, MD 20014

L. Mastroianni, Jr.
Department of Obstetrics and Gynecology
University of Pennsylvania School of Medicine
Philadelphia, PA 19104

S. M. McCann
Department of Physiology
The University of Texas Health Science Center
Dallas, TX 75235

Charles E. McCormack
Department of Physiology
Chicago Medical School
2020 W. Ogden Ave.
Chicago, IL 60612

Anne McLaren
M.R.C. Mammalian Development Unit
University Hospital
Wolfson House
4 Stephenson Way
London NW1 2HE England

Daniel R. Mishell, Jr.
Department of Obstetrics and Gynecology
University of Southern California School of Medicine
Los Angeles, CA 90033

John McLean Morris
Yale University School of Medicine
New Haven, CT 06510

F. Naftolin
Department of Obstetrics and Gynecology
McGill University/Royal Victoria Hospital
Montreal, Quebec H3A 1A1
Canada

A. V. Nalbandov
Department of Animal Science
University of Illinois
Urbana, IL 61801

William B. Neaves
Department of Cell Biology
The University of Texas Health Science Center
Dallas, TX 75235

Bert W. O'Malley
Department of Cell Biology
Baylor College of Medicine
Houston, TX 77030

Harold Papkoff
University of California, San Francisco
San Francisco, CA 94143

C. Alvin Paulsen
Department of Medicine
University of Washington School of Medicine
Box 3145
Seattle, WA 98114

D. G. Porter
Department of Anatomy
The Medical School
Bristol BS8 1TD England

Peter W. Ramwell
Department of Physiology and Biophysics
Georgetown Medical Center
Washington, D.C. 20007

Ralph M. Richart
College of Physicians and Surgeons
Columbia University
New York, NY 10032

G. T. Ross
Reproductive Research Branch
National Institute of Child Health and Human
Development
National Institutes of Health
Bethesda, MD 20014

Robert J. Ryan
Mayo Clinic
Rochester, MN 55901

Hilton Salhanick
Department of Obstetrics and Gynecology
Harvard Medical School
Boston, MA 02115

C. H. Sawyer
Department of Anatomy
The University of California Health Science Center
Los Angeles, CA

Neena B. Schwartz
Department of Biology
Northwestern University
2153 Sheridan Road
Evanston, IL 60201

Sheldon J. Segal
Biomedical Division, The Population Council
Rockefeller University
New York, NY 10021

B. P. Setchell
Department of Biochemistry
Agricultural Research Council
Institute of Animal Physiology
Babraham, Cambridge CB2 4AT, England

R. V. Short
M. R. C. Unit of Reproductive Biology
Edinburgh, Scotland

Emil Steinberger
Department of Reproductive Medicine and Biology
The University of Texas Medical School at Houston
Houston, TX 77025

Ronald S. Swerdloff
Department of Medicine
University of California at Los Angeles
Harbor General Hospital Campus
Torrance, CA 90509

Howard J. Tatum
Biomedical Division, The Population Council
Rockefeller University
New York, NY 10021

Christopher Tietze
The Population Council
245 Park Ave.
New York, NY 10017

R. Utiger
Department of Medicine
University of Pennsylvania School of Medicine
Philadelphia, PA 19174

Paul W. Waltz
Equation Model Associates
Chicago, IL

Darrell N. Ward
M. D. Anderson Hospital and Tumor Institute
Houston, TX 77025

H. G. Williams-Ashman
University of Chicago
Chicago, IL 61637

Richard J. Wurtman
Department of Nutrition
Massachusetts Institute of Technology
Cambridge, MA 02142

R. Yanagimachi
John A. Burns School of Medicine
University of Hawaii
1960 East-West Road
Honolulu, HI 96822

S. S. C. Yen
Department of Reproductive Medicine
University of California, San Diego
P.O. Box 109
La Jolla, CA 92093

Preface

This volume of essays covering most of the major areas of research on the reproductive process and its control is part of a survey of research and funding in this area sponsored by the Ford Foundation. The primary aim was to obtain from active investigators personal assessments of where their fields stand in respect to major accomplishments, knowledge gained, and concepts formulated. The essayists were also asked to point out the possibilities for interfering with the reproductive process and to identify problems in urgent need of intensive study and early solution. We felt it to be of equal importance to specify what is not known as well as what is known, since the unknown will provide a challenge both to established investigators and to young persons seeking to contribute to the solution of this topmost social problem—population growth and the assurance of reproductive excellence.

The essays were solicited in 1973, and most were submitted in 1974. Progress since then has made some of the details reported obsolete or incomplete, and the contributions should be considered "state-of-the-art" only as of 1974. In its broad outlines, however, the territory surveyed in this collection has not changed.

The essayists were requested not to prepare either the customary annotated bibliography or the conventional review of the literature, both of which specify who did what when. We were especially interested in content and readability but realized that some helpful guidance to the literature was essential, especially for the uninitiated reader. In addition to the literature sources provided by the essayists, many key references will be found in the historical charts.

Inasmuch as the topics to be developed are of widely varying scope, those of modest proportions were prepared by a single author, whereas those covering broad areas were assigned to teams. These teams of scientists met one or more times to pool their knowledge and organize the undertaking.

These papers are essays in the true sense; they express the views, summations, and evaluations by the persons preparing the essays, all of whom are outstanding authorities in their special fields. A unique feature of this series of papers is that the approach used is, in each instance, the one preferred by and therefore best suited to the author or team of authors to present a narrative account of their particular field of scientific research. Although the format of the essays is not uniform, we find this diversity advantageous for the purpose at hand. It heightens interest and fosters a feeling of personal communication with the author(s). We have, therefore, dared break with tradition and have allowed the essays to stand essentially as they were submitted.

We have included a number of historical charts, each covering a broad area of research on the female or male reproductive systems. These were developed with the help of the related essays and other reviews. Although the preparation of each summary table was spearheaded by a single individual, they were all reviewed in detail by a group of active workers and checked by one or more clinicians for interference points of immediate or potential contraceptive significance. The charts scan the major discoveries before and after 1960 and reveal the tremendous intensification of research activity and acceleration of progress that has occurred over the past two decades. While this step-up in the tempo of progress coincides with the gains in funding that occurred during this same period, it is also true that a background of three decades of pioneering research helped pave the way for these extremely fruitful years. These correlations are recorded and discussed in detail in the companion volume, entitled *Reproduction and Human Welfare: A Challenge to Research.*

It is a pleasure to express our gratitude to the many scientists who have contributed essays or helped with the preparation of the summary tables for this book. We are also much indebted to Jacki Ans, Joyann Brody, and Ardell Wilbur for their aid in assembling this material for publication, and to Dallas Galvin and Judy Kelso for their help with the historical charts.

Roy O. Greep
Marjorie A. Koblinsky

Frontiers in Reproduction
and Fertility Control

1 The Gonadotropic Hormones, LH (ICSH) and FSH

Harold Papkoff, Robert J. Ryan, and Darrell N. Ward

1.1 Introduction

Early in this century the pituitary gland was discovered to be intimately associated with processes of reproduction. The classic experiments of P. E. Smith in the 1920s on the hypophysectomy of the rat showed clearly that removal of the pituitary gland led to gross reproductive dysfunction. Immature hypophysectomized rats of either sex failed to mature sexually, and mature, sexually functioning rats underwent atrophy of the gonads and cessation of reproductive function. Injections of homogenates and extracts of pituitary glands into suitable animals profoundly affected many of the organs and tissues, particularly the gonads and sex accessory organs.

With the recognition that the pituitary gland possessed several hormonal substances, efforts in the 1930s emphasized the development of methods for extracting and purifying the pituitary hormones and the design of procedures for qualitatively and quantitatively assessing the various hormones present. Progress was slow, since the biological and chemical aspects were very interdependent, and both sciences lacked the sophistication of expertise and methodology that exists today. Nevertheless, during this period the pituitary hormones were found to be protein or polypeptide in nature, and—with respect to reproductive biology—evidence showed two hormones, not one, which acted upon the gonads and regulated reproductive function. These hormones are today known as follicle stimulating hormone (FSH) and luteinizing hormone (LH). LH is synonomous with interstitial cell stimulating hormone (ICSH). In addition to the knowledge of the two gonadotropins, investigators learned that they contained carbohydrate and are thus classified chemically as glycoproteins. One other pituitary hormone, thyrotropin (TSH), is also a glycoprotein and in recent years has been shown to be chemically closely related to both LH and FSH.

Substantial progress in purifying the pituitary hormones waited until the 1950s. During this period many of the modern methods of protein and polypeptide chemistry were developed, such as ion exchangers, various types of preparative electrophoresis, and gel filtration media, all of which were capable of providing the chemist with superior techniques for the purification of proteins. These techniques, coupled with meth-

ods of analysis for amino acids, molecular weights, and amino acid sequences were soon applied to the pituitary hormones, resulting in the astonishing progress of the last 20 years. The preparation of the first pituitary gonadotropin in highly purified form was achieved by two separate laboratories in the same year—1959. Both Squire and Li (Berkeley) and Ward and colleagues (Houston) announced the isolation of LH from extracts of sheep pituitaries and determined some of its properties. Within a few years, methods were improved in various laboratories to give better yields of ovine LH, setting the stage for intensive studies on its chemical nature. In addition, other species of LH (bovine, porcine, rat, and human, among others) were isolated. Although the 1960s featured slower progress than the 1950s, highly purified preparations of ovine and human FSH became available.

The availability of these highly purified gonadotropin preparations opened the way for the progress of the past 10 years. With preparations of high purity, unambiguous biological studies could be performed; radioimmunoassays could be developed; and the chemistry of the gonadotropins could be realistically studied.

1.2 Major Advances in the Last Decade on the Chemistry of the Gonadotropins

Isolation of Highly Purified Gonadotropins from the Pituitary Gland

Early studies on isolation and purification of the pituitary gonadotropins—conducted over a period ranging from the 1920s to the 1950s—probed the solubility and stability properties of the gonadotropins. Two types of fractionation approach evolved: aqueous ammonium sulfate fractionation techniques and buffered ethanolic precipitation techniques. Concomitantly, suitable bioassay techniques were developed to define the gonadotropic activities of the pituitary gland. Although these bioassay techniques are crucial to the isolation of the pituitary gonadotropins, they will not be considered further in this statement on the chemistry of the gonadotropins.

In the late 1950s new methodologies for protein purification were applied to the pituitary gonadotropin isolations. Examples of the technology available to the protein chemist at that time include the cellulose ion-exchange materials, the molecular exclusion processes, the subsequent combination of the ion-exchange and molecular exclusion, starch gel electrophoresis, polyacrylamide disc-gel electrophoresis, and, more recently, isoelectric focusing. With the application of these new methodologies, problems relating to the purification of the pituitary gonadotropins could be defined: the carbohydrate heterogeneity relative to the carbohydrate moieties on these glycoproteins; protein heterogeneity as it relates particularly to the carboxyl and amino terminal heterogeneity that has often been encountered in the products obtained; and—from chemical studies that have accumulated on the glycoprotein hormones—the loss of amides, which contributes to the electrophoretic heterogeneity. These problems are in part artifacts of the isolation techniques, but apparently are also attributable in part to the nature of the source—the pituitary gland—and to the relationship of the hormone contained therein to biosynthesis in the pituitary gland. Although the powerful tools available to the protein chemist allow one to deal with the heterogeneity problems relating to the glycoprotein hormones of the pituitary gland now as never before, in very few instances have the studies actually been carried to the molecular level for the definition of the type of difficulties one may encounter. With the establishment of amino acid sequences of the glycoprotein hormones, these problems can be handled better than before.

Reasonably pure LH preparations from the pituitary gland have been obtained from ovine, bovine, human, rat, rabbit, porcine, and equine pituitary glands. A few laboratories have also considered the isolation of gonadotropins from the pituitary glands of nonmammalian species. LH has been found to have relatively good stability in the species so far investigated, particularly the mammalian species; thus, difficulties in isolating it have been largely restricted to problems of procurement of adequate quantities of the required pituitary glands.

Isolating highly purified FSH, however, has been fraught with many difficulties (as yet unidentified). Most success has been obtained with the human follicle stimulating hormone (hFSH), which appears to have a somewhat better stability for the isolation techniques employed than other FSH activities. Reasonably high-potency ovine, equine, and rat FSH preparations have been obtained. The porcine FSH has been studied, although its degree of purity has not seemed to be high. In the case of the bovine FSH, the product seems to be either very low-potency material or highly labile in terms of the activity. The success obtained with the isolation of rat FSH has contributed considerably to knowledge of the physiology of this hormone in the laboratory rat.

Although gonadotropic activity can be detected in urine under a variety of physiological conditions, the only one that can—apparently—be isolated as a well-characterized chemical identity from this source would be the chorionic gonadotropin (CG) from the urine of pregnant donors. Consideration of this material will be the subject of a separate report.

The closely related (physiologically) gonadotropin in the serum of pregnant mares (PMSG) can also be isolated in high purity and in good yields. This material, since it is not of pituitary origin, will not be considered further in the present report.

Gonadotropin Subunits

A significant contribution to our understanding of the chemistry of the pituitary gonadotropins came with the observation in 1964 by Li and Starman that ovine LH (ICSH) sedimented as a molecule with a molecular weight of 30,000 daltons at neutral pH; at acidic pH (1.3), however, the molecule sedimented as if it had a molecular weight of 15,000 daltons. These observations, as well as others that were subsequently made in various laboratories, could be interpreted as a monomer-dimer dissociation, but in 1966, Ward and colleagues were able to propose a dissimilar-subunit model based on chemical evidence. Shortly thereafter, Papkoff and Samy were able to report a countercurrent distribution procedure that separated the subunits. These findings were subsequently extended to other species of LH and to the other glycoprotein hormones (such as TSH, CG, FSH, and PMSG).

Although the separation procedure devised by Papkoff and Samy is perhaps the most widely applied in the subunit separations for the various gonadotropins, it has not proven universally applicable; in certain instances, other approaches were necessary to obtain adequate subunit separation. The modifications that have been devised in various laboratories to achieve subunit separation may be classified into three major categories: first, variation of the type of countercurrent distribution system (for example, the procedure of Ward and colleagues for separation of human LH subunits); second, dissociation in a medium such as propionic acid or urea, followed by molecular exclusion or ion-exchange chromatography (for example, the TSH subunit separation procedure of Pierce and colleagues; the hCG subunit separation procedure of Bahl and colleagues or Canfield and colleagues); third, the preparation of subunit derivatives, generally derivatizing the disulfide bond by reduction-alkylation or reduction thiolation (for example, the procedure of Ward and colleagues for ovine LH, Canfield and colleagues for hCG, or Gospodarowicz for PMSG). The latter procedures, employing derivatives of subunits, are adequate for chemical studies but do not serve for physiological studies involving subunit recombination.

Recently Gospodarowicz has reported a procedure for the isolation of highly purified LH preparations using affinity chromatography. In this procedure an antibody to the LH desired (generally employing a more readily available LH preparation that cross-reacts with a species of LH for which pituitary materials are in short supply) is affixed to a Sepharose column and the desired LH is selectively adsorbed. After removal of impurities, the desired gonadotropin is desorbed from the antibody column. Since the binding affinity of an LH preparation to its antibody is stronger than the subunit-subunit binding affinity, such a desorption procedure results in the dissociated subunit, and recombination must be employed to obtain biologically active material. Despite this disadvantage, this procedure, as a general approach to the isolation of gonadotropins from pituitary glands obtainable only in very short supply, may be anticipated as a widely applicable technique for future studies.

The knowledge that the gonadotropins are comprised of dissimilar subunits has opened many new approaches to the study of both the chemistry and physiology of the gonadotropins. In chemical studies the possibility of isolating dissimilar subunits as discrete molecular entities greatly accelerated the determination of the amino acid sequence of the gonadotropins for which sequences have already been presented (vide infra). In physiological studies this knowledge has greatly accelerated the understanding of the degree of cross-reactivity and the chemical source for this cross-reactivity among the various glycoprotein hormones. In specific instances the cross-reactivity specificity has been used advantageously to discriminate, for example, between hLH and hCG or monkey LH or monkey CG, with significant implications for the study of pregnancy.

A number of studies reported recently have taken advantage of the dissimilar-subunit nature of LH to prepare derivatives on selected functional groups of either the alpha or beta subunits or both, and then to study the effects of these substitutions on the biological properties of the recombined derivative molecules. Thus the signal observations of Li and Starman on the dissociation of luteinizing hormones into subunits have provided the informational base for a significant expansion of knowledge of both the chemical nature and the physiological function of the gonadotropins.

The recombination of dissimilar subunits of the gonadotropins to obtain a biologically active molecule requires expanded technology. In general, studies have employed recombination for periods of time ranging from 2 to 16 hours at neutral pH, to obtain a biologically active product. Nevertheless, since the biological activity recovered is usually less than anticipated com-pared to that of the native hormone from which the subunits were obtained, this recombination may not occur in exactly the proper conformation for the required biological activity. Studies of this point and of the actual binding strength involved in the recombination of the subunits have been hampered by inadequate kinetic procedures. Recently, Ingham and colleagues at the National Institutes of Health have reported the use of fluorescent probes for determining the reassociated form of the hormones. These studies provide the first information about the kinetic aspects of the recombination process or, conversely, the dissociation of the subunits. Study results promise to have considerable impact on knowledge both of the physiological state and metabolism of gonadotropins as well as of the chemistry and particularly the comparative biochemistry of gonadotropins isolated from different species.

Amino Acid Sequence Determinations

Progress toward elucidation of the amino acid sequence followed rapidly on the heels of the isolation of the subunits of LH. Bovine TSH was sequenced in the laboratory of J. G. Pierce, and ovine LH was sequenced independently in two laboratories, that of D. N. Ward in Houston and that of C. H. Li in Berkeley. The principal investigators—Liao and Pierce; Sairam, Papkoff, and Li; and Liu and colleagues—published findings about these basic sequences that have led to realization of the extensive body of homology in this series of glycoprotein hormones. With these pioneering studies on the amino acid sequences of the glycoprotein hormones, plus the demonstration that the dissimilar-subunit model extended to all of the various species of glycoprotein hormones—in particular, gonadotropic hormones from the pituitary gland—amino acid sequence data accumulated rapidly from 1970 to 1974.

Initially the α subunits were shown to be identical in sequence, but as the phylogenetic diversity for the species was broadened, the identity was not maintained, although a considerable constancy of structure was apparent. Sequence identity is approximately 75 percent between ovine or bovine LHα and human LHα for example. The identities between ovine LHα and porcine LHα are approximately 95 percent. (See Figure 1.1 for a comparative summary of the amino acid sequences of the α subunit of LH.)

A notable feature of the α subunit sequence is the conservation of the amino acid sequence around the C-terminal end, which appears important for the maintenance of biological activity in its interaction with the β subunit. Another notable feature for the α subunit sequence is the constancy of placement of half-cystine and probably of the disulfide bond cross-linkages (al-

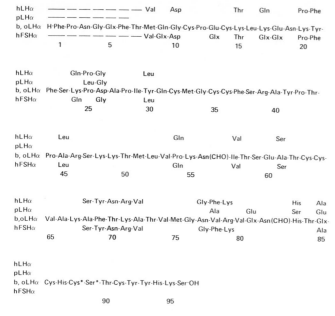

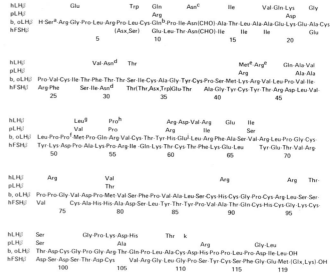

Figure 1.1 Comparative amino acid sequences of LHα and FSHα. Positions 88-89 (Cys-Ser) are given as Ser-Cys in the oLHα sequence reported by Sairam, Papkoff, and Li [57, 63].

Figure 1.2 Comparative amino acid sequences of LHβ and FSHβ. After this figure was compiled, Keutmann et al. published a paper [68] that clarifies a number of points relative to the hLHβ sequence. Their studies included the following portions of the molecule: residues 1-19 from the intact subunit and residues 38-45, 46-57, 60-64, 65-72, 87-93, and 109-113 as partial sequence determinations on the chymotryptic peptides. (The numbering is that used in our figure; numbering may vary slightly among the publications referenced, according to the number of insertions or deletions noted below that have been adopted.) All sequences in the paper by Keutmann et al. are in accord with those given here, with the following additions or clarifications:
Position 10 His (Shome and Parlow [65] and Sairam and Li [67] agree. The figure is in error in lacking this residue)
Position 13 Asn in good yield (i.e., no carbohydrates attached)
Position 19 Glu (Gln is a typographical error)
Positions 40-42 Thr-Met-Met
Position 52 Leu
Positions 109-113 Keutmann et al. agree with Shome and Parlow for this position of the C-terminal peptide, but they have not identified the residue at position 112. They also isolated two C-terminal peptides with this N-terminal sequence.

though this latter point has not been established experimentally). This constant position has been true for the subunits from all species examined in sufficient detail so far.

Interesting homologies occur between the α subunit of CG and the sequences shown in Figure 1.1; further comment on this aspect of the homology and the interrelationships of the elucidation of these sequences is in another section on CG.

The sequence of the β subunit, or—as it has come to be known—the hormone-specific subunit, is presented in Figure 1.2. In Figures 1.1 and 1.2 the human sequences are identical with the ovine and bovine LH sequence, unless a different amino acid is indicated along the line designated. The position of the NH₂-terminal amino acid in other sequences was established by aligning the first half-cystine residue in each sequence. All half-cystine residues are aligned throughout the sequences except the hFSHβ sequence of Shome and Parlow. In that instance, after the third half-cystine residue all subsequent residues in their sequence are displaced four residues relative to the LH sequences. The sources for Figures 1.1 and 1.2 are indicated in Table 1.1.

Although the β subunit is responsible for determining the type of biological activity obtained, in combination with the α subunit, the variability in amino acid sequence is greater among the different species than that of the α subunit. For example, the ovine sequence has about a 65 percent identity with the human amino acid sequence.

[a] Ward and co-workers for oLHβ and bLHβ and Maghuin-Rogister and co-workers for pLHβ and bLHβ provide indirect evidence that the NH₂-terminal Ser is partially acylated, although the nature of the blocking group is not established.
[b] This residue is Glu in the oLH sequence of Sairam et al. [58].
[c] Closset et al. [66] place a carbohydrate moiety at residue 13 in hLHβ, as is found in pLHβ, bLHβ, and oLHβ. Neither Sairam and Li [67] nor Shome and Parlow [65] indicate such a moiety at this position of hLHβ.
[d] Residue 30 in hLHβ (or residue 24 in the hFSHβ sequence) carries a carbohydrate moiety.
[e] Sairam and Li [67] have the sequence Met-Arg-Val-Leu, as shown; Shome and Parlow [65] have Arg——Val-Leu, and Closset et al. [66] propose Arg-(Met)-Leu-Leu for this portion of the hLHβ sequence.
[f] Sairam et al. [58] insert an additional Pro residue in the oLHβ sequence at this point.
[g] Closset et al. [66] have Val instead of Leu at this position of hLHβ.

[h]This Pro residue is deleted in the hLHβ sequences of Shome and Parlow [65] and Sairam and Li [67].

[j]Gln in the oLHβ sequence of Sairam et al. [58].

[k]Beyond the last Cys residue in hLHβ the COOH-terminal peptide is variously reported as follows:
Cys-Asp-Pro-Gln-His-Ser-Gly·OH by Sairam and Li [67]
Cys-Asx-Glx-Pro-His-(Ser-Lys-Gly)·OH by Shome and Parlow[65]
Cys-(Glx-Asx-Ser-Lys)-Gly·OH by Closset et al. [66].

Table 1.1 Sources for the sequences in Figures 1.1 and 1.2

Sequence	Sources[1]	Sequence	Sources[1]
oLHα	55, 57	oLHβ	56, 58
bLHα	62, 64	bLHβ	60, 62, 64
hLHα	63	hLHβ	65, 66, 67
pHLα	59	pLHβ	59
hFSHα	69	hFSHβ	70

[1]Numbers refer to the reference list at the end of the chapter.

Among the important points of identity in the various species of LH sequenced is the placement of the half-cystine residues—and presumably the disulfide bonds in the molecule—in a constant position relative to the rest of the amino acid sequence.

The aspects of the structure that are identically conserved from one species to another might reasonably be suspected to be most essential for the establishment of the biological activity of both the α and β subunits; however, critical demonstration of this at the molecular level or in a chemical sense requires extended study.

Less than five years have elapsed since the presentation of the first amino acid sequence for a pituitary gonadotropin (LH), and the number of sequences represented in Figures 1.1 and 1.2 indicates the rapid advances in this field. The impact of this information on the study of the physiological role of these molecules has been impressive. As one knows more precisely the molecule one is dealing with, one can more precisely define the experiments and the experimental conditions one imposes on his test systems. Returns of this sort are continually accruing, and though a final evaluation cannot yet be made of the contribution of this structural knowledge to the understanding of reproductive biology, its current value cannot be overstated.

In 1974 Shome and Parlow reported on the amino acid sequence of the hFSH subunits. These results await confirmation, but the work is of great significance and will make possible comparisons among LH, FSH, and TSH. As suspected, the amino acid sequence of hFSHα is identical to both hLH and hTSHα, thus confirming the generalization of the common subunit among the pituitary glycoprotein hormones. A preliminary appraisal of the structure of FSHβ, as reported by Shome and Parlow, show it to possess areas of homology to both LHβ and TSHβ as well as to each of these subunits. The suggestion that all three pituitary glycoprotein hormones evolved from a common ancestral molecule appears to be well supported.

1.3 Major Advances Resulting from the Availability of Highly Purified Gonadotropins

Development of Radioimmunoassays

The development of radioimmunoassays (RIAs) for hLH and hFSH followed shortly after the development of methods for purifying these glycoprotein hormones. The development of these RIAs led to the discovery that the human glycoprotein hormones—LH, FSH, hCG, and TSH—shared common antigenic determinants. During this same time period, subunit structures were recognized in both ovine and human LH and human FSH. The common antigenic determinants of the glycoprotein hormones were clarified when sequence data revealed a common α subunit and a hormone-specific β subunit.

Despite the presence of common antigenic determinants, specific RIAs were developed, but up to the present time, all assays for hFSH require the removal of cross-reacting antibodies by absorption with hCG. The purification of the β subunits of these glycoproteins should allow the preparation of highly specific antisera and assays; indeed, this is already demonstrated in the preparation of antisera to hCGβ that distinguish this hormone from native hLH or hLHβ, despite considerable homology in the primary sequences of the β subunits of these two hormones.

Experience with RIA showed clear immunologic differences between pituitary and urinary hLH and hFSH. These differences determine the choice of standards appropriate for assay of gonadotropins in pituitary extracts and urine, but as yet no data determine the requirements for a standard for serum LH or FSH.

Following the development of RIAs for human gonadotropins, assays were developed for FSH and LH from a variety of species. Homologous assays relied on purified gonadotropins from several species but more prominently upon the development of heterologous systems wherein the labeled tracer was a hormone from a species different from that used as an immunogen.

A quantitative appraisal of the impact of the development of these RIAs on biomedical research can be seen in Table 1.2.

A qualitative appraisal of the impact of the development of RIAs can be judged from three factors: first,

Table 1.2 Medline Citations[1]

Key Words	1970	1971	1972	1973[2]
RIA LH	102	170	238	250
RIA FSH	60	114	146	141
Blood LH	141	217	336	415
Blood FSH	73	125	180	187

[1]Subject matter key words; data base 1200–1500 journals.
[2]1973 Medline plus Sideline Retrieval File (January and February 1974).

enhanced understanding of the physiology of gonadotropins (see below); second, facilitation of the purification, assay, and understanding of the physiology of releasing factors; and third, routine clinical use of these assays in the differential diagnosis and treatment of human disorders of reproduction.

Biological Roles of LH and FSH

Although considerable data had been obtained in the bioassay era concerning hormonal events in the human menstrual cycle and mammalian estrous cycle, the application of RIAs substantiated these data, filled in the missing details, and allowed definition of events that were previously unrecognized. Both the steroid and gonadotropin RIAs contributed to these developments. FSH, in human serum, is elevated at the onset of the follicular phase; it falls to a nadir, rises to a midcycle peak, and declines to its lowest level during the luteal phase of the cycle. Serum LH, in menstruating women, rises slowly during the follicular phase, increases markedly 24 to 36 hours prior to ovulation (midcycle surge), and declines to its lowest levels during the luteal phase. Serum estradiol rises during the follicular phase, peaks about one day prior to the midcycle LH peak, drops, and then rises to a second midluteal peak. Serum progesterone does not increase until after the midcycle LH surge. Similar types of observations have been made for the estrous cycles of rhesus monkey, chimpanzee, rat, rabbit, sheep, cow, and dog.

Such observations have led to much interesting work. Consequences include the following:

1. A rising serum concentration of estrogen rather than progesterone is the signal for the ovulatory surge of LH.

2. A high-frequency (15 to 60 minute) low-amplitude pulsatile pattern of LH release has been recognized in the monkey, rat, human, and bull. These pulses are accentuated after castration and suppressed by estrogen.

3. FSH and LH are measurable in serum and urine prior to the onset of puberty—and indeed there is evidence for cyclic release in the female infant chimpanzee and human. A synchronization of LH release with sleep appears to be an early pubertal event, as is the release of LH induced by clomiphene citrate.

Although important new information concerning the biological role of LH and FSH has come from the application of RIAs, relatively little has been derived from administration of chemically pure preparations during the past six to eight years. This relates in part to the long unavailability of biologically (at least relatively pure) preparations of LH and FSH. Some data of significance have appeared concerning the circulatory half-life of LH and FSH, the role of sialic acid residues in metabolic clearance of the hormones, the lack of a role for sialic acid residues in tissue binding and in vitro activity, at least for hCG, and the absence of biological activity of the isolated subunits of the gonadotropins.

Mode of Action of Gonadotropins

The current conceptualization concerning the action of LH and FSH involves the following sequence of events: plasma membrane binding; activation of adenylate cyclase; increased intracellular cAMP; binding of cAMP to a protein kinase and activation of that kinase; phosphorylation of an intracellular protein; production of a product (such as progesterone or testosterone) or function (luteinization or spermatogenesis).

Although the availability of purified LH and FSH has contributed to the study of all of these processes, they have been absolutely essential for study of plasma membrane binding and thus the identification and characterization of gonadotropin receptors. These studies of receptors require labeling a pure gonadotropin with an isotope under conditions that preserve biological activity and incubating the labeled hormone with the target tissue (ovary or testis).

Binding of radioiodinated LH or hCG or both has been shown to occur to corpora lutea or luteinized granulosa cells of rats, pigs, cows, humans, and monkeys. Binding has also been demonstrated in rat Leydig cells using ^{125}I hCG and in Leydig cell tumors using unlabeled LH. This binding is principally, if not entirely, localized to the plasma membranes, as evidenced by subcellular fractionation techniques and EM autoradiography.

In vitro experiments with a crude particulate fraction from luteinized rat ovaries indicate that binding of labeled LH or hCG is specific for hormones with LH or hCG activity and is a saturable process dependent upon time, temperature, pH, and molarity of salts. Binding is of high affinity ($K_d = 10^{-11}$ M), and Hill plots indicate binding of one mole of hormone to one mole of receptor. The binding affinity is high enough to be relevant to the physiological concentration of the hormone in the circulation. The rat Leydig cell receptor appears to have similar properties.

Kinetic analysis of binding of radioiodinated hLH and hCG with rat luteal receptors indicate an association rate constant of $2.5–5.7 \times 10^{-6} M \ sec^{-1}$ and a biphasic dissociation with rate constants of $1.4–2.4 \times 10^{-4} M \ sec^{-1}$ and $4.7–6.7 \times 10^{-6} M \ sec^{-1}$. The dissociation rate constants, at least, are temperature-dependent. The biphasic dissociation suggests the possibility that the native LH or hCG molecules are bound to the receptor at more than one site on the molecule. Data are available indicating that the isolated α and β subunits do not bind to the receptor and do not compete with the native molecule for binding.

LH-hCG, when incubated with rat luteal tissue, becomes inactivated in the sense that the unbound hormone is no longer capable of binding to a fresh batch of receptor. The unbound LH-hCG remains intact, as evidenced by gel filtration and immunoprecipitability, and thus the inactivation is more analogous to the inactivation of glucagon than to the inactivation of insulin on exposure of these hormones to liver cell membranes.

The LH-hCG receptors from rat luteal tissue and rat Leydig cells have been solubilized with Triton X-100 and Luberol-PX. The solubilized luteal receptor has a lower binding affinity ($K_d = 10^{-10} M$) than the particulate receptor. The physical properties of the solubilized rat luteal and Leydig cell receptors are very similar, and both have a molecular weight of approximately 220,000 daltons.

The LH-hCG receptor has been purified from rat luteal tissue, using affinity chromatography. The eluted receptor maintained its specificity for LH, had a binding affinity of $10^{-10} M$, showed a single band on disc-gel electrophoresis under several conditions, and antisera prepared against it yielded a single precipitin arc when tested against purified receptor and crude Triton X-100 extracts of ovarian tissue. But the antisera also showed a single precipitin arc when tested against crude detergent extracts of liver, spleen, and kidney, which are not thought to be target organs for LH-hCG. Further, disc-gel electrophoresis of detergent extracts of these tissues showed a protein band with the same mobility as purified ovarian receptor, and purification of the liver extract by affinity chromatography yielded a protein with similar binding affinity and specificity as the purified ovarian receptor. These data suggest that tissue specificity is not determined solely by the presence or absence of receptor but rather by some masking process that renders the receptor active or inactive.

Data have been presented indicating that specific FSH receptors exist in rat ovarian follicles and testicular tubules. Because of the limited binding of labeled FSH, most likely due to damage during the radioiodination procedure, valid conclusions concerning binding kinetics are not yet possible.

These studies of gonadotropin receptors have a number of interesting implications for the future. First, the receptors can and are being used as methods for the assay of LH and FSH. The receptor assays have the advantage of reflecting biologically active molecules rather than antigenic determinants that may not be related to biological activity. Second, the use of receptor assays will greatly facilitate efforts to define the biologically active site on the LH (and FSH) molecule and thus lead to synthesis of agonistic and antagonistic molecules. Since the receptors are reflected on the external surface of the plasma membrane, it should be possible to affect LH and FSH action without disturbing intracellular events. This approach to contraception should be safer than currently available techniques, particularly when applied to an expendable cell such as the luteal cell. Third, the phenomenon of receptor masking (and unmasking) represents another level of control that may have broad biological significance.

Selected References to Gonadotropin Studies

This compilation of references is not intended to provide a detailed and comprehensive documentation of the published work relating to this report. Rather, our major goal, in addition to providing a number of key references, has been to illustrate the scope of the studies, the many investigations involved, and the progress that has been made in the past 10 to 15 years. The references have been grouped into a number of general sections, but in many cases a given reference will relate to more than one of these areas.

General Review Articles and Symposia

1. Ryan, R. J., N. S. Jiang, and S. Hanlan. Some physical and hydrodynamic properties of human FSH and LH. Rec. Prog. Horm. Res. 26:105, 1070.

2. Pierce, J. G., T. H. Liao, S. M. Howard, B. Shome, and J. S. Cornell. Studies on the structure of thyrotropin: Its relationship to luteinizing hormone. Rec. Prog. Horm. Res. 27:165, 1971.

3. Ward, D. N., L. E. Reichert, Jr., W.-K. Liu, H. S. Nahm, J. Hsia, W. M. Lamkin, and N. S. Jones. Chemical studies of luteinizing hormone from human and ovine pituitaries. Rec. Prog. Horm. Res. 29:533, 1973.

4. Papkoff, H., M. R. Sairam, S. W. Farmer, and C. H. Li. Studies on the nature and function of interstitial cell hormone. Rec. Prog. Horm. Res. 29:563, 1973.

5. Rosenberg, E., ed. *Gonadotropins*. Los Angeles: Geron-X, 1968.

6. Butt, W. R., A. C. Crooke, and M. Ryle, eds. *Gonadotropin and ovarian development*. London: E. and S. Livingston, 1971.

7. Margulies, M., and F. Greenwood, eds. *Protein and polypeptide hormones*, Parts I and II. Excerpta Med. Intern. Congr. Ser. No. 241, 1971–1972.

8. Saxena, B. B., C. G. Beling, and H. M. Gandy, eds. *Gonadotropins*. New York: John Wiley & Sons, 1972.

9. Li, C. H., ed. *Hormonal proteins and peptides*. New York: Academic Press, 1973.

10. Mougdal, N. R., ed. *Gonadotropins and gonadal function*. New York: Academic Press, 1974.

11. Bishop, W. H., A. Nureddin, and R. J. Ryan. Pituitary luteinizing and follicle stimulating hormones. In *Peptide hormones*, ed. J. Parson. New York: Macmillan, 1974.

12. Diczfalusy, E., ed. *Immunoassay of gonadotropins*. Acta Endrocrinol. Suppl. 142, 1969.

Purification and Properties of Gonadotropins

13. Squire, P. G., and C. H. Li. Purification and properties of interstitial cell stimulating hormone from sheep pituitary glands. J. Biol. Chem. 234:520, 1959.

14. Ward, D. N., R. F. McGregor, and A. C. Griffin. Chromatography of luteinizing hormone from sheep pituitary glands. Biochem. Biophys. Arch. 32:305, 1959.

15. Reichert, L. E., Jr. Preparation of purified bovine luteinizing hormone. Endocrinology 71:729, 1969.

16. Squire, P. G., C. H. Li, and R. N. Andersen. Purification and characterization of interstitial cell stimulating hormone. Biochemistry 1:412, 1962.

17. Reichert, L. E., Jr. Purification of porcine luteinizing hormone. Endocrinology 75:970, 1964.

18. Reichert, L. E., Jr., and A. F. Parlow. Partial Purification and separation of human pituitary gonadotropins. Endocrinology 74:236, 1964.

19. Papkoff, H., D. Gospodarowicz, A. Candiotti, and C. H. Li. Preparation of ovine interstitial cell stimulating hormone in high yield. Arch. Biochem. Biophys. 111:431, 1965.

20. Jutisz, M., C. Hermier, A. Colonge, and R. Courrier. Purification, physicochemical, and biological properties of sheep FSH. Ann. Endocrinol. (Paris) 26:670, 1965.

21. Hartree, A. S. Separation and partial purification of the protein hormones from human pituitary glands. Biochem. J. 100:754, 1966.

22. Papkoff, H., D. Gospodarowicz, and C. H. Li. Purification and properties of ovine follicle stimulating hormone. Arch. Biochem. Biophys. 120:434, 1967.

23. Ward, D. N., M. Adams-Mayne, N. Ray, D. E. Balke, J. Coffey, and M. Showalter. Comparative studies of luteinizing hormone from beef, pork, and sheep pituitaries. I: Purification and properties. Gen. Comp. Endrocrinol. 8:44, 1967.

24. Saxena, B. B., and P. Rathnam. Purification of follicle stimulating hormone from human pituitary glands. J. Biol. Chem. 242:3769, 1967.

25. Papkoff, H., L.-J. Mahlmann, and C. H. Li. Some chemical and physical properties of human pituitary follicle stimulating hormone. Biochemistry 6:3976, 1967.

26. Ryan, R. J. On obtaining luteinizing and follicle stimulating hormone from human pituitaries. J. Clin. Endocrinol. Metab. 28:886, 1968.

27. Reichert, L. E., Jr., R. H. Kathan, and R. J. Ryan. Studies on the composition and properties of immunochemical grade human pituitary follicle stimulating hormone (FSH): comparison with luteinizing hormone (LH). Endocrinology 82:109, 1968.

28. Roos, P. *Human follicle stimulating hormone*. Acta Endocrinol. Suppl. 131, 1968.

29. Peckham, W. D., and A. F. Parlow. Solution from human pituitary glands of three discrete electrophoretic components with high luteinizing hormone activity. Endocrinology 85:618, 1969.

30. Peckham, W. D., and A. F. Parlow. On the isolation of human follicle stimulating hormone. Endocrinology 84:953, 1969.

31. Barker, S. A., C. J. Gray, J. F. Kennedy, and W. R. Butt. Evaluation of human FSH preparations. J. Endocrinol. 45:275, 1969.

32. Rathnam, P., and B. B. Saxena. Isolation and physicochemical characterization of luteinizing hormone from human pituitary glands. J. Biol. Chem. 245:3725, 1970.

33. Braselton, W. E., Jr., and W. H. McShan. Purification and properties of follicle stimulating and luteinizing hormones from horse pituitary glands. Arch. Biochem. Biophys. 139:45, 1970.

34. Sherwood, O. D., H. J. Grimck, and W. H. McShan. Purification and properties of follicle stimulating hormone from sheep pituitary glands. J. Biol. Chem. 245:2328, 1970.

35. Amir, S. M., and A. F. Parlow. Amino acid composition and molecular weight of human follicle stimulating hormone. Proc. Soc. Exp. Biol. Med. 139:1120, 1972.

Subunit Nature of Gonadotropins

36. Li, C. H., and B. Starman. Molecular weight of sheep pituitary interstitial cell stimulating hormone. Nature 202:291, 1964.

37. Ward, D. N., M. Fujino, and W. M. Lamkin. Evidence for two carbohydrate moieties in ovine LH. Fed. Proc. 25:348, 1966.

38. Papkoff, H., and T. S. A. Samy. Isolation and partial characterization of polypeptide chains of ovine interstitial cell stimulating hormone. Biochim. Biophys. Acta 147:175, 1967.

39. de la Llossa, P., and M. Jutisz. Reversible dissociation into subunits and biological activity of ovine luteinizing hormone. Biochim. Biophys. Acta 181:426, 1969.

40. Reichert, L. E., Jr., M. A. Rasco, D. N. Ward, G. D. Niswender, and A. R. Midgley, Jr. Isolation and properties of subunits of bovine pituitary luteinizing hormone. J. Biol. Chem. 244:5110, 1969.

41. Liao, T.-H., and J. G. Pierce. The presence of a common type of subunit in bovine thyroid stimulating and luteinizing hormone. J. Biol. Chem. 245:3275, 1970.

42. Lamkin, W. M., M. Fujino, J. D. Mayfield, G. N. Holcomb, and D. N. Ward. Separation of the subunits of ovine luteinizing hormone by a chromatographic procedure and

comparison with a counter current distribution procedure. Biochim. Biophys. Acta 214:290, 1970.

43. Ward, D. N., L. E. Reichert, Jr., B. A. Fitak, H. S. Nahn, C. M. Sweeney, and J. D. Neill. Isolation and properties of subunits of rat pituitary luteinizing hormone. Biochemistry 10:1796, 1971.

44. Hennen, G., Z. Prusik, and G. Maghuin-Rogister. Porcine luteinizing hormine and its subunits. Eur. J. Biochem. 18:376, 1971.

45. Hartree, A. S., M. Thomas, M. Brakevitch, E. T. Bell, E. W. Christie, G. V. Spaull, R. Taylor, and J. G. Pierce. Preparation and properties of subunits of human luteinizing hormone. J. Endocrinol. 51:169, 1971.

46. Ryan, R. J. Stokes radius of human pituitary hormones and demonstration of dissociation of luteinizing hormone. Biochemistry 8:495, 1969.

47. Reichert, L. E., Jr., A. R. Midgley, Jr., G. D. Niswender, and D. N. Ward. Formation of a hybrid molecule from subunits of human and bovine luteinizing hormone. Endocrinology 87:534, 1970.

48. Papkoff, H., and M. Ekblad. Ovine follicle stimulating hormone: Preparation and characterization of its subunits. Biochem. Biophys. Res. Commun. 40:614, 1970.

49. Saxena, B. B., and P. Rathman. Dissociation phenomenon and subunit nature of follicle stimulating hormone from human pituitary glands. J. Biol. Chem. 246:3549, 1971.

50. Reichert, L. E., Jr., and D. N. Ward. On the isolation of the alpha and beta subunits of human pituitary follicle stimulating hormone. Endocrinology 94:655, 1973.

51. Parlow, A. F., and B. Shome. Specific homologous radioimmunoassay of highly purified subunits of human pituitary follicle stimulating hormone. J. Clin. Endocrinol. Metab. 39:195, 1974.

52. Landefeld, T. D., and W. H. McShan. Equine luteinizing hormone and its subunits. Isolation and physicochemical properties. Biochemistry 13:1389, 1974.

53. Landefeld, T. D., and W. H. McShan. Isolation and characterization of subunits from equine pituitary follicle stimulating hormone. J. Biol. Chem. 249: 3527, 1974.

54. Grimek, H. J., and W. H. McShan. Isolation and characterization of highly purified ovine follicle-stimulating hormone. J. Biol. Chem. 249:5725, 1974.

Amino Acid Sequence Analysis of LH and FSH

55. Liu, W.-K., H. S. Nahm, C. M. Sweeney, W. M. Lamkin, H. N. Baker, and D. N. Ward. The primary structure of ovine luteinizing hormone. I. The amino acid sequence of the reduced and s-aminoethylated s-subunit (LH-α). J. Biol. Chem. 247:4351, 1972.

56. Liu, W.-K., H. S. Nahm, C. M. Sweeney, G. N. Holcomb, and D. N. Ward. The primary structure of ovine luteinizing hormone. II. The amino acid sequence of the reduced, s-carboxymethylated A-subunit (LH-β). J. Biol. Chem. 247:4365, 1972.

57. Sairam, M. R., H. Papkoff, and C. H. Li. The primary structure of ovine interstitial cell stimulating hormone. I. The α-subunit. Arch. Biochem. Biophys. 153:554, 1972.

58. Sairam, M. R., T. S. A. Samy, H. Papkoff, and C. H. Li. The primary structure of ovine interstitial cell stimulating hormone. II. The β-subunit. Arch. Biochem. Biophys. 153:572, 1972.

59. Maghuin-Rogister, G., Y. Combarnous, and G. Hennen. The primary structure of the porcine luteinizing hormone α-subunit. Eur. J. Biochem. 39:255, 1973.

60. Maghuin-Rogister, G., and G. Hennen. Luteinizing hormone: The primary structures of the β-subunit from bovine and porcine species. Eur. J. Biochem. 39:235, 1973.

61. Tertrain-Clary, C., P. de la Llosa, M. Hurolt, C. Courti, and M. Jutisz. Quelques points de structure de l'hormone luteinsante bovine comparison avec l'hormone luteinsante ovine. Biochim. Biophys. Acta 263:115, 1972.

62. Ward, D. N., and W.-K. Liu. The chemistry of ovine and bovine luteinizing hormone. In *Protein and polypeptide hormones*, eds. M. Margoulies and F. Greenwood. Part II. Excerpta Med. Intern. Congr. Ser. No. 241, 1972.

63. Sairam, M. R., H. Papkoff, and C. H. Li. Human pituitary interstitial cell stimulating hormone: Primary structure of the α-subunit. Biochem. Biophys. Res. Commun. 48:530, 1972.

64. Ward, D. N., L. E. Reichert, Jr., W.-K. Liu, H. S. Nahm, and W. M. Lamkin. Comparative studies of ovine, bovine and human LH. In *Gonadotropins*, eds. B. B. Saxena, C. G. Beling, and H. M. Gandy. New York: John Wiley & Sons, 1972.

65. Shome, B., and A. F. Parlow. The primary structure of the hormone-specific β-subunit of human pituitary luteinizing hormone. J. Clin. Endocrinol. Metab. 36:618, 1973.

66. Closset, J., G. Hennen, and R. Lequin. Human luteinizing hormone: The amino acid sequence of the β-subunit. FEBS Letters 29:97, 1973.

67. Sairam, M. R., and C. H. Li. Internat. Res. Commun. Syst., Biochemistry of Hormones (73–11) 3–5–17, November 1973.

68. Keutmann, H. T., J. W. Jacobs, W. H. Bishop, and R. J. Ryan. Human luteinizing hormone: amino-terminal sequence analysis of the β-subunit using (^{35}S) phenylisothiocyanate. Hoppe-Seyler's Z. Physiol. Chem. 355:935, 1974.

69. Shome, B., and A. F. Parlow. Human follicle stimulating hormone (hFSH): First proposal for the amino acid sequence of the α-subunit (hFSHα) and first demonstration of its identity with the α-subunit of human luteinizing hormone (hLHα). J. Clin. Endocrinol. Metab. 39:199, 1974.

70. Shome, B., and A. F. Parlow. Human follicle stimulating hormone: First proposal for the amino acid sequence of the hormone-specific, β-subunit (hFSHβ). J. Clin. Endocrinol. Metab. 39:203, 1974.

Gonadotropin Radioimmunoassay Studies

71. Diczfalusy, E., ed. *Immunoassay of gonadotropins* Acta Endocrinol. Suppl. 142, 1969.

72. Kirkham, K. E., and W. M. Hunter, eds. *Radioimmunoassay methods*. Edinburgh: Churchill Livingstone, 1971.

73. Midgley, A. R., Jr. Radioimmunoassay: A method for human chorionic gonadotropin and human luteinizing hormone. Endocrinology 79:10, 1966.

74. Odell, W. D., G. T. Ross, and P. L. Rayford. Radioim-

munoassay for luteinizing hormone in plasma or serum. Physiological studies. J. Clin. Invest. 46:248, 1967.

75. Bagshawe, K. D., C. E. Wilde, and A. H. Orr. Radioimmunoassay for human chorionic gonadotropin and luteinizing hormone. Lancet 1:1118, 1966.

76. Faiman, C., and R. J. Ryan. Radioimmunoassay for human luteinizing hormone. Proc. Soc. Exp. Biol. Med. 125:1130, 1967.

77. Faiman, C., and R. J. Ryan. Radioimmunoassay for human follical stimulating hormone. J. Clin. Endocrinol. Metab. 27:444, 1967.

78. Midgley, A. R., Jr. Radioimmunoassay for human follicle stimulating hormone. J. Clin. Endocrinol. Metab. 27:295, 1967.

79. Rosselin, G., and J. Dolais. Dosage de l'hormone folliculo-stimulante humaine (HFSH) par la methode radioimmunologique. Presse Med. 75:2027, 1967.

80. Albert, A., E. Rosemberg, G. T. Ross, C. A. Paulsen, and R. J. Ryan. Report of the National Pituitary Agency Collaborative Study on the Radioimmunoassay of FSH and LH. J. Clin. Endocrinol. Metab. 28:1214, 1968.

81. Schlaff, S., S. W. Rosen, and J. Roth. Antibody to follicle stimulating hormone: Cross-reactivity with three other hormones. J. Clin. Invest. 47:1722, 1968.

82. L'Hermite, M., and A. R. Midgley, Jr. Radioimmunoassay of human follicle stimulating hormone with antisera to the ovine hormone. J. Clin. Endocrinol. Metab. 33:68, 1971.

83. Hendrick, J. C., J. J. Legros, and P. Franchimont. Le dosage radioimmunologique de la FSH de rat et etude radioimmunologique de la reaction croisee entre la FSH de rats monton, et de pare. Ann. Endocrinol. (Paris) 32:241, 1971.

84. Midgley, A. R., Jr., G. D. Niswender, V. L. Gay, and L. E. Reichert, Jr. Use of antibodies for characterization of gonadotropins and steroids. Rec. Prog. Horm. Res. 27:286, 1971.

85. Vaitukaitis, J. L., G. D. Braunstein, and G. T. Ross. A radioimmunoassay which specifically measures human chorionic gonadotropin in the presence of human luteinizing hormone. Am. J. Obstet. Gynecol. 113:751, 1972.

86. Franchimont, P., H. Burger, and J. J. Legros. Impact of radioassay techniques on the field of sex hormones. Metabolism 22:1003, 1973.

Gonadotropin Receptor Studies

87. Lee, C. Y., and R. J. Ryan. The uptake of human luteinizing hormone (hLH) by slices of luteinized rat ovaries. Endocrinology 89:1515, 1971.

88. de Kretser, D. M., K. J. Catt, and C. A. Paulsen. Studies on the *in vitro* testicular binding of iodinated luteinizing hormone in rats. Endocrinology 88:332, 1971.

89. Moudgal, N. R., W. R. Moyle, and R. O. Greep. Specific binding of luteinizing hormone to Leydig tumor cells. J. Biol. Chem. 246:4983, 1971.

90. Dufau, M. L., K. J. Catt, and T. Tsuruhara. Retention of in vitro biological activities by desialylated human luteinizing hormone and chorionic gonadotropin. Biochem. Biophys. Res. Commun. 44:1022; 1971.

91. Lee, C. Y., and R. J. Ryan. Luteinizing hormone receptors: Specific binding of human luteinizing hormone to homogenates of luteinized rat ovaries. Proc. Natl. Acad. Sci. USA 69:3520, 1972.

92. Kammerman, S., R. E. Canfield, J. Kolena, and C. P. Channing. The binding of iodinated hCG to porcine granulosa cells. Endocrinology 91:65, 1972.

93. Means, A. R., and J. Vaitukaitis. Peptide hormone "receptors": Specific binding of ^{3}H–FSH to testis. Endocrinology 90:39, 1972.

94. Lee, C. Y., and R. J. Ryan. Interaction of ovarian receptors with human luteinizing hormone and human chorionic gonadotropin. Biochemistry 12:4609, 1973.

95. Lee, C. Y., C. B. Coulam, N. S. Jiang, and R. J. Ryan. Receptors for human luteinizing hormone in human corpora luteal tissue. J. Clin. Endocrinol. Metab. 36:148, 1973.

96. Gospodarowicz, D. Properties of the luteinizing hormone receptors of isolated bovine corpus luteum plasma membranes. J. Biol. Chem. 248:5042, 1973.

97. Reichert, L. E., Jr., F. Leidenberger, and C. G. Trowbridge. Studies on luteinizing hormone and its subunits: Development and application of a radioligand receptor assay and properties of the hormone-receptor interaction. Rec. Prog. Horm. Res. 29:497, 1973.

98. Bhalla, V. K., and L. E. Reichert, Jr. Properties of follicle-stimulating hormone-receptor interactions. Specific binding of human follicle-stimulating hormone to rat testis. J. Biol. Chem. 249:43, 1974.

2 The Chemistry and Biology of Human Chorionic Gonadotropin and Its Subunits

Om P. Bahl

Introduction

Exciting developments have recently occurred in the field of gonadotropins in general and of human chorionic gonadotropin (hCG) in particular. The most striking among these is the availability of simple methods for their large-scale preparation, recognition of the two noncovalently bonded subunits and their dissociation and separation, and the elucidation of the sequences of amino acids in the polypeptide chains of hCG and of luteinizing (LH), follicle stimulating (FSH), and thyroid stimulating (TSH) hormones. The sequence of monosaccharides has been established in hCG only. A great deal of progress has also been made in understanding the nature of their binding to the target tissue receptors and the solubilization and characterization of the receptors. Rapid and specific radioimmunoassays and radioligand-receptor assays have been developed. Finally, investigations on structure and function relationships have been initiated. Some interesting concepts regarding the role of carbohydrate in the function of the hormones are beginning to emerge. Nevertheless, knowledge in the area of structure and function and molecular mechanisms of gonadotropic action is still in its infancy.

One encouraging consequence of these basic advances, particularly in the area of hCG, has been the realization of their potential in clinical areas, such as the early detection of normal and ectopic pregnancies by radioimmunoassay, based on the use of anti-hCGβ or radioligand-receptor assay, and the possible use of hCGβ, or its appropriate fragment, linked to a hapten or a carrier protein, in fertility regulation by active immunization.

Covalently bonded carbohydrate forms about 30 percent of the molecule of hCG, a glycoprotein hormone. It is produced by syncytiotrophoblast in placenta, and its maximum level in the urine or serum is reached during the first trimester of pregnancy. Its chemical and biological properties closely resemble those of LH. Its function in the ovary is to maintain the corpus luteum and thereby to stimulate the synthesis of progesterone, which prepares the endometrium for implantation and its subsequent maintenance. Because of its LH-like action, hCG also stimulates the synthesis of testosterone in the interstitial tissues of the testis, although this is obviously not its physiological function. This report deals with the progress made in recent years in the chemistry and biology of hCG.

2.2 Purification

Purification of hCG

Earlier attempts to purify hCG resulted in preparations of biological activity not exceeding 8000–9000 IU/mg (Li 1949). The first successful attempt to obtain a homogeneous preparation of hCG with an activity of 12,000 IU/mg from the pregnancy urine was made by Got and Bourillon (1960a, b). Since then, several workers have obtained hCG with potencies up to 19,000 IU/mg from patients with trophoblastic tumors (Reisfeld and Hertz 1960; Wilde and Bagshawe 1965). Recently, commercial preparations of hCG with biological activity of 2500–3000 IU/mg have been employed by several investigators (Bahl 1969a; Chang et al. 1967; van Hell et al. 1968; Bell et al. 1969; Mori 1970; Ashitaka et al. 1970; Canfield et al. 1971; Graesslin et al. 1970, Merz et al. 1974) in obtaining preparations with potencies of 12,000 to 18,000 IU/mg.

The various procedures for isolation of the hormone from commercial preparations are based on the use of ion-exchange chromatography of one type or another, molecular sieving, electrophoresis in supporting media, and isoelectric focusing. A simple and reproducible procedure that is routinely followed in our laboratory involves three chromatographic steps (Bahl 1969a): (1) chromatography on DEAE-Sephadex using stepwise linear salt gradient; (2) chromatography on DEAE-Sephadex using continuous linear salt gradient; (3) gel permeation on Sephadex G–100. This procedure yields a preparation with potency of over 12,000 IU/mg (Bahl 1969a). Isoelectric focusing provides a powerful tool and is capable of further fractionating preparations of 12,000 IU/mg into several components having biological activity as high as 16,000 IU/mg (Qazi et al. 1974; Merz et al. 1974).

Whereas a number of methods are available for the purification of hCG from trophoblastic tumors, the reports of its isolation from normal or diseased chorionic tissue are limited (Ashitaka 1970; Ashitaka et al. 1972). Ashitaka (1970) has been able to obtain a preparation of hCG from first-trimester tissues with biological activity of 18,000–20,000 IU/mg. It would be interesting to know whether or not the tissue hCG is chemically and biologically identical to urinary hCG. The preliminary data of Ashitaka indicate significant differences in both amino acid and carbohydrate compositions, although these results await confirmation by other investigators.

Preparation of the Subunits

It is well established that hCG consists of two dissimilar, noncovalently bonded subunits commonly designated as α and β. The initial attempt to dissociate hCG into subunits was made by Bahl (1969a) and Bell et al. (1969), using sedimentation equilibrium and gel filtration of the reduced and alkylated hCG. The nonidentity of the polypeptide chains was recognized when electrophoresis in polyacrylamide gel of the reduced and alkylated hCG yielded two bands (Canfield et al. 1970). The question of whether the polypeptide chains were noncovalently or disulfide linked, however, was not resolved until separation of the subunits from native hCG was achieved by Swaminathan and Bahl (1970) and confirmed by Morgan and Canfield (1971).

The procedure developed in our laboratory is simple, involving dissociation of the subunits with 8 M urea, followed by their separation by chromatography on DEAE-Sephadex. The individual subunits are further purified by reincubation of individual subunits from DEAE-Sephadex with 8 M urea followed by gel filtration on Sephadex G–100. Interestingly, this procedure for the purification of hCG subunits is equally effective in the preparation of subunits of other gonadotropins such as human LH (Rathnam and Saxena 1971) and FSH (Saxena and Rathnam 1971; Reichert and Ward 1974), equine LH (Landefeld and McShan 1974b) and FSH (Grimek and McShan 1974), and pregnant mare serum gonadotropin, PMSG (Bahl 1974; Papkoff 1974).

Microheterogeneity

Microheterogeneity is very common in glycoproteins. Accordingly, hCG and its subunits show polymorphism, as reflected by their behavior on electrophoresis, in polyacrylamide or starch gel, isoelectric focusing, and on ion-exchange chromatography (Bahl 1969a; van Hell et al. 1968; Goverde et al. 1968; Graesslin et al. 1972, 1973; Merz et al. 1974). Their electrophoretic patterns are characterized by broad or multiple bands. All forms have almost identical amino acid compositions, with variation in their carbohydrate portion, especially in the sialic acid content.

Microheterogeneity comes from the degradation of the polypeptide or the polysaccharide or both chains during renal clearance, from the introduction of artifacts during isolation, or from the incomplete synthesis of the carbohydrate chains. The deamidation of asparagine and glutamine, oxidation of methionine,

and loss of labile sialic acid residues have been frequently encountered. Methionine sulfoxide is commonly present in highly purified hCG preparations (Carlsen and Bahl 1974).

Whereas the various polymorphic forms of hCG differ in their biological potencies (Brossmer 1971a, b; Graesslin et al. 1972), the immunological properties are unaltered, as shown by immunoelectrophoresis and immunodiffusion. Hilgenfeldt et al. (1972) have examined the spectral properties of the various forms of hCG and have found them to be unchanged also. The discrepancy in the biological activities has been attributed to their plasma half-life. The removal of sialic acid, which occupies the nonreducing terminal positions in the carbohydrate chains, exposes the adjoining galactose residues and results in rapid metabolic clearance (Morell et al. 1971).

The amino acid sequences of hCGα (Bahl et al. 1972; Bellisario et al. 1973) and ovine LH (Liu et al. 1972a, b; Sairam et al. 1972a) indicate microheterogeneity in the amino terminal region. Similarly, hCGβ and LHβ reveal carboxyterminal microheterogeneity (Liu et al. 1972b; Sairam et al. 1972b). Our recent studies on the carbohydrate sequences in both subunits indicate that whereas the asparagine-linked carbohydrates in hCGβ are almost identical in structure, the two carbohydrate units of hCGα show minor differences. Similar differences have been discovered in the serine-linked carbohydrate units of hCGβ (Marz and Bahl 1975).

2.3 Properties

Physicochemical Properties

With a value of 0.69 used for the partial specific volume, hCG has a sedimentation constant of 2.89S and a molecular weight of about 40,000 daltons by sedimentation equilibrium (Bahl 1973). This value is in good agreement with the molecular weight calculated from the amino acid sequences of the α and β subunits and from their carbohydrate compositions (Bellisario et al. 1973; Carlsen and Bahl 1973; Bahl 1973). The molecular weights of the α and β subunits are 14,000 and 24,000 daltons, respectively. The molecular weights of hCG and the subunits determined by gel filtration on Sephadex G–100 are erroneously high (Bahl 1969a; Bell et al. 1969). Even the SDS gel electrophoresis yields higher values on the order of 18,000 and 28,000 daltons for the α and β subunits, respectively (Morgan et al. 1974; Canfield et al. 1971; Reichert and Lawson 1973a, b).

Since it has a low isoelectric point of 2.9, hCG is highly charged at physiological pH (Got and Bourillon 1960a). The $E^{1\%}$ 278 nm values for hCG, hCGα, and hCGβ are 3.88 (Bahl 1969a), 4.3, and 2.1, respectively

(Morgan et al. 1974). The molar extinction coefficients from their molecular weights are 1.48×10^4, 0.64×10^4, and 0.56×10^4 M^{-1} cm^{-1}, respectively.

Like human LH (Rathnam and Saxena 1972) and ovine LH (Bewley and Li 1973), hCG and its subunits do not display any α helix or antiparallel β-pleated-sheet structure (Mori and Holland 1971; Hilgenfeldt et al. 1972), since they do not exhibit a negative cotton effect at 220 nm—not even a shoulder—and no positive cotton effect can be detected in the far ultraviolet region. A drastic change in the secondary structure of the hormone can be observed at high concentrations of hexafluoropropanol, however. In this solvent the hormone and its subunits convert to an ordered structure that contains only α-helix components (Hilgenfeldt et al. 1974).

The circular dichroic (CD) spectrum of the native hCG shows two negative cotton effects at 207 and 196 nm and has significant differences from those of the α and β subunits. While the CD spectrum of the β subunit is similar to that of the native hCG, the α subunit has only one cotton effect at 195 nm and a plateau between 205 and 202 nm. The CD spectra of the hormone and the subunits are not greatly affected by pH and protein concentration (Hilgenfeldt et al. 1974).

Dissociation and Reassociation of the Subunits
A systematic investigation of the optimum conditions for the dissociation and association of the subunits by urea has been carried out by Aloj et al. (1973). The dissociation and association is followed flurometrically, using 1,8 anilino naphthalene sulfonate. This dye interacts with intact hCG and not with the subunits, resulting in a large increase in quantum yield. The rate of dissociation of hCG is a function of the urea concentration, pH, and temperature. The optimum conditions for the dissociation have been found to be 8 to 10 molar urea at pH 7.4 or 4.8 at 25° or preferably at 37° for one to two hours. Similarly, the rate of association is also dependent on the ionic strength of the buffer, pH, and temperature. Obviously, low ionic strength and high pH and temperature favor association.

The dissociation and association can also be followed by immunodiffusion, radioimmunoassay, bioassay (Merz et al. 1974), polyacrylamide gel electrophoresis (Pierce et al. 1971), gel filtration, radioligand-receptor assay (Reichert et al. 1973), and finally by circular dichroic measurements (Merz et al. 1974).

Biological and Immunological Properties
Whereas the highly purified hormone preparations show biological potencies of 12,000–19,000 IU/mg by the usual bioassays such as the ventral prostate method, the α and β subunits have activities less than 1 percent in the same system (Pierce et al. 1971; Morgan

and Canfield 1971; Catt et al. 1973; Bahl et al. 1973; Morgan et al. 1974). The question still remains to be answered as to whether this in vivo activity represents slight contamination by the undissociated hormone or is an intrinsic property of the subunits, particularly when the half-life of the subunits is 5 to 8 percent that of the native hCG (Braunstein et al. 1972). In vitro and in vivo studies of the binding of ^{125}I- or ^{3}H-labeled hormone or its subunits further confirm the bioassay results—the subunits have little if any biological activity (Kammerman and Canfield 1972; Lee and Ryan 1972). The subunits neither bind nor compete with the labeled hormone for binding to more than 1 percent; hCGα has been found to be 0.9 percent, and hCGβ 0.7 percent, as potent as native hCG in inhibiting LH uptake in vitro (Lee and Ryan 1973a). Finally, the subunits lack the ability to stimulate testosterone synthesis in rat Leydig cells (Catt et al. 1973). They recombine to yield 60–85 percent of the biological activity, indicating that the biologically active parts of the molecule must be derived from both subunits and are dependent on conformation of hCG (Pierce et al. 1971; Morgan and Canfield 1971; Aloj et al. 1973; Donini et al. 1973; Merz et al. 1974). This is further supported by the circular dichroic spectrum, which reflects conformational changes when hCG undergoes dissociation. Although the subunits have little biological activity in the above systems, they may be active in other biological systems (Gospodarowicz 1971; Licht and Papkoff 1971; Yang et al. 1972; Rao and Carmen 1973; McKerns 1973).

The plasma half-life of hCG is much greater than that of LH; this is attributed to its higher sialic acid content. The subunits of hCG have a plasma half-life 5 to 8 percent that of native hCG (Braunstein et al. 1973). The hybrids of hCG with complementing LH subunits have a greater biological activity than LH. For instance, the hCGα and bLHβ hybrid has been found to be 1.6 fold more active than the bLHα and bLHβ hybrid (Vaitukaitis et al. 1973). The greater biological activity is probably due to longer plasma half-life of the hybrid preparation, which would be conferred by hCGα. The sialic acid content of hCGα is 30 percent that of hCG, and it alone is more than LH.

Investigators have found hCG to have blood group A-like activity. Surprisingly, this activity resides in the α subunit, which lacks N-acetylgalactosamine, the immunodominant sugar for blood group A activity. A similar situation exists in the carcinoembryonic antigen (März et al. 1973). Thyrotropic activity has also been shown in hCG (Nisula et al. 1974). The physiological significance of these unusual activities is not clear at present.

The immunological activities of the highly purified hCG preparations range between 6500–7000 IU/mg

(Bahl and Agrawal 1969; Donini et al. 1973). The activities of the α and β subunits are about 5–10 percent of the native molecule in hCG–anti-hCG system (Donini et al. 1973; Bahl et al. 1974). The recombination of the subunits restores about 70–90 percent of the immunological activity (Donini et al. 1973).

One of the exciting developments has been the finding that all gonadotropins share a common, interchangeable α subunit. It is the β subunit that confers hormonal specificity (Pierce et al. 1971; Vaitukaitis and Ross 1972). It is interesting that TSH, though functionally unrelated to gonadotropins, also shares this common α subunit. Apparently, the immunological cross-reactivity of the glycoprotein hormones is due largely to the α subunit. Antiserum raised to hCGα has almost similar affinity for the other glycoprotein hormones, whereas the anti-hCGβ displays incomplete cross-reactivity with the other hormones (Vaitukaitis and Ross 1972). Consequently, the antisera to the β subunits are more specific and, therefore, are better suited for radioimmunoassays of the hormones (Vaitukaitis and Ross 1972; Donini et al. 1973).

Antisera against the subunits have been exploited to determine the degree of homology between hormones from different species as well between different hormones from the same species. According to Vaitukaitis et al. (1972b), whereas ovine, bovine, and rat LHα fail to yield inhibition in anti-hLHα radioimmunoassay system, hFSHα and hCGα show complete cross-reactivity with hLHα. Ovine, bovine, and rat LHβ do show complete cross-reactivity with hLHβ in the anti-hLHβ radioimmunoassay system; however, hCG and its β subunit show incomplete cross-reactivity. These results indicate that (1) interspecies cross-reactivity resides in the β subunit of the hormone, and (2) within species, cross-reactivity resides in the α subunit.

With antisera against hCGα or hCGβ used in homologous radioimmunoassay systems, chimpanzee and gorilla chorionic gonadotropins (chCG, gorCG) show complete cross-reactivity, indicating that both α and β subunits of chCG and gorCG have a high degree of homology with hCG (Hodgen et al. 1973). Surprisingly, the rhesus monkey does not show cross-reactivity with hCG in any of the systems.

2.4 Chemistry

Chemical Composition

There is a striking agreement between the amino acid compositions of hCG reported from several laboratories (Bahl 1969a; Bell et al. 1969; Mori and Holland 1971). The hormone shows an unusually high content of proline, probably second to collagen, which indicates that the molecule probably has little or no α helical content. In fact, circular dichroic measurements

indicate the virtual absence of α helix or β structure. The hormone has a fairly large number of serine and disulfide bonds. Contrary to earlier reports, amino acid sequence studies on hCGα and hCGβ indicate the absence of tryptophan. Among all the glycoprotein hormones so far analyzed, hLHβ is the only one that has one residue of tryptophan.

The amino acid compositions of the subunits show that while the α subunit contains considerably higher amounts of lysine, histidine, glutamic acid, methionine, tyrosine, and phenylalanine residues, the β subunit is rich in arginine, proline, isoleucine, and leucine.

Among all gonadotropins, hCG has the second-highest proportion of carbohydrate, approximately 30 percent (Got 1965; Bahl 1969b); PMSG has 40 percent carboydrate (Gospodarowicz 1972). The carbohydrate moiety is made up of L-fucose, D-galactose, D-mannose, 2-acetamido-2-deoxy-D-glucose, 2-acetamido-2-deoxy-D-galactose, and sialic acid. The L-fucose component accounts for less than 1 percent, while neutral sugars, hexosamines, and sialic acid range between 9–11 percent each. The carbohydrate content of the subunits is about 30 percent each (Bahl 1973).

The monosaccharide compositions of hCGα and hCGβ show marked differences. Whereas N-acetylgalactosamine and fucose are present in hCGβ, they are virtually absent from hCGα. In addition, compared with hCGα, the number of sialic acid and galactose residues is much higher in hCGβ.

Amino Acid Sequence

Amino acid sequences of both subunits of hCG have been completed (Bahl et al. 1972; Morgan et al. 1973). The amide groups and positions of the disulfide bonds remain to be assigned. Whereas there is almost complete agreement on the sequence of the α subunit, there are minor differences between the amino acid sequences of hCGβ reported by two laboratories (Bahl et al. 1972; Bellisario et al. 1973; Carlsen et al. 1973; Morgan et al. 1973).

The sequence of hCGα, which contains 92 amino acids, is shown in Figure 2.1; it is almost identical with human LHα (Sairam et al. 1972a), except that hCGα has three additional residues at the N-terminus. In addition, residues 84 and 85 of serine and half-cystine seem to be inverted.

According to Bahl et al. (1973), hCGβ has 147 amino acid residues; Morgan et al. (1973) propose 145. The amino acid sequence of hCGβ is shown in Figure 2.2. A few discrepancies between this sequence and that proposed by Morgan et al. (1973) still remain to be resolved. Most of the differences lie in the carboxy-terminal region, with one additional dispute at position 55. Canfield's proposal has one additional serine residue at position 121, Ser instead of Pro at position 137, and three fewer residues at the carboxy end. Another difference between the two proposals resides in the placement of the serine-linked carbohydrate units.

A comparison of amino acid sequences of hCGα and hCGβ with LH, FSH, and TSH subunits is shown in Figures 2.1 and 2.2. The amino acid differences among the various α subunits and those in the β subunits are summarized in Tables 2.1 and 2.2. They show that while the hCGα is almost identical to those of hLHα (Sairam et al. 1972a) and hFSHα (Shome and Parlow 1974a; Rathnam and Saxena 1975), hCGα has as many as 25 residue differences from LHα and TSHα of other species; hCGβ, on the other hand, has much greater variation from the other β subunits, hLHβ being the closest with 49 residue differences (Closset et al. 1973; Shome and Parlow 1973a) and hFSHβ being the furthest with 105. It is not surprising, therefore, that the β subunits are immunologically more specific than the α subunits, and that they have the unique structural features that confer hormonal specificity. It is also possible, on the basis of the extent of the structural homology, to predict the degree of immunological cross-reactivity among the various glycoprotein hormones.

Table 2.1 Amino acid residue differences between hCGα and the α subunits of other glycoprotein hormones

	hCGα[1]	o/bLHα[2]	bTSHα	Total residues
hLHα[3]	2 (2.2)*	24 (26.9)	29 (32.5)	89
pLHα[4]	25 (27.7)	5 (5.5)	11 (12.2)	90
hFHSα[5]	0	25 (27–28)	25 (27–28)	89, 92
bTSHα[6]	25 (26.0)	0		96

*Figures in parentheses represent percentage differences from hCGα, based on 92 residues.

[1]Bellisario et al. 1973. Bahl et al. 1972.
[2]Sairam and Papkoff 1974.
[3]Sairam et al. 1972a.
[4]Maghuin-Rogister et al. 1972.
[5]Shome and Parlow 1974a; Rathnam and Saxena 1974.
[6]Liao and Pierce 1971.

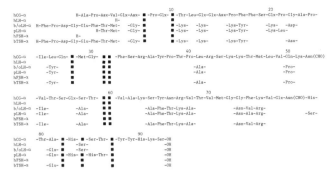

Figure 2.1 Amino acid sequences of the α subunits. See the notes to Table 2.1 for references. Solid squares represent the positions of the cysteine residues.

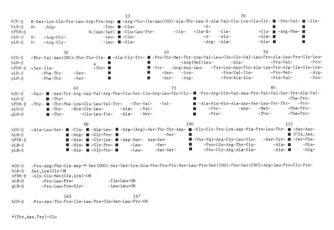

Figure 2.2 Amino acid sequences of the β subunits. See the notes to Table 2.2 for references. Solid squares represent the positions of the cysteine residues.

Table 2.2 Amino acid residue differences between hCGβ and the β subunits of other glycoprotein hormones

	hCGβ[1]	b/oLHβ	bTSHβ	Total residues
hLHβ[2]	49 (33.3)*	43	63	115
b/oLHβ[3]	72 (48.9)		87	119
pLHβ[4]	75 (51.0)	18	84	120
hFHSβ[5]	105 (71.2)	78	75	115
hTSHβ[6]	100 (68.0)	84	32	114
bTSHβ[7]	100 (68.0)	87		113

*Figures in parentheses represent percentage differences from hCGβ, based on 147 residues.

[1]Carlsen and Bahl 1973.
[2]Closset et al. 1973.
[3]Sairam and Papkoff 1974.
[4]Maghuin-Rogister and Dockier 1971.
[5]Shome and Parlow 1974b.
[6]Shome and Parlow 1973b.
[7]Liao and Pierce 1971.

Carbohydrate Sequence

There are two distinct types of carbohydrate-protein linkages in the hCG molecule (Bahl 1969a). There are four asparagine-linked multiple-branched complex heteropolysaccharide units, two in the α at residues 52 and 78 (Bellisario et al. 1973) and two in the β at residues 13 and 30 (Carlsen et al. 1973). In addition, the β subunit has three simple serine-linked oligosaccharide units near the C-terminus of the molecule at positions 118, 129, and 131. In this regard, hCG is different from other glycoprotein hormones which have only one type of protein-carbohydrate linkage: the asparagine type, with two units in the α and one in the β subunit (hFSHβ is an exception with two carbohydrate units).

The monosaccharide sequence of hCG has been determined by sequential degradation of hCG and the individual glycopeptides (Bahl 1969b; März and Bahl 1975) with specific exoglycosidases (Bahl 1973), neuraminidase, β galactosidase, β N-acetylglucosaminidase (Agrawal and Bahl 1968; Bahl and Agrawal 1969), α mannosidase (Matta and Bahl 1972), and α N-acetylgalactosaminidase (McDonald and Bahl 1972). The enzymes hydrolyze carbohydrate chains from the nonreducing ends and were used serially in different combinations. The proposed sequences of the aspargine- and serine-linked carbohydrate units are shown in Figure 2.3 (Bahl 1969b; Bahl 1973).

2.5 Interaction with Target Tissues

Binding

A great deal of attention has been focused on understanding the molecular mechanisms of gonadotropin

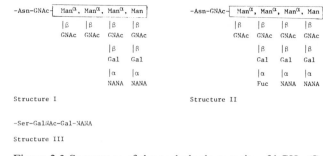

Figure 2.3 Structures of the carbohydrate units of hCHα (I), hCGβ (II), and (III).

action. The approach has been threefold: first, to determine the primary site of action; second, to elucidate the nature of the initial interaction with cellular receptors by binding studies using labeled hormone and by the actual isolation of the receptor molecule; and third, to investigate the effect of structural alterations of the hormone and the receptors on the hormone-receptor interaction and subsequent biological phenomena. The ultimate goal, of course, is to unravel all the biochemical steps beginning with the initial interaction between hormone and receptor and ending eventually in protein synthesis. Despite the work of many investigators in this field, the progress so far has been limited.

Specific uptake of labeled gonadotropins by testis (Catt et al. 1972a; Catt and Dufau 1973b; Leidenberger and Reichert 1972) and ovary has been demonstrated by autoradiography and by binding studies in vitro and in vivo (Presl et al. 1972; Rajaniemi and Vanha-Perttula 1972; Braendle et al. 1973; Cole et al. 1973; Rajaniemi et al. 1974; Lee and Ryan, 1973a; Danzo et al. 1972; Danzo 1973; Kammerman and Canfield 1972; Ashitaka et al. 1973; Ashitaka and Koide 1974). Thus highly specific binding sites of hCG and LH are present in these tissues. Both hormones compete for the same receptor sites in testis and ovary. Furthermore, no species difference appears (Bellisario and Bahl 1975), although these studies have thus far been confined to rat testis and ovary, bovine and human corpus luteum (Lee and Ryan 1971; Lee et al. 1973, Goldenberg et al. 1973), and porcine granulosa cells (Channing and Kammerman 1973). Binding of various subcellular fractions with the labeled hormone, followed by radioactivity measurement or autoradiography (Han et al. 1974) or by the use of immobilized hormone, has established that the binding sites or receptors are located on the plasma membranes. Although there is a high degree of specificity of binding to testis and ovary, some binding does take place to liver and kidney and other subcellular sites, such as cytoplasm (Midgley 1972), mitochondria, and microsomes (Rao et al. 1972). The studies conducted in our laboratory, which take advantage of the chromatographic behavior of the hormone-receptor complex and specific binding of desialyzed hCG to rat testis, show that the binding to tissues other than the target organs is nonspecific (Bellisario and Bahl 1975).

The binding sites in testis and ovary are limited in number, approximately 6000 per cell. The binding of hCG-LH is dependent on time, temperature, and pH and is saturable. It is characterized by a high affinity constant of the order of 10^{10} M^{-1} (Lee and Ryan 1972; Lee and Ryan, 1973a), which is concordant with the circulating levels of luteinizing hormone in plasma of various species and with concentrations of LH and hCG (10^{-1} to 10^{-12} M) required to activate steroidogenesis in vitro (Catt et al. 1972a). The degree of total binding suggests that only a small portion of the binding sites need to be occupied by gonadotropins in order to elicit a maximum physiological response; this possibility is supported by studies correlating hormone binding, cyclic AMP formation, and steroidogenesis (Catt and Dufau 1973a; Moyle et al. 1975).

The association rate constant for LH and hCG binding to the receptors at 25° is 3.5×10^6 M^{-1} sec^{-1}. In the dissociation of LH-hCG receptor to rat ovarian tissue in vitro, two different complexes dissociate at different rates, fast and slow; the dissociation rate constants are 1.4×10^{-3} sec^{-1} and 8×10^{-5} sec^{-1}. The dissociation rate is temperature-dependent. The association constant obtained from the rate constant is similar to the one obtained from equilibrium data (Lee and Ryan 1973b). It has been observed that hCG dissociated from the membranes at low pH has higher biological activity than the starting material, suggesting that hCG does not undergo any molecular alteration on binding to the receptors (Dufau et al. 1972).

Solubilization of the Receptors
The LH-hCG receptors from interstitial tissue of rat testis (Dufau and Catt 1973; Bellisario and Bahl 1975; Dufau et al. 1973) and rat and bovine ovaries can be solubilized by nonionic detergents, Triton X–100, Emulphogene, Luberol WX, Luberol PX, sodium deoxycholate, sodium dodecyl sulfate, and guanidine hydrochloride (Dufau et al. 1974a; Haour and Saxena 1974). The detergent-solubilized receptors bind specifically to LH or hCG and exhibit properties similar to those of membrane-bound receptors. Guanidine hydrochloride–solubilized receptor, on the other hand, is inactive, but the activity is claimed to be restored by incubation, with the total lipid fraction indicating that the lipid is essential for the binding activity (Haour and Saxena 1974). The initial rate of binding of the hormone to the testicular soluble receptor is dependent on temperature; it is higher at 37°C than at 24°C and 4°C, but degradation of the receptors occurs at higher temperatures than that (Dufau et al. 1973; Bellisario and

Bahl 1975). The association constant of the soluble receptor varies between 5 and 10 M^{-1} and is lower than the membrane receptor (Dufau et al. 1973; Bellisario and Bahl 1975).

The protein nature of the receptors is evidenced by their inactivation by trypsin and pepsin (Dufau et al. 1973; Haour and Saxena 1974; Rao 1974; Bellisario and Bahl 1975). Like the membrane receptors, the binding of the hormone to the soluble receptors is inhibited at high concentrations of NaCl, $MgCl_2$, urea, and guanidine hydrochloride (Bellisario and Bahl 1975; Haour and Saxena 1974). Conflicting reports have appeared about the effect of lipases C and A on the soluble receptor (Dufau et al. 1973; Saxena et al. 1974; Rao 1974).

Sucrose gradient centrifugation yields a value of 6.5S for the testicular soluble receptors and 7.5S for the hCG-soluble receptor complex. The S-value of the complex extracted from the prelabeled testis by binding with the labeled hormone with Triton X–100 is 8.8S. The sedimentation behavior of the receptor has been found to be dependent on the detergent used for its extraction. When the hormone-receptor complex is extracted from the prelabeled tissue with Lubrol PX and Lubrol WX, the value of sedimentation constant is 7S, indicating that either a different degree of association of the detergent occurs with the receptor or that the receptor occurs in polymorphic forms (Charreau et al. 1974). The molecular weights of the receptor and the hormone-receptor complex determined by density gradient centrifugation are 194,000 and 224,000 daltons, respectively (Dufau et al. 1973). These values may not be reliable because of the interaction of the detergent with the receptors, resulting in a change in their density and thus in their sedimentation behavior. The molecular weight of the bovine corpus luteum receptor has been reported to be 30,000 to 70,000 daltons by SDS gel electrophoresis and by gel filtration (Haour and Saxena 1974).

Labeling of LH-hCG Receptor
One of the major problems in the isolation and characterization of LH-hCG receptor has been its presence in extremely low amounts in the tissues. The availability of radioactively labeled receptor would certainly facilitate the investigation. Two approaches have been followed to this end: these involve the incorporation of ^{14}C-labeled N-acetylglucosamine or a ^{131}I label in the membrane receptor for LH-hCG. The incorporation of ^{14}C has been effected by pulse labeling the hCG-primed ovaries from immature rats in vitro with N-acetylglucosamine. The incorporation of the label in the receptor has been established by its isolation by chromatography on Sepharose 6B, by affinity chromatography on hCG-Sepharose complex, and by gel elec-

trophoresis (Bahl et al. 1974). This approach is based on the assumptions that, first, the receptor is a glycoprotein, since it is located on the plasma membranes that have glycoproteins as one of their major components, and second, the synthesis of the receptor is stimulated by hCG and FSH.

The ^{131}I label has been incorporated in the receptor in the plasma membranes from bovine corpora lutea by a four-step procedure: first, protection of the receptor sites with unlabeled hCG; second, labeling the membrane protein with unlabeled NaI using glucose, glucose oxidase, and lactoperoxidase method; third, removal of the hCG by rabbit anti-hCG; and fourth, labeling with Na^{131}I as in the second step. The incorporation of the label in the receptor has been shown by its isolation as outlined above (Pandian et al. 1975).

2.6 Structure and Function Relationships

Early work in the study of hCG has been limited to a few areas such as the effect of urea, acetylation, reduction (Li 1949), and hydrolysis with neuraminidase (Whitten 1948) and proteases (Li 1949). Only recently has highly purified hormone become available and the primany structure of the hormone been elucidated. As a consequence, a great deal of interest has been generated in the structure and function relationships. Since hCG is a glycoprotein hormone, structural alterations have been attempted in the protein or the carbohydrate moiety or both. The effects of a specific modification on its physicochemical, conformational, and biological properties have been studied to determine the essential components of the structure related to that property; that is, attention has been focused on the parts of the molecule involved in the subunit interaction, in conformation, in binding to the receptor, in cyclic AMP stimulation and steroidogenesis, and in protein synthesis and biological and immunological activities. A similar approach in the case of other polypeptide hormones, including glucagon and ACTH, has provided an insight into the molecular mechanisms of their action. Detailed evaluation of the various modified forms, particularly the polypeptide part of the hormone, has not been carried out extensively so far, although some interesting information has emerged from a study of the carbohydrate-degraded hormone derivatives.

Brossmer et al. (1971b) have obtained several hormone derivatives by the modification of the polypeptide portion by acetylation, succinylation, carbamylation, deamidation, nitration, and polymerization, under rather exhaustive conditions. No detailed characterization of the derivatives was attempted to determine the site(s) of alterations. The various derivatives were tested for their biological activity only by the rat

prostate method. Succinylation and acetylation of up to three amino groups did not show an effect on the biological activity. Similarly, one-third of the tyrosine residues are not involved in the biological activity. Polymerization with glutaraldehyde, benzodiazobenzidine, and Woodward reagent K results in no loss in activity when the degree of polymerization is between one and two (i.e., the molecular weight of the polymer varies between 40,000 and 80,000 daltons) (Brossmer et al. 1971b). Carlsen and Bahl (1974) and Bahl et al. (1974) have performed several modifications, such as maleylation, alkylation of methionine, photo-oxidation of histidine, and blocking of carboxyl groups. All of these reactions have been carried out under exhaustive conditions, and all of the derivatives are biologically inactive and lose their ability to bind to the receptor. No attempt has been made to characterize the derivatives.

Two laboratories carried out detailed investigations of the role of tyrosyl residues in the biological activity of hCG, in the subunit interaction, and in binding to the receptor sites. The conductometric titrations and the spectral studies show that about 50 percent of the tyrosyl residues (about four out of seven) are exposed to the solvent, and some of these may be involved in binding to the receptor. Urea unfolds the molecule, and two more tyrosines become accessible to the perturbant molecule. One tyrosyl residue, however, is still incompletely exposed (Mori and Holland 1971). The nitration of hCG and of the subunits under controlled or exhaustive conditions or both have led to the following conclusions: the tyrosyl 88 or 89 of hCGα is the most susceptible residue to nitration; although these residues are not involved in the subunit interaction, they may play a role in binding to the testicular receptor, since the binding affinity of the mononitro-hCG is about 50 percent of the hormone. Residue 65 of hCGα is involved neither in binding to hCGβ nor in binding to the receptor. Residue 37 of hCGα seems to be involved in binding to the β subunit. The tyrosyl residues at positions 37 or 59 of hCGβ are involved in binding to hCGα and do not play a role in the biological activity. Tyrosyl 82 of the β subunit is apparently not involved in either subunit interaction or the hormone receptor interaction (Carlsen and Bahl 1976). These results are somewhat in disagreement with those of Hum et al. (1974).

The disulfide bonds of the hormones are essential for binding to the receptor (Schlumberger 1968; Bahl et al. 1974; Dufau et al. 1974b) and also play a role in subunit interaction. Bellisario and Bahl (1975) and Carlsen and Bahl (1974) have examined all of the tryptic and chymotryptic peptides from the reduced and alkylated hCGα and hCGβ for immunological and binding activity. None of them show any immunological or receptor binding activity, even at 10,000 fold concentrations. Thus the biologically active parts of the molecule are derived from both subunits, and the conformational integrity of the molecule is mandatory for the hormone activity (Bahl et al. 1974).

A great deal of work has been done to evaluate the role of carbohydrates in the physicochemical, immunological, and biological properties of hCG-induced cyclic AMP stimulation and steroidogenesis.

The removal of sialic acid by neuraminidase increases the isoelectric point of hCG, and the acid-base titration curves are different; the differences correspond to a loss of strongly acidic groups, the number of which equals that of the neuraminic acid residues (Mori and Holland 1971). The circular dichroic spectra of hCG and asialo-hCG do not show any significant conformational change. Intrinsic viscosities of hCG and asialo-hCG are 3.4 and 3.2, respectively. The asialo-hCG is biologically inactive, probably due to shorter plasma half-life (Van Hall et al. 1971a; Ross et al. 1972), but immunologically it is equally active (Van Hall et al. 1971b). The desialyzation of hCG results in an almost twofold increase in the binding to the plasma membrane receptor in testis or ovary. Whereas the ability of the hormone to stimulate steroidogenesis remains unaltered, its ability to stimulate hormone-induced cyclic AMP accumulation is considerably impaired (Moyle et al. 1975).

The removal of about 60 percent galactose, 55 percent N-acetylglucosamine, and 20 percent mannose residues from asialo-hCG can be effected by specific exoglycosidases. The cleavage of galactose, N-acetylglucosamine, and mannose residues result in about 10–20 percent loss of immunological activity but almost complete loss of biological activity. The antigenic determinants apparently do not reside in the carbohydrate part of the molecule (März et al. 1973).

The asialo-agalacto hCG (NG-hCG), asialic-agalacto-aglucosaminyl hCG (NAG-hCG), bind as well as native hCG. On removing mannose residues from NGA-hCG (NGAM-hCG), however, the binding to the rat testicular receptors is drastically reduced; the loss is proportional to the mannose removed (März et al. 1973). All of these derivatives not only fail to stimulate cyclic AMP formation, but act as competitive inhibitors. Furthermore, all of them can stimulate steroidogenesis maximally, but the relative potency of the derivatives is considerably reduced—that is, a much larger dosage of the derivatives than hCG is required for stimulation to the same extent (Bahl et al. 1974; Moyle et al. 1975). These results on the biological properties of asialo-hCG and asialo-agalacto-hCG are in agreement with those obtained by Tsuruhara et al. (1972a, b). Thus the studies on the carbohydrate part of hCG suggest that the carbohydrate has a biological

function in contrast to the glycoenzymes, where the catalytic activity of the enzyme does not seem to be affected by the removal of the carbohydrate.

2.7 Clinical Applications

Because of the structural similarity between hCG and LH, they share common biological properties and show immunological cross-reactivity; anti-hCG fails to discriminate between LH and hCG. But hCGβ, on the other hand, has some unique structural features that render its antibody quite specific—it reacts with hCG but not significantly with LH. This fact has been used to develop a radioimmunoassay that measures hCG specifically (Vaitukaitis et al. 1972b). The assay is sufficiently sensitive and can measure as low as 5 mIU (0.2 ng) of hCG in 200 μl of the serum sample. It can distinguish hCG from follicular or luteal phase LH levels. The specificity of the assay is ideal both for diagnosing and following the course of disease among patients undergoing chemotherapy for hCG-secreting tumors and for following serum-hCG levels in patients after termination of molar pregnancies. The assay is also quite useful in the detection of pregnancy at an early stage.

The specificity of hCGβ has also been exploited in preliminary studies on fertility regulation. Structural alterations of an antigen, by coupling to a hapten or a carrier protein such as tetanus or diphtheria toxoid, not only enhance its antigenicity but also impair its cross-reactivity with homologous endogenous antigens. In addition, the secretion of the autologous antigen does not "boost" antibody levels (Stevens 1973; Talwar and Bahl 1974). The use of hCGβ or any of its carboxy-terminal fragments after conjugation with hapten or a carrier protein offers a potentially promising approach to the problem of fertility regulation. A limited number of trials using hCGβ-tetanus toxoid have been performed in humans of reproductive age (three cases of experimental and three of control women). It is claimed that the antibody to hCGβ-tetanus toxoid conjugate does not cross-react with hLH, despite a considerable homology in the 115 amino-terminal residues of hLHβ and hCGβ. Whether this is true or not remains to be established by further human experimentation. Removal of the maximum portion of the polypeptide from the amino-terminus with retention of some immunogenicity in the residual carboxy-terminal peptide or a modified hCGβ may prove to be more suitable than hCGβ.

Radioligand-receptor assay for LH or hCG (Catt et al. 1971; Catt et al. 1972b) has been applied to the early detection of pregnancy, ectopic pregnancy, and spontaneous abortion, with a high degree of reliability (Saxena et al. 1974; Landesman and Saxena 1974). The radioligand-receptor assay has permitted the detection of a gonadotropinlike material in the rabbit blastocyst, which may have important implications in the area of reproduction (Haour and Saxena 1974). The assay has several advantages: it measures the biologically active species, it is rapid, and it can be performed on urine or serum without prior extraction.

It has already been noted that the carbohydrate-degraded hCG derivatives lose their ability to stimulate the hormone-induced accumulation of cyclic AMP and are less potent in stimulating testosterone biosynthesis. Consequently, these derivatives appear able to bind to the target tissue membranes as well as does the native hormone, but with little or no biological response. It would be interesting to know if they suppress ovulation in vivo or prevent or terminate pregnancy in animals.

An unbalanced synthesis of the subunits of hCG occurs in the presence of certain neoplasms. This may help in the diagnosis of certain types of malignancies (Weintraub et al. 1973; Braunstein et al. 1973).

2.8 General Considerations

Several aspects of the chemistry and biology of hCG and its subunits have been considered, such as isolation, physicochemical and biological properties, amino acid and carbohydrate structure and its relationship to biological function, and interaction of the hormone with target tissue receptors. Other developments in the field—the most significant being the radioimmunoassay of hCG—have not been covered. The biochemical mechanisms of hormone action at cellular and molecular levels are not well understood and therefore have not been discussed. Only selected references on the reviewed areas have been cited.

The areas of future fundamental investigations from the biochemical standpoint include, particularly, the fine details of the carbohydrate structure and the effect of this structure on biological and immunological properties and on the subunit interaction and conformation of hCG. Some of the other areas of fundamental interest include elucidation of the structure and function relationships, at the molecular level, of the biochemical mechanisms underlying various events from the initial hormone-receptor interaction to the protein synthesis, and the isolation and characterization of the hCG-LH receptor. Little is known about the biosynthesis of hCG and its regulation. Most importantly from the standpoint of clinical application, the use of carboxy-terminal fragments in the detection and control of fertility needs further investigation. Finally, it should be possible to undertake the study of diseased state hCG from patients with hydatidiform mole and choriocarcinomas now that the structure of the normal hCG is known.

References

Agrawal, K. M. L., and O. P. Bahl. Glycosidases of Phaseolus vulgaris. II. Isolation and general properties. J. Biol. Chem. 243:103, 1968.

Aloj, S. M., H. Edelhoch, K. C. Ingham, F. J. Morgan, R. E. Canfield, and T. R. Grief. The rates of dissociation and reassociation of the subunits of human chorionic gonadotropin. Arch. Biochem. Biophys. 159:497, 1973.

Ashitaka, Y. Studies on the biochemical properties of highly purified human chorionic gonadotropin extracted from chorionic tissue. Acta Obstet. Gynecol. Jap. 17:124, 1970.

Ashitaka, Y., Y. Tokura, M. Tane, M. Mochizuki, and S. Tojo. Studies on the biochemical properties of highly purified hCG. Endocrinology 87:233, 1970.

Ashitaka, Y., M. Mochizuki, and S. Tojo. Purification and properties of chorionic gonadotropin from the trophoblastic tissue of hydatidiform mole. Endocrinology 90:609, 1972.

Ashitaka, T., Y. Y. Tsong, and S. S. Koide. Distribution of tritiated human chorionic gonadotropin in superovulated rat ovary. Proc. Soc. Exp. Biol. Med. 142:395, 1973.

Ashitaka, Y., and S. S. Koide. Interaction of human chorionic gonadotropin with rat gonads. Fertil. Steril. 25:177, 1974.

Bahl, O. P. Human chorionic gonadotropin. I. Purification and physico-chemical properties. J. Biol. Chem. 244:567, 1969a.

Bahl, O. P. Human chorionic gonadotropin. II. Nature of the carbohydrate units. J. Biol. Chem. 244:575, 1969b.

Bahl, O. P., and K. M. L. Agrawal. Glycosidases of aspergillus niger. I. Purification and characterization of α- and β-galactosidases and β-N-acetylglucosaminidase. J. Biol. Chem. 244:2970, 1969.

Bahl, O. P. Some of the problems related to the primary structure of glycoprotein hormones. In Structure-activity relationships of protein and polypeptide hormones, eds. M. Margoulies, and F. C. Greenwood, Excerpta Med. Intern. Congr. Ser. No. 241, 1971.

Bahl, O. P., R. B. Carlsen, R. Bellisario, and N. Swaminathan. Human chorionic gonadotropin: Amino acid sequence of the α and β subunits. Biochem. Biophys. Res. Commun. 48:416, 1972.

Bahl, O. P., R. B. Carlsen, and R. Bellisario. Human chorionic gonadotropin. Amino acid sequence of the α and β subunits and the nature and location of the carbohydrate units. In Proceedings of the Fourth International Congress of Endocrinology, eds. R. O. Scow, F. J. G. Ebling, and I. W. Henderson. Amsterdam: Excerpta Medica, 1973.

Bahl, O. P. Chemistry of human chorionic gonadotropin. In Hormonal Proteins and Peptides, ed C. H. Li. New York: Academic Press, 1973.

Bahl, O. P., L. März, and W. R. Moyle. The role of the carbohydrate in the biological function of human chorionic gonadotropin. In *Hormone binding and target cell activation in the testis*, eds. M. L. Dufau, and A. R. Means. New York: Plenum Press, 1974.

Bahl, O. P. Unpublished work, 1974.

Bahl, O. P., M. R. Pandian, W. R. Moyle, and Y. Kobayashi. Chemistry of human chorionic gonadotropin and fertility regulation. In *Advances in fertility regulation through basic research*, eds. W. A. Sadler, and S. Segal. New York: Plenum Press, 1974.

Bell, J. J., R. E. Canfield, and J. J. Sciarra. Purification and characterization of human chorionic gonadotropin. Endocrinology 84:298, 1969.

Bellisario, R., R. B. Carlsen, and O. P. Bahl. Human chorionic gonadotropin: Linear amino acid sequence of the α subunit. J. Biol. Chem. 248:6796, 1973.

Bellisario, R., and O. P. Bahl. Human chorionic gonadotropin: V. Tissue specificity of binding and partial characterization of soluble hCG-receptor complexes. J. Biol. Chem. 250:3837, 1975.

Bewley, T. A., N. R. Sairam, and C. H. Li. Circular dichroism of ovine interstitial cell stimulating hormone and its subunits. Biochemistry 11:932, 1972.

Braendle, W., M. Breckwoldt, D. Graesslin, and H. Weise. Distribution and binding of I-131-human chorionic gonadotropin (hCG) in different organs of pseudopregnant female rats. Fertil. Steril. 24:126, 1973.

Braunstein, G. D., J. L. Vaitukaitis, and G. T. Ross. The *in vivo* behavior of human chorionic gonadotropin after dissociation into subunits. Endocrinology 91:1030, 1972.

Braunstein, G. D., J. L. Vaitukaitis, P. P. Carbone and G. T. Ross. Ectopic production of human chorionic gonadotropin by neoplasms. Ann. Intern. Med. 78:39, 1973.

Brossmer, R., M. Dorner, U. Hilgenfeldt, F. Leidenberger, and E. Trude. Purification and characterization of human chorionic gonadotropin. FEBS Letters 15:33, 1971a.

Brossmer, R., M. Dorner, U. Hilgenfeldt, F. Leidenberger, and E. Trude. Chemical modification of human chorionic gonadotropin and its biological and immunological characterization. FEBS Letters 15:36, 1971b.

Canfield, R. E., G. M. Agosto, and J. J. Bell. Studies of the chemistry of human chorionic gonadotropins. In *Gonadotropins and ovarian development*, eds. W. R. Butt, A. C. Crooke, and M. Ryle. Edinburgh: E. & S. Livingstone, 1970.

Canfield, R. E., F. J. Morgan, S. Kammerman, J. J. Bell, and G. M. Agosto. Studies of human chorionic gonadotropin. Recent Prog. Horm. Res. 27:121, 1971.

Carlsen, R. B., O. P. Bahl, and N. Swaminathan. Human chorionic gonadotropin: Linear amino acid sequence of the β subunit. J. Biol. Chem. 248:6810, 1973.

Carlsen, R. B., and O. P. Bahl. Unpublished work, 1973.

Carlsen, R. B., and O. P. Bahl. The reaction of tetranitromethane with human chorionic gonadotropin. Arch. Biochem. Biophys. 175:209, 1976.

Catt, K. J., M. L. Dufau, and T. Tsuruhara. Studies on a radioligand-receptor assay system for luteinizing hormone and chorionic gonadotropin. J. Clin. Endocrinol. Metab. 32:860, 1971.

Catt, K. J., T. Tsuruhara, and M. L. Dufau. Gonadotropin binding sites of the rat testis. Biochim. Biophys. Acta 279:194, 1972a.

Catt, K. J., M. L. Dufau, and T. Tsuruhara. Radioligand-receptor assay of luteinizing hormone and chorionic gonadotropin. J. Clin. Endocrinol. Metab. 34:123, 1972b.

Catt, K. J., M. L. Dufau, and T. Tsuruhara. Absence of intrinsic biological activity in LH and hCG subunits. J. Clin. Endocrinol. Metab. 36:73, 1973.

Catt, K. J., and M. L. Dufau. Interactions of LH and hCG with testicular gonadotropin receptors. In *Receptors for reproductive hormones*, eds. B. W. O'Malley, and A. R. Means. New York: Plenum Press, 1973a.

Catt, K. J., and M. L. Dufau. Spare gonadotropin receptors in rat testis. Nature New Biol. 244:219, 1973b.

Chang, Y., E. H. Wiseman, and R. Pinson. The purification of human chorionic gonadotropin on DEAE-Sephadex. J. Chromatog. 28:104, 1967.

Channing, C. P., and S. Kammerman. Effects of hCG, asialo hCG, and the subunits of hCG upon luteinizing of monkey granulosa cells in culture. Endocrinology 92:531, 1973.

Charreau, E. H., M. L. Dufau, and K. J. Catt. Multiple forms of solubilized gonadotropin receptors from the rat testis. J. Biol. Chem. 249:4189, 1974.

Closset, J., G. Hennen, and R. M. Lequin. Human luteinizing hormone. The amino acid sequence of the β-subunit. FEBS Letters 29:97, 1973.

Cole, F. E., J. C. Weed, G. T. Schneider, J. B. Holland, W. L. Geary, and B. F. Rice. The gonadotropin receptor of the human corpus luteum. Am. J. Obstet. Gynecol. 117:87, 1973.

Danzo, B. J., A. R. Midgley, Jr., and L. J. Kleinsmith. Human chorionic gonadotropin binding to rat ovarian tissue *in vitro*. Proc. Soc. Exp. Biol. Med. 139:88, 1972.

Danzo, B. J. Characterization of a receptor for human chorionic gonadotropin in luteinizing rat ovaries. Biochim. Biophys. Acta 304:560, 1973.

Donini, S., V. Oliveri, G. Ricci, and P. Donini. Subunits of human chorionic gonadotropin: An immuno-chemical study. Acta Endocrinol. 73:133, 1973.

Dufau, M. L., K. J. Catt, and T. Tsuruhura. Biological activity of human chorionic gonadotropin released from testis binding sites. Proc. Natl. Acad. Sci. USA 69:2414, 1972.

Dufau, M. L., and K. J. Catt. Extraction of soluble gonadotropin receptors from rat testis. Nature New Biol. 242:246, 1973.

Dufau, M. L., E. H. Charreau, and K. J. Catt. Characteristics of a soluble gonadotropin receptor from rat testis. J. Biol. Chem. 248:6973, 1973.

Dufau, M. L., E. H. Charreau, D. Ryan, and K. J. Catt. Soluble gonadotropin receptors of the rat ovary. FEBS Letters 149, 1974a.

Dufau, M. L., D. Ryan, and K. J. Catt. Disulfide groups of gonadotropin receptors are essential for specific binding of human chorionic gonadotropin. Biochim. Biophys. Acta 343:417, 1974b.

Goldenberg, R. L., E. O. Reiter, J. L. Vaitukaitis, and G. T. Ross. Hormonal factors influencing ovarian uptake of human chorionic gonadotropin. Endocrinology 92:1565, 1973.

Gospodarowicz, D. Lipolytic activity of the luteinizing hormone (LH) and of its two subunits. Endocrinology 89:571, 1971.

Gospodarowicz, D. Purification and physicochemical properties of the pregnant mare serum gonadotropin (PMSG). Endocrinology 91:101, 1972.

Got, R., and R. Bourrillon. Nouvelle methode de purification de la gonadotropine choriale humaine. Biochim. Biophys. Acta 42:505, 1960a.

Got, R., and R. Bourrillon. Nouvelles donnés physiques sur la gonadotropine choriale humaine. Biochim. Biophys. Acta 39:241, 1960b.

Got, R. Physicochemical properties of chorionic gonadotropins. Eur. Rev. Endocrinol. Suppl. 1:191, 1965.

Goverde, B. C., F. J. Veenkamp, and J. D. Homan. Studies on human chorionic gonadotropin. II. Chemical composition and its relation to biological activity. Acta Endocrinol. 59: 105, 1968.

Graesslin, D., Y. Yaoi, and G. Bettendorf. Purification of human pituitary FSH and LH controlled by disc electrophoresis and carbohydrate analysis. In *Gonadotropins and ovarian development*, eds. W. R. Butt, A. C. Crooke, and M. Ryle. Edinburgh: E. & S. Livingstone, 1970.

Graesslin, D., H. C. Weise, and W. Braendle. The microheterogeneity of human chorionic gonadotropin (hCG) reflected in the β-subunits. FEBS Letters 31:214, 1973.

Grimek, H. J., and W. H. McShan. Isolation and characterization of the subunits of highly purified ovine follicle-stimulating hormone. J. Biol. Chem. 249:5725, 1974.

Han, S. S., H. J. Rajaniemo, M. I. Cho., A. N. Hirshfield, and A. R. Midgley, Jr. Gonadotropin receptors in rat ovarian tissue. II. Subcellular localization of LH binding sites by electron microscope radioautography. Endocrinology 95:589, 1974.

Haour, F., and B. B. Saxena. Characterization and solubilization of gonadotropin receptor of bovine corpus luteum. J. Biol. Chem. 249:2195, 1974.

Haour, F., and B. B. Saxena. Detection of a gonadotropin in rabbit blastocyst before implantation. Science 185:444, 1974.

Hilgenfeldt, V., W. E. Merz, and R. Brossmer. Circular dichroism studies of human chorionic gonadotropin and its subunits. FEBS Letters 26:267, 1972.

Hilgenfeldt, V., W. E. Merz, and R. Brossmer. Circular dichroism of human chorionic gonadotropin; A study of the structural characteristics of the hormone and its subunits under various conditions. Hoppe-Seyler's Z. Physiol. Chem. 355:1051, 1974.

Hodgen, G. D., W. E. Nixon, J. L. Vaitukaitis, W. W. Tuller, and G. T. Ross. Neutralization of primate chorionic gonadotropin activities by antisera against the subunits of human chorionic gonadotropin in radioimmunoassay and bioassay. Endocrinology 92:705, 1973.

Hum, G. V., J. E. Knipfel, and K. J. Mori. Human chorionic gonadotropin. Reaction with tetranitromethane. Biochemistry 13:2359, 1974.

Kammerman, W., and R. E. Canfield. The inhibition of binding of iodinated human chorionic gonadotropin to mouse ovary *in vivo*. Endocrinology 90:384, 1972.

Landefeld, T. D., and W. H. McShan. Equine luteinizing hormone and its subunits. Isolation and physicochemical properties. Biochemistry 13:1389, 1974a.

Landefeld, T. D., and W. H. McShan. Isolation and characterization of subunits from equine pituitary follicle-stimulating hormone. J. Biol. Chem. 249:3527, 1974b.

Landesman, R., and B. B. Saxena. Radioreceptor assay of human chorionic gonadotropin as an acid in miniabortion. Fertil. Steril. 25:1022, 1974.

Lee, E. Y., and R. J. Ryan. The uptake of human luteinizing hormone (hLH) by slices of luteinizing rat ovaries. Endocrinology 89:1515, 1971.

Lee, C. Y., and R. J. Ryan. Luteinizing hormone receptors: Specific binding of human luteinizing hormone to homogenates of luteinized rat ovaries. Proc. Natl. Acad. Sci. USA 69:3520, 1972.

Lee, C. Y., C. B. Coulam, N. S. Jiang, and R. J. Ryan. Receptors for human luteinizing hormone in human corpora luteal tissue. J. Clin. Endocrinol. Metab. 36:148, 1973.

Lee, C. Y., and R. J. Ryan. Luteinizing hormone receptors in luteinized rat ovaries. In *Receptors for reproductive hormones*, eds. B. W. O'Malley and A. R. Means. New York: Plenum Press, 1973a.

Lee, C. Y., and R. J. Ryan. Interaction of ovarian receptors with human luteinizing hormone and human chorionic gonadotropin. Biochemistry 12:4609, 1973b.

Leidenberger, F., and L. E. Reichert, Jr. Evaluation of a rat testis homogenate radioligand receptor assay for human pituitary LH. Endocrinology 91:901, 1972.

Leidenberger, F., and L. E. Reichert, Jr. Species differences in luteinizing hormone as inferred from slope variations in a radioligand receptor assay. Endocrinology 92:646, 1973.

Li, C. H. The chemistry of gonadotropic hormones. Vitamins and Hormones I. p. 223, 1949.

Liao, T. H., and J. G. Pierce. The primary structure of bovine thyrotropin. II. The amino acid sequences of the reduced, s-carboxymethyl α and β chains. J. Biol. Chem. 246:850, 1971.

Licht, P., and H. Papkoff. Gonadotropic activities of the subunits of ovine FSH and LH in the lizard *Anolis carolinensis*. Gen. Comp. Endocrinol. 16:586, 1971.

Liu, W.-K., H. S. Nahm, C. M. Sweeney, W. H. Lamkin, H. N. Baker, and D. N. Ward. Primary structure of ovine luteinizing hormone. I. The amino acid sequence of the reduced and s-aminoethylated s-subunit (LH-α). J. Biol. Chem. 247:4351, 1972a.

Liu, W.-K., H. S. Nahm, C. M. Sweeney, G. N. Holcomb, and D. N. Ward. Primary structure of ovine luteinizing hormone. II. The amino acid sequence of the reduced s-carboxymethylated A-subunit (LH-β). J. Biol. Chem. 247:4365, 1972b.

Maffezzoli, R. D., G. N. Kaplan, and A. Chrambach. Fractionation of immunoreactive human chorionic gonadotropin and luteinizing hormone by isoelectric focusing in polyacrylamide gel. J. Clin. Endocrinol. Metab. 34:361, 1972.

Maghuin-Register, G., Y. Combarnous, and G. Hennen. Porcine luteinizing hormone. The amino acid sequence of the α subunit. FEBS Letters 25:57, 1972.

Maghuin-Register, G., and A. Dockier. The amino acid sequence of the bovine luteinizing hormone β subunit. FEBS Letters 19:209, 1971.

März, L., O. P. Bahl, and J. F. Mohn. Blood-group activity of human chorionic gonadotropin. Biochem. Biophys. Res. Commun. 55:717, 1973.

März, L., and O. P. Bahl. Unpublished work, 1975.

Matta, K. L., and O. P. Bahl. Glycosidases of *Aspergillus niger*. IV. Purification and characterization of α-mannosidase. J. Biol. Chem. 247:1780, 1972.

McDonald, M. J., and O. P. Bahl. α-N-Acetylgalactosaminidase from *Aspergillus niger*. In *Methods in enzymology*, ed. V. Ginsburg. New York: Academic Press, 1972.

McKerns, K. W. Gonadotropin regulation of nucleotide biosynthesis in corpus luteum. Biochemistry 12:5206, 1973.

Merz, W. E., V. Hilgenfeldt, M. Dorner, and R. Brossmer. Biological, immunological, and physical investigations on human chorionic gonadotropin. Hoppe-Syeler's Z. Physiol. Chem. 355:1035, 1974.

Midgley, A. R., Jr. Gonadotropin binding to frozen sections of ovarian tissue. In *Gonadotropins*, eds. B. B. Saxena, C. G. Beling, and H. M. Gandy. New York: John Wiley & Sons, 1972.

Morell, A. G., G. Gregoriadis, I. H. Scheinberg, J. Hickman, and G. Ashwell. The role of sialic acid in determining the survival of glycoproteins in the circulation. J. Biol. Chem. 246:1461, 1971.

Morgan, F. J., and R. E. Canfield. Nature of the subunits of human chorionic gonadotropin. Endocrinology 88:1045, 1971.

Morgan, F. J., S. Birken, and R. E. Canfield. Human chorionic gonadotropin—A proposal for the amino acid sequence. Mol. Cell Biochem. 2:97, 1973.

Morgan, F. J., R. E. Canfield, J. L. Vaitukaitis, and G. T. Ross. Properties of the subunits of human chorionic gonadotropin. Endocrinology 94:1601, 1974.

Mori, K. F. Antigenic structure of human gonadotropins: Importance of protein moiety to the antigenic structure of human chorionic gonadotropin. Endocrinology 86:97, 1970.

Mori, K. F., and T. R. Holland. Physicochemical characterization of native and asialo human chorionic gonadotropin. J. Biol. Chem. 246:7223, 1971.

Moyle, W. R., O. P. Bahl, and L. März. Role of the carbohydrates of human chorionic gonadotropin in the mechanism of hormone action. J. Biol. Chem., 250:9163, 1975.

Nisula, B. C., F. J. Morgan, and R. E. Canfield. Evidence that chorionic gonadotropin has intrinsic thyrotropic activity. Biochem. Biophys. Res. Commun. 59:86, 1974.

Pandian, M. R., O. P. Bahl, and S. J. Segal. Labeling of LH/hCG receptor in rat ovaries. Biochem. Biophys. Res. Commun. 64:1199, 1975.

Papkoff, H. Chemical and biological properties of the subunits of pregnant mare serum gonadotropin. Biochem. Biophys. Res. Commun. 58:397, 1974.

Pierce, J. G., O. P. Bahl, J. S. Cornell, and N. Swaminathan. Biologically active hormones prepared by recombination of the α chain of human chorionic gonadotropin and the hormone-specific chain of bovine thyrotropin or of bovine luteinizing hormone. J. Biol. Chem. 246:2321, 1971.

Presl, J., J. Pospisol, V. Figarova, and V. Wagner. Development changes in uptake of radioactivity by the ovaries, pituitary and uterus after 125 I-labelled human chorionic gonadotrophin administration in rats. J. Endocrinol. 52:585, 1972.

Qazi, M. H., G. Mukherjee, K. Javidi, A. Pala, and E. Diczfalusy. Preparation of highly purified human chorionic gonadotrophin by isoelectric focusing. J. Biochem. 47:219, 1974.

Rajaniemi, H. J., and T. Vanha-Perttula. Specific receptor for LH in the ovary: Evidence by autoradiography tissue and fractionation. Endocrinology 90:1, 1972.

Rajaniemi, H. J., A. N. Hirshfield, and A. R. Midgley, Jr. Gonadotropin receptors in rat ovarian tissue. I. Localization of LH binding sites by fractionation of subcellular organelles. Endocrinology 95:579, 1974.

Rao, Ch. V. Properties of gonadotropin receptors in the cell membranes of bovine corpus luteum. J. Biol. Chem. 249:2864, 1974.

Rao, Ch. V., and L. B. Carmen. Stimulation of ovarian cyclic guanosine 3', 5'-monophosphate levels by the subunits of human chorionic gonadotropin. Biochem. Biophys. Res. Commun. 54:744, 1973.

Rao, Ch. V., B. B. Saxena, and H. M. Gandy. Subcellular distribution of hCG in rat corpus luteum. In *Gonadotropins*, eds. B. B. Saxena, C. G. Beling, and H. M. Gandy. New York: John Wiley & Sons, 1972.

Rathnam, P., and B. B. Saxena. Subunits of luteinizing hormone from human pituitary glands. J. Biol. Chem. 246:7087, 1971.

Rathnam, P., and B. B. Saxena. Subunits of FSH from human pituitary glands. In *Gonadotropins*, eds. B. B. Saxena, C. G. Beling, and H. M. Gandy. New York: John Wiley & Sons, 1972.

Rathnam, P., and B. B. Saxena. Primary amino acid sequence of follicle-stimulating hormone from human pituitary glands. I. α subunit. J. Biol. Chem. 250:6735, 1975.

Reichert, L. E., Jr., F. Leidenberger, and C. G. Trowbridge. Studies on luteinizing hormone and its subunits: Development and application of a radioligand receptor assay and properties of the hormone receptor interaction. Recent Prog. Horm. Res. 29:497, 1973.

Reichert, L. E., Jr., and G. M. Lawson, Jr. Molecular weight relationships among the subunits of human glycoprotein hormones. Endocrinology 92:1034, 1973a.

Reichert, L. E., Jr., and G. M. Lawson, Jr. Influence of alpha- and beta-subunits on the kinetics of formation and activity of native and hybrid molecules of LH and human chorionic gonadotropin. Endocrinology 93: 938, 1973b.

Reichert, L. E., Jr., and D. N. Ward. On the isolation and characterization of the alpha and beta subunits of human follicle-stimulating hormone. Endocrinology 94:655, 1974.

Reisfeld, R. A., and R. Hertz. Purification of chorionic gonadotropin from the urine of patients with trophoblastic tumors. Biochim. Biophys. Acta 43:540, 1960.

Ross, G. T., E. V. Van Hall, J. L. Vaitukaitis, G. D. Braunstein, and P. L. Rayford. Sialic acid and the immunologic and biologic activity of gonadotropins. In *Gonadotropins*, eds. B. B. Saxena, C. G. Beling, and H. M. Gandy. New York: John Wiley & Sons, 1972.

Sairam, M. R., and H. Papkoff. Chemistry of the gonadotropins. In *Handbook of physiology*, Section 7: Endocrinology, Volume IV, eds. E. Knobil and W. Sawyer. Baltimore: Williams & Wilkins, 1974.

Sairam, M. R., H. Papkoff, and C. H. Li. The primary structure of ovine interstitial cell-stimulating hormone. I. The α-subunit. Arch. Biochem. Biophys. 153:554, 1972a.

Sairam, M. R., T. S. A. Samy, H. Papkoff, and C. H. Li. The primary structure of ovine interstitial cell-stimulating hormone. II. The β-subunit. Arch. Biochem. Biophys. 153:572, 1972b.

Saxena, B. B., S. H. Hasan, F. Haour, and M. Schmidt-Gollwitzer. Radioreceptor assay of human chorionic gonadotropin: Detection of early pregnancy. Science 184:793, 1974.

Saxena, B. B., and P. Rathnam. Dissociation phenomenon and subunit nature of follicle-stimulating hormone from human pituitary glands. J. Biol. Chem. 246:3549, 1971.

Schlumberger, H. D. Physikalische, chemische und biologische Charakterisierung von menschlichem Choriongonadotropin. Z. Naturforschg 23b:1412, 1968.

Shome, B., and A. F. Parlow. The primary structure of the hormone-specific, beta subunit of human pituitary luteinizing hormone (hLH). J. Clin. Endocrinol. Metab. 36:618, 1973a.

Shome, B., and A. F. Parlow. Human TSH subunits: Radioimmunoassay and primary strucutre of the beta-subunit. The Endocrine Society, Program of the Fifty-Fifth Annual Meeting, June, 1973b.

Shome, B., and A. F. Parlow. Human follicle stimulating hormone (hFSH): First proposal for the amino acid sequence of the α-subunit (hFSHα) and first demonstration of its identity with the α-subunit of human luteinizing hormone (hLHα). J. Clin. Endocrinol. Metab. 39:199, 1974a.

Shome, B., and A. F. Parlow. Human follicle stimulating hormone: First proposal for the amino acid sequence of the hormone-specific β subunit (hFSHβ). J. Clin. Endocrinol. Metab. 39:203, 1974b.

Stevens, V. C. Immunization of female baboons with hapten-coupled gonadotropins. J. Obstet. Gynecol. 42:496, 1973.

Swaminathan, N., and O. P. Bahl. Dissociation and recombination of the subunits of human chorionic gonadotropin. Biochem. Biophys. Res. Commun. 40:422. 1970.

Talwar, G. P., and O. P. Bahl. Unpublished work, 1974.

Tsuruhara, T., M. L. Dufau, J. Hickman, and K. J. Catt. Biological properties of hCG after removal of terminal sialic acid and galactose residues. Endocrinology 91:296, 1972.

Tsuruhara, T., E. V. Van Hall, M. L. Dufau, and K. J. Catt. Ovarian binding of intact and desialylated hCG *in vivo* and *in vitro*. Endocrinology 91:463, 1972.

Vaitukaitis, J. L., and G. T. Ross. Antigenic similarities among the human glycoprotein hormones and their subunits.

In *Gonadotropins*, eds. B. B. Saxena, C. G. Beling, and H. M. Gandy. New York: John Wiley & Sons, 1972.

Vaitukaitis, J. L., G. T. Ross, L. E. Reichert, Jr., and D. N. Ward. Immunologic basis for within and between species cross-reactivity of luteinizing hormone. Endocrinology 91: 1337, 1972a.

Vaitukaitis, J. L., G. D. Braunstein, and G. T. Ross. A radioimmunoassay which specifically measures human chorionic gonadotropin in the presence of human luteinizing hormone. Am. J. Obstet. Gynecol. 113:751, 1972b.

Vaitukaitis, J. L., G. T. Ross, and L. E. Reichert, Jr. Immunologic and biologic behavior of hCG and bovine LH subunit hybrids. Endocrinology 92:411, 1973.

van Hell, H., R. Matthijsen, and J. D. H. Homan. Studies on human chorionic gonadotropin. I. Purification and some physicochemical properties. Acta Endocrinol. 59:89, 1968.

Van Hall, E. V., J. L. Vaitukaitis, and G. T. Ross. Effects of progressive desialylation on the rate of disappearance of immunoreactive hCG from plasma in rats. Endocrinology 89: 11, 1971a.

Van Hall, E. V., J. L. Vaitukaitis, and G. T. Ross. Immunological and biological activity of hCG following progressive desialylation. Endocrinology 88:456, 1971b.

Whitten, W. K. Inactivation of gonadotropins. Aust. J. Sci. Res. k:388, 1948.

Weintraub, B. D., and W. W. Rosen. Ectopic production of the isolated beta subunit of human chorionic gonadotropin. J. Clin. Invest. 52:3135, 1973.

Wilde, C. E., and K. D. Bagshawe. The purification of chorionic gonadotropin. In *Gonadotropins*, eds. G. E. W. Wolstenholme and J. Knight. Boston: Little, Brown, 1965.

Yang, W. H., M. R. Sairam, H. Papkoff, and C. H. Li. Ovulation in hamster: induction by β-subunit of ovine interstitial cell stimulating hormone. Science 175:637, 1972.

3 Prolactin

Henry G. Friesen

3.1 Introduction

This essay will be concerned with recent advances in the chemistry, physiology, and pathology of prolactin, with particular emphasis on aspects related to reproductive biology. Undoubtedly one of the most significant advances has been the identification and purification of human prolactin, along with the development of methods for measuring human prolactin in serum samples. These discoveries have provided a tremendous impetus to the entire field. As recently as four years ago, opinion was divided about the existence of a separate human prolactin, but now that human prolactin concentrations can be measured in serum, a great amount of research is underway to gain a better understanding of the role of human prolactin in human reproduction. Thus far the available studies suggest great similarity between the factors controlling prolactin secretion in rodents and man. Major differences in the comparative physiology of prolactin have been noted, however, especially in the area of reproduction. As is true of so much research in reproductive biology, much more information is available on the role of prolactin in female than in male reproductive processes.

Although no hormone is secreted or acts in isolation, it is worth emphasizing in the case of prolactin that many of its effects result from interaction with other hormones. Indeed, some investigators have suggested that the principal role of prolactin may be the modulation of other hormonal effects.

Endocrinologists generally agree that the measurement of the serum concentration of a hormone is not the sole determinant of its biological effectiveness. Other factors are involved, such as binding to serum proteins, metabolic clearance rate, and tissue responsiveness. The state and number of target tissue receptors may also play a key role in determining the type and degree of activity of a hormone. Recent studies identify receptors for prolactin in a number of tissues, some of which had not been recognized as target tissues for prolactin. These observations suggest that prolactin may have several as yet unrecognized biological effects. Not only is the distribution of tissue receptors for prolactin interesting, but studies in our laboratory have revealed that the number of tissue receptors for prolactin varies under different physio-

logical circumstances, suggesting that the action of prolactin itself may be modulated by changes in tissue receptors. As yet, nothing is known about these phenomena in human tissues.

3.2 Prolactin and the Pituitary

Prolactin has been identified in a great many species ranging from teleosts to humans. The hormone is synthesized in a specific cell type sometimes referred to as the lactotrope. This cell type can be identified with specific histological staining techniques or with immunochemical localization procedures. The number of lactotropes increases greatly during pregnancy and lactation in several species. Erdheim and Stumme reported this change in human pituitary glands as early as 1909, long before prolactin was recognized as a hormone. Not only does the number of lactotropes increase, but prolactin content also increases during pregnancy. In human subjects this increase is presumably mediated by the increase in estrogen secretion during pregnancy; however, the mechanism for the increase in prolactin content is still unclear in species such as the rhesus monkey, where estrogen secretion does not change dramatically throughout pregnancy. Electron microscopists have provided descriptions of the appearance of the lactotrope and have emphasized the characteristic polymorphic appearance of the storage granules.

No evidence has been reported of synthesis of a large prohormone prolactin molecule. Several recent reports have appeared, however, in which a large molecular weight (40,000 daltons) species of prolactin was identified in the serum of a patient with a prolactin-secreting pituitary adenoma. In a careful study on human serum samples, 10–20 percent of prolactin in serum appears to be of this form, the majority species having a molecular weight of 20,000 daltons. More data are required to establish the precise form in which prolactin is synthesized, stored, and secreted.

Kaplan et al. (1976) have reported a fascinating study of the ontogenesis of prolactin-containing cells and the secretion of prolactin in human fetuses. The investigation is particularly valuable because they have examined the pituitary content and blood levels not only of prolactin but also of growth hormones and gonadotropins (FSH and LH). Each hormone has its own particular developmental pattern. In some cases major differences in secretory patterns are observed between male and female fetuses, suggesting that the secretion of each hormone and its biological effect form a carefully controlled and integrated process. Moreover, this research suggests that prolactin and other pituitary hormones may have an extremely important role in fetal development, perhaps inducing enzymes or initiating developmental changes. It now becomes mandatory to examine tissue receptors for prolactin at comparable stages of fetal development.

3.3 The Chemistry of Prolactin

Prolactin has been purified in bulk from only a few species, including sheep, pig, beef, rat, and mouse. More recently, human and monkey prolactin have been purified in limited amounts. Isolated reports have appeared of the purification of goat and dog prolactin, but relatively little is known of the chemistry of those preparations. The entire amino acid sequence is known for only two prolactin preparations, namely, sheep and pig prolactin. The partial amino acid sequence is available for human and bovine prolactin. Comparisons of the amino acid sequences of prolactins, placental lactogens, and growth hormones have proved interesting because bovine, porcine, and human prolactins demonstrate considerable homology with preparations of human growth hormone and human placental lactogen. The latter preparations have both growth-promoting and lactogenic activities in a number of assays.

In addition, the studies of Niall et al. (1973) at the Massachusetts General Hospital have also indicated a close homology between sheep or pig prolactin and human prolactin. The studies of Niall and Li, the two investigators who have carried out most of the studies on the chemistry of these hormones, have emphasized not only the external homology that exists among several prolactin and growth hormone preparations but also the internal homology of four peptide sequences consisting of 15 to 20 amino acid residues within each molecule (see Wolstenholme and Knight 1972). One possible explanation for this repeating sequence is that the original primordial prolactin or growth hormone molecule was a relatively small structure, compared with the present-day prolactin or growth hormone molecule. It has been suggested that these molecules have evolved to their present size by gene reduplication. If this is the case, only a comparatively small portion of the entire molecule might have intrinsic biological activity. All attempts to identify such fragments have been rather unsuccessful, however. The attempts

to pinpoint the precise minimal sequence required for biological activity should be encouraged because they may ultimately offer clues as to the precise reaction of the active site of the hormone with the tissue receptors for prolactin.

3.4 Assays of Prolactin

As in so many other areas of endocrinology, progress in understanding prolactin has hinged upon the development of suitable, sensitive, and specific assays for the hormone. For many years the standard bioassay for prolactin was the pigeon cropsac assay. While this has proved satisfactory for measuring relatively large amounts of the hormone, it lacks the necessary sensitivity for measuring prolactin levels in blood. The second bioassay that has been used extensively depends on inducing a lactational response in pseudopregnant rabbits following the intraductal administration of prolactin. This assay is even more crude and less sensitive than the pigeon cropsac assay, and the results obtained by the two assay procedures do not agree necessarily in all circumstances. For example, human growth hormone or human placental lactogen are as potent in the pseudopregnant rabbit assay as purified sheep prolactin, whereas in a pigeon cropsac assay the former are much less potent.

Other forms of in vitro assays have also been used. In general, these depended upon histological assessment of cellular development or alveolar secretion of midpregnant mouse or rabbit mammary gland tissue. Alternatively, biochemical end points such as P 32 incorporation or N-acetyllactosamine synthetase activity were monitored. These assays brought major advances in understanding human prolactin physiology, but their procedures were costly and time-consuming, and hence only a modest number of samples could be assayed at any one time.

Many of the advances in understanding endocrine physiology have resulted from the application of radioimmunoassays for the measurement of hormones in blood samples. Immunoassays for prolactin also have been developed from many species, including sheep, goat, beef, rat, and mouse. Many of these studies were made possible by the Hormone Distribution Program sponsored by the National Institute of Arthritis and Metabolic Diseases. NIH provides hundreds of investigators with radioimmunoassay kits for prolactin and other hormones, and this provision has dramatically increased the research carried out not only on prolactin but also on other hormones involved in reproduction, such as FSH and LH.

A major problem that stymied investigators for at least a decade was the failure to separate human or monkey prolactin from growth hormone. Only in the primate does the growth hormone have both growth-promoting and lactogenic activities; hence, attempts at separation, which depended upon a bioassay, invariably ended in failure. With the recognition that growth hormone and prolactin differ immunologically, a procedure could be developed for separating the two hormones. Once the separation procedures were developed and human prolactin was purified, a radioimmunoassay could be developed for human and monkey prolactin. Since 1971, when the first radioimmunoassay became available, literally hundreds of papers have appeared on the measurement of human prolactin under a great variety of different circumstances. For the first time, critical studies began to deal with the relationship of human prolactin to reproductive processes in both the male and the female.

Evidence is growing that, under a number of circumstances, the immunological and biological activities of the hormone can be dissociated. Because radioimmunoassays ultimately determine the immunological activity of a hormone, they can reveal very high concentrations of a hormone even when bioassay indicates little activity. Bioassays are generally limited in terms of sensitivity and specificity.

The radioreceptor assay may represent a compromise between a bioassay and immunoassay. It depends on specific binding sites on the plasma membrane of a target tissue in the case of protein hormones, or on cytoplasmic or nuclear binding sites in the case of steroids. These binding sites or receptors have great specificity and affinity for the hormone; hence one can develop a specific assay procedure. Although radioreceptor assays are technically somewhat more difficult to perform than are radioimmunoassays, they are advantageous for measuring the biologically active site of a hormone. In addition, while most radioimmunoassays tend to be species-specific, most radioreceptor assays, including those for prolactin, are not species-specific but measure all biologically related substances—that is, all substances that have prolactinlike or lactogenic activity. In many situations, radioreceptor assays may begin to replace or at least supplement radioimmunoassays for the study of prolactinlike materials.

Using a rabbit mammary gland receptor, we have developed a radioreceptor assay for prolactin. This assay can measure human growth hormone, human prolactin, and human placental lactogen, all of which are equipotent in the rabbit. Moreover, pituitary prolactin preparations obtained from species as different as birds and humans appear to react similarly in this system. Hence the comparative endocrinology of prolactin is much easier to study with this type of assay procedure.

3.5 The Control of Prolactin Secretion

Present concepts of the regulation of prolactin secretion are derived in large measure from studies in rodents. More recently, with the availability of specific and sensitive radioimmunoassays for human prolactin, many similar studies have been carried out in humans. A comparison of results obtained from these studies with those obtained in rodents leads to the conclusion that in general the control mechanisms regulating prolactin secretion are very similar in primates and in rodents. Even in animal studies, however, the data on which the concepts are based are often not as direct and straightforward as one would like. For example, the hypothalamus contains a prolactin-inhibiting factor (PIF) that appears to be of prime importance in tonically suppressing prolactin secretion. Yet very little information is available regarding its chemistry, its site of production, or its secretory rate. Similarly, PIF secretion is allegedly under the influence of dopaminergic fibers in the hypothalamus. Again, this suggestion is based on experiments in which pharmacological agents that influence biogenic amine levels have been used to alter prolactin secretion. When changes are observed, they are usually ascribed to alterations in PIF secretion, but no one has actually measured secretory rates of PIF in either the hypothalamus or the portal circulation.

Prolactin secretion appears to be controlled by both inhibitory and stimulatory signals from the hypothalamus. In mammalian species, prolactin synthesis and release is primarily under tonic hypothalamic inhibition. Along with this inhibitory control, the existence of a stimulatory prolactin-releasing factor (PRF) has been reported. Both PIF and PRF appear to be controlled by hypothalamic biogenic amines. Any condition that interferes with the synthesis or the release of these neurotransmitters, with their actions at the synaptic level, or with the transport of the inhibiting or releasing factors to the pituitary, will induce an alteration in serum prolactin concentrations.

Experimental evidence from morphological and histochemical studies in rats suggests that dopamine is the major catecholamine present in the tuberoinfundibular neurons, the cell bodies of which are found mainly in hypothalamic nuclei. Because both dopamine and norepinephrine cause an inhibition of prolactin release, the possibility exists that dopamine itself may directly control prolactin secretion. But recent studies demonstrating the presence of dopaminergic receptors in the pituitary raise serious questions about the conventional interpretation of many previous studies that relied on pharmacological agents which affected dopamine receptors. In the past it was thought that if prolactin increased or decreased after the administration of these compounds, the change was mediated via dopaminergic receptors in the hypothalamus, but this is now in doubt. A series of elegant experiments in which dopamine was infused into the portal vessels directly but had no effect on prolactin secretion seemed to provide fairly direct evidence that dopamine itself or dopaminergic receptors may not be primary factors controlling pituitary secretion of prolactin (Kamberi et al. 1971). Other investigators have failed to confirm these results (Takahara et al. 1974). The nature of PIF remains a puzzle.

A variety of pharmacological agents that alter dopamine levels have been used to increase or suppress prolactin secretion. L-DOPA was among the first agents reported to suppress prolactin secretion. This drug is converted into dopamine after it passes through the blood-brain barrier. Presumably, stimulation of PIF secretion lowers prolactin levels.

A relationship exists not only between effective dopamine levels in the hypothalamus and prolactin secretion, but also between prolactin levels and the dopamine turnover rate in tuberoinfundibular neurons. When prolactin is implanted into the median eminence, a decrease in pituitary prolactin secretion follows, suggesting a short feedback loop by which prolactin controls its own secretion. Since prolactin affects dopamine turnover in the hypothalamus and PIF secretion is dopamine-dependent, the effect of prolactin on PIF secretion may be partly indirect, by a change in monoamines. It has been reported that FSH and LH releasing hormone as well as PIF is present in portal blood after the infusion of dopamine into the third ventricle, suggesting a dopamine-mediated reciprocal relationship between prolactin and gonadotropins. This reciprocal relationship might explain the frequent association of galactorrhea and elevated prolactin levels and amenorrhea in human subjects. This mechanism may also account for the frequent association of galactorrhea and amenorrhea in patients taking drugs such as reserpine or phenothiazines.

The mechanism by which steroids affect prolactin secretion has not been completely defined, but it is clear that estrogen acts at the hypothalamic level and also by a direct pituitary effect to augment prolactin secretion. At the hypothalamic level, PIF secretion is suppressed either directly or by influencing monoamine concentrations in the hypothalamus.

Although considerable evidence points to the existence of a hypothalamic factor that inhibits prolactin secretion, only limited evidence substantiates the existence of a prolactin-releasing factor. One candidate—TRH—has emerged recently; in a number of species and particularly in primates, TRH is a very potent releaser of prolactin. Careful dose-response curves demonstrate that after the administration of TRH, pro-

lactin release is seen at every point where TSH is released. On the other hand, in many situations one can demonstrate independent release of prolactin without TSH and vice versa. At present, an additional prolactin-releasing factor other than TRH may have to be postulated.

An acute elevation in prolactin is seen immediately after the onset of nursing or after breast stimulation; this is more likely due to the release of a prolactin-releasing factor than to inhibition of PIF secretion, although animal data on this point are contradictory. If one postulates that suckling both induces the release of PRF and suppresses PIF, then one must postulate the existence of a neurotransmitter that is capable of a dual-control mechanism. The observation that serotonin has no direct action on pituitary lactotropes, whereas it elicits prolactin release when injected into the third ventricle, suggests that serotonin stimulates prolactin secretion either by triggering the release of PRF or by inhibiting PIF secretion. That both mechanisms may be operative is suggested by the recent demonstration of complete inhibition of prolactin release following suckling in rats that have been pretreated with an inhibitor of serotonin synthesis. Recent human data have shown the involvement of serotonin secretion on other anterior pituitory hormones, and in at least one study in which 5 OH tryptophan was administered orally, large increases in prolactin secretion were noted.

Knowledge of the multifactorial control mechanisms regulating prolactin secretion is obviously still very limited. Prolactin secretion appears to be regulated from moment to moment by two major regulatory systems, monoaminergic and serotoninergic. Activation of either system can alter prolactin secretion by stimulating the release of one and inhibiting the secretion of the opposing factor. It will be a major undertaking to validate this hypothesis.

3.6 Physiological Factors That Influence Prolactin Secretion

My studies have focused primarily on factors that influence the secretion of human prolactin; hence these will be emphasized, though attention will occasionally be drawn to the variations in the control of prolactin secretion in different species. The average concentration of human prolactin in adult males is 5–8 ng/ml; in females it ranges from 8 to 10 ng/ml. When large numbers of samples from both sexes are analyzed, a statistically significant difference emerges between the two sexes, though these differences are not nearly as large as in some other species, such as the rat or mouse, that have been studied.

As is true for secretion of many pituitary hormones,

the secretion of prolactin appears to be episodic—short bursts of prolactin secretions occur at intervals ranging from 20 to 30 minutes. These pulsatile release patterns are not as apparent as they are for LH or FSH. There is a well-described diurnal variation in prolactin secretion, maximal concentrations occurring some six to eight hours after the onset of sleep. This peak extends over a period of hours, as compared to the short-lived growth hormone peak, which is observed one to two hours after the onset of sleep and is of much shorter duration. The diurnal variation in prolactin secretion is sleep-related; if sleep is delayed, the prolactin peak is correspondingly delayed.

Prolactin has a very rapid half-time disappearance in the circulation, varying between 15 and 20 minutes. A number of physiological conditions lead to changes in prolactin concentrations. In the immediate newborn period, the concentrations are maximal, ranging from 100 to 500 ng/ml. Over a period measured in weeks rather than in days, prolactin concentrations gradually decline, reaching adult levels by two to three months. Slight sex differences first appear at the time of puberty.

In view of the luteotropic role of prolactin in several species, many studies have been conducted to determine whether an increase in prolactin concentration occurs during the luteal phase of the menstrual cycle. The results of several such studies disagree. In our own studies samples were taken at daily intervals and no increase occurred in prolactin concentrations in the luteal phase; however, the variance of prolactin concentrations in the luteal phase was greater than that observed in the follicular phase. Other investigators have observed a modest increase in prolactin around the time of ovulation, especially in the luteal phase.

These same investigators have also demonstrated an estrogen-induced increase in prolactin, particularly in postmenopausal women. The administration of pharmacological doses of estrogen for a period of several weeks resulted in a three to four fold increase in prolactin levels. In human subjects as in the rodents, estrogen administration thus apparently leads to an increase in prolactin secretion. During pregnancy, prolactin levels gradually increase, reaching maximal levels just before delivery. At this time concentrations range between 100 and 400 ng/ml.

The mechanism leading to the increase in prolactin concentrations throughout pregnancy may be related to the increase in estrogen secretion. In rhesus monkeys, for example, no major increase occurs in secretion of estrogen in pregnancy, and prolactin levels remain in the nonpregnant range throughout most of gestation. In the last week prior to delivery prolactin levels dramatically increase; this persists for only a day or two postpartum. In human subjects the postpar-

tum period shows gradual decline in prolactin levels, which return to the nonpregnant range by three weeks postpartum in those subjects who do not lactate.

In subjects who breastfeed, the pattern in prolactin secretion is quite different. In the initial phase the prolactin levels remain elevated. Following suckling by the infant, prolactin levels increase, reaching maximal levels within 30 minutes of the onset of nursing. The concentrations then gradually decline but remain elevated. In an intermediate phase—one week to three months—the basal prolactin levels are somewhat elevated, but a dramatic increase occurs with each episode of nursing, with concentrations rising from 30 to 300 ng/ml. In several subjects studied throughout a 24-hour period, this increment occurred with each episode of nursing. At a later stage—somewhere beyond three to four months postpartum—basal prolactin levels return to the nonpregnant range, and there is no additional increase in prolactin with each episode of nursing. Despite these low prolactin concentrations, adequate milk is produced. (This changing pattern of prolactin in the postpartum period was first described by Tyson et al. in 1972.) These observations are very important because a relative period of infertility coincides with the intermittent surges of prolactin that occur with breastfeeding. Our thesis is that the intermittent elevations of prolactin block the cyclic release of LH and FSH from the pituitary, leading to anovulatory cycles. If this hypothesis is correct, it suggests that the period of breastfeeding is an extremely important natural contraceptive process.

Unfortunately, with the modern trend toward bottle feeding, this period of infertility is shortened or eliminated. In developing countries this may well have devastating consequences. The introduction of bottle feeding has in some cases taken place before there is adequate knowledge of personal hygiene; a high infant mortality rate then results from diarrheal diseases introduced by poorly cleaned bottles. In addition, with the decline in breastfeeding, women in the postpartum period begin to ovulate earlier and increase the risk of pregnancy.

The mechanism by which elevated prolactin levels induce anovulatory cycles is not clear, but several possible explanations have arisen. The elevated prolactin levels may in some as yet unknown manner inhibit the cyclic discharge of LHRH from the hypothalamus. In addition, the intermittent peaks of prolactin may blunt the pituitary responsiveness to LHRH. Indeed, after the administration of LHRH to women in the postpartum period, we have noted a major difference between the responses of the pituitary in women who are breastfeeding, and in those who are not. Subjects who are breastfeeding show a markedly inhibited response to LHRH for a much longer period of time postpartum—six to eight weeks. The return of the LHRH response occurs at approximately the time when ovulatory cycles begin to return. Previous investigations suggest that in the postpartum period the ovary is refractory to the exogenous administration of pituitary gonadotropins. The intermittent elevations of prolactin levels during this period may be responsible for this phenomenon.

An important avenue of exploration would involve a detailed comparison of hormonal patterns in the postpartum period between subjects who are breastfeeding and those who are not. This type of study would be most appropriately carried out in those societies where breastfeeding is still the norm and is exclusively relied upon for providing nutrition for the young. In North America the easy substitution of bottle feeding when any problems of breastfeeding arise makes this type of study very difficult to perform.

Two additional bits of information support the hypothesis that the intermittent surges of prolactin in some way alter the normal cyclical pattern of gonadotropin release. The first line of evidence is derived from a study of patients with microadenomas of the pituitary gland. These tumors can be relatively small in size, ranging from 10 to 20 mg in a 500 mg pituitary gland. Characteristically these patients have amenorrhea, galactorrhea, and elevated prolactin. Gonadotropin levels appear to be only slightly, not dramatically, reduced. Amenorrhea and galactorrhea disappear when the elevated prolactin levels are returned to the normal range either by microsurgery of the pituitary gland, with careful selective enucleation of the adenoma, or by pharmacological means, with the administration of drugs such as ergocryptine (CB154). The major hormonal manipulation appears to be a reduction in prolactin levels, which is followed by the normal cyclical pattern of gonadotropin release.

The second line of evidence suggesting that elevated prolactin levels may alter the normal midcycle LH release is derived from studies in which TRH was administered to primates, baboons, or rhesus monkeys throughout a normal menstrual cycle. The daily administration of TRH, which results in intermittent surges of prolactin, abolished the normal midcycle peak and ovulation and menses. In addition, Bohnet et al. (1976) have found that prolonged hyperprolactinemia leads to an abolition of episodic secretion of LH. Thus several lines of evidence suggest an intimate relationship between prolactin levels and the normal hypothalamic mechanisms that control cyclic discharge of LH. Still, the precise mechanisms involved are not well defined and require future investigation.

In addition to the diurnal changes in prolactin, in some species, particularly the cow, one can see seasonal changes in prolactin levels. These seasonal changes may be partly responsible for the well-known seasonal variations in response to prolactin that are observed in both the pigeon and the rabbit.

The changes in prolactin concentration have been described in some detail in human subjects. Changes in prolactin have also been studied in sheep, in goats, and in cows, but particularly in the rat, both male and female. Careful studies have been carried out in relation to the normal estrous cycle by numerous investigators during proestrus as well as during pseudopregnancy. The precise role of prolactin at each of these stages is not well understood, although in the case of the rat, there is abundant evidence that prolactin is important in the maintenance of the corpus luteum, which in this species is necessary for maintenance of pregnancy. The diurnal variations that have been observed in human prolactin are also found in rat prolactin. Major changes occur with the highest levels observed during the night. These diurnal variations appear to be magnified at different phases of the cycle and are noted particularly during periods of pseudopregnancy.

A variety of other stimuli may lead to increases in prolactin concentration. These include stressful situations, such as surgery, strenuous exercise, or insulin-induced hypoglycemia. In some but not all female subjects, nipple stimulation leads to an increase in prolactin concentration, whereas in the male this rarely occurs. Sexual intercourse in some subjects leads to an increase in prolactin concentration. Changes in osmolality may also produce changes in prolactin concentrations; decreasing serum osmolality by ingestion of large amounts of water leads to suppression of prolactin levels, whereas the infusion of hypertonic saline will lead to an increase in prolactin concentration. These changes may in part relate to the well-recognized effects of prolactin on regulating salt and water metabolism in amphibians. Recent attempts to confirm the effects of a water load on lowering prolactin have been negative.

The highest concentration of prolactin in any biological fluid is observed in the amniotic fluid in primates. Concentrations of prolactin in amniotic fluid are 10 to 100 times greater than those found in maternal or fetal blood samples. Prolactin may play an extremely important role in regulating amniotic fluid osmolality or salt and water transport. The site of production of amniotic fluid prolactin is not established. Minimal transfer of prolactin into amniotic fluid was noted when radioactively labeled prolactin was administered to the mother or the fetus. One practical advantage of this observation is that a suitable alternative source for the purification of human prolactin is available. Methods have been developed for purifying amniotic fluid prolactin.

3.7 Biological Effects of Prolactin

In an extensive review of the comparative biology of prolactin, Nicoll 1974 has identified more than eighty effects of this hormone and has grouped them into five major categories. Historically the most widely known effects of prolactin relate to reproductive processes. In the females of some species, prolactin is critical for development and maintenance of the corpus luteum and continued progesterone secretion; this role of prolactin is not at all clear for human females, in whom no large increase in prolactin is observable in the luteal phase. Second, when women were placed on CB154 and prolactin levels were reduced to less than 3 ng/ml throughout the cycle, no influence on menses was observed. In rhesus monkeys similar treatment resulted in a major decrease in progesterone levels.

Attempts to demonstrate binding of prolactin to human ovarian tissue by radioautography have thus far been negative. When receptor studies were performed on human ovarian tissue, however, a modest degree of prolactin binding was noted. In culture of granulosa cells, prolactin stimulated progesterone secretion. Prolactin obviously has a definite effect on the human ovary, but low levels may be adequate for maintaining activity. Not only does prolactin have a luteotropic role in some species, but it also is luteolytic in some. This phenomenon has been studied extensively by Meites and his colleagues (for review see Meites and Clemens 1972).

No attempts have been made to examine prolactin effects on vaginal or uterine secretions in human subjects. It is well known that in rodents prolactin promotes progesterone secretion, which brings about the release of accumulated uterine fluid.

The only action of prolactin that is well documented in humans is the effect on milk production. If prolactin is reduced to low levels with CB154 or if the peripheral action of prolactin on the breast is blocked with estrogen, milk production is totally inhibited. The biochemical mechanism accounting for this effect is not known.

In males only a few effects of prolactin have been reported, and some of these are poorly documented. Prolactin influences prostatic growth and the growth of the seminal vesicles in rats. The mechanism may be mediated by an increased uptake of testosterone, which may be mediated in turn by a prolactin-induced increase in cytoplasmic binding protein for testosterone. This may be similar to the increase in estrogen binding protein in the uterus and mammary tissue that occurs after the administration of prolactin. Indeed, this may be the biochemical basis of the synergism, which has been frequently observed when prolactin and steroids are administered simultaneously.

In men with prolactin-secreting tumors and grossly elevated serum prolactin concentrations, an extreme loss of libido has been observed. The decrease in libido is out of proportion to the minimal decrease found in testosterone levels. In rats with mammotropic tumors, testicular size decreases as prolactin levels increase. In rats small amounts of prolactin affect cholesterol poolsize in the testes.

Prolactin has important effects on maternal behavior in many species. These effects have been reviewed by Nicoll (1974) and will not be described here. It is not known if prolactin has a similar role in primates.

3.8 Mechanism of Action

Although a number of effects of prolactin on reproductive processes are documented, very little information is available on the precise mechanism of action. In some systems prolactin effects are known to be mediated by specific recognition sites for prolactin on the plasma membrane of the cell. These specific hormone binding sites have been referred to as hormone receptors. As a first step in identifying the site of action of prolactin, we have examined numerous tissues to determine which ones have receptor sites for prolactin; the assumption is that the hormone may have an action in the tissues where prolactin receptors exist. Receptors have been studied in 14 tissues from six species. Our hypothesis is that the tissues with large numbers of receptors for prolactin may be more responsive to the action of prolactin. As a result of our research program several tissues have been identified with large numbers of prolactin receptors. In some cases such as the sheep uterus, we found a significant number of prolactin binding sites. Of great interest was the observation that the receptor population in the same tissue is not static but in a state of flux, varying in number depending on the hormonal milieu. Thyroidectomy, oophorectomy, hypophysectomy, and estrogen administration all influence the prolactin receptor population.

These observations are extremely important, because they indicate that the action and effectiveness of prolactin in a given tissue may vary enormously, depending on the state and number of tissue receptors. Perhaps this is the first clue to explaining the point emphasized by Nicoll (1974) and Meier (1972) that there are temporal variations in responsiveness of tissues to prolactin. Moreover, phasing of tissue responsiveness could also be accounted for by this mechanism.

The prolactin receptor from rabbit mammary glands has been purified by affinity chromatography. Antibodies to the receptor have been generated in guinea pigs. These antibodies will inhibit the binding of prolactin to the mammary gland and also specifically inhit the action of prolactin on a number of biochemical events in the mammary gland.

The concept of temporal interactions between hormones is often not given due consideration because endocrinologists are accustomed to thinking of one hormone = one action when considering endocrine-related processes. In the future, investigators should pay special attention to the interaction of various hormones, taking into account temporal variations.

3.9 Conclusion

I have reviewed highlights of prolactin physiology, with special emphasis on reproductive processes. I have concentrated on the many findings related to human prolactin, but it must be emphasized that research in this field has been profoundly dependent on prior knowledge of the role of prolactin in other species. The availability of this information has clarified the approach to be utilized for studies on human prolactin and thus has facilitated the task of defining the role of human prolactin in human reproduction.

Major Reference Papers and Reviews

Bern, A., and S. Nicoll. The comparative endocrinology of prolactin. Recent Prog. Horm. Res. 24:681, 1968.

Bohnet, H. G., H. G. Dahlen, W. Wuttke, and H. G. P. Schneider. J. Clin. Endocrinol. Metab. 42:132, 1976.

Cowie, A. T., and J. S. Tindal. *The physiology of lactation*. Monograph of the Physiological Society No. 22, 1971.

Frantz, A. G., D. L. Kleinberg, and G. E. Noel. Studies on prolactin in man. Recent Prog. Horm. Res. 28:527, 1972.

Friesen, H., and P. Hwang. Human prolactin. Ann. Rev. Med. 24:251, 1973.

Horrobin, D. F. *Prolactin: Physiology and clinical significance*. Lancaster, Eng.: Medical and Technical Publishing Co., 1973.

Kamberi, I. A., R. Mical, and J. C. Porter. Effect of anterior pituitary perfusion and intraventricular injection of catecholamines on prolactin release. Endocrinology 88:1012, 1971.

Kaplan, S. L., M. M. Grumbach, and M. L. Auber. The ontogenesis of pituitary hormones and hypothalmic factors in the human fetus. Recent Prog. Horm. Res. 32:161, 1976.

Kelly, P. A., B. I. Posner, T. Tsushima, and H. G. Friesen. Studies of insulin, growth hormone and prolactin binding: Ontogenesis of receptors. Endocrinology 95:532, 1974.

Kelly, P. A., B. I. Posner, and H. G. Friesen. Effects of hypophysectomy, ovariectomy, and cycloheximide on specific binding sites for lactogenic hormones in rat liver. Endocrinology 97:1408, 1975.

Martini, L., F. Fraschini, and M. Mott. Neural control of anterior pituitary functions. Recent Prog. Horm. Res. 24:439, 1968.

Martini, L., and W. F. Ganong, eds. *Frontiers in neuroendocrinology*. New York: Oxford University Press, 1971.

Meier, A. H. Gen. Comp. Endocrinol. Suppl. 3:499, 1972.

Meites, J., and J. A. Clemens. Hypothalamic control of prolactin secretion. Vitam. Horm. 30:165, 1972.

Meites, J., K. H. Lu, W. Wuttke, C. W. Welsch, H. Magasawa, and S. Quandri. Recent studies on function and control of prolactin secretion in rats. Recent Prog. Horm. Res. 28:471, 1972.

Niall, H. D., M. L. Hogan, G. W. Tregear, G. V. Segre, P. Hwang, and H. Friesen. The chemistry of growth hormone and the lactogenic hormones. Recent Prog. Horm. Res. 29: 387, 1973.

Nicoll, C. S. Problems in interpreting the physiological significance of results obtained with exogenous prolactin and with data on endogenous circulating levels of the hormone. In *Lactogenic hormones, fetal nutrition and lactation*, J. B. Josimovich, M. Reynolds, and E. Cobo, eds. New York: John Wiley & Sons, 1974.

Pasteels, J. L., and C. Robyn, eds. *Human prolactin*. Amsterdam: Excerpta Medica, 1973.

Posner, B. I., P. A. Kelly, and H. G. Friesen. Induction of a lactogenic receptor in rat liver: Influence of estrogen and the pituitary. Proc. Natl. Acad. Sci. USA 71:2407, 1974.

Posner, B. I., P. A. Kelly, R. P. C. Shiu, and H. G. Friesen. Studies of insulin, growth hormone and prolactin binding: Species variation and effect of sex and pregnancy. Endocrinology 95:521, 1974.

Riddle, O. Prolactin in vertebrate function and organization. J. Cancer Inst. 31:1039, 1963.

Shiu, R. P. C., P. A. Kelly, and H. G. Friesen. Radioreceptor assay for prolactin and other lactogenic hormones. Science 180:968, 1973.

Takahara, J., A. Arimura, and A. V. Schalley. Endocrinology 95:462, 1974.

Tyson, J. E., H. G. Friesen, and M. S. Anderson. Science 117:897, 1972.

Wolstenholme, G. F. W., and J. Knight, eds. *Lactogenic hormones*. The Ciba Foundation. London and Edinburgh: J. & A. Churchill and E. & S. Livingstone, 1972.

4 Steroid Hormone Secretions

Seymour Lieberman, Erlio Gurpide, Mortimer Lipsett, and Hilton Salhanick

4.1 Introduction

The exact nature of the principal steroids synthesized by the endocrine glands and by the placenta has been known for decades. In this review we have emphasized those features of steroid hormone secretion uncovered in the last ten years that we, in our collective judgment, consider to be of special importance. We have assumed a familiarity with the body of knowledge that bears on the chemistry of the steroid hormones and the physiological roles they play in reproductive processes.

4.2 Anatomical Considerations

Cellular Compartmentalization in Steroid-Secreting Glands

In each gland the specific steroid-synthesizing capacity is relatively localized in discrete cell types. Evidence accumulated over the past 20 years indicates that each steroidogenic endocrine gland may be considered a composite of different, but possibly interacting, steroidogenic cell types.

In the testis, results obtained during the past decade have suggested that the seminiferous tubule has the capacity to synthesize testosterone. The isolated tubule can use labeled C_{21}-steroid precursors, beginning with pregnenolone, to make the androgen; the tubule, however, in contrast to the Leydig cell, apparently cannot convert cholesterol into testosterone under the conditions employed. Although the amount of testosterone synthesized by the tubule was shown to be negligibly small compared to the amount synthesized by the Leydig cell, the tubular synthesis of even small amounts of testosterone may nevertheless be significant for some as yet unknown aspect of seminiferous tubule function. The specific cell within the tubule that engages in these steroid conversions is unidentified. The Sertoli cell, however, is known to contain rough endoplasmic reticulum associated with the microsomal enzymes catalyzing the conversion of pregnenolone to testosterone. In contrast, one recent paper describes testosterone synthesis by free-floating spermatocytes. Questions badly in need of clarification in this area are the quantitative aspects and physiological significance of tubular testosterone synthesis and of the cell types involved. Although at this time there is no reason to doubt the homogeneity of the tubular preparations

used, further clear demonstrations of the absence of contaminating Leydig cells would be highly desirable.

Steroid hormone receptors are localized in several cell types in the testes. The Leydig cell contains a cytoplasmic receptor that binds estradiol avidly. Its function is unknown. The tubule contains an androgen cytosol receptor having physical chemical characteristics similar to those of the receptor present in the prostate and the seminal vesicles. This supports the hypothesis that the tubule is a target tissue for testosterone. The tubule also has a 5 alpha-reductase, capable of converting testosterone to dihydrotestosterone, and another reductase, which can convert the latter compound into androstane–3 alpha, 17 beta diol.

The testicular enzymes responsible for the aromatization of testosterone to estrogens are also probably located in a specific cell of the testis. Recent data suggest that cells in the tubule synthesize estradiol in vitro at a rate considerably greater than that characterizing the Leydig cell, which is also able to aromatize.

In the ovary, compartmentalization involves the follicle, the corpus luteum, the stroma, and often the Leydig cells in the hilus. In the follicle, most hormone formation, especially that of estrogens, occurs in the theca interna, with the granulosa making minor contributions. Furthermore, since the corpus luteum is formed from both the theca interna and the granulosa, the compartmentalization that exists in the follicle may carry over to the more morphogenetically developed cells. The theca externa and ovarian stroma ordinarily do not secrete significant amounts of steroids, but under certain conditions (such as hyperthecosis), abnormal secretion from these sources may dominate the steroid profile. Steroid synthesis attributed to the stroma may be caused by thecal cells scattered in the stroma.

In the placenta, the question of compartmentalization has not been examined sufficiently.

In the adrenal gland, cellular compartmentalization of the biosynthetic capabilities for steroid hormones has not been demonstrated in humans, except for the formation of aldosterone. Since the adrenal cortex is not normally involved in the reproductive process, this issue is not further pursued here.

Subcellular Compartmentalization in Steroid-Hormone-Producing Cells

In the last decade considerable attention has been

given to the subcellular compartmentalization of the enzymes involved in the steroid-hormone-producing processes. The rough endoplasmic reticulum in all secretory cells has been found to be the site of most sterol and steroid oxidations. Cholesterol side-chain cleavage, 11 beta hydroxylation, and a few other hydroxylations (for example, at C_{18}) have been localized on the inner membrane of the mitochondria. Each of the relevant enzymes appears to be localized consistently in the same subcellular pattern in different secreting tissues. For example, the cholesterol side-chain cleavage system has been found in the mitochondria of the ovary, adrenal gland, testis, and placenta. These mitochondria have been characterized morphologically as containing tubular membranes in addition to the usual septal types of membranes.

The microsomal and mitochondrial compartments each contain different electron transport systems: the microsomal system is composed of a flavoprotein, NADPH reductase, and the substrate-specific cytochrome P-450. The mitochondrial system, on the other hand, requires an iron sulfur protein to transfer electrons from the NADPH reductase to the cytochrome P-450. Thus there is specificity in the terminal oxidase not only for the substrate but for the intermediate electron donor. The substrate specificity of the reductase has yet to be established.

Each cell type in an organ or tissue has a characteristic enzyme pattern that determines its secretory products. Thus the cholesterol side-chain cleavage system is located in the mitochondria of the placental cell, and the aromatization system appears in both the microsomal and mitochondrial components. This latter finding presents a good example of the ever-present possibility that fractionated cells or subcellular particles are not homogeneous. Interpretations of functions based on experiments using such fractionated units may be faulty, being either too simplistic or unnecessarily complicated. Furthermore, in glandular cells capable of many different oxidations (such as those of the adrenal gland), subcellular organelles from different cell types of that gland are probably not identical. It is also almost certain that subcellular fractions isolated with present techniques from the same cell are not homogeneous.

The Biosynthetic Particle

In the past few years results obtained with synthetic analogs of steroid hormone precursors have revealed that many of the traditionally conceived pathways of biosynthesis are simplistic. Doubt has been cast on the concept that cholesterol or cholesterol sulfate is converted into the various steroid hormones by reactions that involve discrete, stable, isolatable intermediates, most of which are products formed by specific hydroxylases. The evidence suggests that the true intermediates in these conversions are more likely to be transient, reactive complexes, composed of the steroidal precursor, oxygen, and the appropriate metalloenzyme. Hydroxylated "intermediates" that can be isolated from in vitro experiments of one kind or another, or metabolites that are often found in body fluids (blood or urine), particularly in pathological circumstances, are, in this view, inadvertent products caused either by the artificiality of the experimental conditions, by "leakage" from the complex, or by pathology.

These findings have led to the hypothesis that the enzyme components required for the steroidogenic processes are fixed on some superstructure or subcellular particle (as opposed to existing in a random state in some medium), and that, by a concerted series of reactions, the precursor is rapidly transformed through a preferred route into the product, without the involvement of free, isolatable intermediates. According to this view, each hormonal product is produced by its own multienzyme system, which resides on a particular subcellular particle. These biosynthetic particles may be thought of as functional units, which are characterized by organized arrangements of their enzyme components. In the past, thinking has been strongly influenced by the existence of minor amounts of intermediates; in this postulate they are accounted for by leakage from the complexes. This manner of considering steroidal hormone biosynthesis from precursors may be closer to actuality than is the traditional conception, which usually results in two-dimensional presentation of the series of reactions leading from cholesterol to cortisol, aldosterone, testosterone, and estradiol. In this display, cholesterol is shown as being transformed by stepwise reactions through discrete intermediates until the desired hormone is biosynthesized. Some of the intermediates are considered to be involved in the formation of more than one hormone. Clearly, if the traditional two-dimensional scheme is assumed to be the model characterizing the pathways of steroidogenesis, experiments based on it are doomed to yield erroneous interpretations.

In addition, the biosynthetic particle may contain, in close proximity, an organized aggregation of terminal-substrate-linked oxidases as well as the electron transport enzymes. As stated above, these include in mitochondria a flavoprotein reductase, an iron-sulfur protein, and a terminal oxidase (cytochrome P-450).

The concept of a biosynthetic particle is further complicated by consideration of the utilization of cofactors, NADPH and oxygen. Presumably, a lipid site exists on the terminal oxidase for the accumulation of an oxygen pool. It is also known that electrons from NADPH are transported to the terminal oxidase by flavin or iron-containing enzymes or both. The necessarily close proximity of these enzymes must convey to the biosynthetic particle a three-dimensional component.

The sequence of molecular events involved in steroid oxidations has been worked out: the substrate combines with oxidized cytochrome P-450, which is then reduced by NADPH-generated electrons transported through the electron chain. The combination of electrons, oxygen, and substrate-enzyme complex leads rapidly to oxidation, hydroxylation, or carbon-carbon cleavage. Fission of C_{27} precursors (to C_{21}-products) or C_{21}-precursors (to C_{19}-products), as well as aromatization of a C_{19}-precursor (to a C_{18}-estrogen) occurs, presumably, as a set of concerted reactions.

Since the solubilization and separation of the various enzymes of the biosynthetic unit are achieved only with great difficulty—and in some instances not at all—the physical cohesiveness of the unit remains a challenge for future exploration.

4.3 Chemical Considerations

Conversions and Interconversions

About 10 years ago some steroids secreted by endocrine glands were discovered to undergo transformations peripherally, and the products formed possessed different chemical and hormonal characteristics than the secreted precursors from which they were derived. Moreover, the amount of hormone produced in this way was physiologically significant. For example, dehydroisoandrosterone sulfate or its unconjugated form, dehydroisoandrosterone, both biologically inactive compounds secreted by the adrenal cortex, could, by peripheral conversion, be transformed into the potent androgen, testosterone (or androstenedione). This does not occur normally; but in the notable instance of a masculinizing tumor, the androgen principally responsible for the virilizing symptom—testosterone—was entirely derived by peripheral conversions from dehydroisoandrosterone sulfate, a conjugate produced in huge amounts by the tumor itself. The most consequential finding in this area was that dehydroisoandrosterone sulfate secreted by the adrenal glands of the fetus was the principal steroidal precursor of estradiol (or estrone) made by the placenta in the latter part of pregnancy. The placenta was long known to be the source of huge amounts of estrogens during pregnancy, but this finding gave important experimental support for the notion that it is an incomplete endocrine gland. The placenta is now thought to depend upon the secretion of C_{19}-steroid by the maternal adrenal gland (in the first trimester) or by the fetal adrenal gland (in the second and third trimesters) for the precursor it uses to synthesize estradiol. This fact provides the most significant support for the recently popularized concept of the placenta and the fetus functioning as an endocrinological unit.

Of importance for the reproductive processes are several peripheral conversions that have been characterized and quantified. The following conversions occur at rates that result in production of physiologically effective amounts of hormone in the blood:

testosterone → estradiol (liver, fat, brain)

androstenedione → testosterone (liver, skin, other tissues)

androstenedione → estrone (liver, fat, brain)

testosterone → dihydrotestosterone (liver, skin, prostate)

The tissues given in parentheses are the extraglandular sites where the conversions have been demonstrated.

Another interesting finding is that in tissues that respond to androgen by growth and secretion (such as the prostate, seminal vesicles, hair follicles, and sebaceous glands), the effective intracellular androgen is dihydrotestosterone. This steroid is synthesized from circulating testosterone or androstenedione by a 5 alpha-reductase and a 17 oxosteroid reductase in the target cell. The 5 alpha-reduced steroid, dihydrotestosterone, is presumably transported into the nucleus in association with a receptor protein present in the cytosol. The moiety in the nucleus appears to be the active species that initiates the biochemical events that are recognized as the endocrinological response.

Other conversions that occur in target tissues and that must be considered in relation to the expression of hormonal activity are:

estradiol → estrone (endometrium, myometrium, skin, mammary gland)

estrone sulfate → estrone (endometrium, pituitary)

testosterone → androstane–3 alpha, 17 beta diol (hypothalamus and pituitary)

progesterone → 5 alpha dihydroprogesterone (endometrium)

androstenedione → testosterone (prostate)

testosterone → estradiol (hypothalamus)

Although these conversions are not reflected by increased concentration of blood-borne products, they nevertheless can influence the response of the target tissue to the hormone. For instance, the extent of conversion of estradiol to estrone in human endometrium varies during the menstrual cycle, and this phenomenon influences the intracellular level of estradiol, the component responsible for hormonal action.

The Nature of Hormonal Precursors

Cholesterol is generally considered to be the principal steroidal precursor of the steroid hormones. Not all precursor cholesterol molecules have the same origin; some are derived from acetate by de novo synthesis in the endocrine cell, some constitute the active cholesterol pool present in the cell, some originate by hydrolysis from endogenous cholesterol fatty acid esters, and some enter the cell from perfusing blood. Some molecules of cholesteral are present in the cell membranes and other structural elements of the cell and are probably not available for steroid synthesis. The enumeration of these sources does not imply complete or certain knowledge of the true nature of the steroidal precursors of the steroid hormones.

Another recently uncovered facet of steroid hormone biosynthesis and secretion relates to steroidal sulfates as precursors of the steroid hormones. The role of these conjugates in physiological processes remains to be elucidated. In steroid-producing endocrine glands, enzymes that catalyze the conversion of a C_{27}-sterol into the various steroid hormones appear to recognize two kinds of substrates: those that are free or unconjugated and those that are conjugated with sulfuric acid. Whether there are two sets of enzymes, one for the conjugated and one for the unconjugated substrates, or whether one set is unable to discriminate one kind of substrate from the other, is not yet established. Nor is it known whether one kind of precursor serves one function and the other, another purpose. Nevertheless, there can be little doubt that enzymatic processes that use sulfates as substrates exist in endocrine glands and that these glands, particularly the adrenal glands and the testes, secrete sulfated steroids into their effluent.

Control of Steroidogenesis

The secretory products from steroidogenic tissues are subject to both exogenous and endogenous controls. The trophic hormones interact with membrane receptor sites and presumably activate, directly or indirectly, nucleotide messengers, which in turn lead to an increase in steroid synthesis. Other external controls that can be identified are blood flow and the rates of transport of precursors and of oxygen. Internally, an intricate network of electron donors and transport mechanisms leads to the reduction of NADP, the electron source of the terminal chain. The electrons may be derived by reverse transport through the conventional electron transport chain or through shunts such as that involving the malic enzyme. Other control factors that have been revealed include the availability of oxygen, the hypothetical mitochondrial-activating factor, and certain carrier proteins for sterols.

The rates of synthesis of complex molecules may be affected by transport within the cell. For example, since hydroxylations on the side chain occur in the endoplasmic reticulum, and nuclear hydroxylations (such as 11 beta) occur in the mitochondrion, the rate of cortisol synthesis (and indeed the ratio of cortisol to 11-deoxycortisol) might well be determined by transport rates concerned with the movement of pregnenolone from the mitochondrion, where it is synthesized, to the cytoplasm, where isomerization and 17 and 21 hydroxylation take place. Obviously, many factors might affect such transport, and they are virtually undefined.

Among the internal controls of steroidogenesis are the hormones themselves. Not only is there end-product inhibition of certain enzymes, but more generalized effects than that may also occur. Estrogens have long been known to enhance gonadotropic stimulation of follicular growth, development, and secretion, and recent data indicate that androgens may promote atresia. Understanding of these cellular and intracellular actions is particularly important for the understanding of some of the actions of steroidal contraceptives.

Secretion

Nature of the process In contrast to the complex but identifiable steps in the secretion of peptide hormones, no specific secretory process for steroid hormones has been found. Of interest, however, is the finding that interference with microtubules in the adrenal cortex promotes steroid secretion. Steroid secretion seems to be a process of passive diffusion whose velocity depends on the blood-cell gradient of diffusible molecules. No evidence exists that the effective response to the trophic hormones is due to a process other than an increase in the intracellular concentration.

Rapid changes in the blood levels of hormones have been detected by frequent sampling at short time intervals. The physiological significance—if any—of these fluctuations is not known.

Ovary With respect to steroid hormones, the ovary secretes two important hormones, estradiol and progesterone. The rates of secretion of these hormones vary with the phase of the menstrual cycle.

In the early follicular phase, estradiol secretion is about 50 μg per day. The blood production rate of estrone is similar, but less than 50 percent is derived from ovarian secretion; the rest originates by conversion from estradiol and androstenedione. Androstenedione is a secretory product of both the ovary and the adrenal cortex. Progesterone secretion during this phase is low, probably less than 1 mg per day.

As the dominant follicle grows, the theca interna differentiates, and just before ovulation, estradiol secretion rises to about 400 μg per day. At this time estrone production rates are about 200 μg per day, of which about half is secreted by the ovary. Immediately after ovulation, estrogen secretion falls. During the midluteal phase, however, estradiol and estrone secretion rates, as well as their production rates, are only slightly lower than those during the preovulatory period. With ovulation, luteinization of granulosa and thecal cells takes place. The granulosa cells of the emerging corpus luteum secrete up to 30 mg of progesterone per day until its secretion rate begins to fall off, at about 11 to 12 days after ovulation. The origin of estradiol during the luteal phase is not certain, although it has been proposed that persisting luteinized thecal cells are the source of this estrogen.

Of all the estrogen moieties present in blood, estrone sulfate exists in highest concentration, but most if not all of it is produced by sulfaction of estrone outside the ovary. The significance of this plasma estrogen precursor is unknown, but the endometrium has been shown to rapidly hydrolyze it to estrone.

Testosterone and androstenedione, which are biosynthetic precursors of estradiol and estrone, are also secreted by the ovary. Ovarian stroma containing interstitial and thecal cells has been shown to be capable of synthesizing androgens. In women, ovarian androstenedione secretion rates during the follicular phase are about 1 mg per day and are somewhat increased during the luteal phase; testosterone secretion rates are less than 100 μg per day. Although in these amounts androgens may have little biological effect, intrafollicular androgen may exert significant influences on the processes of follicular maturation and atresia.

Testis The outlines of the secretory pattern in this gland have been known for 10 years. Leydig cells, under the influence of LH, secrete about 7 mg testosterone per day. There are recent findings of considerable interest concerned with the intratesticular effect of testosterone. For normal spermatogenesis, testosterone must be present in testicular interstitial fluid at high concentrations. Testosterone has been shown to diffuse into the tubule and to be metabolized to dihydrotestosterone and androstane–3 alpha, 17 beta–diol. The presence of a cytosol receptor for androgen in the tubule is further evidence that the tubule is a target organ for androgens. Administration of exogenous androgen, including testosterone, suppresses spermatogenesis by lowering LH secretion. The resulting decrease in the secretion of testosterone by the Leydig cell causes the intratesticular concentration of testosterone to fall.

The recent identification of another androgen-binding protein (ABP) in rete testis fluid and in the epididymis may give a clue to another role for testosterone. ABP resembles plasma-binding proteins such as TEBG more closely than it resembles androgen cytosol receptor. It is probably synthesized in the Sertoli cell, enters the tubular fluid, and is then carried to the epididymis with its charge of testosterone. This may be a delivery system for the androgen required for the maintenance of the caput epididymis, or it may be concerned with Sertoli cell function. The synthesis of ABP is stimulated by FSH; this suggests the manner by which this pituitary hormone influences testicular function.

The capacity for steroid synthesis by the tubule is limited (see above), even though an ample supply of precursors from the Leydig cell may be available. Thus it is unknown whether androgens found in the tubules are synthesized in situ or whether they diffuse into the tubules from the Leydig cell.

Evidence that high intratesticular androgen concentrations are necessary for spermatogenesis makes interesting the finding that the testosterone concentration in the testicular artery is higher than that in peripheral arterial blood. The transfer of testosterone from spermatic vein to spermatic artery has been shown and probably results from the close proximity of these vessels in the rete testis. The proposed countercurrent mechanism thus serves to increase the testosterone concentration of blood entering the testis.

In men, about one-third of the 40 μg of estradiol entering the general circulation daily is secreted by the testis. Whether this amount of estradiol exerts a physiological effect in men on hypothalamic or other receptors has yet to be fully defined. No evidence exists for separate regulatory mechanisms for testosterone and estradiol synthesis. Some data suggest that estradiol may have direct effects on the tubule quite distinct from those inhibiting gonadotropin secretion. If this is so, then local stimulation of estrogen secretion could inhibit spermatogenesis without significant peripheral effects.

4.4 Methodological Considerations

The recent development of radioligand assays for the measurement of hormones has had a strong impact in the estimation of rates of hormone production. Gonadal steroids can now be easily measured in plasma of men and nonpregnant women, as well as in target tissues.

Advances in the theory of tracer methods led to a large number of quantitative studies of secretion, metabolism, distribution, and fetomaternal transfers of hormones. The simultaneous administration of two steroids labeled with different isotopes was successfully used to evaluate the extraglandular formation of hormones under physiological conditions. The new concepts used for the design of in vivo tracer experiments were applied to in vitro studies involving the superfusion of tissues with mixtures of metabolically related radioactive hormones.

Progress has also been made in the application of computer techniques to define models of endocrine systems, to facilitate the interpretation of data related to studies on hormone production and metabolism, and to perform calculations involved in hormonal assays. The contribution of system analysis to the advance of knowledge in endocrinology is difficult to assess. Although tangible results may not be evident yet, incorporation of computer techniques into hormone research may prove to be a very significant advance initiated during the past decade.

Possibilities for Contraception
After identifying the landmark discoveries of the past ten years, we have been asked to attempt to expose the "gaps" in our knowledge of steroid hormone secretions.

It is our understanding that the main purpose of this exercise is to allow the reader to focus better on those facets of the subject that seem to give promise for the development of new and presumably superior fertility controlling agents. While such an exercise appears to have merit, we hesitate to play this game because it has, in our opinion, a phantasmagoric quality. To begin with, pinpointing promising areas for future effort presupposes a precognitive capability we are reluctant to lay claim to. It would be wrong to give either scientists or nonscientists the impression that we arrogate to ourselves this predictive skill. The most trenchant reason for shrinking from this exercise, however, is that we do not want to appear to lend support to the notion that science proceeds by such a process. Experts know the limitations of their knowledge and will easily, if so disposed, disclose their ignorance. But the identification of a gap or an unexplored area is of limited value unless appropriate techniques for the scientific examination of the question exist. To identify a gap, in the absence of acceptable methods for its exploration, can do little to advance our knowledge of a scientific area. In science, method is an essential attribute of question, and without method, the substance of the puzzle is only words.

At another level, it may be possible that methods and questions do not come together because those in possession of one are unaware of the other. In the event that the imagination of some endocrine biochemists and physiologists could be stimulated by our comments, we have made some efforts to reveal, in what follows, some thoughts about the possibilities for contraception that might result from the filling of the lacunae of our present knowledge

The possibilities for contraception based upon present knowledge depend upon either accelerating or in-

hibiting known processes. The concept is a simple one and is only broadly conceived because our knowledge of physiological processes is not profound enough to be more specific. It becomes clear that research into the fundamentals of these processes must proceed not only on a broad front but also in detailed depth.

Ovary Both estradiol and progesterone are required for the transport of the egg in the Fallopian tube and for conditioning the uterus to accept the fertilized ovum and support its development; therefore, any means of effectively inhibiting the production of ovarian hormones is potentially of interest in contraception. Furthermore, disturbances in the timing as well as in the amount of hormone secretion may hinder the reproductive process. Purposeful alteration of the normal sequence of ovarian secretory events may achieve this goal.

More information about the control of steroidogenesis and the secretion of steroids is required before attempts to inhibit hormone production can be intelligently pursued. Intimate knowledge of these events may permit us to devise chemical inhibitors, modifiers, and accelerators of synthesis. If, for example, the secretion of progesterone were prevented by an inhibitor, the progesterone-sustained activities, including the secretory endometrium and the pregnancy, might be terminated. This might lead to a once-a-month type of contraception or a chemical means of terminating pregnancy. Similar but more complicated cases for estrogen biosynthesis can be conceived.

Inhibitors of hormone production may be used as contraceptives at particular times during the cycle rather than on a continual basis. For instance, opportune interruption of the secretion or action of progesterone during a short period may result in endometrial shedding. Furthermore, inhibitors of these types can be used after conception, since ovarian progesterone is necessary to maintain the conceptus for six to eight weeks after implantation. Inhibitors of binding of pituitary gonadotropins to ovarian receptors, which may possibly be obtained by modifying chemically the gonadotropins to destroy their activity while preserving their ability to bind, might suppress gonadotropin stimulation. Thus blockage of gonadotropins at the ovarian level represents another approach to the regulation of estradiol and progesterone production.

Blocks might theoretically be made to occur at several other sites, for example, the multienzyme system that synthesizes progesterone or the transport mechanisms. Even degradative processes might be accelerated.

The safety of an inhibitor depends upon its specificity. Some available inhibitors act on the cytochromes that oxidize or hydroxylate steroid molecules. These inhibitors reduce ovarian and placental steroidogenesis, but there is a chance that they may, in large concentrations, also affect the secretion of cortisol. Thus compounds of high specificity are desirable. The ovarian aromatase system, which converts androgens to estrogens, is present in ovaries and placentas but not in adrenal glands; this constitutes another attractive target for specific inhibitors.

Testis At every organizational level, from its effects on behavior to its action in the cell to its role in spermatogenesis, knowledge of androgen is incomplete. Further broad explorations are obviously necessary. A way is needed to alter sperm production selectively without impairing the ability to secrete or utilize androgen. Among several conceivable ways of doing this, one is related to the transport of androgen into the cells of the seminiferous tubule. Research on the characteristics of the transport system may permit synthesis of hormonally inactive compounds that bind tightly to the testicular androgen-binding protein and thereby prevent the transport of testosterone. Knowledge of the biochemistry of the action of androgen and estrogen on the cells of the seminiferous tubule may reveal methods of interrupting this essential mechanism.

Sperm production requires that the Leydig cells of the testis synthesize testosterone; this function cannot be replaced by oral administration of androgens. Thus if it were possible to interrupt with steroids the secretion of LH by the pituitary gland, thereby causing cessation of Leydig cell secretion and decreased spermatogenesis, another approach to contraception might be achieved. Replacement of the androgenic secretions of the Leydig cell that are required for anabolic processes might then be accomplished with oral medication. An equally valid approach to inhibition of spermatogenesis would entail the selective inhibition of one key step in the biosynthetic process by which testosterone is made, without interfering with pituitary function. It would, of course, still be necessary to use replacement doses of androgen for spermatogenesis and virilization.

It has been suggested that estrogens can directly suppress tubular function. If this is so, is it possible to increase selectively the aromatizing capacity of the testis? Will some of the low-activity estrogens, such as the impeded estrogens, retain their effects at the level of the tubule?

The synthesis of ABP is a relatively unknown area. If it is solely tubular in origin and is regulated by FSH, then selective manipulation of FSH release by steroids or the tubular factor would effect an ideal suppression of tubular function without interference with Leydig cell function.

The development of drugs invokes the problems of toxicity. In general, it can be stated that toxicity relates to specificity. There are two ways to understand specificity; the classical and still necessary approach is trial and error, often over a long period of time. The more modern, perhaps quicker, approach is to understand a site of action as a means to achieving a high degree of specificity. While this latter approach does not eliminate the need for prolonged studies, it increases the probability of success, especially when one searches for a new drug.

Historically, drug discovery has depended most often upon association of a known drug with an understanding of a disease mechanism. Now the search for a "magic bullet" is being repeated. We have the disease and need the drug for it, but we are uncertain of the mechanisms involved.

The steps to an effective, safe contraceptive are fraught with uncertainty, and a case may be made for a serendipitous discovery as well as for a planned effort. Nevertheless, one aspect is certain: more research is needed because neither planned nor serendipitous discoveries occur in a vacuum. The balance between, and indeed the definitions of, applied and basic research are moot.

The solution to our dilemma is to study as many approaches as possible, in as much depth as possible.

5 Hormonal Regulation of the Development, Maturation, and Ovulation of the Ovarian Follicle

J. M. Bahr, G. T. Ross, and A. V. Nalbandov

Even though the endocrinology of the ovary in general and of the ovarian follicle in particular have been studied by endocrinologists for about 45 years, knowledge of the hormonal basis of ovarian function remains fragmentary. We have collected a few of the facts about the ovary and about follicular development and have suggested areas requiring further research. In our opinion gaps in the fundamental understanding of follicular function must be filled before the follicular function can be controlled.

Gametogenesis (ovulation) and the secretion of sex steroids are interdependent processes requiring coordinate interactions of ovarian components responsive to hormonal stimulation. An orderly progression of changes, including enlargement of the oocyte and proliferation and alteration in the appearance of granulosa cells, occurs within the limiting membrane and results in progressively enlarging follicles.

Not all of the enlarging follicles are destined to ovulate; many of them die and degenerate, that is, become atretic. Atresia appears to be a normal process that occurs in all species studied, especially between birth and puberty. Both the basis for selection of a cohort of follicles destined to begin maturation and the causes of atresia remain unknown.

After the differentiation of the theca from surrounding stroma, the next alteration in the morphology consists in the appearance and accumulation of a fluid-filled cavity, the antrum. The volume of this fluid increases with progressive increase in the diameter of maturing follicles. Analysis of this fluid reveals that it contains estrogens, androgens, and progestogens in concentrations exceeding those found in simultaneously collected peripheral blood specimens. In addition, the antral fluid contains low molecular weight plasma proteins and some other macromolecules, which are secretory products of the granulosa cells.

We do not know whether the gonadal steroids found in the follicular fluid have a physiological function or whether they are secreted into the fluid because they are no longer required in the follicular or ovarian endocrine economy. When gonadotropic hormones are injected into females, a great and almost immediate outpouring of gonadal steroids can be demonstrated in the ovarian vein. Whether these steroids are mobilized from the follicular fluid or from the theca cells forming part of the follicular wall remains to be determined.

Atresia could be ascribed to inadequate hormonal stimulation or to an incorrect ratio of gonadotropins; however, some atresia continues after puberty has been reached and is not of uniform intensity during the cycle. The rate of atresia appears to increase toward the time when ovulation occurs. Possibly this could be ascribed to the finite amount of trophic hormone available for the entire ovary, since injection of exogenous gonadotropins or the removal of one ovary greatly reduces the number of atretic follicles in ovaries remaining in situ. Why certain follicles are selected to mature in preference to others is unknown. Possibly this selection is determined by blood supply; follicles that have a poor blood supply do not get the necessary hormonal stimulus, and they die. The role of the vascular supply in follicular growth and maintenance is very sketchily known and deserves intensive study.

Another puzzle involving follicular growth concerns the species in which only one follicle matures and ovulates. How is this one follicle chosen? An obvious possibility again involves the blood supply. Some maturing follicles may have a choicer location in the vascular bed than others have. Some follicles would then be close to blood vessels that carry the nutrients and trophic hormones essential for follicular growth and ovulation. This idea may have merit and deserves study. For instance, in monotocous females such as women, it remains unknown whether the ovary containing the follicle destined to ovulate has an increased blood flow compared to the ovary that does not contain such a follicle. As yet unpublished studies show this possibility in sheep; the ovary containing the corpus luteum receives significantly more blood than the other ovary receives. The same study (by Reimers and Niswender) also shows that this increased blood flow, in the case of the corpus-luteum-containing ovary, is regulated by LH.

Previous studies of ovarian vascular changes have demonstrated adaptational changes in ovarian arteries associated with the growth of Graafian follicles, ovulation, and development of corpora lutea. We do not know what changes occur in microcirculation during these times or what changes occur in vascularity from the preovulatory to the postovulatory follicle.

Further explanation must be applied to one of the first effects of gonadotropins on ovarian tissue, which is a significantly increased blood supply and flow. The suspicion that hormones such as FSH and LH may affect the vascular bed more than the follicle itself remains just that—a suspicion. A more likely assumption is that both the vascular bed and the cellular components of the follicle may be target tissues, but at present, few research workers would consider that the primary action of gonadotropins could be on the vascular bed; this does not mean that they are right.

One of the most puzzling aspects of follicular growth lies in the fact that toward the end of the follicular phase of the cycle, growth rate accelerates and culminates in a phenomenal increase, which is often called the ovulatory spurt. While these events occur, the gonadotropic hormones that cause follicular growth are barely detectable by radioimmunoassay in the bloodstream of a large variety of females. In women, FSH levels decrease in the bloodstream at the very time when follicular growth rate accelerates. An explanation for this paradox is not presently available. The two most plausible explanations involve the possibility that follicular growth is due to the cumulative effect of constant, albeit low, levels of gonadotropins or that as follicles approach ovulation they acquire increasing numbers of so-called binding sites, which are frequently invoked as being essential for the recognition of specific hormones and for the translation of their message into visible physiological effects such as growth. What causes the induction of increasing numbers of binding sites is presently unknown. It could be the gonadotropins, the steroids made by the follicle, or a delicate interaction between the gonadotropins and follicular steroids. Variable sex steroid hormone concentrations in antral fluid might possibly determine the response of an individual follicle to gonadotropins. Assays have been developed that are sufficiently sensitive to permit measurements of sex steroid hormone concentrations in antral fluid from individual follicles, and techniques have been developed for direct instillation of gonadotropins into single follicles. These developments should make it possible to characterize these interactions more definitively than before. Some of these questions are now under study, but much additional work will be required before we gain complete understanding of the mechanism involved.

If the sex steroids are involved in the genesis of binding sites for gonadotropins, some of the ovarian components may plausibly have binding sites for steroid hormones—a possibility that has not yet been studied. Another hiatus in our knowledge concerns the degree of binding of steroids contained in the follicular fluid.

One of the difficulties involved in the study of follicular development lies in the present trend of studying levels of gonadotropic hormone by radioimmunoassay (RIA). Not everyone is convinced that these assays accurately reflect hormone levels. Bits of evidence now emerging should encourage in-depth studies of what exactly RIAs measure in comparison to bioassays. Some of the recent findings may be summarized briefly. Two RIAs can be used to detect rhesus monkey plasma LH. One is called O-O RIA and uses labeled anti-ovine LH; the other is called hCG-Rh RIA and uses labeled antirhesus hCG. Both assay systems detect LH in adult rhesus plasma, for instance, the ovulatory peak. In infant monkeys, however, the O-O RIA detects large quantities of a substance that behaves like the LH of adult monkeys, while the hCG-Rh RIA detects no LH in infants. In a study in women, plasma LH levels were compared in an RIA system and a highly sensitive bioassay system. In all subjects (postmenopausal women as well as women with normal cycles), the bioassay detected from 2 to 14 times more LH in the plasma than the RIA detected. In chickens, the ovarian ascorbic acid depletion (OAAD) assay detects at least two peaks of plasma LH during the ovulatory cycle, both accompanied by significant increases in steroid synthesis in the follicles. In contrast, RIA detects only one LH peak, which coincides with one of the peaks found by OAAD. These examples (which could be multiplied) cause concern and raise the question whether RIA has earned the confidence of investigators studying gonadotropins.

Finally, while the present RIA methods measure FSH and LH separately, under normal conditions both hormones are present simultaneously, and previous data have repeatedly shown that these two hormones synergize. The old bioassay systems were not able to detect the two gonadotropins in reasonable volumes of plasma, but they could measure the pituitary gland content of these hormones. In assays of the pituitary gland, the changes in the total hypophysial gonadotropin concentration correspond to ovarian development and to follicular growth much better than do the RIA studies on the plasma of rats, women, and pigs.

All of these problems raise the question whether the RIA studies are suitable to enlarge understanding of the endocrine interrelation between the ovary and the hypophysis. Unfortunately, the ease with which RIAs can be performed and the rapidity with which results can be obtained has blinded many investigators to the constant necessity of running parallel checks with bioassay. Several highly sensitive in vitro bioassay systems have recently become available, at least for LH.

Not even the nature of the ovulation-inducing hormone (OIH) is definitely known. It is known that LH in small doses or FSH in large doses will cause follicular rupture; however, it is also known that if the two hormones are given together in proper ratios, the dose of either one can be reduced below the level at which either hormone alone can induce ovulation. Furthermore, in most animals studied, both hormones are released together. They form the so-called ovulatory peak just prior to ovulation. All of this would argue that the physiological OIH is a mixture of FSH and LH. Against this is incomplete and not totally convincing evidence that ovulation can be prevented by the injection (at appropriate times) of antibodies to LH but not of those to FSH. On the other hand, injection of anti-FSH decreases the number of ovulatory follicles in the next cycle. Again more work is needed to decide whether the experiments with FSH or LH antibodies are faulty or whether the ovulatory process operates on a redundancy principle under which, in a pinch, LH alone can accomplish follicular rupture.

Variable sex steroid hormone concentrations in antral fluid provide a second plausible basis for factors that might operate locally to determine the fate of individual follicles undergoing maturation. Estrogens have long been known to stimulate growth of follicles in the absence of gonodatropins and to enhance follicular growth in response to gonadotropins in hypophysectomized immature female rats. In contrast to the stimulatory effects of estrogens, androgens inhibit the follicle-stimulating effects of both estrogens and gonadotropins and enhance atresia in this model.

Neurogenic stimuli provide the basis for a third factor that might operate locally to determine follicular responses. The ovaries of mammalian and avian females are innervated by adrenergic nerves. Preliminary data show that injections of antiadrenergic drugs decrease steroid hormone concentrations in ovarian venous effluent and block ovulating responses to exogenous gonadotropins. The potential of these drugs for use in control of ovulation should be further explored.

A considerable body of circumstantial evidence implicates the oocyte in determining responses of the follicular complex to stimuli. This provides the basis for a fourth factor that might operate as a local determinant of follicular maturation. For example, it has been postulated that death of the oocyte initiates atresia. Furthermore, fragmentary data support the contention that the follicle does not luteinize as long as it contains an oocyte. In addition, some experimental evidence suggests that the luteostatic properties of the ovum are somehow transferred to the follicular fluid.

An excellent example of the role of the oocyte on the fate of the follicle can be found in the rabbit. This species is unusual but not unique in that a major portion of ovary consists of the so-called interstitial gland, which is steroidogenially active (it secretes 20 alpha hydroxyprogesterone in contrast to the corpus luteum, which secretes progesterone). The cells comprising the interstitial gland in the rabbit bear a very close histological resemblance to luteal tissue. While it is well established that luteal tissue is formed from follicular granulosa cells after ovulation, it is less commonly realized that the interstitial tissue is also formed from follicles—but only those which become atretic. Thus in the progress of follicular atresia in rabbit ovaries, as soon as an oocyte shows signs of degeneration (recognizable by its staining properties), the theca and granulosa cells surrounding it show signs of luteinization. After complete degeneration and disappearance of the ovum, the former follicle is completely transformed into a structure like corpus luteum, which now joins and fuses with the pool of the interstitial gland formed by follicles that had become atretic earlier. While interstitial tissue is most conspicuous in lower vertebrates such as rabbits and raccoons, it is found in all species, including primates. Its endocrine role, if any, remains to be elucidated. Past as well as recent data suggest that high doses of LH increase the total proportion of interstitial tissue significantly in immature hypophysectomized rats, without appreciably altering the histological appearance of other ovarian components. It is unknown whether in species with less prominent interstitial glands, the interstitial tissue is also from atretic follicles.

In the experiments of nature in which either very few or no oogonia are produced, the resultant gonad contains neither oocytes nor follicles, and the remaining cells function inefficiently, if at all, in the biosynthesis and secretion of sex steroid hormones. Surgical removal of the oocyte from a follicle results in morphological alterations in the remaining granulosa cells and changes in the quality of secreted steroid hormone. Similarly, the destruction of oocytes with ionizing radiation or with drugs, or the spontaneous depletion of these cells with aging, all result in significant alteration in the quantity and quality of ovarian sex steroid hormone secretion. Steroid hormone production varies, depending upon whether microsurgical transplants of granulosa cells contain theca cells as well. The evidence, then, is consistent with interaction among oocytes, granulosa cells, and thecal cells during follicular maturation and sex steroid hormone secretion. The mediators of these interactions remain to be determined. The ovary of the woman in menopause is an excellent example of altered ovarian steroid metabolism in the absence of a normal complement of follicles and hence of oocytes.

The roles of estrogen and progesterone in female reproduction have been correctly associated with the development and function of the reproductive duct system and the breasts. However, practically nothing is known about the role played by androgen even though the ovarian follicles of some species synthesize it in quantities larger than those of the other two steroids. The role of follicular androgen in the reproductive physiology of females is much less clear, mostly because until recently, few endocrinologists had been aware of its prominence. Follicular androgen may be made simply because it is one of the steps in the metabolic pathway from progesterone to estrogen, or it may have other functions, such as participation in the hypothalamo-hypophyseal-ovarian feedback system. Some inconclusive data on women suggest that it may be the hormone responsible for female concupiscence. Castrated rabbit females implanted with testosterone exhibit normal mating behavior when the plasma testosterone levels are at physiological levels normal for intact females.

Follicular steroids may also be necessary to establish an optimal intragonadal hormonal milieu that is involved in the follicular development and in the modulation of the response of follicles to gonadotropins. One totally uninvestigated area is the possible role of gonadal steroids in the maturation of the oocyte.

Several other aspects of the internal hormonal environment of the follicle are inadequately understood. While we know that follicles contain large quantities of all three sex steroids, we do not know whether they are released constantly during follicular maturation or whether there is a storage phase and a release phase. We need to understand the hormonal stimuli involved in steroid synthesis (perhaps without major release) and the stimuli required for release. For instance, it is now well established that a major peak of estrogen of follicular origin occurs in the bloodstream of females and acts on the hypothalamo-hypophyseal system, causing release of peaks of the gonadotropic hormones required for ovulation. What we need to know is the cause of this massive estrogen release in the face of unchanging concentration of trophic hormones in the peripheral circulation. Major releases of follicular steroids are caused by both gonadotropic hormones, implying that they are required not only for synthesis of the steroids but also for their release. If the ovarian blood vessels of females are cannulated and ovarian blood is collected, animals injected with gonadotropins show an almost instantaneous very large increase in the concentration of all three steroids in the ovarian blood. Are these increased steroid levels due to an instant increase in the rate of steroid synthesis or are they due to the ability of FSH or LH or both to cause the release of steroids stored in the follicle (fluid or cells or both)? Still more confusing is the preliminary information that the release rates of the steroids vary; we need to know whether any one of the three steroids can be released alone without the other two, and if so, how this is controlled hormonally.

One of the reasons for the inadequacy of our knowledge of what is happening at the ovarian level (with follicles and corpora lutea) is that hitherto endocrino-logists have been largely concerned with the interrelation between the hypothalamo-hypophyseal system and the ovary, treating the ovary as primarily a target organ. We are now technically ready to focus attention on the ovarian structures and to study their responses to the stimuli normally impinging on them.

For each of the four potential locally active control mechanisms we have discussed, the possibility of pharmacological intervention exists. For example, the identification and synthesis of analogs with inhibitory properties, a highly developed technology in experimental pharmacology, might be expected to result from defining the mediators of vasomotor and neurogenic stimuli. It is possible, then, to envision development of substances with minimal systemic effects, allowing for control of ovulation while reducing the hazards of untoward reactions such as those accruing from the systemic administration of synthetic sex steroid hormones. The experimental pharmacologist and the endocrinologist should work collaboratively in such a manner that each exploits the insights and technology of both disciplines.

A considerable amount of basic research in mammals (including humans) needs to be done to establish the normative and to work out appropriate models. Throughout the course of our deliberations, however, we have become increasingly aware of the difficulties inherent in determining the roles of local ovarian processes for control of ovulation in women. Gross inspection of human ovaries cannot be accomplished without anesthesia, and when ovarian function is normal, rarely are there ethically justifiable indications for such an examination, exclusively for this purpose. Recovery of sufficient ovarian tissue for meaningful microscopic examination is even more complicated than gross inspection and is associated with additional, albeit minimal, morbidity. Such examinations of normal ovarian tissue are restricted to abdominal surgery for other reasons or to surgical procedures in women being evaluated for infertility where the lesion is in gonaducts rather than ovaries. Furthermore, governmental regulations concerning human experimentation are becoming increasingly restrictive, further reducing the likelihood that scientifically adequate clinical studies can be performed in the United States.

Although we are aware of the difficulties inherent in assuming that results obtained in other species will be valid for man, basic experimentation in animal models remains the only viable basis for further progress. The insights gained from these experiments should facilitate design of ethically acceptable, low-risk human experimentation, if not in the United States, then in other countries with less restrictive regulations.

6 The Endocrinology of Ovulation and Corpus Luteum Formation, Function, and Luteolysis in Women

D. T. Baird and R. V. Short

6.1 Introduction

The ever-increasing need to regulate the rate of human reproduction is focusing attention on the reproductive processes that are most amenable to intervention. High on this list comes ovulation and the formation, function, and regression of the corpus luteum. A wealth of data is now available about animals, but a marked dichotomy appears to exist between primates and laboratory and domestic animals. These differences are reflected principally in the mechanisms responsible for the regression of the corpus luteum at the end of a nonpregnant cycle and for prolongation of the life of the corpus luteum in the event of a pregnancy (l).

We concentrate here on the evidence available about humans and primates, and we refer to other animal experiments only when they seem particularly relevant to the human situation.

Of the theoretical possibilities for interfering with reproduction, the female presents more promise than the male; ovulation is a discrete process occurring only once a month, whereas spermatogenesis is a continuous process. The time lag between the initial stimulus for ovulation and the actual event is a matter of days, whereas many weeks must elapse between the initiation of spermatogenesis and ejaculation of mature spermatozoa. It should be easier to prevent the monthly shedding of one egg than the daily production of millions of spermatozoa.

If contraception is to be achieved by controlling some phase of the menstrual cycle, thought must be given to the reproductive state of the woman induced by the contraceptive regime. We do not know whether it is better to superimpose a cyclical form of therapy in an attempt to reproduce the menstrual cycle or to aim for continuous ovarian suppression with consequent amenorrhea.

6.2 Normal Follicular Development

The present consensus of opinion is that follicular development is a continuous process (2). Once initiated in early childhood it goes on continuously throughout the menstrual cycle, pregnancy, and the postpartum period. In animals, the early stages of follicular development appear to be largely independent of gonadotropic control, but in humans we do not have adequate evidence on this point. There is no doubt, however, that the final stages of follicular development leading up to ovulation are entirely dependent on gonadotropic support.

In women, the final stage of follicular growth is probably initiated by the rise of FSH and LH, which occurs at the end of the luteal phase of the previous cycle as a result of the declining secretion of estradiol and progesterone from the regressing corpus luteum (3). The high peripheral levels of gonadotropin result in a selective transport of FSH (but not LH) into the follicular fluid of a number of developing follicles (4). Presumably this entry of FSH stimulates mitosis in the granulosa and thecal cells of these follicles. Soon after the entry of FSH, the concentrations of estradiol begin to rise in the follicular fluid. By day 7, the developing follicle is clearly established as a major source of estrogen production in the ovary, as indicated by the higher concentration of estradiol in the vein draining the ovary that contains the developing follicle, compared to that in the vein draining the other ovary (5). This rise in the estradiol secretion inhibits FSH secretion from the pituitary by negative feedback, so that the concentration of this gonadotropin falls progressively in the peripheral blood (3). The growth of the Graafian follicle is maintained, however, since its FSH concentration within the follicular fluid remains relatively constant, and this, together with the extremely high concentrations of estradiol in the follicular fluid, probably sensitizes the cells to FSH and LH (6). Thus the follicle that is secreting estradiol stimulates its own growth while at the same time inhibiting the growth of other developing follicles, which therefore become atretic.

While the FSH concentration in peripheral blood is beginning to fall, the concentration of LH is actually rising slightly (3). The reason for this is obscure, but it may be a result of differential hypothalamic-pituitary sensitivity to the negative feedback effects of gonadal steroids (7). This rise in basal LH secretion is probably important for maintaining estradiol secretion by the theca interna cells of the follicle.

There is now good evidence that in women, once the secretion of estradiol has reached a certain critical level (about 200 μg per day), it triggers a reflex discharge of LH and FSH from the pituitary (8). This midcycle surge in gonadotropin secretion is responsible for inducing ovulation 24 to 36 hours later. An immediate consequence of the LH surge is that this gonadotropin enters the follicular fluid of the preovulatory follicle, initiating oocyte maturation and preovulatory progesterone secretion by the granulosa cells (4, 9). The concentration of estradiol in the peripheral blood declines abruptly at the time of the LH peak, due to decreased secretion by the preovulatory follicle (10). Morphological studies suggest that this is due to an inhibition of the theca interna cells by high levels of LH (9).

Although the maturation of the oocyte and the commencement of progesterone secretion by the granulosa cells are initiated by LH, we do not understand in detail how these changes are brought about. For example, it has been postulated that the oocyte may inhibit the luteinization of the granulosa cells (11), and that the follicular fluid may contain a meiotic inhibitor (12). But perhaps these effects could be equally well explained by the changes in the gonadotropin concentration in follicular fluid. Evidence in the rhesus monkey suggests that one of the actions of FSH is to stimulate the production of new LH receptors in the granulosa cells, and this may be important for their subsequent secretory activity after luteinization (12). The metabolic requirements of the granulosa cells and the oocyte are presumably high and may account for the relatively low oxygen tension within the follicle (13). While the declining oxygen tension in the developing follicle may be necessary for oocyte maturation (14), the concomitant fall in prolactin concentration may be necessary for progesterone secretion by the granulosa cells (15).

We still do not understand what actually causes mechanical rupture of the follicle; the steriods present in follicular fluid may play a role (16). Evidence in the rabbit and the rat suggests that prostaglandins E_2 and $F_{2\alpha}$ are present in high concentrations in the preovulatory follicle, and local inhibition of their synthesis will prevent follicular rupture (17).

6.3 Formation, Function, and Regression of the Corpus Luteum

It is important to remember that the endocrine events preceding ovulation probably influence the subsequent secretory activity of the corpus luteum throughout its lifespan (3). The human corpus luteum is unusual in that it contains a large component of morphologically distinct thecal cells in addition to the luteinized granulosa cells (18). This is perhaps the most plausible explanation for the relatively large amounts of estrogen secreted by the gland. The combined secretion of estrogen and progesterone is undoubtedly responsible for the decline in FSH and LH secretion during the lu-

teal phase of the menstrual cycle, and this is reflected in the increased proportion of atretic follicles in the ovaries at this time (19).

Evidence about the nature of the pituitary luteotropic stimulus in women is scanty and difficult to obtain. The studies in hypophysectomized patients leave little doubt that LH is one of the essential factors (8). However, since measurable amounts of prolactin are present in the peripheral blood of all hypophysectomized patients (20), this hormone may also play a permissive role in luteal maintenance, as it does in most other mammalian species. Human granulosa cells in tissue culture require prolactin for normal progesterone secretion, although supraphysiological levels of the hormone are inhibitory (15).

The corpus luteum of the cycle normally starts to regress about 10 days after its formation, and contrary to the situation in other species, this is not due to any luteolytic activity coming from the uterus (21). In the species with a uterine luteolysin, little doubt remains that the active substance is in fact prostaglandin $F_{2\alpha}$ (22, 23). Evidence about the luteolytic activity of intravenously administered prostaglandin $F_{2\alpha}$ in women is equivocal, but this may stem from the difficulty of delivering adequate amounts to the ovary through this route (21). Intra-aortic infusion of prostaglandin $F_{2\alpha}$ is known to depress progesterone secretion by the corpus luteum in rhesus monkeys (24), and in humans prostaglandin receptors are known to be present in luteal tissue (25). Thus women may have a local intra-ovarian luteolytic mechanism. In this regard it seems significant that local injections of estradiol into the corpus luteum will provoke luteal regression in women (26), and irradiation of the ovaries in the luteal phase of the cycle, with destruction of all the follicles, will apparently prolong the functional life of the corpus luteum (27). Although the concentrations of pituitary gonadotropins are at their lowest at the time of luteal regression, luteolysis seems unlikely to result solely from the withdrawal of pituitary gonadotropic support. There is no doubt, however, that placental luteotropins are responsible for the continued maintenance of luteal activity seen at the commencement of pregnancy (28).

6.4 Possibilities for Clinical Intervention

Stimulation of Follicular Development
Follicular growth can be stimulated either by the administration of exogenous gonadotropins or by the stimulation of endogenous release. Gonadotropin therapy appears to work by reducing the incidence of atresia in large developing follicles, rather than by stimulating an excessive number of new developing follicles (29). In view of the complex sequence of changes initi-

ated by gonadotropins in the follicular phase of the cycle, it is hardly surprising that these are difficult to mimic therapeutically. For example, a single injection of LH-RH will not induce ovulation except when given at a time of the cycle when the follicle is already matured (30). The relative success of clomiphene therapy for the induction of ovulation is probably due to the fact that it acts at a hypothalamic rather than at a pituitary or ovarian level (31). Thus the developing follicle is given time to regulate the secretion of pituitary gonadotropins and, in particular, to initiate its own ovulatory surge of LH and FSH.

Further improvements in the induction of ovulation will be dependent upon increased understanding of the critical sequence of events occurring in the normal preovulatory follicle.

Inhibition of Follicular Development

Follicular development can be suppressed by inhibiting endogenous pituitary gonadotropin secretion. The conventional combined contraceptive pill containing both estrogen and progestogen suppresses LH and particularly FSH to levels below which normal follicular development cannot occur (32). Estrogen alone in large doses will also inhibit follicular development. On the other hand, progesterone itself has little if any negative feedback effect and does not suppress the basal secretion of FSH and LH (33). It does, however, inhibit the ability of estradiol to provoke an ovulatory surge of gonadotropins, and hence it can block ovulation. Many of the synthetic gestagens used for contraception do have the ability to suppress basal levels of FSH and LH, so that follicular development is impaired (32). In low-dose continuous gestagen therapy, progestogen may be insufficient to block ovulation, and the contraceptive effect is due to actions elsewhere in the reproductive tract.

Although conventional steroidal contraceptives are highly effective and relatively safe, they do have a number of well-recognized drawbacks that prevent widespread acceptance. Apart from the serious medical hazards that occur in a small minority of patients, the irritating minor symptomatic complaints, coupled with the inconvenience of daily medication, result in a high dropout rate (32). It is difficult to see how many of these drawbacks can be overcome. Although the long-acting injectables may overcome some of the problems of medication, they have the added disadvantage of causing menstrual irregularities during and after therapy (34).

Advances in immunization schedules have now made it possible to immunize animals experimentally not only against pituitary gonadotropins but also against hormones of low molecular weight that are not naturally antigenic, such as hypothalamic releasing hormones, steroids, and prostaglandins. Although these active immunization techniques offer a novel and interesting way of interfering with fertility, the difficulties of assessing the possible long-term consequences of active immunization against naturally occurring hormones in humans makes it unlikely that they will find practical application in the near future. In the short term, however, passive immunization or use of synthetic inhibitors or competitive antagonists may neutralize the effects of endogenous hormones. For example, in marmoset monkeys, passive immunization against hCG appears to induce abortion (35); some synthetic polypeptides structurally similar to LH-releasing hormone can apparently inhibit ovulation in rats (36); inhibitors of prostaglandin synthesis can likewise inhibit ovulation in rats and rabbits, apparently by preventing rupture of the follicle (17). If prostaglandin production by the endometrium is involved in the normal mechanism of menstruation, prostaglandin inhibitors might disturb the critical synchronization between ovary and uterus that is essential for normal implantation (37, 38). We may even discover other nonsteroidal pituitary inhibitors without the toxic side effects of such compounds as methallibure.

Interference with Luteal Function

We have already pointed out that the secretory activity of the corpus luteum is partially determined by endocrine events taking place prior to ovulation. For example, it has been suggested that an "inadequate" luteal phase in women is due to disturbed gonadotropin secretion in the early proliferative phase of the cycle (3). Thus pharmacological manipulation at any stage of the menstrual cycle may lead to disturbance of luteal function. In this section, however, we confine ourselves to substances that act on the fully formed corpus luteum.

Both synthetic estrogens and gestagens administered in high doses during the luteal phase of the cycle depress progesterone secretion by the human corpus luteum (39–42); the disadvantages of this approach as a potential form of contraception are obvious. While clinical trials of the naturally occurring prostaglandins have failed to provide convincing evidence of luteolytic activity, there is a real possibility that some of the newer synthetic analogs with longer biological half-lives in the systemic circulation and more selective action on the ovary could be used as inducers of luteolysis (43, 44).

6.5 Summary

It is clear from this review that the manipulation of ovarian function is still likely to be one of the most fruitful areas for future contraceptive development. Our ability to translate concepts into practice is severely hampered by our lack of fundamental understanding of normal human ovarian physiology.

The following lists summarize our views about areas of fundamental research where more information is required, and about areas of present clinical practice that are based on insufficient factual information. Much of our knowledge of ovarian function has inevitably been derived from animal experimentation, and now we need to verify these findings in humans.

Fundamental Aspects

1. The dynamics of follicular growth and atresia in the human ovary.

2. The mechanism of follicular rupture.

3. The luteotropic control of the human corpus luteum.

4. The mechanism of human luteal regression and its prevention in early pregnancy.

5. The biochemistry of the human endometrium, and the mechanism of menstruation.

Clinical Aspects

1. The merits and disadvantages of cyclical as opposed to continuous ovarian suppression as a form of contraception.

2. The medical control of menstruation and an assessment of the morbidity caused by disorders of menstruation.

References

1. The corpus luteum. Biol. Reprod. 8:128, 1973.

2. Pederson, T. Follicle growth in the mouse ovary. In *Oogenesis*, eds. J. D. Biggers and A. W. Schuetz. Baltimore: University Park Press, 1972.

3. Ross, G. T., C. M. Cargille, M. B. Lipsett, P. L. Rayford, J. R. Marshall, C. A. Shott, and D. Rodbard. Pituitary and gonadal hormones in women during spontaneous and induced ovulatory cycles. Recent Progr. Horm. Res. 26:1, 1970.

4. McNatty, K. P., W. M. Hunter, A. S. McNeilly, and R. S. Sawers. Changes in the concentrations of pituitary and steroid hormones in the follicular fluid of human Graafian follicles throughout the menstrual cycle. J. Endocrinol. 64:555, 1975.

5. Baird, D. T., and I. S. Fraser. Concentration of oestrone and oestradiol-17β in follicular fluid and ovarian venous blood of women. Clin. Endocrinol. 4:259, 1974.

6. Goldenberg, R. L., J. L. Vaitukaitis, and G. T. Ross. Oestrogen and follicle stimulating hormone interactions on follicle growth in rats. Endocrinology 90:1492, 1972.

7. Vaitukaitis, J. L., J. A. Bermudez, C. M. Cargille, M. B. Lipsett, and G. T. Ross. New evidence for an anti-oestrogenic action of clomiphene citrate in women. J. Clin. Endocrinol. Metab. 32:503, 1971.

8. Vande Wiele, R. L., J. Bogumiel, I. Dyrenfurth, M. Ferin, R. Jewelewicz, M. L. Warren, T. Rizkallah, and G. Mikhail. Mechanisms regulating the menstrual cycle in women. Recent Prog. Horm. Res. 26:63, 1970.

9. Delforge, J. P., K. Thomas, F. Roux, J. Carneiro de Siqueira, and J. Ferin. Time relationships between granulosa cells growth and luteinization, and plasma luteinizing hormone discharge in humans. I. A morphometric analysis. Fertil. Steril. 23:1, 1972.

10. Baird, D. T., and I. S. Fraser. Blood production and ovarian secretion rates of oestradiol-17β and oestrone in women throughout the menstrual cycle. J. Clin. Endocrinol. Metab. 38:779, 1974.

11. El-Fouly, M., B. Cook, M. Nekola, and A. V. Nalbandov. Role of the ovum in follicular luteinization. Endocrinology 87:288, 1970.

12. Channing, C. P., and S. Kammerman. Binding of gonadotrophins to ovarian cells. Biol. Reprod. 10:179, 1974.

13. Fraser, I. S., D. T. Baird, and F. Cockburn. Ovarian venous blood PO_2, PCO_2 and pH in women. J. Reprod. Fertil. 33:11, 1973.

14. Gwatkin, R. B. L., and A. A. Haidri. Oxygen requirements for the maturation of hamster oocytes. J. Reprod. Fertil. 37:127, 1974.

15. McNatty, K. P., R. S. Sawers, and A. S. McNeilly. A possible role for prolactin in control of steroid secretion by the human Graafian follicle. Nature 250:653, 1974.

16. Rondell, P. Role of steroid synthesis in the process of ovulation. Biol. Reprod. 10:199, 1974.

17. Tsafriri, A., H. R. Lindner, U. Zor, and S. A. Lamprecht. Physiological role of prostaglandins in the induction of ovulation. Prostaglandins 2:1, 1972.

18. Corner, G. W., Jr. The histological dating of the human corpus luteum of menstruation. Am. J. Anat. 98:377, 1956.

19. Block, E. Quantitative morphological investigation of the follicular system in women. Acta Endocrinol. (Kbh.) 8:33, 1951.

20. McNeilly, A. S. Personal communication, 1974.

21. Henzl, M. R. Luteolysis in humans and subhuman primates. Research in Prostaglandins 1:1, 1972.

22. Goding, J. R., I. A. Cumming, W. A. Charnley, J. M. Brown, M. D. Cain, J. C. Cerini, M. E. D. Cerini, J. K. Findlay, J. D. O'Shea, and D. H. Pemberton. Prostaglandin $F_{2\alpha}$: "the" luteolysin in the mammal? Hormones and antagonists. Gynecol. Invest. 2:73, 1972.

23. Hansel, W., P. W. Concarron, and J. H. Lukaszewska. Corpora lutea of the large domestic animals. Biol. Reprod. 8:222, 1973.

24. Auletta, F. J., L. Speroff, and B. V. Caldwell. $PGF_{2\alpha}$ induced steroidogenesis and luteolysis in the primate corpus luteum. J. Clin. Endocrinol. Metab. 36:405, 1973.

25. Powell, W. S., S. Hammarström, B. Samuelsson, and B. Sjöberg. Prostaglandin $F_{2\alpha}$ receptor in human corpora lutea. Lancet 1:1120, 1974.

26. Hoffman, F. Untersuchungen über die hormonale Beeinflussing der lebensdauer des corpus luteum im zyklus der frau. Geburtsch. Frauenheilk 20:1153, 1960.

27. Rivera, A., and A. I. Sherman. Prolongation of the survival time of the corpus luteum. Am. J. Obstet. Gynecol. 103:986, 1969.

28. Short, R. V. Implantation and the maternal recognition of pregnancy. In *Foetal Anatomy*, Ciba Foundation Symposium, eds. G. E. W. Wolstenholme and M. O'Connor. London: J.&A. Churchill, 1969.

29. Peters, H., A. G. Byskov, and R. Himelstein-Brau. The control of ovarian structure. Follicle growth: The basic event in the ovary. Proceedings of a Symposium on the Functional Morphology of the Ovary, Glasgow, September 1974. J. Reprod. Fertil. (in press).

30. Schally, A. V., A. J. Kastin, and A. Arimura. The hypothalamus and reproduction. Am. J. Obstet. Gynecol. 114: 423, 1972.

31. Greenblat, R. B., A. Zarate, and V. B. Mahesh. Stimulation of gonadal function by clomiphene citrate. In *Clinical endocrinology II*, eds. E. B. Astwood and C. E. Cassidy. New York: Grune & Stratton, 1968.

32. Klopper, A. Developments in steroidal hormonal contraception. Br. Med. Bull. 26:39, 1970.

33. Franchimont, P. The regulation of follicle stimulating hormone and luteinizing hormone secretion in humans. In *Frontiers in Neuroendocrinology*, eds. L. Martini and W. F. Ganong. New York: Oxford University Press, 1971.

34. Shearman, R. P. Recent advances in contraceptive technology. Med. Gynaecol. Androl. Sociol. 6:11, 1972.

35. Hearn, J. P., R. V. Short, and S. F. Lunn. The effects of immunizing marmoset monkeys against the β subunit of HCG. In *Physiological effects of immunity against reproductive hormones*, eds. R. G. Edwards and M. H. Johnson. London: Cambridge University Press, 1976.

36. Debeljuk, L., A. Arimura, and A. V. Schally. Stimulation of release of FSH and LH by infusion of LH-RH and some of its analogues. Neuroendocrinology 11:130, 1973.

37. Pickles, V. R. A plain-muscle stimulant in the menstruum. Nature 180:1198, 1957.

38. Downie, J., N. L. Poyser, and M. Wunderlich. Levels of prostaglandins in human endometrium during the normal menstrual cycle. J. Physiol. 236:465, 1974.

39. Jewelewicz, R., I. Dyrenfurth, M. Warren, U. Joshi, and R. L. Vande Wiele. Factors involved in the maintenance and regression of the corpus luteum of women. In *Le Corps Jaune*, eds. R. Denamur and A. Netter. Paris: Masson et Cie, 1973.

40. Klaiber, E. L., M. R. Henzl, C. W. Lloyd, and E. J. Segre. Corpus luteum inhibiting action of oxymethalone. J. Clin. Endocrinol. Metab. 36:142, 1973.

41. Johansson, E. D. B., and C. Gemzell. Plasma levels of progesterone during the luteal phase in normal women treated with synthetic oestrogens (RS 28 74, F6103 and ethinyl oestradiol). Acta Endocrinol. 68:551, 1971.

42. Johansson, E. D. B. Depression of progesterone levels in women treated with synthetic gestogens after ovulation. Acta Endocrinol. 68:779, 1971.

43. Southern, E. M., ed. *The Prostaglandins: Clinical Application in Human Reproduction*. Papers and edited discussion from Brook Lodge Symposium, Augusta, Michigan. Mount Kisco, N.Y.: Futura Publishing Co., 1972.

44. Binder, D., J. Bowler, E. D. Brown, N. S. Crossley, J. Hutton, M. Senior, L. Slater, P. Wilkinson, and N. C. A. Wright. 16-Aryloxyprostaglandins: A new class of potent lutolytic agent. Prostaglandins 6:87, 1974.

7 Induction of Ovulation — Carl Gemzell

7.1 Introduction

Ovulation involves at least three major processes: the ripening of a follicle, the rupture of the follicle with discharge of an oocyte, and the transformation of the ruptured follicle into a corpus luteum. Ovulation is under the control of two gonadotropic hormones from the anterior pituitary—follicle-stimulating hormone (FSH) and luteinizing hormone (LH). The first stage of the development of the Graafian follicle includes oogenesis, organization of the granulosa and theca interna, and growth to the formation of the follicular antrum. Under the influence of its own estrogen, the follicle starts to respond to the pituitary gonadotropins. The follicle then increases rapidly in size with marked hypertrophy of the theca interna and the granulosa. During the preovulatory phase a rapid secretion of follicular fluid and hyperemia of the follicle takes place, and, following a sudden increase in the secretion of LH, the follicle ruptures. LH is also responsible for the maintenance of the corpus luteum.

7.2 Physiology of Ovulation

During the process of ovulation an oocyte is released from the ovary and becomes available for conception to occur. The normal human ovary contains about 500,000 oocytes at birth. During a woman's reproductive life less than one per thousand of these are released by the process of ovulation; the others degenerate and become atretic. Once the ovarian cycle has been established at the time of menarche, it goes on uninterrupted until the menopause, when no more oocytes are present in the ovary. Ovulation is interrupted by pregnancy and subsequent lactation. Following termination of pregnancy, the cyclic release of oocytes is resumed, after variable intervals. In women who for various reasons do not ovulate, the degeneration of eggs occurs at an unaltered rate. The administration of oral contraceptives that inhibit ovulation does not seem to influence the rate at which the eggs degenerate.

The number of follicles developing to maturity during each cycle and the rate at which follicles mature seem to be constant for each species. By the administration of exogenous FSH the number of maturing follicles can be increased, but the rate at which they mature is unaltered. Thus in order to deliver a certain number of eggs in a given species, the amount of FSH released from the anterior pituitary must be rather constant.

In the human female, during the early part of each menstrual cycle, a group of follicles start to grow. When they have reached a certain size, only one goes further to full maturation and rupture; the others become atretic. The mechanism behind this selection of a single follicle is not well understood. It may be that the amount of FSH released from the pituitary is only enough to evoke estrogen production in the most receptive follicle. This endocrine response of the follicle may then depress the release of FSH below the reactive threshold of other follicles. An alternative hypothesis is that appreciable amounts of estrogen produced by the dominant follicle may desensitize the other follicles to FSH. Under certain conditions this inborn mechanism of the ovary may be missing. Exogenous FSH administered in excess to a woman with normal ovaries seldom causes superovulation, while superovulation with small amounts of FSH is a common finding in women even with the polycystic ovary syndrome. This discrepancy in sensitivity to exogenous FSH is not well understood and should be further investigated.

7.3 Hormonal Control of Ovulation

The hormonal control of ovulation depends on a complex relationship between the hypothalamus, the pituitary, and the ovary. The gonadotropin-releasing hormones (GnRH) stimulate the synthesis and secretion of FSH and LH that results in ovarian follicular growth and maturation. At about midcycle, under the added influence of a surge of LH, the favored FSH-primed follicle ruptures with discharge of an ovum. The ruptured follicle is then transformed into a corpus luteum in which progesterone and small amounts of estrogen are synthesized. The output of these steroids then inhibits the hypothalamus and the pituitary, with a subsequent lessening of ovarian stimulation. In the absence of ovarian hormones, menstruation follows, the pituitary begins to function again, and the cycle repeats itself.

7.4 Pathophysiology of Ovulation

Failure to ovulate is a major problem in reproductive disorders. It may be the result of dysfunction at any level of a complex system, including higher centers in the brain, the hypothalamic-pituitary-ovarian axis, and the steroid feedback mechanism. It renders the woman infertile, which is the prime reason for attempts at restoration of ovulatory cycles.

Anovulation is the basic deficit in the polycystic ovary syndrome—sometimes called the Stein-Leventhal syndrome—and is followed by amenorrhea, sometimes oligomenorrhea, and even apparently regular cycles. Generally, anovulatory menstruation is associated with recognizable irregularity of the cycle and occurs most frequently in the menarche and in the premenopausal state. In most instances women with regular cycles have sporadic anovulation. In primary or secondary ovarian failure, ovulation has never occurred or has ceased definitely.

Anovulation with amenorrhea may be the first and only sign of a pituitary tumor such as a chromophobe adenoma. Pituitary destruction, due to infarct necrosis at the time of delivery, causes anovulation and amenorrhea but also other signs of grave pituitary insufficiency.

In most cases of anovulation with or without amenorrhea there are no gross organic lesions of the pituitary or the hypothalamus. Ovulation may cease in connection with the discontinuation of oral contraceptive treatment, severe dieting, or emotional disturbances, but also without any obvious signs of hypothalamic dysfunction.

A prerequisite for the induction of ovulation in women who do not ovulate is the presence of normal ovaries with oocytes and follicles. The lack of oocytes, as in women with primary ovarian failure or with premature menopause, renders treatment impossible.

7.5 Treatment of Anovulation

In principle, there are two approaches to ovarian stimulation for induction of ovulation—a hormonal approach with human gonadotropins and a chemical approach with clomiphene citrate. Human gonadotropins act directly on the ovaries, bypassing the pituitary and the hypothalamus, while clomiphene requires for its action an intact pituitary and hypothalamus.

GnRH has been isolated from the hypothalamus and has also been synthesized. It reaches the anterior pituitary via a portal system and releases both FSH and LH. Consequently, it would be an ideal means of stimulating the ovaries in cases of normal pituitary and abnormal hypothalamic function. In women who do not ovulate, GnRH has been shown to increase the release of both FSH and LH from the pituitary, but not sufficiently to stimulate follicular growth or to induce ovulation of mature follicles, even those primed with human gonadotropins. The reason for this is not clear. It may be that the pituitary of an amenorrheic woman is not adequately adapted to GnRH and, following exogenous administration of GnRH, releases an insufficient amount of gonadotropins during too short a time.

Human gonadotropins seem to be the panacea for induction of ovulation, as this method only requires normal ovaries. It is possible with human gonadotropins to induce ovulation in women who have a pituitary tumor or necrosis or have had hypophysectomy. But this method risks the possibility of complications such as overstimulation leading to cyst formation or multiple pregnancies, so human gonadotropins should not be used as the first means of induction of ovulation. Clomiphene citrate is relatively safe to use, and when it is administered in daily doses of 50 to 200 mg for five days, it does not give rise to any serious side effects or complications.

7.6 Gonadotropin Preparations

Extracts from animal pituitaries or pregnant mare serum containing follicle-stimulating activity, in combination with human chorionic gonadotropin (hCG), have received extensive clinical trial in women with menstrual disorders and infertility. Pregnant mare serum gonadotropin (PMS), followed by hCG, increased follicular size, luteinization, and urinary excretion of estrogens. A menstrual period usually appeared two weeks later. In terms of induced ovulation, the results showed a lack of consistency, probably due to the effect of antibodies to FSH from the animal sources.

The gonadotropic hormones are relatively species-specific and are often capable of inducing the formation of antibodies in other species. This is one reason why PMS has failed to become recognized as an effective agent for induction of ovulation in humans. A second treatment often had no effect, and repeated treatments provoked allergic reactions and anaphylactic shock. Gonadotropins from human sources have little tendency to induce the formation of antibodies in the human and are obviously preferable.

It is now well established that in order to induce ovulation in the human, gonadotropins from human sources should be used. They are from two sources: human pituitaries (hPG) obtained at autopsy or the urine of postmenopausal women (hMG). Extracts of different potency and ratio between FSH and LH have been used, and almost all preparations give good results. A widely used preparation of hPG contains 25–30 IU (2nd International Reference Preparation of hMG) of FSH activity and 20–30 IU of LH (2nd IRP-hMG) per mg, with a ratio between FSH and LH of 1:1.

Further purification of this hPG preparation yielded preparations that were clinically less potent, while rather impure preparations with ratio of FSH to LH of 1:6 gave rather good results. Consequently, nothing indicated that hPG preparations with low LH content were superior to those with high LH contamination and that further purification of the pituitary extract gave better clinical results. Some preliminary results seem to indicate, however, that in women with the polycystic ovary syndrome who are very sensitive to hPG, preparations with low LH content are preferable to those with high LH contamination.

Extract from postmenopausal urine (hMG) has been used together with hCG to stimulate the ovaries and induce ovulation and corpus luteum formation. Two commercial preparations are in common use today. They contain about 75 IU of FSH activity per ampule, with a ratio of FSH to LH of 1:1 (Pergonal) or 1:2 (Humegon).

LH from the human pituitary has never been needed for induction of ovulation, thanks to the luteinizing effect of hCG, which is readily extracted from pregnancy urine. Human pituitary LH does not prevent overstimulation. If it is used instead of hCG, repeated doses must be administered, as its biological half-life is shorter than that of hCG.

Several commercial preparations of hCG are available, and these have the same general effect on the primed follicle as natural hCG.

Although pituitary and urinary FSH are chemically different, they seem to have the same clinical effect when preparations with equal FSH activity are used. The two preparations administered to the same women gave similar responses in terms of ovulations, pregnancies, and the rise in total urinary estrogen excretion.

7.7 Clomiphene Citrate

Clomiphene citrate exists as two isomers that have been separated as *cis* and *trans* clomiphene. Although preliminary data suggest that *cis* clomiphene is more potent than *trans* clomiphene in terms of ovulation induction, the two isomers are mixed in the commercial preparation. The mechanism of action of clomiphene is not clear, but it appears to reduce estradiol uptake by the pituitary and anterior hypothalamus. The major stimulus for the ovarian response to clomiphene is probably mediated via the hypothalamus and the pituitary and acts on the release of gonadotropins. Clomiphene also appears to have a direct effect on the ovaries; administered together with hPG, it increases the sensitivity of the ovaries to hPG. Overstimulation is rarely seen with excessive doses of clomiphene.

7.8 Selection of Patients for Induction of Ovulation

In a fertile woman, normal menstruation depends on two basic factors: a patent müllerian duct system with endometrium capable of responding to hormonal stimuli, and normal function of the ovaries with cyclic production of estrogen and progesterone.

Primary amenorrhea may be the result of absence, hypoplasia, or maldevelopment of the müllerian duct system. It may be attributable to a complete lack of oocytes and follicles, as in primary ovarian failure. Alternatively, primary amenorrhea may be caused by pituitary insufficiency and may constitute an important symptom in the clinical entity of hypogonadotropic ovarian failure, complete or partial hypopituitarism or pituitary-hypothalamic dysfunction.

Once a patient has had a spell of cyclic menstrual bleedings, female gonads and an intact müllerian duct system can be taken for granted. Secondary amenorrhea or oligomenorrhea can, therefore, be attributable to lack of oocytes and follicles, as in premature menopause, to a deficient stimulation by gonadotropic hormones, or to a deranged synthesis of steroid hormones within the ovaries.

Pituitary gonadotropic failure can occur with an apparently normal pituitary, with a pituitary that is the site of a tumor or necrosis, or with a primary abnormality in the hypothalamic region. A characteristic finding in these patients is a low level of FSH and LH in serum, although normal levels may not exclude a pituitary insufficiency. Also common in these patients is a low serum level of estrogens or the excretion of total estrogens in urine, indicating inactive ovaries. These patients, without any other symptoms of endocrine disorders or congenital malformations, are suitable for treatment with human gonadotropins.

The ideal patient for treatment with human gonadotropins is under 35 and has nonfunctioning ovaries, primary or long-lasting secondary amenorrhea, normally developed sex organs, and lack of urinary gonadotropins as evidence of pituitary failure. She should be fully investigated, be complaining of infertility, have a normally fertile husband, and show no barriers to conception. Pregnancy should not be contraindicated on medical grounds, and there should be no preferable alternative method.

Clomiphene citrate has proved to be an especially useful drug in patients who do not ovulate because of a hypothalamic dysfunction. The estrogen excretion must be adequate, and the serum-FSH level must be within the normal range. There should be no signs or symptoms of any gross pituitary or hypothalamic changes. The only contraindication to treatment is the presence of ovarian cysts or tumors. Clomiphene should also be used in women who ovulate only two or three times yearly or in women who show persistent anovulatory cycles. Some women have secondary amenorrhea or oligomenorrhea that is attributable to a deficient stimulation by gonadotropic hormones from the pituitary or to deranged synthesis of steroid hormones within the ovaries; these women often exhibit an estrogen production in the normal range. In such cases clomiphene is recommended. Women with amenorrhea following the use of oral contraceptives and women with galactorrhea and amenorrhea belong to this group even if their endogenous estrogen production is low.

7.9 Monitoring Therapy for Induction of Ovulation

The purpose of monitoring gonadotropic therapy is to obtain an ovarian response that compares as closely as possible with ovarian changes taking place during a normal spontaneous ovulation and to avoid overstimulation leading to multiple pregnancies or ovarian cyst formation.

The ovarian changes that take place during a normal ovulatory cycle can be recorded by daily determinations of estrogens and progesterone in blood or urine. The estrogens during the follicular phase reflect the maturation of the follicle; progesterone during the luteal phase reflects the activity of the corpus luteum. By comparing changes in levels of estrogens and progesterone of normal ovulatory cycles with those that follow stimulation with human gonadotropins, information can be obtained about the optimal daily dose of human gonadotropin, the number of days this dose should be administered, when hCG or LH administration should be commenced, if and when ovulation took place, and the hormonal activity of the corpus luteum.

Daily determination of total urinary estrogens (TE) has been used successfully to obtain information about the optimal daily dose of hPG and the number of days this dose should be administered. Increases in plasma progesterone will then confirm the occurrence of ovulation and the activity of the subsequent corpus luteum.

Following an adequate hPG dose is usually a latent period of four to five days without any change in TE. Thereafter TE rises continuously during another period of four to five days, with daily increases of about 50 percent over the previous day. When a suitable level of TE is reached, ovulation is induced by the adminis-

tration of hCG. If the rise in plasma progesterone follows the same course of increase as the one found after a spontaneous ovulation, the risk of overstimulation is limited. If, on the other hand, the rise in plasma progesterone is slow, and menstrual bleeding occurs less than 10 days after the hCG administration, ovulation may be questioned. By nine days after ovulation, the detection of hCG in serum by a radioimmunoassay will confirm conception.

Gross appearance, sialic acid concentration, the arborization pattern and the *spinnbarkeit* of the cervical mucus, and the ability of sperm to penetrate the cervical mucus are other criteria that can be used to assess ovarian response to hPG; however, they are less reliable and sometimes more difficult to evaluate than the TE excretion. Some women display a close correlation between ovarian response and the karyopyknotic index, whereas others, mainly due to vaginitis and coitus, fail to do so.

Clomiphene therapy is much safer than therapy with human gonadotropins and need not be controlled as strictly. Pelvic examination should be performed before and after each course of treatment in order to exclude those who have enlarged ovaries. If enlarged ovaries are detected, the spacing of subsequent treatment should be reconsidered. In order to obtain information about when and if ovulation takes place, the women should record their basal body temperature. Repeated determinations of plasma progesterone can eventually reveal an insufficient corpus luteum.

7.10 Methods of Treatment with Human Gonadotropins (hPG)

One of the difficulties in the treatment with human gonadotropins is individual variations in response. There is no fixed dosage schedule for all patients. Even the response of the same patient to the same dose may differ significantly from one cycle to the next. One woman, having aborted seven fetuses after her first treatment, had a single pregnancy after her second treatment without any change of dosage. Moreover, a very small range exists between a dose that completely fails to stimulate follicle ripening and one that produces overstimulation.

It has been suggested that in a normal spontaneous ovulation a certain amount of endogenous FSH and LH is released from the pituitary, and that in the same woman this amount is rather constant from one cycle to another. The same is true for most anovulatory women who are treated with hPG or hMG, but there are a few exceptions. Some anovulatory women treated over periods of several years require more FSH with time in order to respond, while other women require different amounts of FSH from course to course.

The latter usually show some ovarian activity, so the difference in requirement of hPG is probably due to the endogenous hormones, which may act against or together with the exogenous ones, or to the status of the ovaries at the beginning of the treatment.

The aim of an hPG treatment of an individual woman is to find the hPG dose that produces a change in TE and plasma progesterone that approaches as closely as possible the changes found during the normal ovulatory cycle. If this goal is achieved, chances are good for a normal single conception, and the risk of overstimulation is negligible.

The administration of hPG or hMG can be handled in many different ways, all of which give more or less good results. Divided doses or equal daily doses of human gonadotropins usually give the same rise in urinary estrogens and the same number of conceptions, but the divided doses seem to be more difficult to control and in general require larger amounts of the hormones than the equal doses require. Ovulation is induced by a rather large dose of hCG, which has to be repeated after some days in order to obtain normal length of the luteal phase. The plasma levels of progesterone should be determined at least three times in order to confirm ovulation and to control the activity of the corpus luteum.

7.11 Methods of Treatment with Clomiphene

After full investigation, including assays of FSH and estrogens in serum or urine, doses of 50 mg clomiphene are given for five days, starting on the fifth day of the cycle or, if there is no cycle, on the fifth day after a bleeding induced by progesterone. If after four weeks menstruation has not occurred and the patient is not pregnant, the dose of clomiphene is increased to 100 or 200 mg. If there is no response to the 200 mg dose, treatment is stopped, and eventually human gonadotropins are substituted. If, however, ovulation is induced following any of these courses, clomiphene is continued at the dose level that gave a response for three to four courses of treatment or until conception occurs.

7.12 Results of Treatment

Human gonadotropins (hPG) have been used since 1959 to induce ovulation in infertile women. Since 1968 daily estrogen determinations have been done to monitor the treatment. During an eight-year period (1960–1967) when 290 patients were treated, the pregnancy rate was 45 percent, the multiple-births rate was 33 percent, and the abortion rate was 28 percent. Clinical symptoms of overstimulation leading to hospital care occurred in less than 2 percent of the induced cycles. During a second five-year period (1969–1973) when daily estrogen determinations were done, 351 patients were treated. The pregnancy rate was 41 percent, the multiple-births rate 17 percent, and the abortion rate 19 percent. Only 0.5 percent of the treatments ended with symptoms of overstimulation. Careful monitoring of treatment with daily estrogen determinations clearly lowered the multiple-births rate and probably had some effect on the abortion rate. Most of the multiple pregnancies were twins, and the cases of overstimulation were mild and did not require hospital care.

The second group included women with secondary amenorrhea and quiescent ovaries, women with secondary amenorrhea and active ovaries who were clomiphene failures, and seven women who were hypophysectomized due to a pituitary adenoma. All these women were suitable for hPG therapy, and there was no alternative. Interestingly, 84 percent of the pregnancies occurred following the first two courses of treatment, and an additional 7 percent following the third course. It follows from these results that after three treatments with hPG the chance of conception is rather small and an alternative should be considered. It also shows that the selection of patients is of great importance. The low pregnancy rate might be partially explained by the fact that some women had subfertile husbands with rather poor sperm counts, and that 22 percent of the women were treated only once.

A third group of 15 women with primary amenorrhea were treated during a ten-year period. They were all highly motivated to the treatment, and no alternative method was available. All were primed with cyclic estrogen therapy before treatment with hPG. In view of the infantile form of the genital tract of these patients, it was surprising to find a high rate of conception (87 percent), together with a low rate of abortions (10 percent).

In women with the Stein-Leventhal syndrome, the treatment with hPG gave rather poor results. Many of these patients were "clomiphene failures," and only about 30 percent conceived, usually following the first or second treatment with hPG.

In cases with the Stein-Leventhal syndrome, the treatment with hPG did not give good results. Many of these patients were "clomiphene failures," and only about 10 percent conceived, usually following the first or second treatment with hPG.

During the last five-year period, women with secondary amenorrhea with normal basic estrogen levels, women with oligomenorrhea, and women with anovulatory cycles were treated with clomiphene. The daily dose varied between 50 and 200 mg administered for five days. Ovulation occurred in about 80 percent of the women, but the pregnancy rate was only about 30 percent. In a few cases ovarian enlargement was found following the treatment but disappeared after treatment with synthetic gestagens for three to four weeks.

7.13 Summary

Induction of ovulation with human gonadotropins is not only a valuable means of treatment of infertile women but also a method to elucidate the normal and pathological function of the ovary.

Many gaps persist in our knowledge about the function of the human ovary and its response to gonadotropins. For example, what initiates the first step of development of the primordial follicle, and when does it become dependent on gonadotropic stimulation? Once the ovary is mature and its cyclic pattern is initiated, numerous selected primary follicles are stimulated and enter the growth phase. How are they selected and how are those in storage kept from degenerating? Little is known about this process of degeneration of ovarian follicles. What initiates the process and when does it begin? Other problems awaiting solutions involve the mechanism behind the selection of a single follicle for maturity and rupture during the menstrual cycle and the great differences among ovaries in sensitivity to gonadotropins.

The clinical aspects of ovarian function are relatively simple. A hypophysectomized woman shows no ovarian activity. Following administration of exogenous FSH and LH, the follicles increase in size and number and start to produce estrogens. The mature follicle can then be brought to ovulation by the addition of LH or hCG. Other women with quiescent ovaries respond in a similar way, while anovulatory women with active ovaries are more difficult to treat and respond to gonadotropins in many different ways. This is difficult to understand and will require further study, as will the reason why they respond better to clomiphene.

Abnormal ovarian function, as in the Stein-Leventhal syndrome, can be elucidated by the administration of exogenous gonadotropins, which result in an exaggeration of the abnormal steroid pattern. If the condition is reversible, it may be due to defective gonadotropic stimulation; if it is not reversible, it is probably due to an inherent property of the ovary. Gonadotropins and clomiphene in many cases bring about ovulation, while conception only occasionally takes place. This, too, is an important field for further research.

8 Feedback Regulation of Reproductive Cycles in Rats, Sheep, Monkeys, and Humans, with Particular Attention to Computer Modeling

Neena B. Schwartz,
Donald J. Dierschke,
Charles E. McCormack,
and Paul W. Waltz

8.1 General Introduction to the Concept of Feedback in Endocrinology and Reproductive Biology

Early in the history of physiology it became necessary to postulate that signals were returned to a central place in the body to modulate or regulate physiological responses. This necessity was clearly seen by the Sherringtonian school in studying postural reflexes and by Starling and others in studying cardiovascular reflexes. Only after engineering and systems analysts adopted the term *feedback* did this word come into use in physiology, but the concept was clearly evident before the word.

In the early 1930s, Moore and Price did a series of experiments that revealed the necessity of postulating negative feedback (or *reciprocal inhibition*, as it was then called) in the control of the ovaries. The pioneering work of P. E. Smith in hypophysectomy revealed that gonadal histology, size, and secretion of estrogenic substances regressed after removal of the pituitary gland. Moore and Price then showed that ovarian regression, with sex accessory weight stimulation, occurred in intact rats when estrogens were injected. These experiments were the cornerstone of the negative feedback theory in gonadal control. New experimental evidence in four species completely validates, by a direct methodology, the early findings.

Not only has it been established that negative feedback is the basic mode of control of levels of ovarian steroid hormones in the blood, but other evidence in intervening years has established a similar control of testicular steroid, thyroid hormones, and adrenal cortical steroids. Furthermore, glands such as the pancreas and parathyroids have been shown to be under control of blood levels of nonhormonal substances such as glucose or calcium ion, which serve as feedback signals for the control of insulin and parathormone, respectively.

In the female mammal, it has become necessary to postulate a second type of control of pituitary hormonal secretion rates by gonadal steroids. In every species studied, estrogen appears to cause a short-lived, high-level release of pituitary hormones (especially LH), which then cause ovulation. This has been termed positive or facilitative feedback. This feedback of estrogen appears to be a necessary function to induce ovulation and to maintain cycles in mammals that show spontaneous (non-coitus-induced) reproductive cycles.

Modern endocrinology in general, and reproductive biology in particular, include two levels of intensive study: at the cellular or subcellular level, research concentrates on hormone-receptor interaction; at the whole organism level, research is focused on the control of glandular secretion rates and of gametogenesis. We deal here with the whole organism level.

8.2 Two Methodological Approaches to Steroid Feedback Research: Comparative and Systems Analysis

This section is a general discussion of two methodologies useful in studying steroid feedback mechanisms in reproduction. These general methods are equally appropriate to the study of other areas in reproductive biology.

Comparative Studies

A great deal has been learned in reproductive biology by the use of comparative studies in different species. Some experiments, such as ovariectomy, cannot be carried out on humans without reason, although natural experiments occur, such as Turner's syndrome, where only a gonadal streak is present that does not secrete steroids. By the use of other animals, however, experimental maneuvers such as surgery or injections can be done under carefully controlled circumstances.

When one carries out experiments on animal models with the ultimate view of transferring the information back to humans, how close must the animal model be to humans for it to be satisfactory? Work on only subhuman primates and not on other species turns out to be insufficient for the transfer of observations. For example, in comparative data relevant to steroid feedback mechanisms in four species—humans, monkeys (mainly rhesus), sheep, and rats—*where significant differences existed*, the sheep or rat sometimes turned out to be more satisfactory than the monkey in predictive value for the human. For most data, however, when experiments are done in all four species, it is found that all four respond in a *similar* fashion.

If this is the case, then one must take into account the cost-effectiveness of research in animal models such as sheep or rats, which are considerably cheaper to maintain and purchase than are monkeys. This is particularly true of the rat, which can be housed under virtually any laboratory conditions. Workers using other species may frequently be able to take advantage of preliminary work in the rat in planning their experiments. For example, the recent work from Knobil's and Spies's laboratories on the hypothalamic support of pituitary function in monkeys benefited from previous work on the localization of neural areas that had been carried out in the rat; even if the data prove different from that on the rat, the advantage of knowing where to begin to look is considerable. Furthermore, some of the work in monkeys and sheep was partially based, conceptually, on the rat model; the advantage of the large animal was frequently the number of serial samplings of blood that became possible, rather than any closeness to the human or new experimental design.

The comparative approach is also of intrinsic interest because it elucidates the wide variety of mechanisms used by different species for the same end—reproduction. For example, in the nonmated rat, only a brief luteal phase exists, in contrast to the other three species. A luteal phase, very similar to that seen in primates and sheep, can be induced by sterile mating (pseudopregnancy). The mechanism of maintaining the corpus luteum of the cycle in the rat by prolactin has induced a search in the other three species for a role of prolactin in luteal maintenance. Searches of this kind produce good basic research, even if the mechanisms turn out to be not the same.

Research in the sheep, however, is relevant to human needs other than studies of the processes of reproduction. Breeding sheep for food or wool is impossible throughout the year, because sheep's breeding processes are tied to seasonal factors. A study of the sheep's reproductive biology may well yield the answer to overcoming its strong seasonal ties and thus extending its capabilities as a food source.

Furthermore, the study of reproductive biology of rats—and even of insects—has led to the development of natural means of controlling these predators or pests on the human food supply. For insects, attractant or repellent pheromones may be useful for controlling population distribution. For rodents, vasectomy of males could possibly reduce the population of a given group of wild rats by causing pseudopregnancy in the females.

The Systems Analysis Approach
Systems analysis provides a methodology for dealing with communication and the transmission of information. The system involving the ovaries and the central nervous system–pituitary axis is certainly a system exquisitely adapted for such information transmission, for steroid feedback information as well as for inputs from the environment.

Endocrinologists have always been modelers in the sense that they frequently summarize data and almost always teach by means of diagrams with arrows connecting organs. This informal kind of systems analysis is useful for many purposes, but it is not as powerful as formal modeling. The virtue of the latter approach is the explicit nature of the process, which forces the endocrinologist to choose what he or she regards as the most important parts of the system, forces a choice of hypothesis concerning the causative sequences involved, and then provides a methodology (computer simulation) for testing the choices. In its most sophisticated form, systems analysis and computer simulation can predict data not yet obtained by the investigator; however, no model of the rat or human is as yet mature enough to provide useful predictions.

But this immaturity of modeling in reproductive biology is no reason to stop modeling. The modeling that has already been done, in both rats and humans, has revealed large lacunae in data gathering that need to be filled. This in itself provides a rational approach for the design of new experiments, just as the lacunae revealed by the comparative approach show where experimentation might profitably be carried out in different species.

8.3 The Comparative Approach: Empirical Observations in Rat, Sheep, Subhuman Primate, and Human

This section provides a data base of experimental observations relevant to steroid feedback in four species. The format of the data base is sectional, taking up each topic in turn and contrasting all four species (where information is available) in text and tables. (Tables 8.1 to 8.10 are grouped together at the end of the section.) Blank spots in the tables, indicating no data on a given point in a given species, also represent deficits in the data base that may be seen as potential future experiments.

Six points in the data base show pronounced species differences in important areas: (1) In all four species a pulsatile discharge of LH occurs after ovariectomy, but only in sheep and women has this also been observed in intact individuals. (2) A properly timed injection of progesterone elicits an LH surge in humans and rats, but has not been demonstrated to do so in monkeys and sheep. (3) Seasonal rhythmicities have been demonstrated in ovarian function in sheep and monkeys, but not in humans and laboratory rats. (4) Pentobarbitol can lower the high LH secretion in ovariectomized sheep and rats, but not in monkeys; the experiment has not been done in humans. (5) Castrated male sheep and rats do not demonstrate LH surges after injection of estrogen or progesterone or both; castrated men and monkeys do. (6) The facilitatory response of LH to estrogen during "prepubertal feedback dormancy" can be elicited in sheep and rats, but not in humans or monkeys. Only in the last two observations is the rhesus monkey a better model for human responses than the sheep or rat.

Negative Feedback (See Table 8.1)

The concept of negative feedback is based on the existence of a closed loop relationship between the hypothalamo-hypophyseal complex and the gonad. Thus the gonadotropic hormones (LH and FSH) secreted into the bloodstream by the adenohypophysis have a stimulatory effect upon the gonads (ovaries), resulting in an increased secretion of gonadal steroids (especially estrogens and progesterone). The elevated levels of circulating steroids then "feed back" to the hypothalamo-hypophyseal unit, causing a reduction in gonadotropin secretion by the adenohypophysis. This general relationship has been upheld in all four species—that is, surgical removal of the ovaries or ovarian inactivity (such as in the menopause) results in a hypersecretion of LH and FSH, and the administration of estrogens in small quantities leads to a reduction in the peripheral levels of gonadotropin. Progesterone given alone in physiological quantities is usually not effective in this regard; however, a few reports suggest that progesterone can facilitate the negative feedback effects of small (marginally effective alone) amounts of estrogen in certain experimental situations. Androgenic steroids are surprisingly effective in the negative feedback sense—both testosterone and dihydrotestosterone inhibit LH secretion in the ovariectomized rat, and testosterone (but not dihydrotestosterone) has effects similar to estrogen in the ovariectomized monkey. It has been suggested, but not proved, that such effects may be due to conversion of testosterone to estrogen (T. Yamaji, unpublished observations).

An interesting recent observation in agonadal individ-uals of all four species is that gonadotropic hypersecretion is not stable but pulsatile, with a burst of secretion occurring approximately once an hour. The pulses are abolished by the administration of estrogen, but their regulation and timing in the absence of gonadal steroids is unknown. Similar patterns of pulsatile secretion have been described for intact women and sheep, but not for intact monkeys or rats.

Internal Feedback (See Table 8.2)

Implantation of gonadotropins into the hypothalamus of rats caused a decrease in the rate of gonadotropin secretion by the pituitary. This observation has led to hypotheses that when plasma gonadotropins perfuse the hypothalamus, the secretion of gonadotropin-releasing hormones is suppressed. As might be predicted from this hypothesis, LRF activity was detectable in the plasma of hypophysectomized rats but not in intact rats. Does this internal type of negative feedback play an important physiological role in regulating gonadotropin secretion? Conceivably, in hypogonadal states (such as gonadectomy, gonadal agenesis, menopause), wherein negative feedback from gonadal steroids is deficient or absent, the high rate of gonadotropin secretion might be even more elevated, were it not for internal feedback. Even this "normal" role for internal feedback lacks the support of experimental evidence. For example, intravenous infusion of ovariectomized monkeys and sheep with large quantities of various LH preparations failed to suppress the elevated, pulsatile patterns of endogenous LH in both species. Also, in gonadectomized rats, wherein the levels of gonadotropins are already elevated, nephrectomy (by prolonging the half-life of gonadotropins) causes the gonadotropin level to rise still further. This response would be unlikely if the internal feedback system were operating at a significant level.

Positive (Facilitative) Feedback (See Table 8.3)

During the normal menstrual or estrous cycle, ovulation is precipitated by a large increase (surge) in blood levels of gonadotropic hormones. In order to achieve this result, it is important that the gonadotropin surge not occur before the follicle is capable of ovulating. The proper timing is apparently achieved through the increasing levels of blood estrogen, which arise from the maturing follicle and exert a positive feedback effect upon the hypothalamo-hypophyseal unit. Thus, in all four species, an increase in endogenous estrogen is seen prior to the preovulatory gonadotropin surge; moreover, as shown in studies in monkeys and rats, this surge is prevented by the properly timed administration of estrogen antagonists. On the other hand, the administration of estrogen will elicit "extra" surges in cyclic individuals at various times of the menstrual or estrous cycle or in anestrous or agonadal individuals. In the monkey, the estrogen signal involves a strength/duration component, and elevated levels of estrogen must be present at the end, as well as at the beginning, of the stimulus period.

The role of progesterone in mediating positive feedback has been in dispute during the past decade. While it is recognized that this steroid is capable of inducing surges under certain experimental circumstances in women and that progestins (of ovarian or adrenal origin) may modify the timing, shape, and magnitude of gonadotropin surges, no demonstration has been made of an obligatory role of progesterone in triggering normal preovulatory surges. On the other hand, progesterone seems to be exceedingly effective in blocking spontaneous surges induced by estrogen, especially in intact individuals. A discrepancy exists between the effectiveness of progesterone in blocking the positive feedback regulation of gonadotropin secretion and its relative ineffectiveness on its own in negative feedback systems.

In terms of the negative and positive feedback regulation of gonadotropic hormone secretion by steroids, a potentially important gap in current knowledge relates to the possible role of binding proteins such as testosterone-estrogen binding globulin (TEBG) in the feedback relationships. Studies in the human and monkey show, for example, that the plasma concentration of this protein varies among different reproductive states. Also, most steroids assays in routine use at present do not distinguish between steroids that are bound to TEBG or other circulating proteins and those that are not bound. A changing ratio of bound to unbound steroid may be an important determinant of feedback control in certain reproductive situations (Liao 1975).

Environmental Influences (See Table 8.4)

If steroid regulation of gonadotropin secretion is to benefit the animal optimally, it must operate effectively in the animal's normal environment and yet be capable of modification if the environment changes. In small nocturnal animals, in which predation during the day has made mating contact safe only during the night, the likelihood of conception may be improved by closely linking activity patterns to the onset of the preovulatory gonadotropin surge. To do this, the time of the surge and steroid regulation of the surge are precisely set by environmental (light-dark) cues. In day-active mammals, which are usually larger and faster than nocturnally active species, a close linking of activity patterns with gonadotropin secretion may not be essential for survival.

Because considerable progress has been made in understanding the regulatory role of light-dark cycles on the timing of gonadotropin secretion in the female rat, its special case will be considered first and will provide a basis for comparison with other species. In rats exposed to daily photoperiods of eight to sixteen hours, the preovulatory gonadotropin surge begins two to five hours after the midpoint of the photoperiod. Advancing or delaying the onset of the daily photoperiod (length of photoperiod held constant) produces, within one to two weeks, a corresponding shift in the gonadotropin surge. Exposure to continuous light causes the hour of the onset of the surge to be delayed, and eventually gonadotropin surges and ovulation ceases. Exposure to continuous darkness usually does not interfere with cyclic ovulation. The effectiveness of ovarian steroids in facilitating gonadotropin secretion in rats is also modified by the light-dark cycle. For example, administration of estrogen or progesterone can advance ovulation by twenty-four hours, but only if these steroids are given during certain time intervals on days prior to the normal LH surge.

Less information is available concerning the effect of light-dark cycles on the timing of reproductive events in the sheep, monkey, and human, but light-dark cycles appear to be less important in these species than in the rat. For example, quite unlike rats, behavioral estrus in ewes may begin at any time of the day, and in monkeys the time of the onset of the preovulatory gonadotropin surge showed considerable variation (midnight to 9 A.M.). It is not yet known whether the preovulatory gonadotropin surge in women begins at a particular hour of the day; however, numerous other body functions do display definite daily rhythms (for example, wakefulness, body temperature, glucocorticoid secretion, and sodium excretion). It will be surprising if the timing of an event as important as ovulation is not linked with rhythmic fluctuation of other body functions.

Long photoperiods may influence gonadotropin secretion similarly in sheep and rhesus monkeys, as both display a tendency toward failure of ovulation in the summer. These observations do not rule out the possibility that other seasonal changes in the environment may be acting to synchronize these seasonal reproductive rhythms. Seasonal breeding cycles still appeared in sheep exposed the year around to continuous light, thus refuting the generally accepted theory that day length is the primary determinant of sexual cyclicity and leaving the mechanism for this phenomenon in question. Information regarding the effects of photoperiod length on human reproduction is especially sparse, and that which is available is difficult to tie together.

Anesthetics, Sedatives, Surgical Stress, and Gonadotropin Secretion (See Table 8.5)

In the rat several different types of neurally active drugs (barbiturates, anticholinergics, adrenergic blockers, chlorpromazine, reserpine) block the preovulatory LH surge. In addition, pentobarbital administration markedly lowers the high tonic rate of secretion of LH in ovariectomized rats (other drugs have not yet been tested). Thus in rats both the surge type and the tonic type of LH secretion can be suppressed by neurally active drugs. The results of comparable experiments in rhesus monkeys point up the possibility of significant differences in the control mechanisms for gonadotropin secretion. More specifically, in monkeys, chlorpromazine, haloperidal, and alpha adrener-gic blockers will depress the tonic hypersecretion of LH by castrates, but attempts to block the natural preovulatory LH surge (or estrogen-induced LH surges) with these drugs have been unsuccessful. This has led to speculation that a neurally located "clock" is absent in the monkey and that the pituitary initiates the preovulatory surge after a threshold level of estrogen has been maintained in the blood for an adequate time period. But neural blocking agents prevent preovulatory LH secretion in rats only if given during a short interval preceding the preovulatory surge, so it is possible that the precise time interval has not yet been located in monkeys. This view is made more plausible by the observation that ovulation in baboons can be blocked by pentobarbital administered at an appropriate time on the day before expected ovulation. In sheep the general effect of these drugs is to delay, rather than prevent, ovulation.

In female rats, surgical stress late on the day prior to the preovulatory gonadotropin surge often delays the surge; however, surgical stress early on the day of the preovulatory surge may advance the surge. In both cases the presumed mechanism involves a stress-induced release of corticotropin and a subsequent increased output of adrenal progesterone, which, depending on when it is secreted, can inhibit or enhance gonadotropin secretion. In humans and in monkeys, the stress of daily (or more frequent) blood sampling without the use of anesthesia usually does not interfere with cyclic ovulation and menses.

Neonatal Organization by Androgens of Neural Control of Gonadotropin Secretion (See Table 8.6)
In females of all polyestrous species that have been studied, gonadotropin (usually both LH and FSH) secretion peaks dramatically shortly before ovulation. Similar cyclic peaks in gonadotropin secretion have not been reported for males, and except for possible low-magnitude diurnal fluctuations, both FSH and LH are secreted noncyclically. Why is it that cyclic gonadotropin secretion is seen only in females? Early experiments with rats gave rise to the hypothesis that the hypothalamic-pituitary axis is, at birth, capable of cyclic gonadotropin secretion in both males and females, but neonatal exposure of the brain to testicular androgen in males redirects the axis to secrete gonadotropins noncyclically. Recently, it has been shown that treatment with estrogen and progesterone will elicit a surge in gonadotropin secretion (resembling the preovulatory surge) in intact ovariectomized female rats, unless they are treated with androgen neonatally; however, these facilitative (positive feedback) effects of estrogen and progesterone on gonadotropin secretion are not demonstrable in male rats unless they are cas-

trated—and thus, deprived of neonatal androgen—on the first day after birth.

What is the evidence for or against neonatal organization by androgen of gonadotropin secretion in sheep, monkeys, and humans? First, neonatal or even prenatal treatment of female monkeys and sheep with androgen, or neonatal exposure of girls to androgen (adrenogenital syndrome) does not result in sterility in adulthood, and ovarian cycles appear to be normal. In sheep, however, androgenization of the mother during the first half of pregnancy seems to interfere with the later reproductive performance of the female offspring. Second, treatment with estrogen (or estrogen followed by progesterone) does induce gonadotropin surges in castrated men and monkeys, but not in intact individuals. Thus it seems that the hypothalamic-pituitary axis is capable of secreting a surge of gonadotropin in response to ovarian steroids once the inhibitory effect of testicular androgens is removed by adult castration. Gonadotropin surges have not been induced in intact or castrated male sheep by treatment with estrogen and progesterone; thus, in this respect, the sheep resembles the rat.

Collectively, these observations indicate that neonatal or prenatal androgen secretion is relatively more important for organization of subsequent gonadotropin secretion in sheep and rats than it is in monkeys and humans.

Site(s) of Action of Steroid Feedback (See Table 8.7)
Theoretically, steroids could modify the rate of gonadotropin secretion (1) by acting on receptors in the brain (probably hypothalamus), so that the secretion of gonadotropin-releasing factors is modified, (2) by acting on receptors in the anterior pituitary, either to modify gonadotropin secretion directly or to modify the sensitivity of the pituitary to gonadotropin-releasing factors, or (3) by combinations of the above. The types of experiments that provide information regarding the site of action of steroid feedback fall into four major categories: first, locating possible receptors by administering radiolabeled gonadal steroids; second, observing the effects on gonadotropin secretion of administering steroids directly into the hypothalamus or anterior pituitary; third, observing the effects of hypothalamic lesions on gonadotropin secretion; and fourth, determining changes in the responsiveness of the pituitary to gonadotropin-releasing factor before and after steroid treatment.

Studies with radiolabeled estrogen in rats and monkeys indicate that estrogen receptors are located in the hypothalamus and anterior pituitary, but such studies have not determined which location is most important for steroid regulation of gonadotropin secretion or what the function of the receptors is.

In rats, implantation of estrogen into the medial basal hypothalamus or the anterior hypothalamus leads to gonadal atrophy, indicative of decreased gonadotropin secretion. In ovariectomized monkeys, injecting estrogen into the former region decreased plasma levels of LH. It must not, however, be immediately concluded from these observations that negative feedback of estrogen is acting solely on the hypothalamus; it is possible that the hypothalamic estrogen reaches the anterior pituitary via the blood supply (hypophysial portal vessels). Blood in these vessels traverses first the hypothalamus and then the anterior pituitary. Considerable evidence from implant studies indicates that, at least in rats, estrogen can and does act directly on the pituitary to modify gonadotropin secretion. For example, estrogen implants into the pituitary cause the disappearance of a cell type (castration cells) indicative of hypersecretion of gonadotropins. Direct facilitative effects of estrogen on the pituitary have also been demonstrated: in intact rats, pituitary implants of estrogen were more effective in advancing ovulation (and presumably the LH surge) than were implants of estrogen in the hypothalamus. On the other hand, hypothalamic implants of progesterone were more effective in advancing ovulation than were pituitary implants. Comparable experiments have not yet been performed in sheep, monkeys, or humans.

Experiments in which discrete lesions were placed in the hypothalamus indicate that in the rat the medial basal hypothalamus (MBH) must be connected with the preoptic area (POA)—rostral hypothalamus—for normal cyclic gonadotropin secretion to occur. In some monkeys, cyclic gonadotropin secretion can apparently occur even when the MBH is isolated from all other parts of the brain; in other monkeys, lesions of the POA disturb ovarian cyclicity. These observations suggest that connections between POA and MBH are essential for steroidal facilitation of gonadotropin secretion in the rat but may be less important in the monkey.

Some experimental evidence from rats, monkeys, and women indicates that the pituitary is most responsive to LRF near or during the normal time of the preovulatory gonadotropin surge. Presumably, this increased sensitivity to LRF could be due to the peculiar steroid environment (high estrogen) present at this time. On the other hand, pituitary responsiveness to LRF was increased by ovariectomy in female monkeys and was also increased in women without gonadal function; in both species, administering estrogen lowered the sensitivity of the pituitary to LRF. In rats, ovariectomy may cause a slight decrease in pituitary sensitivity to LRF (as compared to intact proestrous rats), but treatment of the ovariectomized rat with estrogen greatly enhances pituitary sensitivity to LRF—to the point that such rats are far more responsive than are cycling proestrous rats. Treatment of ovariectomized rats with progesterone in the presence or absence of estrogen failed to modify pituitary responsiveness to LRF. Similarly, elevated levels of progesterone in women and monkeys did not modify pituitary sensitivity to LRF, but the effect of progesterone on LRF sensitivity in sheep is ambiguous.

Collectively these observations suggest that at least some feedback control is exerted at the pituitary level, that estrogen can markedly modify (sometimes inhibit and sometimes enhance) pituitary sensitivity to LRF, and that progesterone's facilitative effect on LH secretion is not due to enhanced pituitary sensitivity to LRF.

With the recent development of radioimmunoassays for quantitating circulating levels of GnRH, a new dimension is being added to this area of investigation. For example, Nett et al. (1974) found no significant change in serum concentration of GnRH throughout a sampling period during which ewes were responding to injected estrogen with LH surges; they concluded that increased levels of GnRH in the peripheral circulation were *not* responsible for LH release under these circumstances.

Feedback Dormancy

The characteristics of negative and positive feedback control of gonadotropin secretion, which are evident in the adult and which we accept as "normal," are not necessarily present throughout the lifetime of an individual. For example, certain pubertal changes precede the attainment of full reproductive capability, while periods of relative feedback dormancy are apparent even in the adult, such as during pregnancy and lactation. Several species differences in this regard are rather distinct.

Prepubertal dormancy (see Table 8.8) The negative feedback system seems to develop at an early age in all four species, in that circulating levels of gonadotropin may be suppressed by the administration of estrogen. Indeed, substantial evidence suggests that the prepubertal hypothalamo-hypophyseal unit is more sensitive to the negative feedback effects of estrogen at an early age than in adult life. Ovariectomy (or agonadal conditions in humans) leads to the typically adult hypersecretion of gonadotropins; however, the maximum response is delayed until about the normal time of puberty in humans and monkeys. Sheep and rats, however, are capable of responding to the positive feedback effects of estrogen well before the normal time of puberty. In primates this feedback system is not functional until late in the pubertal sequence (shortly before the time of menarche in humans but not until after menarche in monkeys). GnRH administration to prepubertal humans, monkeys, sheep, and rats results in an increased secretion of LH. In prepubertal humans and monkeys, however, relatively more FSH than LH is secreted, and this ratio is reversed in the adult individual. It has been demonstrated in the monkey that these responses to GnRH are a direct reflection of the quantities of LH and FSH contained in the anterior pituitary.

The pulsatile pattern of LH secretion is present in neonatal ewe lambs and continues into adulthood; this type of gonadotropin secretion does not appear until late in the human pubertal process, when it first becomes evident during sleep. Sleep-associated LH secretion has not been reported for other species.

These findings suggest that prepubertal rats and sheep exhibit less feedback dormancy relative to prepubertal primates and that a major limiting factor in attaining the adult type of positive feedback control in primates may be an inability of their hypothalamo-hypophyseal unit to respond to increased levels of estrogen, even though this unit seems to be very sensitive to the negative feedback effects of estrogen.

Pregnancy and lactational dormancy (see Table 8.9)
The general observation in all four species is that in pregnant individuals, peripheral levels of gonadotropins are low, while steroid levels are high. GnRH administration to pregnant women results in increased secretion of FSH, and pituitary secretions are required in rats for maintenance of the early corpora lutea of pregnancy. It might thus be assumed that the depressed gonadotropic hormone concentrations in the blood during this period simply reflect the negative feedback effects of elevated steroid concentrations and that this situation is rectified upon parturition. This explanation seems to fit the rat, since a postpartum gonadotropin surge and ovulation occur shortly after parturition. Such is not the case, however, in the other three species, where no postpartum ovulation occurs; feedback dormancy persists in varying degrees in all four species during lactation.

Differential Feedback of Gonadal Steroids on LH versus FSH (See Table 8.10)
A long-standing question exists about whether either FSH or LH has its own unique control system or whether each is routinely secreted in response to the same feedback stimuli. This question has been raised anew by the finding that the hypothalamic releasing hormone that was thought to specifically regulate the secretion of LH also induces the secretion of FSH. Indeed, in all physiological conditions investigated, FSH is never secreted without some concurrent LH secretion, and vice versa. Nevertheless, the ratio of FSH to LH in the blood does vary significantly under different circumstances. For example, during the primate menstrual cycle, the levels of these two hormones diverge markedly during the early follicular and late luteal phases. Estrogen, for the primate as well as for sheep, reportedly has a greater negative feedback effect on FSH than on LH, whereas in the rat, more estrogen is required to prevent the postcastration hypersecretion of FSH than that of LH. In the human (in contrast to the monkey) the gonadotropin surges elicited by progesterone in estrogen-treated women involve the secretion of both FSH and LH. In neonatal and peripubertal lambs, the peripheral levels of LH are high and exhibit a pulsatile pattern, while the levels of FSH are low and stable. From this morass of data, one is left with the impression that while the variations in relative amounts of FSH and LH secreted in a given situation are real, they are quantitative rather than qualitative differences. Part of the problem may lie in the emerging problems of separating FSH from LH in abnormal conditions (see Schwartz 1974).

Local (Ovarian) Effects of Steroids on Follicular Growth and Steroidogenesis
In addition to modifying the rate at which the pituitary secretes gonadotropins, estrogen also acts locally within the ovary to facilitate follicular growth. If the estrogen-stimulated follicle increases its rate of estrogen secretion as it grows, then a positive feedback loop is acting locally within the follicle wall. The amount of follicular growth that can be produced in a hypophysectomized rat by administering a given amount of FSH is greatly increased if the rat is pretreated with estrogen or given estrogen simultaneously with the FSH (Bradbury 1961; Smith 1961; Reiter et al. 1972b; Goldenberg et al. 1972).

Takahashi et al. (1975) have shown that large doses of progesterone can actually induce ovulation in rats that have been hypophysectomized shortly after the onset of the preovulatory gonadotropin surge. These findings tend to substantiate early observations of Lostroh (1971) that $20\,\alpha$OH progesterone could induce ovulation in FSH-primed hypophysectomized immature rats. To our knowledge, comparable studies in other species have not been performed.

Comparative Tables
On the following pages will be found tabular comparisons of empirical observations. The following abbreviations are used in the tables:

admin.—administration

AP—anterior pituitary gland

conc.—concentration

E—estrogen

F—female

GnRH—gonadotropin-releasing hormone

GnTH—gonadotropin (FSH plus LH)

LRF—LH-releasing factor (considered by many to be GnRH)

M—male

MBH—medial basal hypothalamus

neg.—negative

ovec.—ovariectomy (or ovariectomized)

P—progesterone

POA—preoptic area

secr.—secretion

Table 8.1 Negative feedback by gonadal steroids

Response Being Compared	Human	Monkey	Sheep	Rat
Ovec. leads to hypersecr. of GnTH in all 4 species	Ostergard et al. 1970; Franchimont 1972; Yen et al. 1974. Hypersecr. also occurs in postmenopausal Fs	Atkinson et al. 1970	Roche et al. 1970a	McCann and Ramirez 1964; Parlow 1964
LH hypersecr. in ovec. Fs is pulsatile in all 4 species	Midgley and Jaffe 1971; Root et al. 1972; Yen et al. 1974. Pulsatile LH secr. occurs in ovec., hypogonadal, and intact Fs	Dierschke et al. 1970; Weick et al. 1973. LH secr. is pulsatile in ovec. but not in intact Fs	Butler et al. 1972. LH secr. is pulsatile in ovec. and intact Fs	Gay and Sheth 1972; Weick 1974. LH secr. is pulsatile in ovec. but not in intact Fs
Admin. of E decreases GnTH hypersecr. and abolishes pulsatile secretory pattern	Franchimont 1972; Yen et al. 1972; Tsai and Yen 1971	Yamaji et al. 1972	Diekman and Malven 1973	McCann and Ramirez 1964
Admin. of P alone in physiological doses does not decrease GnTH hypersecr.	Nillius and Wide 1971; Franchimont 1972; Yen et al. 1974	Yamaji et al. 1972	Diekman and Malven 1973; Scaramuzzi et al. 1971. Exceptions have been noted in anestrous ewes (Davis and Borgen 1974) and in prepubertal F lambs (Foster and Karsch 1975)	McCann and Ramirez 1964; Parlow 1964
Admin. of P with E may exert greater neg. feedback than either alone	Wallach et al. 1970; Yen et al. 1974	Karsch et al. 1973b	Hauger et al. 1975. In another study P with E had no greater effect than E alone (Diekman and Malven 1973)	McCann and Ramirez 1964

Table 8.2 Internal feedback

Response Being Compared	Human	Monkey	Sheep	Rat
Internal neg. feedback (INF): Does the perfusion of plasma GnTH in the hypothalamus inhibit the secr. of GnTH-releasing factor?	Some data suggest that pulsatile secr. of LH may be due to INF (Boyar et al. 1972b; Szontagh 1973)	Data do not support concept of INF: admin. of large amounts of hCG, human LH, or ovine LH had no effect on secr. of endogenous (monkey) LH (Knobil 1974); pulsatile LH secr. occurred during constant infusion of LRF, suggesting that pulsatile mode of LH secr. is inherent to pituitary (Ferin et al. 1973)	Hypothesis of INF refuted by failure of infusion of ovine LH to prevent the secr. of endogenous LH in ovec. sheep (Coppings and Malven 1975)	Data mixed: hypothalamic implants of GnTH inhibit pituitary GnTH secr. (Martini et al. 1968; Corbin and Story 1967); LRF activity is seen in blood of hypophysectomized rats but not in that of intact cycling rats (Nallar and McCann 1965; Corbin and Upton 1973); INF does not prevent nephrectomy from increasing the already elevated serum GnTH levels of gonadectomized rats (Gay 1974).

Table 8.3 Positive (facilitative) feedback by estrogen (E), progesterone (P), and adrenal steroids

Response Being Compared	Human	Monkey	Sheep	Rat
Circulating E rises prior to preovulatory GnTH surge	Vande Wiele and Dyrenfurth 1973; Thorneycroft et al. 1974	Weick et al. 1973	Hansel et al. 1973	Hori et al. 1968; Brown-Grant et al. 1970
Does circulating P rise prior to GnTH surge?	No (Vande Wiele and Dyrenfurth 1973; Thorneycroft et al. 1974)	No (Weick et al. 1973)	No (Hansel et al. 1973)	Ovarian P—no; adrenal P—maybe (Barraclough 1973)
Removal or neutralization of E prevents the GnTH surge	No information found	Properly timed admin. of anti-E drug usually prevented LH surge (Spies and Niswender 1972). Immunization of cyclic Fs against E → *an*ovulation (Ferin et al. 1974a)	Caldwell et al. 1970	Shirley et al. 1968; Ferin et al. 1969
Admin. of E can elicit LH surges	In cyclic Fs (Yen and Tsai 1972; Monroe et al. 1972; Leyendecker et al. 1972). In ovec. or hypogonadal Fs (Yen et al. 1972a; Leyendecker et al. 1972)	In cyclic Fs (Yamaji et al. 1971; Dierschke et al. 1973). In ovec. Fs (Yamaji et al. 1971; Karsch et al. 1973b). Elevated E is required at the onset of GnTH surge (Karsch et al. 1973c)	In cyclic ewes (Bolt et al. 1971; Howland et al. 1971). In ovec. or anestrous ewes (Scaramuzzi et al. 1971; Goding et al. 1969; Beck and Reeves 1973; Reeves et al. 1974; Jonas 1973)	In intact Fs (Krey and Everett 1973). In ovec. Fs (Caligaris et al. 1971a)
Properly timed admin. of P can prevent E from inducing a GnTH surge; and E does not induce GnTH surge during luteal phase	P administration prevents spontaneous preovulatory GnTH surge (Netter et al. 1973)	P or luteal phase prevents spontaneous preovulatory GnTH surge (Spies and Niswender 1972) and E-induced GnTH surge in intact (Dierschke et al. 1973) but not in ovec. monkeys (Clifton et al. 1975)	P or luteal phase usually prevents E-induced GnTH surge in adult ewes (Scaramuzzi et al. 1971; Bolt et al. 1971; Howland et al. 1971) and in prepubertal F lambs (Foster and Karsch 1975), but not always (Yuthasastrakosol 1974)	P given early in estrous cycle delays preovulatory LH surge and ovulation by 24 hr (Zeilmaker 1966)

Table 8.3 (continued)

Response Being Compared	Human	Monkey	Sheep	Rat
Properly timed P admin. elicits or advances the LH surge in some situations, not in others	Injected P induces an LH surge within a few hours of the injection; LH surge following E injection does not occur for 24 hr (Leyendecker et al. 1972; Odell and Swerdloff 1968)	P advanced the time of E-induced LH surge in ovec. but not in intact monkeys (Clifton et al. 1975)	No information found	P given late in estrous cycle advances LH surge and ovulation by 24 hr (Zeilmaker 1966)
Does adrenal steroid (i.e., P) secr. act as an important signal to initiate the preovulatory LH surge?	No information found	In adrenalectomized, ovec. Fs, admin. of E elicited LH surges comparable to those seen in E-treated ovec. Fs; therefore adrenal steroids are not essential as a signal for LH surge (Knobil 1974)	No information found	To produce a normal LH surge in ovec. adrenalectomized Fs, E treatment must be followed with P; i.e., either steroid alone is insufficient (Mann and Barraclough 1973). Ovulation occurs in adrenalectomized Fs, but may be a few hours late (Lawton 1972; Feder et al. 1971; Mann and Barraclough 1973). Antibodies against P do not prevent ovulation (Ferin et al. 1969)

Table 8.4 Environmental influences

Response Being Compared	Human	Monkey	Sheep	Rat
Is the basal level of GnTH secr. significantly higher at one time of the day than at another?	Some say plasma GnTH is highest in morning; others disagree (Curtis 1972). Variations in GnTH secr. may be due to sleep-wake cycles (Kapen et al. 1973)	No information found	No information found	Even during diestrus, plasma LH tends to be higher in afternoon hours than during morning hours (Gay et al. 1970; Legan and Karsch 1975)
Does the spontaneous ovulatory GnTH surge or an E-induced surge begin at a specific time of the day?	No information found	Spontaneous or E-induced LH surges occur at various times of day or night, and timing of the surge can be altered by varying the strength/duration characteristics of the E stimulus (Weick et al. 1973; Karsch et al. 1973c)	Time interval between E injection and LH surge was constant regardless of time of day of E admin. (Jackson and Thurman 1974). Onset of behavioral estrus (and presumably ovulation) occurs at various times of day or night (Robertson and Rakha 1965b)	Spontaneous ovulatory GnTH surge begins 2–5 hr after midpoint of photoperiod (Everett 1970). E-induced LH surges only occur during these same hours (Caligaris et al. 1971a,b). Treatment with E or P can advance ovulation by 24 hr but only if these steroids are given during the morning or early afternoon on days prior to the normal LH surge (Krey and Everett 1973; Weick et al. 1971; Everett and Sawyer 1949)

Table 8.4 (continued)

Response Being Compared	Human	Monkey	Sheep	Rat
Does altering the light-dark (LD) cycle modify the time of the ovulatory GnTH surge?	No information found	Has not been tested, but see above statement (Weick et al. 1973)	Has not been critically tested, but see above statement (Robertson and Rakha 1965b)	Time of ovulatory GnTH surge is shifted by alteration of LD cycle (Everett 1970; McCormack 1973)
Are annual (i.e., seasonal) reproductive activity rhythms present? If so, what is the environmental cue for these rhythms?	Seasonal reproductive rhythms, if present, are not apparent; however, an increase in pregnancies (esp. multiple pregnancies) has been associated with increased day lengths (Timonen and Carpen 1968)	Increased incidence of amenorrhea and anovulation during summer months *even* under conditions of controlled light and temperature (Keverne and Michael 1970; Riesen et al. 1971; Dailey and Neill 1975). But in a long-term longitudinal study, anovulation seemed to be more closely correlated with individual monkeys than with the season (Fritz et al. 1974)	Under natural lighting, seasonal anestrus always occurs during summer months, i.e., with long photoperiods (Robinson 1959); however, even when kept in constant light year-round, ewes showed seasonal breeding patterns (Thibault et al. 1966)	No evidence found for seasonal rhythms in reproductive activity
What is the physiological mechanism for seasonal anestrus?			Both neg. (Deikman and Malven 1973) and positive feedback mechanisms (Goding et al. 1969; Beck and Reeves 1973; Reeves et al. 1974; Jonas et al. 1973) for control of GnTH secr. are functioning or are capable of functioning in anestrus ewes. Pinealectomized ewes maintained normal estrous cycles, LH levels, and seasonal breeding patterns (Roche et al. 1970b) and responded to ovec. by increased secr. of GnTH (Roche et al. 1970a)	
What are the effects of constant light (LL) or constant darkness (DD) on reproductive activity?	Blind girls exhibit menarche at an earlier age than girls with normal vision (Zacharias and Wurtman 1964) or those with less impaired vision (Magee et al. 1970)	No information on exposure of rhesus monkeys to LL; however, baboons continued to show regular menstrual cycles and ovulation after several years of exposure to LL (Hagino 1971)	Sheep exposed to LL displayed normal estrous cycles (Thibault et al. 1966) even when this condition was imposed from birth (Ducker et al. 1973)	Exposure to LL produces persistant vaginal and behavioral estrus. Ovulatory GnTH surges are absent; LH and estradiol are secreted tonically at intermediate levels (Naftolin et al. 1972)

Table 8.5 Effects of neurally active drugs and surgical stress on gonadotropin secretion

Response Being Compared	Human	Monkey	Sheep	Rat
Can the spontaneous preovulatory GnTH surge be blocked with neurally active drugs?	No information found	Chlorpromazine, haloperidol, phentolamine, phenoxybenzamine, and pentobarbital failed to prevent spontaneous or E-induced LH surges in intact monkeys (Knobil 1974). In baboons, pentobarbital admin. in the afternoon, but not in the morning, of the day preceding expected ovulation prevented ovulation (Hagino 1971)	Pentobarbital did not prevent the preovulatory LH surge (Ellicott et al. 1974), but ovulation was delayed (Radford 1966). Pentobarbital delayed the E-induced LH surge in ovec. ewes (Radford and Wallace 1974). Chlorpromazine sedation delayed, but did not prevent, ovulation (Robertson and Rakha 1965a)	Pentobarbital and numerous other sedatives and anesthetics block the LH surge and ovulation if given immediately before the surge (Everett 1964; Schwartz and McCormack 1972)
Can the high rate of GnTH secretion in ovec. Fs be diminished by admin. of neurally active drugs?	No information found	Tranquilizers (chlorpromazine, haloperidol) and α adrenergic blockers (phentolamine, phenoxybenzamine) but not a β adrenergic blocker (propranolol) suppressed GnTH secretion in ovec. Fs (Bhattacharya et al. 1972); pentobarbital anesthesia had no consistent effect (Bhattacharya et al. 1972; Arimura et al. 1973a)	Pentobarbital anesthesia caused the plasma LH conc. of ovec. ewes to decrease significantly (Ellicott et al. 1974)	Pentobarbital anesthesia caused the plasma LH conc. of ovec. rats to decrease significantly (Beattie et al. 1973)
What are the effects of surgical or sampling stress on GnTH secretion?	Circulating levels of GnTH secr. were not altered by surgery in cyclic or postmenopausal women (Charters et al. 1969; Stone et al. 1975)	In monkeys and humans the stress of daily or more frequent blood sampling without anesthesia usually does not interfere with cyclic ovulation and menses (Knobil 1974; Ross et al. 1970)	No information found	Surgical stress under ether, late on the day prior to the ovulatory GnTH surge, delays the surge (Schwartz 1964); surgical stress early on the day of the GnTH surge advances the surge (Nequin and Schwartz 1971; Proudfit and Schwartz 1974)

Table 8.6 Neonatal organization by androgens of gonadotropin secretion

Response Being Compared	Human	Monkey	Sheep	Rat
What are the effects of neonatal androgen (endogenous or exogenous) on the pattern of GnTH secr. in adulthood? Does neonatal treatment of Fs with androgen produce sterility?	No evidence that exposure to androgen at an early age leads to sterility	Testosterone admin. at birth had no effect on adult ovarian or menstrual cycles (Treloar et al. 1972). Testosterone propionate admin. prenatally resulted in birth of pseudohermaphroditic Fs in which menarche was delayed, but subsequent ovarian function was normal (Goy and Resko 1972)	Admin. of testosterone to Fs at birth or *in utero* (12 and 15 weeks) had no effect on adult reproductive function (Przekop et al. 1974), while testosterone given to ewes before day 60 of gestation, but not after day 80, prevented normal estrous cycles in F offspring (Short 1974)	Noncyclic (M) type of GnTH secr. develops if M or F rats are exposed neonatally to endogenous or exogenous androgen. In the absence of neonatal androgen, F (cyclic) type of GnTH secretion develops. Fs treated with androgen neonatally are sterile (Barraclough 1966)
Can the positive feedback effects of E or E plus P be demonstrated in intact adult Ms? in adult Ms castrated in adulthood? in adult Ms castrated neonatally?	In intact Ms, positive feedback responses to exogenous E were reported by some (Kulin and Reiter 1974a; Dörner et al. 1972). Others were unable to elicit positive feedback response to E or P (Odell and Swerdloff 1968; Leyendecker et al. 1971). In castrated Ms, E treatment alone elicited an LH surge (Kulin and Reiter 1974b); P elicited LH surges if GnTH levels were first suppressed by P (Stearns et al. 1973)	In intact Ms, no LH surge was seen following acute E admin. (Yamaji et al. 1971); however, in E-suppressed castrated Ms the acute admin. of E produced distinct LH surges (Karsch et al. 1973a; Steiner et al. 1974)	In intact Ms, LH surges did not occur following admin. of E, P, or testosterone (Bolt 1971). Acute admin. of E to E-suppressed castrated Ms was also ineffective (Karsh and Foster 1975)	Positive feedback effects of E or of E plus P on GnTH secr. are demonstrable in adult ovec. rats, unless these rats are given androgen neonatally. Likewise, admin. of E or E plus P fails to evoke GnTH surges in intact Ms, or in Ms castrated later than 5 days after birth. E admin. does induce LH surges in Ms castrated on the day of birth (Caligaris et al. 1971a,b, 1972, 1973; Neill 1972)

Table 8.7 Site of action of steroid feedback

Response Being Compared	Human	Monkey	Sheep	Rat
Where are E receptors located—the brain, AP, or both locations?	No information found	Binding of radiolabeled E is high in arcuate nucleus of hypothalamus and AP (Eisenfeld 1974)	No information found	Binding of radiolabeled E is high in hypothalamus and AP (Barraclough 1973)
What is the effect on GnTH secr. of admin. of E directly into hypothalamus or AP?	No information found	E injected into several areas of the MBH and fields of Forel, but not in anterior hypothalamus and POA, was followed by a reduction in plasma LH conc. (Ferin et al. 1974c)	Ovarian function was normal in ewes that had E implants in anterior hypothalamus (Przekop and Domanski 1970)	Implants of E in certain areas of hypothalamus cause decreased GnTH secr. (Flerko 1966; Lisk 1967); however, E may be reaching AP by portal vessels. E implants in AP of ovec. rats cause disappearance of "castration cells"; therefore E can act directly on AP to decrease GnTH secr. (Bogdanove 1963). Implants of E into AP can advance ovulation (and presumably the LH surge) by one day; hypothalamic E implants were less effective (Weick and Davidson 1970). Implants of P were more effective in advancing ovulation if placed in MBH than in AP (Döcke and Dörner 1969)
What are the effects of hypothalamic lesions on GnTH secretion? Must the MBH have intact connections with the POA for cyclic GnTH secr. to occur?	No information found	Following surgical isolation of the MBH from the rest of the brain, 3 of 7 monkeys showed spontaneous GnTH surges and ovulation; similar spontaneous feedback responses were noted in 4 of 7 having frontal cuts only. GnTH surges could be induced by admin. of E in 12 of these same 14 Fs (Krey et al. 1975). Placement of electrochemical lesions in the POA caused most monkeys to have irregular ovarian cycles; some were acyclic; some had normal cycles (Spies et al. 1974)	Lesions placed in supraoptic nucleus and in anterior hypothalamic nucleus did not block ovulation (Przekop and Domanski 1970)	MBH must have intact connections with anterior hypothalamic nucleus and POA for cyclic GnTH secr. and ovulation to occur (Koves and Halasz 1970). Lesions that separate POA from MBH produce a state of anovulation and persistent vaginal estrus (Rodgers and Schwartz 1972). Such rats will not ovulate in response to E or E plus P (Barraclough 1973).

Table 8.7 (continued)

Response Being Compared	Human	Monkey	Sheep	Rat
Do gonadal steroids modify the responsiveness of the AP to LRF? If so, then at least part of feedback action of gonadal steroids is exerted directly on the AP	Admin. of E usually results in a decreased response to standard dose of LRF in Fs with or without gonadal function (Yen et al. 1973; Gual et al. 1973; Malacara et al. 1973), but an augmentative effect of E has also been demonstrated (Jaffe and Keye 1974). The pituitary responsiveness to LRF during the luteal phase of the cycle (plasma P is elevated) is equal to (Malacara et al. 1973) or greater than (Yen et al. 1973) the responsiveness during the early follicular phase of the cycle. The greatest increase in circulating levels of LH following LRF admin. (Yen et al. 1973; Saito et al. 1973a) occurred in subjects lacking gonadal function (plasma E very low) or during the midcycle GnTH surge (plasma E elevated) (Yen et al. 1973; Malacara et al. 1973; Saito et al. 1973b); therefore the response to LRF may depend more on conditions within pituitary at time of LRF admin. than on direct effects of steroids on pituitary responsiveness to LRF	Increased levels of circulating E decrease the amount of LH released in response to LRF admin. peripherally (Krey et al. 1973) or directly into the pituitary (Spies and Norman 1975); however, the amount of LH released following LRF admin. at the early follicular (low endogenous E) and the late follicular (high endogenous E) stage of the cycle did not differ significantly (Ferin et al. 1974b). LH release following intraventricular infusion of LRF was not modified by peripheral admin. of E (Spies and Norman 1975). Pituitary responsiveness to LRF was not modified by experimentally altering plasma P conc. (Krey et al. 1973; Spies et al. 1972), and pituitary responsiveness to LRF during luteal phase of cycle is similar to or somewhat greater than responsiveness during follicular phase (Ferin et al. 1974b). The largest responses to LRF were seen when it was given at times when GnTH secr. was already high (i.e., in untreated ovec. Fs or when preovulatory surge of GnTH was already underway) (Krey et al. 1973; Ferin et al. 1974b)	E may augment the release of LH when given in conjunction with LRF (Reeves et al. 1973). In some studies, P had no effect on the amount of LH released by LRF (Reeves et al. 1973; Cumming et al. 1972), while in others P decreased the amount of LH released by LRF (Reeves et al. 1973; Hooley et al. 1974). No distinct differences in LH release following LRF at different stages of the estrous cycle were noted (Symons et al. 1974)	Pretreatment of adult ovec. rat with E increased pituitary responsiveness to injected LRF. P admin. alone, or P given after E, failed to modify responsiveness (Libertun et al. 1974). On the other hand, E decreased responsiveness of AP homografts (under kidney capsule) to LRF (McLean et al. 1975). Cycling proestrous rats are far less responsive to injected LRF than are E or E plus P treated ovec. rats (Libertun et al. 1974; Martin et al. 1974)

Table 8.8 Feedback dormancy—Puberty

Response Being Compared	Human	Monkey	Sheep	Rat
Neg. feedback: When is it first demonstrable, and how does the threshold for E-inhibition of GnTH secr. compare before and after puberty?	Neg. feedback present at early age: circulating GnTH is elevated in agonadal children (Visser 1973; Grumbach et al. 1974; Winter and Faiman 1972) but is even higher in agonadal individuals after puberty (Winter and Faiman 1972). Neg. feedback is more sensitive to E before puberty than in adulthood (Visser 1973; Grumbach et al. 1974)	Following ovec. of premenarchial Fs, plasma GnTH rises, but only after an extended delay (Dierschke et al. 1974a). Suppression of GnTH hypersecr. may be achieved with smaller doses of E in Fs ovec. before menarche as compared with those ovec. as adults (Dierschke et al. 1974a)	Hypersecr. of LH began promptly when ovec. was performed shortly after birth (Liefer et al. 1972) but was delayed following ovec. at a peripubertal age (Diekman and Malven 1973)	Neg. feedback action of E is operational at 15 days of age (Ramirez 1973). Threshold for E-inhibition of GnTH secr. is higher in adults than in prepubertal rats (Ramirez 1973)
Positive feedback effects of gonadal steroids on GnTH secr.: When are they first demonstrable?	The positive feedback response to E is not operational until late in pubertal sequence (Grumbach et al. 1974), but can be demonstrated shortly before menarche (Reiter et al. 1974)	Admin. of E does not elicit LH surges until several months after menarche (Dierschke et al. 1974b). Treatment of premenarchial animals with E, P, or 5α androstane-3β, 17β-diol did not induce precocious puberty (Dierschke et al. 1974a)	Definite LH surges followed admin. of E to lambs as young as 38 days old (Land et al. 1970), and the response gradually increased in magnitude between 7 and 27 weeks of age (Foster and Karsch, 1975)	Facilitative effects of E plus P are demonstrable well before puberty. In 18–24-day-old rats, E must be followed with P to elicit an LH surge (McCormack and Meyer 1964). In 25–32-day-old rats, E alone will induce an LH surge (Caligaris et al. 1972; Ying and Greep 1971)
Pituitary responsiveness to LRF: Is it different before and after puberty?	LRF admin. elicits primarily FSH secr. in prepubertal subjects, whereas after puberty much more LH is secreted (Grumbach et al. 1974)	AP of premenarchial Fs contain large (i.e., adult) quantities of FSH, but less than adult quantities of LH, and the amount of these hormones secreted following LRF admin. reflect pituitary content (Dierschke et al. 1974b)	In response to admin. of GnTH-RF, considerably more LH was secreted by 68-day-old prepubertal Fs than by 3- or 11-day-old Fs (Foster et al. 1972a)	Responsiveness of AP to LRF is greater both with respect to LH and FSH secr. prepubertally than postpubertally (Debeljuk et al. 1972)
Pulsatile pattern of LH secr.: If present in intact members of the species, when does it develop?	Pulsatile pattern of LH secr. was not seen until about the time of puberty, and was associated with periods of sleep when it first appeared (Boyar et al. 1972a)	Pulsatile LH secr. only seen on gonadectomized monkeys (Dierschke et al. 1970; Weick et al. 1973)	Pulsatile pattern of LH secr. is present in neonatal Fs, and this pattern continues without substantial change into adulthood (Foster et al. 1972b)	Pulsatile LH secr. only seen in gonadectomized rats (Gay and Sheth 1972)

Table 8.9 Feedback dormancy—Pregnancy and lactation

Response Being Compared	Human	Monkey	Sheep	Rat
In all 4 species, circulating levels of E plus P are high during pregnancy	Yannone 1972; Csapo et al. 1971	Atkinson et al. 1975; Bosu et al. 1973; Hodgen et al. 1972; Macdonald et al. 1973; Stabenfeldt and Hendrickx 1972, 1973	Stabenfeldt et al. 1972; Chamley et al. 1973b	Morishige et al. 1973; Wayneforth et al. 1972; Pepe and Rothchild 1974
In all 4 species, circulating levels of GnTH are relatively low during pregnancy	FSH is low (Jaffe et al. 1969; Faiman et al. 1969)	FSH and LH are low (Atkinson et al. 1971)	LH is low (Goding et al. 1969)	FSH and LH are low (Morishige et al. 1973; Linkie and Niswender 1972). Some LH is secreted on days 1–12 of pregnancy as prolactin alone will not maintain luteal E plus P production (Nalbandov 1973)
Is responsiveness of AP to injected LRF altered during pregnancy?	LRF admin. produced significant elevation of circulating FSH (Zarate et al. 1973)	No information found	Amount of LH secreted following GnTH-RH decreased throughout pregnancy to none at 18 weeks of gestation (Chamley et al. 1974a,b)	No information found
Does postpartum ovulation occur?	No (Said and Wide 1973; Reyes et al. 1972; Arimura et al. 1973b)	No (Weiss et al. 1973)	No (Chamley et al. 1973a)	Yes, presumably because GnTH secr. is released from steroid suppression (Hoffmann and Schwartz 1965; Hoffman 1973)
Is the return of cyclic ovulation delayed after parturition? If so, is this period of anovulation prolonged by lactation?	A period of amenorrhea usually follows parturition; the length of amenorrhea is prolonged by nursing (Cronin 1968; Reyes et al. 1972; Tolis et al. 1974)	Similar situation to human (Weiss et al. 1973)	A period of anestrus follows parturition, but reports conflict as to whether lactation prolongs the length of this anestrus (Hunter and Van Aarde 1973; Thibault et al. 1966; Shevah et al. 1974)	In nonlactating Fs, cyclic ovulation returns immediately (Rothchild 1960). In lactating Fs, except for the postpartum ovulation, cyclic ovulation is delayed by lactation; the more intense the suckling, the longer the delay (Rothchild 1960)
What are the levels of circulating GnTH after parturition and during lactation? What are the plasma levels of gonadal steroids during lactation?	Circulating levels of GnTH (and ovarian steroids) are low following parturition and remain so for a longer period of time in lactating Fs (Jaffe et al. 1969; Said and Wide 1973; Reyes et al. 1972; Crystal et al. 1973)	Basal secr. of GnTH is low, especially in lactating Fs (Weiss et al. 1972); plasma levels of gonadal steroids are also low (Bosu et al. 1973; Weiss et al. 1973)	LH levels immediately following parturition were similar to the low levels seen in late pregnancy (Chamley et al. 1973b)	Suckling of young inhibits GnTH secr.; the more intense the suckling, the greater the inhibition (Rothchild 1960; Ford and Melampy 1971; Hammonds et al. 1973)
Can the facilitative (positive feedback) effects of E be demonstrated in postparturient Fs or lactating Fs?	Admin. of E to nonlactating Fs during the first postpartum month stimulated GnTH secr. (Crystal et al. 1973)	Admin. of E usually elicited LH surges by the 2d postpartum month in nonlactating Fs, but this response was delayed until 3–9 months postpartum in lactating Fs (Weiss et al. 1973)	Secr. of LH in response to E given at 11–40 days postpartum was usually depressed in lactating ewes (Pelletier and Thimonier 1973; Restall et al. 1972; Lewis et al. 1974)	No information found

Table 8.9 (continued)

Response Being Compared	Human	Monkey	Sheep	Rat
Is pituitary responsiveness to LRF normal in postpartum Fs? Does lactation modify responsiveness to LRF?	Lactating or nonlactating Fs showed no increase in serum GnTH when treated with LRF during the first week postpartum. Full GnTH responses following LRF were noted 15 days to 6 weeks after delivery. The longer recovery times were generally associated with lactation (Arimura et al. 1973; Canales et al. 1974; Nakano et al. 1974; Tolis et al. 1974)	Admin. of LRF to intact or ovec. lactating Fs produced only minor elevations in plasma LH (Weiss et al., unpublished)	Amount of LH and FSH secreted in response to GnTH at 3 or 6 weeks postpartum was less than in cyclic ewes or ewes in early pregnancy, but was equivalent to the response in late pregnancy (Chamley et al. 1974a,b; Rippel et al. 1974)	No information found
Does ovec. produce hypersecr. of GnTH in lactating Fs?	No information found	Hypersecr. of GnTH was delayed in lactating (but not in nonlactating) Fs if ovec. was performed during the first postpartum month (Weiss et al. 1973)	No information found	Intense suckling inhibits the increased secr. of GnTH following ovec. (Rothchild 1960; Ford and Melampy 1971; Hammonds et al. 1973)

Table 8.10 Differential feedback of gonadal steroids on FSH and LH secretion

Response Being Compared	Human	Monkey	Sheep	Rat
Is the secr. of one GnTH more easily suppressed by gonadal steroids than that of the other?	E seems to exert a greater neg. feedback effect on FSH than on LH in cyclic and postmenopausal Fs (Cargille et al. 1973; Tsai and Yen 1971; Vande Wiele et al. 1970)	The ratios of plasma LH and FSH diverge markedly during the early follicular and late luteal phases of the normal menstrual cycle (Karsch et al. 1973d; Krey et al. 1973), but not because of changes in plasma levels of progestogens (Resko et al. 1974)	Plasma FSH levels in anestrous ewes were decreased with smaller doses of E than were necessary to decrease plasma LH (Reeves et al. 1974). Markedly different patterns of plasma FSH and LH were noted at several stages of the estrous cycle (Salamonsen et al. 1973)	More E was necessary to prevent postovec. hypersecr. of FSH than LH (Parlow 1964)
Are the facilitative effects of E on GnTH secr. exerted primarily on LH secr.?	The GnTH surge resulting from E admin. to cyclic women consists primarily of LH with little or no FSH (Yen and Tsai 1974; Monroe et al. 1972); while that resulting from P (following E pretreatment) consists of both LH and FSH (Leyendecker et al. 1972)	Admin. of E causes both LH and FSH secr. to surge (Knobil 1974)	In neonatal and peripubertal lambs, plasma LH is high and variable, while plasma FSH is low and stable (Foster et al. 1972a)	Admin. of E induces LH surge; for an FSH surge, E followed by P may be required (Caligaris et al. 1971a; Taleisnik et al. 1970). FSH surge is normally more prolonged than that of LH; stimulus for prolongation of this surge may be testosterone (Gay and Tomacari 1974)

8.4 The Systems Analysis Approach to Reproductive Biology

Introduction: Why Model?
The inescapable need for making assumptions and devising models

Precisely because living systems are so very complex, one can never expect to achieve anything like a complete mathematical description of their behavior. Before the mathematical analysis itself is begun, it is therefore invariably necessary to reduce the complexity of the real system by making various *simplifying assumptions* about how it behaves. In effect, these assumptions allow us to replace the actual biological system by an imaginary *model* system which is simple enough to be described mathematically. The results of our mathematical analysis will then be rigorously applicable to the model. But they will be applicable to the original biological system only to the extent that our underlying assumptions are reasonable. Hence, the ultimate value of our mathematical labors will be determined in large part by our choice of simplifying assumptions.

In the last three chapters of this book, detailed consideration will be given to making assumptions and devising model systems, but it is important from the very outset for the reader to recognize the *inescapable* need for this approach. Every chapter will deal more or less explicitly with model systems. There is no alternative.(Rigg 1963)

The heuristic value of modeling

The question asked by the endocrinologist at this point must be whether the systems approach has contributed anything to our understanding of the problem of reproductive cyclicity in the rat. I feel that it has and would submit the following arguments in its favor. First, the enormous amount of data . . . seems incomprehensible without some aid to organizing the information. The model . . . provides a storage function and a mnemonic device to permit bringing together of the individual data. Second, the act of developing a model . . . forces the investigator to spell out hypotheses and concepts, rather than keeping these intuitive or implicit. This can be a shaking experience, but a valuable one. Third, the model, because it is explicit in its predictions, permits the designing of critical experiments of a hypothesis-testing nature and discourages semirandom "data gathering." This, of course, means that the modeler must be willing to discard parts of the model as soon as experiments indicate that they do not conform to the real system. Finally, computer simulation of the model provides a means of comparison of model with experimentally generated data, and also can be used to "pretest" experiments in order to see whether they might be of value in testing hypotheses.

The overview provided by the systems analysis approach can be exhilarating. . . . However, as Mesarović . . . has said: "The fundamental question for the community of biologists is whether an explanation on the systems theoretic basis is acceptable as a true scientific explanation in the biological inquiry." (Schwartz 1969)

We feel that the preceding quotations broadly answer the question: Why model? We follow with a documentation of the issues raised in the quotations.

A Dialogue between a Systems Analyst–Amateur Endocrinologist and an Endocrinologist–Amateur Systems Analyst.*

Paul Waltz and Neena Schwartz are meeting to discuss a computer model of the rat reproductive system called Hyperbolic LH Production Model. We have talked for many hours over a number of years about reproduction cyclicity in the rat and computer simulation, and it is difficult for us to retrieve that "first careless rapture" (Noel Coward) that we had in our first few discussions. We try to let the reader share a late dialogue by developing a point-by-point description of what the formulas mean.

SCHWARTZ: Paul, I wonder if you could start by introducing the novice to the sections of the model in Figure 8.1.

WALTZ: There are 36 equations in all in three sections. The first section is lines (1) through (9). The function of its equations is to specify data and parameters, describe what kind of print outputs are desired, and do basic "housekeeping" functions, so that the computer can run the model and supply the appropriate output. The section from (10) to (16) is executed at the beginning of each run. This section resets level variables and does some initial parameter calculations. The rest of the model, lines (17) through (36), calculates the values variables take throughout the run. Lines (17) through (36) really form the most important part of the model and can be thought of as separated into two parts. The first part is from line (18) to line (28); this section deals with the events that take place during the cycle. The rest of the model—line (17) and the lines beyond (28)—describes the continuous changing of the hormone levels and the other variables.

SCHWARTZ: Paul, could you comment further on lines (1) through (6)?

WALTZ: Lines (1) through (6) set the data for the model in the form of parameters and constants. For example, parameter A0 is set in line (2) to the standard value of 156. The difference between a parameter and a constant is that a parameter can be changed from computer run to computer run but is left constant for a given run; whereas the constants are set once and all remain constant at least for the purpose of the runs that we are considering. The constants are thought to be better known than the parameters.

*We acknowledge the support of PHS contract HD 02307, which supported the modeling and simulation described in this section. This model is not yet published.

```
        ∇ESMODEL[□]∇
     ∇ ESMODEL
[1]     'ESMODEL' TITLE 'A MODEL OF THE MAMMALIAN REPRODUCTIVE SYSTEM'
[2]     PARAMETERS 'A0←156, M←0.39, G←.01, AES←4, ALH←10, ATR←.014, A2, A3'
[3]     CONSTANTS 'BETA←2.4, FRCP←3.6, ALPHA2←1.38, LHCP←50, ESCP←15'
[4]     CONSTANTS 'THES←10, CCON←100, FRMIN←.01, TIM0←16, T←1'
[5]     CLDATA←(0 0),(11 0),(12 0.2),(13 0.5),(14 1)
[6]     CLDATA←CLDATA,(17 1),(18 0.5),(19 0.2),(20 0),(24 0)
[7]     METHOD 'TRAPZ, ΔTIME←.25, T0←140'
[8]     5 PRINT 'CTIMF, BLH'
[9]     50 PLOT 'ES, ∊, 0, 50, LH, l, 0, 100, FR, ○, 0, 4, BLH, ⁻, 0, 125'
[10]    MODEL
[11]    →GO
[12]    INITIAL:M←3×N←4
[13]    DEN←A0×ALPHA2÷ALH
[14]    A3←DEN×AES÷A0
[15]    A2←(BETA×ALH×AES)÷A0-BETA×ALH
[16]    LEVELS 'TIME←TIM0, ES←ESCP, LH←LHCP, FR←FRCP'
[17]    EQUATIONS:CTIME←24|TIME
[18]    →APL
[19]    NEWACYCLE:→NXT 1
[20]    →NXT ES<THES
[21]    →NXT ES≥THES
[22]    →NXT 0<CTIME AFGEN CLDATA
[23]    BEGIN:→NXT 0=SURGE←CCON×CTIME AFGEN CLDATA
[24]    OVTIME←TIME+6
[25]    →NXT 1
[26]    →NXT TIME≥OVTIME
[27]    FR←FRMIN
[28]    END:→NEWACYCLE
[29]    FA←C4×FR×FR
[30]    FV←FA×FR÷3
[31]    BLH←SURGE+A0×A2÷A2+ES
[32]    FES←0↑(M×FA)-N×FV
[33]    ΔFR←(-ATR×0⌈FR-FRMIN)+T×G×LH
[34]    ΔLH←(-BETA×LH)+BLH
[35]    ΔES←(-ALPHA2×ES)+T×(A3×LH)+FES
[36]    →CHK 0=4|TIME
     ∇
```

Figure 8.1 Listing of ESMODEL with hyperbolic LH production.

SCHWARTZ: I would like to make some introductory remarks regarding endocrinology of the model, roughly comparable to what Paul has just said about the computer functions. I owe it to my fellow endocrinologists to say why I have decided to try to model certain variables and parameters and not others. If every single variable that has been measured in the rat estrous cycle were to be put into the model, we would have not 36 but thousands of lines. When Paul and I first started, I tried to use only variables that had been measured, directly or indirectly, with some degree of precision, reliability, and frequency. I also stipulated that we should model only variables that have the following two characteristics: (1) I was convinced they were an integral part of the process of cycling, and (2) I understood something about the way in which they were controlled by inputs and the way in which they acted as inputs for other things. It will be recognized that enormous numbers of observations have been left out.

The only variables we are modeling are follicle radius (FR), blood levels of LH (LH), and blood levels of estrogen (ES). At the time we started, these were the only variables we had definite ideas about. Now we could also model the values for serum progesterone, FSH, prolactin, and 20 alpha hydroxyprogesterone, but I am still not sure about all of the physiological causative sequences of these other variables in terms of the two characteristics just outlined. Thus we are still modeling just the variables we started with.

Follicle radius permits us to look at ovulation, the LH is the output from the pituitary that causes secretion of estrogen and ovulation, and estrogen is the only

feedback signal we are dealing with. Thus the rat estrous cycle is seen as an animal model of follicular growth and ovulation, and the termination of the cycle is the event of ovulation, which initiates the next cycle. Essentially, we are looking at a nonpregnant rat, without observing behavior; we are not turning on prolactin and thereby prolonging the lifespan of the corpus luteum, and we are not modeling puberty. We are modeling in the time domain of the adult cycle, and our underlying hope at the beginning was that the variables we were modeling would undergo cycle lengths of four or five days, at a minimum.

WALTZ: Let's start at line (16) of the model, where the initial value of the level variables are being assigned at the start of the run. There are four level variables: time, ES, LH, and FR. The phrase *level variable* comes from analogy with the water level in a tank, which has the properties that it can be directly observed and measured and that the state of the tank may be completely described by giving the value of this level. Equation (16) says that time at the beginning is assigned the value TIM0, ES is assigned the value ESCP, LH is assigned the value LHCP, and FR is assigned the value FRCP. These are the values of the variables at 1600 of the day of proestrus during the critical period (CP).

SCHWARTZ: What is the critical period, and why did we choose that as time zero? That brings us not only to equation (16), but to TIM0 in line (4) and to LHCP, ESCP, and FRCP as defined on line (3). Everett's observations in the late 1940s showed indirectly, but quite conclusively, a critical time period, during the afternoon of the day of proestrus, when luteinizing hormone was released from the pituitary, causing ovulation that night. When Paul and I first started working on the computer model I chose 1600 hours on that day as the initial time, because it was the only time when I knew, or could guess, the values of FR, LH, and ES. Incidentally, FR is in microns, LH is in nanograms per milliliter, ES is in picograms per milliliter, and time is in hours.

WALTZ: Choosing the time during the cycle when variables were changing most quickly did present some problems in getting the model to behave properly, but in the final analysis this starting time was as good as any. In line (16), then, we are dealing with four basic variables in the model. Starting at TIM0, time progresses linearly, and events begin to take place. The reason that time progresses linearly is that the rate of change of time (ΔTIME) is specified as constant in line (7) (a Δ in front of a level variable means its rate of change). Line (7) indicates that we are moving the clock ahead in steps of 0.25 hours or 15 minutes. Since this model is written with a constant derivative of time, we need to specify it only once, and that is why

ΔTIME is specified in the data section, whereas Δ LH, ΔFR, and ΔES are specified in the part of the model that is recalculated throughout the run.

SCHWARTZ: Paul, why are derivatives being used in this at all?

WALTZ: We are dealing with a number of continuous processes in which the variables can be viewed as changing continuously. This is different from a discrete process, in which variables take on a fixed number of values. In that case we would be dealing not with derivatives, but with the increments by which they would change up or down. We are using derivatives here because ES, LH, and FR do change continuously with time, at least to the outside observer of the system.

SCHWARTZ: In equations (33), (34), and (35), what you are calculating is ΔFR, ΔLH, and ΔES; what we want to plot, however, is not the change, but the actual level of the variable at each point of time. Where are the equations that get us back to level?

WALTZ: Once you have the starting value as given in line (16) and the rates of change (33), (34), (35), you can calculate the value of each of these variables at any point in time by adding on or subtracting from equation (16). You start with certain values—for example, time starts at 16 and then at each iteration in the model, 15 minutes is added. As far as the value of estrogen is concerned, it starts as ESCP (defined in line (3) as 15 pg/ml), and its rate of change is determined by equation (35). The actual calculation in which the amount of the change is being added (or subtracted) to the previous value is not explicit in these model equations; internal program parts are doing that work. Another example: line (33) of the model says that the rate of change of follicle radius is given by everything to the right of the left arrow (←); this is the formula that calculates the current rate of change of FR. The expression of this formula is a model-building activity; calculating the new follicle radius, given this rate of change, is a detail best handled by the simulation program. Since what is on the right-hand side of the arrow in (33) is formidable, I think it would be best to skip up to lines (29) and (30), which are simpler to look at. Line (29) reads: the follicle surface area (FA) is given by the sphere formula $4\pi r^2$.

SCHWARTZ: Where is π?

WALTZ: Well, that's what "circle (○) 4" means—○4 reads 4π in this language (APL). Anyway, what we have is ○4 × FR × FR, with FR being one of the basic levels given in line (16). (Incidentally, the way APL language operates is that you specify what the operations are and what variables are needed to make them up. This language executes its statements from right to left; the parentheses do make a difference in terms of

how calculations are executed. What happens in line (29) is that FR is first multiplied by FR, and that is then multiplied by 4, which is then multiplied by π in order to produce the follicle area.) Line (30) follows: the follicle volume is calculated as $(4/3)\pi r^3$.

SCHWARTZ: I would like to make a comment. The reader might well ask, at this point, why we don't use either area or radius as the sole indicator of follicular growth. The answer is complicated. Briefly, in our first modeling we did start out using just follicle radius, because you can stimulate an ovulation by taking a large follicle radius and making it become a small one. But we felt that as a follicle grew, increasing surface area and then volume, some effects on estrogen secretion rate might occur that would be proportional *independently* to surface area and to volume.

WALTZ: Let's return to line (33), where the rate of change of the follicle radius (ΔFR) is calculated as a function of—and here I will go from right to left—LH (the current LH level); G, a constant which has to do with the growth rate of the follicle as a function of the amount of LH; T, which is simply a signal used during runs to turn the effect of LH on follicle radius off or on. (In effect, when T is 1, that part of the equation reads simply G×LH.)

SCHWARTZ: May I interrupt to point out that G and T are defined in lines (2) and (4)?

WALTZ: In line (2), G is a parameter, and it has been permitted to vary over wide ranges during the years that we've been working with the simulation. It has never been measured empirically. For this particular model it is set at 0.01. Back to line (33). After calculating the term T×G×LH, that term is added to everything in parentheses to the left. The next calculation is that the minimum follicle radius (FRMIN) is subtracted from the current follicle radius. The minimum follicle radius is a device by which we simulate the radius associated with the new follicle after ovulation. This new starting radius, defined in line (4), is 0.01 microns: its value is very small, but we have found it more convenient to use it rather than zero; it helps make the rest of the model run and achieve consistent results. If we start at zero, since the follicle growth rate is exponential, small changes in the starting value could achieve fairly significant changes later on; therefore, we start at the value of FRMIN.

SCHWARTZ: Here I will remind Paul that I did not arbitrarily select FRMIN just to please him for the simulation; the very nature of the process by which follicles are produced in the ovary is such that all of the follicles that are ever going to be present in the rat ovary are present at a very small diameter within a couple of days of birth and actually do start out growing at some point at approximately this radius. They are not at zero. What turns out to be convenient for Paul as a systems analyst happens to be true for me as an endocrinologist.

WALTZ: Next in the model is a statement of "loss" of follicle radius due to atresia (ATR). Since we do not expect that the follicle radius will ever get below FRMIN, the loss due to atresia is a function only of the amount by which the present follicle radius exceeds FRMIN (FR−FRMIN).

SCHWARTZ: Are you referring to that zero with the bar ($\lceil$) there? You haven't explained the meaning of that symbol.

WALTZ: It's an APL symbol. Reading from the right, first FRMIN is calculated, then the larger of zero and that quantity is calculated—that is, FRMIN is used as long as it is bigger than zero, but if it is less than zero, "take zero as the value." This symbol ($\lceil$) means maximum. The result of that calculation is then multiplied by the atresia factor (ATR), which in line (2) is assigned the value of 0.014.

SCHWARTZ: The atresia factor is really a loss rate constant for atresia; that may seem funny, since we are used to seeing loss rate constants only for hormone levels in endocrinology. We are using an atresia loss (= 1/72 hr = 0.014) for two reasons, one of which is in the real world, while the other has to do with the modeling. If we had no way in the model to get rid of a follicle once it started growing except by ovulating it, we could get a growth to infinity in the absence of an LH surge. Thus if we were testing a model and not getting an ovulatory surge, we would be in trouble. Now every ovarian physiologist knows that that isn't what happens—follicles growth to a certain size, they mature under the influence of LH (and FSH), and then if the mature follicle is not ovulated by a surge of LH within a few days, it becomes atretic and incapable of responding to a late surge; it starts declining in size and eventually disappears from the ovary. So here is a factor that both is convenient for the model and represents a fact of ovarian physiology.

WALTZ: Summarizing line (33), follicle radius is a function basically of two terms added together: the contribution from the amount of LH that is present and the loss due to atresia. Line (34), where the rate of change of LH is calculated, is a function of two terms also, although the second term, BLH, is actually a composite and is calculated in line (31). BLH, the production or secretion rate of LH, is added to beta×LH (beta is the loss rate constant for LH, having the dimensions of time^{-1}).

Before finishing the three derivatives (ΔFR, ΔLH, ΔES), let me skip up to line (31) and discuss how BLH is calculated. It is a function of two things; the right-hand formula is A0 × A2 divided by A2 + ES. This is a hyperbolic formula for calculating the negative effect of estrogen on LH production. As estrogen levels increase, the denominator term becomes smaller. When estrogen is 0, the expression is A0 × A2 divided by A2, which equals just A0 as the production rate of LH in the absence of estrogen feedback. The first term in equation (31) is the surge, which is zero most of the time (except when it is made to become nonzero and adds to the production rate of LH).

SCHWARTZ: I feel that line (31) is the basic equation of the system in the sense that it is a "feedforward" equation. In its absence the whole system runs down to zero as LH→0; that would be equivalent to taking the pituitary out. The physiological necessity for A0 is as follows: For many years we've known that when one takes the ovary out, estrogen levels approach or reach zero, and there is a high rate of secretion of LH from the pituitary gland because of a positive input or action we have designated A0.

When we first started modeling we felt the need to have a data-based value for A0; the only one we could find was from an article by Gay and Bogdanove (1968) in which they had measured, by bioassay in castrated rats, the blood levels of LH before and after hypophysectomy. Since the animals were castrated, they had no estrogen feedback. Gay and Bogdanove assumed a distribution volume of 10 ml; from blood LH, loss rate constant, and assumed distribution volume, they calculated a basic LH secretion rate by the pituitary of 156 ng/ml/hr.

That was the best figure we had available; as you can see on line (2), that is the value of A0 used at the present time. We knew that estrogen was exerting a negative feedback on LH, because if you inject an excess of estrogen, LH levels go down near zero. Finally, we inserted a surge factor, which added on to the difference between A0 and what was subtracted from the estrogen feedback. The reason for adding a surge was that the maximum value of LH during the surge actually exceeds the values that one finds in the absence of estrogen feedback; that is, the LH value during the surge is equal not to A0 but to a higher value.

When we first began modeling (Schwartz and Waltz 1970), we used a linear equation to describe the relationship between A0 and ES. A0 was put in as the positive factor, and the effect of feedback was calculated as ES times the negative feedback constant, A2. This equation cannot be linear, because with the value A0 = 156, the steady-state values of LH are too high in the linear model, and yet when we took the ovaries out and actually measured the LH production rate, it came remarkably close to this older value of 156. So we have decided that the equation is not linear, and we now represent it as hyperbolic. As Paul just pointed out, in line (31), if ES = 0, then A0 = 156. This is a good representation of the LH secretion rate in the absence of the ovary. Paul, I think you wanted to comment on the hyperbolic form itself.

WALTZ: Yes, because you could a priori choose any mathematical form to represent the effect of estrogen on LH production. We decided that the equation would have to produce LH at the rate A0 in the absence of estrogen LH, but that with the addition of a small amount of estrogen, LH production would become considerably more depressed than it would have been if the formula had been linear (as it was in previous models). A small amount of estrogen depresses LH considerably more than a large amount does, unlike what one would expect from a linear form. The hyperbolic form was chosen only because it appears to have the correct shape. The A2 value in line (31) is the slope of the curve that represents LH as a negative function of estrogen; in the previous linear form, line (31) read SURGE + A0 − (A2 × ES); A2 was the derivative or slope of the LH production curve; it is still the derivative when ES = 0 in line (31). We have not found a value for A2 from the rat literature, so A2 is not a measured parameter of the system (as you can see in line (2), A2 is not specified). It is a parameter, and A2 and A3 (a feedforward constant) are calculated from AES and ALH, which are specified in line (2). Those values are steady-state values of estrogen and LH, reasonably well known from the literature, and are used to calculate the feedback constants A2 and A3 by solving two simultaneous equations, (14) and (15). The calculation of A2 and A3 is in lines (13), (14), and (15) at the beginning of the run, where the basic inputs are the steady-state levels of LH (ALH) and estrogen (AES). These equations are derived by assuming a steady-state—the derivatives of LH and estrogen are 0 in lines (34) and (35)—and then solving two equations with two unknowns.

SCHWARTZ: I would like to add to what Paul said about the calculation of A3 and A2, in terms of the origins of the numbers that go into equations (13), (14), and (15)—that is, which are real values and which are made up? Paul has indicated that A2 and A3 are computed by solving the steady state of (34) and (35). ALPHA2, the loss rate constant for estrogen, comes from Jensen's data. BETA, the loss rate constant of LH, comes from the literature and has also been measured in our laboratory. What Paul means by the steady-state value for LH and estrogen (that is, ALH and AES) is that: (a) if there were no surge LH levels in the blood, LH would be measured around 10 ng/ml (depending on standard used), shown on line (2) as ALH; (b) steady-state values for estrogen tend to remain at the value for AES—4pg/ml—which appears on line (2). To summarize, we are taking some measurements that we know (namely ALPHA2, BETA, ALH, AES, and A0) and using these in two simultaneous equations

to get values that we do not know (namely A2 and A3).

WALTZ: The variable DEN in line (13) is simply being used as an intermediate variable in the calculation —it's a "place" to store a result.

This brings us to line (35), the rate of change equation for estrogen. The first term is ALPHA2 × ES, which computes the loss rate of estrogen. The second term, A3 × LH, is the positive feedforward of LH on estrogen. Both the second and third terms are positive, but we have kept the direct effects of LH, A3 × LH, and the follicle effect (FES) separate, since evidence suggests at least two sources of estrogen production, one from the growing follicle (FES) and one from another compartment of the ovary (A3 × LH). The variable T appears in line (33) and again in (35); T multiplies the sum of FES and A3 × LH in (35). When T = 0, there is no positive effect on estrogen, and ES will decay according to the first term in that equation—to zero, which simulates ovariectomy.

WALTZ: No, T multiplies everything to its right. The product A3 × LH is added to FES, comprising total estrogen production, but the T multiplies all of that. When T = 0, the estrogen secretion rate will immediately go to zero, and ES will also go to zero in the time it takes to decay. When T = 0, the follicle radius will be affected only by atresia, and it will also go to zero (line (33)). The effect of setting T to zero and restarting the simulation is that estrogen, within four hours, goes to a very small value, and the follicle radius decays more slowly.

SCHWARTZ: Paul, would you consider setting T to zero a way of "ovariectomizing" the model?

WALTZ: Yes, except that the follicle is not removed from the system; everything around it is removed!

SCHWARTZ: Yes, but the follicle is simply retained temporarily by its atresia rate constant. That's not biologically correct, of course, because if you take the ovary out—

WALTZ: It's out. But it's a useful sort of ovariectomy, because you can observe the effect of atresia on the follicle at the same time. It's the equivalent of taking the ovary out and putting back the follicle and having it gradually become atretic and disappear —line (33).

So that's the explanation for lines (33), (34), and (35), except for an investigation of where FES comes from. It represents the production of estrogen by the follicle and is calculated on line (32). We have already discussed follicle area and follicle volume. FES is contributed to positively by the surface area of the follicle, but it is suppressed by the volume of the follicle. The equation is (M × FA) − (N × FV). Since FA is proportional to FR × FR, and FV is proportional to FR cubed, as FR grows there will be a point where the negative term of (32) is bigger than the first term.

At that point all the calculations to the right of the maximum sign ($\ulcorner$) will be negative, and no "follicle" estrogen will be produced (FES = 0). But while the follicle radius is small, the M × FA term dominates; then the follicle will secrete estrogen. That seems to correspond reasonably well to observations. (As we originally modeled line (32) it would have read "follicle estrogen is proportional to the first power of follicle radius," but it was very difficult to model the growth of estrogen production by the follicle in that way, because at the beginning of the cycle there was too much estrogen being produced, and at the end, not enough.)

SCHWARTZ: I would like to make a "physiological" comment about equation (32). We started out with a rather simple FES, just a function of follicle radius. Paul was dissatisfied with the outputs because he felt that their "shape" was wrong, and I must confess that I had the same feeling. While we were discussing this, he asked whether there was any reason to think that the effects of follicle growth on estrogen secretion rate might have a greater effect at the beginning than toward the end of follicle growth. As I considered the spherical growth of the follicle and the probable thecal and granulosal sources of estrogen, it occurred to me that as the surface area of the follicle sphere grows, initially the estrogen production is going to be very high; as the volume gets large enough, the follicle probably runs ahead of blood supply; any estrogen produced might have more difficulty getting into the bloodstream and the follicle lumen. This is particularly true, I believe, just after the LH surge has started to act.

Thus here is a case where a systems analyst asks an endocrinologist for some basis on which he can obtain a rather odd-looking formula, and the endocrinologist can think through the ovarian system and see one possibility as to why it might work this way. I feel that a basic strength of the model that we have constructed has been exactly that kind of interactive approach. At no point has either one of us forced the other into an uncomfortable situation just for the purpose of getting a cycle out of the model.

WALTZ: In line (32) M and N are positive and negative feedback constants of follicle area and follicle volume, respectively. Only M needs to be specified as an independent parameter, however. Since eventually the follicle area and follicle volume effects become equal, as soon as we know the follicle radius which that equality corresponds to, we can calculate the other constant. M is specified on line (2) as 0.39. Equation (12) says that N is calculated as 3 × M divided by 4. The 4 here is the radius of the follicle at which the two effects become equal and cancel each other out. The follicle production of estrogen is suppressed when the follicle radius becomes 4 microns.

With respect to parameters M and G, M is used to calculate the positive production of estrogen by the follicle, and G is used to calculate the rate of follicle growth as a function of LH—line (33). Both these parameters were experimented with in modeling for a long time in order to come up with values that made the simulation results look reasonable. Neither has been the result of any empirical experiments.

SCHWARTZ: There is still one parameter whose origin we have not described: the atresia factor. I estimated from the rat literature that if a follicle is mature on the day of proestrus and does not ovulate within three days, it is no longer ovulable. So we calculated the loss rate constant on the basis of 1/72 hours.

The question we are now left with, both physiologically and in the model, is what it is that causes the LH surge and ovulation. The literature on the rat tells us several things about this surge that must be modeled. Everett and Sawyer's (1950) original work using pentobarbital blockade showed that if ovulation were blocked on a day of proestrus, the surge would be released 24 hours late. If it were blocked for a second day, it would be released 24 hours after that. Furthermore, if the lighting conditions around the animal were reversed, the time of surge was reversed. Thus it seemed necessary to postulate a "clock" function in the system that sets a time during the 24 hours when it is "permissible" to have the surge.

The second point that appears to be important physiologically is that the surge did not take place every day, but—under normal circumstances—only once every four or every five days. In a series of empirical experiments, we tried to elucidate the necessary antecedent conditions; it appears from much data that estrogen levels had to reach some threshold value, or a threshold rate of rise, in order for this surge of LH to take place on the afternoon of proestrus. If you blocked the estrogen, you could block the surge.

Thus from experimental data, we came up with two necessary and (we felt) sufficient conditions for triggering an LH surge: (1) estrogen had to exceed a threshold value and (2) the right time of day—some time after 1400—had to be achieved. The third physiological "imperative" was that after the surge was released, a certain latent period had to elapse before ovulation could occur. In ovulation the follicle was, in a sense, wiped out, with a new follicle appearing. These physiological processes are represented in the remaining equations of the model.

Before winding up my contribution to the background for the next section, let me point out that THES—line (4)—is the threshold value for estrogen, which we are assuming has to be achieved; it was empirically determined from data by Brown-Grant et al. (1970). We have assumed that when estrogen hits a value of 10 pg/ml, "something" gets turned on. With respect to the question of a "clock" function, the LH surge under normal conditions appears to be unable to start much before two hours after the midpoint of the light period, which is 1400; it can go on for several hours after that but then fades out. It appears to be difficult, if not impossible, to elicit an LH surge in a rat on any alternating lighting condition much before 1400 or much after 1800. That is what determined our selection of "permissible" times.

WALTZ: The next discussion will concentrate on lines (18) through (28) of the model, together with lines (5) and (6), where a function called CLDATA is inserted in the model in the form of a series of number pairs. The first pair of each number is the clock time, and the second is the value of the function CLDATA. The first pair says that at 0000hr, CLDATA is 0; at 1100 the value is still 0; at 1200 it is 0.2; at 1300 it is 0.5; at 1400 it is 1. It remains 1 through 1700; then at 1800 it begins to fall until at 2000 it is again 0. Equations (18) to (28) constitute a whole and are called an APL section; line (18) reads "branch to APL."

The first time "branch to APL" occurs, the status of the model is set to BEGIN, control is passed to line (23), and the cycle starts. As events take place throughout the cycle the status changes, moving from BEGIN at (23) to the label END (line (28)), then to NEW CYCLE—line (19), and then back down again. The advancing of model status is done statement by statement.

Let's start with line (23), which reads "go to the next (NXT) block," when the surge is equal to zero. The surge is calculated as a function of CLDATA and CTIME. The constant CCON is in line (4) and is set to 100, just for unit purposes. (If we set CCON to 0, it is not possible to have a SURGE, an "experiment" that we have done now and then to simulate the anovulatory state of "persistent estrus.") In line (23) the surge is calculated by the equation CCON×CTIME AFGEN CLDATA. (AFGEN is a linear function interpolator; in case "time" is not one of those times specified in the table—(for example, if it is 1130—it would linearly interpolate the value of the SURGE as between 0 and 12.) In equation (17) CTIME is calculated by linearly advancing the 24-hr clock. Thus the surge is calculated, and if it is positive, the model status is unchanged, starting at line (23), waiting for the surge to finish. Of course, at the start of the model, the surge is not zero because TIM0 is 16—line (4). When the model starts, CLDATA is not zero, and therefore the surge is not zero, so we stay at line (23) and the model continues to advance *in time* until the surge becomes zero. When the surge ends, model status advances to line (24).

At that point OVTIME is calculated. This is the time when ovulation will actually take place and is the cur-

rent time, plus six hours. This is the latent period (six hours from the end of the surge) previously discussed. Since there is no NXT block associated with this calculation, we advance immediately to the next block, and that block says "NXT 1," which always means go to the block or line. This serves the purpose of skipping over the "OVTIME equals TIME plus 6" calculation (if the NXT 1 statement were not there, line (24) might be repeated and the time of ovulation would never be reached). We now enter the block—line (26)—that calculates whether or not the time of ovulation has been reached. As soon as the surge becomes zero, OVTIME is calculated and we move through to line (26); when the time of ovulation is reached, model status again advances and we drop through to the next line (27) which says "reduce the follicle radius to minimum."

In line (27), then, follicle radius is reduced to 0.01. Since there is no NXT block associated with that calculation, we move to line (28), which is an "end" statement and says "back to new cycle"—line (19). This expresses the fact that we have an iterative process that represents itself, and we are always restarting at this point—a new cycle with a follicle reduced to its minimum radius. Line (19) is another NXT block, which only serves to advance the model status to line (20), the NXT block that tests whether or not estrogen is less than threshold. We are presently testing whether or not estrogen has actually gone below threshold (which might be an automatic function in a normal animal), because in some of the "pathological" cases that we've examined with the model, estrogen has stayed above threshold after ovulation; as a result of that, we would get another surge the next day. Thus we wait at line (20) until estrogen goes below threshold, and then we can actually fall through that block and begin testing for increasing estrogen levels—line (21)—in the next cycle.

SCHWARTZ: You are saying that as long as we retain equation (20), we would not be able to use this model to give us repeated surges, although I can tell you, for example, that in ovariectomized animals, given a high dose after a low dose of estrogen, there *can* be repeated surges at 24-hour intervals (Legan and Karsch 1975). At the moment we can't model this, although we know how to change the model in order to model it.

WALTZ: That's right. If no mechanism is testing whether estrogen goes below threshold, repeated surges would be possible, if ES stayed high; or if ES simply dropped slightly below threshold and then came back up, that would do it. Whether or not there is an actual biological mechanism that corresponds to this is, of course, anybody's guess.

So, then, after being assured that estrogen is below threshold at the start of a new cycle, line (21) is entered and begins testing whether or not estrogen has achieved threshold value. The model waits at line (21) until estrogen has achieved threshold in the next cycle. The status then advances to line (22), at which clock time is tested. First estrogen must achieve threshold, then the clock must indicate that it is a possible surge time by seeing whether or not the clock data function, CTIME AFGEN CLDATA, is bigger than zero. This will not occur until about 1100, according to line (5). Shortly after 1100 that calculation will show a positive value and the status advances to line (23), where the surge is calculated—later to be added to line (31)—and we wait until the surge becomes zero again. Thus we drop from line (22) to (23) when the surge becomes positive, and we drop from (23) to (24) when it returns to zero. The entire series of calculations from (18) to (28) describes the events that take place within the cycle, with a sequential "logic" in which the central nervous system–pituitary axis is controlling the cycle.

It seems worthwhile to compare again the types of things that are happening in the discrete section—(18) to (28)—with what happens in the continuous sections, lines (17) and (29) through (31). While the model is in the discrete section it waits at the various statements within it; however, all the calculations in the continuous portion of the model are being done continuously at each ΔT. As the condition that those continuous equations produce causes the next discrete state to be achieved, the discrete section will move to that next state. Thus the interplay between the continuous and the discrete sections is critical to achieving accurate modeling of the whole process. This method of modeling reflects our prejudice that the reproductive cycle really is a series of events that take place on a background of continuously changing hormone levels.

Before discussing the computer print-outs we must discuss several lines—(1), (7), (8), (9), (10), (11), and (36)—which are in the model only as a concession to the computer. Line (1) names the model and has to be executed before the model can be run. Line (7) is a "method" statement, specifying the method used (trapezoidal = TRAPZ) to integrate the derivatives needed in calculating (33), (34), and (35). As discussed before, ΔTIME is the increment of time—0.25 hours. TO is the time at which the simulation stops, 140 hours. Line (8) says which variables we are going to print; 5 specifies how many digits of the answer we want to see. As you can see, we print clock time (CTIME) and BLH, the secretion rate of LH. Line (9) shows the variables that are going to be plotted, defines the symbol to be used for each, and delineates the plot scales. For ES, an example, 50 means "make the plot 50 positions wide and plot ES using a symbol E on a scale from 0 pg/ml to 50 pg/ml." Lines (10) and

(11), always the same for models like this, are the first two statements of the model section. When, in order to make changes, a computer run is stopped in the middle of a run by pressing the attention key on the terminal, generally the model will stop at line (10). Finally, line (36) checks to see whether it is time to print on the terminal. Many calculations are made throughout the cycle when output is not desired; the instruction reads "print the output every four hours" (more precisely it says to calculate whether four evenly divides time; if so, zero does equal four modulo time and there will be a print).

There are three output illustrations; the first (Figure 8.2) shows a run through the whole cycle; Figure 8.3 shows the run with an ovariectomy performed partway through; Figure 8.4 shows an "exploded" time view of the events around the surge and ovulation. Let's take a look at each of these print-outs in turn.

In Figure 8.2 the model has been activated by typing its name—ES model. A list of the parameters is printed, because at the start of each computer run these parameters may be changed for experimentation; it is also useful for documentation purposes later. In this case each of these values is as specified on line (2) of the model in Figure 8.1. A2 and A3 are calculated from other parameters and constants, as explained previously, and are displayed here because, although they

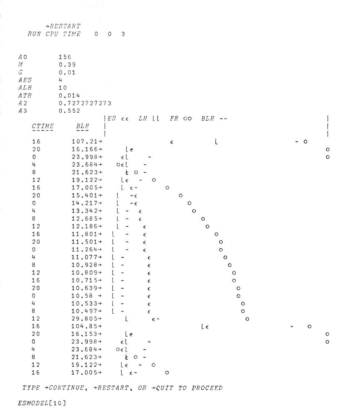

Figure 8.2 Print-out of complete cycle.

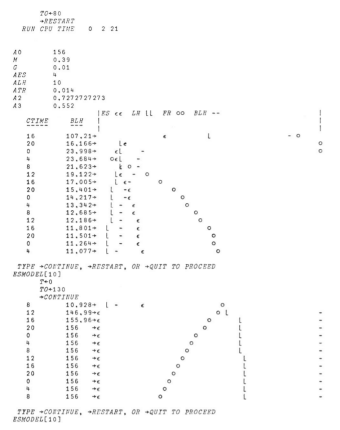

```
        TO←80
       →RESTART
   RUN CPU TIME   0  2 21

A0      156
M       0.39
G       0.01
AES     4
ALH     10
ATR     0.014
A2      0.7272727273
A3      0.552

                 |ES  ϵϵ  LH  LL  FR  OO  BLH --              |
  CTIME     BLH  |                                            |
   ───      ───  |                                            |
   16     107.21→             ϵ         L             - o     |
   20      16.166→    Lϵ                                    o
    0      23.998→   ϵL     -                               o
    4      23.684→    oϵL   -
    8      21.623→    Ł o -
   12      19.122→    Lϵ   -  o
   16      17.005→    L  ϵ-        o
   20      15.401→    L   -ϵ         o
    0      14.217→    L   -ϵ          o
    4      13.342→    L  -  ϵ          o
    8      12.685→    L  -    ϵ         o
   12      12.186→    L  -    ϵ           o
   16      11.801→    L   -    ϵ            o
   20      11.501→    L  -      ϵ             o
    0      11.264→    L   -      ϵ           o
    4      11.077→    L  -       ϵ            o

   TYPE →CONTINUE, →RESTART, OR →QUIT TO PROCEED
ESMODEL[10]
        T←0
       TO←130
      →CONTINUE
    8      10.928→   L  -     ϵ             o
   12     146.99→ϵ                    o  L               -
   16     155.96→ϵ                  o       L            -
   20      156   →ϵ                   o        L         -
    0      156   →ϵ                     o       L        -
    4      156   →ϵ                   o         L        -
    8      156   →ϵ                      o       L       -
   12      156   →ϵ                     o          L     -
   16      156   →ϵ                       o         L    -
   20      156   →ϵ                     o          L     -
    0      156   →ϵ                       o         L    -
    4      156   →ϵ                     o           L    -
    8      156   →ϵ                  o              L    -

   TYPE →CONTINUE, →RESTART, OR →QUIT TO PROCEED
ESMODEL[10]
```

Figure 8.3 Print-out showing ovariectomy partway through run.

```
        T←1
       TO←100
       ∇ESMODEL[36□1]
[36]  →CHK  0=4|TIME
            ///////
[36]  →CHK  0
[37]   ∇
      →RESTART
   RUN CPU TIME   0  1 56

A0      156
M       0.39
G       0.01
AES     4
ALH     10
ATR     0.014
A2      0.7272727273
A3      0.552

                 |ES  ϵϵ  LH  LL  FR  OO  BLH --              |
  CTIME     BLH  |                                            |
   ───      ───  |                                            |
   16     107.21→             ϵ         L             - o     |

   TYPE →CONTINUE, →RESTART, OR →QUIT TO PROCEED
ESMODEL[10]
       ∇ESMODEL[3ϵ□1]
[36]  →CHK  0
[36]  →CHK  0=1|TIME∇
       TO←130
      →CONTINUE
    4      10.533→   L  -      ϵ              o
    5      10.523→   L  -      ϵ              o
    6      10.514→   L  -      ϵ              o
    7      10.505→   L  -      ϵ              o
    8      10.497→   L  -      ϵ              o
    9      10.489→   L  -      ϵ               o
   10      10.482→   L  -      ϵ              o
   11      10.476→   L  -      ϵ              o
   12      29.805→    L         ϵ-            c
   13      57.919→          L   ϵ    -        o
   14     105.94→              Ł        o         -
   15     104.84→                 Lϵ         o-
   16     104.85→                 Lϵ            -  o
   17     105.5 →               ϵ L          -     o
   18      56.694→          Ł       -              o
   19      29.91 →         L  ϵ-                   o
   20      16.153→     Lϵ                          o
   21      23.139→    ϵL   -                       o
   22      24.149→    ϵL   -                       o
   23      24.019→    ϵL   -                       o
    0      23.998→    ϵL   -                       o
    1      24    →    ϵL   -                       o
    2      24    →o   ϵL   -
    3      23.928→ o   ϵL   -
    4      23.684→   oϵL   -
    5      23.296→   ϵL   -
    6      22.802→   ϵ♭   -
```

Figure 8.4 Exploded time view of events around surge and ovulation.

cannot be directly changed, they are a function of A0, ALH, and AES. Then the simulation display appears. On the left, the CTIME and BLH variables are printed; on the right the designated variables are plotted. The plot heading repeats the symbols for the variables. The strokes down the side of the symbols delineate the maximum range; the ranges are not printed, but they were specified in the model at line (9).

On this run, we are starting at CTIME = 16, in the middle of the critical period. Values of follicle radius, estrogen, and LH are high, but they are dropping off rapidly. For the first few hours the follicle radius grows and then drops off, as ovulation takes place between 0000 and 0400 hours. The display proceeds down the page for five days, with ovulation again occurring on the fourth day. The follicle radius, after initially growing and being reduced to a small value, grows again until it achieves its maximum growth during the surge period on the fourth day or proestrus. Estrogen grows in parallel with the follicle radius to a point, but then when the follicle grows very quickly during the surge, the estrogen secreted by the follicle drops out and estrogen levels drop off. LH starts out high in the critical period, drops off to a low value,

seems to fall further during metestrus and diestrus where no "events" are taking place, and then rises during the sixteenth hour when the surge is activated. At the end of the display of the print-out the words *type*, *continue*, *restart*, or *quit to proceed* are printed automatically. The model waits at ES MODEL (10), which is the first statement of the model section (Figure 8.1). If we wish to continue, we type *continue* and the simulation will be carried to more units of time. *Restart* starts the simulation over again, and *quit* enables us to leave the model.

SCHWARTZ: When I first started modeling the rat estrous cycle with Paul, I said that the model had to fit two criteria at a minimum: one was that it had to cycle, and, as we have seen from Figure 8.2, it does indeed provide cyclic output without having cyclic input. The second criterion was that if we did an ovariectomy, estrogen had to go to zero and LH had to rise to maximum values. This "experiment" is performed in the second simulation (Figure 8.3), which goes for 80 hours; at that point T was set to zero. You will see that plasma estrogen drops very quickly, as would be expected from its short half-life; follicle radius goes down slowly (we have already commented on that); and LH rises immediately to a high value. Something is wrong in the rapid rise of LH, since it is not nearly as fast in the female rat. This indicates minimally that a biological time delay is present, which is not in the model. The third simulation (Figure 8.4) simply displays the rapidly changing events of the proestrous critical period on an expanded time scale of one hour. At the start of proestrous (0400) the follicle radius is reasonably high, estrogen levels have already started up, and LH values follow. Actually, estrogen levels have been shown, in our laboratory, to go up somewhat earlier than this, and the LH surge in the simulation is occurring a bit early, but manipulation of the values of G and M would correct these two differences from the empirical evidence. Ovulation takes place early in the morning of estrus (0200), as it does in the real rat.

Empirical LH and Estrogen Curves
The data in Figure 8.5 represent measurements of LH and estrogen (and FSH) during the four-day and five-day estrous cycle. Data are running averages.

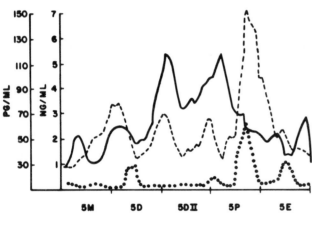

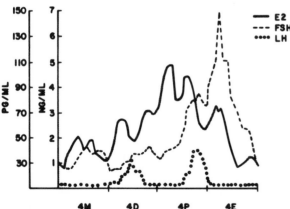

Figure 8.5 Empirical LH and estrogen curves. From Nequin et al. (1975).

References

Arimura, A., H. G. Spies, and A. V. Schally. Relative insensitivity of Rhesus monkeys to LH-releasing hormone (LH-RH). J. Clin. Endocrinol. Metab. 36:372, 1973a.

Arimura, A., M. Saito, Y. Notake, T. Kumasaka, N. Nishi, Y. Yaoi, A. Kato, T. Koyama, A. Horiguchi, T. Kobayashi, and S. Nurayama. Clinical studies with synthetic LH-releasing hormone (LH-RH) in Japan. In *Hypothalamic hypophysiotropic hormones*, eds. C. Gual and E. Rosemberg. Amsterdam: Excerpta Medica, 1973b.

Atkinson, L. E., A. N. Bhattacharya, S. E. Monroe, D. J. Dierschke, and E. Knobil. Effects of gonadectomy and plasma LH concentration in the Rhesus monkey. Endocrinology 87:847, 1970.

Atkinson, L. E., J. Hotchkiss, G. Fritz, A. H. Surve, J. D. Neill, and E. Knobil. Circulating levels of steroids and chorionic gonadotropin during pregnancy in the Rhesus monkey, with special attention to the rescue of the corpus luteum in early pregnancy. Biol Reprod. 12:335, 1975.

Barraclough, C. A. Modification in the CNS regulation of reproduction after exposure of prepubertal rats to steroid hormones. Recent Prog. Horm. Res. 22:503, 1966.

Barraclough, C. A. Sex steroid regulation of reproductive neuroendocrine processes. In *Handbook of physiology*, Section 7, Vol. 2: *Female reproductive system*, ed. R. O. Greep. Baltimore: Williams & Wilkins, 1973.

Beattie, C. W., C. S. Campbell, L. G. Nequin, L. F. Soyka, and N. B. Schwartz. Barbiturate blockade of tonic LH secretion in the male and female rat. Endocrinology 92:1634, 1973.

Beck, T. W., and J. J. Reeves. Serum luteinizing hormone (LH) in ewes treated with various dosages of 17β-estradiol at three stages of the anestrous season. J. Anim. Sci. 36:566, 1973.

Ben-Jonathan, N., R. S. Mical, and J. C. Porter. Superfusion of hemipituitaries with portal blood. I. LRF secretion in castrated diestrous rats. Endocrinology 93:497, 1973.

Beyer, C., R. B. Jaffe, and V. L. Gay. Testosterone metabolism in target tissues: Effects of testosterone and dihydrotestosterone injection and hypothalamic implantation on serum LH in ovariectomized rats. Endocrinology 91:1372, 1972.

Bhattacharya, A. N., D. J. Dierschke, T. Yamaji, and E. Knobil. The pharmacologic blockade of the circhoral mode of LH secretion in the ovariectomized Rhesus monkey. Endocrinology 90:778, 1972.

Bogdanove, E. M. Failure of anterior hypothalamic lesions to prevent either pituitary reactions to castration or the inhibition of such reactions by estrogen treatment. Endocrinology 72:638, 1963.

Bolt, D. J. Changes in the concentration of luteinizing hormone in plasma of rams following administration of oestradiol, progesterone or testosterone. J. Reprod. Fertil. 24:435, 1971.

Bolt, D. J., H. E. Kelley, and H. W. Hawk. Release of LH by estradiol in cycling ewes. Biol. Reprod. 4:35, 1971.

Bosu, W. T. K., E. D. B. Johansson, and C. Gemzell. Patterns of circulating oestrone, oestradiol-17-beta and progesterone during pregnancy in the Rhesus monkey. Acta Endocrinol. (Kbh.) 74:743, 1973.

Boyar, R., J. Finkelstein, H. Roffwarg, S. Kapen, E. Weitzman, and L. Hellman. Synchronization of augmented luteinizing hormone secretion with sleep during puberty. New Engl. J. Med. 287:582, 1972a.

Boyar, R., M. Perlow, L. Hellman, S. Kapen, and E. Weitzman. Twenty-four pattern of luteinizing hormone secretion in normal men with sleep stage recording. J. Clin. Endocrinol. Metab. 35:73, 1972b.

Bradbury, J. Direct action of estrogen on the ovary of the immature rat. Endocrinology 68:115, 1961.

Brown-Grant, K., J. M. Davidson, and F. Greig. Induced ovulation in albino rats exposed to constant light. J. Endocrinol. 57:7, 1973.

Brown-Grant, K., D. Exley, and F. Naftolin. Peripheral plasma estradiol and luteinizing hormone concentrations during the estrous cycle of the rat. J. Endocrinol. 48:295, 1970.

Butler, W. R., P. V. Nalven, L. R. Willeth, and D. J. Bolt. Patterns of pituitary release and cranial output of LH and prolactin in ovariectomized ewes. Endocrinology 91:793, 1972.

Caldwell, B. V., R. J. Scaramuzzi, S. A. Tillson, and I. H. Thorneycroft. Physiologic studies using antibodies to steroids. In *Immunologic methods in steroid determination*, eds. F. G. Peron and B. V. Caldwell. New York: Appleton-Century-Crofts, 1970.

Caligaris, L., J. J. Astrada, and S. Taleisnik. Release of luteinizing hormone induced by estrogen injection into ovariectomized rats. Endocrinology 88:810, 1971a.

Caligaris, L., J. J. Astrada, and S. Taleisnik. Biophasic effect of progesterone on the release of gonadotropin in rats. Endocrinology 89:331, 1971b.

Caligaris, L., J. J. Astrada, and S. Taleisnik. Influence of age on the release of luteinizing hormone induced by oestrogen and progesterone in immature rats. J. Endocrinol. 55:97, 1972.

Caligaris, L., J. J. Astrada, and S. Taleisnik. Development of the mechanisms involved in the facilitatory and inhibitory effects of ovarian steroids on the release of follicle-stimulating hormone in th⁻ immature rat. J. Endocrinol. 58:547, 1973.

Canales, E. S., A. Zarate, J. Garrido, C. Leon, J. Soria, and A. V. Schally. Study on the recovery of pituitary FSH function during puerperium using synthetic LRH. J. Clin. Endocrinol. Metab. 38:1140, 1974.

Cargille, C. M., J. L. Vaitukaitis, J. A. Bermudoz, and G. T. Ross. A differential effect of ethinyl estradiol upon plasma FSH and LH relating to time of administration in the menstrual cycle. J. Clin. Endocrinol. Metab. 36:87, 1973.

Chamley, W. A., J. M. Brown, M. E. Cerini, I. A. Cumming, J. R. Goding, J. M. Obst, A. Williams, and C. Winfield. An explanation for the absence of post-parturient ovulation in the ewe. J. Reprod. Fertil. 32:334 (Abstract), 1973a.

Chamley, W. A., J. M. Buckmaster, M. E. Cerini, I. A. Cumming, J. R. Goding, J. M. Obst, A. Williams, and C. Winfield. Changes in the levels of progesterone, corticosteroids,

estrone, estradiol-17β, luteinizing hormone and prolactin in peripheral plasma of the ewe during late pregnancy and at parturition. Biol. Reprod. 9:30, 1973b.

Chamley, W. A., J. R. Findlay, I. A. Cumming, J. M. Buckmaster, and J. R. Goding. Effect of pregnancy on the LH response to synthetic gonadotropin-releasing hormone in the ewe. Endocrinology 94:291, 1974a.

Chamley, W. A., J. K. Findlay, H. Jonas, I. A. Cumming, and J. R. Goding. Effect of pregnancy on the FSH response to synthetic gonadotropin-releasing hormone in ewes. J. Reprod. Fertil. 37:109, 1974b.

Charters, A. C., W. D. Odell, and J. C. Thompson. Anterior pituitary function during surgical stress and convalescence: Radioimmunoassay measurement of blood TSH, LH, FSH, and growth hormone. J. Clin. Endocrinol. Metab. 29:63, 1969.

Clifton, D. K., R. A. Steiner, and J. A. Resko. Estrogen-induced gonadotrophin release in the ovariectomized Rhesus monkey and its advancement by progesterone. Biol. Reprod. 13:190, 1975.

Coppings, R. J., and P. V. Malven. Rhythmic patterns of endogenous LH release in castrate sheep receiving exogenous LH. Proc. Soc. Exp. Biol. Med. 148:64, 1975.

Corbin, A., and J. C. Story. "Internal" feedback mechanism: Response of pituitary FSH stalk median eminence follicle stimulating hormone–releasing factor to median eminence implants of FSH. Endocrinology 80:1006, 1967.

Corbin, A., and G. V. Upton. Effect of dopaninergic blocking agents on plasma luteinizing hormone releasing hormone activity in hypophysectomized rats. Experientia 29:1552, 1973.

Cronin, T. J. Influence of lactation upon ovulation. Lancet 2:422, 1968.

Crystal, C. D., G. A. Sawaya, and V. C. Stevens. Effects of ethinyl estradiol on the secretion of gonadotropins and estrogens in postpartum women. Am. J. Obstet. Gynecol. 116:616, 1973.

Csapo, A. I., E. Knobil, H. J. Vander Nolen, and W. G. Wiest. Peripheral plasma progesterone levels during human pregnancy and labor. Am. J. Obstet. Gynecol. 110:630, 1971.

Cumming, I. A., J. M. Buckmaster, J. C. Cerini, M. E. Cerini, W. A. Chamley, W. A. Findlay, and J. K. Goding. Effect of progesterone on the release of luteinizing hormone induced by a synthetic gonadotrophin-releasing factor in the ewe. Neuroendocrinology 10:338, 1972.

Curtis, G. C. Psychosomatics and chronobiology: Possible implications of neuroendocrine rhythms. A review. Psychosom. Med. 34:235, 1972.

Dailey, R. A., and J. D. Neill. Seasonal aperiodicity of gonadotropin secretion in monkeys. Proceedings of the annual meeting of the Society for the Study of Reproduction. Abstract #32. 1975.

Davis, S. L., and M. L. Borgen. Dynamic changes in plasma prolactin, luteinizing hormone and growth hormone in ovariectomized ewes. J. Anim. Sci. 38:795, 1974.

Debeljuk, L., A. Arimura, and A. V. Schally. Pituitary responsiveness to LH-releasing hormone in intact female rats of different ages. Endocrinology 90:1499, 1972.

Diekman, N. A., and P. V. Malven. Effect of ovariectomy and estradiol on LH patterns in ewes. J. Anim. Sci. 37:562, 1973.

Dierschke, D. J., A. N. Bhattacharya, L. E. Atkinson, and E. Knobil. Circhoral oscillations of plasma LH levels in the ovariectomized Rhesus monkey. Endocrinology 87:850, 1970.

Dierschke, D. J., T. Yamaji, F. J. Karsch, R. F. Weick, G. Weiss, and E. Knobil. Blockage by progesterone of estrogen-induced LH and FSH release in the Rhesus monkey. Endocrinology 92:1496, 1973.

Dierschke, D. J., F. J. Karsch, R. F. Weick, G. Weiss, J. Hotchkiss, and E. Knobil. Hypothalamic-pituitary regulation of puberty: Feedback control of gonadotropin secretion in the Rhesus monkey. In *The control of the onset of puberty*, eds. M. M. Grumbach, G. D. Grave, and F. Mayer. New York: John Wiley & Sons, 1974.

Dierschke, D. J., G. Weiss, and E. Knobil. Sexual maturation in the female Rhesus monkey and the development of estrogen-induced gonadotrophic hormone release. Endocrinology 94:198, 1974b.

Döcke, F., and G. Dorner. A possible mechanism by which progesterone facilitates ovulation in the rat. Neuroendocrinology 4:139, 1969.

Dörner, V. G., W. Rohde, and L. Krell. Auslösung eines positiven ostrogen feedback effect bei homosexuellen männern. Endokrinologie 60:297, 1972.

Ducker, M. J., J. C. Bowman, and A. Temple, The effect of constant photoperiod on the expression of oestrus in the ewe. J. Reprod. Fertil. Suppl. 19:143, 1973.

Eisenfeld, A. Ontogeny of the estrogen and androgen receptors. In *The control of the onset of puberty*, eds. M. M. Grumbach, G. D. Grave, and F. Mayer. New York: John Wiley & Sons, 1974.

Ellicott, A. R., H. J. Benoit, R. C. Strickler, and C. A. Woolever. Influence of pentobarbital on luteinizing hormone levels in ovariectomized and intact ewes. Biol. Reprod. 9:107 (Abstract #119), 1974.

Everett, J. W. Central neural control of reproductive functions of the adenohypophysis. Physiol. Rev. 44:374, 1964.

Everett, J. W. Photoregulation of the ovarian cycle in the rat. In *La photoregulation de la réproduction chez les oiseaux et les mammifères*. Colloques Internationals du Centre National de la Recherche Scientifique 172:388, 1970.

Everett, J. W., and C. H. Sawyer. A neural timing factor in the mechanism by which progesterone advances ovulation in the cyclic rat. Endocrinology 45:581, 1949.

Everett, J. W., and C. H. Sawyer. A 24-hour periodicity in the "LH release apparatus" of female rats, disclosed by barbiturate secretion. Endocrinology 47:198, 1950.

Faiman, C., R. J. Ryan. S. J. Zwirek, and M. E. Rubin. Serum FSH and hCG during human pregnancy. J. Clin. Endocrinol. Metab. 28:1321, 1969.

Feder, H. H., K. Brown-Grant, and C. S. Corker. Pre-ovulatory progesterone, the adrenal cortex and the "critical period" for luteinizing hormone release in rats. J. Endocrinol. 50:29, 1971.

Ferin, M., P. W. Carmel, E. A. Zimmerman, M. Warren, R. Perez, and R. L. Vande Wiele. Location of intrahypothalamic estrogen-responsive sites influencing LH secretion in the female Rhesus, 1974c.

Ferin, M., A. Tempone, P. Zimmering, and R. L. Vande Wiele. Effect of antibodies to 17β-estradiol and progesterone on the estrous cycle of the rat. Endocrinology 85:1070, 1969.

Ferin, M., S. Kharlaf, M. Warren, I. Dyrenfurth, R. Jewelewicz, W. White, and R. L. Vande Wiele. Effects of continuous infusions of synthetic LH releasing hormone (LRH) in Rhesus monkeys. Proceedings of the annual meeting of The Endocrine Society, Abstract #198, 1973.

Ferin, M., I. Dyrenfurth, S. Cowchock, M. Warren, and R. L. Vande Wiele. Active immunization to 17β-estradiol and its effects upon the reproductive cycle of the Rhesus monkey. Endocrinology 94:765, 1974a.

Ferin, M., M. Warren, I. Dyrenfurth, R. L. Vande Wiele, and W. F. White. Response of Rhesus monkeys to LRH throughout the ovarian cycle. J. Clin. Endocrinol. Metab. 38:231, 1974b.

Flerko, B. Control of gonadotrophin secretion in the female. In *Neuroendocrinology*, eds. L. Martini, and W. F. Ganong. New York: Academic Press, 1966.

Ford, J. J., and R. M. Melampy. Changes in serum and pituitary LH levels following ovariectomy in lactating rats. Fed. Proc. 30:474 (Abstract), 1971.

Foster, D. L., T. A. C. Cruz, G. L. Jackson, B. Cook, and A. V. Nalbandov. Regulation of luteinizing hormone in the fetal and neonatal lamb. III. Release of LH by the pituitary *in vivo* in response to crude ovine hypothalamic extract or purified porcine gonadotrophin releasing factor. Endocrinology 90:673, 1972a.

Foster, D. L., and F. J. Karsch. Development of the mechanism(s) regulating the preovulatory LH surge in female sheep. Proceedings of the annual meeting of the Society for the Study of Reproduction, Abstract #235, 1975.

Foster, D. L., J. A. Lemons, and G. D. Niswender. Sequential patterns of LH/FSH during sexual development of female lambs. Fourth International Congress of Endocrinology, Washington, D. C. Abstract #252, Excerpta Medica Internat. Congr. Ser. #256, 1972b.

Franchimont, P. Human gonadotrophin secretion. J. R. Coll. Physicians Lond. 6:263, 1972.

Fritz, G. R., D. J. Dierschke, R. F. Weick, and E. Knobil. Influence of season on ovulation in the Rhesus monkey in a closed environment. Proceedings of the annual meeting of the American Association for Laboratory Animal Science, Abstract, 1974.

Gay, V. L. Decreased metabolism and increased serum concentrations of LH and FSH following nephrectomy of the rat: Absence of short-loop regulatory mechanisms. Endocrinology 95:1582, 1974.

Gay, V. L., and E. M. Bogdanove. Disappearance of endogenous and exogenous luteinizing hormone activity from the plasma of previously castrated, acutely hypophysectomized rats: An indirect assessment of synthesis and release rates. Endocrinology 82:359, 1968.

Gay, V. L., A. R. Midgley, Jr., and G. D. Niswender. Patterns of gonadotrophin secretion associated with ovulation. Fed. Proc. 29:1880, 1970.

Gay, V. L., and N. A. Sheth. Evidence for a periodic release of LH in castrated male and female rats. Endocrinology 90:158, 1972.

Gay, V. L., and R. L. Tomacari. Follicle stimulating hormone secretion in the female rat: Cyclic release is dependent on circulating androgen. Science 184:75, 1974.

Goding, J. R., K. J. Catt, J. M. Brown, C. C. Kalbenback, I. A. Cumming, and B. J. Mole. Radioimmunossay for ovine luteinizing hormone. Secretion of luteinizing hormone during estrus and following estrogen administration in the sheep. Endocrinology 85:133, 1969.

Goldenberg, R. L., J. L. Vaitukaitis, and G. T. Ross. Estrogen and follicle stimulating hormone interactions on follicle growth in rats. Endocrinology 90:1492, 1972.

Goy, R. W., and J. A. Resko. Gonadal hormones and behavior of normal and pseudohermaphroditic non-human female primates. Recent Prog. Horm. Res. 28:707, 1972.

Grumbach, M. M., J. C. Roth, S. L. Kaplan, and R. P. Kelch. Hypothalamic-pituitary regulation of puberty: Evidence and concepts derived from clinical research. In *The control of the onset of puberty*, eds. M. M. Grumbach, G. D. Grave, and F. Mayer. New York: John Wiley & Sons, 1974.

Gual, C., R. Lichtenberg, A. V. Schally, A. Ortiz, G. Perez-Palacios, and A. R. Midgley, Jr. Effects of sex steroids on the pituitary responsiveness to synthetic LH- and FSH-releasing hormone (LH-RH/FSH-RH) in women. In *Hypothalamic hypophysiotropic hormones*, eds. C. Gual and E. Rosemberg. Amsterdam: Excerpta Medica, 1973.

Hagino, N. Influence of constant light on the hypothalamic regulation of pituitary function in the baboon. Endocrinology 89:1322, 1971.

Hammonds, J., M. Velasco, and I. Rothchild. Effect of sudden withdrawal or increase of suckling on serum LH levels in ovariectomized post parturient rats. Endocrinology 92: 206, 1973.

Hansel, W., P. W. Concannon, and J. H. Lukaszewska. Corpora lutea of the large domestic animals. Biol. Reprod. 8: 222, 1973.

Hauger, R. L., F. J. Karsch, and D. L. Foster. Role of progesterone in the negative feedback inhibition of LH secretion during the estrous cycle of the ewe. Proceedings of the annual meeting of the Society for the Study of Reproduction, Abstract #92, 1975.

Hodgen, G. D., M. L. Dufau, K. J. Catt, and W. W. Tullner. Estrogens, progesterone and chorionic gonadotropin in pregnant Rhesus monkey. Endocrinology 91:896, 1972.

Hoffman, J. C. The influence of photoperiods on reproductive functions in female mammals. In *Handbook of physiology*, Section 7: *Endocrinology*, Vol. 2: *Female reproductive system*, ed. R. O. Greep. Baltimore: Williams & Wilkins, 1973.

Hoffman, J. C., and N. B. Schwartz. Timing of postpartum ovulation in the rat. Endocrinology 76:620, 1965.

Hooley, R. D., R. W. Baxter, W. A. Chamley, I. A. Cumming, H. A. Jonas, and J. K. Findlay. FSH and LH response to gonadotropin-releasing hormone during the ovine estrous cycle and following progesterone administration. Endocrinology 95:937, 1974.

Hori, T., M. Ide, and T. Miyake. Ovarian estrogen secretion during the estrous cycle and under the influence of exogenous gonadotropins in rats. Endocrinol. Japan 15:215, 1968.

Howland, B. E., A. H. Akbar, and F. Stormshak. Serum LH levels at luteal weight in ewes following a single injection of estradiol. Biol. Reprod. 5:25, 1971.

Hunter, G. L., and I. M. R. Van Aarde. Influence of season of lambing on postpartum intervals to ovulation and oestrus in lactating and dry ewes at different nutritional levels. J. Reprod. Fertil. 32:1, 1973.

Jackson, G. L., and J. C. Thurmon. Absence of a critical period in estrogen-induced release of LH in the anestrous ewe. Endocrinology 94:918, 1974.

Jaffe, R. B., and W. R. Keye, Jr. Estradiol augmentation of pituitary responsiveness to gonadotropin-releasing hormone in women. J. Clin. Endocrinol. Metab. 39:850, 1974.

Jaffe, R. B., P. A. Lee, and A. R. Midgley. Serum gonadotrophins before, at the inception of, and following human pregnancy. J. Clin. Endocrinol. Metab. 29:1281, 1969.

Jonas, H. A., L. A. Salamonsen, H. G. Burger, W. A. Chamley, I. A. Cumming, J. K. Findlay, and J. R. Goding. Release of FSH after administration of gonadotrophin-releasing hormone or estradiol to the anestrous ewe. Endocrinology 92: 862, 1973.

Kalra, S. P., K. Ajika, I. Krulich, C. P. Fawcett, M. Quijada, and M. W. McCann. Effects of hypothalamic and preoptic electrochemical stimulation on gonadotropin and prolactin release in proestrous rat. Endocrinology 88:1150, 1971.

Kapen, S., R. Boyar, L. Hellman, and E. D. Weitzman. Episodic release of luteinizing hormone at mid-menstrual cycle in normal adult women. J. Clin. Endocrinol. Metab. 36:724, 1973.

Karsch, F. J., D. J. Dierschke, and E. Knobil. Sexual differentiation of pituitary function: Apparent difference between primates and rodents. Science 179:484, 1973a.

Karsch, F. J., D. J. Dierschke, R. F. Weick, T. Yamaji, J. Hotchkiss, and E. Knobil. Positive and negative feedback control by estrogen of luteinizing hormone secretion in the Rhesus monkey. Endocrinology 92:799, 1973b.

Karsch, F. J., and D. L. Foster. Sexual differentiation of the mechanism controlling the preovulatory discharge of luteinizing hormone in sheep. Endocrinology 97:373, 1975.

Karsch, F. J., R. F. Weick, W. R. Butler, D. J. Dierschke, C. Krey, G. Weiss, J. Hotchkiss, T. Yamaji, and E. Knobil. Induced LH surges in the Rhesus monkey: Strength-duration characteristics of the estrogen stimulus. Endocrinology 92: 1740, 1973c.

Karsch, F. J., R. F. Weick, J. Hotchkiss, D. J. Dierschke, and E. Knobil. An analysis of the negative feedback control of gonadotropin secretion utilizing chronic implantation of ovarian steroids in ovariectomized Rhesus monkeys. Endocrinology 93:478, 1973d.

Keverene, E. B., and R. F. Michael. Annual changes in the menstruation of Rhesus monkeys. J. Endocrinol. Metab. 48: 669, 1970.

Knobil, E. On the control of gonadotropin secretion in the Rhesus monkey. Recent Prog. Horm. Res. 30:1, 1974.

Koves, K., and B. Halasz. Location of the neural structure triggering ovulation in the rat. Neuroendocrinology 6:180, 1970.

Krey, L. C., W. R. Butler, and E. Knobil. Surgical disconnection of the medial basal hypothalamus and pituitary function in the Rhesus monkey. I. Gonadotropin secretion. Endocrinology 96:1073, 1975.

Krey, L. C., W. R. Butler, G. Weiss, R. F. Weick, D. J. Dierschke, and E. Knobil. Influences of endogenous and exogenous gonadal steroids on the actions of synthetic LRF in the Rhesus monkey. In *Hypothalamic hypophysiotropic hormones*, eds. C. Gual and E. Rosemberg. Amsterdam: Excerpta Medica, 1973.

Krey, L. C., and J. W. Everett. Multiple ovarian responses to single estrogen injections early in rat estrous cycles: Impaired growth, luteotropic stimulation and advanced ovulation. Endocrinology 93:377, 1973.

Kulin, H. E., and E. O. Reiter. Delayed sexual maturation with special emphasis on the occurrence of the syndrome in the male rat. In *The control of the onset of puberty*, eds. M. M. Grumbach, G. D. Grave, and F. Mayer. New York: John Wiley & Sons, 1974a.

Kulin, H. E., and E. O. Reiter. Personal communication, 1974b.

Land, R. B., J. Thimonier, and J. Polletier. Possibilité d'induction d'une décharge de LH par une injection d'oestrogene chez l'agnelle femelle en fonction de l'age. C. R. Acad. Sci. Paris, Serie D 271:1549, 1970.

Lawton, E. E. Facilitatory feedback effects of adrenal and ovarian hormones on LH secretion. Endocrinology 90:575, 1972.

Legan, S. J., and F. J. Karsch. A daily signal for the LH surge in the rat. Endocrinology 96:57, 1975.

Lewis, P. E., D. J. Bolt, and E. K. Inskeep. Luteinizing hormone release and ovulation in anestrous ewes. J. Anim. Sci. 38:1197, 1974.

Leyendecker, G., S. Wardlaw, B. Leffek, and W. Nocke. Studies on the function of the hypothalamic sexual centre in the human: Presence of a cyclic centre in a genetic male. Acta Endocrinol. (Kbh.) Suppl. 155:36 (Abstract #36), 1971.

Leyendecker, G., S. Wardlaw, and W. Nocke. Experimental studies on the endocrine regulations during the periovulatory phase of the human menstrual cycle. Acta Endocrinol. (Kbh.) 71:160, 1972.

Liao, S. Cellular receptors and mechanisms of action of steroid hormones. Int. Rev. Cytol. 41:87, 1975.

Libertun, C., K. J. Cooper, C. F. Fawcett, and S. M. McCann. Effects of ovariectomy and steroid treatment on hypophyseal sensitivity to purified LH-releasing factor (LRF). Endocrinology 94:518, 1974.

Liefer, R. W., D. L. Foster, and P. J. Dziuk. Levels of LH in the sera and pituitaries of female lambs following ovariectomy and administration of estrogen. Endocrinology 90:981, 1972.

Linkie, D. N., and G. D. Niswender. Serum levels of prolactin luteinizing hormone, and follicle stimulating hormone during pregnancy in the rat. Endocrinology 90:632, 1972.

Lisk, R. D. Sexual behavior: Hormonal control. In *Neuroendocrinology*, vol. 2, eds. L. Martini and W. F. Ganong. New York: Academic Press, 1967.

Lostroh, A. J. Induction of ovulation with 20α-OH-progesterone in the hypophysectomized rat. Fed. Proc. 30:595 (Abstract #2239), 1971.

Macdonald, G. J. Normal and induced ovulation in simians. In *Handbook of physiology*, Section 7: *Endocrinology*, Vol. 2: *Female reproductive system*, ed. R. O. Greep. Baltimore: Williams & Wilkins, 1973.

Macdonald, G. J., K. Yoshinaga, and R. O. Greep. Progesterone values in monkeys near term. Am. J. Phys. Anthropol. 38:201, 1973.

Magee, K., J. Baisinska, B. Quarrington, and H. C. Stancer. Blindness and menarch. Life Sci. [I] 9:7, 1970.

Mann, D., and C. A. Barraclough. Role of estrogen and progesterone in facilitating LH release in 4-day cyclic rats. Endocrinology 93:694, 1973.

Martin, J. E., L. Tyrey, J. W. Everett, and R. E. Fellows. Variation in responsiveness to synthetic LH-releasing factor (LRF) in proestrous and diestrous—3 rats. Endocrinology 94:556, 1974.

Martini, L., F. Fraschini, and M. Motta. Neural control of pituitary functions. Recent Prog. Horm. Res. 24:439, 1968.

McCann, S. M., and V. D. Ramirez. The neuroendocrine regulation of hypophysial luteinizing hormone secretion. Recent Prog. Horm. Res. 20:131, 1964.

McCormack. C. E., and R. K. Meyer. Minimal age for induction of ovulation with progesterone in rats: Evidence for neural control. Endocrinology 74:793, 1964.

McCormack, C. E. Acute effects of altered photoperiods on the onset of ovulation in gonadotropin-treated immature rats. Endocrinology 93:403, 1973.

McLean, B. K., N. Chang, and Winer-Nikitovitch. Ovarian steroids directly alter luteinizing hormone (LH) release by pituitary homografts. Endocrinology 97:196, 1975.

Midgley, A. R., Jr., and R. B. Jaffe. Regulation of human gonadotropins. X. Episodic fluctuation of LH during the menstrual cycle. J. Clin. Endocrinol. Metab. 33:962, 1971.

Monroe, S. E., R. B. Jaffe, and A. R. Midgley, Jr. Regulation of human gonadotropins. XII. Increase in serum gonadotropins in response to estradiol. J. Clin. Endocrinol. Metab. 34:342, 1972.

Morishige, W. K., G. J. Pepe, and I. Rothchild. Serum luteinizing hormone, prolactin and progesterone during pregnancy in the rat. Endocrinology 92:1527, 1973.

Naftolin, F., K. Brown-Grant, and C. S. Corker. Plasma and pituitary luteinizing hormone and peripheral plasma estradiol concentrations in the normal estrous cycle of the rat and after experimental manipulation of the cycle. J. Endocrinol. 53:17, 1972.

Nakano, R., F. Kayashima, A. Mori, J. Kotsuji, N. Hashiba, and S. Tojo. Gonadotrophin response to luteinizing hormone releasing factor (LRF) in puerperal women. Acta Obstet. Gynecol. Scand. 53:303, 1974.

Nalbandov, A. V. Control of luteal function in mammals. In *Handbook of physiology*, Section 7, Vol. 2: *Female reproductive system*, ed. R. O. Greep. Baltimore: Williams & Wilkins, 1973.

Nallar, R., and S. M. McCann. Luteinizing hormone releasing factor in plasma of hypophysectomized rats. Endocrinology 76:272, 1965.

Neill, J. D. Sexual differences in hypothalamic regulation of prolactin secretion. Endocrinology 90:1154, 1972.

Nequin, L. G., and N. B. Schwartz. Adrenal participation in the timing of mating and LH release in the cyclic rat. Endocrinology 88:325, 1971.

Nequin, L. G., J. A. Alvarez, and N. B. Schwartz. Steroid control of gonadotropin release. J. Steroid Biochem. 6:1007, 1975.

Nett, T. M., A. M. Akbar, and G. D. Niswender. Serum levels of luteinizing hormone and gonadotropin-releasing hormone in cycling, castrated and anestrous ewes. Endocrinology 94:713, 1974.

Netter, A., A. Gorins, K. Thomas, M. Cohen, and J. Joubinzux. Blockage du pic d'ovulation de LH et de FSH par la progesterone à faibles doses chez la femme. Ann. Endocrinol. (Paris) 34:430, 1973.

Nillius, S. J., and L. Wide. Effects of progesterone on the serum levels of FSH and LH in postmenopausal women treated with estrogen. Acta Endocrinol. (Kbh.) 67:362, 1971.

Odell, W. D., and R. S. Swerdloff. Progesterone-induced luteinizing and follicle-stimulating hormone surge in postmenopausal women: A stimulated ovulatory peak. Proc. Natl. Acad. Sci. US 61:529, 1968.

Ostergard, D. R., A. F. Parlow, and D. E. Townsend. Acute effect of castration on serum FSH and LH in the adult woman. J. Clin. Endocrinol. Metab. 31:43, 1970.

Parlow, A. F. Differential action of small doses of estradiol on gonadotropins in the rat. Endocrinology 75:1, 1964.

Pelletier, J., and J. Thimonier. Comparison of the induced preovulatory LH discharge in lactating and dry sheep during seasonal anoestrus. J. Reprod. Fertil. 33:310, 1973.

Pepe, G. J., and I. Rothchild. A comparative study of serum progesterone levels in pregnancy and in various types of pseudopregnancy in the rat. Endocrinology 95:275, 1974.

Proudfit, C. M., and N. B. Schwartz. Reversal by pentobarbital blockage of ovulation after cardiac puncture. Endocrinology 94:526, 1974.

Przekop, F., and E. Domanski. Induction of ovulation in sheep by electrical stimulation of hypothalamic regions. J. Endocrinol. Met. 64:305, 1970.

Przekop, F., B. Skubiszewski, and E. Domanski. Lack of masculinizing effect of testosterone injected pre- and postnatally into the female lambs. Acta Physiol. Pol. 25:555, 1974.

Radford, H. M. Pharmacological blockade of ovulation in the ewe. J. Endocrinol. 34:135, 1966.

Radford, H. M., and A. L. C. Wallace. Central nervous blockade of oestradiol-stimulated release of luteinizing hormone in the ewe. J. Endocrinol. 60:247, 1974.

Ramirez, V. D. Endocrinology of puberty. In Handbook of physiology, Section 7, Vol. 2: Female reproductive system, ed. R. O. Greep. Baltimore: Williams & Wilkins, 1973.

Reeves, J. J., T. W. Beck, and T. M. Nett. Serum FSH in anestrus ewes treated with 17β-estradiol. J. Anim. Sci. 38:374, 1974.

Reeves, J. J., P. K. Chakraborty, T. D. Colter, T. W. Beck, and G. K. Tarnsky. Physiological studies on synthetic LH-RH/FSH-RH in domestic animals. In Hypothalamic hypophysiotropic hormones, eds. C. Gual and E. Rosemberg. Amsterdam: Excerpta Medica, 1973.

Reiter, E. O., R. L. Goldenberg, J. L. Vaitukaitis, and G. T. Ross. Evidence for a role of estrogen in the ovarian augmentation reaction. Endocrinology 91:1518, 1972a.

Reiter, E. O., H. E. Kulin, and S. M. Hamwood. The absence of positive feedback between estrogen and luteinizing hormone in sexually immature girls. Pediat. Res. 8:740, 1974.

Reiter, E. O., H. E. Kulin, and D. Loriaux. FSH suppression during short term hCG administration: A gonadally mediated process. J. Clin. Endocrinol. Metab. 34:1080, 1972b.

Resko, J. A., N. L. Norman, G. D. Niswender, and H. G. Spies. The relationship between progestins and gonadotropins during the late luteal phase of the menstrual cycle in Rhesus monkeys. Endocrinology 94:128, 1974.

Restall, B. J., H. M. Radford, and A. L. C. Wallace. Response of lactating ewes to injection of oestradiol benzoate or testosterone propionate. J. Reprod. Fertil. 28:164 (Abstract), 1972.

Reyes, F. I., J. S. D. Winter, and C. Faiman. Pituitary-ovarian interrelationships during the puerperium. Am. J. Obstet. Gynecol. 114:589, 1972.

Riesen, J. W., R. K. Meyer, and R. C. Wolf. The effect of season on occurrence of ovulation in the Rhesus monkey. Biol. Reprod. 5:111, 1971.

Riggs, D. S. The mathematical approach to physiological problems. Baltimore: Williams & Wilkins, 1963.

Rippel, R. H., R. H. Moyer, E. S. Johnson, and R. E. Mauer. Response of the ewe to synthetic gonadotropin releasing hormone. J. Anim. Sci. 38:605, 1974.

Robertson, H. A., and A. M. Rakha. The timing of the neural stimulus which leads to ovulation in the sheep. J. Endocrinol. 32:383, 1965a.

Robertson, H. A., and H. A. Rakha. Time of onset of oestrus in the ewe. J. Reprod. Fertil. 10:271, 1965b.

Robinson, T. J. The estrous cycle of the ewe and doe. In Reproduction in domestic animals, eds. H. H. Cole and P. T. Cupps. New York: Academic Press, 1959.

Roche, J. F., D. L. Foster, P. J. Karsch, and P. J. Dziuk. Effect of castration and infusion of melatonin on levels of luteinizing hormone in sera and pituitaries of ewes. Endocrinology 87:1205, 1970a.

Roche, J. F., P. J. Karsch, D. L. Foster, S. Takagi, and P. J. Dziuk. Effect of pinealectomy on ostrus, ovulation and luteinizing hormone in ewes. Biol. Reprod. 2:251, 1970b.

Rodgers, C., and N. R. Schwartz. Diencephalic regulation of plasma LH, ovulation, and sexual behavior in the rat. Endocrinology 90:461, 1972.

Root, A., A. DeCherney, D. Russ, G. Duckett, C. R. Garcia, and E. Wallach. Episodic secretion of luteinizing and follicle-stimulating hormones in gonadal and hypogonadal adolescents and adults. J. Clin. Endocrinol. Metab. 35:700, 1972.

Ross, G. T., C. N. Cargille, M. B. Lipsett, P. L. Rayford, J. R. Marshall, C. J. Strott, and D. Rodbard. Pituitary and gonadal hormones in women during spontaneous and induced ovulatory cycles. Recent Prog. Horm. Res. 26:1, 1970.

Rothchild, I. The corpus luteum–pituitary relationship: The association between the cause of luteotrophin secretion and the cause of follicular quiesence during lactation, the basis for a tentative theory of the corpus luteum–pituitary relationship in the rat. Endocrinology 67:9, 1960.

Said, S. A. H., and L. Wide. Serum levels of FSH and LH following normal parturition. Acta Obstet. Gynecol. Scand. 52:361, 1973.

Saito, S., K. Abe, N. Nagata, K. Tanaka, E. Nakamura, and T. Kaneko. Evaluation of pituitary function by use of LH-releasing hormone and thyrotropin-releasing hormone. In *Hypothalamic hypophysiotropic hormones*, eds. C. Gual and E. Rosemberg. Amsterdam: Excerpta Medica, 1973a.

Saito, H., A. Arimura, T. Kumasaka, N. Nishi, K. Kato, Y. Yaoi, and T. Koyama. Effects of administration of synthetic LH-RH at various phases of the menstrual cycle on uringary estrogen, pregnanediol and pregnanetrol excretion and on the subsequent events of the menstrual cycle in normal women. In *Hypothalamic hypophysiotropic hormones*, eds. C. Gual and E. Rosemberg. Amsterdam: Excerpta Medica, 1973b.

Salamonsen, L. A., H. A. Jonas, H. G. Burger, J. M. Buckmaster, W. A. Chamley, I. A. Cumming, J. K. Findlay, and J. R. Goding. A heterologous radioimmunossay for follicle stimulating hormone: Application to measurement of FSH in the ovine estrous cycle and in several other species including man. Endocrinology 93:610, 1973.

Scaramuzzi, R. J., S. A. Tillson, I. H. Thorneycroft, and B. V. Caldwell. Action of exogenous progesterone and estrogen on behavioral estrus and luteinizing hormone levels in the ovariectomized ewe. Endocrinology 88:1184, 1971.

Schwartz, N. B. Acute effects of ovariectomy on pituitary LH, uterine weight, and vaginal cornification. Am. J. Physiol. 207:1251, 1964.

Schwartz, N. B. A model for the regulation of ovulation in the rat. Recent Prog. Horm. Res. 25:1, 1969.

Schwartz, N. B. Mechanisms controlling ovulation in small mammals. In *Handbook of physiology*, Section 7: *Endocrinology*, Vol. 2: *Female reproductive system*, ed. R. O. Greep. Baltimore: Williams & Wilkins, 1973.

Schwartz, N. B. The role of FSH and LH and of their antibodies on follicle growth and on ovulation. Biol. Reprod. 10:236, 1974.

Schwartz, N. B., and C. E. McCormack. Reproduction, gonadal function and its regulation. Ann. Rev. Physiol. 34:425, 1972.

Schwartz, N. B., and P. Waltz. Role of ovulation in the regulation of the estrous cycle. Fed. Proc. 29:1907, 1970.

Shevah, Y., W. J. M. Black, W. R. Carr, and R. B. Land. The effect of lactation on the resumption of reproductive activity and the preovulatory release of LH in Finn × Dorset ewes. J. Reprod. Fertil. 38:369, 1974.

Shirley, B., J. Wolinsky, and N. B. Schwartz. Effects of a single injection of an estrogen antagonist on the estrous cycle of the rat. Endocrinology 82:859, 1968.

Short, R. V. In *The sexual endocrinology of the perinatal period*, eds. M. G. Forest and J. Bertrand. Collogue International INSERM, 1974.

Smith, B. The effect of diethylstilbesterol on the immature rat ovary. Endocrinology 69:238, 1961.

Spies, H. G., and G. D. Niswender. Effect of progesterone and estradiol on LH release and ovulation in Rhesus monkeys. Endocrinology 90:257, 1972.

Spies, H. G., and R. L. Norman. Interaction of estradiol and LHRH on release in Rhesus females: Evidence for a neural site of action. Endocrinology 97:685, 1975.

Spies, H. G., R. C. Franz, and G. D. Niswender. Patterns of luteinizing hormone in serum following administration of stalk-median eminence extracts to Rhesus monkeys. Proc. Soc. Exp. Biol. Med. 140:161, 1972.

Spies, H. G., J. A. Resko, and R. L. Norman. Evidence of preoptic hypothalamic influence on ovulation in the Rhesus monkey. Fed. Proc. 33 (Part I):222 (Abstract), 1974.

Stabenfeldt, G. H., M. Drost, and C. E. Franti. Peripheral plasma progesterone levels in the ewe during pregnancy and parturition. Endocrinology 90:144, 1972.

Stabenfeldt, G. H., and A. G. Hendrickx. Progesterone levels in the Bonnet monkey (*Macaca radiata*) during the menstrual cycle and pregnancy. Endocrinology 91:614, 1972.

Stabenfeldt, G. H., and A. G. Hendrickx. Progesterone studies in the *Macaca fascicularis*. Endocrinology 92:1296, 1973.

Stearns, E. L., J. S. D. Winter, and C. Faiman. Positive feedback effect of progestin upon serum gonadotropins in estrogen-primed castrate men. J. Clin. Endocrinol. Metab. 37:635, 1973.

Steiner, R. A., D. K. Clifton, H. G. Spies, and J. A. Resko. Feedback control of LH by estradiol in female, male and female pesudohermaphroditic Rhesus monkeys. Proceedings of the annual meeting of the Endocrine Society, Abstract #280, 1974.

Stone, S. C., R. P. Dickey, and A. Mickal. The acute effect of hysterectomy on ovarian function. Am. J. Obstet. Gynecol. 121:193, 1975.

Symons, A. M., N. F. Cunningham, and N. Saba. The gonadotrophic hormone response of anoestrous and cyclic ewes to synthetic luteinizing hormone-releasing hormone. J. Reprod. Fertil. 39:11, 1974.

Szontagh, F. E. Short-loop ("internal") pituitary-hypothalamus gonadotropin feedback in the human. Endocrinol. Exp. 7:65, 1973.

Takahashi, M., J. J. Ford, K. Yoshinaga, and R. O. Greep. Induction of ovulation in hypophysectomized rats by progesterone. Endocrinology 95:1322, 1975.

Taleisnik, S., L. Caligaris, and J. J. Astrada. Positive feedback of progesterone on the release of FSH and the influence of sex in rats. J. Reprod. Fertil. 22:89, 1970.

Thibault, C., M. Courot, L. Martinet, P. Mauleon, F. Mesnil du Buisson, R. Ortavant, J. Pelletier, and J. P. Signoret. Regulation of breeding season and estrous cycles by light and external stimuli in some mammals. In *Environmental in-*

fluences on reproductive processes, J. Anim. Sci. 25 Suppl.:119, 1966.

Thorneycroft, I. H., B. Sribyatta, W. K. Tom, R. M. Nakamura, and D. R. Mishell, Jr. Measurement of serum LH, FSH progesterone, 17-hydroxy-progesterone and estradiol-17β levels at 4-hour intervals during the periovulatory phase of the menstrual cycle. J. Clin. Endocrinol. Metab. 39:754, 1974.

Timonen, S., and E. Carpen. Multiple pregnancies and photoperiodicity. Ann. Chir. Gynaecol. Fenn. 57:135, 1968.

Tolis, G., H. Guyda, R. Pillorger, and H. G. Friesen. Breastfeeding: Effects on the hypothalamic pituitary gonadal axis. Endocrinol. Res. Commun. 1:293, 1974.

Treloar, O. L., R. C. Wolfe, and R. K. Meyer. Failure of a single neonatal dose of testosterone to alter ovarian function in the Rhesus monkey. Endocrinology 90:281, 1972.

Tsai, C. C., and S. S. C. Yen. Acute effects of intravenous infusion of 17β-estradiol on gonadotropin release in pre- and post-menopausal women. J. Clin. Endocrinol. Metab. 32:766, 1971.

Vande Wiele, R. L., J. Bogumil, I. Dyrenfurth, N. Ferin, R. Jewelowicz, M. Warren, T. Rizkallah, and G. Mikhail. Mechanisms regulating the menstrual cycle in women. Recent Prog. Horm. Res. 26:63, 1970.

Vande Wiele, R. L., and I. Dyrenfurth. Gonadotropin-steroid interrelationships. Pharmacol. Rev. 25:189, 1973.

Visser, H. K. A. Some physiological and clinical aspects of puberty. Arch. Dis. Child. 48:169, 1973.

Wallach, E. E., A. W. Root, and C. R. Garcia. Serum gonadotropin responses to estrogen and progesterone in recently castrated human females. J. Clin. Endocrinol. Metab. 31:376, 1970.

Wayneforth, H. B., G. S. Pope, and Z. D. Hosking. Secretion rates of oestrogens into the ovarian venous blood of pregnant rats. J. Reprod. Fertil. 28:191, 1972.

Weick, R. F. Acute and chronic effects of gonadal steroids on pulsatile discharges of LH in the castrate rat. Fed. Proc. 33 (Part I):231 (Abstract), 1974.

Weick, R. F., and J. M. Davidson. Localization of the stimulatory feedback effect of estrogen on ovulation in the rat. Endocrinology 87:693, 1970.

Weick, R. F., E. R. Smith, R. Dominquez, A. P. S. Dhariwal, and J. M. Davidson. Mechanism of stimulatory feedback effect of estradiol benzoate on the pituitary. Endocrinology 88:293, 1971.

Weick, R. F., D. J. Dierschke, F. J. Karsch, W. R. Butler, J. Hotchkiss, and E. Knobil. Periovulatory time courses of circulating gonadotropic and ovarian hormones in the Rhesus monkey. Endocrinology 93:1140, 1973.

Weiss, G., D. J. Dierschke, F. J. Karsch., J. Hotchkiss, W. R. Butler, and E. Knobil. The influence of lactation on luteal function in the Rhesus monkey. Endocrinology 93:954, 1973.

Winter, J. S. D., and C. Faiman. Serum gonadotropin concentrations in agonadal children and adults. J. Clin. Endocrinol. Metab. 35:561, 1972.

Yamaji, T., D. J. Dierschke, J. Hotchkiss, A. N. Bhattacharya, A. H. Surve, and E. Knobil. Estrogen induction of LH release in the Rhesus monkey. Endocrinology 89:1034, 1971.

Yamaji, T., D. J. Dierschke, A. N. Bhattacharya, and E. Knobil. The negative feedback control by estradiol and progesterone of LH secretion in the ovariectomized Rhesus monkey. Endocrinology 90:771, 1972.

Yannone, M. E. Hormonal changes in pregnancy. MCV Quart. 8:43, 1972.

Yen, S. S. C., and C. C. Tsai. Acute gonadotropin release induced by exogenous estradiol during the mid-follicular phase of the menstrual cycle. J. Clin. Endocrinol. Metab. 34:298, 1974.

Yen, S. S. C., C. C. Tsai, G. Vandenberg, and R. Rebar. Gonadotropin dynamics in patients with gonadal dysgenesis: A model for the study of gonadotropin regulation. J. Clin. Endocrinol. Metab. 35:897, 1972a.

Yen, S. S. C., G. Vandenberg, R. Rebar, and Y. Ehara. Variation of pituitary responsiveness to synthetic LRF during different phases of the menstrual cycle. J. Clin. Endocrinol. Metab. 35:931, 1972b.

Yen, S. S. C., R. Rebar, G. Vandenberg, F. Naftolin, H. Judd, Y. Ehara, K. J. Ryan, J. Rivier, M. Amoss, and R. Guillemin. Clinical studies with synthetic LRF. In *Hypothalamic hypophysiotropic hormones*, eds. C. Gual and E. Rosemberg. Amsterdam: Excerpta Medica, 1973.

Ying, S.-Y., and R. O. Greep. Effect of age of rat and dose of a single injection of estradiol benzoate (EB) on ovulation and the facilitation of ovulation by progesterone (P). Endocrinology 89:785, 1971.

Yuthasastrakosol, P., B. E. Howland, S. Simaraks, and W. M. Palmer. Estrogen-induced LH release in progesterone-treated ovariectomized ewes. Can. J. Anim. Sci. 54:565, 1974.

Zacharias, L., and R. J. Wurtman. Blindness: Its relation to age of menarche. Science 144:1154, 1964.

Zarate, A., E. S. Canales, J. Soria, C. MacGregor, P. J. Naneiro, and A. V. Schally. Pituitary responsiveness to synthetic luteinizing hormone-releasing hormone during pregnancy: Effect of follicle-stimulating hormone secretion. Am. J. Obstet. Gynecol. 116:1121, 1973.

Zeilmaker, G. H. The biphasic effect of progesterone on ovulation in the rat. Acta Endocrinol. (Kbh.) 51:461, 1966.

9 Secretion of Gonadotropins

Roger Guillemin, S. M. McCann,
C. H. Sawyer, and J. M. Davidson

9.1 Nature of Hypothalamic Hypophysiotropic Hormones Controlling the Secretion of Gonadotropins

The most important development in this area over the past decade was the final characterization—in brain extracts from two different species—of LRF, the hypothalamic controller of the secretion of luteinizing hormone (LH). Demonstrations of the existence in hypothalamic extracts of a substance stimulating the secretion of LH was reported by McCann et al. (1960), Harris (Campbell et al. 1961), and Guillemin (Courrier et al. 1961), then at Collège de France in Paris. The criteria involved in these early studies were laborious when specificity was of the essence.

The first partial purification of LRF was reported by Guillemin et al. (1962) with methods eventually used in the final isolation of LRF. Following these early studies, considerable difficulties were encountered in attempts to isolate LRF; it became rapidly obvious that the isolation of LRF would be an enormous undertaking, as only infinitesimal quantities of the (hypothetical) substance appeared to be present in each hypothalamic fragment. Also, simpler types of assays would have to be developed, assays more easily amenable to screening large numbers of fractions during any purification procedure, while retaining high specificity and characteristics relating linearly log doses to response.

Essentially two laboratories took up the challenge: Guillemin's group, at Baylor College of Medicine, collected some 5 million sheep hypothalamic fragments over four years, and Schally's group, at the Veterans Administration Hospital in New Orleans, collected some 2.5 million porcine hypothalamic fragments.

Considerable confusion prevailed in the literature until 1970, ranging from reports that an FSH-releasing factor had been separated from an LH-releasing factor and was one of the polyamines (Schally et al. 1968), to claims that the LH-releasing factor was not a polypeptide (White 1970).

Not until 1969 was an assay reported for gonadotropin-releasing factors, with all the necessary characteristics described above, based on the measurement by radioimmunoassay of the plasma levels of gonadotropins LH or FSH or both in normal male rats or, using an earlier preparation then designed for bioassays, in gonadectomized rats treated with estrogen and progesterone.

Meanwhile, in 1968, ovine thyrotropin-releasing factor (TRF) was isolated, and its structure was established the following year (Burgus et al. 1969) as that of the tripeptide pGlu-His-Pro-NH$_2$. This in itself was of significance for the efforts to characterize the gonadotropin-releasing factor: one of the hypothalamic releasing factors had been unquestionably characterized as an oligopeptide, thus removing to some extent the cloud of doubts which so far had accompanied the "elusive" hypothalamic hormones.

Highly purified ovine LRF was obtained and described in 1970 as a small polypeptide with a pGlu N-terminal residue (Amoss et al. 1970). Then early in 1971, both Schally's group (Schally et al. 1971a) and Guillemin's group (Amoss et al. 1971) reported simultaneously that porcine and ovine LRF had been isolated as a nonapeptide, either preparation (of porcine or ovine origin) containing the residues Glu 1, His 1, Ser 1, Leu 1, Gly 2, Arg 1, Thr 1, Pro 1. Schally's laboratory realized and reported a few months later (Matsuo et al. 1971) that porcine LRF was actually a decapeptide containing Trp 1 over and above the amino acids reported previously; furthermore, the same paper put forth a tentative proposal for a sequence of porcine LRF as pGlu-His-Trp-Ser-Tyr-Gly-Leu-Arg-Pro-Gly-NH$_2$, with the statement that a synthetic replicate of that sequence had biological activity. A few months later, ovine LRF was shown to have the same composition and sequence as porcine LRF (Burgus et al. 1971, 1972), the pure synthetic replicate having the full biological activity of LRF qualitatively and quantitatively (Monahan 1971).

The structure of porcine LRF was proposed and obtained on about 200 nanomoles of the peptide; that of ovine LRF was ascertained on less than 40 nanomoles—stressing the ingenuity and methodological extremes that had been necessary to attain this new knowledge.

It was also obvious that pure LRF, either of native or of synthetic origin, was stimulating the secretion of both LH and FSH, though with considerably different potencies, LRF releasing more LH than FSH in most systems studied. This led Schally et al. (1971b) to reverse their earlier position and to propose that the decapeptide LRF is the sole hypothalamic controller of the secretion of both gonadotropins.

By 1974 the synthetic LRF was available throughout

the world, in practically unlimited quantities. The synthetic material is highly active in humans to stimulate secretions of both gonadotropins LH and FSH. Synthetic LRF is widely used as a diagnostic tool to ascertain hypophyseal secretory ability for the gonadotropins. It is also used as a therapeutic agent in certain types of (hypothalamic) amenorrheas, oligospermia, or specific gonadotropic deficiencies; the therapeutic use of LRF is still in its infancy. Of importance for such uses will be the development of long-acting analogs or preparations of LRF, as the synthetic replicate of the native sequence has a very short biological half-life (a few minutes).

Structural analogs of LRF have been devised and synthesized with much greater specific activity than the native molecule, two of the more interesting types of these super-LRFs having one of several possible D-amino acids substituted for the Gly residue in position 6 (Monahan 1973) or a modified C-terminal residue or both (Fujino et al. 1972).

Analogs of LRF have been devised and synthesized that act as partial agonists and even as true competitive antagonists of LRF (Vale et al. 1972). Though the LRF antagonists designed and available so far are still of relatively low potency, they are of obvious interest as a totally novel approach to fertility regulation and contraception.

The possible existence of an FSH-releasing factor (FRF) different from the decapeptide LRF has recently been subjected to review by a group of investigators claiming to have purified from hypothalamic extracts a fraction that preferentially releases FSH over LH (Bowers et al. 1973). Other laboratories have not been able to confirm this proposal so far. The proof will involve elucidation of the primary sequence of the material reported as FRF, its confirmation by synthesis, and the consensus of the scientific community about its reported biological activity.

Evidence regarding the mode of action of LRF at the cellular level shows that the peptide is recognized by pituitary receptors located in the plasma membrane of the gonadotrophs. It is likely, though not conclusively proven, that the binding of LRF to pituitary receptors involves Ca^{2+} and the adenyl cyclase, cAMP system, to be followed by secretion of the gonadotropins LH or FSH or both (Grant et al. 1973). The peptide stimulates the secretion of already formed pituitary hormones, and its secretory activity is not modified by inhibitors of ribosomal protein synthesis (cycloheximide, puromycin) or of DNA-directed mRNA synthesis (actinomycin D) (Baulieu 1972). The inhibitory effects of gonadal steroids on the secretion of gonadotropins (negative feedback), for the part that involves the pituitary response to LRF, call upon entirely different mechanisms, in keeping with the current concepts of the mechanism of action of steroids (Baulieu 1972).

Though localization of the LRF-secreting (neuronal) elements within the hypophysiotropic area of the hypothalamus appears to point to the arcuate nucleus and the median eminence (McCann et al. 1974a), the exact nature of the cellular elements involved in the synthesis of LRF has not been determined any more than have the biosynthetic pathways that lead to manufacturing (and storage?) of LRF.

To sum up, then, after 10 years of efforts and handling of enormous quantities of brain tissues as starting material, the hypothalamic releasing factor (LRF) for the gonadotropin luteinizing hormone (LH) was characterized in 1971 as a decapeptide. The substance has been reproduced by total synthesis and is now available in practically unlimited quantities. Synthetic LRF is highly active in humans and stimulates the secretion of both gonadotropins LH and FSH (follicle stimulating hormone). Synthetic LRF is already widely used throughout the world as a diagnostic tool to ascertain pituitary secretory ability for gonadotropins; the therapeutic use of LRF to correct various types of infertility in men or women is in its early stages. Synthetic analogs of LRF have been prepared that are more potent than the native substance; other analogs act as competitive inhibitors of LRF, thus opening a new approach to contraceptive medication.

9.2 Mechanisms of Central Nervous Control of Pituitary Gonadotropic Functions in Mammals

Fundamental knowledge of the reciprocal relations between functions of the central nervous system and the secretion of gonadotropins has reached a rather high level of sophistication over the past 20 years.

In terms of their heuristic value, the three most significant achievements of this period are the following:

1. Demonstration of a sexual dimorphism in the neuronal architecture of the anterior hypothalamus that is, at one time during ontogeny, sensitive to male steroid hormones.

2. Characterization in hypothalamic tissues and reproduction by synthesis of a polypeptide molecule, which constitutes the ultimate information whereby the central nervous system positively drives the release of pituitary gonadotropins, thus leading to ovulation or testicular activity. This substance, luteinizing-hormone-releasing factor (LRF), is highly active in humans to stimulate secretion of luteinizing hormone and follicle-stimulating hormone.

3. The demonstration in laboratory animals that the hypothalamic peptide LRF, characterized by its hypophysiotropic activity, can increase mating behavior through mechanisms not involving the pituitary gland and gonadal steroid secretion, thus pointing to the existence of neuronal receptors for the peptide in parts of the central nervous system that are related to sexual behavior.

In terms of fertility regulation and control, available industrial synthesis of the hypothalamic peptide LRF may well have far-reaching significance, though it is early for long-range assessment of the results. Because it is active in humans in microgram quantities, LRF can be used to induce or restore fertility in patients, men or women, whose normal secretion of the hypothalamic releasing factor is deficient. Furthermore, it is possible to design and actually synthesize molecular analogs of the peptide LRF whose structure is so modified that they will act as competitive inhibitors of endogenous LRF. Several such molecules have recently been described by Guillemin's research group; they inhibit ovulation in laboratory animals by competitive inhibition of LRF. Clinical testing of such analogs has begun. Much more work is necessary, however, to design and obtain such inhibitory molecules with enough biological activity to be of practical use in humans, as a possible means of routine fertility control.

Availability of LRF raises another possibility. We know that LRF, acting directly at the level of the pituitary cells that are secreting gonadotropins, can stimulate release of the pituitary hormones in spite of the presence of large concentrations of (ovarian) steroids, which normally inhibit ovulation. In some perhaps not too distant nor too Orwellian future, where either voluntary or compulsory negation of fertility would be obtained by long-term implantation of steroids, administration of LRF could be used to reestablish fertility by triggering secretion of the gonadotropins, even in the presence of the steroids.

We have only just started to understand the significance of most of this new fundamental knowledge in terms of clinical applications to human psychology, human reproductive medicine, and regulation of human fertility. Over the next few years expanding programs should be oriented toward the goal of elucidating those outstanding problems in human reproductive biology that could not be approached until the fundamental knowledge described in this chapter had been obtained. Obviously, competitive inhibitors of LRF could not be devised and synthesized prior to the discovery of the structure of LRF, to cite one example. A great deal of the activity in the next few years in this field will be basic research, but research oriented toward understanding or influencing specific questions concerning physiological or biochemical events involved in the processes of human reproductive biology.

9.3 The Nature of the Neurotransmitters Involved in the Control of Secretion of the Gonadotropin-Releasing Factors

Discovery of the gonadotropin-releasing factors aroused interest in examining putative synaptic transmitters that might influence the release of these factors into the hypophysial portal vessels. Here we shall examine (1) the areas of the preoptic-hypothalamic region involved in control of FSH and LH secretion, the localization of the gonadotropin-releasing factors, and the localization of the various monoamines as possible neurotransmitters, and (2) the current experimental evidence for participation by these transmitters in hypothalamic control of pituitary gonadotropic functions. Finally, we shall attempt to summarize the current status of this rather controversial field.

Localization of Gonadotropin-Controlling Centers

On the basis of both stimulation and lesion experiments, LH release appears to be controlled by a medial basal region of the brain, which extends from the preoptic region rostrally through the anterior hypothalamus to the median eminence–arcuate region caudally. The region controlling FSH release overlaps that concerned with LH release, but its rostral extent appears to be slightly more caudal, extending only as far forward as the anterior hypothalamic area (McCann et al. 1974b). The localization of LRF activity corresponds quite closely to the region just described as involved in the control of LH release. LRF can be extracted from a medial basal region extending from the preoptic area to the median eminence–arcuate region. This distribution of LRF has been determined on the basis of bioassay in vivo, bioassay in vitro with measurement of hormone release from pituitaries by bioassay or immunoassay, and, most recently, by radioimmunoassay for the decapeptide LRF (McCann et al. 1974a). FSH-releasing activity is also present throughout this region; however, it is always less than the LH-releasing activity and can be accounted for by the intrinsic FSH-releasing activity of the decapeptide. Thus, though these experiments bring no evidence for a separate FSH-releasing factor, we still believe that such a factor probably exists on the basis of the lesion and stimulation experiments, which point to a localization of the centers controlling FSH more caudal than those controlling LH. In addition, in many physiological conditions, the release of FSH and LH can be dissociated and partial separations of FSH-RF and LRF have been reported.

In early experiments carried out in McCann's laboratory and also that of Mess and Martini, suprachiasmatic lesions led, on measurement sometime later, to a reduction in LRF stored in the median eminence. In McCann's experiments, this was true in both intact and castrate animals. The castrate animals were used to eliminate the possible influence of altered negative feedback of gonadal steroids on the results. These data were interpreted to mean that LRF neurons, with cell bodies located in the suprachiasmatic region and axons that projected to the median eminence, had been destroyed by the lesions. Since LRF activity did not disappear from the median eminence, it was postulated that other LRF neurons had cell bodies located more caudally.

Recent studies in which antibodies to the decapeptide have been localized in hypothalamic structures by immunofluorescence or immunoperoxidase techniques have led to conflicting results. Some authors find LRF in ependymal cells, lending some credence to the theory of ependymal origin of releasing factors, while others find it only in terminals of neurons projecting to the external layer of the median eminence. One group has localized LRF to cell bodies of neurons in the preoptic region, an area that contains radioimmunoassayable LRF (Stumpf 1974).

It is important to compare the localization of monoamines in the hypothalamus with that of LRF. The localization of these putative transmitters has been vastly facilitated by the use of the immunofluorescence technique of Falk and Hillarp (see Fuxe and Hökfelt 1969). Using this technique and also chemical determination of the amines, investigators found that terminals of norepinephrine-containing neurons are present in the preoptic–anterior hypothalamic area, thought also to contain cell bodies of the LRF neurons. In addition, norepinephrine-containing terminals are found in the median eminence–arcuate region, a probable source of cell bodies and a certain source of axon terminals of the LRF neurons.

In addition, the evidence is now overwhelming for the existence of a tuberoinfundibular dopaminergic pathway; the cell bodies of these neurons lie in the arcuate nucleus, and their axons project to the external layer of the median eminence. Thus dopamine also could serve as a transmitter to release LRF by axo-axonal transmission.

Serotonin is also found widely throughout the hypothalamus. High concentrations are present in the suprachiasmatic nucleus and also in the median eminence region. Cholinergic terminals appear to be widely distributed throughout the hypothalamus, and recently, choline acetyl transferase has been found in abundance in the median eminence. Thus, on anatomical grounds, there are abundant opportunities for synapses between monoaminergic neurons on the one hand and the gonadotropin-releasing neurons on the other.

Effects of Administered Catecholamines on Gonadotropin Release

One approach to examining the possible role of these agents in controlling the release of gonadotropins is to inject the amines and determine the effect on gonadotropin release by measurement of plasma titers of radioimmunoassayable FSH and LH. In these experiments the substances are usually injected into the third ventricle or into the hypothalamus itself, in order to circumvent the blood-brain barrier. They have also been injected into cannulated portal vessels to perfuse the anterior pituitary directly. In early experiments intraventricular injection of dopamine was found to increase plasma LH in ovariectomized, estrogen-progesterone-primed rats, very sensitive test animals for the effects of LRF, and in animals on diestrus day 2 or on proestrus. Dopamine had a slight effect in males but was ineffective in ovariectomized animals or in females on diestrus day 1 or on estrus. An increase in LRF was found in circulating plasma of hypophysectomized animals following the intraventricular injection of dopamine (McCann et al. 1974b). In other experiments in male rats, intraventricular dopamine was found to increase plasma LH and FSH and to elevate the gonadotropin-releasing activity of portal blood (Porter et al. 1972). In all of these experiments norepinephrine and epinephrine were less effective than dopamine or had no effect.

In later experiments it has been difficult to confirm the gonadotropin-releasing action of dopamine in male rats (Cramer and Porter 1973); in ovariectomized rats primed with a relatively small dose of estrogen, no effect on FSH and LH release was observed, even though intraventricular dopamine substantially reduced plasma prolactin (Ojeda et al. 1974).

In proestrous rats in which the preovulatory discharge of LH was blocked by Nembutal, intraventricular epinephrine was found to be the most effective agent in releasing LH, whereas norepinephrine and dopamine had little effect (Rubenstein and Sawyer 1970). In the rabbit, recent evidence suggests that intraventricular dopamine can actually block the ovulatory surge of gonadotropins (Sawyer et al. 1974). In the experiments in which dopamine stimulated LH release, the stimulatory action could be blocked by alpha but not beta blocking agents—a surprising response, since the actions of dopamine are usually not antagonized by alpha blockers.

The Effects of Catecholamines on the Release of Gonadotropins In Vitro

The effects of catecholamines have also been evaluated using in vitro systems in which the amines are added either to pituitaries incubated alone or to pituitaries incubated together with ventral hypothalamic fragments. In these systems little effect was obtained from catecholamines added to pituitaries alone; however, a dose-related increase in LH and FSH release was reported when dopamine was added to the coincubates. Since the catecholamines did not alter the response to FSH- and LH-releasing factors, release of these factors was assumed to have occurred in response to dopamine.

Both in vivo and in vitro estrogen could block the response to dopamine. In vitro, the blockade could be reversed by inhibitors of protein synthesis, such as puromycin or cyclohexamide. This suggested that negative feedback by estrogen might be mediated in part by the formation of an inhibitory peptide or protein, which antagonized the ability of dopamine to stimulate release of the gonadotropin-releasing factors (Schneider and McCann 1970). This would be analogous to the inhibitory peptide or protein thought to be formed in the pituitary in response to thyroxin (Vale et al. 1968).

Evidence Based on the Use of Adrenergic Blocking Drugs and Drugs Modifying Catecholamine Synthesis

The first experiments along these lines were performed by Sawyer and Everett many years ago (for review, see Everett 1964). They found that the alpha blocker, phenoxybenzamine, could block ovulation. More recent studies have confirmed the ability of alpha blockers to interfere with the postcastration rise in gonadotropins in the rat (Ojeda and McCann 1973) and to inhibit circhoral LH release in ovariectomized monkeys (Bhattacharya et al. 1972).

Blockade of catecholamine synthesis using alpha methyltyrosine, an inhibitor of tyrosine hydroxylase, has been found capable of blocking the postcastration rise in gonadotropins and the stimulation of gonadotropins that can be evoked in estrogen-primed animals by both estrogen and progesterone (McCann et al. 1974b). Furthermore, large doses of alpha methyltyrosine can also block ovulation when administered on proestrus. Reinitiation of catecholamine synthesis by administration of L-DOPA to such animals is associated with reversal or partial reversal of the blockade. When norepinephrine synthesis is selectively blocked by drugs such as diethyldithiocarbamate or U-14624 to inhibit dopamine beta hydroxylase, blockade of the gonadotropin responses to the above stimuli is also produced; these blocks can be reversed either totally or partially by the administration of dihydroxyphenylserine to re-

verse the blockade of norepinephrine synthesis. The dopamine receptor blocker, pimozide, did interfere significantly with the postcastration rise in FSH. Thus these studies with adrenergic blocking drugs and drugs that alter catecholamine synthesis point clearly to catecholaminergic control over both negative and positive feedback mechanisms. The preponderance of evidence would favor a role for norepinephrine in mediating these responses, but there is some evidence that dopamine may be involved as well.

McCann's group attempted to localize the presumed noradrenergic synapse by evaluating the effects of drugs that block catecholamine synthesis on the response to preoptic stimulation (Kalra and McCann 1973). Alpha-methyltyrosine or diethyldithiocarbamate could inhibit this response, and the inhibition could be reversed by the administration of precursors that bypassed the block. On the other hand, when the median eminence–arcuate region was stimulated, the blockers were without effect. Presumably, in the former situation the stimulation was presynaptic, and when norepinephrine synthesis was blocked, synaptic transmission was prevented. On the other hand, stimulation in the median eminence–arcuate region presumably involved the axons of the LRF neurons themselves. The localization of a noradrenergic synapse in the preoptic–anterior hypothalamic area is consistent with the presence of noradrenergic terminals in this region. Presumably, increased impulse traffic across this noradrenergic synapse would bring about increased release of LRF.

Turnover of Catecholamines in the Hypothalamus

Studies of turnover of catecholamines lend further support for the role of norepinephrine in the control of gonadotropin release. There is increased turnover of norepinephrine following castration and during proestrus (see McCann et al. 1974a, b for references). On the other hand, dopamine turnover studies are consistent with an inhibitory role for dopamine in release of gonadotropins, since dopamine turnover is increased in situations in which gonadotropin release is inhibited (Fuxe and Hökfelt 1969). The proper means for assessing catecholamine turnover is under considerable dispute. Furthermore, the turnover measured is that of a large population of neurons, which may be involved in different functions: consequently, turnover of dopamine in the population could give misleading results.

Possible Role of Acetylcholine in Stimulating the Release of Gonadotropin-Releasing Factors

Sawyer and Everett (see Everett 1964) showed many years ago that large doses of atropine given subcutaneously could block ovulation. Recently it has been shown that the subcutaneous or intraventricular administration of atropine can block the preovulatory discharge of FSH, LH, and prolactin and can interfere with the postcastration rise in gonadotropins (Libertun and McCann 1973). On the other hand, intraventricular injection of carbachol, a cholinergic agonist, had quite small immediate effects on gonadotropin release. This is surprising if acetylcholine is playing a role, since carbachol administered intraventricularly can trigger release of neurohypophyseal hormones; however, acetylcholine has been found to evoke release of gonadotropin-releasing factors from ventral hypothalami incubated together with pituitaries in vitro (Martini 1974). Thus there is some suggestion of a cholinergic control of gonadotropin release, but the situation has not yet been clarified.

Possible Role of Serotonin and Melatonin in Control of Gonadotropin Release

The intraventricular injection of serotonin has been reported to inhibit FSH and LH release (Schneider and McCann 1970; Porter et al. 1972). Studies with inhibitors of serotonin synthesis have not yielded conclusive evidence for a role for serotonin in the normal control of gonadotropins, but this possibility warrants further investigation. Similarly, the pineal indole, melatonin, can inhibit gonadotropin release and may play a role in mediating the antigonadotropic effects of the pineal. Again, the exact role of melatonin under physiological conditions remains to be established.

Role of Prostaglandins in the Release of Gonadotropin-Releasing Factors

Although prostaglandins are not thought at the present time to be synaptic transmitters, they do appear to be involved in the releasing process. Intraventricular injection of prostaglandin E_2 is a potent stimulus to LH and—to a lesser extent—FSH release in ovariectomized rats. If the animals are under the influence of estrogen, prostaglandin E_1 also is effective, although less so. Prostaglandins $F_{1\alpha}$ and $F_{2\alpha}$ have been without effect (Harms et al. 1974). In evaluating the possible site of action of prostaglandins in stimulating release of LRF, McCann's group has administered various blocking drugs. It has not been possible to block the stimulatory action of prostaglandin E_2 utilizing effective doses of alpha or beta blockers, of pimozide, of atropine, or of serotonin-blocking drugs. Prostaglandins apparently act directly in the LRF neuron and not transsynaptically to promote release of the releasing factor.

Conclusions

From the evidence reviewed above, release of gonadotropin releasing factors is clearly under catecholaminergic control. The preponderance of evidence fits with a stimulatory role for norepinephrine in the process, but some evidence implicates dopamine as well. Although serotonin and melatonin can inhibit gonadotropin release, their physiological significance has yet to be established. Relatively large doses of atropine are known to block gonadotropin release; however, in view of the relative inefficacy of cholinergic agonists, further work will be necessary to establish cholinergic control over gonadotropin release. Adrenergic blocking drugs could possibly be used as a means of fertility control, though the broad action of these drugs makes this approach risky. This approach could be made practical only by using a drug with action limited primarily to the hypothalamus.

9.4 Anatomical Structures Involved in CNS Control of Gonadotropin Secretion

Anatomical Aspects

Progress during the past 10 years will be described in this section largely by reference to books and symposia, including the names of the major investigators sometimes but excluding specific titles or page numbers of individual contributions.

In the late 1960s two authoritative volumes updated anatomical relationships of the hypothalamus, with consideration given to pituitary gonad function: *Hypothalamic control of the anterior pituitary* by J. Szentágothai, B. Flerko, B. Mess, and B. Halász (Akademiai Kiadó, Budapest, 3rd edition, 1968) and *The hypothalamus* by W. Haymaker, E. Anderson, and W. J. H. Nauta (C. C Thomas, Springfield, Illinois, 1969). In the first of these treatises Szentágothai et al. introduced the concept of an hypophysiotropic area, a region extending from in front of the paraventricular nuclei back to the basal premammillary region, in which hypothalamic factors are produced that stimulate and inhibit anterior pituitary function. Basophilic granulation was maintained in pituitary tissue transplanted into this region but not into other parts of the brain. To study the degree of independence maintained by the hypophysiotropic area, Halász devised a stereotaxic knife for deafferenting the region—removing input from the rest of the brain. Gonads were partially maintained by the isolated hypophysiotropic area ("hypothalamic island"), but cyclic phenomena such as ovulation did not occur. As a Ford Fellow working with Gorski at UCLA, Halász extended the deafferentation studies and found that influences important for ovulation entered the hypophysiotropic area from rostral regions such as the preoptic region.

In the volume by Haymaker et al., Nauta and Haymaker give a beautiful description of hypothalamic nuclei and their fiber connections, including such neuroendocrinologically interesting pathways as the medial cortico-hypothalamic tract in the rat, which carries impulses from the hippocampus to the region of the arcuate nucleus. The whole array is related to Nauta's previously presented concept of limbic midbrain and limbic forebrain systems. The effects of localized hypothalamic stimuli and lesions and exteroceptive factors on reproductive function are reviewed in chapters by Green, Sawyer, and Desclin.

In *Frontiers in neuroendocrinology, 1969* edited by W. F. Ganong and L. Martini (Oxford University Press, 1969), Halász expands the scope of his rat deafferentation studies and describes large anterior cuts (work with Köves) in which the preoptic region and hypothalamus were isolated as a unit that permitted ovulation to occur—that is, the timing mechanism for cyclic ovulation may reside in the preoptic region. Knobil reports (Recent Prog. Horm. Res. 30:1, 1974) that ovulation can occur in the monkey with only a small hypothalamic island in contact with the pituitary. In the 1969 *Frontiers*, Fuxe and Hökfelt gave the first comprehensive neuroendocrine overview of the catecholaminergic systems they had been mapping with the Hillarp histofluorescence technique. They described a noradrenergic system, projecting from the midbrain rostrally, and two dopaminergic (DA) systems: nigrostriatal and tuberoinfundibular (TIDA), with cell bodies of TIDA neurons lying in the arcuate nucleus. They suggested that the TIDA system was inhibitory to gonadotropic secretion. Also in this volume, Beyer and Sawyer reviewed electrophysiological methods of mapping sites of hormonal feedback action on the brain, including the multiple unit method and the microiontophoretic technique introduced by Ruf and Steiner (Science 156:667, 1967), who applied dexamethasone by multibarreled pipettes to neurons from which they were recording unit activity. The steroid slowed the firing rate of these cells, which could be marked with dye and localized histologically.

In *Steroid hormones and brain function*, edited by C. H. Sawyer and R. A. Gorski (University of California Press, 1971), reporting a 1970 symposium, Steiner demonstrated that his microiontophoretic technique would also deliver peptide hormones to localizable neurons. The ontogenetic effects of gonadal steroids on brain function and sterility were widely discussed by Gorski and Barraclough and their colleagues, and Flerko proposed that early androgen treatment reduced the number of estrogen receptors in the brain. Both Stumpf and Pfaff mapped the distribution of estradiol-concentrating neurons in the periventricular brain by autoradiographic methods; both also described heavy concentrations in the region of the arcuate nucleus.

In a symposium on brain-endocrine interactions organized by Sawyer for the American Association of Anatomists (Am. J. Anat. 129:193, 1970), Stumpf elaborated his concept of the periventricular brain and the inclusion of amygdalo-hypothalamic neurons and pathways in the estrogen-concentrating system. Raisman described projections from the limbic system to the hypothalamus delineated by nerve degeneration techniques and visualized by light and electron microscopic (EM) methods. On the basis of deafferentation and EM studies, Knigge and Scott proposed that releasing factors might be secreted into the third ventricle and picked up by the portal system in the median eminence. As a discussant, Harris questioned the evidence for this system.

In *Frontiers in neuroendocrinology, 1971*, edited by Martini and Ganong (Oxford University Press, 1971), Raisman and Field presented a superb structural-functional analysis of relations between the hypothalamus and such limbic structures as hippocampus, amygdala, septum, and pyriform cortex, and between the preoptic region and hypothalamus. They employed deafferentation, silver, and EM techniques to trace the projections.

In *The neurobiology of the amygdala*, edited by B. E. Eleftheriou (Plenum Press, New York, 1972), Raisman and Field reviewed their brilliant study originally announced in Science (173:731, 1971), in which a sexual dimorphism in the preoptic region of the rat brain was discovered by electron microscopy. Preoptic neurons in the female brain have about twice as many dendritic spines as in the male, and a large proportion of the dendritic spine synapses are of amygdaloid origin. Early androgen treatment morphologically masculinizes the female's preoptic neuron pattern. The book contains several excellent morphological and electrophysiological analyses of dorsal and ventral amygdalofugal fibers and their neuroendocrine implications. Amygdalo-hypothalamic fibers facilitatory to gonadotropin release run largely in the dorsal *stria terminalis* pathway.

In *Brain-endocrine interaction*, edited by K. M. Knigge, D. E. Scott, and A. Weindl (S. Karger, Basel, 1972), the median eminence was explored by EM, autoradiographic, fluorescence, histochemical, deafferentation, and vascular perfusion techniques, and its capacity to absorb substances from the third ventricle for transmission to the pituitary was debated. Halász maintained that projections from the preoptic region must synapse in the arcuate nucleus before reaching the median eminence. Weiner, Gorski, and Sawyer reported, on the basis of deafferentation cuts and chemical assays, that noradrenergic fibers enter the hypothalamus from a rostrolateral direction, a finding confirmed by Hökfelt and Fuxe with their fluorescence technique and later by Cuello, Weiner, and Ganong (Brain Res. 59:191, 1973) by EM methods.

In *Hormones and brain function*, edited by K. Lissak (Plenum Press, New York, 1973), Taleisnik and Carrer reviewed their evidence that the midbrain contains areas stimulatory and others inhibitory to pituitary-gonadal function. The stimulatory projections appear to utilize the amygdala–*stria terminalis* route, and the inhibitory pathways project via the hippocampus–medial corticohypothalamic route. Kawakami and his colleagues also used deafferentation, stimulation, and electrical recording techniques combined with radioimmunoassay of pituitary hormones to explore limbic-hypothalamic projections.

In *Frontiers in neuroendocrinology, 1973*, edited by Ganong and Martini (Oxford University Press, 1973), Cross gives an excellent account of the electrophysiological antidromic firing technique of identifying and localizing neurons projecting to the basal hypothalamus. Combined with the microiontophoretic method of applying transmitters, releasing factors, and even pituitary trophins to the living yet localizable neurons and observing effects on their firing rates, the technique promises to give valuable information on the anatomy and physiology of brain pituitary mechanisms.

Finally, in *Anatomical neuroendocrinology*, edited by W. E. Stumpf and L. G. Grant (S. Karger, Basel, 1975), several investigators, notably Kozlowski, Hökfelt, and Kordon, present immunohistochemical evidence of this localization of LRF, principally in the lateral external zone of the median eminence. Nerve cell bodies appearing to contain the factor were described in the preoptic region, diagonal band, and nucleus of the *stria terminalis* and other regions, but caution was expressed about specificity—the possibility is great of artifacts giving false positive results.

9.5 Behavioral Components of Gonadotropin Secretion

The title of this section refers to behavioral influences on gonadotropin secretion. Since CNS regulation of gonadotropin secretion presents many analogies to hormonal control of behavior, some comments on research in the latter area are also included. Although no reviews directed specifically at the primary area are available, references and discussions can be found in Bermant and Davidson (1974, primarily chap. 6) and to some extent in Davidson (1972) and Davidson and Levine (1972).

Behavioral Influences on Gonadotropin Secretion
Aggressive behavior and stress Increased LH release (OAAD assay) has been reported in mice defeated in aggressive encounters (Eleftheriou and Church 1967), but such changes may simply be manifestations of general stress effects—that is, nonspecific stimuli of the type that activate the pituitary-adrenal system. Such influences can have facilitatory or inhibitory effects on gonadotropin secretion, depending on circumstances (Ajika et al. 1973; Guiliani 1969). No safe generalizations can yet be made about what determines the sign of these effects.

A recent development of considerable interest is the stress-induced suppression of circulating testosterone levels (rats: Bardin and Peterson 1967; rhesus monkeys: Rose et al. 1972; humans: Monden et al. 1972). This effect is apparently not mediated by gonadotropin release (Monden et al. 1972), and it is of considerable interest to determine its mechanism and the consequences for gonadotropin feedback. The negative relationship between blood testosterone and social dominance in rhesus monkeys (Rose et al. 1972) may be related to this phenomenon.

Sexual behavior and ovulation It has been known for many years that mating can precipitate ovulation in spontaneously ovulating species, but only in recent years has the phenomenon been properly studied. Coitus-induced ovulation has been demonstrated in rats when spontaneous ovulation is blocked by hormonal or pharmacological means or by environmental manipulations (see references in Brown-Grant et al. 1973). The most detailed endocrinologic analysis has been performed in constant light-exposed rats (Brown-Grant et al. 1973; Davidson et al. 1973b; Smith and Davidson 1974) and in estogren-treated rats (Aron et al. 1968; Davidson and Smith 1974). The effects reported include hypothalamic LRF depletion, plasma LH and prolactin increases, and only a slight rise in FSH level. The CNS pathway for this neuroendocrine reflex apparently enters the hypothalamus from its anterior aspect (Kalra and Sawyer 1970).

In male rats, several laboratories have failed to show acute postcoital gonadotropin increases (Spies and Niswender 1971; Davidson et al. 1973a). Nevertheless, much indirect evidence indicates that repeated cohabitation has chronic proandrogenic effects in male rats that tend to retard senile atrophy of the reproductive system (Drori and Folman 1964). Recently, acute release of testosterone following coitus in male rats has been reported (Purvis and Haynes 1974).

A belief long held by clinicians that coitus-induced (paracyclic) ovulation can occur in humans is based largely on anecdotal evidence. An exhaustive study on one subject (Fox and Fox 1971) and other marginally convincing reports (such as Ismail and Harkness, 1967) claim postcoital testosterone increases in the human male. Negative reports are available on FSH and LH (Stearns et al. 1973) and on FSH, LH, and testosterone (Davidson and Trupin 1974), but more exhaustive study is required. Postcoital elevation of blood prolactin accompanying orgasm has been reported in some women (Noel et al. 1972).

Progestational effects of behavioral stimuli In rodents, coitus provides stimuli that are necessary for normal gestation. The usual model for study of this process is the state of pseudopregnancy, which results from sterile mating. Increased prolactin and progesterone blood levels (Wuttke and Meites 1970; Bartosik and Szarowski 1973) are related to the behavioral activation of the corpus luteum. The physiological importance of this type of effect was clearly demonstrated by Wilson et al. (1965); ejaculation resulted in successful pregnancy only when accompanied by an adequate number of intromissions providing sufficient genital stimulation. The mechanisms involve both enhanced sperm transport and luteal activation (Chester and Zucker 1970; Adler 1970). This phenomenon is under further study in the laboratory of Norman Adler (University of Pennsylvania).

Pheromones Behavioral-social effects on reproduction may be mediated by chemical agents sensed via olfactory (or gustatory) routes (reviewed by Bronson 1968; Whitten 1974; Bermant and Davidson 1974). Those acting on the endocrine system are termed primer pheromones, as opposed to the signaling type (sex attractants). The most studied species is the laboratory mouse, in which these processes (including the Bruce, Whitten, and Lee-Boot effects) are prominent and apparently rather important. The phenomena include abortion induced by an alien male and estrus induced or blocked by exposure to males or females, respectively. The onset of puberty is also affected by pheromonal stimuli (Vandenbergh 1969).

Little is known of primer pheromones in other mammalian species, though suggestive but indirect evidence for synchronization of menstrual cycles in young women, possible via pheromones, has been reported (McClintock 1971) and accorded some publicity. The chemical nature of a mammalian primer pheromone has yet to be elucidated, but structures are known for several signaling pheromones. These are the 3-OH-5 androst-16-one derivative in the boar (Patterson, Signoret), which induces sexual receptivity in the sow; cis-4-OHdodeca-6-enoic acid lactone in the black-tailed deer (Muller-Schwarze); and the vaginal "cocktail" of short chain fatty acids in the rhesus monkey (Michael). Signaling pheromone effects of vaginal secretions have also been demonstrated for dogs (Beach). Pheromonal effects involving both promotion and inhibition of aggression in mice have been reported (Mugford and Nowell). References to the above work can be found in Bermant and Davidson (1974, pp. 175–176) and the other reviews mentioned above. Interesting speculations on the possible physio-

logical importance and practical applications of mammalian pheromones are presented by Comfort (1971).

Effects of Hormones on Reproductive Behavior
The following developments of the last decade are chosen for the analogies that they show to demonstrated processes of importance in the CNS control of gonadotropin secretion. In some experimental situations the behavioral model provides an excellent instrument for experimentation on reproductive neuroendocrinology (for example, in studying effects of hormones on brain); the advisability of supporting research in behavioral endocrinology derives in part from its potential for providing leads for research on reproductive neuroendocrinology in general.

An area of active research has been the investigation of the "organizational" effects of perinatal androgen on adult sexual behavior (see reviews by Beach 1971; Gorski 1971; and Goy and Resko 1972). The period during which exposure to androgen causes permanent behavioral masculinization is prenatal in species with young born at a more advanced stage of development and neonatal in species like the rat, mouse, and hamster, in which the newborn are relatively undeveloped. The critical periods and amounts of androgen required for behavioral and physiological (gonadotropic) masculinization differ to some extent (Gorski 1971). It is important to extend this research into different species, since almost the only work available outside rodents and monkeys is that of Beach's group on dogs. In the primate, Goy and Phoenix's group has studied this problem. Interestingly, no effects of the prenatal androgen exposure on reproductive cycles have yet been found in primates.

The last decade has also seen extension of the concept of steroid receptors in the hypothalamus involved in activation of sexual behavior. Androgen implants in the anterior hypothalamic-preoptic area restore copulatory behavior in castrated male rats (Davidson 1966). Hart and Haugen (1968) have demonstrated stimulatory effects of steroid hormones implanted into the spinal cord on male sexual reflexes. Effects of estrogen on the peripheral nervous system have also been recently studied: in the laboratories of Komisaruk and of Pfaff, estrogen was found to increase the sensory field of nerves supplying the perineal-genital region (Komisaruk et al. 1973). Quite recently it was discovered in two laboratories (Moss and McCann; Pfaff) that LRF could replace progesterone in the facilitation of sexual receptivity in female rats. The effect is apparently not mediated by pituitary or adrenal hormones, and the intriguing implication is that LRF, released in a preovulatory surge, diffuses directly to adjacent diencephalic areas regulating sexual behavior (see Pfaff 1973).

Following initial work by Meyerson (1964), investigation of the involvement of biogenic monoamines in control of sex behavior has become an active area. A conference devoted largely to this subject was held in June 1974 in Sardinia (Sandler and Gessa 1975; see also Davidson and Levine 1972; Janowsky et al. 1971). The best evidence from this work is for a serotoninergic involvement in the inhibition of female sexual receptivity in rodents; a similar pathway has been proposed for the male. Recent work also points to the possible involvement of norepinephrine, dopamine, and cholinergic mechanisms in the control of sexual behavior.

With the hypothalamic control of male and female sexual behavior well established, some recent work has concentrated on extrahypothalamic mechanisms, particularly olfactory and limbic structures. Removal of the olfactory bulbs in male and female rodents has been found to modulate sexual behavior, while destruction of the septum and structures near the hypothalamic-mesencephalic junction increases it in male and female rats; these experiments point to the existence of CNS inhibitory mechanisms (Lisk 1973; Nance et al. 1974).

Analogous to the effects of gonadotropin secretion, progesterone has been shown to have biphasic-facilitatory followed by inhibitory effects on sexual receptivity in several species (see Bermant and Davidson 1974). The interactions between these two processes and coitus-induced gonadotropin release have been considered (Davidson et al. 1973b; Davidson and Smith 1974).

Recently several studies have been devoted to structure-function relationships with regard to the perinatal organizational and adult activational effects of different steroids. Among the more interesting findings have been the discovery that dihydrotestosterone (the "active androgen" of peripheral tissues) is relatively or totally ineffective on male sexual behavior, depending on the species (see Johnston and Davidson 1972; Sandler and Gessa 1975). This has led to the hypothesis that behavioral (and other) effects of androgen on the brain are mediated by aromatization to estrogen (Naftolin et al. 1972). This hypothesis, not yet verified despite suggestive evidence, is presently under active study in several laboratories (K. Larsson, Göteborg; L. Clemens, East Lansing; C. Beyer, Mexico City). The ineffectiveness of the two most potent antiandrogens on sexual behavior of male rodents is one of several differences which exist between feedback and behavioral receptors for androgen (Davidson et al. 1973a). Cyproterone acetate is becoming used on a fairly widespread scale in Germany for treatment of criminal and other sexual offenders (Laschet 1973). Unfortunately, adequate endocrine and behavioral studies have not yet been conducted, and the possibility remains that the effects of cyproterone are a combination of placebo effects and gonadotropic inhibition, leading to functional castration. Reliable studies on this compound are much needed.

Finally, it should be emphasized that there is a lack of progress in understanding the relationship between hormones and human sexual behavior. One of the few interesting studies in recent years was that of Masters's group (Kolodny et al. 1971), purportedly demonstrating a positive correlation between serum testosterone and male homosexuality. Several groups have failed to confirm this work (for example, Tourney and Hatfield 1973), and more work is needed. Almost the only consistent and serious investigator in behavioral reproductive endocrinology is John Money. His studies on the long-lasting effects of elevated perinatal androgen have not demonstrated major changes in sexual behavior or orientation, although subtle effects on sexuality and personality were found in a variety of congenital or iatrogenic conditions involving aberrant androgen levels in early development (Money 1972). There is great need for large-scale studies on the activational and organizational effects of hormonal changes in human sexual behavior.

References

Adler, N. T. Effects of the male's copulatory behavior on successful pregnancy of the female rat. J. Comp. Physiol. Psychol. 69:613, 1969.

Ajika, K., S. P. Kalra, C. P. Fawcett, L. Krulich, and S. M. McCann. The effect of stress and nembutal on plasma levels of gonadotropins and prolactin in ovariectomized rats. Endocrinology 90:707, 1972.

Amoss, M., R. Burgus, R. Blackwell, W. Vale, R. E. Fellows, and R. Guillemin. Purification, amino acid composition and N-terminus of the hypothalamic luteinizing hormone releasing factor (LRF) of ovine origin. Biochem. Biophys. Res. Commun. 44:205, 1971.

Amoss, M., R. Burgus, D. N. Ward, R. E. Fellows, and R. Guillemin. Evidence for a pyroglutamic acid (PCA) N-terminus in ovine hypothalamic luteinizing hormone-releasing factor (LRF). The Endocrine Society, June 10, 1970.

Aron, C., J. Roos, and G. Asch. New facts concerning the afferent stimuli that trigger ovulation by coitus in the rat. Neuroendocrinology 3:47, 1968.

Bardin, C. W., and R. E. Peterson. Studies of androgen production by the rat: Testosterone and androstenedione content of blood. Endocrinology 80:98, 1967.

Bartosik, D., and D. H. Szarowski. Progravid phase of the rat reproductive cycle: Day to day changes in peripheral plasma progestin concentrations. Endocrinology 92:949, 1973.

Baulieu, E. E. A 1972 survey of the mode of action of steroid hormones. In Endocrinology, ed. R. O. Scow. Amsterdam: Excerpta Medica, Elsevier, 1972.

Beach, F. A. Hormonal factors controlling the differentiation, development and display of copulatory behavior in the Ramstergig and the related species. In *Biopsychology of development*, eds. L. Aronson and E. Tobach. New York: Academic Press, 1971.

Bermant, G., and J. M. Davidson. A possibility of medical treatment of sexual deviation and perversion in man. In *Biological bases of sexual behavior*, eds. G. Bermant and J. M. Davidson. New York: Harper & Row, 1972.

Bhattacharya, A. N., D. J. Dierschke, T. Yamaji, and E. Knobil. The pharmacologic blockade of the circhoral mode of LH secretion in the ovariectomized rhesus monkey. Endocrinology 90:778, 1972.

Bowers, C. Y., B. L. Currie, K. N. G. Johansson, and K. Folkers. Biological evidence that separate hypothalamic hormones release the follicle stimulating and luteinizing hormones. Biochem. Biophys. Res. Commun. 50:20, 1973.

Bronson, F. H. Pheromonal influences on mammalian reproduction. In *Perspectives in reproduction and sexual behavior*, ed. M. Diamond. Bloomington, Ind.: Indiana University Press, 1968.

Brown-Grant, K., J. M. Davidson, and F. Greig. Induced ovulation in albino rats exposed to constant light. J. Endocrinol. 57:7, 1973.

Burgus, R., M. Butcher, M. Amoss, N. Ling, M. Monahan, J. Rivier, R. Fellows, R. Blackwell, W. Vale, and R. Guillemin. Structure moléculaire du facteur hypothalamique (LRF) d'origine ovine contrôlant la sécrétion de l'hormone gonadotrope hypophysaire de lutéinisation (LH). C.R. Acad. Sci. (Paris) 273:1611, 1971.

Burgus, R., M. Butcher, M. Amoss, N. Ling, M. Monahan, J. Rivier, R. Fellows, R. Blackwell, W. Vale, and R. Guillemin. Primary structure of ovine hypothalamic luteinizing hormone-releasing factor (LRF). Proc. Natl. Acad. Sci. USA 69:278, 1972.

Burgus, R., T. F. Dunn, D. N. Ward, W. Vale, M. Amoss, and R. Guillemin. Dérivés polypeptidiques de synthèse doués d'activité hypophysiotrope TRF. C.R. Acad. Sci. (Paris) 268:2116, 1969.

Campbell, H. T., G. Feuer, J. Garcia, and G. W. Harris. The infusion of brain extracts into the anterior pituitary gland and the secretion of gonadotropic hormone. J. Physiol. 157:30, 1961.

Chester, R. V., and I. Zucker. Influence of male copulatory behavior on sperm transport, pregnancy and pseudopregnancy in female rats. Physiol. Behav. 5:35, 1970.

Comfort, A. Likelihood of human pheromones. Nature (London) 230:432, 1971.

Courrier, R., R. Guillemin, M. Jutisz, E. Sakiz, and P. Ascheim. Présence dans un extrait de l'hypothalamus d'une substance qui stimule la sécrétion de l'hormone antéhypophysaire de lutéinisation. C.R. Acad. Sci. (Paris) 253:922, 1961.

Cramer, O., and J. C. Porter. Catecholamines and the control of prolactin secretion in humans. In *Progress in brain research: Drug effects on neuroendocrine regulation*, eds. E. Zimmerman, B. H. Marks, and D. deWied, 39:311. New York: Elsevier, 1973.

Davidson, J. M. Activation of the male rat's sexual behavior by intracerebral implantation of androgen. Endocrinology 79:783, 1966.

Davidson, J. M. Hormones and reproductive behavior. In *Reproductive biology*, eds. H. Balin and S. Glasser. Amsterdam: Excerpta Medica, 1972.

Davidson, J. M., C. Cheung, E. R. Smith, and P. Johnston. Feedback regulation of gonadotropins in the male. Adv. Biosci. 10:63, 1973a.

Davidson, J. M., and S. Levine. Endocrine regulation of behavior. Ann. Rev. Physiol. 34:375, 1972.

Davidson, J. M., and E. R. Smith. Gonadotropin release as a function of mating and steroid feedback in the female rat. Horm. Behav. 5:163, 1974.

Davidson, J. M., E. R. Smith, and C. Y. Bowers. 1973b. Effects of mating on gonadotropin release in the female rat. Endocrinology 93:1185, 1973b.

Davidson, J. M., and S. Trupin. In *Sexual behavior: Pharmacology and biochemistry*, eds. M. Sandler and G. L. Gessa. New York: Raven Press, 1974.

Drori, D., and Y. Folman. Effects of cohabitation on the reproductive system, kidneys and body composition of male rats. J. Reprod. Fertil. 8:351, 1964.

Eleftheriou, B. E., and R. L. Church. Effects of repeated exposure to aggression and defeat on plasma and pituitary levels of luteinizing hormone in C57BL-6J mice. Gen. Comp. Endocrinol. 9:263, 1967.

Everett, J. W. Central neural control of reproductive functions of the adenohypophysis. Physiol. Rev. 44:373, 1964.

Fox, C. A., and B. Fox. A comparative study of coital physiology, with special reference to the sexual climax. J. Reprod. Fertil. 24:319, 1971.

Fujino, M., S. Kobayashi, M. Obayashi, T. Fukuda, S. Shinagawa, I. Yamazaki, R. Nakayama, W. White, and R. H. Rippel. Structure-activity relationships in the C-terminal part of luteinizing hormone releasing hormone (LH-RH). Biochem. Biophys. Res. Commun. 49:863, 1972.

Fuxe, K., and T. Hökfelt. Catecholamines in the hypothalamus and the pituitary gland. In *Frontiers in neuroendocrinology*, eds. L. Martini and W. F. Ganong. New York: Oxford University Press, 1969.

Giuliani, G. Studies on gonadotropin release during stressful situations and the role of the central nervous system. In *Physiology and pathology of adaptation mechanisms*, ed. E. Bajusz, Oxford: Pergamon Press, 1969.

Gorski, R. A. Effect of pituitary hormones on pituitary weight. In *Frontiers in neuroendocrinology*, eds. L. Martini and W. F. Ganong. New York: Oxford University Press, 1971.

Goy, R. W., and J. A. Resko. Gonadal hormones and behavior of normal and pseudohermaphroditic nonhuman female primates. Recent Prog. Horm. Res. 28:707, 1972.

Grant, G., W. Vale, and J. Rivier. Pituitary binding sites for [^{3}H]-labelled luteinizing hormone releasing factor (LRF). Biochem. Biophys. Res. Commun. 50:771, 1973.

Guillemin, R., M. Jutisz, and E. Sakiz. Purification partielle d'un facteur hypothalamique (par LRF) stimulant la sécrétion de LH. C. R. Acad. Sci. (Paris) 256:504, 1963.

Harms, P. G., S. R. Ojeda, and S. W. McCann. Prostaglandin-induced release of pituitary gonadotropins: Central nervous system and pituitary sites of action. Endocrinology 94:1459, 1974.

Hart, B. L., and C. M. Haugen. Activation of sexual reflexes in male rats by spinal implantation of testosterone. Physiol. Behav. 3:735, 1968.

Ismail, A. A. A., and R. A. Harkness. Urinary testosterone excretion in men in normal and pathological conditions. Acta Endocrinol. 56:469, 1967.

Janowsky, D. S., W. E. Fann, and J. M. Davis. Monoamines and ovarian hormone-linked sexual and emotional changes: A review. Arch. Sexual Behav. 1:205, 1971.

Johnston, P., and J. M. Davidson. Intracerebral androgens and sexual behavior in the male rat. Horm. Behav. 3:345, 1972.

Kalra, S. P., and S. M. McCann. Effect of drugs modifying catecholamine synthesis on LH release induced by preoptic stimulation in the rat. Endocrinology 93:356, 1973.

Kalra, S. P., and C. H. Sawyer. Blockade of copulation-induced ovulation in the rat by anterior hypothalamic differentiation. Endocrinology 87:1124, 1970.

Kolodny, R. C., W. H. Masters, J. Hendryx, and G. Toro. Plasma testosterone and semen analysis in male homosexuals. New Engl. J. Med. 285:1170, 1971.

Komisaruk, B., N. Adler, and J. Hutchison. Genital sensory field enlargement by estrogen treatment in female rats. Science 178:1295, 1972.

Laschet, U. Medical News Schering (Berlin) 2:11, 1973.

Libertun, D., and S. M. McCann. Blockade of the release of gonadotropins and prolactin by subcutaneous or intraventricular injection of atropine in male and female rats. Endocrinology 92:1714, 1973.

Lisk, R. D. Hormonal regulation of sexual behavior in polyestrous mammals common to the laboratory. In Handbook of physiology, eds. R. O. Greep and E. B. Astwood, p. 223. Baltimore: Williams & Wilkins, 1973.

McCann, S. M., L. Krulich, M. Quijada, J. Wheaton, and R. L. Moss. Gonadotropin releasing factors: Sites of production, secretion, and action in the brain. In Anatomical neuroendocrinology, eds. W. Stumpf and L. G. Grant. Basel: S. Karger, 1974a.

McCann, S. M., S. R. Ojeda, C. P. Fawcett, and L. Krulich. Catecholaminergic control of gonadotropin and prolactin secretion with particular reference to the possible participation of dopamine. In Advances in neurology, vol. 5, eds. F. McDowell and A. Barbeau. New York: Raven Press, 1974b.

McCann, S. M., S. Taleisnick, and H. M. Friedman. LH-releasing activity in hypothalamic extracts. Proc. Soc. Exp. Biol. Med. 104:432, 1960.

McClintock, M. K. Menstrual synchrony and suppression. Nature (London) 229:244, 1971.

Martini, L. Cholinergic mechanisms and the control of gonadotropin releasing hormone secretion. In Anatomical Neuroendocrinology, eds. W. Stumpf and L. G. Grant. Basel: S. Karger, 1974.

Matsuo, H., R. M. G. Nair, A. Arimura, and A. V. Schally.

Structure of the porcine LH- and FSH-releasing hormone: The proposed amino acid sequence. Biochem. Biophys. Res. Commun. 43:1334, 1971.

Meyerson, B. J. Central nervous monoamines and hormone induced estrus behavior in the spayed rat. Acta Physiol. Scand. 63 (Suppl. 241):1, 1964.

Monahan, M., M. Amoss, H. Anderson, and W. Vale. Synthetic analogs of the hypothalamic luteinizing hormone releasing factor with increased agonist or antagonist properties. Biochemistry 12:4616, 1973.

Monahan, M., J. Rivier, R. Burgus, M. Amoss, R. Blackwell, W. Vale, and R. Guillemin. Synthèse totale par phase solide d'un décapeptide qui stimule la sécrétion des gonadotropines hypophysaires LH et FSH. C.R. Acad. Sci. (Paris) 273:508, 1971.

Monden, Y., K. Koshiyama, H. Tanaka, S. Mizutani, T. Aono, Y. Hamanaka, T. Vozumi, and K. Matsumoto. Influence of major surgical stress on plasma testosterone, plasma LH and urinary steroids. Acta Endocrinol. 69:542, 1972.

Money, J. Clinical aspects of sexually dimorphic behavior. In Steroid hormones and brain function, eds. C. H. Sawyer and R. A. Gorski. Los Angeles: University of California Press, 1972.

Naftolin, R., K. J. Ryan, and Z. Petro. Aromatization of androstenedione by the anterior hypothalamus of adult male and female rats. Endocrinology 90:295, 1972.

Nance, D. M., J. Shryne, and R. A. Gorski. Septal lesions: Effects on lordosis behavior and pattern of gonadotropin release. Horm. Behav. 5:1, 1974.

Noel, G. L., H. K. Sun, G. Stone, and A. G. Frantz. Human prolactin and growth hormone release during surgery and other conditions of stress. J. Clin. Endocrinol. Metab. 35:840, 1972.

Ojeda, S. R., and S. M. McCann. Evidence for participation of a catecholaminergic mechanism in the post-castration rise in plasma gonadotropins. Neuroendocrinology 3:34, 1973.

Ojeda, S. R., P. G. Harms, and S. M. McCann. Effect of blockade of dopaminergic receptors on prolactin and LH release: Median eminence and pituitary sites of action. Endocrinology 94:1650, 1974.

Pfaff, D. Luteinizing hormone-releasing factor potentiates lordosis behavior in hypophysectomized ovariectomized female rats. Science 182:1148, 1973.

Porter, J. C., I. A. Kamberi, and J. G. Ondo. Role of biogenic amines and cerebrospinal fluid in the neurovascular transmittal of hypophysiotrophic substances. In Brain-endocrine interaction. Median eminence: Structure and function, eds. K. M. Knigge, D. E. Scott, and A. Weindl. Basel: S. Karger, 1972.

Purvis, K., and N. B. Haynes. Short-term effects of copulation. Human chorionic gonadotrophin injection and non-tactile association with a female on testosterone levels in the male rat. Endocrinology 60:429, 1974.

Rose, R. M., T. P. Gordon, and I. S. Bernstein. Plasma testosterone levels in the male rhesus: Influences of sexual and social stimuli. Science 178:643, 1972.

Rubenstein, L., and C. H. Sawyer. Role of catecholamines in stimulating the release of pituitary ovulating hormone(s) in rats. Endocrinology 86:988, 1970.

Sandler, M., and G. L. Gessa. *Sexual behavior: Pharmacology and biochemistry*. New York: Raven Press, 1975.

Sawyer, C. H., J. Hilliard, S. Kanematsu, S. Scaramuzzi, and C. A. Blake. Effects of intraventricular infusions of norepinephrine and dopamine on LH release and ovulation in rabbits. Neuroendocrinology 15:328, 1974.

Schally, A. V., A. Arimura, Y. Baba, R. M. G. Nair, H. Matsuo, T. W. Redding, L. Debeljuk, and W. F. White. Isolation and properties of FSH- and LH-releasing hormone. Biochem. Biophys. Res. Commun. 43:393, 1971a.

Schally, A. V., A. Arimura, C. Y. Bowers, A. J. Kastin, S. Jawana, and T. W. Redding. Hypothalamic neurohormones regulating anterior pituitary function. Recent Prog. Horm. Res. 24:497, 1968.

Schally, A. V., A. Arimura, A. J. Kastin, H. Matsui, Y. Baba, T. W. Redding, R. M. G. Nair, and L. Debeljuk. Gonadotropin-releasing hormone: One polypeptide regulates secretion of luteinizing and follicle-stimulating hormones. Science 173:1036, 1971b.

Schneider, H. P. G., and S. M. McCann. Dopamine pathways and gonadotropin releasing factors. In *Aspects of neuroendocrinology*, eds. W. Bargmann and B. Scharrer. Berlin: Springer-Verlag, 1970.

Smith, E. R., and J. M. Davidson. Luteinizing hormone releasing factor in rats exposed to constant light: Effects of mating. Neuroendocrinology 14:129, 1974.

Spies, H. G., and G. D. Niswender. Levels of prolactin, LH and FSH in the serum of intact and pelvic-neurectomized rats. Endocrinology 88:937, 1971.

Stearns, E. L., J. S. D. Winter, and C. Faiman. Positive feedback effect of progestin upon serum gonadotropins in estrogen-primed castrate men. J. Clin. Endocrinol. Metab. 37:635, 1973.

Stumpf, W., and L. G. Grant, eds. *Anatomical neuroendocrinology*. Basel: S. Karger, 1974.

Tourney, G., and L. M. Hatfield. Androgen metabolism in schizophrenics, homosexuals, and normal controls. Biol. Psychiatry 6:23, 1973.

Vale, W., R. Burgus, and R. Guillemin. On the mechanism of action of TRF: Effects of cycloheximide and actinomycin on the release of TSH stimulated *in vitro* by TRF and its inhibition by thyroxine. Neuroendocrinology 3:34, 1968.

Vale, W., J. Grant, J. Rivier, M. Monahan, M. Amoss, and R. Blackwell. Synthetic polypeptide antagonists of the hypothalamic luteinizing hormone releasing factor. Science 176:933, 1972.

Vandenbergh, J. C. Male odor accelerates female sexual maturation in mice. Endocrinology 84:658, 1969.

White, W. Chemistry of hypophysiotropic hormones. Discussion in *Hypophysiotropic hormones of the hypothalamus: Assay and chemistry*, vol. I., ed. J. Meites, p. 248. Baltimore: Williams & Wilkins, 1970.

Whitten, W. K., and A. K. Champlin. The role of olfaction in mammalian reproduction. In *Handbook of physiology*, Section 7, vol. 5, eds. R. O. Greep and E. B. Astwood. Baltimore: Williams & Wilkins, 1973.

Wilson, J. R., N. Adler, and B. Le Boeuf. The effects of intromission frequency on successful pregnancy in the female rat. Proc. Natl. Acad. Sci. USA 53:1392, 1965.

Wuttke, W., and J. Meites. Induction of pseudopregnancy in the rat with no rise in serum prolactin. Endocrinology 90:438, 1972.

10 Brain Neurotransmitters and the Hypothalamic Control of Pituitary Gonadrotropin Secretion

Richard J. Wurtman

10.1 Introduction

The major factors controlling the secretion of the pituitary gonadotropins FSH, LH, and prolactin are thought to be hypothalamic hormones, the releasing factors. These compounds, presumably liberated by modified neurons within the medial basal hypothalamus and median eminence, are delivered to the anterior pituitary via its "private" portal circulation. Although considerable progress has been made toward elucidating the chemical structures of some of these releasing factors, it has not yet been possible to identify their specific cells of origin or even to establish beyond question that the hypothalamus is the unique locus of these cells.

Even in the absence of a method for positively identifying the cells that secrete hypothalamic releasing factors, there is considerable evidence that these cells are typical neuroendocrine transducers, in that the primary physiological stimuli that cause them to secrete are neurotransmitter molecules impinging upon them at synapses. A syllogism outlining this view (and some of the evidence supporting it) can be constructed as follows:

1. Signals originating within the nervous system can influence gonadotropin secretion and are probably necessary for physiological ovulation and lactation. (Thus light, acting via the eyes, controls the timing of the "critical period"; rabbits ovulate in response to an interoceptive input, stimulation of the cervix; suckling accelerates prolactin secretion and facilitates lactation; the destruction of neuronal inputs to the hypothalamus by a Halász knife cut blocks ovulation.)

2. In the mammalian brain, communications between neurons and neurons, or between neurons and neuroendocrine transducers, are, in general, mediated by neurotransmitters.

3. Drugs known to modify the release or actions of certain brain neurotransmitters markedly alter gonadal function and lactation by modifying the secretion of pituitary hormones. (For example, reserpine and tetrabenazine, which deplete the brain of catecholamines, can suppress spontaneous ovulation; chlorpromazine and other drugs that block central dopamine receptors initiate prolactin secretion and can cause lactation.)

This report briefly examines available information concerning the role of particular brain neurotransmitters in the control of pituitary gonadotropin secretion. My bias is that strategies designed to modify the metabolism of brain monoamines, and perhaps of other central neurotransmitters, will eventually have considerable value in the control of reproductive function. But the potential utility of this approach will not be fully realized until there is a major increase in the number of investigators trained to integrate the two different and difficult disciplines involved—neuroendocrinology and neurotransmitter pharmacology.

10.2 Hypothalamic Releasing-Factor Cells as Neuroendocrine Transducers

Mammalian cells utilize two types of signals for communicating with each other: hormones and neurotransmitters. Hormones include members of a number of chemical families: they can be water-soluble (adrenocorticotropin; epinephrine) or lipid-soluble (steroids; melatonin); they can range in size from amino acids (thyroxine) to peptides (thyrotropin-releasing factor) to proteins (insulin) to glycoproteins (FSH, LH, and hCG). In contrast, neurotransmitters tend to be low-molecular-weight, water-soluble amines or amino acids that are charged at the pH of body fluids and perhaps peptides. The best-studied transmitters are the catecholamines dopamine, norepinephrine, and epinephrine; the indoleamine serotonin; acetylcholine; and gamma amino butyric acid. Hormones are distributed ubiquitously by the circulation and attain "privacy" only because they must be "decoded" by tissue-specific receptors; thus even though virtually every cell in the body is bathed with circulating luteinizing hormone, only the cells of the ovary or testis contain the decoding apparatus needed to enable this organ to respond to the pituitary hormone. In contrast, neurotransmitters are distributed to only a very small number of cells—those that receive synapses from the neuron releasing the neurotransmitter; "privacy" thus derives from anatomic considerations.

Theoretically, four types of specialized communications cells could exist, differentiable by their use of hormones or neurotransmitters as input and output signals. These are endocrine cells, which both respond to and emit hormonal signals (the thyroid, gonads, and adrenal cortex); true neurons, which both respond to and emit neurotransmitters; neuroendocrine transducer cells, which respond to neurotransmitter inputs by releasing hormones into the circulation; and an unnamed fourth category of cells, which respond to circulating hormones by releasing more or less of a neurotransmitter at synapses. No examples of this last category have yet been positively identified; however, it can be presumed that such cells do exist, inasmuch as the brain can be shown experimentally to contain "sensors," probably neurons, which respond to changes in the plasma concentrations of certain hormones (for example, estradiol) by changing the secretion of the hypothalamic releasing factors. The carotid body, which provides the brain with information about circulating oxygen, pH, and carbon dioxide levels, may also constitute such a humoral-neural transducer.

The identification of a cell or organ as a neuroendocrine transducer requires two kinds of evidence: first, the cell must be shown by electron microscopic techniques to receive synapses; second, the capacity of the cell to secrete appropriate quantities of its hormone must be shown to be lost when its innervation is interrupted. (Thus, for example, the adrenal medullary chromaffin cells fail to secrete epinephrine in response to insulin-induced hypoglycemia when the adrenal is transplanted or when its preganglionic cholinergic nerves are transected.) By application of these criteria, neuroendocrine transducer cells have been identified both within and outside of the brain. Examples within the brain are the magnocellular hypothalamic neurons of the supraoptic and paraventricular nuclei, which liberate the polypeptides oxytocin and vasopressin into the portal circulation and the systemic blood, and the modified hypothalamic neurons that secrete releasing factors into the portal blood vessels supplying the anterior pituitary. (Since these cells cannot be identified by available histologic approaches, it has not been possible to obtain histologic evidence concerning their synaptic inputs.) Examples of neuroendocrine transducer cells outside the brain include: the pineal organ, which synthesizes and secretes its hormone melatonin in response to the release of norepinephrine from sympathetic neurons; the adrenal medulla, which secretes epinephrine in response to acetylcholine released from preganglionic cholinergic neurons; the renal juxtaglomerular cells, which secrete renin in response to norepinephrine released from sympathetic neurons; and, perhaps, the beta cells of the pancreas, which release less insulin in response to circulating glucose when suppressed by the norepinephrine released from adjacent sympathetic neurons.

All of these neuroendocrine transducer cells are influenced by hormonal as well as neuronal inputs—thus epinephrine synthesis is controlled by glucocorticoid hormones; insulin secretion depends on circulating glucose; hyperkalemia stimulates renin se-

cretion; some steroid hormones probably feed back directly on hypothalamic releasing factor cells; and so forth. What makes these cells special, however, is their capacity to transduce synaptic to humoral signals. Some of the neuroendocrine transducer cells —for example, those of the magnocellular nuclei —contain distinct neurosecretory granules that aid in their histologic identification. Unfortunately, the presence of secretory granules is not characteristic of all such transducer cells and has not facilitated the identification of releasing factor cells. Whether or not a secretory cell happens to store its hormone in granules seems to depend upon the chemical nature of the hormone; for example, proteins, large peptides, and amines are stored, while lipid-soluble compounds are not.

10.3 Monoamine Neurotransmitters in the Hypothalamus

The hypothalami of virtually all mammals studied contain relatively high concentrations of the monoamines norepinephrine, dopamine, and serotonin, and lesser quantities of epinephrine. On the basis of histochemical fluorescence and immunochemical observations, it seems that most, if not all, of the norepinephrine, serotonin, and epinephrine is present within the terminals of neurons whose cell bodies lie within the upper brain stem. Some of the dopamine in the hypothalamus may be localized within neurons wholly contained within the hypothalamus itself.

Considerable information is now available concerning the biochemistry and pharmacology of these compounds in peripheral tissues and in other brain regions; presumably, the same processes occur within monoaminergic neurons in the hypothalamus. The catecholamines dopamine, norepinephrine, and epinephrine are synthesized from the amino acid tyrosine. The rate-limiting step in this synthesis, the conversion of tyrosine to dopa, is catalyzed by the enzyme tyrosine hydroxylase. The in vivo activity of this enzyme is enhanced when the neuron containing it increases its firing rate; this enhancement is mediated by accelerated synthesis of the enzyme and by lessened end-product inhibition of tyrosine hydroxylase by its neurotransmitter products. The rate at which brain neurons synthesize catechols also may depend on the availability of tyrosine to the neuron.

Catecholamines are stored within characteristic vesicles at the presynaptic portion of the neuron; it is not presently clear whether the molecules that are actually released into synapses when the neuron fires consist of the contents of one or more storage vesicles ("quantal" release), or whether this release comes from a small intracytoplasmic pool. Once within the

synaptic cleft, the catecholamine molecules can interact with postsynaptic receptors (presumably altering
the ionic fluxes and bioelectric activities of the postsynaptic neurons), or they can be inactivated, primarily by the process of "reuptake," in which neurotransmitter molecules reenter their cells of origin. Most of
the catecholamine molecules formed within brain neurons apparently never are released into synapses; instead they are metabolized intraneuronally, by the
enzyme monoamine oxidase.

The indoleamine serotonin (5-hydroxytryptamine) is
synthesized from the amino acid tryptophan; the initial
process in this synthesis, catalyzed by the enzyme
tryptophan hydroxylase, appears to be very largely
under the control of intraneuronal tryptophan levels.
Since various foods and hormones, by changing the
levels of tryptophan and other neutral amino acids in
the plasma, can modify brain tryptophan levels, serotonin neurons can act as "sensors," providing the
brain with information about peripheral metabolic
state. Serotonin may also be stored within presynaptic
vesicles. Once liberated into brain synapses, this neurotransmitter is probably also inactivated by reuptake;
it may also be metabolized by a special monoamine
oxidase.

10.4 The Use of Drugs to Modify Brain Monoamine Neurotransmitters and Reproductive Function

Many drugs are available that act with some specificity
at particular steps in the synthesis, release, metabolic
fates, or physiological effects of the monoamine neurotransmitters. (The word *some* should be emphasized; numerous neuroendocrinologists who have used
these drugs have subsequently learned to their dis-
may that a widely used, allegedly specific inhibitor of
serotonin synthesis may also affect catecholamine formation, that reserpine depletes the brain of *all* of the
monoamines, and so forth.) From the standpoint of
neuroendocrinology, the important considerations
about these drugs would appear to be: (1) Probably
none of them is truly specific, but some are more specific than others. Thus the dopamine-receptor blocking agents (such as haloperidol and pimozide) exhibit
considerable specificity, while the synthetic amino
acids (such as PCPA or alpha methyl paratyrosine) affect the uptake of natural amino acids into the brain
and are thus rather nonspecific in their effects on monoamines. (2) The use of drugs to demonstrate the
involvement of a given monoamine in controlling the
secretion of a particular gonadotropin increases in effectiveness in rough proportion to the number of drug
types tested (for example, drugs to block dopamine
synthesis or storage; drugs to destroy dopaminergic
neurons; drugs to stimulate or block dopamine recep-

tors; drugs to block dopamine release; "control"
drugs that should affect noradrenergic but not dopaminergic neurons). (3) New drugs come along with surprising frequency, thereby increasing the power of this
research tool. (4) No multisynaptic pathway of brain
neurons seems to utilize only a single neurotransmitter. Hence it can be anticipated, for example, that the
neurotransmitters involved in mediating the passage of
the ovulatory signal from the preoptic region to hypothalamic luteinizing-hormone-releasing factor (LRF)
cells might include most of the five listed above, plus
other, presently unidentified neurotransmitters.
Hence a bewildering array of drugs might be expected
to have some effect on ovulation. (5) "Molecular tin-
kering" with the basic catecholamine and serotonin
molecules has already met with enormous success in
the development of new drugs, and there is every reason to hope that this tradition will carry over to reproductive neuroendocrinology. For reasons that are not
entirely clear, minor modifications in the dopamine
molecule have yielded drugs that act with remarkable
specificity—and benefit—on the heart, the blood vessels, the mucous membranes of the upper pharynx, the
menstrual uterus, "satiety centers" in the brain, and
so forth. One would feel safe in predicting that, if future research indicates that a central noradrenergic
agonist might be useful in, for example, accelerating
pubescence, an array of such compounds will be synthesized, identified by screening procedures, and
made available within a short time.

10.5 Dopamine and Prolactin Secretion

Probably the best-analyzed mechanism relating a brain
monoamine neurotransmitter to the secretion of a pituitary gonadotropin hormone is the apparent inhibition
by hypothalamic dopamine of prolactin secretion. I
shall summarize here some of the studies that have established and characterized this relationship in humans and rats, which I hope constitute a paradigm for
further research.

Although experiments using cropsac assays and other in vivo biological assays had succeeded in showing
that the brain influenced (that is, tonically inhibited)
prolactin secretion, it was not until Frantz, Friesen,
and others developed more sensitive assay methods in
1970 to 1972 that it became practical for investigators
to perform detailed analyses of the neurotransmitters
involved in mechanisms controlling prolactin secretion. Very soon thereafter it was shown by Frantz that
(1) suckling rapidly stimulates prolactin secretion, especially in postpartum women; (2) plasma prolactin
levels (and, presumably, the secretion of the hormone
from the pituitary) rise during the sleep period, remaining elevated for much of the night, in a rhythm not

directly correlated with the electroencephalogram; (3) prolactin is a "stress" hormone, its secretion and plasma levels rising during surgery and general anesthesia; (4) estrogen administration causes a two- to threefold rise in plasma prolactin levels in males; and (5) plasma prolactin levels may also be increased by hypoglycemia or during sexual intercourse.

The administration of a number of neuroleptic drugs had been shown by Sulman and others to cause prolactin release in animals. The drugs involved included compounds known to exert a number of effects on brain monoamines—for example, reserpine, which blocks the storage of all of the monoamines; phenothiazines such as chlorpromazine, which antagonize dopamine and norepinephrine receptors but also exert numerous other effects; and butyrophenones like haloperidol and pimozide, which are fairly specific blockers of dopamine receptors. Subsequent studies by Frantz and his collaborators showed that administration of the dopamine precursor L-DOPA could block the chlorpromazine-induced rise in plasma prolactin. That the locus at which the dopamine acted was the pituitary itself, and not at synapses on the hypothalamic cells secreting PIF (prolactin-inhibiting factor), was suggested by in vitro studies on the effects of dopamine on rat pituitaries (Birge et al. 1970; MacLeod et al. 1970), and by Frantz's observation that L-DOPA also blocks the acute prolactin response to thyrotropin-releasing factor, presumably a direct pituitary effect.

One complication encountered by investigators attempting to analyze the role of monoamine neurotransmitters in the control of pituitary secretion is the tendency of the organism to use these compounds as signals at multiple loci. Thus if a drug that acts, for example, by blocking dopamine receptors is shown to affect the secretion of a pituitary hormone, this finding provides no insights as to whether it is interfering with the flux of signals within the hypothalamus (for example, with the response of PIF cells to presynaptic dopamine), within the pituitary itself (for example, with the response of prolactin cells to dopamine secreted by the hypothalamus into the pituitary portal blood), or even elsewhere in the brain (for example, with a limbic dopaminergic region that influences neuroendocrine function). This difficulty is compounded by methodological limitations, such as the great difficulty faced in collecting pituitary portal blood and assaying its monoamine concentrations or the tendency of catecholamines to auto-oxidize during in vitro incubations with pituitary tissue.

While it is still not possible to claim with certainty that the role of dopamine in prolactin secretion is to serve as the unique PIF (that is, to act physiologically on the pituitary to suppress prolactin secretion), the most likely explanation (at least to this observer) for the effects of L-DOPA and of such dopamine-receptor blockers as the butyrophenones on prolactin secretion is that inhibitory dopamine receptors are present on pituitary cells that secrete prolactin. This hypothesis has been buttressed by additional data from Shaar and Clemens (1974) showing that: (1) the PIF activity of hypothalamic extracts is lost when catecholamines are removed from these extracts (either by passing them over alumina columns or by exposing them to purified monoamine oxidase) but not when they are incubated with proteolytic enzymes; (2) drugs known to activate dopamine receptors (such as apomorphine, ET-495) can override the stimulation of prolactin secretion caused by low doses of butyrophenones or phenothiazines; drugs that interact with norepinephrine or serotonin receptors fail to affect prolactin secretion.

At the present time, numerous investigators in academic and industrial institutions are attempting to apply their knowledge of dopamine-prolactin interactions to the search for new therapeutic agents for diseases that may involve prolactin, such as metastatic breast carcinoma and idiopathic and drug-induced galactorrheas. I view these developments with optimism.

10.6 Conclusions and Recommendations

There is compelling evidence that brain neurons utilizing known neurotransmitters (such as the catecholamines, serotonin, acetylcholine, GABA) participate in the control of gonadotropin secretion from the anterior pituitary gland. Moreover, a considerable amount of information is available concerning the biochemistry and pharmacology of these neurotransmitters—especially the monoamines, and many diseases are now effectively treated by drugs specifically designed to modify neurotransmitter metabolism. I hope to see the development of agents that, by acting selectively on brain synapses, will accelerate or suppress the secretion of specific gonadotropic hormones.

The first such set of drugs may well be those designed to suppress prolactin secretion by exploiting the relationship between dopamine receptors (possibly located within the pituitary itself) and inhibition of prolactin secretion.

A large number of investigators are now working on various aspects of neurotransmitter-pituitary interactions. Most are either varying hormonal state (as after hypophysectomy) and measuring the synthesis, fate, etc., of brain monoamines, or doing the reverse —giving drugs that modify brain monoamines and examining alterations in neuroendocrine function. Unfortunately, much of this work appears to be of poor quality. The most significant problem retarding the development of this field is the fact that both neuroendocrinology and neurotransmitter pharmacology are difficult fields, whose practitioners require considerable training. Few scientists are equally at home in both fields, with the result that the endocrine-neuroendocrine literature overflows with articles manifesting surprising neuropharmacologic naivete (often illustrated by the assumption that all of the drugs being used have only a single effect). (The reverse is less often seen, probably because, even now, only a relatively few neuropharmacologists appear to be working on endocrine problems.) The most likely solution to this problem would be the development of training programs to generate neuroendocrinology-neuropharmacology hybrids.

References

Anton-Tay, R., and R. J. Wurtman. Brain monoamines and endocrine function. In *Frontiers in neuroendocrinology*, eds. L. Martini and W. F. Ganong. New York: Oxford University Press, 1971.

Birge, C. A., L. S. Jacobs, C. T. Hammer, and W. H. Daughaday. Catecholamine inhibition of prolactin secretion by isolated rat adenohypophyses. Endocrinology 86:120, 1970.

Frantz, A. G. Catecholamines and the control of prolactin secretion in humans. Prog. Brain Res. 39:311, 1973.

Frantz, A. G., and D. L. Kleinberg. Prolactin: Evidence that it is separate from growth hormone in human blood. Science 170:745, 1970.

Friesen, H., H. Guyda, P. Hwang, J. E. Tyson, and A. Barbeau. Functional evaluation of prolactin secretion: A guide to therapy. J. Clin. Invest. 51:706, 1972.

Hwang, P., H. Guyda, and H. Friesen. A radioimmunoassay for human prolactin. Proc. Natl. Acad. Sci. USA 68:1902, 1971.

MacLeod, R. M., E. H. Fontham, and J. E. Lehymeyer. Prolactin and growth hormone production as influenced by catecholamines and agents that affect brain catecholamines. Neuroendocrinology 6:283, 1970.

Shaar, C. J., and J. A. Clemens. The role of catecholamines in the release of anterior pituitary prolactin in vitro. Endocrinology 95:1202, 1974.

Sulman, F. G. *Hypothalamic control of lactation*. New York: Springer, 1970.

Wurtman, R. J. Brain catecholamines and the control of secretion from the anterior pituitary gland. In *Hypophysiotropic hormones of the hypothalamus: assay and chemistry*, ed. J. Meites. Baltimore: Williams & Wilkins, 1970.

Wurtman, R. J. Neuroendocrine transducer cells in mammals. In *The neurosciences: Second study program*, ed. F. O. Schmitt. New York: Rockefeller University Press, 1970.

Wurtman, R. J. Brain monoamines in endocrine function. Neurosci. Res. Program Bull. 9(2). Reprinted in *Neurosciences Research Symposium Summaries*, vol. 6, eds. F. O. Schmitt, G. Adelman, T. Melnechuk, and F. G. Worden. Cambridge, Mass.: MIT Press, 1972.

11 Hypothalamic Influences on Pituitary Function in Humans

S. S. C. Yen, F. Naftolin, A. Lein, D. Krieger, and R. Utiger

11.1 Introduction

History and Background

The control of the adenohypophysis (anterior pituitary) and, through it, control of the thyroid, gonads, and adrenal cortex by the central nervous system (CNS) were recognized conceptually long before the relevant morphological and physiological pathways were delineated. The influence of emotional problems on gonadal and adrenal cortical function in humans and the effect of environmental factors on female reproductive cycles in many lower mammals required postulating some neural control of pituitary function. The anterior pituitary, although arising embryologically from ectodermal epithelium in an area destined to become the mouth, migrates toward that part of the primitive brain which ultimately forms the hypothalamus and the neurohypophysis (posterior pituitary). The proximity of the anterior pituitary to the hypothalamus would lead one to suspect that this part of the brain may be involved in pituitary regulation; however, investigators were faced with the troublesome finding that the anterior pituitary has virtually no nerve supply. Direct neurosecretory control thus seemed highly unlikely.

Another anatomical relationship between the hypothalamus and the anterior pituitary was reported in 1930 by Popa and Fielding, who described the vascular network between the hypothalamus and the anterior pituitary now known as the hypothalamic-hypophyseal portal system. Several years later (1937), Wislocki confirmed the presence of this portal system and further suggested that the blood flows from the median eminence toward the anterior pituitary. Very little further research on this system was reported over the next decade, until Green and Harris (1947) reexamined the brain-pituitary relationship in a number of different species of laboratory animals and found the hypothalamic-hypophyseal portal system in all of them. This work marked the beginning of an intensive investigation of this vascular network as the pathway by which the hypothalamus regulates anterior pituitary function. The hypothalamus was postulated to produce substances that are delivered directly to the anterior pituitary by the portal system and that control hormone secretion by the anterior pituitary. This hypothesis was soon validated, and, indeed, several such substances have now been isolated and characterized, and some of them have been synthesized. Thus the hypothalamus must now be defined as an endocrine gland whose principal function is the control of the anterior pituitary; when the vascular connections between the hypothalamus and the pituitary are severed, regulation of pituitary function is significantly disrupted.

In recent years other parts of the brain have been found to be involved in the regulation of endocrine activity. The brain appears to be a master gland, which not only exerts profound effects on pituitary activity (and on other endocrine glands) but also responds to the feedback effect of hormones of the target glands. These hormones may have important effects on the brain, some permanent, some transient; the gonadal steroids, for example, not only control sexual differentiation and initiate puberty but, through their action on the brain, regulate sexual behavior and modulate gonadotropin secretion. The recent demonstration of specific receptors or binding sites in brain tissue for gonadal steroids suggests that distinctive areas of the brain have specific neuroendocrine functions. Furthermore, the brain, particularly the hypothalamus, possesses the capacity for steroid modifications, such as the conversion of androgens to estrogens, the hydrolysis of estrone sulfate, the interconversion of estradiol and estrone, and most importantly, the 2-hydroxylation of estrogens to form catechol estrogens.

The brain not only reacts to and acts on target gland hormones but also performs de novo synthesis and secretion of several peptide hormones. Studies of the hypothalamic peptides TRF, LRF, and somatostatin, all of which regulate secretion of anterior pituitary hormones, have suggested that these peptides are synthesized by neurosecretory neurons. The recent identification of these peptides in the nerve terminals of many regions of the CNS has led to the postulation of a system of peptidergic neurons in the brain, analogous to the catecholaminergic systems, with axon terminations on the pituitary portal system. This hypothesis reaffirms the significance of these peptide hormones in the regulation of biological rhythms by the brain.

Communication among the billions of neurons in the brain requires the production of interneuronal neurotransmitters. Many neurotransmitters have been identified in the CNS: the catecholamine system (dopamine and norepinephrine), the indoleamines (serotonin and its derivative melatonin), acetylcholine, histamine, and gamma aminobutyric acid (GABA). The catecholamines appear to be the most important of the neurotransmitters in the neuroendocrine function of the brain and are particularly significant in determining or modulating hypothalamic endocrine functions. Thus some endocrine disorders ascribed to hypothalamic dysfunction may not represent a primary defect in the hypothalamic neurosecretory cells but may be attributable to disturbances of antecedent catecholamine systems. At any rate, the brain, in addition to all of its other functions, is clearly an important endocrine gland, producing and secreting hormones and responding, through classical feedback mechanisms, to peripheral target gland hormones.

Clinical Investigation

Hypothalamic involvement in the control of the anterior pituitary is more easily definable in lower mammals than in the human. In the female rabbit and cat, for example, ovulation normally occurs reflexly following coitus; this ovulation involves neural pathways in the spinal cord with input to the hypothalamus, which probably releases LRF and thereby induces LH release by the pituitary and ovulation. In the rat, LH release is correlated with the diurnal cycling of environmental illumination. In this case the optic nerves serve as pathways for neural impulses that finally reach the hypothalamus; blinded rats or those kept in total darkness lose their ability to ovulate and have no periods of sexual receptivity. Human release of LRF and ovulation depend neither on coitus nor on light-dark cycles. The hypothalamic and hypophyseal precursors to ovulation occur spontaneously, and blinded women, as well as sexually inactive women, exhibit normal ovarian cycles, suggesting that they possess normally operating hypothalami. On the other hand, emotional problems sometimes have significant impact on the menstrual cycle in women. A noteworthy example, of course, is pseudocyesis (false pregnancy), in which the anterior pituitary, presumably driven by the hypothalamus, produces hormones in a pattern and amount similar to that occurring in early pregnancy.

Until recently, most of the information concerning the hypothalamic control of the adenohypophysis in humans was extrapolated from the results of animal experimentation principally in rodents and later in infrahuman primates. This early work provided the basis for recent studies of the neuroendocrine regulation of reproductive cycles in the human. The advent of radioimmunoassays made possible a renewed effort to investigate quantitatively the hormonal basis for control of the menstrual cycle in the human. The results of these investigations disclosed a general scheme of gonadotropin rhythm from birth to old age (Figure 11.1),

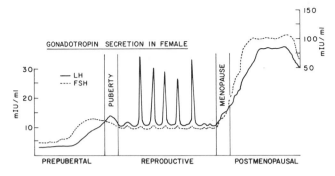

Figure 11.1 An overview of the life cycle of gonadotropin secretory patterns in the human female (from Yen).

the pulsatile pattern of release of gonadotropins, the peculiar relationship of sleep to pituitary function, and the fundamental role of the hypothalamus. Synthetic hypothalamic hormones (or factors) led to the design and execution of quantitative studies on hormonal factors influencing the response of the pituitary to the hypothalamus. Although limited by the kinds of experimental manipulations that may be performed in human subjects, much information has been generated concerning the operating characteristics of the hypothalamic-hypophyseal system.

The CNS-hypothalamic complex may be regarded as a signal generator, the pituitary may be seen as a decoder and signal transmitter, and a responding tissue or organ that in most cases serves also as a signal modulator. Investigators dealing with the neuroendocrine control of reproductive function, today and in the future, must know that normal operation of this three-faceted system requires not only the appropriate LRF-gonadotropin activity but also the integrity and interplay of other hypothalamic-pituitary functions, such as CRF-ACTH and TRF-TSH prolactin systems. Special emphasis must be given to the hypothalamic regulation of prolactin secretion and the influence of prolactin on endocrine function in general and on the output and action of gonadotropin in particular.

11.2 Control of Gonadotropin Secretion

The CNS-Hypothalamic Complex

Although the hypothalamus is recognized as the center in the CNS from which immediate control of anterior pituitary function emanates, input to the hypothalamus from other parts of the brain is known to be involved in the hypothalamic regulation of pituitary gonadotropin secretion.

Pattern of LRF release The principal hypothalamic hormone (or factor) determining gonadotropin hormone release by the pituitary is known as LRF (or LHRF), the luteinizing-hormone-releasing factor.

LRF is a decapeptide; it has been synthesized, and the naturally occurring and synthetic hormones are equally potent in inducing LH and FSH release from the pituitary. Bioassayable circulating LRF has been found to fluctuate in short pulses similar to the pulses of gonadotropin, and the administration of small amounts of LRF every two hours for a 10-hour period to eugonadal males is found to produce pulses of gonadotropin similar to those found in normal females. Such experiments have shown also that the pituitary is able to detect small increments or decrements in the amount of LRF and to respond accordingly. Thus it seems likely that the pulsatile character of gonadotropin secretion is dependent on pulses of LRF and that the amplitude and frequency of the pulses of gonadotropin may be determined by the amplitude and frequency of the pulsed release of LRF by the hypothalamus.

Biosynthesis and the site of LRF production The biosynthetic pathway for LRF has not yet been established, although experiments have shown that hypothalamic tissue (of the rat) is able, during incubation in vitro, to incorporate labeled arginine into a polypeptide with the same mobility as LRF. Present knowledge is limited concerning the precise site(s) of origin of LRF in the hypothalamus and the mechanism of delivery to the hypothalamic-hypophyseal portal system. Such information could be of considerable importance to our understanding of the hypothalamic-hypophyseal control mechanisms. For example, the hypothalamus probably has more than a single store of LRF, these stores may be functionally and morphologically distinct, and they may require different inputs to mobilize and release their contents. Although some evidence may be derived indirectly from the results of experiments using hypothalamic lesions, such studies have the common shortcoming that they do not distinguish between the destruction of an LRF-producing area and the interruption of a pathway involved in conveying LRF from the site of production to the site of release. Similar difficulties of interpretation apply also to data obtained in experiments employing electrical stimulation of hypothalamic structures.

Through the use of recently developed immunochemical methods of identifying LRF, immunoreactive LRF has been found in the median eminence (in processes near portal capillaries), in the perikarya of neurons scattered throughout the medial basal hypothalamus, and in the cytoplasm of tanycytes in the median eminence. Immunoreactive LRF has been found also in the arcuate nucleus.

Of considerable significance is the failure to detect LRF along the axons known to run from the neuronal cell bodies of the arcuate neurons to the hypothalamic capillary bed of the portal system. Although the functional significance of the observed LRF distribution is not clear in these preliminary studies, they do suggest that LRF may be synthesized in arcuate neurons and delivered to the tanycytes, which may concentrate and store LRF and ultimately deliver LRF, as required, to the portal system. The release of tanycyte LRF may be determined in part by the direct effect of gonadal steroids or by catecholamines, which are known to have profound effects on the subcellular morphology of tanycytes. Of interest in this connection is the observation that dopaminergic neurons frequently terminate on tanycytes.

Regulation of LRF secretion The hypothalamus may be considered an endocrine gland in which the production and release of LRF is regulated by several inputs, including neural signals arising in higher centers in the brain. The neural signals to the hypothalamus are apparently transmitted by humoral mediators; a number of catecholamines have been implicated for this function.

The precise neurons, the particular catecholamines involved, and the mechanisms of action remain unclear at the present time; however, dopamine and noradrenalin are present in well-defined neuronal pathways in the brain. For example, a prominent dopaminergic system has been described as consisting of small neurons located in the arcuate nucleus and axons projecting to the external layer of the median eminence. Preliminary studies have also revealed the occurrence of noradrenalin, together with dopamine, in the basal hypothalamus.

Several mechanisms have been proposed for the release of LRF in response to catecholamines. An attractively simple mechanism is represented by the suggestion that adrenergic control of local blood flow increases permeability of the portal vascular system, permitting the entry of increased amounts of LRF. A particularly interesting alternative suggestion for the role of catecholamines in the control of LRF secretion arises from the observation that the tanycytes in the median eminence, which connects the floor of the third ventricle with the portal vessels, possess microvilli on the surface facing the ventricle and abundant microtubules and microfilaments on the surfaces in juxtaposition with the portal vessels. A transport mechanism appears to exist, since compounds with protein-sized molecules can be recovered in the portal vessels after they have been injected into the third ventricle. Good evidence supports a role for catecholamines in this process: injection of dopamine into the third ventricle (but not into the general circulation) is found to induce a rapid increase in LRF and PIF (prolactin-inhibiting factor) activity in the portal blood, obviously suggesting the presence of a dopamine-mediated LRF and PIF control mechanism.

Studies of this aspect of hypothalamic function have

involved adrenergic blocking agents, and pulsatile LH release was found to be abolished by α (phentolamine) but not by β (propanolol) blocking agents in the ovariectomized rhesus monkey. This was not found in humans, but although the doses of α and β blocking agents used in the human studies were pharmacological (as indicated by the cardiovascular effects), they were only one-tenth of those used in the monkey experiments. Consequently, it is not certain whether this discrepancy between the rhesus monkey and humans is related to dosage or to species differences. Another possible explanation for the negative findings in humans is a partial blood-brain barrier for phentolamine, with the result that effective concentrations in the hypothalamus may not have been reached. Attempts to increase hypothalamic dopamine via the administration of L-DOPA or dopamine infusion in humans have provided evidence indicating that dopamine significantly inhibits LH release. Although the physiological significance of these findings is as yet undetermined, they are consistent with the results of animal studies and imply a role for catecholamines in the regulation of hypothalamic LRF release.

In view of the neuronal input to the hypothalamic LRF secreting mechanisms, it is not surprising to find changes in the LH pulses associated with certain emotional states. A marked increase in the amplitude of LH pulses is observed in patients with pseudocyesis, whereas a decrease is found in patients with anorexia nervosa. Certain hypothalamic lesions also result in decreased LH pulses. All of these observations, together with the sleep-related increase in LH pulses in puberty, support the concept that the frequency and amplitude of LH pulses are determined in part at least by neuronal rhythms.

LRF secretion is also regulated by another input to the hypothalamus, an input represented by blood plasma ovarian hormone concentration. Both estradiol and progesterone are involved. In much of the work on gonadal regulation of hypothalamic function, the effects on LRF secretion have been inferred from measurements of circulating pituitary gonadotropin levels. More recently, however, LRF bioassay and radioimmunoassay methods have been developed, and these permit direct measurement of the influence on LRF secretion of the manipulation of various regulatory inputs.

Assays of LRF in the portal blood of rats, performed by superfusing rat hemipituitaries, disclosed that castration causes an increase in the LRF concentration in hypothalamic-hypophyseal portal blood. Similar results are found in humans—bioassayable LRF concentration is significantly elevated in plasma of postmenopausal women as compared with the plasma levels obtained in premenopausal women, indicating

an inhibitory action on LRF secretion by gonadal steroids. Further measurements in women indicate that gonadal steroids may exert both an inhibitory and a facilitory effect (negative and positive feedback) on hypothalamic LRF secretion. As examples of the latter, increased levels of circulating bioassayable or radioimmunoassayable LRF are found at midcycle in normally cycling women and in women and in castrated men following treatment with estrogens. The feedback effect (both positive and negative) of gonadal steroids on LRF secretion is particularly significant in the maintenance of menstrual cycles and the timing of ovulation.

Metabolism of LRF   Nothing is known of the metabolism or transport characteristics of LRF between the time it leaves the hypothalamic neurons and the time it reaches the adenohypophysis. Specific binding proteins have not been demonstrated, although an estrogen-sensitive carrier (neurophysin) has been found in the portal blood of the rhesus monkey. This has not been shown to be a carrier for releasing factors, and one is tempted to question the need for a carrier protein for hypothalamic hypophysiotropic factors, since the delivery channels, the hypothalamic-hypophyseal portal vessels, provide direct transport to the pituitary without dilution by the systemic circulation and without the danger of prior loss or inactivation by the kidneys or liver.

The availability of isotopically labeled forms of LRF and the development of a specific radioimmunoassay for LRF have afforded the necessary tools for examining the metabolic fate of administered LRF. Administered LRF (labeled with tritium or with iodine 125) initially distributes in a space that approximates plasma volume and disappears from the plasma rapidly, exhibiting two components, an initial disappearance curve with a $t_{1/2}$ of about four minutes and a subsequent slower curve with a $t_{1/2}$ of about 50 minutes. Several tissues appear to be able to pick up and concentrate LRF; among them are the liver, kidney, posterior and anterior pituitary, and pineal gland. One hour after the injection of tritium-labeled LRF, a marked accumulation of radioactivity, as indicated by an elevated tissue to plasma (T/P) ratio, is found in the kidney ($T/P = 21.9$), the posterior pituitary ($T/P = 15.1$), the pineal ($T/P = 11.6$), the liver ($T/P = 2.5$), and the anterior pituitary ($T/P = 2.1$). The anterior pituitary, of course, is the accepted respondant to LRF, and its elevated T/P ratio is to be expected; the liver and the kidney in particular are probably important sites for the inactivation of LRF. One hour and 24 hours after the injection of labeled LRF, 48 percent and 73 percent, respectively, of the administered radioactivity is found in the urine. The urinary excretion products of LRF are biologically inactive, and some 80 to 90 percent of the radioactivity in the urine, after injecting labeled LRF, is found to be associated with a dipeptide, pyroglutamyl histidine. One of the mechanisms for inactivation of LRF, therefore, may be the cleavage of this dipeptide moiety from the N-terminus of LRF.

The high T/P ratio observed in the posterior pituitary and more particularly in the pineal is surprising. The pineal has recently been shown to contain 20 times more LRF than the hypothalamus contains. Whether this high concentration of LRF in the pineal represents accumulated LRF or LRF synthesized de novo is of primary importance; in any case, these findings implicate the pineal gland in the regulation of hypothalamic LRF and consequently in reproductive function. It seems possible that the pineal gland, tanycytes, and cerebrospinal fluid may be components in another pathway (circumventricular) for regulation of the adenohypophysis.

The Adenohypophysis
Pattern of gonadotropin secretion Gonadotropin secretion by the pituitary appears to consist of two components—a relatively constant basal secretion and, superimposed on it, an episodic or pulsatile release. Levels or concentrations of circulating gonadotropins are determined by the rate of release from the pituitary, the plasma dilution volume, and the rate of loss (clearance) from the circulating plasma. Since, under usual circumstances, the basal secretion rate, the clearance rate, and dilution volume in a given individual do not vary widely or rapidly, short-term changes in plasma concentration of gonadotropins are largely a reflection of the frequency and amplitude of the pulsed release from the pituitary. The hypothalamus and the pituitary form a closely coupled functional unit, and hypothalamic LRF is the chemical link between these two structures. A pulsatile release of hypothalamic LRF may be responsible for pulsed pituitary gonadotropin release, and the finding of episodic fluctuations of bioassayable circulating LRF in (hypogonadal) women adds credence to this assumption. Additional support is provided by a recent study using repeated injections of LRF (five times) at two-hour intervals, with large (150 μg), small (10 μg), incremental (10–300 μg), and decremental (300–10 μg) doses, to observe the effect on the pattern of gonadotropin release in eugonadal males with a relatively stable hypothalamic-pituitary-gonadal system. This experimental design was employed in order to simulate a pulsatile hypothalamic LRF input assumed to be immediately responsible for the pulsatile pituitary gonadotropin output and to determine whether the pituitary detects small incremental and decremental changes of LRF input at two-hour intervals. With repeated constant doses of LRF, the rates at which serum LH increases and decreases ap-

pear remarkably similar to those of spontaneous pulses in normal male subjects. The pituitary apparently can detect relatively small increments or decrements of LRF, as reflected by corresponding changes in circulating LH concentrations. The data obtained indicate that graded doses of LRF induce a graded variation in the quantity of LH released, and these data suggest, as indicated earlier, that variations in the amount of LRF delivered represent a significant factor in the control of the pituitary gonadotropin output.

Since the pituitary is able to respond repeatedly to moderate stimulation without reduction in the apparent amount of LH secreted and is able to follow changes in the dose of LRF even after several hours of repeated stimulation, either the pituitary has a large reserve of LH or it is able to synthesize and release new LH rapidly. Although the synthesis of new LH must be closely coupled to release, the immediate effect of LRF may be the release of stored pituitary hormone.

Pulsatile gonadotropin release is not modified by sleep and general anesthesia in normal adult females or by electrical shock therapy in psychiatric patients. On the other hand, modifications of the pulsatile gonadotropin rhythms can be found in patients with hypothalamic or suprahypothalamic dysfunction. A marked exaggeration of the amplitude of pulses is seen in patients with pseudocyesis, and a virtual absence of pulses is found in certain patients with anorexia nervosa, hypothalamic lesions, and in selected patients with hypogonadotropic "hypothalamic amenorrhea" or isolated gonadotropin deficiency.

Mechanism of the pituitary response to LRF Currently available evidence indicates that pituitary cells respond directly and acutely to LRF by releasing stored hormone, both LH and FSH. In fact, all of the hypothalamic hypophysiotropic hormones (HHH) appear to act directly on pituitary cells, as indicated by the release of the appropriate pituitary hormone when pituitary cells in vitro are exposed to a given hypothalamic factor. Thus the addition of LRF to cultured pituitary cells results in a high rate of gonadotropic hormone secretion that remains constant for at least a four-hour period. The initial pituitary response to HHH seems to involve the release of stored hormones. Short-term pretreatment of the pituitary with puromycine or cyclohexamide does not decrease the amount of pituitary hormone secreted in response to HHH, indicating that continuous de novo synthesis of the appropriate pituitary hormone is not *required* for the acute release in response to HHH.

Synthesis of new gonadotropic hormone is also stimulated by LRF, however; whether this is a direct LRF effect or secondary to the loss of hormone is not clear. Addition of nanogram amounts of LRF to female rat anterior pituitary cultures not only increases the release of both LH and FSH, but also increases the total content of LH and FSH in the culture. Similar evidence has been obtained in vivo during chronic administration of LRF to hypophysectomized rats bearing pituitary grafts. Chronic treatment with LRF stimulates production of FSH and LH in both sexes. As suggested above, this may not be a direct effect on synthesis; recently the adenyl cyclase and cyclic AMP system has been implicated as the mediator of the action of LRF.

The structure of LRF may be modified without eliminating its full biological expression; some changes may even enhance its activity. Large numbers of LRF analogs have been synthesized and tested. Deletion of one amino acid from the structure of native LRF results in a substantial, if not a complete, loss of biological activity. On the other hand, some substitutions of amino acids increase LRF activity; for example, (DAla^6) LRF has a potency of four to five times that of LRF, and des-Gly-amide^{10}-(Pro N ethyl amide^9) possesses three to five times more activity and longer action than native LRF. Analogs with antagonistic action to LRF have also been described; des-his^2-LRF, with low activity, does bind to the LRF receptor, as evidenced by its inhibition of LRF-induced LH release. This suggests that although histidine is required for stimulation of pituitary hormone secretion, it is not required for receptor recognition. Thus des-his^2-LRF behaves as a competitive antagonist, with its inhibiting effect overcome by increasing doses of LRF. Incorporating the D-Ala^6 modification or des-Gly^{10} proethylamide^9 modification into des-his^2-LRF enhances its antagonist potency threefold, but these antagonists are still rather weak inhibitors; a 700-fold molar excess of des-his^2-LRF is required to inhibit in vitro LH secretion by 50 percent. This line of investigation deserves considerable emphasis, since the future discovery of more potent LRF antagonists could represent a major advance in fertility control.

Using (^{3}H-Pro^9) LRF with high specific activity, two populations of binding sites have been found in the rat pituitary cells; one has a high affinity but low capacity, while the other is characterized by low affinity and high capacity for binding LRF. The high-affinity receptor is more specific than the other but nevertheless binds LRF, LRF agonists, and LRF antagonists, even in the presence of an excess of inactive LRF analogs saturating the low-affinity binding sites. Thus the limiting factor for biological activity of LRF and its analogs appears to be binding to the high-affinity LRF receptor.

Specificity of LRF action on the pituitary in humans
Until recently, a "unitary" concept of the relationship between hypothalamic factors and pituitary hormones held that each hypothalamic factor controls release of a single pituitary hormone. During the past three years, exceptions have been found for all three synthetic hypothalamic hormones: thyrotropin-releasing factor (TRF) releases prolactin as well as TSH, LRF releases FSH as well as LH, and somatostatin inhibits the release of TSH as well as growth hormone. In addition, somatostatin has been shown to inhibit the α and β cell function of the pancreas. Like the native hypothalamic decapeptide, synthetic LRF stimulates a greater release of LH than FSH in all species studied. The identification of but a single gonadotropin-releasing factor (LRF) has led to some difficulties in understanding the control of the changing levels of the two gonadotropins, FSH and LH, especially the changes occurring during the menstrual cycle. Two possibilities have been given consideration. A separate FSH-releasing factor (FRF), which causes release of FSH more effectively than release of LH, has been suggested, but its existence has not been demonstrated. Another possibility is that LRF serves as a releasing factor for both LH and FSH and that the kind and concentration of circulating gonadal steroids determine whether LRF will act mainly on one or the other of the two gonadotropins. Of interest in this connection is the histoimmunological evidence that LH and FSH are contained in the same cells of the human adenohypophysis.

Responses of the adult male pituitary to LRF In order to avoid the cyclic variation inherent in female reproductive function, some of the pharmacological and physiological properties of synthetic LRF have been studied in normal eugonadal males. Based on the dose response studies of LRF-induced LH release, 100–150 μg of LRF given intravenously are found to represent a near maximal stimulating dose, and 10 μg may be regarded as a threshold dose. Using either 10 μg or 150 μg doses of LRF, reasonably constant responses to LRF may be obtained in subjects with an intact hypothalamic-hypophyseal-testicular axis. An increase in circulating levels of LH occurs within two minutes after intravenous LRF administration. The maximal increments are greater and are achieved sooner for LH (25 minutes) than for FSH (45 minutes). The decline in gonadotropin concentration following the peak response to LRF is relatively slow and approximates a logarithmic decay curve with a mean $t_{1/2}$ of 92 minutes for LH and 450 minutes for FSH. These rates of disappearance are two to three times longer than those previously determined following hypophysectomy; this disparity is probably the result of a continued basal secretion of gonadotropin in the intact human, absent of course in the hypophysectomized individual. In any event, gonadotropin (LH) levels return to normal within six hours after LRF administration; no changes in circulating levels of TSH, prolactin, or growth hormone are observed, thus indicating the specificity of LRF on gonadotropin release. A consistent testicular response, as indicated by an increase in circulating testosterone, is not found following LRF administration, probably because of the short duration of the LH response and the already pulsatile character of testosterone secretion.

Routes of administration of LRF   The response to 100 μg of synthetic LRF given intravenously, intramuscularly, or subcutaneously appears to be independent of the route of administration. The release of LH and FSH is quantitatively similar with respect to magnitude and time course for all three routes. A more sustained LH and FSH release can be achieved by intravenous infusion of LRF over a given time period.

Intranasal application of a single dose of synthetic LRF dissolved in saline induces LH release, but the potency of LRF by this route is much lower than for the other routes of administration. In view of the efficacy of a 100 μg dose given subcutaneously, self-administration at six-hour intervals by the patient who requires chronic treatment appears to be a reasonable procedure until a long-acting preparation can be developed.

The Ovary

Cyclic changes in the release of gonadotropins   During their reproductive years, women exhibit a cyclic release of gonadotropin with a monthly periodicity. Both the tonic or basal secretion of gonadotropin and pulsatile release are involved, and this cycle, correlated with the menstrual cycle, appears to be consequent to the cyclicity inherent in the secretory and gametogenic aspects of ovarian function. When repeated small doses of LRF or constant infusions of LRF are administered, the induced pulses of LH in the plasma (ΔLH) increase in amplitude progressively through the follicular phase and into the midluteal phase of the cycle.

The pattern of serum LH response to both pulsed and continuous LRF stimulation in women supports the concept of the presence of two pools of releasable LH in the anterior pituitary, one immediately releasable and the other requiring continued stimulus input (Figure 11.2). A similar phenomenon has been reported for men and for pubertal (but not prepubertal) children. Thus the biphasic response to continued LRF infusion strongly suggests that the rapid rise in serum LH during the first 30 minutes results from release of the first pool, and that, with continued LRF stimulation, the second or reserve pool is tapped, with a secondary rise in serum LH concentration. In the case of pulsed LRF administration, the first pulse would appear to induce LH release from the first pool, and the increased release from subsequent pulses of LRF may be a result of activations of the reserve pool of LH.

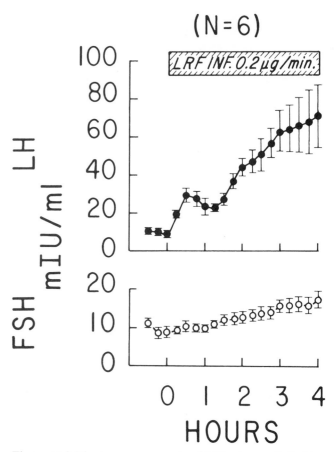

Figure 11.2 The two components of LH release elicited by constant LRF infusion in subjects during the early follicular phase of the cycle (mean ± SE).

The functional expression of these two components of gonadotropin release exhibited profound changes during the menstrual cycle and were in synchrony with the cyclicity of ovarian steroid levels (Figure 11.3); during the early follicular phase, both sensitivity and reserve were at a minimum, but increasing levels of E_2 brought about a preferential increase in reserve than in sensitivity ($P < 0.005$). In the late follicular and particularly in the early to midluteal phases of the menstrual cycle, the second and subsequent gonadotropin responses to pulsed LRF always exceed the response to the first pulse (Figure 11.4). Perhaps the first pulse not only induces release from the first pool but also activates the reserve pool, so that subsequent pulses of LRF may induce release of stored or reserve gonadotropin. The pattern of gonadotropin release during LRF infusion agrees with this concept. This self-priming effect of LRF occurs only during those phases of the menstrual cycle when the serum E_2 concentration is high; it can be produced in hypogonadal women through estrogen treatment. Although the physiological significance of the self-priming effect of LRF is not clear, it probably serves to activate the reserve pool and render its gonadotropin more readily releasable;

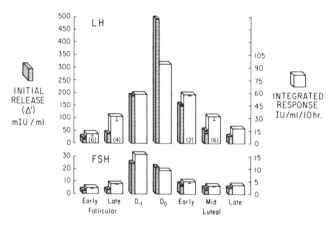

Figure 11.3 Analyses of the changes in pituitary sensitivity (Δ^i) and reserve (integrated response) elicited by pulses of LRF during different phases of the menstrual cycle (mean ± SE).

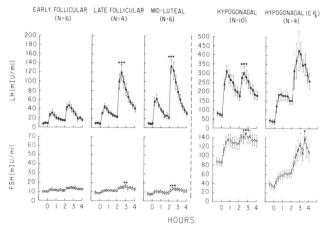

Figure 11.4 Quantitative and qualitative comparison between gonadotropin release to the first and second pulses of LRF (10 μg) during the low (early follicular) and high estrogen phases (late follicular and midluteal) of the cycle. Also, the effect of estrogen treatment in hypogonadal subjects (** = P < 0.01; *** = P < 0.005).

this is then revealed as an increase in sensitivity. The finding of a more rapid increase in sensitivity than in reserve from the late follicular phase to the midcycle surge is consistent with this postulate and is evidenced by a dramatic and stepwise increase in pituitary sensitivity on the day prior to and during the midcycle surge. This confirmation of changes in pituitary function may play an important role in the development of the midcycle surge.

Although both sensitivity and reserve increased dramatically near the midcycle, the relative change in these two components were reversed from the late follicular phase to the midcycle surge. This phenomenon may be causally related to the development of a self-priming effect of LRF at this time, as evidenced by an augmentation of gonadotropin release to the second pulse of LRF. Thus a buildup in pituitary store consequent to the greater increase in reserve than in sensitivity, together with the appearance of the self-priming effect of LRF induced by progressively rising levels of E_2, may constitute the essential dynamics required for the development of the midcycle gonadotropin surge. Pituitary sensitivity and reserve continue to be high during the early luteal phase but fall off progressively thereafter. In all studies, FSH responses are less obvious but show remarkable parallelism to the pattern of LH responses.

The foregoing discussion suggests that the functional state of the gonadotrops, as a target cell, is ultimately determined by the combined inputs of the hypophysiotropic effect of LRF and the modulating effect of ovarian steroids through their influence on sensitivity and reserve.

The feedback loop Modulation of the LH pulses is ac-

complished by the cycling concentration of ovarian sex steroids. The ovary appears to be an inherently cycling organ, producing and releasing mature ova and two principal hormones, estradiol and progesterone, in response to the pituitary gonadotropins. These ovarian hormones modulate the production of LRF by the hypothalamus and the pituitary LH response to LRF; thus they constitute a feedback loop in the regulation of hypothalamic-hypophyseal function. The feedback effect on pituitary function is apparently accomplished largely by modification of pituitary sensitivity to LRF.

An obvious means of studying the feedback regulation of the pituitary is to determine the pattern and amount of gonadotropin release after disruption of the feedback loop. Accordingly, circulating LH and FSH concentrations have been measured at frequent intervals in hypogonadal women with no preexisting feedback and after bilateral ovariectomy in premenopausal women. In the latter case, gonadotropin concentrations were found to rise over a three-week postoperative period to reach maximum levels about 10 times higher than the initial concentrations. Similar high concentrations of gonadotropins are found in hypogonadal patients, in whom no feedback loop exists, and in postmenopausal women, in whom ovarian aging has removed the feedback mechanism. In all of these women the FSH increase is higher than that for LH, but this probably happens not because of a greater secretory response for FSH, but because FSH is lost from the blood much more slowly than LH is and consequently accumulates to achieve a higher steady-state concentration. The important finding in these women is the constant observation that when the sex steroids are withdrawn, the release of gonadotropins from the pituitary is increased and the pulsatile pattern persists. The decreased concentration or virtual absence of estradiol is largely responsible for the elevated gonadotropin in each of these subjects, and ovarian steroids may thus be regarded as the feedback agents. Treatment of postmenopausal, hypogonadal, or ovariectomized women with estradiol reduces the LH and FSH output, and thus estradiol may be said to exert negative feedback.

The increased levels of gonadotropins in the absence of the normal feedback loop may be attributed in part to the elevated hypophysiotropic effect of increased LRF secretion; this has been observed both in the laboratory rat and in humans. Another important effect of ovarian steroid withdrawal is an increased sensitivity of the pituitary to LRF. Thus the action of administered estradiol in diminishing LH secretion in hypogonadal and in ovariectomized women may result from a combination of decreased LRF release and lowered responsiveness of the pituitary to LRF.

Frequency as well as amplitude of gonadotropin pulses is modulated by the feedback action of ovarian steroids. Hypogonadal women exhibit high-amplitude, high-frequency pulses, and both are reduced following administration of estrogen. Normally cycling women exhibit a pattern of high-frequency, low-amplitude pulses during the follicular phase. This pattern is modified during the luteal phase to a lower frequency and higher amplitude, thus suggesting that progesterone as well as estradiol exerts a modulating feedback effect on pulsed release of gonadotropin.

Progesterone plays other significant roles in regulating hypothalamic-hypophyseal function. It can trigger an acute surge of both LH and FSH after estrogen priming in humans; this effect has recently been demonstrated during the follicular phase in normally cycling women. Progesterone administered during the late follicular phase has been found to induce a relatively brief (12-hour) surge of LH and FSH. This progesterone activity is not demonstrable in the low-estrogen phase of the cycle, but in the high-estrogen phase it appears to be operative in relatively low serum concentrations. Of additional interest is the fact that 17α hydroxyprogesterone has no such effect. Since plasma progesterone concentration has been shown to be significantly elevated at the time of the midcycle LH surge, progesterone may act synergistically with estrogen.

Negative versus positive feedback When the role of estradiol as a feedback modulator of LH release is studied through the administration of this hormone to otherwise normal women, something puzzling occurs: whereas estradiol inhibits the pituitary response to LRF in hypogonadal women, in normal women the response of the pituitary to LRF is enhanced. Thus ovar-

ian steroids are said to exert both negative and positive feedback on gonadotropin secretion, and for many years numerous attempts were made to sort out and explain these effects. Until the advent of radioimmunoassay methods, however, methodological inadequacies limited the kinds of studies that might yield necessary information on this issue. The results of a series of recent investigations, in which estrogen was employed and circulating gonadotropin concentrations were measured, suggest that the feedback action of estradiol is not interrupted but can be represented by a U-shaped curve (Figure 11.5). Moderate concentrations of estradiol, such as are found in the early follicular phase of the menstrual cycle, inhibit gonadotropin output, but a change in estradiol concentration in either direction tends to diminish that inhibition and permit increased activity of the hypothalamic-hypophyseal complex. The normal, unopposed hypothalamus-pituitary system (as in the hypogonadal ovariectomized woman) produces gonadotropin at a relatively high rate; small amounts of estradiol suppress the gonadotropin output, but when the estradiol concentration is further elevated, the ability to suppress the gonadotropin release is reduced and the hypothalamic-hypophyseal complex begins again to function in a relatively unopposed manner.

When the response to LRF is measured in normal women during the first half of the menstrual cycle (follicular phase), the sensitivity of the pituitary to LRF increases progressively from the early to late follicular phase as the plasma estradiol concentration increases. Thus the effect of a range of estradiol concentrations

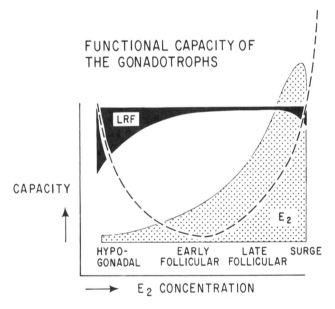

Figure 11.5 The relationship between the functional capacity (sensitivity and reserve) of the gonadotrophs and E_2 as a function of concentration and time. The rationalization of the endogenous LRF input is also depicted (from Yen).

has been observed, extending from the very low levels found in ovariectomized women to the relatively high levels found in normal women in the late follicular phase of the menstrual cycle, and the pituitary sensitivity to LRF as a function of estradiol concentration appears to follow the U-shaped curve mentioned above. This is not a unique situation; many bivariate relationships in biology seem to follow a similar pattern, and molecular explanations have been proposed.

Pituitary content of gonadotropin, as well as rate of release, appear to be determined in part by circulating estrogen concentration. This may be of considerable importance, since the content represents a reserve supply of gonadotropin, potentially available for release. The estrogen effect on pituitary gonadotropin reserve seems to approximate the same U-shaped curve presented above. These formulations may provide a basis for rationalizing the hypothalamic component in the operating characteristics of the pituitary. During the late follicular and midluteal phases of the cycle, when sensitivity and reserve are high and the self-priming effects of LRF are at a maximum, the relatively low basal gonadotropin secretion normally found requires that endogenous LRF release be very low. The modest increase in basal LH secretion observed just prior to the onset of the midcycle surge may reflect the beginnings of incremental LRF secretion; increased amounts of LRF have been found at the time of the midcycle surge in the portal blood of rhesus monkeys and in the peripheral blood of humans. The increased pituitary sensitivity and reserve, the development of the self-priming effect of LRF, and the increments in LRF release may represent the essential combination required to induce the stepwise release of LH at the time of the midcycle surge.

A progressive decrease in sensitivity and reserve characterizes pituitary function from the midluteal to late luteal phases and into the early follicular phase of an ensuing cycle. This probably results largely from the progressive decline in concentration of ovarian steroids on which sensitivity and reserve appear to be dependent; however, the elevation in basal LH and FSH release—in the face of reduced sensitivity and reserve—observed during the early follicular phase requires that an increased LRF release be postulated for this period of the cycle. Additionally, a decrease in the speculated ovarian inhibitory factor with preferential action on FSH secretion should be considered, in order to account for the higher levels of FSH than of LH seen at this time.

Mechanism of feedback action of ovarian steroids
Although the mechanism and sites of steroid feedback action are poorly understood, knowledge in this area is rapidly expanding. A clear and coherent pic-

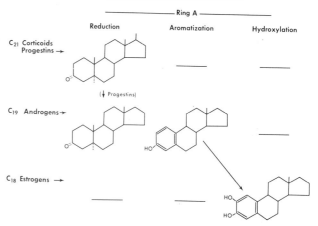

Figure 11.6 The metabolism of steroids by hypothalamic tissue (from Naftolin).

ure has not yet emerged, but a brief review may be appropriate.

The hypothalamus, pineal, and pituitary pick up and concentrate the radiolabel after injection of radioactive estrogen and progesterone. Cytosol binding of estrogens by pituitary and hypothalamic tissues has been clearly demonstrated, but nuclear binding in these tissues has not been well established.

Brain and pituitary tissues have been shown to be highly active in steroid metabolism (Figure 11.6). Three pathways are of particular interest, since they furnish active compounds that may play a cellular and/or synaptic role in brain-hypophyseal function: (1) Ring A Reduction—Reduction of androgens, corticoids, and progesterone occurs actively in the brain and pituitary, and the compounds formed may be considered to be equally or less active than the parent steroids in affecting hypothalamic-pituitary function. (2) Ring A Aromatization—The formation of estrogens from C_{19} and 19-norandrogen prehormones in the brain (and much less so in the pituitary gland) has been demonstrated in humans and experimental animals. Although the conversion rate (0.01–3.0 percent) is low, the compounds produced are far more active than the parent androgens. One is tempted to consider the possibility that local estrogens are important in hypothalamic regulation even in the male. (3) Ring A Hydroxylation—When considered on the basis of tissue weight, the hypothalamus has been shown to be the most active source of 2-hydroxylated estrogens in the body. Though poorly active in estrogenic secondary sexual effects, 2-hydroxy estrogens interfere with active-amine metabolism and can be active in influencing gonadotropin levels.

The significance of these metabolic pathways for steroids in the hypothalamus or pituitary is not yet understood. Suffice it to state for the moment that estrogens play a critical role in determining the function of the hypothalamic-hypophyseal complex, possibly in the male as well as in the female, and that the action of estrogen at the cellular level almost certainly involves both binding to specific receptors and metabolic changes in the structure of the estrogen, either before or after binding at the action site.

Transport of ovarian steroids Gonadal steroids circulate in the plasma, tightly bound to specific carrier proteins and loosely bound to albumin. Recent advances in our knowledge of these binding proteins have contributed significantly to our understanding of sex hormone metabolism and action. One such protein, sex-hormone-binding globulin (SHBG), is known to bind both testosterone (T) and E_2 reversibly, and changes in SHBG concentration then significantly affect the ratio of bound to unbound T and E_2 in plasma. Of interest here is the observation that estrogen and androgen have opposing effects on SHBG synthesis by the liver, with estrogen promoting and androgen suppressing synthesis.

Progesterone also circulates bound to a specific protein, in this case the same protein that transports cortisol and is known as corticosteroid-binding globulin (CBG), even though the association constant between progesterone and CBG is higher than that between cortisol and CBG. Another plasma protein with a high binding affinity for progesterone is α 1-acid glycoprotein (AAG), present in human serum at a concentration of about 750 mg/l.

Several possible roles have been proposed for plasma-steroid-binding proteins. The protein binding in plasma may play a buffering role, stabilizing the unbound steroid concentrations and minimizing extensive swings in concentration of steroid for reliable "monitoring" by the hypothalamic-pituitary system. Further, protein binding reduces the metabolic clearance rate of steroids; this may have "economic" value, in that the protein-bound steroids represent a circulating reservoir of sex hormone, protected, partially at least, from inactivation and excretion. Still another possibility is that the carrier protein is required for translocation of the steroid from the blood to the first binding site in the target tissue. In this case, one is led to question whether the physiologically significant moiety of circulating gonadal steroid is the protein-bound fraction or the free, unbound hormone. At any rate, it seems evident that the steroid-binding proteins play an important part in the regulation of the hypothalamic-hypophyseal-gonadal system in humans.

The Integrated Hypothalamic-Hypophyseal-Gonadal System
The menstrual cycle and ovulation Function of the normal, intact hypothalamic-hypophyseal-gonadal system is characterized in part at least by the occurrence of a menstrual cycle, which includes ovulation as one of its important events. The foregoing discussion shows that much progress has been made in our understanding of the operating characteristics of the components of this system, and we are ready to attempt to synthesize these components into an operational system. The ovary, inherently a cycling organ, in a sense supports its own monthly cycle through the feedback modulation of its steroids on the hypothalamus and pituitary. In the first half of the cycle—the follicular phase—estradiol output slowly increases in response to gonadotropin stimulation. The rising estradiol concentration seems to increase the magnitude of three variables: pulsed LRF output, pituitary sensitivity to LRF, and pituitary reserve. These combine to induce even greater output of gonadotropin, which in turn results in still higher estradiol concentration. This represents a classical example of positive feedback, and, as is typical of positive feedback, the system must place a limit on the rapidly developing responses, to avoid marked instability. In this case, when the three variables reach a given maximum, a paroxysmal release of LH occurs (the LH surge), which is responsible, some 12 hours later, for ovulation.

At the time of the LH surge and the consequent ovulation, important morphological and functional changes occur in the ovary. It begins to secrete progesterone in addition to estradiol, and these two hormones, acting together, possibly synergistically, maintain the pituitary sensitivity at a relatively high level. Some evidence has been presented to indicate the progesterone levels in the blood are already elevated in the late follicular phase, so this steroidal hormone may represent still another component in the simultaneous inputs that lead to ovulation.

An example of "local" positive feedback is found in the evidence that LRF appears not only to stimulate the secretion of pituitary gonadotropin but also to prime the adenohypophysis, so that further exposure to LRF results in an enhanced LH response. This priming effect of LRF appears to be operative only after sufficient exposure to rising concentrations of estradiol, either during the late follicular phase of the cycle or after appropriate administration of estradiol, and occurs normally at or near midcycle. It may be a major link between the augmented pituitary reserve and the onset of midcycle surge, and it may be critical in determining the timing and amplitude of that surge.

Manipulation of the system with drugs In normally cycling women the administration of estradiol and small amounts of progesterone increases the LH response to LRF; moreover, LH may be regarded as the "ovulation" hormone. By what mechanism, then, do estrogens block ovulation when administered in contraceptive pills? In women and other primates, cycling is determined by the functional characteristics of the ovary; in lower animals, on the other hand, the primary cycling organ may be the hypothalamus. In women, the ovary is itself an inherently cycling organ, with cycles created by the "time constants" for ovarian response to pituitary gonadotropins. The peculiar timing of these responses induce secondary cycling of the hypothalamus and pituitary through feedback mechanisms. Steroids administered in contraceptive pills override the cyclic feedback of ovarian steroids and, in effect, impose an externally determined cycle on the hypothalamic-hypophyseal complex, a cycle that does not include the ingredients required for ovulation. A clinical model for acyclicity is found in patients with polycystic ovaries. The ovaries in these patients are not able to cycle but do secrete a large and relatively steady amount of estradiol. The hypothalamic-hypophyseal mechanism responds appropriately, with an amplified pulsed output of LH at a relatively high but steady level; it retains the pulsatile pattern, since this is of hypothalamic origin, but it does not exhibit monthly cycles because it lacks the cyclic feedback input normally provided by the ovary. Although LH production is high in these women, the usual surge, required for ovulation, does not occur. A self-sustaining acyclicity is thus perpetuated, with acyclic ovaries creating acyclicity in the hypothalamic-pituitary system, which then maintains the ovaries in a noncycling state. If this system can be disturbed so that the ovaries are induced to cycle just once, the system may and frequently does begin to cycle spontaneously.

The effect of administration of clomiphene may also be rationalized in terms of the proposed system. This compound, an antiestrogenic material, apparently competes with estradiol for estrogen-binding sites in the hypothalamus and pituitary. Since clomiphene itself is a very weak estrogen, the hypothalamus and pituitary "see" a lack of estrogen, and they function much as they would in a hypogonadal woman. In terms of the U-shaped curve of Figure 11.6, the operating characteristics of the system move to the far left; gonadotropin output is increased, and if the ovaries are able to respond, follicular maturation and ovulation may be induced.

Analogs of LRF and their interaction with the pituitary have been briefly discussed above. Only two analogs of LRF have been studied in humans for their ability to inhibit secretion of gonadotropin; further investigation is of great potential importance. An analog able to reduce gonadotropin release could represent a significant advance in our methods of fertility control. Such LRF analog activity is based on the principle that structurally related compounds devoid of biological (LRF-like) activity may compete for the receptor sites normally occupied by the native, biologically active

LRF and displace it. The process is presumed to be reversible, and the magnitude of the physiological effect is a function of the fraction of the total number of active sites occupied by the analog. An analog with a minimum of biological activity and with a high binding affinity is required. At this time, however, the lack of clear understanding of basic hormone-receptor dynamics in the hypothalamus and the pituitary gland seems to constitute a major limitation in the application of LRF analogs to fertility control.

Maturation of the system: The onset of puberty The mechanism responsible for the onset of puberty has been, until recently, an unsolved puzzle. The enigma involved the apparent development of secondary sex characteristics prior to the detection of an increase in plasma levels or sex steroids. But the recent disclosure of a sleep-associated increase in pulsatile pituitary LH secretion at the time of puberty has advanced our understanding of the basis for sexual maturation. A progressive increase in the pulsed release of LH during sleep occurs in females from puberty stage I through stage V, and a temporally associated nocturnal testosterone secretion in males is also found.

Since this progressive augmentation of LH release during sleep appears to precede gonadal activity and does not seem to require sex hormone production, a "CNS program" may account for the pubertal activation of the hypothalamic-pituitary system. The concept of a CNS program is supported by the finding that release of LH following the administration of LRF is minimal in prepubertal children but increases markedly at puberty. Thus puberty appears to be initiated by a preprogrammed development or maturation of the CNS-hypothalamic-hypophyseal complex that is manifested only during sleep in the pubertal child. More information is certainly required about this entire phenomenon.

11.3 Control of Prolactin Secretion

The major role of prolactin in human physiology appears to be as a stimulator of lactation. Other actions of prolactin—in stimulating growth, in stimulating either maintenance of the corpus luteum of the ovary or its degeneration, and in regulating water and salt balance—have been described in experimental animals. Little evidence of these actions of prolactin has been demonstrated in humans, but studies of prolactin actions have not been extensive. Despite the seeming paucity of prolactin actions in humans, abundant evidence now suggests that prolactin secretion fluctuates widely in normal individuals, that it can be altered by a wide variety of physiological events and pharmacological agents, and that the major, if not only, control of its secretion is exerted by hypothalamic hormones.

Prolactin Secretion in Normal Individuals

Under ordinary circumstances, prolactin secretion appears primarily to be tonically inhibited by the hypothalamus. Perhaps the major evidence for this in humans is that separation of the vascular connections between the hypothalamus and pituitary gland result in increased prolactin secretion. This type of observation has led to suspicion of a hypothalamic prolactin-inhibiting hormone (PIH). Other studies have yielded evidence of a hypothalamic prolactin-releasing hormone (PRH) or hormones, a PRH having been partially isolated from animal hypothalamic tissue.

Prolactin secretion in normal subjects occurs in a pulsatile fashion; there is a superimposed diurnal rhythm. No major differences in plasma prolactin concentrations are found between prepubertal and postpubertal subjects. Nor are any significant differences in serum prolactin levels found between men and women, or among women in various phases of the reproductive cycle. During pregnancy, however, plasma prolactin concentrations progressively increase. Serum prolactin concentrations remain elevated during lactation, especially in its earlier phases. Moreover, breastfeeding is associated with striking increases in plasma prolactin concentrations.

Ovarian hormones are known to increase prolactin secretion, at least when administered in pharmacological doses for relatively long periods. Such hormones, no matter what their site of action, could be responsible, at least in part, for the augmented prolactin secretion occurring during normal pregnancy.

Pharmacological Effects on Prolactin Secretion

A variety of pharmacological agents cause major changes in prolactin secretion. These agents almost certainly exert their actions in the hypothalamus. Agents such as L-DOPA that lead to increased brain dopaminergic activity also cause reduced prolactin secretion. This is thought to be due to increased PIH secretion, but it could be as well explained by decreased secretion of a PRH. Inhibitors of adrenergic or dopaminergic neurotransmitter formation or action, such as various antihypertensive and tranquilizing agents, generally result in increased prolactin secretion.

Prolactin Secretion in Disease

A number of diseases appear to produce discrete hypothalamic lesions and result in chronically increased prolactin secretion. These disorders supposedly result in impairment of PIH secretion, but since in many of these situations the increased prolactin secretion can be reduced substantially by administration of L-DOPA, it is equally plausible that the initial abnormality is an increase in PRH secretion.

Direct Pituitary Modifiers of Prolactin Secretion

Thyrotropin-releasing hormone (TRH) is such a potent direct stimulator of prolactin secretion that appreciably smaller doses of it are required to stimulate prolactin secretion than are required to stimulate TSH secretion; this leads to the suggestion that TRH may be a physiologically important hypothalamic PRH. This action of TRH can be abolished by administration of L-DOPA; it can also be modified to some extent by thyroid hormones, increased quantities reducing the prolactin response to TRH and decreased quantities increasing the response. Indeed, reduced plasma thyroid hormones concentrations are occasionally associated with increased basal prolactin secretion. Since breastfeeding does not result in increased TSH secretion, the prolactin increase is probably not mediated by TRH secretion.

Summary

Alterations in prolactin secretion clearly occur with great frequency and rapidity, and a multiplicity of physiological and pharmalogical events result in altered prolactin secretion. Most if not all of these events alter prolactin secretion by actions on hypothalamic hormones. The ease with which prolactin secretion is altered indicates that virtually any CNS active agent may affect prolactin secretion in one or another way. What is uncertain are the physiological consequences of chronically increased or decreased prolactin secretion. Does the former only result in lactation in the postpartum woman and occasionally also in other subjects? Is it possible that the increased prolactin secretion occurring in the postpartum period results in the decreased pituitary gonadotropin secretion and acyclic ovarian function during this period? Curiously, no target organ product has been identified from the breast, gonad, or anywhere else that serves as a feedback regulator of prolactin secretion. These and many other problems, such as the chemistry of PRH and PIH, await further study.

11.4 Control of Thyrotropin Secretion

Thyroid hormones have a profound effect on the growth, development, and metabolism of virtually all tissues. The major, if not only, physiological action of TSH is to maintain the synthesis and secretion of the two thyroid hormones, thyroxine and triiodothyronine. Secretion of TSH from the pituitary is regulated by two major control mechanisms. One of these, the circulating concentration of the thyroid hormones, thyroxine and triiodothyronine, acts directly in the pituitary to inhibit TSH secretion. When circulating thyroid hormone concentrations are reduced, TSH secretion is increased. This is one of the best-known negative feedback control systems. The second regulator of TSH secretion is the hypothalamic hormone TRH, which stimulates TSH secretion. Abundant evidence indicates that, of these, the plasma thyroid hormone concentrations are the most important determinants of TSH secretion. The role of the hypothalamic hormone is generally considered, though hardly adequately established, to determine the rate of secretion of TSH occurring in the presence of normal plasma thyroid hormone levels and to render the TSH-secreting cells of the pituitary more sensitive to fluctuations in plasma thyroid hormone concentrations. Since TRH originates in the hypothalamus, which is richly interconnected with other areas of the CNS, a pathway is available for neural activation of TRH and thus for TSH and thyroid hormone secretion.

Thyroid Hormone Regulation of TSH Secretion

By far the greatest changes in TSH secretion occur when plasma thyroid hormone concentrations fall as a result of some intrinsic thyroidal abnormality. In many instances, if the thyroid gland is not irreversibly damaged and the thyroid secretory tissue mass is not too small, the increase in TSH secretion results in sufficient thyroidal stimulation to restore plasma thyroid hormone concentrations to near normal levels. At least theoretically, but probably also in fact, temporary reductions in serum thyroid hormone concentrations available to tissues could result from increases in thyroid hormone degradation, increases in thyroid hormone binding in serum, or decreases in peripheral generation of triiodothyronine from thyroxine. In such situations, increased TSH secretion should be at least temporarily required to restore the plasma thyroid hormone concentrations to normal.

Conversely, elevations in serum thyroid hormone concentrations result in prompt reduction in TSH secretion and therefore in plasma TSH concentration that persists as long as the TSH-secreting cells are exposed to the increased plasma thyroid hormone concentrations.

From a large number of observations based both on findings in patients with various diseases and on the results of a number of physiological experiments, the TSH-secreting mechanisms appear to be exquisitely sensitive to very small changes in plasma thyroid hormone concentrations. These changes in thyroid hormone concentrations are often too small to be recognized by any means other than direct measurement of TSH.

Thyrotropin-Releasing Hormone (TRH)

The structure of porcine and ovine TRH is known to be pyroglutamylhistidyl-prolineamide. TRH has been found in human hypothalamic extracts; its structure is presumed but not proved to be the same. No data are available concerning the regional distribution of TRH in the human hypothalamus. Similarly little information is available concerning the neurotransmitters involved in TRH secretion.

Hypothalamic Inhibition of TSH Secretion

Recent studies have shown that exogenously administered somatostatin (SRIH) inhibits the TSH response to TRH. Thus SRIH may be a physiologically important hypothalamic inhibitor of TSH secretion.

TRH Physiology in Humans

The requirement for TRH in humans is based primarily on the finding that thyroid deficiency occurs in human subjects with either or both hypothalamic damage and low plasma TSH levels that increase after exogenous TRH administration. No direct measurements of TRH physiology are as yet available. Sensitive and specific TRH radioimmunoassays have been developed, but endogenous TRH concentrations have not yet been measurable either, because of insufficient assay sensitivity or because of the presence in plasma of one or more enzymes that rapidly destroy TRH.

A number of physiological events not preceded by alterations in plasma thyroid hormone concentrations have been shown to result in changes in plasma TSH concentrations; they are presumed to occur as a result of altered TRH secretion. These events include:

1. Diurnal variation—Diurnal variations in plasma TSH concentrations have been demonstrated by some, but not all, investigators. When variations have been found, the higher plasma TSH levels have generally occurred in the late evening or early morning, and peak TSH concentrations are no more than twice those at other times of the day.

2. Neonatal TSH secretion—A striking increase in plasma TSH concentration occurs in the first minutes after birth. Since this occurs in the presence of reasonably normal plasma thyroid hormone concentrations, it presumably results from increased TRH secretion. The initiating physiological event is not known.

3. Steroid hormones, both of adrenal and ovarian origin, may under certain circumstances alter thyroid and TSH secretion, probably as a result of hypothalamic effects.

4. Modest changes in TSH secretion in humans have been observed in a few stressful situations, both environmental and psychological, unassociated with changes in plasma thyroid hormone levels.

The alterations in TSH secretion described above are in general of small magnitude and of very limited duration. Only in the instance of the newborn infant have these changes been shown to result in significant changes in thyroid secretion. Considerable experimental evidence indicates that sustained increases in TRH secretion would not result in significant sustained increases in TSH secretion, and therefore in thyroid secretion, due to the primacy of thyroid hormone control of TSH secretion.

The above comments avoid consideration of the possibility that the alterations in TSH secretion which follow alterations in plasma thyroid hormone concentrations are mediated by effects of thyroid hormones on TRH secretion, rather than by direct thyroid hormone action on TSH secretion. No direct evidence of this possibility is available in humans, but the known effects of thyroid hormones or their deficiency on the TSH responses to exogenously administered TRH in humans suggest that a hypothalamic action of thyroid hormones need not be postulated to explain any feature of the control of TSH secretion.

Pharmacological Effects of TRH
TRH was the first of the hypothalamic hormones to become available for use in humans, and in just a few years a large body of data has been accumulated about the effects of exogenously administered TRH in humans. TRH is now known to have four actions, at least when administered in pharmacological amounts. They are: stimulation of TSH release, stimulation of prolactin release, stimulation of growth hormone release, and perhaps psychotropic actions.
Stimulation of TSH release Administration of TRH to normal subjects results in prompt increases in TSH secretion. When maximally effective doses are given, plasma TSH concentrations generally rise 5- to 20-fold within 20 to 30 minutes if the TRH is given intravenously and within two to four hours if it is given orally. Minor differences have been observed in responses, depending on the age and sex of the recipient or the time of day or phase of the menstrual cycle, but the significance of these differences, if any, is unknown.

Several factors modify the TSH response to TRH. By far the most important are diseases of the thyroid and pituitary gland. When plasma thyroid hormone concentrations are low as a result of thyroid disease, not only are resting plasma TSH concentrations elevated but the increase in plasma TSH after TRH administration is exaggerated. This exaggeration may be observed even when plasma thyroid hormone concentrations are not unequivocally low or plasma TSH concentrations unequivocally high. Thus exaggerated plasma TSH increases after TRH administration may be the most sensitive of all indicators of intrinsic thyroid disease. Patients who have thyroid deficiency as a result of TSH deficiency usually have no TSH response to TRH. The same lack of response is observed in patients who are TSH-deficient but not thyroid-deficient. Such patients are said to have decreased pituitary TSH reserve.

Plasma TSH response after exogenous TRH administration usually does not occur in patients with elevated plasma thyroid hormones concentrations. This is the case not only in patients who have obvious excess secretion of thyroid hormones, but also in patients with various thyroid diseases or patients receiving exogenous thyroid hormone, in whom the plasma thyroid hormone concentrations are well within the normal range.

In normal subjects the TSH response to a dose of TRH can result in a small rise in plasma thyroid hormone concentration; however, if the TRH is administered repetitively for a day or two, the plasma TSH increase is considerably less. The implication of these findings is that marked sustained elevations in plasma TSH and thyroid hormone concentrations are not likely to result from prolonged TRH administration (or prolonged increases in endogenous TRH secretion), since the increased thyroid hormone secretion occurring in response to early TRH-induced TSH secretion inhibits the TSH responses to later TRH administration.

These results again indicate the great sensitivity of the TSH secretory mechanism to minor alterations in plasma thyroid hormones, which regulate TSH secretion primarily, if not entirely, by a pituitary, not a hypothalamic, action.
Stimulation of prolactin release Administration of TRH also results in prompt increases in prolactin secretion. Details concerning this action of TRH and its physiological significance are covered in another section of this report.
Stimulation of growth hormone release Transient increases in plasma growth hormone concentrations have been found after TRH administration in a few patients with growth-hormone-secreting pituitary tumors and chronic renal disease. The significance of these observations is obscure, but they clearly do not apply to normal individuals.
The psychotropic actions of TRH Some evidence has been accumulated that TRH, when administered to both normal and depressed subjects, has an antidepressant and mood-elevating effect. It has also been shown to have "antischizophrenic" actions. These observations raise many questions: Is this a pharmacological action of TRH, or is TRH involved in normal brain functions? Is this action of TRH useful in the long-term therapy of human psychiatric disease? Is TRH a neurotransmitter? That TRH may have widespread CNS physiological functions is suggested by re-

cent studies that show immunoreactive TRH widely distributed throughout the brain of experimental animals.

Summary

The evidence outlined in this section indicates that TSH secretion from the pituitary is very closely regulated by thyroid hormones. Since in few if any situations are increased tissue concentrations of thyroid hormone acutely required for survival or even normal physiological adaptations, it is perhaps not surprising that nonthyroidal events, such as increased TRH secretion, do not result in sustained increases in TSH secretion. Therefore, disrupting the function of the hypothalamic-pituitary thyroid axis by augmenting the production of either TSH or TRH will not likely lead to sustained or significant thyroidal hypersecretion, unless the stimulation, whether of TSH or TRH secretion, is marked and/or cannot be overcome by the pituitary inhibitory effects of the thyroid hormones. On the other hand, reduction of TSH or TRH secretion, or reduction of the ability of the pituitary to increase TSH secretion in response to thyroid hormone deficiency, may result in significant thyroid deficiency. This might occur as a result of reduced TRH secretion, increased production of a hypothalamic TSH-inhibiting hormone, if such exists, or direct reduction of TSH secretion. Thus thyroid secretion could be reduced in numerous ways, chronically or transiently, by physiological or pharmacological stimuli. The available evidence suggests the system is well protected against centrally acting events or agents that might increase thyroid secretion and is less well protected against reduced secretion of its components.

11.5 Control of ACTH Secretion

ACTH is stimulatory to the adrenal cortex. The adrenal cortex produces three types of hormones: glucocorticoids, which are of major importance in an individual's stress responses; mineralocorticoids, which regulate salt and water balance; and androgens, which may play a role in some of the events leading to puberty. Large doses of salt may to some extent replace the mineralocorticoid function of the adrenal. The absence of glucocorticoids (cortisone) causes inability to meet stressful situations (such as infections, traumas, and marked emotional upsets); in situations such as these in patients with adrenocortical insufficiency, death usually occurred before the isolation of cortisone. Overactivity of the adrenal cortex is most commonly manifested as Cushing's syndrome, which is usually a mixture, in varying proportions, of glucocorticoid and androgen excess; overproduction of mineralo-

corticoids has been implicated in some varieties of hypertension.

CNS Regulation of Secretion

At least three different aspects of ACTH release are generally accepted: basal, circadian, and stress-related. Each of these aspects may be modulated via separate anatomical and/or neurophysiological pathways. The hypothalamus is considered to be a final relay station, receiving neural input superiorly from the cortex, anteriorly and laterally from the limbic system (which is believed to be involved in emotional behavior), and posteriorly from the median forebrain bundle and reticular activating system (providing input from the vascular system as well as peripheral pain receptors, etc.). These pathways may utilize different neurotransmitter substances (such as acetylcholine, noradrenalin, or serotonin), one or more of which are released in the final synapse that activates the hypothalamic neurosecretory cell that produces corticotropin(ACTH)-releasing factor. Although this has not yet been isolated, it may be similar to vasopressin, which can stimulate the pituitary directly to secrete ACTH; however, vasopressin itself may cause the release of corticotropin-releasing factor. As yet, there is no evidence of a corticotropin-inhibiting factor.

The circadian periodicity of ACTH appears to be different from that of the other pituitary hormones in that it is not locked into the sleep-wake cycle. (It may persist in the absence of sleep, although in a person with a normal sleep-wake cycle the time of the major circadian rise always occurs up to four hours prior to awakening.) Light-dark influences also appear to play a minor role in the regulation of this periodicity in humans (Figure 11.7).

Feedback Regulation of ACTH Secretion

The circadian periodicity of ACTH secretion is assumed to be independent of feedback regulation, since such periodicity persists in the absence of the adrenal gland. Termination of stress-induced adrenal secretion (once this became appropriate) is probably by way of steroid (cortisone) feedback, suppressing ACTH output; an additional component of ACTH itself may be acting to reduce release and/or synthesis of corticotropin-releasing factor.

Evidence also exists that ACTH or fragments of it may alter behavior via a direct action on the CNS. The major site of steroid feedback has not been established for certain; in part this is because studies have been done with both naturally occurring steroids and with synthetic steroids, and there is evidence that uptake by the pituitary and CNS (the two sites favored by different proponents as being the loci of feedback) differs

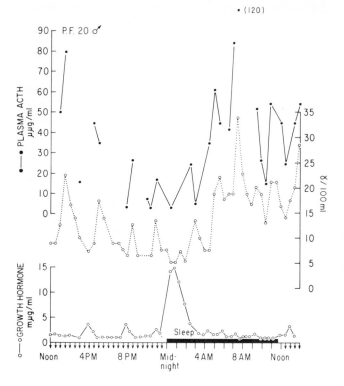

Figure 11.7 The pulsatile and circadian periodicity of ACTH secretion in humans (from Krieger).

for these two types of steroids. At present strong evidence suggests that native steroids act in a large part on a CNS locus, whereas synthetic steroids (for example, dexamethasone) may act on the pituitary.

Action of Nonadrenal Hormones on CNS Regulation of ACTH

Progesterone has been reported to suppress the ACTH release that normally occurs following the lowering of plasma corticosteroid levels. There is some evidence that free cortisol rises during pregnancy, so possibly greater than normal suppression of ACTH release might occur in response to stress.

In rats estradiol is reported to stimulate adrenal corticosterone production and inhibit 5α reductase activity, presumably by synergizing the action of ACTH on the adrenal cortex. Prolactin may reverse the stimulating effects of ACTH on adrenal function, and in rats it is also reported to decrease pituitary-adrenal responsiveness to stress.

Integration of the Gonadal and Adrenal Cortical System at the CNS Level

Several of the lines of investigation designed to develop contraceptive agents may involve changes in parameters that affect the hypothalamic regulation of ACTH. Some of the agents used may alter CNS content (generalized or in specific areas) of various neu-

rotransmitter agents; the neurotransmitter agents believed to regulate gonadotropin release (namely, dopamine and norepinephrine) have also been suggested to be involved in ACTH regulation. The effect of gonadal steroids (in excessive amounts) on circadian periodicity and stress responsiveness has not been systematically investigated.

Methodology Available for the Investigation of Hypothalamic Regulation of ACTH Release

Because of the relative insensitivity of previously available bioassays and limited access to sufficiently sensitive antisera with which to measure plasma ACTH levels, much of the investigative work in this field has relied on the measurement of plasma cortisol levels as an endpoint. This may not be a totally valid indicator, since similar increments in plasma cortisol levels may occur in response to stimuli that produce different increments in plasma ACTH levels. Radioimmunoassay of ACTH with some antisera measures a "big" ACTH with equal affinity to that of "normal," "little" ACTH; the "big" ACTH has, however, only 4 percent the potency of the "little" ACTH. The availability of sensitive bioassays for the determination of plasma ACTH that can be done concomitantly with that of radioimmunoassayable ACTH should clarify the nature of the ACTH response to various stimuli, as well as the nature of the ACTH secreted in disease states such as Cushing's disease.

Since a CRF has not been identified, clinical testing of pituitary response, similar to that performed with TRF or LRF, has not been possible. Vasopressin, however, may be used as a prototype of CRF. Thus far, no evidence exists of an isolated ACTH deficiency that may be secondary to lack of releasing factor stimulation.

11.6 Control of Growth Hormone Secretion

Growth hormone (GH) action sites are ubiquitous: GH does not have a specific target "gland" as is the case for the adrenal and ACTH. GH is essentially an anabolic hormone, in contrast to ACTH, which is a catabolic hormone. GH action is believed to be mediated by somatomedin (of which there may be several forms). Somatomedin is a protein believed to be synthesized in the liver and perhaps in the kidney, which is responsible for most, if not all, of the observed metabolic effects of GH. In the absence of GH in childhood, the most outstanding abnormality is lack of linear growth; occasionally hypoglycemia may occur or sexual development may be delayed. In the adult, lack of GH secretion is not accompanied by major clinical abnormalities. Excess GH secretion in the prepubertal individual is associated with giantism, in the adult with acromegaly, occasionally hypertension, and a diabetic glucose tolerance curve.

CNS Regulation of Secretion

The precise neural substrate involved in GH regulation has not been defined. The medial basal hypothalamus and the limbic system have been shown to play a regulatory role. Basal release, stress-induced release, and sleep-associated release have also been defined. The latter is not a true circadian periodicity, since it is tightly locked to the sleep cycle, the major growth peak occurring 90 minutes after sleep (whether sleep occurs by day or night). No agents affecting neurotransmitter levels have been effective in blocking the sleep-associated rise in plasma GH levels. Stress release of GH is believed to be mediated via α adrenergic pathways; there is also some evidence that serotonin and dopamine may both be stimulatory to basal GH release. The identity of the postulated GH-releasing factor, produced within the CNS, has not been clarified. In addition, there is a suggestion of regulation by a GH-inhibiting factor of CNS origin, somatostatin. This inhibits release of GH during sleep as well as under stress. The specificity of this inhibitory action is currently under study. The current concept of neuroendocrine regulation of GH secretion is shown in Figure 11.8.

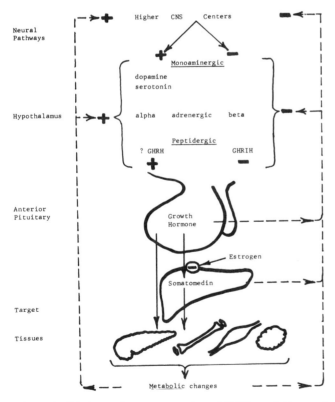

Figure 11.8 Schematic representation of CNS regulation and modulating factors of growth hormone secretion by the pituitary (from Krieger).

Feedback Regulation of GH Secretion

Some of the substrates upon which GH acts have been demonstrated to have feedback effects on GH secretion. Glucose and free fatty acids will inhibit GH release, probably by an action on the CNS releasing factor, although the role of somatostatin has not been investigated. There is also some evidence that GH may suppress its own secretion, presumably acting upon the CNS loci that effect its release. At present there is no evidence for a pituitary site of feedback.

Action of Other Hormones on CNS Regulation of GH

Estrogens increase GH levels, though they may block its action by interfering with somatostatin generation. (Increased GH levels have been reported following the administration of oral contraceptives.) Large doses of progesterone are reported to suppress GH secretion, though whether this is maintained on a long-term basis remains to be ascertained. Progesterone has been suggested as a therapeutic agent for acromegaly.

Integration of GH and Gonadal Hormone Secretion at the CNS Level

Some of the neurotransmitters involved in gonadotropin regulation are also involved in the regulation of GH secretion. Investigators have not tested the effect of chronic steroid treatment in unphysiological doses on GH secretion in response to stress.

Methodology Available for the Investigation of Hypothalamic Regulation of GH Release

The advent of the radioimmunoassay for the determination of plasma GH levels has contributed enormously to the understanding of the factors involved in GH release. Application of some of these studies to humans has been somewhat confused by the observation that many of the stimuli that normally occasion GH release in humans do the reverse in rats, which have been the experimental animals most used in such studies. Like ACTH, GH may exist in the circulation in "big" forms, the nature of which (prohormone or aggregates of "little" GH) is not clear. The presence of normal or elevated levels of GH in some subjects manifesting evidence of GH deficiency and a lack of responsiveness to exogenous GH would imply a defect of GH receptors in these cases. Since, as noted above, many of the biological actions of GH are secondary to GH stimulation of somatomedin, characterization and development of assays for such substance(s) will aid in the clarification of GH regulation.

Since a GH-releasing factor has not been identified, it can only be postulated that some cases of idiopathic GH failure are secondary to lack of stimulation by such a releasing factor. Although somatostatin (GH-inhibiting factor) has been shown to inhibit GH release in vitro, as well as stress-induced and sleep-aroused GH, its demonstrated effectiveness in blocking TRF stimulation of TSH release, as well as its effectiveness in blocking insulin and glucogon release, raise some questions as to the mode of the specificity of its inhibitory action.

It should also be noted that patients with GH-secreting tumors (acromegaly) have abnormal responses to the known releasing factors: TRF and LRF both release GH as well as their specific pituitary target hormones. This may imply some abnormality in the receptors present in such tumors. Abnormal responses to L-DOPA, which normally increases GH levels, have also been noted in these patients.

Although GH-releasing factor is not available for testing, it has been noted that the GH responsiveness, in patients with GH-secreting tumors, to stimuli believed to act via the CNS (hypoglycemia, hyperglycemia) suggests that such tumors may not be autonomous.

Selected Bibliography

Arimura, A., L. Debeljuk, and A. V. Schally. Stimulation of FSH release *in vivo* by prolonged infusion of synthetic LH-RH. Endocrinology 91:529, 1972.

Arimura, A., A. J. Kastin, and A. Schally. Immunoreactive LH-releasing hormones in plasma: Midcycle elevation in women. J. Clin. Endocrinol. Metab. 38:510, 1974.

Ben-Jonathan, N., R. S. Mical, and J. Porter. Superfusion of hemipituitaries with portal blood. I. LRF secretion in castrated and diestrous rats. Endocrinology 93:497, 1973.

Blake, C. A., and C. H. Sawyer. Effects of hypothalamic deafferentation on the pulsatile rhythm in plasma concentrations of luteinizing hormone in ovariectomized rats. Endocrinology 94:730, 1974.

Bogdanove, E. M. Direct gonad-pituitary feedback: An analysis of effects of intracranial estrogenic depots on gonadotropin secretion. Endocrinology 73:696, 1963.

Boyar, R. M., J. W. Finkelstein, H. Roffwarg, S. Kapen, E. D. Weitzman, and L. Hellman. Twenty-four-hour luteinizing hormone and follicle stimulating hormone secretory patterns in gonadal dysgenesis. J. Clin. Endocrinol. Metab. 37:521, 1973.

Ferin, M., A. Tempone, P. E. Zimmering, and R. L. Vande Wiele. Effect of antibodies to 17β-estradiol and progesterone on the estrous cycle of the rat. Endocrinology 85:1070, 1969.

Ferin, M., I. Dyrenfurth, S. Cowchock, M. Warren, and R. L. Vande Wiele. Active immunization to 17β-estradiol and its effects upon the reproductive cycle of the rhesus monkey. Endocrinology 94:765, 1974.

Fishman, J., and B. Norton. Catechol estrogen formation in the central nervous system of the rat. Endocrinology 96:1054, 1975.

Fuxe, K., and T. Hökfelt. Catecholamines in the hypothalamus and the pituitary gland. In *Frontiers in neuroendocrinol-*

ogy, eds. W. F. Ganong and L. Martini. New York: Oxford University Press, 1969.

Green, J. D., and G. Harris. The neurovascular link between the neurohypophysis and adenohypophysis. J. Endocrinol. 5:136, 1947.

Halász, B. Hypothalamic mechanisms controlling pituitary function. Prog. Brain Res. 38:97, 1972.

Harris, G. W. The induction of ovulation in the rabbit by electrical stimulation of the hypothalamo-hypophysial mechanism. Proc. Roy. Soc. Lond. [Biol.] 122:374, 1937.

Harris, G. W., and F. Naftolin. The hypothalamus and control of ovulation. Br. Med. Bull. (Control of Human Fertility) 26:3, 1970.

Haterius, H. O., and A. J. Derbyshire, Jr. Ovulation in the rabbit following upon stimulation of the hypothalamus. Am. J. Physiol. 119:329, 1937.

Hohlweg, W., and K. Junkmann. Die hormonal-nervöse regulierung des funktion des hypophysenvorderlappens. Klin. Wschr. 11:321, 1932.

Hohlweg, W. Veränderungen des hypophysenvorderlappens und des ovariums nach behandlung mit grossen dosen von follikel-hormon. Klin. Wschr. 13:92, 1934.

Kastin, A. J., C. Gual, and A. V. Schally. Clinical experiences with hypothalamic releasing hormones. Part 2. Luteinizing hormone-releasing hormone and other hypophyseiotropic releasing hormones. Recent Prog. Horm. Res. 28:201, 1972.

Knobil, E. On the control of gonadotropin secretion in the rhesus monkey. Recent Prog. Horm. Res. 30:1, 1974.

Korenman, S. G., and B. M. Sherman. Further studies of gonadotropin and estradiol secretion during the preovulatory phase of the human menstrual cycle. J. Clin. Endocrinol. Metab. 36:1205, 1973.

Lasley, B. L., C. F. Wang, and S. S. C. Yen. The effects of estrogen and progesterone on the functional capacity of the gonadotrops. J. Clin. Endocrinol. Metab. 41:820, 1975.

Malacara, J. M., L. E. Seyler, Jr., and S. Reichlin. Luteinizing hormone releasing factor activity in peripheral blood from women during the midcycle luteinizing hormone ovulatory surge. J. Clin. Endocrinol. Metab. 34:271, 1972.

Midgley, A. R., Jr., and R. B. Jaffe. Regulation of human gonadotropins: X. Episodic fluctuation of LH during the menstrual cycle. J. Clin. Endocrinol. Metab. 33:962, 1971.

Naftolin, F., S. S. C. Yen, and C. C. Tsai. Rapid cycling of plasma gonadotropins in normal men as demonstrated by frequent sampling. Nature; New Biol. 236:92, 1972.

Naftolin, F., K. J. Ryan, I. J. Davies, V. V. Reddy, F. Flores, Z. Petro, and M. Kuhn. The formation of estrogen by central neuroendocrine tissue. Recent Prog. Horm. Res. 31:295, 1975.

Nikitovitch-Winer, M., and J. W. Everett. Functional restitution of pituitary grafts re-transplanted from kidney to median eminence. Endocrinology 63:916, 1958.

Nillius, S. J., and L. Wide. Variation in LH and FSH response to LH-releasing hormone during the menstrual cycle. J. Obstet. Gynaecol. Br. Commonw. 79:865, 1972.

Odell, W. D., and R. S. Swerdloff. Progestogen-induced luteinizing and follicle-stimulating hormone surge in postmenopausal women: A simulated ovulatory peak. Proc. Natl. Acad. Sci. USA 61:529, 1968.

Popa, G. T., and U. Fielding. Hypophysio-portal vessels and their colloid accompaniment. J. Anat. 67:227, 1933.

Porter, J. C., R. S. Mical, N. Ben-Jonathan, and J. D. Ondo. Neurovascular regulation of the anterior hypophysis. Recent Prog. Horm. Res. 29:161, 1973.

Rebar, R., H. L. Judd, S. S. C. Yen, J. Rakoff, G. Vanden Berg, and F. Naftolin. Characterization of the inappropriate gonadotropin secretion in polycystic ovary syndrome. J. Clin. Invest. 57:1320, 1976.

Redding, T. W., A. J. Kastin, D. Gonzalez-Barcena, E. J. Coy, D. S. Schalch, and A. V. Schally. The half-life, metabolism and excretion of tritiated luteinizing hormone-releasing hormone (LH-RH) in man. J. Clin. Endocrinol. Metab. 37: 626, 1973.

Ross, G. T., C. M. Cargille, M. B. Lipsett, P. L. Rayford, J. R. Marshall, C. A. Strott, and D. Rodbard. Pituitary and gonadal hormones in women during spontaneous and induced ovulatory cycles. Recent Prog. Horm. Res. 26:1, 1970.

Santen, R. J., and C. W. Bardin. Episodic luteinizing hormone secretion in man. Pulse analysis, clinical interpretation, physiologic mechanisms. J. Clin. Invest. 52:2617, 1973.

Sawyer, C. H., J. E. Markee, and W. H. Hollinshead. Inhibition of ovulation in the rabbit by the adrenergic-blocking agent dibenamine. Endocrinology 41:395, 1947.

Seyler, L. E., Jr., and S. Reichlin. Luteinizing hormone-releasing factor (LRF) in plasma of postmenopausal women. J. Clin. Endocrinol. Metab. 37:197, 1973.

Seyler, L. E., Jr., and S. Reichlin. Episodic secretion of luteinizing hormone-releasing factor (LRF) in the human. J. Clin. Endocrinol. Metab. 39:471, 1974.

Seyler, L. E., Jr., and S. Reichlin. Feedback regulation of circulating LRF concentrations in men. J. Clin. Endocrinol. Metab. 39:906, 1974.

Siler, T. M., and S. S. C. Yen. Augmented gonadotropin in response to synthetic LRF in hypogonadal state. J. Clin. Endocrinol. Metab. 37:491, 1973.

Vanden Berg, G., and S. S. C. Yen. Effect of anti-estrogenic action of clomiphene during the menstrual cycle: Evidence for a change in the feedback sensitivity. J. Clin. Endocrinol. Metab. 37:356, 1973.

Vanden Berg, G., G. De Vane, and S. S. C. Yen. Effects of exogenous estrogen and progestin on pituitary responsiveness to synthetic luteinizing hormone-releasing factor. J. Clin. Invest. 53:1750, 1974.

Vande Wiele, R. L., J. Bogumil, I. Dyrenfurth, M. Ferin, R. Jewelewicz, M. Warren, T. Rixkallah, and G. Mikhail. Mechanisms regulating the menstrual cycle in women. Recent Prog. Horm. Res. 26:63, 1970.

Wang, C. F., B. L. Lasley, A. Lein, and S. S. C. Yen. The functional changes of the pituitary gonadotrops during the menstrual cycle. J. Clin. Endocrinol. Metab. 42:718, 1976.

Wang, C. F., and S. S. C. Yen. Direct evidence of estrogen modulation of pituitary sensitivity to luteinizing hormone releasing factor during the menstrual cycle. J. Clin. Invest. 55:201, 1975.

Wisloki, G. B., and L. S. King. The permeability of the hypophysis and hypothalamus to vital dyes, with a study of the hypophyseal vascular supply. Am. J. Anat. 58:421, 1932.

Yen, S. S. C., and C. C. Tsai. The effect of ovariectomy on gonadotropin release. J. Clin. Invest. 50:1149, 1971.

Yen, S. S. C., G. Vanden Berg, R. Rebar, and Y. Ehara. Variation of pituitary responsiveness to synthetic LRF during different phases of the menstrual cycle. J. Clin. Endocrinol. Metab. 35:931, 1972.

Yen, S. S. C., C. C. Tsai, F. Naftolin, G. Vanden Berg, and L. Ajabor. Pulsatile patterns of gonadotropin release in subjects with and without ovarian function. J. Clin. Endocrinol. Metab. 34:671, 1972.

Yen, S. S. C., C. C. Tsai, G. Vanden Berg, and R. Rebar. Gonadotropin dynamics in patients with gonadal dysgenesis: A model for the study of gonadotropin regulation. J. Clin. Endocrinol. Metab. 35:897, 1972.

Yen, S. S. C., and C. C. Tsai. Acute gonadotropin release induced by exogenous estradiol during the mid-follicular phase of the menstrual cycle. J. Clin. Endocrinol. Metab. 34:298, 1972.

Yen, S. S. C., R. Rebar, G. Vanden Berg, and H. Judd. Hypothalamic amenorrhea and hypogonadotropinism: Responses to synthetic LRF. J. Clin. Endocrinol. Metab. 36: 811, 1973.

Yen, S. S. C., G. Vanden Berg, C. C. Tsai, and T. Siler. Causal relationship between the hormonal variables in the menstrual cycle. In Biorhythms and human reproduction, eds. M. Ferin et al. New York: John Wiley & Sons, 1974.

Yen, S. S. C., G. Vanden Berg, C. C. Tsai, and D. Parker. Ultradian fluctuations of gonadotropins. In Biorhythms and reproduction, eds. M. Ferin et al. New York: John Wiley & Sons, 1974.

Yen, S. S. C., G. Vanden Berg, and T. M. Siler. Modulation of pituitary responsiveness to LRF by estrogen. J. Clin. Endocrinol. Metab. 39:170, 1974.

Yen, S. S. C., R. Rebar, and W. Quesenberry. Pseudocyesis: Neuroendocrine assessments. J. Clin. Endocrinol. Metab., in press.

Yen, S. S. C., B. L. Lasley, C. F. Wang, H. Leblanc, and T. M. Siler. The operating characteristics of the hypothalamic-pituitary system during the menstrual cycle and observations of biological action of somatostatin. Recent Prog. Horm. Res. 31:321, 1975.

12 Reproductive Immunology K. A. Laurence

12.1 Introduction

The science of reproductive immunology has not yet reached the age of maturity, even though it is an old and established discipline dating back to the turn of the century (1). Immunologic techniques, as they may relate to the study of reproduction, have recently been receiving an ever increasing amount of attention, which is an indication of renewed interest in the potential of immunology to throw light on the sequential events of reproduction.

As an example, the World Health Organization devoted its 1969 and 1974 Karolinska Symposia on Research Methods in Reproductive Endocrinology entirely to discussions of immunology techniques in reproductive endocrinology (2,3). Moreover, three recent international congresses have also been entirely devoted to immunological phenomena and reproduction (4,5,6).

The proceedings of all of these symposia reflect the progress that has occurred in the last decade. They also reflect a change in the attitude of the scientific community toward the applicability of immunologic procedures to the regulation of the fertility processes in man and other animals.

The first Karolinska Symposium (2) dealt entirely with discussions of immunoassay of gonadotropins. The deliberations, purely technical, included immunization techniques, affinity and specificity of antisera, types of immunologic reactions (complement fixation, radioimmunoassay), and correlation studies of biologic and immunologic estimations of gonadotropins in body fluids.

Five years later, the discussions at the seventh symposium were much more concerned with immunologic interference with fertility, using specific immune responses to specific antigens, and the long-term hazards that might be associated with such procedures. This is an indication of the increasing interest in the physiological application of immunology to the study of reproduction.

Whether immunologic techniques will ever reach their potential as fertility-regulating methods for the human is, as yet, a moot point. Nevertheless, immunology may still serve an important role aside from its potential application to the control of fertility. Its techniques may serve as a selective tool to further the understanding of the specific steps of the reproductive process that cannot be accomplished by other techniques. These procedures may in turn shed some light on other means by which fertility can be increased or decreased.

Almost every major laboratory in the world concerned with reproduction—including such diverse fields as endocrinology, obstetrics and gynecology, infertility, urology, clinical pathology, or animal husbandry—already employs, to some extent, immunologic techniques as tools for specific areas of reproductive research. Several procedures developed within the last decade have now become standard for hormone level determinations in biologic fluids, replacing the traditional but less sensitive bioassay techniques of the past. There can be little doubt that many of the still perplexing problems of reproduction will be resolved through the application of immunologic procedures.

If immunology is to contribute to a major breakthrough in fertility control, progress must be made in other disciplines. To be sure, immunologic procedures themselves will be improved, and other techniques will be developed as the need arises; but it will be alongside developments in the fields of endocrinology, physiology, histology, and the multifaceted discipline of chemistry that reproductive immunology should come of age in the next few years.

This is not to say that immunology has yet to make a major contribution to the field of reproduction. In fact there have been at least three contributions of major importance: the development of adjuvant techniques that enhance the antigenicity of substances which ordinarily have not been considered as potential immunogens (7), the rendering of the steroid molecule antigenic (8), and the technical development of radioimmunoassay (9,10).

The introduction of adjuvant procedures that enhance antibody formation and potentiate antigenicity of minute quantities of low-molecular-weight substances of homologous and heterologous origin was a necessary step for the development of reproductive immunology. Without it, studies on allergic aspermatogenesis, on antigenicity of protein and steroid hormones, and on hypothalamic releasing hormones probably would not have occurred (7).

The second giant step forward was the finding that

the steroid molecules could be rendered antigenic by simply coupling specific steroid molecules to a protein carrier of proven antigenic quality (8). This finding was to play a major role in demonstrating the ability of specific antibodies to combine with the steroid molecules in a specific and predictable manner. This technical breakthrough paved the way for immunologic measurement of peripheral, circulating levels of estrogen and progesterone in humans and experimental animals.

This step forward was quickly followed by the development and use of radioimmunoassays for measurement of insulin and growth hormone. Given this procedure, radioimmunoassays for gonadotropins and steroid hormones soon followed (9,10).

These technical advances were the foundations on which the present structure of reproductive immunology were secured.

12.2 Contributions in the Past Decade

Although reproductive immunology in its formative years provided only substantiation of already existing knowledge of the reproductive processes from a different vantage point, it is presently emerging as a formidable tool for expanding such studies.

It has progressed, in fact, to a stage of physiological application. Today its comparatively simple techniques are being used to extend the understanding of the interrelationship of the hypothalamic releasing hormones, the gonadotropins, and the steroid hormones to normal and abnormal menstrual cycles, to normal and abnormal pregnancies, or to cases of male or female infertility—a task of Herculean proportions, which would not even have been suggested just a few years ago. Techniques are available to measure blood levels of all hormones, to identify and locate hormone-producing cells and the site of hormone action at the target organ, and to discriminate the actions of hormones by specific sequestration of their responses in cells, tissues, organs, and on reproduction itself (11,12). Antibodies to specific hormones (LH, FSH, estrogen) at given times of the reproductive sequence can prevent ovulation, delay or prevent nidation, or terminate pregnancies. Antibodies to ICSH can interfere with testosterone production, affect libido, and inhibit spermatogenesis. Immunologic techniques are now being employed to discriminate specific hormone action on spermatogenesis and spermiation.

Immunology is being more extensively used to evaluate the medical sequelae of vasectomy. It is used to evaluate the occurrence and the significance of antibodies that agglutinate or immobilize spermatozoa and the ability of this immune system to interfere with restoration of fertility (13,14).

Similarly, cases of spontaneous infertility in the male may be related to the occurrence of an antibody formation to sperm that in some way lowers fertility. In some cases of infertility in the female, a correlation has been noted between antibody to spermatozoa and reduced fertility (15). Today any case of infertility, whether attributable to the male or to the female, is routinely examined immunologically for the presence of antibodies to sperm and correlated with the state of primary or secondary infertility (16).

The phenomenon of allergic aspermatogenesis has been extensively studied during the past decade and continues to attract attention around the world as a potential birth control method for the male (17,18). Immunization with spermatozoa of the female perhaps holds some promise as a basic method to regulate fertility; however, more recent studies on chorionic gonadotropin as a potential immunogen in humans appear to offer the most promising of all the potential applications of immunology to the regulation of fertility.

Because of advances in our knowledge of the chemistry of chorionic gonadotropins and pituitary gonadotropins, a new immunologic approach to neutralizing the hormonal action of chorionic gonadotropins is now possible.

Human chorionic gonadotropin (hCG) is chemically and immunologically similar to pituitary LH. Because of this similarity, it is possible to initiate antibody production against hCG that would cross-react with LH in urine. Such an antibody can then be utilized to detect levels of LH in the urine of nonpregnant women on a daily basis during a normal menstrual period and to detect the dramatic rise in hCG accompanying pregnancy (19).

Under a different set of circumstances, there is no question that antibody to hCG raised in rabbits or other laboratory animals can neutralize the hormonal action of exogenously administered hCG in test animals. The anti-hCG has little or no adverse effect on the endogenous hormone within the animal so immunized, however, because of the lack of antigenic identity or similarity of rabbit pituitary gonadotropins and the hCG molecule. Immunization of the human female with this hormone of pregnancy could theoretically result in antibody formation that could neutralize the hormonal action in very early pregnancy and thus prevent its continuation.

For several reasons, however, the utilization of hCG as an immunogen for fertility regulation may prove impossible. The hCG molecule would not be likely to stimulate antibody formation because its antigenic and molecular configuration is similar to the LH molecule, to which the human body has already created a condition of immunologic tolerance. If by chance the condition of immunologic tolerance could be overcome and an antibody could be produced, then there would be a strong possibility that neutralization of both hCG and LH, leading to interference of normal ovarian function, would most probably occur.

Stevens has already observed that the immunologic tolerance can be broken by altering the hCG molecule slightly (20). He accomplished this by using hapten-coupled hCG as an antigen. Antibody was produced that reacted with both hCG and human LH.

The problem then presents itself of finding a method to neutralize hCG but not LH. The biochemists have perhaps provided an answer—the observation that the hCG molecule is composed of two subunits, alpha and beta. The alpha subunit is similar to the alpha subunit of other gonadotropins, including LH, but the beta subunit is different (21). This offers an opportunity to elicit the formation of antibodies to the beta subunit, which would combine with and neutralize the native hormonal activity of the hCG molecule, without neutralizing endogenous LH activity.

Since antibody raised against the beta subunit of hCG has a high degree of specificity for hCG and there is a radioimmunoassay sensitive to hCG and not LH, it might be possible to develop a procedure to use the beta subunit of hCG as an immunogen in humans. The basic problem now is to find a procedure by which the immunologic tolerance can be overcome in humans.

Recently, Talwar and co-workers conjugated the beta hCG subunit to a second co-antigen, tetanus toxoid, and were able to demonstrate in monkeys, rabbits, and goats that antibody was formed which reacted with and neutralized the hormonal action of native hCG (22, 23). In a small series, women immunized with the beta hCG–tetanus toxoid conjugate responded with antibodies that combine with hCG. The immunized women reported normal menstrual cycle activity for more than one year following the administration of this immunogen. The long-term effects must still be evaluated, however, before extensive field trials can be made. If the safety of these procedures can be assured in primate experiments by establishing that there is no tissue damage or immune complex disease, and if it is effective in preventing pregnancy and can be reversed, this line of research may soon yield a new method of fertility control.

12.3 Potential Studies

The final product of reproduction is, after all, the set of all of its fractional steps. Without one member of the set, even if it is a subfraction, the final product is never viable or achieved. Each of these fractional sets in reproduction possesses at least potential antigenic prop-

erties and is thus vulnerable to immunologic attack. If one fraction of the sequential set is immunologically impaired, reproduction in its final form is prevented. Immunologic sequestration of pituitary LH, for example, either through active immunization with LH or through passive immunization with preformed specific anti-LH antibodies, can eliminate all the remaining members of the set between ovulation, nidation, and/or pregnancy maintenance. But between these major events there exist subfractional steps that are subject to impairment. The sequestration of LH most likely prevents the release of estrogen and thus ovulation and implantation. Impairment of estrogen action can accomplish the same result. But even further, estrogen action in the uterus is mediated through receptor sites. Might it be possible to stimulate the formation of specific, unique antibodies to estrogen receptors and thus prevent the hormonal action of this steroid at this level? If it were possible, gonadotropin release, estrogen synthesis, and ovulation would not be prevented; only the hormonal action necessary for implantation would be eliminated. Progesterone action can perhaps be neutralized in a similar fashion. The effect on the intricate feedback mechanisms would, of course, require attention. Nonetheless, steroid-receptor antibodies might allow us to learn more about how hormones elicit responses at the cellular and subcellular level and how the intermediate stages of reproduction can be successfully interfered with, without disrupting the overall process of hormone production and release.

Similarly, immunologic systems can interfere with the sequential events that lead to spermatogenesis, spermiation, and fertilization. Studies to date, however, have not advanced to the stage where it is practical to regulate fertility in the human male. Allergic aspermatogenesis, although simple, fast, and long-lasting, has disadvantages. First, the paraffin oil adjuvants necessary for stimulation of the reaction cause severe cutaneous lesions at the site of the injection. Second, the gonads atrophy to a psychologically unacceptable size. What is required is a method that does not interfere with spermatogenesis but simply prevents the spermatozoa from achieving the capacity to fertilize an ovum. There must be changes on the chemical surface of the sperm that allow sperm to penetrate an available ovum. Such changes, if known, might allow development of antibodies to prevent fertilization. It might even be possible to utilize the capacitation factor as an antigen in women, to prevent capacitation of sperm within their reproductive organs. Additionally, enzymes within the sperm may prove sufficiently specific and antigenic to produce a long-lasting infertility in immunized females. The studies of Goldberg on antibodies to LDH-X look promising in this area (24).

References

1. Tyler, A. Approaches to the control of fertility based on immunologic phenomena. J. Reprod. Fertil. 2:473, 1961.

2. Diczfalusy, E. Immunoassay of gonadotrophins. Acta Endocrinol. Suppl. 142, 1969.

3. Diczfalusy, E. Immunological approaches to fertility control. Acta Endocrinol. Suppl. 194, 1974.

4. Bratanov, K., V. H. Vulchanov, V. Dikon, V. K. Dokov, and S. Somlev, eds. *Immunology of spermatozoa and fertilization*. Sofia: Bulgarian Acad. Sci. Press, 1969.

5. Bratonov, K., ed. *Immunology of reproduction*. Sofia: Bulgarian Acad. Sci. Press, 1973.

6. Bratanov, K., ed. *Third International Symposium on Immunology of Reproduction: Abstracts of Papers*. Sofia: Bulgarian Acad. Sci. Press, 1975.

7. Freund, J., M. Lipton, and G. E. Thompson. Aspermatogenesis in the guinea pig induced by testicular tissue and adjuvants. J. Exp. Med. 97:711, 1953.

8. Lieberman, S., B. F. Erlander, S. M. Beiser, and F. G. Agate, Jr. Aspects of steroid chemistry and metabolism. Steroid conjugates: Their chemical immunochemical and endocrinological properties. Recent Prog. Horm. Res. 15:165, 1959.

9. Yalow, R. S., and S. A. Berson. Immunoassay of endogenous plasma insulin in man. J. Clin. Invest. 39:1157, 1960.

10. Hunter, W. M., and F. C. Greenwood. A radioimmunoelectrophoretic assay for growth hormone. Biochem. J. 85:39, 1962.

11. Laurence, K. A., and H. Hassouna. Immunologic studies of the endocrine system in relation to reproduction. *Handbook of physiology*, section 7, vol. 2, part 2. Baltimore: Williams & Wilkins, 1973.

12. Laurence, K. A. Bibliography on biological actions of antibodies to gonadotropins. Bibliography Reprod. 18:325, 1971.

13. Ansbacher, R. Vasectomy: Sperm antibodies. Fertil. Steril. 24:788, 1973.

14. Shulman, S. *Reproductive and antibody response*. Cleveland, Ohio: CRC Press, 1975.

15. Isojima, S., T. S. Li, and Y. Ashitaka. Immunologic analysis of sperm immobilizing factor found in sera of women with unexplained sterility. Am. J. Obstet. Gynecol. 101:677, 1968.

16. Fjallbrant, B., and O. Obrant. Clinical and seminal findings in men with sperm antibodies. Acta Obstet. Gynecol. Scand. 47:451, 1968.

17. Katsh, S., A. R. Aguirre, F. W. Leaver, and G. F. Katsh. Purification and partial characterization of aspermatogenic antigen. Fertil. Steril. 23:644, 1972.

18. Mancini, R. E., J. A. Androda, D. Saraceni, A. Bachmann, J. C. Lavierei, and M. Nemcrovsky. Immunological and testicular response in man sensitized with human testicular homogenate. J. Clin. Endocrinol. Metab. 25:859, 1965.

19. Wide, L., and C. Gemzell. Immunological determinations of pituitary luteinizing hormone in the urine of fertile and postmenopausal women and adult men. Acta Endocrinol. 39:539, 1962.

20. Stevens, V. C. Fertility control through active immunization using placenta proteins. Acta Endocrinol. Suppl. 194: 357, 1974.

21. Ross, G. T., J. L. Vaitukaitis, and J. B. Robbins. In *Structure-activity relationships of protein and polypeptide hormones*, eds. M. Margoulies and F. C. Greenwood. Excerpta Med. 241:153, 1972.

22. Talwar, G. P., S. K. Dubey, M. Salahuddin, N. C. Sharma, C. Das, S. Ramakrishnan, N. Shastri, S. Kumar, and V. Hingorani. Antiplacental immunological approaches for control of fertility: A potential antipregnancy vaccine. In *Third International Symposium on Immunology of Reproduction: Abstracts of Papers*, no. 144, ed. K. Bratanov. Sofia: Bulgarian Acad. Sci. Press, 1975.

23. Talwar, G. P. Contraception 13:125–285, 1976.

24. Goldberg, E. Effects of immunization with LDH-X on fertility. Acta Endocrinol. Suppl. 194:202, 1974.

13 The Oviduct

R. J. Blandau, B. Brackett,
R. M. Brenner, J. L. Boling,
S. H. Broderson, C. Hamner, and
L. Mastroianni, Jr.

13.1 Transport Mechanisms

Overview of Gamete Transport

The role of the oviductal cilia   In mammals the direction of ciliary beat throughout the oviduct was first assumed to be toward the uterus. We now know that a significant variation occurs in the direction of ciliary beat in the different subdivisions of the oviducts of various mammals. Such differences in the direction of beat may play an important role in the transport of spermatozoa to the site of fertilization and in the transport of eggs through the oviducts and into the uterus.

Ciliary activity is primarily responsible for the transport of freshly ovulated eggs in cumulus over the surface of the fimbria into the ostium of the oviduct and down the first few millimeters of the ampulla (Gaddum-Rosse and Blandau 1973; Gaddum-Rosse et al. 1973; Harper 1961). Thus in all animals so far examined (rat, guinea pig, cat, rabbit, pig, sheep, cow, monkey, and human), irrespective of the anatomical configuration of the fimbriae of the infundibulae of the oviducts, the programmed beat of the cilia plays the primary role in egg transport from the surface of the ovary and into the oviduct.

Egg transport through the ampulla   In all animals studied, the mucosal folds of the ampulla are much more extensive and complicated in their configuration than those of the isthmus. Approximately 50 percent of the surface cells lining the mucosa of the ampulla are ciliated. In all animals studied, including women, all of the cilia lining the ampulla appear to beat in the direction of the ampullar-isthmic junction.

The specific role of cilia in the transport of cumulus masses containing the ovulated eggs varies in different animals (Blandau 1973). In the rat and rabbit, egg transport through the ampulla is effected primarily by localized, segmental, peristaltic muscular contractions that compress the cumulus mass and "milk" it forward. Cilia may play an indirect role in holding the egg mass in place. In contrast, direct observations of the transport of freshly ovulated cumulus masses through the monkey ampulla reveal that the unidirectional ciliary beat is primarily responsible for their transport to the ampullar-isthmic junction. In vivo monkey preparations in which egg transport is observed directly and continuously have yielded no evidence that muscle contractions play any role in transport through this segment. It remains to be determined whether still other mechanisms transport the egg through the ampulla in different animals.

The ampullar-isthmic junction and egg retention   In all animals that have been studied in detail, a physiological stricture appears at the ampullar-isthmic junction at about the time of ovulation that prevents the cumulus masses from entering the isthmus before the eggs are fertilized and the follicular cells are dispersed. How spermatozoa are able to pass through the lumen of this stricture to enter the ampulla and effect fertilization is unknown. We know neither the nature of the constriction, when it first appears in the cycle, nor the factors responsible for its relaxation. Nothing is known concerning its neuropharmacology or its endocrinology (Brundin 1965). From 15 to 18 hours after ovulation, the cells comprising the cumulus and corona radiata have dispersed from the egg, possibly due to enzymes present in the oviductal fluids and the action of the sweep of the cilia lining the oviduct, "brushing off" the cells.

Egg transport through the isthmus   It normally requires 36 to 48 hours for eggs to be transported through the isthmus. Because of the thickness of the muscular walls of the isthmus, it is not possible to observe either the spermatozoa or eggs within the lumen of this segment of the oviduct. If stained cumulus masses, black polystyrene microspheres, or oils saturated with lampblack or Sudan dyes are inserted into the lumen of the isthmus, their transport can be followed by critical transillumination.

The pattern of intraluminal transport varies, depending upon when in the cycle the preparation is examined. During the preovulatory and early postovulatory periods in both the rabbit and the pig, the luminal contents of the isthmus are propelled rapidly toward the ampullar-isthmic junction. If stained oils are injected into the junctura region of the isthmus, small amounts of it, similar to a "bolus," are pinched off and carried toward the ovaries by a series of contraction waves that move sequentially from the uterotubal junction to the ampulla. The circular muscles contract so vigorously as to completely occlude the lumen as each wave of contraction progresses toward the ampulla (Blandau and Gaddum-Rosse 1974).

The contraction pattern of the isthmus changes dramatically 24 to 48 hours after ovulation. Then each loop or segment contracts in an undulatory pattern, so that the luminal contents are buffeted backward and forward. How the denuded eggs eventually reach the junction is not known for any mammal. Nothing is yet known regarding the endocrinology and neuropharmacology of the isthmus that could explain the changes in the muscular contractile pattern in the course of the cycle.

Direction of cilia beat in the isthmus Dual ciliary currents have now been described in the isthmi of rabbit and pig oviducts. Pro-ovarian ciliary currents carry particulate matter toward the ampullar-isthmic junction. These currents are particularly strong in the pig isthmus and to a lesser degree in the rabbit. Just how these pro-ovarian currents may assist sperm in their movements through this segment of the oviduct has not been resolved. The dual ciliary currents in the isthmus may also rotate the eggs during their passage through the upper part of the isthmus and may be responsible for the even deposition of the oolemmal membrane.

No dual ciliary pathways have been observed in carefully examined fresh isthmi of sheep, cows, monkeys, or women. Transport of particulate matter was consistently toward the uterine end in all regions of the oviducts (Gaddum-Rosse et al. 1973).

Studies Needed on Gamete Transport
Many unresolved problems remain regarding gamete transport within the oviducts of mammals. The following are some of the areas of observation and experimentation that would help to clarify the mechanism of gamete transport in this tubular system.

The uterotubal junction
1. There is no information regarding the manner in which spermatozoa pass through the uterotubal junction to enter the isthmus of the oviduct.

2. We need to know if and how the junction functions as a unidirectional valve to control the movement of fluids and gametes through this segment.

3. Nothing is known regarding the endocrinology and neuropharmacology of the junction.

4. The cytological changes in its epithelium need to be studied at the levels of light and electron microscopy at various times in the cycle.

5. Species differences in its function and physiology need to be evaluated.

6. The patterns of its muscular contractions, particularly during the preovulatory period, need to be studied.

The isthmus of the oviduct
1. The direction of ciliary beat needs to be studied on a comparative basis to obtain a better understanding of its role in sperm transport.

2. Very little is known regarding the cyclic changes in the pattern of muscle contractions of the isthmus in any animal.

3. The endocrinology and neuropharmacology of muscle contraction need to be explored and related to both sperm and egg transport through this segment of the oviduct.

4. It is important to determine whether the direction of ciliary beat can be reversed and/or the rate of beat controlled by chemical or pharmacological means.

5. No information exists on the mechanism of egg transport through the isthmus.

6. In certain animals an oolemmal membrane is deposited upon the zona pellucida as the egg passes through the isthmus. Investigations are needed on the mechanism by which this membrane is deposited so evenly.

The ampullar-isthmic junction
1. The mechanism effecting the physiological stricture of this segment of the oviduct is not known for any animal.

2. There is no information on how spermatozoa are transported through this narrow bottleneck.

3. Its endocrinology and neuropharmacology have not been explored in any animal.

4. It is important to determine whether it acts as a selective valve in controlling the number of spermatozoa that enter the ampulla.

The ampulla
1. The mechanisms of egg transport, and particularly the roles of muscle and cilia, need to be determined on a comparative basis.

2. We need to learn how spermatozoa are transported through the ampulla to escape into the peritoneal cavity.

The autonomic nervous system and gamete transport in the female In considering factors significant in the transport of the ovum in the mammalian oviduct, reviewers agree that the activity of the autonomic nervous system is highly instrumental in regulating the contractile patterns in the oviductal smooth muscle. These contractions, in turn, are believed to be important in gamete transport (Bell 1972; Marshall 1973; Black 1974). Another general consideration is that the hormonal state of the animal seems highly important in determining both the response of smooth muscle to autonomic stimulation and the concentration of neurotransmitter in the tissue. Both of these parameters —autonomic control and hormonal modification—are very poorly understood but are amenable to investigation with current techniques.

It seems almost axiomatic that one piece of information fundamental to a thorough understanding of the effect the autonomic nervous system has on the smooth muscle of the oviduct is a precise map of the entire tube, showing the complete distribution of autonomic nerves serving the various muscle layers. This information is not available. Classical descriptions of the innervation of the oviduct (Harting 1929) were derived for the most part from examination of material specially treated with silver stains. The architecture of the peripheral nerve networks and their termination can be elegantly displayed with such techniques, and counts of the absolute number of nerve fibers in different portions of the oviduct could be obtained.

The distribution of amine-containing nerve fibers, which are believed to be most important in oviductal contractions, may also be determined by employing the formaldehyde-induced fluorescence methods for the demonstration of biogenic amines (Falck and Owman 1965). Recent studies with this technique have clearly shown that the oviducts of several species, including the human, are abundantly supplied with adrenergic nerves and that norepinephrine is the major neurotransmitter present (Brundin 1965; Sjöberg 1967, 1968; Owman and Sjöberg 1972; Cottle and Higgs 1973). Several workers have reported their impressions concerning the relative density of fluorescent fibers in the ampulla and isthmus of the oviduct, and they concur that the isthmus contains the largest number of fibers. This latter finding has led Brundin (1965) and others to suggest that the isthmus may act as a sphincter in arresting the movement of the ovum at the ampullary-isthmic junction. Pauerstein et al. (1970) have suggested that such contractions of the isthmus are all-important in "tubal-locking" actions. No detailed description has yet been published of the precise density of adrenergic nerve fibers in the oviductal wall. A quantitative evaluation of the actual density of adrenergic nerve fibers, the number of nerve fibers in relation to the amount of smooth muscle present, would provide a detailed map of the pattern of innervation of the oviduct. The attractive features of a project such as this are that local differences in the density of innervation of various portions of the oviduct would be accurately documented and that innervation patterns of different species could be compared. Variations in contractility among species may, in part, be correlated with differences in innervation.

Studies employing fluorescence methods for localizing biogenic amines offer two distinct features that have not been fully exploited in studies relating to the oviduct. The first is that the biogenic amine may be positively identified by its emission spectrum; the second is that the amount of biogenic amine present may be quantitatively determined (Jonsson 1969; Sachs and Jonsson 1973). These useful techniques could be employed to quantitate differences in the density of adrenergic neurons and in the catecholamine content

of the neurons. Some studies point to the importance of being able to do this. Steroid hormones appear to be involved in modulating catecholamine levels and oviduct contractility (Bodkhe and Harper 1973). Combined histochemical and chemical analyses of the oviduct of the rabbit have shown that fluctuations in catecholamine levels are related to the differences in the hormonal state of the animal, reflected as greater or lesser flourescence in individual adrenergic neurons. Administration of estrogenic substances causes an irregular but detectable increase in norepinephrine concentration and in the number of observed adrenergic nerve fibers. When estrogenic substances combined with progesterone are given after estrogen priming, catecholamine levels fall and fewer flourescent fibers are seen (see Sjöberg 1969). These interesting findings suggest that the hormonal state of the animal is in some important way regulating neuron catecholamine concentration.

Data from studies of distribution patterns of the adrenergic nerves of the oviducts from animals and humans in various hormonal states should yield valuable information concerning regional or localized shifts in detectable catecholamine due to hormonal differences. Such studies would assume a special importance if the adrenergic nerve patterns and neuronal catecholamine levels could be shown to relate in some manner to the pharmacological evidence available, which indicates that the smooth muscle of the oviduct contracts upon stimulation with adrenergic drugs but is more susceptible to inhibitory stimulation when dominated by progesterone (Bell 1972).

The best electron-microscopic investigations to date of the relationship between the smooth muscle of the oviduct and the autonomic nerves of the tube have been carried out in Hervonen's laboratory. This group has examined the isthmus of the rabbit exclusively; otherwise, information is essentially lacking. Hervonen has observed two types of nerves associated with the smooth muscle of the rabbit oviducts. One has the morphological characteristics associated with catecholamine-containing adrenergic nerves, and the other type of nerve is most probably not adrenergic (Hervonen and Kanerva 1972, 1973). The adrenergic fibers probably correspond to the nerve fibers seen by fluorescence microscopy after treatment with formaldehyde gas.

Thorough studies of the relationship of adrenergic nerves to smooth muscle are required for all portions of the oviduct. Results of such studies might lead to a general understanding of the different contractile activities in the ampulla and isthmus. Along this line, Burnstock (1970) has suggested that several anatomical features may be employed to differentiate spontaneous, slowly contracting smooth muscle from non-spontaneous, relatively quickly contracting smooth muscle. The distinction involves differences in the distance separating the nerve from the muscle cell and in the degree of communication between muscle cells, as judged by the presence of tight junctions.

Hervonen has also described ultrastructural changes in the adrenergic nerves of the rabbit oviduct after treatment with estrogen (Hervonen et al. 1972, 1973). Although the exact significance of the findings is not immediately forthcoming, these studies show how labile the ultrastructure of adrenergic nerves is to hormonal manipulation. Accordingly, it might be fruitful to document the normal neuromuscular relationships in the oviducts of animals and humans after experimental manipulations with various pharmacological agents known to affect oviductal contractions. The benefit might be that alterations in ultrastructural morphology—for example, degranulation of adrenergic nerves—could be correlated with functional differences in contractility.

General comments All morphological investigations should be accompanied by chemical confirmation of the concentration of neurotransmitters in normal and experimental situations. At this time there is no information about the metabolism or utilization of catecholamine by adrenergic fibers in the oviduct; this is another obvious area for investigation.

The protocol of any experiment—morphological, chemical, or physiological—should be designed to include parallel studies precisely defining hormone levels in blood and tissues to ensure that data obtained from various experiments in different laboratories are directly comparable.

Combined morphological, chemical, and physiological investigations would clarify the highly complex relationships involving gamete transport, intrinsic smooth muscle activity, neuronal modification of smooth muscle activity, hormonal modification of intrinsic smooth muscle activity, and hormonal effects on neuronal modification of smooth muscle activity.

Definitive description of ampullar smooth muscle
No adequate description of the muscle layers of the ampullar wall exists for any mammalian species, let alone a meaningful comparison between species. No major contribution in this area of investigation has been published recently. In general, descriptions in the literature are cursory and appear as adjuncts to reports of studies of oviductal functions, which are the major interest of the investigators. No clear descriptions can be found for intercellular relations and precise arrangements in gross features such as circular or longitudinal fibers or layers. An understanding of these cellular relations is essential if the contractile behavior of the smooth muscle of the ampulla is to be understood.

Methods must be found for separating the exquisitely thin layers of muscle from the mucosa, which comprises as much as 95 percent of the mass of some regions of the ampullar wall. This is essential before accurate biochemical studies can be made on the muscle layer.

An adequate description of the muscle and nerve cell relationships in such regions as the ampullar-isthmic junction would be extremely helpful in attempts to understand the manner in which this physiological sphincter functions. Attempts to determine such a relationship have been published (Brundin 1969).

Transport of cumulus and contained egg through the ampulla of the oviduct For at least 75 years investigators have been acutely aware of the need in mammalian reproductive physiology to determine precisely the manner in which eggs and cumuli are transported through the ampulla, the regulating factors such as hormones, and the total time involved. Significant observations have been difficult because available observation techniques have interfered unpredictably and seriously with normal physiological processes. When the literature related to egg transport through the ampulla was reviewed by Blandau (1961), the best published information indicated that eggs passed through the rabbit ampulla in two hours or less (Greenwald 1959) or in 30 to 45 minutes (Zimmermann 1959).

In 1961 M. J. K. Harper reported ingenious in vivo studies in which he observed that vitally stained cumuli and eggs reached the ampullar-isthmic junction of lightly anesthetized does 4 to 12 minutes after they had been placed in the ostium of the oviduct by means of a fine pipette. The oviducts were periodically exteriorized through an abdominal incision and placed on moist cotton, where they could be observed and events recorded cinematographically.

Subsequently, a technique was developed that allows oviducts of anesthetized rabbits and monkeys to be bathed continuously in a warm physiologically balanced salt solution, where they may be observed and photographed while vitally stained cumulus egg masses are transported through the ampullae under various normal and experimental hormonal states (Blandau 1971). Innervation and blood vascular supplies are essentially intact. With caution, observations can be made continuously over periods of several hours, apparently without serious interference with normal transport mechanisms. The ease with which the reproductive cycle may be manipulated in the rabbit makes this species a reasonable choice for an experimental model. Preliminary observations show that similar techniques can be applied to the pigtail monkey, making it an excellent subhuman subject.

Observations performed with Blandau's "open

dish" technique have yielded the following information:

1. Egg and cumulus transport is more rapid at the time of ovulation in the rabbit than during estrus (prior to coitus or stimulation with an exogenous gonadotropin). Recent data in the literature indicate that estrogens are dominant in the estrous rabbit and that progestins are released following mating or an ovulation-inducing injection of luteinizing hormone (Hilliard et al. 1969).

2. The patterns of contractility of ampullar muscle are better programmed during egg transport in rabbit ampullae under the influence of estrogen followed by progesterone than under the influence of estrogen alone. No similar observations have been reported for other mammals.

3. The cumulus masses have been held at the ampullar-isthmic junction at the end of ampullar transport in the rabbit when estrogens and progestins have been present in physiologically balanced quantities.

4. At the end of ampullar transport in the rabbit, ova have been observed to pass directly through the region of the ampullar-isthmic junction when an antiestrogen (C1-628) has been previously injected.

5. It is now possible to record cinematographically the "pendulumlike" movements of the cumulus masses as they are transported through the entire ampulla. These movements, which are apparently induced by muscle contractions, vary characteristically in various segments of the ampulla and under various hormonal influences. Initial computer analysis of data taken from the cinematographs have shown distinct differences. These analyses are being continued, with the expectation of significant correlations and/or distinctions between egg movements and muscle and ciliary action.

6. Ampullar transport at a relatively normal rate occurs in the rabbit when ampullar muscle contractions have been inhibited by such agents as isoproterenol and Acepromazine Maleate (Ayerst). Under these circumstances transport is apparently accomplished by means of cilia. This distinct separation of the effects of muscle and cilia on egg transport in the same segment of the ampulla is being carefully studied in order to determine any significance it may have for the effective control of ovum transport.

7. The transport of ova through the ampulla of the pigtail monkey is apparently accomplished by ciliary action alone. This observation was not anticipated. It is being carefully repeated and analyzed, as it may be potentially useful in suggesting studies of ampullar transport in women.

8. Mean postovulatory transport time in both the pigtail monkey and the rabbit is more rapid than mean preovulatory transport time. The significance of this difference is not presently clear, but it seems likely to be associated with a change in estrogen and progestin levels.

9. Mean postovulatory ampullar transport time is shorter in the rabbit than in the pigtail monkey (6.1 ± 1.5 minutes vs. 17.8 ± 4.4 minutes), even though the rabbit ampulla is longer.

10. By means of observations of oviducts in the "open dish" preparation, it has been possible to critically assay the usefulness of two separate transducers designed to be implanted into rabbits and monkeys to monitor oviductal activity in freely moving, awake rabbits or monkeys. The first is a miniature optical cuff, which fits snugly about the ampulla or isthmus, holding a light-emitting diode on one side of the oviduct and a light-sensing element on the opposite side of the oviduct. Cuffs implanted in rabbits did not interfere with mating, pregnancy, and delivery of normal young. Unstained cumulus masses have been detected as they have passed between the prongs of cuffs in rabbits and monkeys. This makes the cuffs a potentially useful device for determining the rate of transport and also the time of ovulation, since the cumulus masses move through the ampullae within minutes after ovulation in both rabbits and monkeys. The optical sensor also detects muscle contractions in a manner as yet unexplained. These studies are continuing. A second transducer employs mutually inductive miniature coils, which are applied to the opposite sides of the ampulla or isthmus by means of a nontoxic, nonirritating tissue glue. These transducers are able to detect small changes in oviductal diameter and thus indicate patterns of muscle contractility at the point of coil application.

A limited portion of the data reviewed above has been published (Boling and Blandau 1971a,b); the balance of the work will be published as rapidly as feasible.

Other devices for monitoring oviductal muscle contractions Two recent publications have described methods of monitoring patterns of muscle contractility in awake, intact mammals: Garcia et al. (1974) report muscle contractions detected by means of a strain gauge transducer placed on the isthmus of rabbits or monkeys; Larks et al. (1971) record electrical potentials associated with oviductal muscle contractions. In view of the rate at which developments are occurring in bioengineering methods, unique and improved devices are anticipated for monitoring oviductal muscle contractions.

Influence of hormones on egg and blastocyst transport The role of estrogens and progestins in regulating the rate of ovum transport through the various segments of the oviduct is not clearly defined at this time. Reviews (Boling 1969; Coutinho 1973) and individual publications (Bastians 1973) have indicated that, depending on dosages given, manner of administration, and times at which effects are observed, estrogens and progestins may either accelerate or inhibit the rate of transport. Additional carefully planned observations are urgently needed.

The place of prostaglandins in studies of fertility has received considerable attention during the past decade. The literature is filled with many reports that have not been satisfactorily correlated. Swtantarta et al. (1974) report that prostaglandin $F_2\alpha$ levels are higher in human oviductal fluid than those normally found in circulating serum and that the concentration of this material varies in given oviductal tissues during the menstrual cycle. Ingelman-Sundberg et al. (1971) note that up to 1971 no publications had appeared describing studies related to the influence of prostaglandins on egg transport through oviducts. The data on prostaglandins seem pertinent enough to the subject of oviductal ovum transport to merit the design of definitive research methods for use initially in such mammalian models as the rabbit.

The Biology of Oviductal Cilia

Throughout the biological world, cilia and flagella play enormously important roles. Motility in many single-celled organisms, nutrition in fluid-feeders, excretion in organisms with primitive kidneys, and movement of mucus over respiratory passages are a few of the processes that involve the coordinated activity of these ancient structures—ancient, because evolutionary theory suggests that the first cells were motile, flagellated organisms. Cilia and flagella also play key roles in reproduction. Gametes are usually ciliated or bear one or two long flagella. In mammals, only the male gamete is flagellated, but the movements of the mammalian ovum still depend on cilia, because after ovulation the egg in its cumulus mass comes into immediate contact with a luxurious carpet of highly motile cilia that line the surface of the Fallopian tube. Caught up by the cilia, the cumulus mass is transported over the surface of the fimbria and enters the oviductal ostium. In primates (human and nonhuman), ciliary action within the oviduct provides the key propulsive force that moves the egg toward the ampullar-isthmic junction, where it is normally fertilized. In other mammals that have been studied in depth (rabbit, rat), vigorous contractions of the oviductal musculature "milk" the cumulus mass down the length of the tube (Blandau 1973).

In 1928 Edgar Allen began a series of classic studies of the hormonal regulation of the female reproductive tract in what was then a rare laboratory animal—the rhesus monkey. He made the extraordinary observations that, after ovariectomy, the cilia that line the Fallopian tube disappear and that injection of ovarian extracts into spayed monkeys causes a regeneration of the ciliated epithelium (Allen 1928).

In 1973 Brenner reviewed his own studies of the effects of castration and estrogen replacement therapy on the oviduct of the rhesus monkey (Brenner and Anderson 1973). Allen's findings were confirmed and extended by electron microscopy. The cilia of the rhesus monkey oviduct (especially in the fimbria) disappear within a few weeks of ovariectomy. The entire organ becomes atrophied, and the ciliated cells shrink and either fall out or shed their cilia. Treatment with estradiol for five to seven days stimulates cellular hypertrophy, mitosis, and a complex series of cytoplasmic events that culminate in the production of 200 to 300 motile cilia on the surface of each ciliated oviductal cell. Brenner further reported that a cyclic loss and regeneration of oviductal cilia occurred during the natural menstrual cycle and that this cycle could be mimicked in spayed monkeys by sequential treatment with an estradiol-progesterone regimen. Progesterone clearly is the factor that normally opposes the action of estradiol on the oviduct and leads to oviductal atrophy and deciliation during the luteal phase (Brenner et al. 1974).

In humans the oviduct undergoes similar atrophy and hypertrophy during the menstrual cycle, but the degree of deciliation appears to be much less extensive than in the rhesus monkey (Patek 1974). Considerable conflict exists in the literature over this point, and the matter deserves further study. In rabbits, ovariectomy is followed by a very slow process of atrophy and deciliation that is only partially complete after six months. Estrogen treatment of long-term spayed rabbits leads to an unusual phenomenon, however; the epithelial cells of the oviduct hypertrophy, lose whatever cilia remain, and then regenerate a new, vigorous crop of cilia (Odor and Blandau 1973).

When eggs in cumulus are placed on the surface of the fimbriae of long-term castrate rabbits, transport occurs, but at a slower rate than in normal animals. During the first few days of estrogen treatment of such spayed rabbits, however, when the cilia disappear, the ability of the fimbriae to transport eggs also disappears. As the cilia slowly grow back, the rate of transport also slowly increases until normal values are approached (Odor and Blandau 1973).

Fimbriae from women at midcycle are heavily ciliated and transport eggs rapidly. Very slow transport occurs over the atrophied, sparsely ciliated fimbriae of postmenopausal women (Gaddum-Rosse et al. 1973).

These studies document clearly the crucial role played by cilia in ovum transport. Many pertinent questions cry out for answers: Can the rate of ciliary activity be manipulated pharmacologically? Can the synthesis of new cilia be blocked? What are the normal variations in the rate of ciliary activity during the cycle? Are these rates hormonally influenced? What regional differences exist throughout the oviduct in the rate and pattern of ciliary beat?

Organ and tissue cultures are powerful tools that have provided new insights into the complex phenomena of cellular behavior.

Oviducts have been maintained successfully in vitro, and the cilia will beat for many days (Anderson and Brenner 1974; Rumery 1969), but the oviducts of primates are extraordinarily nonresponsive to estradiol in vitro. For example, spayed monkeys must be primed with three days of estrogen treatment in vivo before their oviducts will develop cilia in vitro. This failure to respond to estradiol in culture may be due to the instability of the cytoplasmic estradiol receptor. Uterine tissues also fail to respond to estradiol in culture, and the estrogen receptor quickly disappears when rat uteri are placed in culture (Peck et al. 1973).

Efforts must be continued to find culture conditions that support the estrogen receptor system and that permit a continued estrogen effect in vitro.

If we could provoke the oviduct to respond to estradiol in culture, various experiments that now require several animals could be performed on the tissues of one animal. How much simpler it would be to test 10 drugs in 10 dishes than in 10 monkeys! Unfortunately, few guidelines can be offered to the experimentalist striving to grow estrogen-sensitive tissues in culture.

We lack information on the accumulation of estradiol and progesterone by oviductal cells. Fortunately, techniques are now available to measure the tissue content of endogenous estradiol and progesterone by radioimmunoassay (Wiest 1973) and to observe the cellular distribution of labeled estradiol and progesterone by autoradiography (Stumpf 1968). For example, preliminary measurements suggest that when the content of cytoplasmic estradiol receptor in oviductal fimbriae is suppressed by progesterone, the tissue levels of estradiol are also suppressed (Brenner et al. 1974). These kinds of data are essential for a fuller understanding of the regulation of oviductal growth and function. For example, most species show a dramatic preovulatory surge of estradiol in plasma, followed by a precipitous fall. This surge presumably triggers the release of ovulatory quantities of LH. But what effect do the surge and the fall have on the tissues of the reproductive tract? What happens to the estrogen receptor during this period? Is there a parallel rise and fall in tissue levels of estradiol? Do these sudden shifts affect the oviductal musculature or the action of the cilia?

There is good evidence that estrogen withdrawal stimulates the rate of contraction of the oviductal musculature in the rabbit (Boling and Blandau 1971a,b). What are the changes in tissue levels of estradiol (and progesterone) in the periovulatory period in the rabbit? What percent of these sex steroids are bound within the smooth muscle cells versus the epithelial cells? Is estradiol driven into target cell nuclei during the preovulatory surge? Are hormones concentrated differently in the different regions of the oviduct? Autoradiographical studies hold great promise for the elucidation of such questions.

Fascinating differences have been observed between the oviducts of different species. In cats ciliary action provides the major propulsive force for egg transport throughout the length of the oviduct (Blandau 1973). In this respect, cats resemble primates more than any other species. Cats also provide a good model for the study of hormonal regulation of cilia; ovariectomy causes complete deciliation a few weeks after surgery, estradiol therapy restores the ciliated epithelium to normal, and progesterone antagonizes this effect of estradiol (Verhage et al. 1974). In dogs the oviduct is similarly regulated by the ovarian steroids (Verhage et al. 1973a,b).

In the oviducts of pigs an extraordinary adovarian ciliary current has been discovered in the region of the isthmus. Particles and fluid boluses are moved from the isthmus into the ampulla and are occasionally even expelled into the peritoneal cavity. These adovarian currents may be very important for sperm transport in pigs (Blandau and Gaddum-Rosse 1974). A similar adovarian current has been observed in the oviduct of the rabbit (Blandau 1973). More species should be examined in this fashion, because comparative anatomy teaches us so much about the evolution of biological mechanisms.

The ubiquitous cilia of the mammalian reproductive tract beat vigorously on. They pose many riddles to the investigator concerned with the movements of eggs, sperm, and blastocysts. Primitive organisms developed cilia as their primary means of locomotion; in advanced organisms, including primates, fertilization depends in part on their controlled, vigorous action. We should pay serious attention to these minute structures, small though they are, for the consequences of their action have been profound, for other species and for ourselves.

13.2 Oviductal Physiology

The Tubal Environment

Several laboratories in the United States and abroad have recently been concerned strictly with oviductal function, while others are studying the oviduct in connection with other aspects of reproduction, especially early reproductive processes.

It is now recognized that the contents of the oviduct are important in reproductive processes, and many constituents of oviductal fluid (the tubal environment) have been cataloged and evaluated. Oviductal fluid has been identified as a secretion as well as a transudate. Specifically, bicarbonate, pH, calcium ion, lactate, pyruvate, and oxygen tension have been identified as important factors in the maintenance of optimal development. Much of this work has been made possible by the development of means for continuous collection of fluid in such species as the rabbit, the sheep, and the monkey.

Hormonal regulation of fluid production has also been assessed, and the relationship between hormonal status and levels of the components of tubal fluid has been explored. To various degrees, these changes have been shown to influence such important processes as capacitation, fertilization, and early embryogenesis. Capacitation occurs optimally during estrus and immediately after ovulation. The environment for fertilization is best after the time of ovulation, whereas early embryogenesis proceeds best in oviductal fluid collected from the second day after ovulation up to the time of implantation.

Oviductal Function

The fluid contained within the oviductal lumen constitutes the milieu in which spermatozoa, ova, and the recently fertilized ovum survive and function. The biological processes known to occur at the oviductal level include capacitation of spermatozoa, fertilization, and cleavage. Thus, over and above its ability to transport gametes, the oviduct functions to provide an appropriate environment for the gametes, for the fertilization process, and for the fertilized ovum during the early stages of development. These environmental influences have not as yet been adequately assessed in laboratory species; and certainly in the primate, both monkey and human, there are glaring deficiencies in our knowledge.

In the rabbit, in vitro fertilization has been accomplished in a chemically defined medium with ova and spermatozoa that have not been exposed to the tubal environment (Seitz et al. 1970). With standard techniques, the fertilization process in vitro is not distinguishable morphologically from that observed in vivo; yet consistently lower proportions of in vitro fertilized and cultured rabbit embryos develop to term following transfer to surrogate dams than develop in the normal situation (Mills et al. 1973). Thus a chemically defined medium that will support fertilization and ear-

ly cleavage may not provide all that is necessary for subsequent normal development.

Conversely, tubal fluid constitutes a satisfactory medium for in vitro fertilization (Suzuki and Mastroianni 1968). Rabbit tubal fluid has also been shown to support early in vitro embryonic development, provided the samples are obtained subsequent to ovulation (Kille and Hamner 1973). Among primate species, in vitro fertilization of human ova has been accomplished, and development through the blastocyst stage has been documented. Yet there is no assurance that such embryos are capable of proceeding through implantation and normal development. The possibility remains that factors provided by tubal fluid are lacking or that a delicate balance of environmental factors should first occur in the Fallopian tube. It is also possible that there is nothing essential or unique about the tubal environment.

Collection of oviductal fluid In 1956 Bishop cannulated the fimbriated end of the rabbit oviduct and measured secretory pressure manometrically. Through his experiments, the feasibility of collection of oviductal fluids via the fimbria was established, and the way was paved for development of various methods for continuous collection of oviductal fluid. For this purpose, cannulae from the oviduct are connected to a collecting chamber located within or outside of the abdominal cavity (Clewe and Mastroianni 1960; Mastroianni et al. 1961a,b; Mastroianni and Wallach 1961; Sugawara and Takeguchi 1964; Hamner and Williams 1963, 1965). Refrigeration of an external collecting device enables short-term storage of the fluid at $+2$ to $+4°C$, thereby retarding enzymatic digestion or bacterial breakdown of the fluid, which may occur more rapidly at higher temperatures (Holmdahl and Mastroianni 1965). Others have cannulated the fimbriated oviductal ends and recovered fluid directly from silastic tubing secured over the back (Feigelson and Kay 1972). Brunton and Brusilow (1972) have recently conducted studies on small volumes (around $50\mu l$) of fluid collected by cannulation over intervals of 1 to 2 hours.

Composition of oviductal fluid Oviductal fluid is formed through the processes of transudation and secretion. Under natural conditions at ovulation, oviductal fluid may be a combination of fluids with contributions from the oviduct itself, the peritoneal fluid, uterine fluid, and follicular fluid. Information is sketchy concerning the specific mechanisms whereby the fluid reaches the lumen of the oviduct. The proportion of the total volume of oviductal fluid produced by transudation and active secretion varies under hormonal influence. In future research efforts one must be aware of this relationship, and any descriptions of oviductal fluid constituents must include an assessment of the endocrine status of the individual donor of the fluid.

Many inorganic and biochemical components of oviductal fluid have been identified. Unique protein components have been reported in oviductal fluid. These experiments have been carried out primarily in three species: the rabbit, the sheep, and the rhesus monkey. Additional data are available on the composition of oviductal fluid in cows and in humans. (See the reviews cited at the end of this chapter.)

Significance of studies on oviductal fluid composition
Many of the constituents that have been identified in oviductal fluids of mammalian species have been shown to be important in events of early reproduction. Bicarbonate ion in appropriate concentrations has been shown to stimulate sperm respiration and may play a role in conditioning the male gamete prior to fertilization (Hamner and Williams 1964).

The fluids of the female reproductive tract have many constituents supporting spermatic metabolism. Glucose, lactate, inositol, hexosamines, several free amino acids and phospholipids, as well as oxygen and carbon dioxide, are available to support oxidative respiration (Bishop 1969). Bicarbonate ensures an alkaline medium and furnishes a source of carbon for metabolic pathways (Hamner and Williams 1964). Amylase is present to digest glycogen, and a diesterase that hydrolyzes glyceryl phosphorylcholine from the seminal plasma is secreted by the female genital tract and may be important in uterus-inseminated species (White and Wallace 1961). The environment of the female reproductive tract surrounding the sperm probably is important in maintaining the proper oxidative state, pH, and osmolarity to prevent spermatic agglutination and promote capacitation (Austin 1970; Bishop 1969).

Developing mouse embryos are capable of carbon dioxide fixation (Graves and Biggers 1970); also bicarbonate can effect the dispersal of the corona radiata cells surrounding the rabbit ovum (Stambaugh et al. 1969). Corona cell dispersion is inhibited in vivo by acetazolamide, a carbonic anhydrase inhibitor (Noriega and Mastroianni 1969). Treatment of does with acetazolamide also caused a delay in cleavage of rabbit ova when given within 10 hours following coitus. A pH within the range of 7.5 to 8.0, resulting from the presence of bicarbonate in a 5 percent CO_2 in air atmosphere, has been found to favor the in vitro fertilization process of rabbit (Brackett and Williams 1968) and hamster (Bavister 1969) gametes. An oxygen tension comparable to that found within the oviduct favors in vitro fertilization and early ovum development (Brackett and Williams 1968; Whitten 1970).

Calcium ions are essential to the fertilization process in the mouse (Iwamatsu and Chang 1971). Wales (1970) reported potassium and calcium ions to be es-

sential for development of two-cell mouse embryos in culture. Daniel and Millward (1969) found calcium but not potassium to be essential for in vitro development of rabbit embryos. Whitten and Biggers (1968) found that mouse embryos could be cultured from the one-cell stage to blastocysts in a medium with an osmolarity reduced by lowering the sodium chloride content.

Utilization of glucose by embryos has been associated with certain stages of development that vary in different species (Brinster 1965; Daniel 1967). Pyruvate and lactate function as substrates for early embryonic development before embryos are capable of using glucose. Reinius (1970) has demonstrated large concentrations of glycogen in the isthmal region of the mouse oviduct, and the possibility exists that such reserves provide a source of glucose for the use of embryos as they pass through this part of the oviduct. Certain of the free amino acids are thought to be essential for embryonic development (Daniel and Olson 1968; Brinster 1970). In the mouse, Glass (1969) has reported that macromolecules are transferred from the bloodstream to the oviductal epithelium, into the lumen, and ultimately into the embryo. Such transfer is selective as to molecular species, oviductal region, and age and hormonal status of the animals in which it occurs.

Knowledge of the composition of oviductal fluid is of fundamental importance to efforts designed to duplicate in vitro the physiological conditions for gamete conditioning, fertilization, and early development and to alter the environments to which the gametes and the cleaving ova are exposed. Both lines of experimentation might lead to development of useful procedures for overcoming infertility or excessive fertility of various mammalian species.

Much progress has been made in defining minimal essential in vitro conditions for many of the important events that normally occur within the oviduct. Thus sperm capacitation, fertilization, and preimplantational embryonic development can take place, at least for a few species, in vitro and under conditions that are sufficiently similar to those provided in vivo. Improvement in the in vitro accomplishment of these processes can be expected as the physiologically correct environment is more closely approximated. This has been demonstrated in experiments of Kille and Hamner (1973), in which rabbit oviductal fluid, recovered eight and nine days after ovulation, provided a medium for optimal development of rabbit zygotes into completely hatched blastocysts, while development was not supported by oviductal fluid obtained from estrous does. In other experiments, Tervit et al. (1972) have been able to overcome the in vitro block to development of sheep and cattle embryos (Wintenberger et al. 1953) by composing a medium of a composition more closely approximating that provided by the oviduct. Efforts need to be continued in understanding the normal environmental conditions to which the gametes and developing embryos are exposed. Further understanding of these physiological conditions should provide greater insight regarding the possibility of manipulating or controlling reproductive processes at the oviductal level.

The oviduct functions obviously and subtly in the early development of the embryo. That the oviduct is responsible for the pickup and transport of the ovum to the uterus has been known for a long time; however, we have recently gained an appreciation for the environment of the oviduct and for specific functions of the various segments of the oviduct. Oviductal fluid is derived by transudation from the blood and secretory activity within the epithelium. Progesterone depresses fluid production and causes release of secretory materials from the epithelial cells. Except for the period three to six days after ovulation, when as much as 30 percent of the liquid passes into the uterus, the fluid flows toward the abdominal cavity.

Oviductal fluid from six mammalian species has been biochemically analyzed. The hormonal state of the female influences the electrolyte content of oviductal fluid. This response varies considerably among species. Specific proteins, which arise from secretory cells of the oviductal epithelium and serum proteins, are present in oviductal fluid. Estrous oviductal fluid stimulates maximal spermatic metabolism. Several constituents, including glucose, pyruvate, lactate, bicarbonate, and an unidentified, nondialyzable, heatlabile constituent, are responsible for the stimulation of respiration and glycolysis.

The contents of oviductal fluid important to fertilization and early development of the embryo have been elucidated by biochemical analysis and in vitro fertilization studies. Minimal requirements include a simple salt solution (280–300 mOsm), protein for macromolecular support, pyruvate or lactate as an energy source, bicarbonate for buffering, a reduced oxygen tension (5–8 percent), and an alkaline pH (7.4–7.8). Mucoproteins secreted by the oviductal epithelium appear to be needed for development and expansion of the blastocyst before its implantation.

Gaps in Our Knowledge
Physiological role of the oviduct in sperm capacitation From recent studies in the mouse and rabbit it appears that the mechanism of sperm capacitation involves removal of seminal plasma components, including decapacitation factor, from the surface of the sperm. We need to know: (1) What is the chemical nature of these adhering substances? (2) What oviduct factors and mechanisms (hormonal, and so on) are involved in

their removal? (3) How can the oviductal mechanisms be altered to produce a contraceptive effect?

Capacitation is probably associated with increased metabolic activity of sperm, but clear evidence of a direct association has not been provided. Questions that remain unanswered are: (1) What metabolic pathway is involved? (2) How is it activated? (3) What oviductal factors are responsible? (4) Can they be controlled?

Sperm transport is important with regard to capacitation because an oviduct with sperm has an adverse effect on capacitation as compared to the normal situation. (1) How does the oviduct control sperm numbers that are transported? (2) What are the hormonal mechanisms involved? (3) Are muscle activity and ciliary activity independently or jointly important, or are they important at all? (4) Can transport be controlled for contraception?

Physiological role of the secretory products of the oviduct The oviduct clearly produces specific secretory material, but our knowledge of its chemical nature and function is shamefully limited. Only the rabbit has been more than superficially studied, although similar secretory material has been noticed in many mammalian species, including monkeys and humans. (1) Are the secretory products necessary? Why? (2) What is their chemical makeup? (3) Can they be altered or eliminated specifically? The physiological and biochemical roles of these substances need to be defined because their regulation might lead to a fertility control method that is specific to the oviductal level.

Role of the oviduct in continued embryonal survival This broad area involves mechanisms through which oviductal environment can involve timing of fertilization, the fertilization process, early cleavage and information on development and storage, or regulation that may control postoviductal embryonic stages. The presence of trypsin inhibitors may influence fertilization timing to prevent the fertilization of the "overripe" or late ovulated egg. (1) What is the role of trypsin inhibitors? (2) Can they be controlled, and will their control be useful in contraception?

There are cleavage-inhibiting agents in preovulatory oviductal fluid of the rabbit. (1) Are such agents responsible for the specific timing of embryo cleavage? (2) Are they found in other species, especially humans? (3) Are they specific to each species, or are they universal inhibitors? (4) What is the mechanism of their inhibition? (5) What is their chemical nature? (6) Can they be induced to remain at high levels in the oviduct for contraceptive activity?

The embryo must be delivered to the uterus at exactly the right time. (1) Are the fluid constituents so programmed that small or great alterations are required to impede normal development? (2) What are

the most crucial constituents? (3) How are they produced or regulated? Can they be altered?

**Effect of the recently ovulated ovum on oviductal
function** The biochemical relationship between the
zygote and oviductal function in the proximity of the
zygote is just beginning to be studied; however, very
preliminary work—anatomical observations and thymidine incorporation—suggests that important communication processes are at work. (1) What mediates
messages between the embryo and oviduct? (2) What
is produced or released by the embryo? (3) What is
produced (and how) by the oviduct, and how is it released? (4) What possible constraints could be directed
at either the embryo or oviduct?

Pharmacological influences on oviductal function
Several pharmacological agents are capable of traversing into the oviductal lumen environment, but many
others are not. If agents are to be used to control oviductal secretions or embryonal development, we have
to know about the mechanism of transport of agents
from the blood to the fluid. (1) What local delivery systems could be developed? (2) What agents are most
likely to be effective?

**Understanding of oviductal function in subhuman
primates and in humans** Little information is available on the oviductal environment of homo sapiens.
All questions asked so far in this section apply especially to humans. Some information is available in the
subhuman primate, but many of the essential processes are not known. (1) Are oviductal functions of
primates similar to that of lower animals? (2) Do they
have species-specific essential mechanisms at work?

**Effect of oviductal fluid on gamete and embryo
transport** Although this subject is largely covered in
the chapter on gamete transport, we need to emphasize the relationship between fluid flow and transport.
(1) Would alteration of fluid flow affect embryo transport? (2) What role do fluid dynamics play in gamete
transport? (3) Would alteration of fluid flow cause ectopic pregnancy? (4) What pharmacological agents
would alter fluid flow?

Review Articles

Blandau, R. J. Gamete transport in the female mammal. In
Handbook of physiology, section 7: *Endocrinology*, vol. 2,
part 2, eds. R. O. Greep and E. B. Astwood. Baltimore: Williams & Wilkins, 1973.

Brenner, R. M. Endocrine control of ciliogenesis in the primate oviduct. In *Handbook of physiology*, section 7: *Endocrinology*, vol. 2, part 2, eds. R. O. Greep and E. P.
Astwood. Baltimore: Williams & Wilkins, 1973.

Hafez, E. S. E. Endocrine control of the structure and function of the mammalian oviduct. In *Handbook of physiology*,
section 7: *Endocrinology*, vol. 2, part 2, eds. R. O. Greep
and E. B. Astwood. Baltimore: Williams & Wilkins, 1973.

Harper, M. J. K., and C. J. Pauerstein, eds. *Ovum transport
and fertility regulation*. Copenhagen: Scriptor, 1976.

Johnson, A. D., and C. W. Foley. *The oviduct and its functions*. New York: Academic Press, 1974.

References

Allen, E. Further experiments with an ovarian hormone in
the ovariectomized adult monkey, *Macacus rhesus*, especially the degenerative phase of the experimental menstrual
cycle. Am. J. Anat. 42:467, 1928.

Anderson, R. G. W., and R. M. Brenner. Estrogen-stimulated oviducts of the rhesus monkey in organ culture. In *Cytological manifestations of secretion: Ultrastructure of endocrine and reproductive organs*, ed. M. Hess. New York:
John Wiley & Sons, 1974.

Austin, C. R. Sperm capacitation: Biological significance in
various species. In *Advances in biosciences*, vol. 4, ed.
G. Raspe. New York: Pergamon Press, 1970.

Bastiaans, L. A. Effecten van Enkele Oestrogene en Proges-
tatieve Stoffen op Ovumtransport en Zwangerschap bij de
Goudhamster, *Mesocricetus auratus* (Waterhouse). Gebr.
Janssen (Nijmegen, Netherlands), p. 1, 1973.

Bavister, B. D. Environmental factors important for in vitro
fertilization in the hamster. J. Reprod. Fertil. 18:544, 1969.

Bell, C. Autonomic nervous control of reproduction: Circulatory and other factors. Pharmacol. Rev. 24:657, 1972.

Bishop, D. W. Active secretion in the rabbit oviduct. Am. J.
Physiol. 187:347, 1956.

Bishop, D. W. Sperm physiology in relation to the oviduct.
In *The mammalian oviduct*, eds. E. S. E. Hafez and R. J.
Blandau. Chicago: University of Chicago Press, 1969.

Black, D. L. Neural control of oviduct musculature. In *The
oviduct and its functions*, eds. A. D. Johnson and C. W. Foley. New York: Academic Press, 1974.

Blandau, R. J. Biology of eggs and implantation. In *Sex and
internal secretions*, ed. W. C. Young. Baltimore: Williams &
Wilkins, 1961.

Blandau, R. J. Gamete transport—Comparative aspects. In
The mammalian oviduct, eds. E. S. E. Hafez and R. J. Blandau. Chicago: University of Chicago Press, 1969.

Blandau, R. J. Methods of observing ovulation and egg
transport. In *Methods in mammalian embryology*, ed. J. C.
Daniel, Jr. San Francisco: W. H. Freeman, 1971.

Blandau, R. J. Gamete transport in the female mammal. In
Handbook of physiology, section 7: *Endocrinology*, vol. 2,
part 2, eds. R. O. Greep and E. B. Astwood. Baltimore: Williams & Wilkins, 1973.

Blandau, R. J., and P. Gaddum-Rosse. Mechanisms of
sperm transport in pig oviducts. Fertil. Steril. 25:61, 1974.

Bodkhe, R. R., and M. J. K. Harper. Mechanism of egg
transport: Changes in amount of adrenergic transmitter in
the genital tract of normal and hormone-treated rabbits. In
The regulation of mammalian reproduction, eds. S. J. Segal,
R. Crozier, P. A. Corfman, and P. G. Condliffe. Springfield,
Ill.: Charles C Thomas, 1973.

Boling, J. L. Endocrinology of oviductal musculature. In

The mammalian oviduct, eds. E. S. E. Hafez and R. J. Blandau. Chicago: University of Chicago Press, 1969.

Boling, J. L., and R. J. Blandau. Egg transport through the ampullae of the oviducts of rabbits under various experimental conditions. Biol. Reprod. 4:174, 1971a.

Boling, J. L., and R. J. Blandau. The role of estrogens in egg transport through the ampullae of oviducts of castrate rabbits. Fertil. Steril. 22:544, 1971b.

Brackett, B. G., and W. L. Williams. Fertilization of rabbit ova in a defined medium. Fertil. Steril. 19:144, 1968.

Brenner, R. M., and R. G. W. Anderson. Endocrine control of ciliogenesis in the primate oviduct. In *Handbook of physiology*, section 7: *Endocrinology*, vol. 2, part 2, eds. R. O. Greep and E. B. Astwood. Baltimore: Williams & Wilkins, 1973.

Brenner, R. M., J. A. Resko, and N. B. West. Cyclic changes in oviductal morphology and residual cytoplasmic estradiol binding capacity induced by sequential estradiol-progesterone treatment of spayed rhesus monkeys. Endocrinology 95:1094, 1974.

Brinster, R. L. Studies on the development of mouse embryos in vitro. II. The effect of energy source. J. Exp. Zool. 158:59, 1965.

Brinster, R. L. Culture of two-cell rabbit embryos to morulae. J. Reprod. Fertil. 21:17, 1970.

Brundin, J. An occlusive mechanism in the fallopian tube of the rabbit. Acta Physiol. Scand. 61:219, 1964.

Brundin, J. Distribution and function of adrenergic nerves in the rabbit fallopian tube. Acta Physiol. Scand. 66(Suppl. 259):1, 1965.

Brundin, J. Pharmacology of the oviduct. In *The mammalian oviduct*, eds. E. S. E. Hafez and R. J. Blandau. Chicago: University of Chicago Press, 1969.

Brunton, W. J., and S. Brusilow. Personal communication, 1972.

Burnstock, G. Structure of smooth muscle and its innervation. In *Smooth muscle*, eds. E. Bulbring, A. F. Brading, A. W. Jones, and T. Tomita. Baltimore: Williams & Wilkins, 1970.

Clewe, T. H., and L. Mastroianni, Jr. A. method for continuous volumetric collection of oviduct secretions. J. Reprod. Fertil. 1:146, 1960.

Cottle, M. K., and G. W. Higgs. Adrenergic innervation of the fallopian tube of the monkey. Histochem. J. 5:143, 1973.

Coutinho, E. M. Hormonal control of tubal musculature. In *The regulation of mammalian reproduction*, eds. S. J. Segal, R. Crozier, P. Corfman, and P. G. Condliffe. Springfield, Ill.: Charles C Thomas, 1973.

Daniel, J. C., Jr. The pattern of utilization of respiratory metabolic intermediates by preimplantation rabbit embryos in vitro. Exp. Cell. Res. 47:619, 1967.

Daniel, J. C., Jr., and J. T. Millward. Ferrous iron requirement for cleavage of rabbit eggs. Exp. Cell. Res. 54:135, 1969.

Daniel J. C., Jr., and J. D. Olson. Amino acid requirements for cleavage of rabbit ovum. J. Reprod. Fertil. 15:543, 1968.

Falck, B., and C. Owman. Detailed methodological description of the fluorescence method for the cellular demonstration of biogenic monoamines. Acta Univ. Lund Sect. 2, No. 7, 1965.

Feigelson, M., and E. Kay. Protein patterns of rabbit oviductal fluid. Biol. Reprod. 6:244, 1972.

Gaddum-Rosse, P., and R. J. Blandau. In vitro studies of ciliary activity within the oviducts of the rabbit and pig. Am. J. Anat. 136:91, 1973.

Gaddum-Rosse, P., R. J. Blandau, and J. B. Thiersch. Ciliary activity in the human and *Macaca nemstrina* oviduct. Am. J. Anat. 138:269, 1973.

Garcia, C.-R., E. Fromm, D. Jeutter, J. Aller, and J. Harrison. Present status of chronic monitoring of tubal muscular activity. Fertil. Steril. 25:301 (Abstract), 1974.

Glass, L. E. Immunocytological studies of the mouse oviduct. In *The mammalian oviduct*, eds. E. S. E. Hafez and R. J. Blandau. Chicago: University of Chicago Press, 1969.

Graves, C. N., and J. D. Biggers. Carbon dioxide fixation by mouse embryos prior to implantation. Science 167:1506, 1970.

Greenwald, G. S. Tubal transport of ova in the rabbit. Anat. Rec. 133:386 (Abstract), 1959.

Hamner, C. E., and W. L. Williams. Effect of the female reproductive tract on sperm metabolsim in the rabbit and fowl. J. Reprod. Fertil. 5:143, 1963.

Hamner, C. E., and W. Williams. Identification of sperm stimulating factor of rabbit oviduct fluid. Proc. Soc. Exp. Biol. Med. 117:240, 1964.

Hamner, C. E., and W. L. Williams. Composition of rabbit oviduct secretions. Fertil. Steril. 16:170, 1965.

Harper, M. J. K. The mechanism involved in the movement of newly ovulated eggs through the ampulla of the rabbit Fallopian tube. J. Reprod. Fertil. 2:522, 1961a.

Harper, M. J. K. Egg movement through the ampullar region of the Fallopian tube of the rabbit. In *Proceedings of the Fourth International Congress on Animal Reproduction*, ed. N. V. Drukkerij Trio. The Hague, 1961b.

Harting, K. Ueber die feinere innervation der Tube. Z. Zellforsch. 9:544, 1929.

Hervonen, A., and L. Kanerva. Adrenergic and noradrenergic axons of the rabbit uterus and oviduct. Acta. Physiol. Scand. 85:139, 1972.

Hervonen, A., and L. Kanerva. Fine structure of the autonomic nerves of the rabbit myometrium. Z. Zellforsch. 136:19, 1973.

Hervonen, A., L. Kanerva, R. Lietzen, and S. Partanen. Ultrastructural changes induced by estrogen in the adrenergic nerves of the rabbit myometrium. Acta Physiol. Scand. 85:283, 1972.

Hervonen, A., L. Kanerva, and R. Lietzen. Histochemically demonstrable catecholamines and cholinesterases of the rat uterus during estrous cycle, pregnancy and after estrogen treatment. Acta Physiol. Scand. 87:283, 1973.

Hilliard, J., H. G. Spies, and C. H. Sawyer. Hormonal factors regulating ovarian cholesterol mobilization and progestin secretion in intact and hypophysectomized rabbits. In

The gonads, ed. K. W. McKerns. New York: Meredith Corp., 1969.

Holmdahl, T. H., and L. Mastroianni, Jr. Continuous collection of rabbit oviduct secretions at low temperature. Fertil. Steril. 16:587, 1965.

Ingelman-Sundberg, A., F. Sandberg, and G. Rydén. The effect of prostaglandins on the uterus and Fallopian tube. In *Pathways to conception*, ed. A. I. Sherman. Springfield, Ill.: Charles C Thomas, 1971.

Iwamatsu, T., and M. C. Chang. Factors involved in the fertilization of mouse eggs in vitro. J. Reprod. Fertil. 26:197, 1971.

Jonsson, G. Microfluorometric studies on the formaldehyde-induced fluorescence of noradrenaline in adrenergic nerves of rat iris. J. Histochem. Cytochem. 17:714, 1969.

Kille, J. W., and C. E. Hamner. The influence of oviductal fluid on the development of one-cell rabbit embryos in vitro. J. Reprod. Fertil. 35:415, 1973.

Larks, S. D., G. G. Larks, R. E. Hoffer, and E. J. Charlson. Electrical activity of oviducts in vivo. Nature (London) 234:556, 1971.

Marshall, J. M. Effects of catecholamines on the smooth muscle of the female reproductive tract. Ann. Rev. Pharmacol. 13:19, 1973.

Mastroianni, L., Jr., and B. G. Brackett. Environmental conditions within the fallopian tube. In *Progress in infertility*, eds. S. J. Behrman and R. Kistner. Boston: Little, Brown, 1968.

Mastroianni, L., Jr., W. Forrest, and W. W. Winternitz. Some metabolic properties of the rabbit oviduct. Proc. Soc. Exp. Biol. Med. 107:86, 1961a.

Mastroianni, L., Jr., U. Shah, and R. Abdul Karim. Prolonged volumetric collection of oviduct fluid in the rhesus monkey. Fertil. Steril. 12:417, 1961b.

Mastroianni, L., Jr., and R. C. Wallach. Effect of ovulation and early gestation on oviduct secretions in the rabbit. Am. J. Physiol. 200:815, 1961.

Mills, J. A., G. G. Jeitles, Jr., and B. G. Brackett. Embryo transfer following in vitro and in vivo fertilization of rabbit ova. Fertil. Steril. 24:602, 1973.

Noriega, C., and L. Mastroianni, Jr. Effect of carbonic anhydrase inhibitor on tubal ova. Fertil. Steril. 20:799, 1969.

Odor, D. L., and R. J. Blandau. Egg transport over the fimbrial surface of the rabbit oviduct under experimental conditions. Fertil. Steril. 24:292, 1973.

Olds, D., and N. L. Van Demark. Composition of luminal fluids in bovine female genitalia. Fertil. Steril. 8:345, 1957.

Owman, C., and N.-O. Sjöberg. The importance of short adrenergic neurons in the seminal emission mechanism of rat, guinea-pig and man. J. Reprod. Fertil. 8:63, 1972.

Patek, E. The epithelium of the human fallopian tube. Acta Obstet. Gynaecol. Scand. 53(Suppl. 31), 1974.

Pauerstein, C. J., D. D. Fremming, and J. E. Martin. Estrogen-induced tubal arrest of ovum: Antagonism by alpha adrenergic blockade. Obstet. Gynecol. 35:671, 1970.

Peck, E. J., Jr., J. DeLibero, R. Richards, and J. H. Clark. Instability of the uterine estrogen receptor under in vitro conditions. Biochemistry 12:4603, 1973.

Reinius, S. Morphology of oviduct, gametes, and zygotes as a basis of oviductal function in the mouse. I. Secretory activity of oviductal epithelium. Int. J. Fertil. 15:91, 1970.

Rumery, R. E. The fetal mouse oviduct in organ and tissue culture. In *The mammalian oviduct*, eds. E. S. E. Hafez and R. J. Blandau. Chicago: University of Chicago Press, 1969.

Sachs, C., and G. Jonsson. Quantitative microfluorometric and neurochemical studies on degenerating adrenergic nerves. J. Histochem. Cytochem. 21:902, 1973.

Seitz, H. M., Jr., B. G. Brackett, and L. Mastroianni, Jr. In vitro fertilization of ovulated rabbit ova recovered from the ovary. Biol. Reprod. 2:262, 1970.

Sjöberg, N.-O. The adrenergic transmitter of the female reproductive tract: Distribution and functional changes. Acta Physiol. Scand. 72(Suppl. 305):5, 1967.

Sjöberg, N.-O. Increase in transmitter content of adrenergic nerves in the reproductive tract of female rabbits after oestrogen treatment. Acta Endocrinol. (Kbh.) 57:405, 1968.

Sjöberg, N.-O. New considerations on the adrenergic innervation of the cervix and uterus. Acta Obstet. Gynaecol. Scand. 48(Suppl. 3):28, 1969.

Stambaugh, R., C. Noriega, and L. Mastroianni, Jr. Bicarbonate ion: The corona cell dispersing factor of rabbit tubal fluid. J. Reprod. Fertil. 18:51, 1969.

Stumpf, W. E. Subcellular distribution of ^{3}H-estradiol in rat uterus by quantitative autoradiography: A comparison between ^{3}H-estradiol and ^{3}H-norethynodrel. Endocrinology 83:777, 1968.

Sugawara, S., and S. Takeguchi. Identification of a volatile fatty acid in genital tract of female rabbit. Jap. J. Zool. Tech. Soc. 35:283, 1964.

Suzuki, S., and L. Mastroianni, Jr. In vitro fertilization of rabbit follicular oocytes in tubal fluid. Fertil. Steril. 19:716, 1968.

Swtantarta, S. O., K. T. Kirton, T. B. Tomasi, and J. Lippes. Prostaglandins in the human Fallopian tube. Fertil. Steril. 25:250, 1974.

Tervit, H. R., D. G. Whittingham, and L. E. A. Rowson. Successful culture in vitro of sheep and cattle ova. J. Reprod. Fertil. 30:493, 1972.

Verhage, H. G., J. H. Abel, Jr., W. J. Tietz, Jr., and M. D. Barrau. Development and maintenance of the oviductal epithelium during the estrous cycle in the bitch. Biol. Reprod. 9:460, 1973a.

Verhage, H. G., J. H. Abel, Jr., W. J. Tietz, Jr., and M. D. Barrau. Estrogen-induced differentiation of the oviductal epithelium in prepubertal dogs. Biol. Reprod. 9:475, 1973b.

Verhage, H. G., N. B. West, and R. M. Brenner. Progesterone antagonism of estrogen-driven ciliogenesis in the cat. Paper presented at the 7th Annual Meeting of the Society for the Study of Reproduction, Abstract 125, 1974.

Wales, R. G. Effects of ions on the development of preimplantation mouse embryo in vitro. Aust. J. Biol. Sci. 23:421, 1970.

White, I. G., and J. C. Wallace. Breakdown of seminal glycerylphosphorylcholine by secretions of the female reproductive tract. Nature (London) 189:843, 1961.

Whitten, W. K. Nutrient requirements for the culture of preimplantation embryos. In *Advances in biosciences*, vol. 6, ed. G. Raspe. New York: Pergamon Press, 1970.

Whitten, W. K., and J. D. Biggers. Complete development in vitro of the preimplantation stages of the mouse in a simple chemically defined medium. J. Reprod. Fertil. 17:399, 1968.

Wiest, W. G. DCR sensitivity related to uterine estradiol (E_2), progesterone (P), and 20 α-OH-P. Endocrinology 92 (Suppl.):65, 1973.

Wintenberger, S., L. Dauzier, and C. Thibault. Le developpement in vitro d l'oeuf de la brebis et de celui de la chèvre. C. R. Soc. Biol. (Paris) 147:1791, 1953.

Zimmermann, W. Untersuchungen uber den Ort der Besamung transplantierter und nichttransplantierter Kanincheneier. Zool. Anz. (Suppl. 23):91, 1959.

14 The Biology of the Uterus   D. G. Porter and C. A. Finn

14.1 Introduction and Summary

The uterus can be divided into two organs, the uterine muscle—the myometrium—and the glandular lining —the endometrium.

Our understanding of the myometrium has greatly improved over the past decade, but a unifying concept of the basic regulatory mechanisms still eludes us. A major gap in our understanding is that we do not know what inhibits the human myometrium during pregnancy and so prevents premature expulsion of the fetus. There are good grounds for skepticism over the extrapolation of the progesterone-block theory, established in rabbits, to the human female or even other laboratory species. The resolution of this problem could lead to improved abortifacients and to better control over premature or abnormal labor and dysmenorrhea.

The problem could be tackled in two ways: First, by parallel endocrinological studies of human subjects and sheep, in which major advances have been made recently in unraveling the hormonal changes that precede parturition. Second, by continuation of studies of myometrial regulation in laboratory and farm animals that have already pointed to hitherto unsuspected control mechanisms. Only if such mechanisms can be elucidated and shown to have interspecies applicability would tests for their existence be justified in human subjects. Immediate, direct studies to discover the basic regulatory mechanisms in women are impracticable, owing to the ethics of such experimentation and also to the interpretational problems of present methods of recording myometrial activity in women.

With regard to the endometrium, antifertility advances will most likely come from studies on the factors responsible for inducing the state of refractoriness to implantation, which pertains through much of the cycle. Suppressing the monthly period of endometrial receptivity would be a very effective contraceptive method.

Another approach is to interfere with the sequence of events following the attachment of a fertilized ovum to the endometrial epithelium. This is dependent upon more fundamental studies of the endometrium and particularly on the application of cell contact physiology and molecular biological approaches to the problem.

Yet another line of research with potential antifertil-

ity applications involves raising antibodies to decidual tissue specifically. These could then be employed as an abortifacient against early pregnancies, with little harm to other systems.

The cervix, because of its key position in the route of sperm ascent, is capable of profoundly affecting human fertility. Further study of the structure, composition, and mode of secretion of mucus by the cervix could lead to the development of drugs to alter the mucus so that it prohibits the passage of sperm through the cervix. Such a method might be relatively free of side effects, but at this time it is not certain that a very high degree of effectiveness could be achieved.

14.2 The Myometrium

The study of the myometrium is in a very exciting phase. Our understanding of parturition has probably advanced little from Hippocrates to Corner and Allen, but the discovery of progesterone and the subsequent studies of Allen, Knaus, Reynolds, and Csapo opened a new era in myometrial physiology, during which the problems have been defined more precisely, quantitative techniques of recording myometrial activity have been introduced, and misleading techniques have been discarded. Significant advances have been made in our understanding of the manner in which the myometrium is regulated. Paradoxically, during the 40 or so years since the discovery of progesterone, an ongoing controversy has raged over applying the knowledge from experimental studies to the human female. Although the controversy still rages, recent advances—such as the work on parturition in sheep, studies on the mechanism of smooth muscle contraction, advances in our understanding of steroid-hormone receptor mechanisms, and the new concepts of myometrial regulation in other species—suggest that it may soon be resolved.

Basic Studies

The last decade has generated a clarification of the action on the rabbit myometrium of progesterone, which the earlier studies of Corner, Allen, and Reynolds had established as the basis of the defence mechanism of pregnancy. The work of Csapo and his school has promoted the concept of an active myometrium, spontaneously contractile, which is restrained during pregnancy. Little support has followed for the view that the uterus is an inert organ that must be activated into labor. The studies on the action of progesterone on the rabbit myometrium have supported its activity. Thus the steroid elevates the resting membrane potential of the uterine muscle cells and impairs electrocoupling between them. The consequence is that coordination of contractile activity in the uterine horn is impaired, so that its tension-generating capabilities are reduced. This accounts for the amplitude-reducing effect on intrauterine pressure cycles of progesterone when given to nonpregnant rabbits. The hyperpolarization explains the refractoriness of the myometrium to oxytocin during pregnancy. This work has led to the progesterone-block theory of pregnancy maintenance, which claims that a "withdrawal" of the effects of progesterone is a prerequisite for labor. This model has proved valuable in the rabbit, and only recently has the suggestion been made that additional myometrial inhibitory factors might be involved. Thus it is now well documented by steroid determinations that progesterone levels rise during the first half of pregnancy in the rabbit and then decline steadily to term, reaching low levels at the time of parturition. Removal of the source of progesterone, the corpus luteum, terminates pregnancy, whereas prevention of the normal withdrawal, by exogenous administration of the steroid, suppresses parturition.

General Applicability of the Basic Concept

The progesterone-block theory enjoys a wide currency today. Indeed it could be said to have achieved the status of a dogma almost unparalleled in modern biological thought. Ironically, while it has become so firmly rooted in our thinking, evidence against it has been accumulating in humans and other species. There are several reasons for this. One lies in the difficulty of separating artifact from truth in studies of the myometrium. Another is the lack of an alternative to the very clear picture in the rabbit, which could claim any body of experimental data. It is of course possible that progesterone will eventually be shown to be an important regulator of the myometrium in women, but the evidence against this concept, together with recent information on other species, demands that a search be made for alternative mechanisms.

The human female Attempts have been made to demonstrate an effect of exogenously administered progesterone on myometrial activity in women in labor. These attempts have consistently failed, despite the use of heroic doses and even the injection of the steroid directly into the uterine muscle. Furthermore, unimpeachable double-blind trials have failed to demonstrate that progesterone is any more effective than a placebo in salvaging pregnancies from threatened premature labor.

The plasma progesterone titers during pregnancy in women also differ remarkably from the pattern and absolute values seen in the rabbit. In women they continue to rise during pregnancy at the same time that myometrial activity is increasing. There is some debate over whether progesterone levels fall before labor, but two recent studies have documented that they do. The fall would appear to be about 30 percent over the last five weeks of pregnancy, so that labor begins at a plasma concentration of about 100–140 ng/ml. Even with such a fall, the human uterus goes into labor in the presence of relatively high plasma progesterone titers; thus there is no withdrawal, as occurs in the rabbit.

Although there is a lack of substantive evidence of an action of progesterone on the human myometrium, the compelling deductive argument was often used that since progesterone acted in all other species (although in fact evidence was conclusive only in the rabbit), it must a priori act in the human. This argument is no longer tenable, since progesterone has been shown to have no inhibitory action on the myometrium of one species (the guinea pig) and probably none on that of another (the rat).

Forty years of controversy and investigation have failed to resolve this problem. The first attempt to modify the block theory suggested that the supply of progesterone to the myometrium becomes a local one from the placenta once dependence on the systemic supply from the corpus luteum is over. As a consequence, the uterus becomes nonuniformly supplied with progesterone, and the areas overlying the placental bed receive a rich supply of progesterone and collect it in extremely high concentrations. Increasingly high concentrations are necessary to block the myometrium, it is argued, because the stretch to which the muscle cells are subjected as a consequence of the growing conceptus elevates their requirement for the steroid. Thus the ratio of myometrial progesterone concentration to cell stretch (i.e., uterine volume) is the final determinant of myometrial activity.

This theory is highly controversial. It raises important questions concerning the mechanisms of action of progesterone and of stretch. Certainly recent studies have shown that stretch, when applied acutely to the myometrium, is a stimulant to uterine activity, probably through the agency of prostaglandin synthesis and release. What is not clear is whether or not the increasing passive tension to which the uterine muscle is subjected with the progress of pregnancy and the growth of the conceptus have a similar stimulatory effect. The rate of change in tension is gradual and the effects might be offset by several mechanisms, for example, by accomodation. Furthermore, it has been suggested recently that the action of progesterone on the myometrium is determined by the concentration of cytoplasmic protein receptors for the steroid in its muscle cells. If it is, then this parameter should change during human pregnancy. Estimations of the concentration of cytoplasmic protein receptors in the myometrium in the rat during pregnancy have suggested that they do decline prior to delivery. This is difficult to reconcile with the observation that prepartum administration of progesterone will prolong pregnancy in the rat.

Clearly this is an important field, which should yield much information on the regulatory mechanisms of the myometrium, and further research is essential. If progesterone has other routes by which it affects the smooth muscle cells, then it is necessary to demonstrate the effect of chronic incremental change in cell length on myometrial cell activity under conditions of constant progesterone concentration. The unequivocal demonstration of an action of the hormone on the human myometrium under any given circumstances is a prerequisite for further models of its action.

Intrauterine pressure recordings It might be thought that a study of the behavior of the human myometrium during pregnancy and the menstrual cycle might shed some light on the progesterone problem, but it has not. Intrauterine pressure provides an indirect measure of myometrial tension, which is the principal parameter of interest in a study of myometrial regulation. Thus tension (T) is related to pressure (P) by the Laplace equation, $T = PR/2w$ (where R is the radius of the uterus and w is the wall thickness). In the gravid uterus, which is a Pascalian system if there are no leaks, the extent and the changes in the activity of the myometrium are generally agreed upon. The myometrium appears to be active throughout pregnancy, since the earliest recordings, made at seven weeks, reveal pressure cycles of low amplitude occurring with high frequency (132/hr). Thereafter amplitude gradually increases and frequency decreases until about the 36th week, after which both parameters increase until the spontaneous activity merges with that of the first stage of labor. This pattern of activity represents a further divergence from the rabbit model, since recent studies on it have shown that very little myometrial activity exists up to moments before the delivery of the first fetus. Again, unlike the rabbit, the human uterus will respond to oxytocin and other pharmacological agents, such as prostaglandins, throughout most of pregnancy. The response is, however, very much reduced in early pregnancy. Thus much more prostaglandin is required to induce abortion in the first trimester than in later pregnancy. These facts support the basic premise that the myometrium is under restraint during pregnancy in the human as in the rabbit.

Unfortunately, opinions differ on what constitutes the normal activity of the myometrium during the menstrual cycle. This is almost certainly due to the use of a variety of different techniques to record intrauterine pressure, ranging from small balloons of differing shapes, sizes, and materials, to catheters with open ends, diaphragms, or sponge tips. Different methods produce different intrauterine pressure records and thus different conclusions on the issue of whether progesterone exerts an inhibitory effect. In general, one school claims that progesterone reduces the frequency and increases the amplitude of contractions (or pressure cycles), while the other school claims that it reduces amplitude, as in the rabbit. Both groups substantiate their claims with recordings obtained during the luteal phase of the cycle and from women treated with progestational steroids. The crux of the problem is that the physics of the recording device *in utero* is not fully understood. Thus with an open-ended catheter, it is difficult to see how the Laplace relationship is preserved, and then what does P represent in terms of myometrial activity? With a balloon, the experimenter imposes his own Pascalian system in which the relationship between P and T is preserved, but, as critics argue, this produces an artifactual situation, since the uterus normally has only a potential lumen during the major part of the menstrual cycle. A very careful mathematical and physiological analysis of these recording systems is essential to avoid still further confusion in the literature.

The Prostaglandins and Myogenic Activity
Undoubtedly the greatest advance in the field of fertility control involving the myometrium has been the development of the prostaglandins (PGs) as abortifacients. Since PGs are generally smooth-muscle stimulants, systemic administration is attended by side effects, which, although seldom dangerous, are unacceptable. Intrauterine administration reduced this problem but prevented the method from being self-applied. The intravaginal route offers this possibility and is presently under trial. PGs have also been employed to induce labor at term and have been found to be almost as efficacious as oxytocin, although dissimilarities in the intrauterine pressure cycle characteristics with the two agents have suggested that oxytocin-induced labor is more nearly normal. On the other hand, the combination of the two agents for induction is proving very acceptable. An extensive literature is developing on the obstetrical applications of PGs.

In view of their oxytocic activity and the demonstrations that PGs increase in plasma and amniotic fluid during labor, are PGs an essential component of the contractile mechanism of the uterine smooth-muscle cell? In the rat, suppression of PG synthesis by indomethacin has been reported to result in dystocia, and in the human female it has been reported to prolong the instillation-abortion interval in hypertonic saline-induced abortion. Although suggestive, these findings do not prove that PGs play an obligatory role. Some progress in our understanding of this problem has been made recently. PGs inhibit the ATP-dependent binding of Ca^{++} ions by the smooth endoplasmic reticulum (SER) isolated from myometrial cells. Since the SER has been suggested to serve the same calcium storage and release function in smooth muscle as the sarcoplasmic reticulum in striated muscle, PGs may act at a fundamental level of muscle contraction. The part played by $3'5'$ cAMP in this awaits clarification. Energy-dependent Ca^{++} binding is increased in smooth muscles when cAMP levels are elevated, thus leading to relaxation. Paradoxical findings have been reported, however, for elevated cAMP levels can coexist in the myometrium with undiminished contractile activity. PGs may also simultaneously increase intracellular cAMP and contractile activity.

Whatever the mechanism of action of PGs on the uterine muscle cell, it is clear that other factors may interfere with it. Thus it has been shown that the response to PGs is greatly reduced in the rabbit and the nonpregnant ewe by prior treatment with progesterone. Since progesterone appears to act solely on the electrical events of the plasmalemma during contraction, it is difficult to see how it might prevent the action of PGs, unless it also affected the SER. Further research is imperative in this important area.

Returning to the question of abortion, no satisfactory answer can be given as to how PGs interrupt pregnancy. Undoubtedly stimulation of the myometrium is an important component, but is it solely a mechanical process? Or does the mechanical activity of the uterine muscle, perhaps through disrupting blood flow to the placenta, cause damage to the conceptus, thus causing abortion? Endocrinological studies have shown that the steroid and protein hormone output of the conceptus falls during the course of PG-induced abortion. Although it is tempting to conclude that the waning progesterone titers permit the expulsion of the fetus, the foregoing discussion indicates that this conclusion is premature. Certainly the possibility should be entertained that the conceptus produces other factors that may inhibit the myometrium and that it is the loss of those, occurring concomitantly with the fall in progesterone production, that is the direct cause of abortion.

Hypertonic Saline-Induced Abortion

This technique, which was first introduced before the war, received considerable attention during the 1960s and has been established as a reliable and relatively safe method for the interruption of pregnancy after the fourth month. Once again our lack of understanding of the fundamental mechanisms regulating the human myometrium has frustrated our attempts to explain how this method induces abortion. A direct action of saline on the myometrium appears to have been ruled out by experimental and clinical studies, but the increase in amniotic fluid volume that follows the introduction of the hypertonic solution may contribute, by causing stretch of the uterine muscle. Acute stretch, a well-established activator of smooth muscle, has been shown to result in the release of PGs in the uterus.

It seems likely, however, that the major factor causing the abortion is the damage the saline inflicts upon the placenta and fetus. Studies have invariably revealed histological damage to the placenta, and the falling steroid and protein hormone output that follows the treatment attests to the biochemical damage. Thus a key to the mechanism would seem to lie in the failing ability of the endocrine output of the conceptus to support pregnancy, but more specific explanations are not possible at this time.

Fetal Role in Parturition

Until quite recently the timing of parturition was generally assumed to be determined solely by maternal and placental factors and not at all by the fetus. A major advance came when experiments based upon reports of prolonged gestation in cattle and sheep in the veterinary literature showed that destruction of the pituitary gland in fetal lambs *in utero* suspended parturition indefinitely. Subsequent studies have shown that the key organ is the adrenal cortex, since the administration of ACTH or glucocorticoids to fetal lambs is followed by premature labor. Evidence of a role for corticosteroids in the initiation of labor has also been obtained in goats, cows, and rabbits, but not in guinea pigs. Supporting this concept is the finding that adrenocortical activity in fetal lambs is increased prepartum in normal pregnancies, although the reason for this is not known.

Despite these important findings, uncertainty still permeates our understanding of the manner in which the changes in fetal adrenocortical activity are translated into the increased myometrial activity of labor. It is known that progesterone levels normally fall during the latter part of pregnancy in sheep and that, in glucocorticoid-induced labor, there is also a decline in progesterone titers. Another similarity is a rise in estrogen levels.

Since PG concentration in the maternal placenta increases during glucocorticoid induction, a tentative hypothesis may be advanced. Glucocorticoids may interfere with progesterone synthesis in the placenta, so that a progesterone withdrawal occurs. Increasing estrogen secretion, perhaps based upon a richer supply of C19 precursors from the fetal adrenal, stimulates PG synthesis in the maternal placenta and results in activation of the unblocked myometrium.

This is probably an oversimplification. This model posits that glucocorticoid-induced labor can take place if a decline in progesterone titers is prevented by exogenous steroid administration. Studies on normal delivery yielded the paradoxical results that while daily administration of progesterone to late pregnant ewes failed to prolong pregnancy, a single dose administered at the very onset of labor apparently did so. Finally the literature nowhere demonstrates that progesterone inhibits myometrial activity in the ewe. And once again, evidence that progesterone is essential to maintain pregnancy is not evidence that progesterone per se acts on the myometrium.

The implications that these studies have for human labor are not yet clear. The major advances made in fetal endocrinology in the 1960s, however, have pointed to the fetus as the regulator of estrogen secretion by the placenta, by virtue of its production of C19 estrogen precursors. Since more recent studies suggest a negative correlation between estrogen excretion rates in late pregnancy in women and the ultimate length of their gestations, the possibility must be entertained of a role for the fetal adrenal in the induction of human labor. A parallel study of the endocrinology of labor in both human and ovine subjects is a potentially valuable approach to the problem.

Control of Premature Labor
Although work had been done before the 1960s both in vitro and in vivo on the action of the catecholamines on the human uterus, not until then were their effects in vivo clarified, and adrenalin was found to inhibit and noradrenalin to stimulate the human myometrium at term. Since the inhibitory action of adrenalin may be ascribed to its action on the β receptors, a search has been continuing for β-mimetic agents that would be of use in controlling premature labor. Agents such as orciprenaline and Ritodrine are employed in the management of premature labor and of term labor associated with excessive uterine activity. The use of these drugs seems to be valuable since they are rapidly cleared from the circulation, enabling the obstetrician to exercise close control over the uterine activity. The disadvantages are cardiovascular effects on both the mother and the fetus, but these may possibly be reduced with the development of new β mimetics.

Another method of reducing myometrial activity that has been applied to the problem of premature labor is the administration of ethyl alcohol. Studies begun in 1967 and subsequently confirmed showed that in about 67 percent of women with threatened premature labor, provided their membranes were intact,

pregnancy could be maintained if they were given ethanol (0.8 G/min) intravenously. Once again, it is not certain how this treatment brings about the change in myometrial activity. Possibilities being investigated are the suppression of neurohypophyseal secretion, stimulation of adrenalin release, and inhibition of PG release or synthesis. The first possibility is prompted by evidence that ethanol inhibits oxytocin release in suckling animals, together with the knowledge that the polypeptide is a potent myometrial stimulant. But determining if it is the mechanism of action of ethanol in the pregnant woman is complicated by our lack of knowledge of the role of oxytocin in either normal labor or threatened abortion. Earlier bioassay data suggested that oxytocin was released during the expulsive phase of delivery, although there was considerable scatter in the results. A more recent study using a radioimmunoassay for oxytocin failed to demonstrate oxytocin in maternal peripheral blood at any stage of labor, although it was found in fetal arterial blood. Whether the mechanism of action is one of inhibiting fetal oxytocin secretion is speculative. The other two possibilities are also difficult to evaluate, since evidence for them is equivocal.

Experimental Studies
The foregoing account has documented the major developments in myometrial physiology that have immediate relevance to human clinical problems. Following is a brief account of recent advances in basic myometrial physiology, which, although they may ultimately influence clinical thought, do not warrant immediate extrapolation.
Electrophysiology In the last decade or so, the first intracellular electrode recordings have been made from myometrial cells. This, together with other technical advances in the electrophysiology of the smooth muscle, has yielded a substantial literature.

Confirmation has developed as to the importance of estrogen to the uterine smooth-muscle cell in maintaining its ability to generate action potentials and to contract. Also strengthened is the view that myometrial electrical activity is myogenic and not dependent on innervation. The ease with which action potentials can be generated depends on the relatively low resting membrane potential of smooth-muscle cells, which appears to be due to the contribution of sodium and chloride ions to the equilibrium.

Once again progesterone is the center of controversy. Several studies claim that in the rabbit, rat, and mouse, progesterone causes hyperpolarization of the myometrial cell membranes. Other studies have failed to confirm this. There seems to be general agreement that uterine muscle is hyperpolarized during pregnancy but no unanimity over what is responsible for this.

Action of catecholamines It has been known for most of this century that stimulation of the hypogastric nerve elicits a response in the uterus that depends upon the reproductive state of the animal. Thus the uterus of the pregnant cat responds with contraction and that of the nonpregnant cat with relaxation, the phenomenon being known as pregnancy reversal.

Studies have now shown that this reversal can be attributed to the action of the ovarian steroids in altering the ratio of α and β receptors in or on uterine muscle cells. Thus estrogen in rats alters the ratio in favor of α receptors, and the addition of progesterone to the estrogen treatment shifts the ratio in favor of β receptors.

Evidence also indicates that adrenalin causes relaxation of the uterus through hyperpolarization of the muscle cells. This hyperpolarization is probably due in part to an increase in potassium permeability, which results in a shift in the resting membrane potential toward the potassium equilibrium potential. There is good evidence that an increase in intracellular cAMP is also a component of catecholamine-induced relaxation.

The physiological role of the uterine innervation is still poorly understood and should be studied further. Since the changes in uterine activity that the nerve supply mediates appear to be subtle, they probably play only a minor role in labor but may be important during gamete transport and implantation. We know very little about the behavior of the myometrium during these crucial stages of reproduction in any species. Since interfering with zygote-endometrial synchrony is a possible antifertility technique, much more work on this topic is warranted.

Alternative Mechanisms of Myometrial Regulation
As mentioned above, substantial evidence now exists that progesterone has no inhibitory action on the guinea pig myometrium. There are also reports that the hormone may have little effect on the uterine activity of the rat, a species hitherto believed to behave according to the rabbit model.

In the guinea pig the character of uterine activity during pregnancy does not resemble that of the rabbit, since the myometrium, although less active than in the nonpregnant animal, is not completely inhibited. The reduction in activity appears to be accomplished by frequency rather than amplitude modulation, and recent work has suggested that relaxin or a relaxinlike substance may be an important regulator of the myometrium in this species. The demonstration that a similar factor may participate with progesterone in the maintenance of pregnancy in the rabbit has suggested that this may not be a mechanism peculiar to the guinea pig.

That relaxin inhibits myometrial activity in vitro and in situ in a number of species has been known for many years, but only recently has a role been postulated for it as a physiological regulator of uterine activity. It is hoped that the development of a radioimmunoassay for relaxin will expand our knowledge of this elusive hormone. Following the surge of clinical interest in relaxin in the late 1950s, virtually nothing has been learned of the role, if any, that this hormone plays in human pregnancy. Since the clinical trials of the 1950s did not conclusively eliminate the possibility that relaxin is an important hormone of human pregnancy, the subject might be profitably reopened.

14.2 The Endometrium

The roles of the endometrium in the reproductive life of mammals may be defined as (1) preparation for implantation, and (2) participation in implantation and formation of the maternal placenta.

Preparation for Implantation
Although the structure and function of the endometrium has been known for years to be dependent upon ovarian endocrine activity, only during the last decade have major advances been made in delineating the mechanism of action of the ovarian hormones on the endometrium. The atrophic endometrium of the castrate animal responds to estrogen by proliferation, hypertrophy, edema, and an increase in metabolic activity. Edema occurs very rapidly (4–6 hr) and has been used as a bioassay.

Edema is thought to be a consequence of increased capillary permeability, which follows the appearance of pores in the endothelia of endometrial capillaries and has been demonstrated by electron microscopy. Recent studies have linked the very early responses of the endometrium to estrogen to the massive influx of eosinophils. Whether the alterations of the vascular dynamics of the uterus are a cause or a consequence of the increased permeability is uncertain, but recent studies using modern methods of measuring blood flow have substantiated earlier reports that estrogen increases uterine blood flow.

Of significance for implantation is the observation that microvilli increase in number and length and become invested in a denser coat of "fuzz" or glycocalyx under the stimulus of estrogen. The fuzz is apparently secreted by the epithelial cells, being exported via the Golgi apparatus.

Evidence of protein synthesis, an increase in ribosomes, is reflected in the increased activity of many enzyme systems such as those of the carbohydrate oxidative system and, more specifically, of alkaline phosphatase and carbonic anhydrase.

Progesterone alone has very little action, although it has very definite effects on the estrogen-stimulated endometrium. This is a fundamental aspect of endometrial function in that it is modulated by a very complex pattern of endocrine influences in which both estrogen and progesterone exert precise actions, both temporally and quantitatively. This very aspect has made difficult the interpretation of the effects of exogenous hormone administration, since physiological amounts of hormone are often uncertain, and, where known, the effects they produce vary greatly with respect to previous hormone administration and duration of action or to variations in endogenous hormone levels. Improvement in hormone assay methods is helping to resolve this, since better methods enable researchers to have a more precise knowledge of the normal physiology and to approximate it more closely in their experiments.

Plasma estrogen levels are elevated during proestrus in rodents and thus stimulate mitosis in the surface epithelium (DNA replication occurring about 14 hours after estrogen administration in ovariectomized animals) and prime the endometrium, significantly modifying later proliferative responses to hormonal or blastocystic stimuli. Thus the important shift of mitotic activity from glandular to stromal cells, which occurs between days 3 and 4 of pregnancy in mice and provides a template of endometrial fibroblasts for decidual cell transformation, appears to be dependent upon the priming effect of estrogen secreted during proestrus.

Decidualization The ability of the uterus to undergo decidualization has been accepted as evidence of a receptive state of the endometrium, that is, a state in which it will permit implantation. The endocrine requirements for optimum decidualization have been carefully defined. A decidual response can be evoked by gross trauma (such as crushing) in ovariectomized rats and mice treated with progesterone only. If an intraluminal stimulus (such as oil) is employed, however, a small dose of estrogen is required as well, administered about seven hours prior to the oil injection. Since this resembles the normal hormonal requirements for implantation, such methods have been assumed to present a more physiological stimulus to the endometrium. In both the rat and mouse the estrogen requirements are critical, since low or high doses inhibit the decidual response. Furthermore, the time interval between the estrogen administration and the application of a decidualizing stimulus is critical—four to eight hours in the mouse. Even the duration of progesterone treatment is important, since no response was obtainable when only two days of progesterone treatment preceded the administration of estrogen, only a limited response was obtainable with three, six,

or seven days, and a maximal response with four or five days. Thus the decidual response clearly requires precise endocrine influence on the endometrium, not only in terms of amount but also in terms of timing. Biochemical studies have revealed increases in histamine, DNA, glycogen, and water in the endometrium during decidualization.

It appears that proteins specific to decidual cells are elaborated following transformation of the stromal cells. This raises the possibility that an antiserum specific to decidual tissue could be raised that might have an abortifacient action. Such a serum has been shown to interrupt pregnancy in rats. Further research along these lines should be profitable.

The function of the deciduum is still debated. It may be a line of defense against trophoblastic invasion, a source of nourishment for the conceptus, or a region for placental dehiscence at term.

Decidualization occurs to a certain extent in the late secretory phase of the human menstrual cycle as well as during implantation. Whether the prerequisites for this transformation are similar to those in rodents is uncertain, and it is difficult to see how such information might be obtained, unless recourse is made to studies on the anthropoid apes.

Both oral contraceptives and the IUD are suspected to cause premature decidualization in women. The significance of this and its relevance, if any, to subsequent pathological change is unknown, but it underscores the importance of careful surveillance of women on contraceptive therapy.

Participation in Implantation
During most of the reproductive cycle in mammals the endometrium is refractory to implantation. Thus the uterus will permit the blastocyst to implant only for very brief periods, during which it is said to be sensitive or receptive. The hormonal requirements for sensitivity are well known and are similar to those for decidualization, except that, as with oil-induced deciduomata, estrogen is essential in most species for the blastocyst to implant. Thus ovariectomy performed the day before implantation occurs, and followed by progesterone treatment, results in delayed implantation. A subsequent injection of estrogen is followed by implantation. That this represents the physiological situation is supported by recent estimations of estrogen in the plasma of rats, which demonstrated a rise in estrogen titers around midday on day 4 (about 24 hours prior to implantation).

Ultrastructural studies have revealed that the lumen of the uterus is lost due to close apposition of the microvilli-coated epithelial surfaces (first stage of closure). On certain epithelial cells, a mushrooming of the plasmalemma occurs and may represent a specialization for the initial contact with the blastocyst. Within 24 hours the microvilli but not the "mushrooms" are lost, and the lumen is represented by a narrow complex channel.

It seems inescapable that the apposition of trophoblast and epithelial plasmalemmas initiates the orderly program of events that constitute the endometrial contribution to implantation. The nature of the stimulus that results from that initial contact remains a crucial unsolved problem, but the application of advances in the field of cell-to-cell contact and membrane science should greatly aid our understanding of the early events in nidation. Also, the information for the orderly sequence of changes in the endometrium that ensue from that event must be encoded in the genome. The challenge of elucidating the mechanism by which this information is transcribed in response to the hormonal and other stimuli of implantation can be met only by the application of modern molecular biological techniques to the endometrium. But a major obstacle has greatly handicapped the interpretation of most biochemical studies on both the endometrium and the myometrium—the problem of separating tissue and cell types. A technical advance here is a prerequisite for advances in the biology of the endometrium. Too many studies in the past have utilized homogenates of whole uteri, or in the cases where separation of myometrium from the endometrium has been attempted, the results have been interpreted without reference to the three major cell types of the endometrium.

The search for pharmacological agents could be given a rational basis as our understanding of the individual subcellular events of the implantation sequence improves. Thus the ideal pharmacological interference would interrupt one key step in the implantation process, and the search for such an agent could be added to the present necessarily empirical approach.

The first stage of closure is dependent upon progestin, and the second stage requires an estrogenic stimulus superimposed upon the progestational background. It has been established, though, that at least 48 hours of progestational influence are essential for estrogen to induce receptivity to the blastocyst or sensitivity to decidualization. Whether or not these changes occur in women is not known, and this information is needed to help determine whether or not the extensive information on rodents can be extrapolated to the human subject.

Thus the endocrinological requirements for uterine receptivity have been carefully determined. The key question is: What is the mechanism by which receptivity is established? This problem is challenging and offers exciting prospects for fertility control. Three basic mechanisms seem likely: either the epithelium secretes a substance that activates the blastocyst to implant, or the epithelium ceases to synthesize a substance that prevents nidation, or the blastocyst in some way provokes receptivity in the endometrium. There have been reports recently of proteins secreted by the endometrium that stimulate blastocyst development, for example, blastokinin and uteroglobulin in rabbits, but their general importance is in doubt. They appear to stimulate blastocyst expansion, but this has also been achieved in vitro in very simple media. Moreover, their relevance is obscure for blastocysts that do not expand markedly prior to nidation, such as in humans.

On the other hand, there is promising evidence from at least two laboratories that implantation is prevented by the elaboration of an inhibitory substance. Thus the administration of actinomycin D, which blocks nuclear transcription and hence protein synthesis, actually stimulates blastocyst implantation in mice exhibiting delayed implantation following ovariectomy and progesterone treatment. It is thus likely that both estrogen and actinomycin D stimulate implantation by preventing the elaboration of an inhibitory substance.

Unfortunately there is reason to doubt that the mechanism is that simple. Evidence has been obtained that estrogen stimulates RNA synthesis in the endometrium of ovariectomized animals, both alone and after progesterone treatment. Indeed the maximal RNA synthetic response occurs if estrogen is given after 48 hours of progesterone treatment—that is, at a time corresponding to maximal sensitivity for decidualization or receptivity to blastocysts. As might be predicted, actinomycin D inhibits the decidual response.

It may be that implantation follows the following sequence: estrogen priming → progestational changes → estrogenic action: inhibitory factor synthesis † suppressed → sensitization → stimulus from blastocyst *(positive pontamine sky blue reaction; edema) * → degeneration of epithelial cells † → transfer of information to stromal cells *? → stromal cell transformation (that is, to decidual cell), † and so on. In this sequence * signifies that no transcription is involved, and † signifies that transcription is involved and that the step is sensitive to actinomycin D.

Support for the concept of an implantation inhibitor has come from studies of the action of uterine flushings, taken from animals in differing reproductive states, on the uridine uptake of blastocysts. Flushings from ovariectomized (untreated or progesterone-treated) and one to four day pregnant rats inhibited uridine incorporation into TCA-soluble RNA, while flushings taken one hour after estrogen administration to ovariectomized progesterone-treated rats had no inhibitory action.

While the studies with actinomycin D suggest that

the postulated inhibitory factor may be a protein, one laboratory has failed to identify any active protein fraction isolated from inhibitory flushings but finds such activity in lipid-containing alcoholic extracts. Indirect evidence supporting this view is the presence of abundant lipid in the basal cytoplasm of the endometrial epithelium, which is dispersed at ovoimplantation.

Clearly this aspect of endometrial physiology is of considerable interest from the point of view of fertility control. It may be possible one day to artificially provoke a refractory state to implantation in the uterus, perhaps through the placement of a capsule providing for a slow release of an inhibitory substance.

14.4 Cervix and Vagina

Studies on the cervix and vagina over the last decade have been generally sporadic rather than systematic, although there are signs that increasing attention is now being directed to the cervix.

All the functions of the cervix are not clearly understood, but several roles have been assigned to it: (1) the secretion of mucus; (2) a mechanical role in pregnancy that prevents premature rupture of the fetal membranes; and (3) possibly together with the vagina, an important sensory role as the afferent limb of the neurohumoral reflex, which provokes the release of oxytocin.

Secretion of Mucus

The anatomy of the cervical "glands" responsible for the secretion of mucus has been studied both histologically and ultrastructurally. It appears that the glands are in fact crypts that are lined by mucous and ciliated cells of the endocervical epithelium. The mucous cells have numerous microvilli on their free borders and contain large numbers of PAS positive secretory granules in their apical cytoplasm that displace the nuclei to the basal region of the cells. The secretory activity of these cells is no longer believed to be apocrine; it is affected by the circulating levels of ovarian hormones, so that mucus of differing properties is secreted at different times in the menstrual cycle. The dependence on ovarian steroids, however, appears to be less than that exhibited by the endometrial or vaginal mucosa. Thus the degree of atrophy observed in these tissues following menopause is not seen in the cervical crypts. The ciliated cells have both microvilli and cilia on their free borders, and the cilia appear to beat, together with kinocilia, which may be present occasionally, toward the vagina. Their action appears to generate a flow of mucus to the vagina but not to transport sperm. They may, however, remove immotile sperm. The absence of secretory granules in the cytoplasm of the ciliated

cells has been interpreted to mean that they contribute little to the cervical mucus.

The quantity of cervical mucus produced daily varies from individual to individual and with the cycle in a given individual. There are normally about 100 aggregations of mucus-secreting crypts in the cervix, and except at midcycle they secrete up to 60 mg of wet mucus per day. At midcycle, probably as the result of increasing estrogenic stimulation, there is about a 10-fold increase in secretion rate, together with a change in the physical properties of the mucus. This phenomenon has been suggested as a means of predicting ovulation. Women can readily recognize the change in the consistency of mucus that apparently begins, on average, 6.2 days prior to ovulation. Further studies are needed to prove whether or not this method is reliable.

Sperm that reach the egg after normal intercourse have to first negotiate the cervix by passing through the mucus. The importance of the mucus in human fertility is therefore considerable. It is known now that during much of the cycle the mucus is hostile to sperm —that is, it impedes sperm migration through it. This appears to be due to an increase in viscosity, protein content ($> 12.5 \mu g/g$ wet weight), and lencocyte content of the mucus, compared with the low-viscosity, low-protein ($< 1.5 \mu g/mg$ wet weight), more hydrated mucus produced at midcycle, which favors sperm penetration. The former type of mucus has been termed G (gestagen) and the latter E (estrogenic) type. The ultrastructure of the mucus is important since its macromolecular configuration may impede or facilitate sperm progression. At midcycle (it has been suggested) the glycoprotein fibrils are arranged in parallel array, whereas during the rest of the cycle a meshwork is produced. It is believed that sperm migrate along the channels between adjacent glycoprotein fibrils and are therefore impeded by a meshwork arrangement. How much the proteolytic enzymes of sperm and seminal plasma aid sperm migration, since they are known to reduce mucus viscosity and gel structure, is not known, nor is the extent to which the α_1 antitrypsin of cervical mucus counteracts this process.

Ultrastructural studies of the mucus weft, however, using transmission and scanning electron microscopy, have failed to yield consistent results; much uncertainty, largely attributable to the difficulties in preparing artifact-free specimens, exists over the true structure of mucus. Since cervical mucus is a heterogeneous substance, it is not surprising that some reports find that the weft configuration varies from area to area in the same sample and also from crypt to crypt in the same woman. Clearly more research is needed, but even more apparent is the importance of developing superior techniques of fixation and preparation.

The chemistry of cervical mucus has been studied.

Its water content rises at midcycle to about 98 percent. Salts, principally sodium chloride, amount to about 1 percent, but there are also traces of other anions and cations. It is known that women bearing the copper IUD have elevated cervical mucus copper levels, although the significance of this for sperm transport is uncertain. Copper has been shown to cause loss of *Spinnbarkeit* and to reduce the sperm penetrability of cervical mucus, possibly through breakage of the disulphide bonds between glycoprotein molecules, but the relation between these two observations is not certain. Sperm penetrability may have been impaired by direct toxic effects of copper on the sperm.

Much is known of the glycoprotein structure in cervical mucus; it may prove possible to pharmacologically influence its configuration and hence the sperm penetrability of mucus. There is evidence, although not uncontested, that the minipills act in part by reducing sperm penetrability of cervical mucus. The extent to which fertility can be reduced by altering the characteristics of cervical mucus alone is uncertain, but it is an important theoretical consideration. An antifertility method directed solely at the cervical mucus might have considerable advantages in being free of side effects. From an a priori viewpoint, however, it is difficult to see how an altered cervical mucus could ever confer the high degree of protection demanded by modern contraception.

This broad area deserves continued support. The approach might be twofold. Continued study of the structure, chemistry, and manner of synthesis and secretion of cervical mucus should be paralleled by studies on its pharmacology, with the view to artificially stimulating the production of hostile mucus. The latter could be supported by studies in suitable experimental models of the potential efficacy of a cervical method of contraception.

The cervical mucus contains immunoglobulins that appear to enter the mucus from the cervix. Cytotoxic antisperm antibodies as well as blood group antibodies have been detected in the cervical mucus of infertile women. Since local antibody production in response to challenge of the cervix with antigen has been reported in cattle, and since human antisperm autoantibodies added to mucus can impair both sperm motility and sperm penetration, the possibility exists of an immunological method of contraception aimed at the cervix. The practical problems, however, are considerable.

Mechanical Role in Pregnancy
Follow-up studies on women who have undergone abortions in which dilatation of cervix was performed have suggested that the midterm abortion rate is increased above normal. The damage caused to the cervix at abortion appears to be the key factor. Incom-

petence of the cervix is a cause of premature labor. These findings point to an important mechanical role for the cervix in preventing abnormal prolapse and rupture of the fetal membranes, which in turn results in abortion. Encouragement should be given to the development of abortifacient techniques that cause little trauma to the cervix, such as the administration of $PGF_{2\alpha}$ intraluminally or suction via a small caliber catheter. A high success rate is imperative, since the necessity for subsequent dilatation and curettage would defeat the purpose.

Neurohumoral Reflex
Recently a number of studies in domestic animals have established the existence of a neurohumoral reflex, activated by distension of the vagina or cervix or both, that culminates in the release of oxytocin from the neurohypophysis. The reflex appears to be seasonally variable and to be depressed by progesterone and augmented by estrogen treatment.

In view of the uncertainties over whether or not maternal oxytocin plays a role in labor, the relevance of this reflex to human obstetrics remains obscure. With radioimmunoassays available for oxytocin, this problem should be reinvestigated.

Miscellaneous
Several other possible functions of the cervix are poorly understood. The cervix has been shown to contain smooth muscle and to contract spontaneously in vitro. Apparently it is stimulated by oxytocin and inhibited by PGE_2. The physiological significance, if any, of these findings is obscure.

Sperm storage may be a function of the cervix, since the gametes can enter the crypts, where they might remain for long periods. A recent study reported that sperm persisted in cervical mucus for up to nine days after coitus. Whether sperm retained in the cervix for these long periods are capable of ascending the uterus and tubes and of fertilizing ova is unknown.

Studies of the vagina have been sparse. Several recent clinical trials have been reported in which contraceptive steroids have been administered by vaginal pessary. This seems to be an effective route and has the advantage of long intervals between administrations. The vagina is also of interest as a route, possibly for self-administration, for PGs in the induction of abortion; pH changes in the vagina have been measured during coitus.

The vagina, except for the mechanical prevention of sperm transport, does not seem to offer the potential of a highly effective contraceptive method. The use of spermicidal agents may be valuable as a supportive method, but since the cervix is bathed in semen following coitus, vaginal methods seem destined to be relatively inefficient.

Acknowledgment

In assembling this report we have consulted with and gained helpful information and suggestions from Professor T. K. A. B. Eskes (Nijmegen, Holland), Dr. F. Leroy (Brussels), Dr. A. Psychoyos (Paris), and Professor A. Turnbull (Oxford).

Recommended Reviews

Myometrium
Bergstrom, S., ed. *Advances in biosciences: International Conference on Prostaglandins*. Oxford: Pergamon Press, 1973.

Csapo, A. I. The diagnostic significance of the intrauterine pressure. Obstet. Gynecol. Survey 25:403, 515, 1970.

Eskes, T. K. A. B. The influence of β-mimetic catecholamines upon the uterine activity in human pregnancy and labor. In *Uterine contraction: Side effects of steroidal contraceptives*, ed. J. B. Josimovich. New York: John Wiley & Sons, 1973.

Finn, C. A., and D. G. Porter. *Handbooks of reproductive biology: The uterus*. London: Paul Elek Ltd., 1974.

Fuchs, A. R., and F. Fuchs. Possible mechanisms of the inhibition of labor by ethanol. In *Uterine contraction: Side effects of steroidal contraceptives*, ed. J. B. Josimovich. New York: John Wiley & Sons, 1973.

Liggins, G. C., S. A. Grieves, J. Z. Kendall, and B. S. Knox. The physiological roles of progesterone, oestradiol-17β and prostaglandin $F_{2\alpha}$ in the control of ovine parturition. J. Reprod. Fertil. (Suppl. 16):85, 1972.

Endometrium
De Feo, V. J. Decidualization. In *Cellular biology of the uterus*, ed. R. M. Wynn. New York: Appleton-Century-Crofts, 1967.

Hubinot, P. O., F. Leroy, C. Robyn, and P. Leleux, eds. *Ovo-implantation, human gonadotropines and prolactin*. Basel: S. Karger, 1970.

Finn, C. A., and D. G. Porter. *Handbooks of reproductive biology: The uterus*. London: Paul Elek Ltd., 1974.

Marcus, E. J., and M. C. Schelesnyak. Steroids in nidation. In *Advances in steroid biochemistry and pharmacology*, ed. M. H. Briggs. New York: Academic Press, 1970.

McLaren, A. Blastocyst activation. In *The regulation of mammalian reproduction*, eds. S. J. Segal et al. Springfield, Ill.: Charles C. Thomas, 1973.

Psychoyos, A. Hormonal control of ovoimplantation. Vitam. Horm. 31:281, 1974.

Symposium Report No. 3: Implantation. J. Reprod. Fertil. 39:173, 1975.

Cervix
Blandau, R. J., and K. Moghissi. *The biology of the cervix*. Chicago: University of Chicago Press, 1973.

Cervical mucus in human reproduction (WHO Colloquium, Geneva, 1972). Copenhagen: Scriptor, 1973.

Moghissi, F. S. The function of the cervix in fertility. Fertil. Steril. 23:295, 1972.

15 Embryogenesis

Anne McLaren

The use of human embryos for research raises both ethical and practical problems. Fortunately, the available evidence suggests that all mammals share a basic developmental pattern and that in studying the causal factors which operate in early embryogenesis, use of animal models may provide information relevant to the human situation. In the present discussion I confine myself to this early period of development, up to the formation of the primitive streak and the appearance of mesoderm.

The study of mammalian development during early embryogenesis can be divided into three phases. The first phase, that of morphological description, began around 1900 and is still continuing—for example, with sophisticated ultrastructural studies. The description of early acting genetic defects falls largely into this phase. The second phase, which began in the late 1950s and is also still continuing, has been characterized by concentration on in vitro cultivation of embryos and has included both biochemical description and the introduction of manipulative techniques. Culture methods are now being extended later in development, biochemical analyses are proceeding at an ever more refined level, and the range of studied species is gradually broadening. The third phase, to me the most exciting, began in the late 1960s but is only now gaining momentum. It involves use of existing knowledge and technical expertise to attempt some causal analysis of mammalian development.

15.1 Morphology

The year 1973 marked the seventieth anniversary of the publication of a classic work by Sobotta in which the early development of the mouse was meticulously described and illustrated. The drawings in Figure 15.1, taken from Sobotta (1902, 1911), cover the period with which this chapter is concerned, the first week of life. As far as we know, human embryos during this period develop in essentially the same way as mouse embryos, though they take a few days longer to reach the same stage of development. We cannot be sure of all

Reprinted with permission from E. M. Coutinho and F. Fuchs, eds., *Physiology and genetics of reproduction* (Part B), New York: Plenum Publishing Corp., 1974.

similarities, since investigators during the last 70 years have seen a million or so early mouse embryos but no more than a few dozen human embryos.

In all mammals fertilization is followed first by cleavage and then by the appearance of an internal fluid-filled cavity, the blastocoele, shown in Figure 15.1 (1). By this stage the first cellular differentiation has taken place; the outer trophoblast cells are morphologically and physiologically different from those of the inner cell mass. The mouse blastocyst implants with its abembryonic pole at the antimesometrial end of the uterine lumen: the zona pellucida disappears; trophoblast cells enlarge and begin to invade the uterine epithelium and stroma, engulfing epithelial cells and anything else in their path; and at the same time the decidual cell reaction begins to develop in the neighboring regions of the uterus. In the embryo a layer of endoderm cells differentiates from the rest of the inner cell mass (2) and grows round the inner surface of the trophoblast shell, while the inner cell mass elongates into the blastocoele to form the egg cylinder (3). Within the egg cylinder embryonic and extraembryonic ectoderm separate (4). A cavity forms, single at first, the proamniotic cavity (5), then divided by the amniotic folds (6) into amniotic cavity, exocoelom, and ectoplacental cavity (7). With the formation of the primitive streak a third layer, the mesoderm, appears. Trophoblast cells proliferate and enlarge to form the ectoplacental cone, which together with the developing allantois (7) gives rise to the fetal component of the chorioallantoic placenta.

This brief description of an immensely complex process of embryogenesis contains nothing that would have been unfamiliar to Sobotta.

For the next 50 years the embryo remained tucked away in cosy inaccessibility, in spite of sporadic attempts at in vitro culture (Brachet 1912; Waddington 1933; Hammond 1949). The single available approach to the unraveling of the causal mechanisms underlying early development appeared to be through the study of mutant genes acting during the first week of life.

Genetics
Mutant genes are sometimes described as "Nature's experiments." As applied to embryos in the period of organogenesis, the study of genetic defects has provided a powerful tool for analyzing mechanisms of

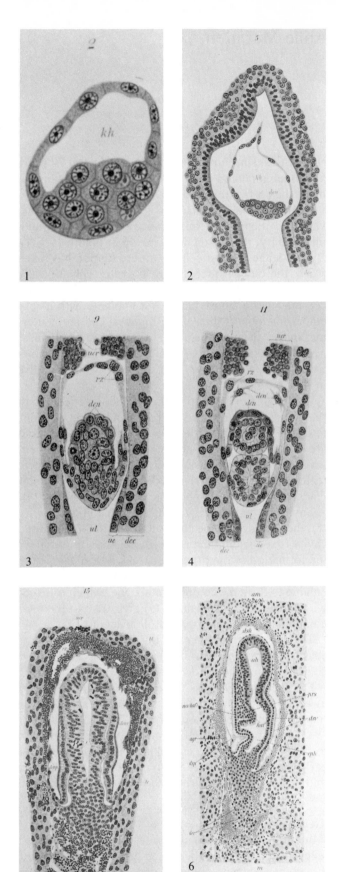

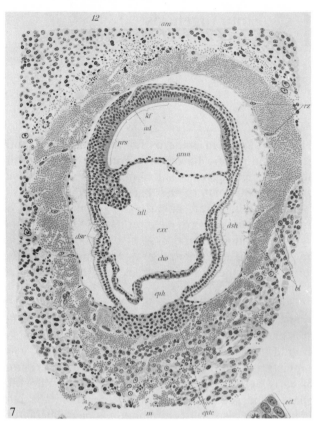

Figure 15.1 Median longitudinal sections of mouse embryos: 1 to 5 from Sobotta (1902); 6 and 7 from Sobotta (1911). The originals, based on camera lucida drawings, are in color. Labels have been added. Magnifications: ×330(1); ×105(2); ×150(3); ×130(4); ×90(5); ×20(6,7).

1. Blastocyst at the end of the fourth day of pregnancy. (bc, blastocyst cavity; tr, trophoblast; icm, inner cell mass)

2. Blastocyst in the uterus at the end of the fifth day of pregnancy. The decidual reaction is already beginning in the uterine stroma. The gap between blastocyst and uterine epithelium is now known to be due to fixation shrinkage. (e, endoderm; ue, uterine epithelium; ul, uterine lumen)

3. Embryo late on the sixth day of pregnancy. Distal endoderm is spreading around the inner surface of the trophoblast. The uterine epithelium has broken down around the embryo, and trophoblast is invading the uterine stroma. (ec, egg cylinder)

4. Embryo early on the seventh day of pregnancy. The ectoderm has differentiated into two parts. (ee, embryonic ectoderm; exe, extraembryonic ectoderm)

5. Embryo later on the seventh day of pregnancy. The proamniotic cavity has appeared. (pc, proamniotic cavity; d, decidual reaction in uterine stroma)

6. Embryo early on the eighth day of pregnancy. The proximal endoderm has differentiated into an embryonic and extraembryonic region. (de, distal endoderm; pe, proximal endoderm; af, amniotic fold; ep, ectoplacental cone)

7. Embryo late on the eighth day of pregnancy. (ps, primitive streak; amn, amnion; al, allantois; ac, amniotic cavity; exc, exocoelom; epc, ectoplacental cavity; mb, maternal blood)

development. For example, the inductive interaction between notochord and neural ectoderm in the development of the mammalian nervous system and the role of organizer phenomena in controlling axis development in the embryo were uncovered in the course of studies on lethal homozygotes for mutant genes in the ninth linkage group of the mouse (Gluecksohn-Waelsch 1953). Again, the realization that normal development of the tail of the mouse depends on the presence of an unassuming embryonic structure, the ventral ectodermal ridge, followed from the observation that the structure was absent in the homozygous vestigial tail mutant (Grüneberg 1956).

Several mutant genes are known (Table 15.1) whose effects in homozygous form are evident during the first week after conception. All are lethal as homozygotes, and most are being actively studied at present.

So far none of the known early lethals has contributed markedly to our understanding of the developmental process. Partly this is because the period between first manifestation and death is very short in early development, since with so few tissues present, each tends to be necessary for survival. In the midterm fetus, if cartilage fails to form normally or indeed if the entire head region fails to develop, the fetus still survives to birth. At implantation, on the other hand, if trophoblast fails to develop normally, death comes quickly. There is thus little time for Grüneberg's "pedigree of causes" to unfold. If a biochemical defect antedating the first morphological abnormality could be uncovered in any of the lethal homozygotes, it might prove illuminating. The most promising approach so far appears to be the analysis of embryonic cell surface antigens, including those of t-series mutants (Bennett et al. 1971; Artzt et al. 1973).

Some hopeful leads may prove to be blind alleys. In homozygous t^{12}/t^{12} embryos, the nucleoli appear abnormal, both at the level of light microscopy (Smith 1956) and at that of electron microscopy (Calarco and Brown 1968). RNA concentration is low (Smith 1956), and the preliminary DNA/RNA hybridization results of Klein and Raska (1968) suggested that t^{12} might involve some deletion of a nucleolar organizer region. But nucleolar abnormalities now appear to be signs of retardation or degeneration (Hillman et al. 1970), and since RNA synthesis and processing are normal for 4s, 18s, and 30–32s RNA (Hillman and Tasca 1973), it seems unlikely that nucleolar function is defective. Again, the trophoblast defect in A^y/A^y embryos may not be primary, as suggested by Eaton and Green (1963); it may be a sign of some more general retardation or degeneration (L. C. Dunn, personal communication). A^y/A^y homozygotes can now be identified as early as the morula stage in embryos cultured from the two-cell stage (Pedersen 1973).

15.2 In Vitro Techniques

In the 1950s research on mammalian reproduction and development was stimulated by an increasing awareness of the social importance of fertility regulation. During this same period the availability of antibiotics, introduced during World War II, led to an uprush of enthusiasm for in vitro techniques. The cultivation of mouse embryos in chemically defined media for up to two days (Whitten 1956), from the eight-cell to the blastocyst stage, was soon followed by a demonstration that embryos treated in this way could grow into normal fertile mice (McLaren and Biggers 1958). Culture methods have since been devised for preimplantation embryos of several other mammalian species, including man (Steptoe et al. 1971). Only in the mouse, however, have the specific requirements for preimplantation development in vitro been defined. In vitro methods are also being devised for the period of implantation (e.g., Grant 1973), for postimplantational development (e.g., Hsu 1972; New 1971), and for the study of trophoblast growth and differentiation (Gwatkin 1966).

The increasing success of culture techniques, combined with the introduction of micromethods of chemical analysis, led to striking advances in our knowledge of the biochemistry of preimplantation development. Some significant differences have been found between mouse and rabbit embryos, suggesting a need for more comparative investigations in this field.

In the mouse, studies of carbohydrate metabolism have revealed a changing pattern of energy sources that can be used by the embryo, perhaps related to a change in the morphology of the embryonic mitochondria (Biggers 1971). RNA synthesis has been extensively examined (Graham 1973); synthesis of ribosomal and transfer RNA can be detected at the four-cell stage, and messenger RNA is thought to be produced soon after. Rabbit transfer RNA becomes extensively demethylated during the transition from morula to blastocyst (Manes and Sharma 1973). Protein synthesis, in common with other metabolic processes, multiplies several times between the eight-cell and the blastocyst stage (Brinster 1973). Paternal gene action has been demonstrated in the blastocyst (Chapman et al. 1971), and recent studies using a highly sensitive assay system for β-glucuronidase suggest that the paternal genome may be expressed as early as the eight-cell stage (L. Wudl and V. M. Chapman, personal communication).

The other field that has been opened up by the increasing success of in vitro techniques is the experimental manipulation of mammalian embryos. In the last few years the technical armamentarium of the mammalian developmental biologist has expanded

Table 15.1 Genetic defects in mouse embryos, manifesting before 7.5 days postcoitum (p.c.)

Locus	Mutant Gene	Defect in Homozygote	References*
Oligosyndactylism	Os	Some cells abnormal at 64-cell stage (3.5 days p.c.). Dead 24 hr later. Decidual reaction normal.	Van Valen (1966)
Velvet coat	Ve	Endoderm normal; ectoderm deficient at 5 days p.c. Dead by 8 days p.c.	Diwan and Stevens (personal communication)
Blind or dysoptic	Bld, Dys	Growth of egg cylinder greatly retarded, endoderm abnormal, no primitive streak. Dead by 7–8 days.	Vankin (1956), Watson (1966)
Agouti	A^y	Cells abnormal at implantation, perhaps earlier. Gene expression restricted to trophoblast? Most dead by egg cylinder stage. Decidual reaction abnormal.	Kirkham (1916), Robertson (1942), Eaton and Green (1963)
	A^x	Looks similar to A^y.	Dunn (personal communication)
Albino	c^{6H}, c^{25H}	Dead in early egg cylinder stage (4.5–5 days p.c.).	Thorndike et al. (1973), Gluecksohn-Waelsch (personal communication)
Hydrocephalus-1	hy-1	(extinct) Claimed to manifest first as trophoblast defect at 4–6 days p.c.	Bonnevie (1944)
Tailless	t^1	(extinct) Death probably before implantation.	Gluecksohn-Schoenheimer (1938)
	t^{12}	Development stops at about 30-cell stage, at morula or early blastocyst. RNA content low.	Smith (1956), Hillman et al. (1970)
	t^0, "t^1"	Prevents segregation of egg cylinder into embryonic and extraembryonic portions. No primitive streak. Dead 5–6 days p.c.	Gluecksohn-Schoenheimer (1940)
	t^{w5}, t^{w17}, etc.	Embryonic ectoderm degenerates from 6.5 days p.c., leaving only extraembryonic. Dead by 8–10 days p.c.	Bennett and Dunn (1958)
	t^4, t^9	Egg cylinder abnormal histologically (6 days p.c.). Head neural folds overdeveloped at 8 days p.c. Dead by 9.5 days p.c.	Moser and Gluecksohn-Waelsch (1967)
	t^{w18}	Movement of cells through primitive streak affected, causing overgrowth.	Bennett and Dunn (1960)
Unidentified factor in DDK strain	—	Incompatibility of DDK cytoplasm with heterozygous nucleus leads to abnormality and death at 4–5 days p.c.	Wakasugi et al. (1967), Wakasugi (1973)

*This list is not intended to include all publications on each defect.

dramatically. Single blastomeres of mouse or rabbit can be separated to develop as "half" or "quarter" embryos (Tarkowski 1959; Moore et al. 1968); two or more embryos from the same or related species can be aggregated to form composites (Tarkowski 1961; Mintz 1965; Zeilmaker 1973); one or more cells can be injected into the blastocyst (Gardner 1968); trophoblast and inner cell mass from different individuals can be reassembled (Gardner and Johnson 1972); and inner cell mass can be differentially destroyed to leave only trophoblast (Snow 1973a). Parthenogenetically activated eggs will develop as haploids, diploids, or haplodiploid mosaics (Graham 1970; Tarkowski et al. 1970); cytochalasin-treated embryos can develop as viable tetraploids (Snow 1973b). Various substances, including radioactive isotopes and DNA, can be microinjected into the embryo or incorporated from the culture medium (Lin and Monie 1973; Snow 1973a; Snow and McLaren 1974).

15.3 Analysis

Descriptions of normal development, whether morphological or biochemical, can never reveal underlying causal mechanisms. To achieve even a glimmer of causal insight, we must modify development, either by experimental manipulation or by genetic means. As we have seen, genetic modifications, in the form of mutant genes, have not yet increased much our understanding of early development in mammals; therefore it is fortunate that a wide range of techniques now exists for experimental manipulation.

The earliest differentiation seen in the mammalian embryo is the distinction between inner cell mass and trophoblast, first apparent in the mouse at about the 16-cell stage. The outer cells (trophoblast) become flattened and connected to one another by tight junctions; they pump fluid and show no tendency to aggregate if isolated in vitro. The inner cells, in contrast, are rounded and only loosely associated, but they can aggregate readily with similar cell groups.

One theory postulated the initial differentiation of the cytoplasm of the fertilized egg, so that the cytoplasm is allocated to the different regions of the embryo in accordance with its developmental potential. Tarkowski and Wroblewska (1967) observed that when cell number was reduced by the destruction of one blastomere at the two-cell or three at the four-cell stage, all the remaining cells usually differentiated as trophoblast, producing "trophoblastic vesicles." From this evidence they argued that their internal position led some cells to develop as inner cell mass, while those on the outside, after three to four cell divisions, became trophoblast. When cell number was re-

duced, all the cells were on the outside, and all became trophoblast.

This environmental, "inside-outside" theory was tested more rigorously by Hillman et al. (1972), using combinations of isotopically or enzymically marked embryos. When the separated blastomeres of a four-cell embryo were placed on the outside of other four-cell embryos, their progeny were found almost entirely in the outer layer of the blastocyst, and at a later stage, they were found in the ectoplacental cone and yolk sac rather than in the embryo. Conversely, when a four-cell embryo was entirely surrounded by other blastomeres, its progeny were always found in the inner cell mass and lacked the capacity to pump fluid. Thus at this early stage the location of cells within the embryo appears to determine their developmental fate.

McLaren (1973) documented the great increase of metabolic activity as the blastocyst stage approaches, and the subsequent decline to a state of dormancy if implantation is delayed. Evidence is growing for a uterine inhibitor during delay, but the question remains open. Another unsolved problem in the area of implantation is the exact nature of the signal that passes from blastocyst to uterus to induce the localized decidual reaction in the estrogen-sensitized endometrium. Probably some low-molecular-weight byproduct of the embryo's increased metabolic activity is involved, since in the mouse the decidual reaction can be stimulated experimentally by injecting into the uterus an appropriate concentration of carbon dioxide. Steroid production on the part of the embryo may also play a role, since Perry et al. (1973) have demonstrated that the pig blastocyst is able to synthesize estrogen in vitro.

In the estrogen-sensitized uterus of the mouse, lysis of the zona pellucida occurs, probably through the action of a uterine protease or possibly through some localized pH effect. Trophoblast invades between the cells of the uterine epithelium and into the stroma, but the actual breakdown of the epithelium in the neighborhood of the embryo is now known to occur spontaneously as part of the decidual reaction; it is not brought about by the invading trophoblast.

Trophoblast Giant Cell Transformation
The enormous size to which trophoblast cells and their nuclei grow has been known since the time of Sobotta. Recent observations by microdensitometry have established that up to a thousand times the haploid DNA content can be found after the so-called trophoblast giant cell transformation has taken place (Barlow and Sherman 1972). The transformation is not dependent on the uterine environment, since it occurs similarly in the uterus, in ectopic sites (e.g., in blastocysts

transferred under the kidney capsule), and in vitro and it is not dependent on loss of the zona pellucida. The initial primary trophoblast invasion and transformation involves all the outer cells of the blastocyst with the exception of the cells overlying the inner cell mass. These remain small and continue to proliferate, and only as the ectoplacental cone grows are the secondary trophoblast giant cells formed around its periphery.

When the inner cell mass is eliminated, either by microsurgery (Gardner and Johnson 1972) or by culture in tritiated thymidine (Ansell and Snow 1975), a vesicle consisting only of trophoblast cells develops. Whether transferred to the uterus or maintained in vitro, all the cells of the vesicle appear to undergo giant cell transformation, and no cell proliferation or ectoplacental cone formation takes place. Suspecting that the ectoplacental cone might, contrary to traditional belief, develop from the inner cell mass, Gardner and his colleagues refurnished each of a series of trophoblastic vesicles with an inner cell mass of a contrasting enzyme type and examined the ectoplacental cones that subsequently formed (Gardner et al. 1973). No evidence could be found that the inner cell mass contributed directly to the ectoplacental cone. Presumably, therefore, the relationship is an inductive one: trophoblast cells proliferate to form an ectoplacental cone only in the presence of an inner cell mass. One hypothesis is that the proximity of the inner cell mass inhibits the overlying trophoblast from undergoing the giant cell transformation, and this allows the trophoblast to continue proliferating until its cells are no longer within range of the inhibitory influence.

It has been suggested that the accumulation of DNA in trophoblast giant cells arises through the fusion of trophoblast cells, either with one another or with decidual cells of maternal origin. Both these possibilities have been rendered unlikely by recent studies in the mouse, using the enzyme marker glucose phosphate isomerase (Chapman et al. 1972). When two genetic variants of this dimer are synthesized in the same cell, as in a heterozygote or a product of cell fusion, electrophoresis reveals a hybrid enzyme band. Aggregation of two eight-cell stages of contrasting enzyme type, or transfer of embryos of one type into a recipient female of the other type, did not result in the appearance of any hybrid enzyme in giant trophoblast cells of the ectoplacental cone or in giant cells differentiating in vitro; hence, giant cells probably do not arise through fusion.

The other possibility—repeated replication of the genome within the cell in the absence of cell division —raises the question of whether the entire genome is replicated in trophoblast giant cells or whether some DNA sequences are amplified at the expense of others. In the giant nuclei of *Drosophila* salivary glands, differential amplification has been demonstrated, with repeated DNA sequences underrepresented. No such effect could be detected in mouse trophoblast giant cells (Sherman et al. 1972).

Regulation of Growth and Differentiation

While the trophoblast cells are enlarging around the periphery of the blastocyst, the inner cell mass is proliferating and growing down into the blastocyst cavity to form the egg cylinder. Nothing is known of how this growth process is regulated. Recently we have compared the size of the inner cell mass and egg cylinder in control "single" mouse embryos and in "double" embryos formed from the aggregation of two eight-cell stages (Buehr and McLaren 1974). Before and during implantation and during the formation of the egg cylinder, doubles were at least twice the size of singles. Once the proamniotic cavity had appeared (i.e., from about 5.5 days p.c.), however, no difference in size was detected. Whatever the nature of the regulatory process, it appears to operate rapidly and accurately, at a critical point in development, when the anteroposterior axis of the embryo is being established and the primitive streak is about to form.

Thus when cell number is increased in the early embryo, growth regulation is completed before organogenesis begins. We are attempting now to examine, by inducing tetraploidy, the consequences for subsequent growth of increasing cell size in the early embryo.

Triploidy is one of the most frequent aberrations seen in early human embryos, affecting about 1 percent of all conceptuses. Most triploids die and are spontaneously aborted during the first trimester, though the cause of death remains unknown. There are indications that the incidence of triploidy may be even higher than 1 percent in women who stop taking oral contraceptives shortly before the beginning of pregnancy (Carr 1970). In a strain of mice that showed a high frequency of spontaneous triploidy, the triploid conceptuses all showed the so-called triploid syndrome, in which the extraembryonic part of the egg cylinder develops more or less normally to form the fetal membranes, but little or no development of the embryonic portion takes place (Wroblewska 1971).

Spontaneous tetraploidy, on the other hand, is rare in both mice and men, but recently a technique has been devised for inducing tetraploidy in a high proportion of mouse blastocysts by treatment with cytochalasin-B at the two-cell stage (Snow 1973b). Cell and nuclear volume in the tetraploid embryos is twice that of control diploid material. Most of the embryos die at or soon after implantation, but about 10 percent develop more or less normally at least up to term. On the other hand, tetraploid embryos produced by a similar technique in a different strain of mice all showed the triploid syndrome (J. Wroblewska and A. K. Tarkowski, personal communication). Preliminary analysis of the tetraploid embryos that have entered the period of organogenesis suggest that body size and organ size are twice that of diploid controls (M. H. L. Snow, personal communication), so that the number of cells involved in any structure is halved.

At the time when the proamniotic cavity first appears, the mouse or rat egg cylinder consists of two layers only, ectoderm and endoderm. With the formation of the primitive streak, a third layer appears, mesoderm. The developmental potentialities of these germ layers have recently been explored. The layers are separated by microdissection and transplanted under the kidney capsule. After a month or more the derivatives of the transplant are analyzed histologically.

In the rat (Levak-Švajger et al. 1969; Levak-Švajger and Švajger 1971; N. Skreb, personal communication), endoderm taken from a two-layered egg cylinder (8.5 days p.c.) fails to grow under these conditions, but ectoderm from the same embryo gives rise not only to ectodermal but also to mesodermal and endodermal derivatives. This observation raises the question of whether the endoderm that covers the egg cylinder at this stage contributes to the definitive endoderm of the fetus. A day later (9.5 days p.c.), the egg cylinder is three-layered, with mesoderm split off from part of the ectodermal layer of the previous day. Ectoderm now transplanted under the kidney capsule gives rise to ectodermal and mesodermal, but no longer endodermal, derivatives. Endoderm on its own still fails to grow, but in combination with mesoderm it gives rise to both endodermal and mesodermal derivatives. Mesoderm on its own, however, gives nothing but brown adipose tissue. Perhaps the development of mesodermal derivatives such as bone, cartilage, and skeletal muscle requires some inductive influence from either ectoderm or endoderm.

In the mouse the germ layers have not been separated, but transplants of whole egg cylinders under the kidney capsule develop, as in the rat, into teratomas containing various types of fully differentiated adult tissues. When two-layered and early three-layered egg cylinders (6–7 days p.c.) of some strains (C3H, CBA, Swiss) are used (Solter et al. 1970; Damjanov and Solter 1974), nearly half the transplants develop into malignant teratocarcinomas, containing nests of undifferentiated tissue as well as differentiated elements. Transplantation of somewhat older embryos (8–9 days p.c.), in which organogenesis is beginning, never results in teratocarcinomas (Damjanov et al. 1971). Similar teratocarcinomas occur spontaneously in the testis

of 129-strain mice and have been reported by Stevens (1970a, b) to develop from mouse preimplantation stages and 11 to 13 day p.c. genital ridges transplanted to the testis and other scrotal sites. C57BL egg cylinders give rise to very few teratocarcinomas if transplanted to C57BL kidneys, but on transplantation to (C3H × C57BL) F$_1$ kidneys they produce the same proportion of teratocarcinomas and teratomas as do, for example, C3H egg cylinders transplanted to isologous hosts (Damjanov and Solter 1974).

The undifferentiated embryonic carcinoma cells are thought to derive from embryonic ectoderm, which they resemble in various ways. Malignant transformation of embryonic ectoderm cells in the mouse has also been reported for lethal t^{w18}/t^{w18} embryos (see Table 15.1) by Artzt and Bennett (1972). The differentiation of embryonic ectoderm into mesoderm in the primitive streak region appears to be blocked, so that excessive undifferentiated primitive streak material accumulates, resembling a rapidly growing tumor bulging into the proamniotic cavity. Transplantation of the material into adult testes frequently results in histologically malignant growths resembling neuroblastomas, whereas grafts from normal littermates give rise only to benign teratomas.

The teratocarcinomas produced by Solter et al. (1970) and by Stevens (1970a, b) contained derivatives of all three germ layers. In contrast, the t^{w18}/t^{w18} tumors were almost exclusively ectodermal, consisting largely of immature neural tissue. This suggests that the genetic defect blocks the differentiation of mesoderm and that this in turn severely restricts the developmental pathways open to ectoderm cells. Such an interpretation is consistent with the view of Bennett (1964) that each of the lethal t alleles interferes with development at a point where some "switch mechanism" normally operates to achieve a new and more complex degree of differentiation; t^{12} affects the morula-blastocyst transition, t^0 the differentiation into embryonic and extraembryonic ectoderm, t^{w18} the development of mesoderm, and so on.

Prospect

In the human species the embryo is attracting an increasing amount of attention. With the decline in neonatal mortality due to infections, congenital malformations are responsible for an even higher proportion of mortality and morbidity among the newborn. Similarly, as other forms of pregnancy wastage are successfully tackled, emphasis is moving to the etiology of early abortion and to the origin of the chromosomal abnormalities so prevalent among early abortuses. Amniocentesis and fetoscopy may become routine screening procedures. Within a decade or two, even egg transfer is likely to be adopted as a standard treatment for certain types of infertility. Gene therapy by various means, including the injection of cells into embryos, is already under discussion.

Studies of the causal factors underlying early embryogenesis in animal models may provide a developmental basis for assessing the various procedures likely to be attempted on human embryos in the future. Such studies could also throw light on the etiology of congenital defects and on early embryonic mortality. In particular, now that appropriate techniques are being devised to allow the in vitro development of postimplantation embryos, more analytical investigations may be conducted during the period immediately following implantation, when the basic architecture of the embryo is being established. The next 10 years may see as much progress in this crucial but hitherto inaccessible area as has been achieved in the last 10 years in our understanding of events in the preimplantation embryo.

References

Ansell, J., and M. H. L. Snow. The development of mouse trophoblast giant cells in the absence of inner cell mass. Exp. Morphol. 33:117, 1975.

Artzt, K., and D. Bennett. A genetically caused embryonal ectodermal tumor in the mouse. J. Natl. Cancer Inst. 48:141, 1972.

Artzt, K., P. Dubois, D. Bennett, H. Condamine, C. Babinet, and F. Jacob. Surface antigens common to mouse primitive teratocarcinoma cells in culture and cleavage embryos. Proc. Natl. Acad. Sci. USA 70:2988, 1973.

Barlow, P. W., and M. I. Sherman. The biochemistry of differentiation of mouse trophoblast: Studies on polyploidy. J. Embryol. Exp. Morphol. 27:447, 1972.

Bennett, D. Abnormalities associated with a chromosome region in the mouse. II. Embryological effects of lethal alleles in the t-region. Science 144:263, 1964.

Bennett, D., E. A. Boyse, and L. J. Old. Cell surface immunogenetics in the study of morphogenesis. Lepetit Symposium, London, 247, 1971.

Bennett, D., and L. C. Dunn. Effects on embryonic development of a group of genetically similar lethal alleles derived from different populations of wild house mice. J. Morphol. 103:135, 1958.

Bennett, D., and L. C. Dunn. A lethal mutant t^{w18} in the house mouse showing partial duplications. J. Exp. Zool. 143:203, 1960.

Biggers, J. D. Metabolism of mouse embryos. J. Reprod. Fertil. Suppl. 14:41, 1971.

Bonnevie, K. Hereditary hydrocephalus in the house mouse. III. Manifestation of the *hy* mutation in embryos 9–11 days old, and younger. Norske Vid. Akad. Skr. 1, 1944.

Brachet, A. Developpement *in vitro* de blastomères et jeunes embryons de mammifères. C. R. Acad. Sci. (Paris) 155:1191, 1912.

Brinster, R. L. Protein synthesis and enzyme constitution of the preimplantation mammalian embryo. In *The regulation of mammalian reproduction*, eds. S. J. Segal, R. Crozier, P. A. Corfman, and P. G. Condliffe. Springfield, Ill.: Charles C Thomas, 1973.

Buehr, M., and A. McLaren. Size regulation in chimaeric mouse embryos. J. Embryol. Exp. Morphol. 31:229, 1974.

Calarco, P. G., and E. H. Brown. Cytological and ultrastructural comparisons of t^{12}/t^{12} and normal mouse morulae. J. Exp. Zool. 168:169, 1968.

Carr, D. H. Chromosome studies in selected spontaneous abortions. I. Conception after oral contraceptives. Canad. Med. Ass. 103:343, 1970.

Chapman, V. M., J. D. Ansell, and A. McLaren. Trophoblast giant cell differentiation in the mouse: Expression of glucose phosphate isomerase (GPI-1) electrophoretic variants in transferred and chimeric embryos. Dev. Biol. 29:48, 1972.

Chapman, V. M., W. K. Whitten, and F. H. Ruddle. Expression of paternal glucose phosphate isomerase (GPI-1) in preimplantation stages of mouse embryos. Dev. Biol. 26:53, 1971.

Damjanov, I., and D. Solter. Host related factors determine the outgrowth of teratocarcinoma from mouse egg cylinders. Z. Krebsforsch. 81:63, 1974.

Damjanov, I., D. Solter, and N. Skreb. Teratocarcinogenesis as related to the age of embryos grafted under the kidney capsule. Wilhelm Roux' Arch. 167:288, 1971.

Eaton, G. J., and M. M. Green. Giant cell differentiation and lethality of homozygous *yellow* mouse embryos. Genetica 34:155, 1963.

Gardner, R. L. Mouse chimaeras obtained by the injection of cells into the blastocyst. Nature 220:596, 1968.

Gardner, R. L., and M. H. Johnson. An investigation of inner cell mass and trophoblast tissues following their isolation from the mouse blastocyst. J. Embryol. Exp. Morphol. 28:279, 1972.

Gardner, R. L., V. E. Papaioannou, and S. C. Barton. Origin of the ectoplacental cone and secondary giant cells in mouse blastocysts reconstituted from isolated trophoblast and inner cell mass. J. Embryol. Exp. Morphol. 30:561, 1973.

Glucksohn-Schoenheimer, S. Time of death of lethal homozygotes in the T (Brachyury) series of the mouse. Proc. Soc. Exp. Biol. Med. 39:267, 1938.

Glucksohn-Schoenheimer, S. The effect of an early lethal (t⁰) in the house mouse. Genetics 25:391, 1940.

Glucksohn-Waelsch, S. Lethal factors in development. Q. Rev. Biol. 28:115, 1953.

Graham, C. F. Parthenogenetic mouse blastocysts. Nature 226:165, 1970.

Graham, C. F. Nucleic acid metabolism during early mammalian development. In *The regulation of mammalian reproduction*, eds. S. J. Segal, R. Crozier, P. A. Corfman, and P. G. Condliffe. Springfield, Ill.: Charles C Thomas, 1973.

Grant, P. S. The effect of progesterone and oestradiol on blastocysts cultured within the lumina of immature mouse uteri. J. Embryol. Exp. Morphol. 29:617, 1973.

Grüneberg, H. A ventral ectodermal ridge on the tail in mouse embryos. Nature 177:787, 1956.

Gwatkin, R. B. L. Amino acid requirement for attachment and outgrowth of the mouse blastocyst in vitro. J. Cell. Physiol. 68:335, 1966.

Hammond, J., Jr. Recovery and culture of tubal mouse ova. Nature 163:28, 1949.

Hillman, N., R. Hillman, and G. Wileman. Ultrastructural studies of cleavage stage t^{12}/t^{12} mouse embryos. Am. J. Anat. 128:311, 1970.

Hillman, N., M. I. Sherman, and C. Graham. The effect of spatial arrangement on cell determination during mouse development. J. Embryol. Exp. Morphol. 28:263, 1972.

Hillman, N., and R. J. Tasca. Synthesis of RNA in t^{12}/t^{12} mouse embryos. J. Reprod. Fertil. 33:501, 1973.

Hsu, Y. Differentiation in vitro of mouse embryos beyond the implantation stage. Nature 239:200, 1972.

Kirkman, W. B. Embryology of the yellow mouse. Anat. Rec. 11:480, 1916.

Klein, J., and K. Raska. Deficiency of "ribosomal" DNA in t^{12} mutant mice. Proc. Twelfth Int. Congr. Genet. 1:149, 1968.

Levak-Švajger, B., and A. Švajger. Differentiation of endodermal tissues in homografts of primitive ectoderm from two-layered rat embryonic shields. Experientia 27:683, 1971.

Levak-Švajger, B., A. Švajger, and N. Skreb. Separation of germ layers in presomite rat embryos. Experientia 25:1311, 1969.

Lin, T. P., and I. W. Monie. The development of mouse blastocysts injected with, or cultured in, trypan blue solution. J. Reprod. Fertil. 32:149, 1973.

Manes, C., and O. K. Sharma. Hypermethylated tRNA in cleaving rabbit embryos. Nature 244:283, 1973.

McLaren, A. Blastocyst activation. In *The regulation of mammalian reproduction*, eds. S. J. Segal, R. Crozier, P. A. Corfman, and P. G. Condliffe, p. 321. Springfield, Ill.: Charles C Thomas, 1973.

McLaren, A., and J. D. Biggers. Successful development and birth of mice cultivated in vitro as early embryos. Nature 182:877, 1958.

Mintz, B. Genetic mosaicism in adult mice of quadriparental lineage. Science 148:1232, 1965.

Moore, N. W., C. E. Adams, and L. E. A. Rowson. Developmental potential of single blastomeres of the rabbit egg. J. Reprod. Fertil. 17:527, 1968.

Moser, G. C., and S. Gluecksohn-Waelsch. Developmental genetics of a recessive allele at the complex T-locus in the mouse. Dev. Biol. 16:564, 1967.

New, D. A. T. Methods for the culture of post-implantation embryos of rodents. In *Methods in mammalian embryology*, ed. J. C. Daniel. San Francisco: W. H. Freeman, 1971.

Pedersen, R. A. In vitro development of lethal yellow (A^{cc}/A^{cc}) mouse embryos. Biol. Reprod. 9:77 (Abstract), 1973.

Perry, J. S., R. B. Heap, and E. C. Amoroso. Steroid hormone production by pig blastocysts. Nature 245:45, 1973.

Robertson, G. G. An analysis of the development of homozygous yellow mouse embryos. J. Exp. Zool. 89:197, 1942.

Sherman, M. I., A. McLaren, and P. M. B. Walker. Studies on the mechanism of DNA accumulation in giant cells of mouse trophoblast. Nature New Biol. 238:175, 1972.

Smith, L. J. A morphological and histochemical investigation of a preimplantation lethal (t^{12}) in the house mouse. J. Exp. Zool. 132:51, 1956.

Snow, M. H. L. The differential effect of ^{3}H-thymidine upon two populations of cells in pre-implantation mouse embryos. In *The cell cycle in development and differentiation*. Br. Soc. Dev. Biol. 1:311, 1973a.

Snow, M. H. L. Tetraploid mouse embryos produced by cytochalasin B during cleavage. Nature 244:513, 1973b.

Snow, M. H. L., and A. McLaren. The effect of exogenous DNA upon cleaving mouse embryos. Exp. Cell Res. 86:1, 1974.

Sobotta, J. Die Entwicklung des Eies der Maus vom Schluss der Furchungsperiode bis zum Auftreten der Amniosfalten. Arch. Mikrosk. Anat. 61:274, 1902.

Sobotta, J. Die Entwicklung des Eise der Maus vom ersten Auftreten des Mesoderms an bis zur Ausbildung der Embryonalanlage und dem Auftreten der Allantois. Arch. Mikrosk. Anat. 78:271, 1911.

Solter, D., N. Skreb, and I. Damjanov. Extrauterine growth of mouse egg cylinders results in malignant teratomas. Nature 227:503, 1970.

Steptoe, P. C., R. G. Edwards, and J. M. Purdy. Human blastocysts grown in culture. Nature 229:132, 1971.

Stevens, L. C. The development of transplantable teratocarcinomas from intratesticular grafts of pre- and postimplantation mouse embryos. Dev. Biol. 21:364, 1970a.

Stevens, L. C. Environmental influence on experimental teratocarcinogenesis in testes of mice. J. Exp. Zool. 174:407, 1970b.

Tarkowski, A. K. Experiments on the development of isolated blastomeres of mouse eggs. Nature 184:1286, 1959.

Tarkowski, A. K. Mouse chimaeras developed from fused eggs. Nature 190:557, 1961.

Tarkowski, A. K., and J. Wroblewska. Development of blastomeres of mouse eggs isolated at the 4- and 8-cell stage. J. Embryol. Exp. Morphol. 18:155, 1967.

Tarkowski, A. K., A. Witkowska, and J. Nowicka. Experimental parthenogenesis in the mouse. Nature 226:162, 1970.

Thorndike, J., N. J. Trigg, R. Stockert, S. Gluecksohn-Waelsch, and C. F. Cori. Multiple biochemical effects of a series of X-ray induced mutations at the albino locus in the mouse. Biochem. Genet. 9:25, 1973.

Vankin, L. The embryonic effects of "blind," a new early lethal mutation in mice. Anat. Rec. 125:648 (Abstract), 1956.

Van Valen, P. Oligosyndactylism, an early embryonic lethal in the mouse. J. Embryol. Exp. Morphol. 15:119, 1966.

Waddington, C. H., and A. J. Waterman. The development in vitro of young rabbit embryos. Am. J. Anat. 67:355, 1933.

Wakasugi, N. Studies on fertility of DDK mice: Reciprocal crosses between DDK and C57BL/6J strains and experimental transplantation of the ovary. J. Reprod. Fertil. 33:283, 1973.

Wakasugi, N., T. Tomita, and K. Kondo. Differences of fertility in reciprocal crosses between inbred strains of mice: DDK, KK, and NC. J. Reprod. Fertil. 13:41, 1967.

Watson, M. L. Further test for the identity of 'dysoptic' with "blind" in mice. Proc. Iowa Acad. Sci. 73:384, 1966.

Whitten, W. K. Culture of tubal mouse ova. Nature 177:96, 1956.

Wroblewska, J. Developmental anomaly in the mouse associated with triploidy. Cytogenetics (Basel) 10:199, 1971.

Zeilmaker, G. Fusion of rat and mouse morulae and formation of chimaeric blastocysts. Nature 242:115, 1973.

16 Clinical and Epidemiological Aspects of Induced Abortion

Christopher Tietze

16.1 Important Developments

Within the past decade abortion laws and practices in a number of countries, including the United States, have been liberalized, making possible the clinical and epidemiological evaluation of the elective termination of pregnancy on a large scale, involving many thousands of essentially healthy women (1, 2). The major result of this research has been an unequivocal recognition of the fact that, in terms of mortality and early morbidity, the medical risks associated with abortion in the first trimester of pregnancy are far lower not only than those associated with second-trimester abortion but also than those ordinarily associated with continued pregnancy and childbirth.

The vacuum aspiration procedure, developed in China in the late 1950s, became popular in the USSR and in other countries of eastern Europe during the early 1960s, and reached western Europe and the United States a few years later (3). It has proven to be a simple and safe procedure for first-trimester abortions, suitable for use by appropriately trained and supervised paramedical workers. In the United States and in a few other countries, first-trimester abortion by vacuum aspiration has been safely performed as an outpatient procedure, under either general or local anesthesia or, in very early gestation, even without anesthesia.

Prostaglandin research has provided a new approach to abortion by chemical means, so far primarily by injection into the amniotic sac during the second trimester. Several other routes of application, possibly useful also in the first trimester, are under investigation.

16.2 Principal Data Sources and Research Centers

Many, but not all, of the countries where abortion laws have been liberalized in recent years collect and publish statistics on abortions performed under these laws. The most comprehensive official data are those from England and Wales (4), Hungary (5), Czechoslovakia (6), and, more recently, Canada (7). In the United States, the Center for Disease Control (CDC) in Atlanta compiles the statistics obtained by an increasing number of state health departments (8). These statistics have been supplemented by surveys conducted by the Alan Guttmacher Institute (9). Individuals who have analyzed these data include Kestelman in London (10), Klinger in Budapest, Mehlan in Rostock, Muramatsu in Tokyo, and Pakter and Tietze in New York.

The Joint Program for the Study of Abortion (JPSA), sponsored by the Population Council, was conducted in 1970/71 as a nationwide survey of early medical complications of legal abortions in the United States, based on 73,000 case histories contributed by 66 institutions in 12 states and the District of Columbia (11). This work is being continued by the CDC. A Pregnancy Termination Study of international scope has been established at the Carolina Population Center in Chapel Hill.

A number of clinical reports involving vacuum aspiration have appeared in the medical literature, including at least three with more than 20,000 cases from a single institution (12–14). The collective JPSA report covers more than 50,000 cases.

The Population Study Center of the Battelle Memorial Institute has been actively involved in the development of "hardware" for the aspiration procedure.

Over the last two or three years a number of authors have reported on very early first-trimester abortions by vacuum aspiration, in some instances under such euphemisms as "menstrual regulation," done prior to the verification of pregnancy by immunological tests. The efficiency, efficacy, and rate of complications of this procedure, compared with vacuum aspiration later in the first trimester, remain to be fully evaluated.

The earliest published report on the use of prostaglandins for the induction of abortion, by Karim at the Makerere University Medical School in Kampala and Filshie at King's College Hospital in London, appeared in Lancet in January 1970 (15). Subsequently, a large number of workers have participated in the clinical evaluation of these compounds. Important centers of research include the Albert Einstein College of Medicine (Saldana, Schulman), the CDC in Atlanta (Cates, Grimes), Cornell University (Laursen, Wilson), the Karolinska Sjukhuset in Stockholm (Bygdeman, Wiqvist), the University of North Carolina (Brenner, Hendricks), the University of Oxford (Embry, Hillier), the University of Pennsylvania (Bolognese, Corson), and Yale University (Speroff). An important controlled comparison of intra-amniotic

PGF$_{2\alpha}$ and hypertonic saline was sponsored by the World Health Organization (WHO) (16). Several international conferences on prostaglandins in fertility control have been held under the auspices of WHO at the Karolinska Institut in Stockholm. For several years the Worcester Foundation for Experimental Biology served as an information center on prostaglandins, published a newsletter, and worked in conjunction with the Population Information Program at the George Washington University Medical Center on a comprehensive bibliography (17, 18).

16.3 Major Gaps in Our Knowledge

We do not yet know enough about the nature and incidence, if any, of late complications and sequelae of abortions performed by trained personnel, especially of repeated abortions; about the specific factors leading to such sequelae; or about the modifications of technique by which their incidence could be minimized.

We have not developed the optimum methods of selecting, training, and supervising medical and paramedical personnel for the performance of legal abortions or the optimum organization for the delivery of legal abortion services to women living in urban or rural areas in a variety of cultural settings.

In the areas of health, education, and organization of services, we do not have effective methods to enable pregnant women to seek and obtain legal abortions at an early stage of gestation, when the risks to their health are lowest.

16.4 Clinical and Epidemiological Aspects

The clinical and epidemiological aspects of induced abortion are only peripherally relevant to the basic understanding of reproductive phenomena. They are highly relevant to the control of human fertility, however.

Because abortion is a curative rather than a preventive measure (the "disease" being unwanted pregnancy), it has been more acceptable to many women throughout the world than the consistent practice of contraception. No population has ever achieved a low birth rate (2–3 children per couple) without substantial utilization of either legal or illegal abortion (19).

The inclusion of legal abortions for the termination of pregnancies resulting from contraceptive failure (or otherwise unplanned) increases the overall effectiveness of any program of fertility regulation. Moreover, legal abortion services made available in a humane and dignified fashion offer an excellent opportunity to recruit new contraceptive users.

16.5 Major Opportunities for Action

Clinical research should clearly continue in this area, involving many procedural details in the performance of first- and second-trimester abortions such as the most suitable means of analgesia and/or anesthesia, methods of dilating the cervical canal that are less traumatic than the customary metal instruments, the application of prostaglandins in the first trimester, the optimal dosage and regimen of intra-amniotic prostaglandin in the second trimester, and the use of mechanical means for the stimulation of uterine contractions. The orderly evaluation of new procedures emerging from the laboratory should, of course, remain a top priority.

Research on late complications and sequelae should also continue, with special emphasis on their etiology and on ways of reducing their incidence. Multipurpose prospective studies of women undergoing legal abortion would be extremely expensive and time-consuming; these studies would also involve major problems in selecting suitable controls and securing the cooperation of participants over a period of 5 to 10 years. As an alternative, a WHO task force has initiated a multicenter study for the evaluation of specific questions, such as the outcome of subsequent pregnancies after legal abortion. Results of these studies, conducted in countries where elective abortion has been legally available for several years, should be forthcoming in late 1977.

Research and, at a later stage, demonstration programs related to the delivery of abortion services should have high priority, especially in countries with high birth rates. Research of this type is constrained by the facts that only a few countries with high birth rates have as yet passed liberal abortion laws, that even fewer have included pregnancy termination in their fertility regulation programs, and that the attitude of the medical profession in most of these countries is quite conservative. Hence funding agencies should be alert and responsive to opportunities for research as they present themselves.

Finally, because abortion has until recently been illegal in most countries and is still illegal in many, a considerable proportion of the medical profession, including even obstetricians and gynecologists, is not well informed about recent advances in the field. A well-defined training program is therefore vitally necessary, including regional conferences, on-site instruction, supervised practice, and translation of the relevant literature.

References

1. Osofsky, H. J., and J. D. Osofsky, eds. *The abortion experience*. New York: Harper & Row, 1973, p. 668.

2. Tietze, C., and M. C. Murstein. Induced abortion: 1975 factbook. Rep. Popul. Fam. Plann. 14:3 (2nd ed.), 1975.

3. Kerslake, D., and D. Casey. Abortion induced by means of the uterine aspiration. Obstet. Gynecol. 30:35, 1967.

4. *The Registrar General's statistical review of England and Wales: Supplement on abortion*. London: Her Majesty's Stationery Office, published annually since 1968.

5. *A Vetélések Adatai*. Budapest: Központi Statisztikai Hital, published 1970–1971 and biennially since 1972–1973.

6. *Potraty*. Prague: Zdravotnická Statistika CSSR, published annually since 1965.

7. *Therapeutic abortions*. Ottawa: Statistics Canada, published annually since 1972.

8. *Abortion surveillance*. Atlanta: Center for Disease Control, published annually since 1970.

9. *Abortion 1974–75: Need and services in the United States, each state & metropolitan area*. New York: Alan Guttmacher Institute, 1976.

10. International Planned Parenthood Federation, Europe Region. *Legal abortion in Britain*. London: IPPF, 1973, p. 33.

11. Tietze, C., and S. Lewit. Joint Program for the Study of Abortion (JPSA): Early medical complications of legal abortion. Stud. Fam. Plann. 3:97, 1972.

12. Beric, B. M., and M. Kupresanin. Vacuum aspiration, using cervical block, for legal abortion as an outpatient procedure up to the 12th week of pregnancy. Lancet 2:619, 1971.

13. Nathanson, B. N. Ambulatory abortion: Experience with 26,000 cases (July 1, 1970–August 1, 1971). New Engl. J. Med. 286:403, 1972.

14. Hodgson, J. E. Major complications of 20,248 consecutive first trimester abortions: Problems of fragmented care. Adv. Planned Parenthood 9:52, 1975.

15. Karim, S. M. M., and G. M. Filshie. Therapeutic abortion using prostaglandin $F_{2\alpha}$. Lancet 1:157, 1970.

16. Task Force on the Use of Prostaglandins, etc. Comparison of intra-amniotic prostaglandin $F_{2\alpha}$ and hypertonic saline for induction of second-trimester abortion. Br. Med. J. 1:1373, 1976.

17. Sparks, R. M., ed. *Prostaglandin abstracts: A guide to the literature*, vol. I, 1906–1970. New York: Plenum Press, 1974.

18. Shalita, R., ed. *Prostaglandin abstracts: A guide to the literature*, vol. II, 1971–1973. New York: Plenum Press, 1975.

19. Tietze, C., and J. Bongaarts. Fertility rates and abortion rates: Simulations of family limitation. Stud. Fam. Plann. 6:113, 1975.

17 Systemic Contragestational Agents

Sheldon J. Segal

17.1 Introduction

Pregnancies can be terminated asurgically through the use of orally active or parenterally administered pharmacological agents. The folklore of many cultures includes descriptions of potions, usually of plant products, that can act as abortifacients. Although these have not been scientifically validated, reports appear persistently in anthropological literature.

Drugs that cause uterine contractions, such as oxytocin, sparteine sulfate, and various ergot alkaloids, have yielded erratic results in attempts to terminate pregnancy. In a controlled study of oxytocin in early pregnancy, for example, the relative insensitivity of the uterus during the first and second trimesters was shown to result in a poor percentage of successful terminations.[24]

The interest in an observation of the 1930s that prostaglandins can cause uterine contractions was revived when chemists found methods to synthesize this naturally occurring class of substituted fatty acids.[26] The unique action of the prostaglandins is to cause contraction of the uterus early in pregnancy, and they are even effective on the nongravid uterus. Thus when the administration of a prostaglandin preparation is effective, the pregnancy is terminated by a process that begins with the initiation of uterine contractions. When the contractions achieve sufficient intensity, separation of the placenta occurs. With the loss of the placental production of progesterone, uterine contractions are intensified, and evacuation of the uterine cavity ensues.[11] Premature contractions of the myometrium have been the only physiological mechanism shown to be definitely applicable as the basis for nonsurgical abortion. A disadvantage of this mechanism is that no agent has yet been discovered that acts selectively on the smooth muscle of the early gravid uterus without affecting the smooth muscle of other organs.

Several other potential mechanisms have emerged from laboratory experiments, and some of them may prove to be useful in humans. Hormonal control is involved in the key postfertilization events of zygote transport through the oviduct, in the secretory function of the oviduct, which assures a proper biochemical milieu for the passage of the zygote, in preparation of the endometrium for nidation, in maintenance of a functional corpus luteum, and in the initiation and continuation of the placentation process. Any intervention that disrupts the proper hormonal balance will, directly or indirectly, have antizygotic, blastotoxic, blastolytic, or abortifacient activity and could appropriately be termed contragestational activity.

Several classes of nonsteroidal compounds, including weak estrogens, antiestrogens, and luteolytic and antimitotic agents, have been tested in the rhesus monkey for contragestational activity (Table 17.1). All of these compounds had first been tested in the rat or mouse, which led to interest in studying them in nonhuman primates.[21,22] The contraceptive activity, or lack thereof, of these agents in the primate as compared to the rodent may in part depend only on timing and dosage requirements. The comparative endocrinology of pregnancy in primates and rodents, however, throws some doubt on the applicability to humans of observations made in the rat, at least for hormonal compounds. For example, plasma estrogen levels are low for a day or two after ovulation in both species, but with the exception of a brief estrogen surge on day 4 of pregnancy, the levels of estrogens remain relatively low and stable in the rat.[62] In contrast, estrogens increase during the luteal phase of the primate cycle and continue to rise as placental production of this steroid increases. Thus while estrogen excess is a nonphysiological situation in rat pregnancy, it is the normal course of the endocrinology of nonhuman and human primate pregnancy.[19,59]

17.2 Postcoital Administration of Estrogens

Ovarian steroid hormones have a major regulatory influence on the transport and normal development of zygotes in the oviduct. Estrogens increase the rate of secretion of tubal fluid,[28] are prerequisites for ciliary growth and movement at the ostial portion of the tube,[6] and tend to increase the frequency and decrease the amplitude of tubal muscle activity.[43] Progesterone, in the presence of estrogen, tends to decrease the frequency of contraction and increase the amplitude.[8] The overall effect of the ovarian steroids is to alter the responsiveness of the tubal musculature to local release of adrenergic agents (norepinephrine) and the posterior pituitary hormone (oxytocin).[9] Upsetting the proper sequence in the hormonal environment can

Table 17.1 Contragestational effectiveness of some nonsteroidal compounds in the female rhesus monkey

Type of Activity and Compounds Tested	Result*	Reference Number
Anti-implantation		
ORF-3858 (2-methyl-3-ethyl-4-phenyl-Δ^4-cyclohexane-carboxilic acid)	+	34
Diethylstilbestrol	+	30
U-11100A (1-(2-(p-(3,4-dihydro-6 methoxy-2-phenyl-1-napthyl) phenoxy) ethyl)-pyrrolidine hydrochloride)	±	32
Clomiphene, MRL 41 1-(p-(β-diethifamino-ethoxy)-phenyl) 1,2-diphenyl-2-chloroethylene	−	32
66/179 (2-phenyl-3-p (β-pyrrolidino-ethoxy)-phenyl-(2:1,b) napthofuran	+	21
DL-cis-bisdehydrodoisynolic acid methyl ether	+	33
H1067 (triphenyl ethylene derivative)	−	50
Centchroman (3,4-trans-2,2-dimethyl-3-phenyl-4-(p-β-pyrrolodinoethoxy)-phenyl)-7-methoxychroman)	+	22
Luteolytic		
Amphenone (U-7256)	−	50
Abortifacient		
Colcemide (desacetylmethyl colchicine)	−	31
BW57-323H (2-amino-6-(1'-methyl-4'-nitro-5' imidazolyl) mercaptopurine	−	31
Triacetyl-6-azauridine	±	60
H1067 (triphenyl ethylene derivative)	±	50
N-desacetyl thiocolchicine	−	50

*+ = positive effect; − = negative effect; ± = marginal effect.

therefore alter motility and disturb the normal passage of cleaving ova in the oviducts.[47] This has been demonstrated by many experiments, but species differences and variations in experimental techniques have made it difficult to construct a unified concept from reported observations.

As early as 1926, Parkes and Bellerby demonstrated the effectiveness of estrogen administered after mating in preventing fertility in the mouse and rat.[38] That observation led to a successful decade of work by Pincus and Kirsh,[39] among others, which established the effect of exogenous estrogen on egg transport in the mouse and rabbit. In 1958 Segal and Nelson reported that a synthetic compound with estrogenic activity prevented pregnancy in the rat if administered during the period of tubal transport of ova.[47] This compound, a triphenylethylene derivative (MER-25), was tested clinically for contraceptive effectiveness. A group of 30 volunteer subjects were placed on an oral regimen of 250 mg daily for 20 days each month, covering with a high level of certainty at least a 10-day postovulatory period. After the third pregnancy had occurred within three months of the trial, further studies were abandoned.

In subsequent laboratory experiments with a related compound, careful ovum counts revealed that the antifertility activity of these weak estrogenic substances, which are at the same time antiestrogenic, could be ascribed to an accelerated passage of tubal ova.[49] This premature expulsion of the ova from the oviducts has been demonstrated with other estrogens in rats and rabbits[16] and in the guinea pig.[13] The effect has now been reported with a variety of synthetic compounds, both steroidal and nonsteroidal, whose common feature is their estrogenicity. Studies with a number of chemical classes of compounds in laboratory rodents led Chang and Yanagimachi to conclude that "any compound with estrogenic activity may have antifertility activity if taken at a particular time soon after mating."[7] The possibility exists, nevertheless, that the contragestational activity of estrogenic compounds may be independent of their general estrogenicity. Thus several attempts have been made to synthesize analogs of synthetic estrogens in an effort to improve the ratio between antifertility action and estrogenicity.[40, 41] In one such program, a series of 94 phenyl-substitute ethylene derivatives were synthesized. Seven of these proved to be effective contragestational agents in rats at the doses tested, but significant estrogenic activity was associated with all of the active compounds. The general structural types of these compounds are indicated in Table 17.2.

The relationship of these findings in animals and in humans is difficult to define. When in the 1930s Pincus and Kirsch reported that estrogenic hormones inter-

Table 17.2 Di- and triphenylethylene derivatives tested for contragestational effects in rats*

Types of Compounds*	Number of Compounds Tested
1,2-Diphenylalkenes	19
1,1-Diphenylalkenes	2
Triphenylpropenes	10
Phenylbornylenes and phenylnorbornylenes	14
Phenoxyalkyl and phenoxyalkenyl acids	22
Styrylpyran-2-ones	4
Naptho-1',2': 2,3-pyridines	5
α-Alkoxyphenyl Δ^9 fluoreneacetonitriles	4
6-Phenylnicotinonitriles	3
Phenylbenzocycloheptenes	2
Phenylbenzoxepines	2
Cycloalken-1-yl-anisoles	2
Triphenyloxiranes	2
1,1-Diphenylpropylene-glycol-2-chloro-benzoates	2
3,4-Dihydronaph (2,1d)isooxazole	1

*These compounds were synthesized and tested for the Population Council by R. Kwok, B. Chamberlain, and D. Hansen of Cutter Laboratories, Berkeley, Calif.

rupted pregnancy in rabbits,[39] considerable excitement ran through both medical circles and the lay press in anticipation that hormonally induced abortion would be among the human applications of the newly discovered ovarian hormones. Although these expectations did not materialize, no systematic study controlling such factors as dose and time of administration was ever launched to test the possibility. Paradoxically, in the intervening decades estrogens were used to induce ovulation,[25] to prevent threatened abortion,[23] and even to "improve" placentation through increasing placental vacularization.[54]

Meanwhile some physicians and pharmacists believed that the administration of estrogens in the postcoital period was better than nothing in attempting to prevent a pregnancy from becoming established after a single midcycle exposure to an unwanted fertilization. Diethylstilbestrol has frequently been used in this manner, although until recently it had not been FDA-approved for this purpose. The first published report on the possible effectiveness of stilbestrol (or ethinyl estradiol) taken postcoitally was in 1966,[30] a limited report of retrospective data, cautiously interpreted by the authors. By 1973 sufficient data were available to permit Morris and van Wagenen to review a considerable body of experience on the use of estrogens in hu-

mans to prevent the establishment of pregnancy.[31–34] (They have suggested the term *interception* to describe this phenomenon.)

In an accumulation of 9,000 midcycle treatments with a variety of estrogenic substances such as diethylstilbestrol, stilbestrol diphosphate, ethinyl estradiol, and conjugated estrogens, 29 pregnancies have resulted. These agents are given in doses of 25 to 50 mg per day (ethinyl estradiol is given 5 mg per day) for five days after unprotected midcycle intercourse, with treatment beginning within 72 hours after coitus. A Pearl Index of about 4.0 includes method failures and inadequacies of timing and dosage as far as can be determined. Nausea with or without vomiting occurs in about half the women treated, and other side effects include breast soreness, headache, and menstrual irregularity. Three ectopic pregnancies have been observed.

The routine use of estrogens on a postcoital basis is not feasible. First, these substances are not well tolerated in pharmacological doses. Second, random use throughout the cycle, which would be characteristic of a method linked to coital pattern, would create a myriad of cycle disturbances, including ovulation suppression, breakthrough bleeding, and estrogen-induced irregular bleeding. In short, under conditions of home use, postcoital application of a frank estrogen would bring about a state of endocrinological chaos. A third consideration, which is of particular concern in cases of frequent use of large amounts of estrogen,[9] is the question of their carcinogenic potential. Although in this situation the estrogen is taken to avoid rather than protect a pregnancy, the occurrence of vaginal adenocarcinoma in the daughters of women who received stilbestrol during the first trimester of pregnancy necessitates cautious use in women who suspect they are pregnant.[18] For these reasons, the method should probably be utilized only in emergency situations. This cautionary view is reflected in the wording of a recent decision of the FDA that included postcoital administration to prevent pregnancy in the labeling of diethylstilbestrol.

While this action reflects a movement from the category of hearsay and anecdotal reports to much more acceptable evidence of effectiveness, this judgment of efficacy is based only on retrospective analysis of clinical records; now, almost certainly, controlled prospective studies will be carried out.

We do not know the mechanism by which estrogens prevent implantation in humans when taken postcoitally. Several possibilities can be considered, such as acceleration in tubal transport of ova (as in the rat), a direct blastotoxic effect, suppression of luteal function, or an imbalance in the hormonally directed progression of endometrial changes necessary for implantation. The timing of postcoital estrogen administration would suggest that an altered rate of passage of the fertilized human ovum through the tube is not the basis of activity. Since the journey takes only three days, the egg has probably reached the uterus by the time treatment begins.[10] (In keeping with Morris's terminology, this concept of action might be termed the "down-and-out" theory.) At high doses in vitro estrogens are cytotoxic to developing *Arbacia* eggs,[48] but even if this is applicable to mammalian ova, estrogens given postcoitally can probably not reach these concentrations in the tubal fluid or uterine lumen. Studies of hormonal content of this bodily fluid are lacking, even under normal conditions.

When diethylstilbestrol is given to women several days after ovulation, progesterone production is significantly inhibited.[15] The abnormally low levels of progesterone in concert with unphysiological estrogen activity may so modify the endometrium that it is unable to support nidation. This concept is supported by studies utilizing scanning electron microscopy that reveal obvious changes in the surface of the endometrium when the hormonal pattern is disrupted.[35,36]

17.3 Antiprogestational Compounds

In all species studied, a successful intrauterine pregnancy requires sufficient progestational support of the endometrium, both for preparation for nidation and for maintenance of the placenta. Pregnancy in women requires adequate corpus luteum function in the secretory phase of the cycle in which fertilization occurs as well as for approximately the first five weeks of pregnancy. Afterward placental production of progesterone is capable of maintaining pregnancy in the absence of the ovaries.

Several compounds have been studied for their ability to suppress luteal-phase progesterone levels, thus causing endometrial breakdown and menstrual discharge whether or not fertilization has occurred. The administration of various synthetic progestomimetic compounds during the postovulatory phase of the cycle reduces plasma progestrone levels (Figure 17.1). Plasma concentrations of progesterone are significantly depressed by daily oral administration of norgestrel, norethindrone, chlormadinone acetate, and medroxyprogesterone acetate. The inhibition of progesterone synthesis may occur either as a direct effect on the ovary or indirectly through modification of pituitary gonadotropin secretion. The effect is transient, however, and the corpus luteum is capable of responding to the stimulating effect of chorionic gonadotropin (hCG) almost immediately (Figure 17.2). Thus many if not most fertile cycles would be expected to proceed unaffected by a progestin-induced drop in midluteal-

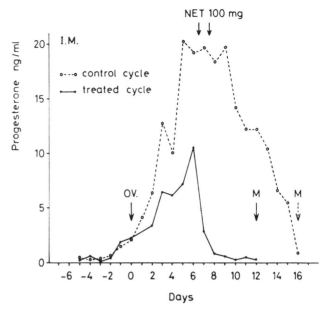

Figure 17.1 Plasma levels of progesterone during the luteal phase of a normal cycle compared to levels during treatment in the same woman with norethindrone (NET) 100 mg daily for two days. Day 0 is the calculated day of ovulation.[20]

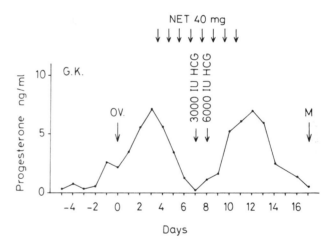

Figure 17.2 Plasma progesterone during the luteal phase of a normal cycle treated with 40 mg norethindrone (NET) daily for eight days. An intramuscular injection of 3000 IU hCG was given on the fourth day of treatment, followed by 6000 IU hCG on the fifth day of treatment. Day 0 is the estimated day of ovulation.[20]

phase plasma progesterone levels. By the time the progestational support of the exogenous progestin recedes, the trophoblast would be producing sufficient hCG to rescue the corpus luteum, preventing a precipitous drop in progesterone and a shedding of the endometrium.

Nevertheless, since timing is a key issue, clinical tests were made of the contragestational effects of progestin-induced reduction in plasma progesterone.[37] Volunteers received a total dose of 200 mg norethindrone between days 19 and 22 of the cycle; 22 pregnancies occurred in 300 treatment cycles. The method appeared to fail either because implantation occurred before treatment or, as in the majority of cases, the corpus luteum responded to hCG from the implanting trophoblast in spite of its previously inhibited condition.

Another approach to reducing progesterone levels during the critical stages of implantation is based on the use of compounds that selectively interfere with a particular enzymatic step in progesterone synthesis. Compounds are known that will prevent the conversion of cholesterol to pregnenolone through their interference with the cytochrome P-450 oxidase system in steroidogenic tissue. Among these are amphenone, glutethimide, metyrapone, and imidazoles.[46] One of the most potent compounds of this series is aminoglutethimide. Experiments in rats demonstrate that the compound will rapidly induce a depression of plasma progesterone, and when administered so that progesterone is continuously depressed, abortion or resorption of fetuses occurs in 72 hours.[14] Clinical experience with aminoglutethimide in women in their second month of pregnancy indicates that as much as 2 g per day for five days will depress progesterone levels about 50 percent, but this will not lead to subsequent abortion. Further experience reveals that progesterone levels must be reduced about 80 to 90 percent for a period of several days for induction of abortion.[45, 46] These findings are encouraging in that they reveal the potential of the method, but they also emphasize the need for an agent that has minimal side effects and is more effective in blocking progesterone synthesis.

In animal studies, progesterone production by the corpus luteum has been suppressed by other agents, such as aminoglutethemide, that would not be acceptable for human use as contragestational drugs because of their pattern of pharmacological activity. A series of amine-oxidase inhibitors with phenylhydrazine structure suppresses progesterone synthesis.[44] In all likelihood, these compounds act by inhibiting the release of luteinizing hormone, which in the rat is required for maintenance of the corpus luteum. Oral administration of compounds in this series terminates pregnancy up to midterm, the time when the pituitary is no longer required for the maintenance of the corpus luteum of pregnancy. The activity may be based on an interference with the step between the neurotransmitter and the synthesis of luteinizing-hormone-releasing factor by the hypothalamus. Little is known of the role of biological amines in pregnancy; exploration of this area could be an especially important pharmacological approach to the study of fertility regulation.

Ergocornine, an antihistamine of the ergot series, has a similar activity. The compound prevents implantation in the rat or mouse when administered during a limited period of tubal transport of fertilized ova.[51] Since progesterone administration reverses the action of the drug, a basic mechanism of the drug action must be to suppress endogenous progestin production. Toxicity was observed at doses required to test effectiveness in humans, however, so further development of this particular compound for contraception is not likely.

The present disappointment notwithstanding, antifertility action through a luteolytic effect of a drug is one of the most intriguing prospects on the research horizon. In theory, an oral preparation active in such a manner could be taken by a woman monthly, at the time of the expected menses, or only on the occasion of a suspected fertile cycle as evidenced by delay in the onset of menstruation.[42]

17.4 Uterine Luteolysin

In some species a humoral luteolytic substance exists that is produced by the uterus and transmitted by tissue diffusion and common blood supply to the ovary.[17] This mechanism does not appear to be operative in controlling the life span of the human corpus luteum. Hysterectomy does not influence the function of the human corpus luteum. Nevertheless, a luteolytic substance recovered from animal uteri would not necessarily be species-specific and could be active in women. The chemistry of uterine luteolysin remains elusive. Studies with uterine flushings from the sow have revealed a high-molecular-weight protein or protein conjugate that has cytolytic effects on granulosa cell cultures that produce mainly progesterone.[52] The uterine material is active if recovered from the late luteal phase but not from the earlier stages in the cycle. The quest for the active cytolytic substance has now turned toward the purification of specific enzymes.[53]

17.5 Immunological and Other Approaches

The key to a possible immunological approach to contragestational activity is the selection of a specific antigen that will not cross-react dangerously with other tissue antigens and that will selectively interfere with a critical event in the reproductive sequence. Through the years, efforts have been made to isolate specific antigens of cervical mucus, uterine or tubal fluid, and ovarian follicular fluid. Although none of these efforts has led to the selection of a specific antigen for purposes of immunization, it would be unwarranted to conclude the infeasibility of the approach. All too often investigators have dropped the topic when difficulties in purification seemed insurmountable, but new methods of protein separation are constantly being developed, and their application in this area of research could eventually prove rewarding.

A specific nonhormonal protein, characteristic of the rabbit uterus in early pregnancy, is uteroglobin (blastokinin),[4] which is said to be completely specific to the pregnant uterus and would therefore appear to be an interesting candidate antigen for active immunization to prevent implantation. Studies of its activity in this context would be of considerable interest.

Other approaches that have been attempted involve the use of hCG, placental lactogen, or other components of the placenta for either active or passive immunization. Animal experiments have demonstrated that injection of antiserum to rhesus monkey placental extracts causes abortion in the species.[3] Similarly, both active and passive immunization of the baboon with human placental lactogen result in abortion during the early months of pregnancy.[55] Given the rapid increase in our knowledge of the structure of hCG,[2] it may prove rewarding to search for specific antibodies to hCG, to one of its subunits, or to a fraction of a subunit that would be able to prevent the continuation of pregnancy at an early time. It is already known that antibodies that inactivate hCG are produced in women actively immunized with a complex antigen consisting of tetanus toxoid linked to the β subunit of hCG or with diazotized hCG.[56,57]

Virtually no research is in progress on chemicals that might be administered safely to women in early pregnancy and that would be selectively toxic to rapidly dividing embryonic cells. Some compounds developed for cancer chemotherapy have been tested in pregnant animals. It is not surprising that oncolytic agents are able to interefere with the growth of embryonic as well as cancer cells. Methotrexate, 6-mercaptopurine, and 6-diazo-5-oxo-L-norleucine (DON) are oncolytic drugs that produce remissions of trophoblastic tumors. This trophoblastolytic action, particularly of methotrexate, suggests the feasibility of using these drugs to terminate normal pregnancies. Although neither the use nor the effectiveness of the drugs has been documented, informal reports and discussions have cited this use of methotrexate as a blastotoxin. Many compounds that act as mitotic poisons, inhibitors of protein synthesis, or antimetabolites will cause resorp-

tion or abortion of implanted embryos in experimental animals.[58] Thiersch's work with 6-thioguanidine suggests that the abortifacient activity can be separated from the general toxic effects these potent cytotoxic agents have on the pregnant female. A serious handicap, however, is the need to achieve a dose that will be completely abortifacient, for insufficient doses could have teratogenic effects without interrupting the pregnancy.[60] All-or-none reactions are difficult to achieve in biological systems, yet nothing short of this would be acceptable in this potential realm of abortion-inducing therapy. Even the availability of surgical abortion, in cases of inadequate response to the drug, would be insufficient security against the hazard of iatrogenic teratogenicity.

17.6 Natural Products

Abortifacient substances distinct from prostaglandin have been found in various plants, yeast extracts, and perhaps marine organisms. Plant products in particular have been studied in this regard, but frequently the abortifacient activity can be ascribed to estrogenicity. This is probably the explanation of the activity of pine needle (*Pinus sylvestris*) extracts and subterranean clover (*Trifolim subterraneum*)[5] in causing fetal resorption in animals. Mexican women are believed to use a brew of a plant called Zoapatle (*Montanoa tuberosa*)[1] to induce abortion. Here again estrogenicity may be involved, but a compound with oxytocic properties may also be present. A yeast product, Malucidin, was reported to induce fetal resorption in dogs, but the activity could not be generalized to other species, and no active constituent was ever isolated in spite of extensive efforts.[27,61]

A substance in bull seminal fluid has been reported that causes fetal resorption in mice.[29] This has been identified as a dimer of ribonuclease.[12]

17.7 Conclusion

What, then, are the prospects for the development of a systemically active, safe, chemical abortifacient, and, indeed, is such a development needed? The low incidence of morbidity with surgical termination of pregnancy, particularly in the first trimester, certainly minimizes a need based solely on the grounds of safety. Surgical abortion, however, involves considerable financial cost to either the community or to the patient, and it requires the time of highly trained surgical personnel and a clinical facility established for surgery and backed up with comprehensive hospital services. It is a procedure that, at best, puts a demanding strain on medical facilities, which in many countries are already stretched near to their limits. Aesthetically, the procedure is not pleasant either for the patient or for the clinic personnel. To the extent that these disadvantages could be overcome by a nonsurgical abortion procedure, the possibilities of developing such a procedure should be encouraged. There is no clear candidate for success on the horizon, although the immunological field could develop most rapidly now that the chemistry of placental hormones is being unraveled, and superantigen techniques of immunization could replace older adjuvant methods.

The case is strong and clear for the development of contragestational agents that would act in the post-fertilization period through the first few days of the first missed period. In a sense, such methodology would be abortion-prevention therapy. While assuring the right of women to have abortions if they choose, is it not the responsibility of medical scientists to provide the advances that will reduce the need for surgical abortions and perhaps even make the procedure obsolete?

References

1. Altschul, S. V. R. *Drugs and foods from little known plants*, p. 318. Cambridge, Mass.: Harvard University Press, 1973.

2. Bahl, O. P. Human chorionic gonadotropin. I. Purification and physiocochemical properties. J. Biol. Chem. 244:567, 1969.

3. Behrman, S. J., and Y. Amano. Monkey antiplacental serum as an abortifacient. Contraception 5:357, 1972.

4. Beier, H. M. Uteroglobin: A hormone-sensitive endometrial protein involved in blastocyst development. Biochim. Biophys. Acta 160:289, 1968.

5. Biely, J., and W. D. Kitts. The antiestrogenic activity of certain legumes and grasses. Can J. Anim. Sci. 44 (3):297, 1964.

6. Brenner, R. M. Biology of oviductal cilia. In *The mammalian oviduct*, eds. E. S. E. Hafez and R. J. Blandau. Chicago: University of Chicago Press, 1969.

7. Chang, M. C., and R. Yanagimachi. Effect of estrogens and other compounds as oral antifertility agents on the development of rabbit ova and hamster embryos. Fertil. Steril. 16:281, 1965.

8. Coutinho, E. M., J. C. De Souza, and A. I. Csapo. Reversible sterility induced by medroxyprogesterone injections. Fertil. Steril. 17:261, 1966.

9. Coutinho, E. M., H. S. Maia, and J. Adeodato-Filko. Responses of the human fallopian tube to adrenergic stimulation. Fertil. Steril. 21:590, 1970.

10. Croxatto, H. B., S. Diaz, B. Fuentealba, H. D. Croxatto, D. Carillo and C. Fabres. Studies on the duration of egg transport in the human oviduct. Fertil. Steril. 23:447, 1972.

11. Csapo, A. I., and W. G. Wiest. An examination of the quantitative relationship between progesterone and the maintenance of pregnancy. Endocrinology 85:735, 1969.

12. D'Alessio, G., A. Parente, C. Guida, and E. Leone. Dimeric structure of seminal ribonuclease. FEBS Letters 27:285, November 1972.

13. Deanesly, R. Further observations of the effects of oestradiol on tubal eggs and implantation in the guinea pig. J. Reprod. Fertil. 5:49, 1963.

14. Glasser, S. R., R. D. Northcutt, F. Chytil, and C. A. Strott. The influence of an anti-steroidogenic drug (aminoglutathimide phosphate) on pregnancy maintenance. Endocrinology 90:1363, 1972.

15. Gore, B. Z., B. V. Caldwell, and L. Speroff. Estrogen-induced human luteolysis. J. Clin. Endocrinol. Metab. 36: 615, 1973.

16. Greenwald, G. S. Interruption of pregnancy in the rabbit by the administration of estrogen. J. Exp. Zool. 135:461, 1957.

17. Hansel, W. Luteotropic and luteolytic mechanisms in bovine corpora lutea. J. Reprod. Fertil. (Suppl.) 1:33, 1966.

18. Herbst, A. L., H. Ulfelder, and D. C. Poskanzer. Adenocarcinoma of the vagina: Association of maternal stilbestrol therapy with tumor appearance in young women. New Engl. J. Med. 284:878, 1971.

19. Hodgen, G. D., M. L. Dufau, and W. W. Tullner. Estrogens, progesterone and chorionic gonadotropin in pregnant rhesus monkeys. Endocrinology 91:896, 1972.

20. Johansson, E. D. B. Depression of the progesterone levels in women treated with synthetic gestagens after ovulation. Acta Endocrinol. (Kbh.) 68:779, 1971.

21. Kamboj, V. P., H. Chandra, B. S. Setty, and A. B. Kar. Biological properties of 2-phenyl-3-p-(beta-pyrrolidinoethoxy)-phenyl-(2:1,b) naphthofuran—A new oral antifertility agent. Contraception 1:29, 1970.

22. Kamboj, V. P., A. B. Kar, S. Ray, P. Grover, and N. Anand. Antifertility activity of 3,4-trans-2, 2-dimethyl-3-phenyl-4-[p-(β-pyrrolidinoethoxy)-phenyl]-7-methoxychroman. Indian J. Exp. Biol. 9:103, 1971.

23. Karnaky, K. J. Estrogenic tolerance in pregnant women. Am. J. Obstet. Gynecol. 53:312, 1947.

24. Kumar, D., and J. J. Russell. Controlled oxytocin infusion as a method of therapeutic abortion in early pregnancy. Bull. Johns Hopkins Hosp. 109:141, 1961.

25. Kupperman, H. S. *Human endocrinology*, p. 249. Philadelphia: A. F. Davis Co., 1963.

26. Kurzrok, B., and C. C. Lieb. Biochemical studies of human semen. Proc. Soc. Exp. Biol. Med. 26:268, 1930.

27. Levi, M. M., J. Manahan, and I. Mandl. Special resorption of the mouse fetus. Obstet. Gynecol. 33:11, 1969.

28. Mastroianni, L., Jr., R. Abdul-Karim, U. Shah, and S. J. Segal. Changes in the secretion rate of the rabbit oviduct following oral administration of 1-(P-2-diethylaminoethoxyphenyl)-1-phenyl-2-p-anisylethanol. Endocrinology 69:396, 1961.

29. Matousek, J., and J. Grozdanovic. Specific effect of bull seminal ribonuclease (as RNAase) on cell systems in mice. Comp. Biochem. Physiol. 46(A):241, 1973.

30. Morris, J. M., and G. van Wagenen. Compounds interfering with ovum implantation and development. III. The role of estrogens. Am. J. Obstet. Gynecol. 96:804, 1966.

31. Morris, J. M., G. van Wagenen, G. D. Hurteau, D. W. Johnston, and R. A. Carlsen. Compounds interfering with ovum implantation and development. I. Alkaloids and antimetabolites. Fertil. Steril. 18:7, 1967.

32. Morris, J. M., G. van Wagenen, T. McCann, and D. Jacob. Compounds interfering with ovum implantation and development. II. Synthetic estrogens and antiestrogens. Fertil. Steril. 18:18, 1967.

33. Morris, J. M., G. van Wagenen, and R. I. Dorfman. The antifertility activity of DL-cis-bisdehydrodisynolic acid methyl ether. Contraception 4:15, 1971.

34. Morris, J. M., and G. van Wagenen. Interception: The use of postovulatory estrogens to prevent implantation. Am. J. Obstet. Gynecol. 115:101, 1973.

35. Nilsson, O., and K. G. Nygren. Scanning electron microscopy of human endometrium. Uppsala J. Med. Sci. 77:3, 1972.

36. Nilsson, O. Personal communication.

37. Nygren, K. G., E. D. B. Johansson, and L. Wide. Postovulatory contraception in women with large doses of norethindrone. Contraception 5:445, 1972.

38. Parkes, A. S., and C. W. Bellerby. Studies on the internal secretions of the ovary. II. The effects of injection of the oestrus-producing hormone during pregnancy. J. Physiol. 62:145, 1926.

39. Pincus, G., and R. E. Kirsch. The sterility in rabbits produced by injections of oestrone and related compounds. Am. J. Physiol. 115:219, 1936.

40. Pincus, G., U. K. Banik, and J. Jacques. Further studies on implantation inhibitors. Steroids 4:657, 1964.

41. Pincus, G. The control of fertility. New York: Academic Press, 1965.

42. Pincus, G. Steroid labile reproductive processes in mammals. Harvey Lect. 62:165, 1968.

43. Pinto, R. M., U. Lerner, and H. Pontelli. In vitro effect of progesterone upon the contractile activity of the three layers of the human pregnant myometrium. Acta Physiol. Lat. Am. 17:333, 1967.

44. Robson, J. M. Br. Med. Abst. 6:489, 1966.

45. Salhanick, H. A. Inhibition of progesterone synthesis. In Endocrinology: Proceedings of the Fourth International Congress of Endocrinology, Washington, D.C. 1972, ed. R. O. Scrow. Amsterdam: Excerpta Medica, 1973.

46. Salhanick, H. A., E. N. McIntosh, V. I. Uzgiris, C. A. Whipple, and F. Mitani. Mitochondrial systems of pregnenolone synthesis and its inhibition. In The regulation of mammalian reproduction, eds. S. J. Segal, R. Crozier, P. A. Corfman, and P. G. Condliffe. Springfield, Ill.: Charles C Thomas, 1973.

47. Segal, S. J., and W. O. Nelson. An orally active compound with antifertility effects in rats. Proc. Soc. Exp. Biol. Med. 98:431, 1958.

48. Segal, S. J., and A. Tyler. Structure-activity-relationships concerning the inhibitory activity of synthetic estrogens and some triphenylethanol derivatives on developing eggs of Arbacia punctulata. Biol. Bull. 15:364, 1958.

49. Segal, S. J., and O. W. Davidson. Prolonged anti-fertility action of clomiphene in delayed implantation. Anat. Rec. 142:278, 1962.

50. Segal, S. J., L. Atkinson, A. Brinson, R. Hertz, W. Hood, A. Kar, L. Southam, and K. Sundaram. Fertility regulation in non-human primates by nonsteroidal compounds. In Proceedings. Symposium on the Use of Non-Human Primates for Research on Problems of Human Reproduction, Sukhumi, USSR. Stockholm: Karolinska sjukhuset, 1972. (Also published as Acta Endocrinol. (Suppl. 116):435, 1972.)

51. Shelesnyak, M. C., and A. Barnea. Studies on the mechanism of ergocornine (ergotoxine) interference with decidualization and nidation. II. Failure of topical application of ergocornine to reveal the site of action of the alkaloid. Acta Endocrinol. 43:469, 1963.

52. Schomberg, W. W., J. A. Campbell, and G. D. Wilbanks. Effects of uterine flushings from pigs on porcine granulosa cells growing in tissue culture. Adv. Biosci. 4:429, 1970.

53. Schomberg, D. W. The regulation of luteal regression. In The regulation of mammalian reproduction, eds. S. J. Segal, R. Crozier, P. A. Corfman, and P. G. Condliffe. Springfield, Ill.: Charles C Thomas, 1973.

54. Smith, O. W., and Smith, G. V. The influence of diethylstilbestrol on the progress and outcome of pregnancy as based on a comparison of treated with untreated primigravidas. Am. J. Obstet. Gynecol. 58:994, 1949.

55. Stevens, V. C., J. E. Powell, and S. J. Sparks. Effects of passive immunizations with antisera against human placental lactogen on gestation in the baboon. (Abstract). Fourth Annual Meeting of the Society for the Study of Reproduction, Boston, June 1971.

56. Stevens, V. C., and C. D. Crystle. Effects of immunization with hapten-coupled hCG on the human menstrual cycle. Obstet. Gynecol. 42:485, 1973.

57. Talwar, G. P., S. K. Dubey, M. Salahuddin, N. C. Sharman, C. Das, S. Kuman, V. Hingorani, and O. P. Bahl. Antiplacental immunological approaches for control of fertility: Development of a potential vaccine for birth control. In Symposium on Development of Contraceptive Technology Through Fundamental Research. New York: Raven Press (in press).

58. Thiersch, J. B. Effects of substituted mercaptopurines on the rat litter in utero. J. Reprod. Fertil. 4:291, 1962.

59. Vande Wiele, R. L., J. Bogumil, I. Dyrenfurth, M. Ferin, R. Jewelewicz, M. Warren, T. Rizkallah, and G. Mikhail. Mechanisms regulating the menstrual cycle in women. Recent Prog. Horm. Res. 26:63, 1970.

60. van Wagenen, G., R. C. Deconti, R. E. Handschumacher, and M. E. Wade. Abortifacient and teratogenic effects of triacetyl-6-azauridine in the monkey. Am. J. Obstet. Gynecol. 108:272, 1970.

61. Whitney, L. F. Malucidin for mismated bitches. Mod. Vet. Pract. 43:76, 1962.

62. Yoshinaga, K., R. A. Hawkins, and J. F. Stocker. Estrogen secretion by the rat ovary in vivo during the estrous cycle and pregnancy. Endocrinology 85:103, 1969.

18 Female Sterilization

Ralph M. Richart and
Katherine F. Darabi

18.1 Introduction

In recent decades a search for the "perfect contraceptive" has led to renewed interest in methods of female sterilization for fertility regulation. Despite increased scientific research and public interest, however, the ideal sterilization procedure has remained elusive, and many of the components of such a technique have seemed to be mutually exclusive. These include:

high rate of effectiveness

low rate of complications and morbidity

short operating time and hospital stay

minimal surgical intervention

ease of teaching and learning

low cost

cosmetic appeal

potential reversibility.

In theory, altering the Fallopian tubes to prevent union of the ovum with the spermatozoa is a simple matter. The tubes can be burned, frozen, irradiated, tied, clipped, excised, plugged, chemically sclerosed, or treated by a combination of some of these. The problem of a delivery system for such methods is somewhat more complex. The tubes can be surgically approached through the abdomen or the vagina, or they can be visualized by either route using fiberoptic endoscopes. Alternatively, a nonsurgical approach can be used to reach the tubes with caustic lavages, or hysteroscopy can be used to guide probes for cautery, cryosurgery, or the placement of plugs and chemicals.

All of these approaches have been advocated and practiced with varying degrees of success. The disagreements over the most effective method and the best means of delivering that method indicate that the ideal procedure has yet to be found. As a consequence, discussions of the relative merits of any procedure frequently digress into arguments over which component of the ideal procedure is most expendable. Should the low materials cost of the traditional abdominal or vaginal tubal ligation be sacrificed for the increased visualization possible with expensive fiber-

optic endoscopes? Should the possibility of reversibility be sacrificed for an increased assurance of contraceptive effectiveness by excision or alteration of large segments of the Fallopian tubes? Is the simplicity of delivery of a toxic lavage that requires repeated instillation preferable to a one-time surgical procedure? Is a more cosmetically appealing procedure preferable to one that requires an abdominal incision, even if it is operationally more difficult?

18.2 Methods of Tubal Closure

Cutting and Tying
One of the long-standing debates involves the relative advantages and disadvantages of different ways of ligating the Fallopian tubes at laparotomy. Recently the same discussion has been extended to ligation procedures at laparoscopy, colpotomy, and culdoscopy. The more extensively the tube is tied, cut, and divided, the lower is the possibility of failure and, concomitantly, the greater is the difficulty of a future reanastamosis procedure. The location of the total injury is also a factor. For example, the Madlener and Pomeroy techniques are more readily reversed than the Kroener procedure.

Technical difficulty is another important consideration, and technical considerations are probably the preeminent factors that have led to the popularity of the Pomeroy technique over the equally successful but technically more complicated Uchida, Aldridge, and Irving methods. Figure 18.1, a chart by Garcia,[10] adapted from Kroener,[15] gives a visual description of several techniques for resection and ligation of the

Reprinted with permission from R. S. Neuwirth, ed., *Hysteroscopy*, Philadelphia: W. B. Saunders, 1975.

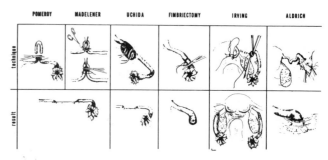

Figure 18.1 Surgical tubal contraceptive procedures.[10]

178   R. M. Richart and K. F. Darabi

Fallopian tubes. Of these, the two that are still significantly employed are the Pomeroy procedure and fimbriectomy.

Electrocoagulation and Cryosurgery

Arguments similar to those outlined for conventional tubal ligation also permeate the literature on electrocautery and cutting the Fallopian tubes. The classic procedure was developed by Palmer and consisted of coagulating and cutting the tubes. Steptoe adopted this technique and carried out the first large-scale clinical trials. In his initial series there was one ectopic pregnancy in approximately 500 patients.[35] Steptoe has continued to use the Palmer technique, and others have modified it. Liston et al.[16] proposed coagulation alone to avoid bleeding, and Semm currently advocates the same procedure. To be effective, this technique requires coagulation of a 1–2 cm length of tube. Failure rates are usually reported to be below 1 percent.

Wheeless adapted the coagulation-alone technique to a single-puncture laparoscopy method using the Palmer-Frangenheim operating laparoscope. He found in his first 1,000 cases that a small cautery burn was associated with failure rates in excess of 1 percent, and he has subsequently advocated a single-puncture technique with coagulation of greater than 1 cm of tube by cauterization of adjacent segments.[40] Other variations include the Siegler technique of using an alligator forceps to coagulate and transect the tube, and the Frangenheim technique of a coagulation-scissor transection of the tube.

All of the electrocautery methods suffer from the risk of bowel burns. This has led to the development of tantalum clips, spring-loaded clips, and Silastic bands to avoid using diathermic cautery. A recent development to meet the same problem is a bipolar electrode to cauterize the tube. This minimizes the risk of bowel burn, and Rioux has reported excellent results in a small series.

Cryosurgery as a method of producing tubal closure has few advocates because of the high cost of the equipment for application transabdominally and the lack of any increased safety. Martens's series showed only 34 percent of the cases had successful closure of the oviducts two months after transcervical cryosurgery.[17] Heat is equally as effective as cold injury and is technically easier and less expensive to deliver.

Experience with the clips and bands is still too limited for failure rates to have been established with certainty. In a comparison of tantalum and spring-loaded clips in animals, Omran and Hulka[22] reported better results for the latter, although both had failures due to clip dislocation. In one study clips were applied

approximately 2 cm from the uterotubal junction in 10 sows, five with tantalum clips and five with spring-loaded clips. Results were compared to five control animals and, over a three month period, pregnancies occurred in three animals with tantalum clips and in three control animals but in none with spring-loaded clips. The tubal lumen remained patent with the rigid clips, but with the spring clips the tubes were completely divided, with necrosis of the musculature and tubal mucosa.[14] Hulka and Omran noted that the design and evaluation of clips requires human trials because of the inadequacy of animal models.[22, 14]

Hulka has now completed a series of 1,000 patients with spring-loaded clips. Some tubes were not closed, and others developed hydrosalpinx early in the series. When two clips were placed close together on the isthmus, rather than one clip on the ampullary tube as before, the early problems appear to have been solved, and good results with no complications have been obtained. Long-term follow-up data are as yet unavailable, however.[13] Hulka no longer claims that the spring-loaded clip is reversible and reports that necrosis occurs when the pressure is adequate for closure.

Gutierrez-Najar has completed a series of 1,112 culdoscopic sterilizations with tantalum hemoclips.[11] Tubal patency was established in nine patients by either Rubin test, hysterosalpingogram, or indigo carmine tests (the author does not specify which tests were used at what intervals, although he mentions that most of the failures occurred early in the series). In addition, three pregnancies occurred, which Gutierrez-Najar attributes to the use of a newly designed forceps. In one case pregnancy resulted from an opening of only 0.25 mm. In 22 cases the clips were removed with no subsequent pregnancies. Gutierrez-Najar advocates the application of two clips spaced 1 mm apart to avoid hydrosalpinx.

Much of the debate on clips centers around the possibility of producing occlusion without necrosis. While many investigators are skeptical about this, Davis claims to have developed a "culdo clip," which, at a specified gap, occludes the tubes without producing necrosis in rabbits.[7] Human trials have not yet been undertaken, however. Hopefully the newly designed clips will not increase the incidence of tubal pregnancies, such as the case reported by Neuwirth et al. with tantalum clips placed at culdoscopy.[20]

Bae Yoon has reported the use of Silastic rubber bands as an alternative to clips.[41] In 147 cases with follow-ups of six months to one year, no pregnancies were reported, and, using hysterosalpingograms in 17 patients, bilateral tubal occlusion occurred at three months in all cases.

If the clips and rubber bands are as effective over

the long term as the short-term experience indicates, they should significantly decrease the incidence of bowel burns associated with cautery, and an increase in their utilization would be anticipated.

Chemical Sclerosing Agents

The use of toxic chemical compounds to occlude the Fallopian tubes is an experimental method that has generated considerable interest in the past few years. The appeal of this approach lies in the possibility of closing the tubes by a simple, nonsurgical, transcervical application of substances that might be effectively applied by paramedical personnel in an outpatient setting. Numerous effective cytotoxic compounds have been identified, but development of an adequate delivery system has been difficult.

In 1941 Salgado published an article describing the effects of repeated injections of tincture of iodine and carbolic acid into the uterine cavities of women.[31] The lavage was administered by local midwives as a temporary method of contraception, but Salgado noted that the instillation resulted in permanent sterilization due to severe scarring of the endometrium and Fallopian tubes. Brazilian midwives stopped using caustic intrauterine injections after Salgado's paper was published.[30]

Recently many compounds have been tested for their tubal-occluding properties, principally in animals. These include:

silver nitrate

zinc chloride

formalin—ethanol

alcohol

copper sulfate pentahydrate

talc suspensions

sodium lauryl sulfate

cadmium

iodoacetate

thio—TEPA

granuloma-producing agents

podophyllin

colchicine

quinacrine

cyanoacrylates.

A number of compounds have been created that utilize inert carriers to bring chemicals into prolonged contact with the tubes. These include agar, carboxymethylcellulose, and polymers such as alginate, gelatin, and tissue adhesives. The chemical agents that have been most commonly used in the compounding include silver nitrate, formalin, paraformaldehyde, quinacrine, and zinc chloride, but others may be equally effective. These studies resulted in the recognition that most of the toxic compounds produce closure only after prolonged exposure.

Zipper et al. have reported a number of animal studies of various chemical agents. In 1969 they published a paper describing a single transcervical instillation of various chemicals into the uterine cavities of rats after exposure of the uterine horns by abdominal incisions.[42] In general, the series showed that single injections of various cytotoxic agents alter the endometrial mucosa and inhibit implantation.[43]

In 1970 Omran and Hulka reported on the treatment of the uterotubal junctions of 12 rabbits and 7 pigs with silver nitrate applicators introduced through a hollow plastic sheath at laparotomy and applied for two minutes.[22] They found that the chemical produced a 3–10 mm × 5 mm lesion, with epithelial destruction also involving the surrounding myometrium. Despite this extensive damage, regeneration of the epithelium was observed after three weeks. All the pigs were subsequently mated, and one conceived.

Neuwirth et al. tested the application of varying concentrations of silver nitrate, zinc chloride, and methyl cyanoacrylate in eight monkeys at laparotomy.[21] At three weeks the treated Fallopian tubes were examined microscopically, and uniform damage was seen. At five weeks active fibroblasts were observed in the tubal lumen, and the tubes treated with silver nitrate were closed. By seven weeks all tubes were closed.

Other compounds that might be used to produce tubal blockage are cyanoacrylate tissue adhesives, which have been used for years in industry and for bone surgery. The tissue adhesives most commonly studied for tubal occlusion are gelatin resorcinol formalin (GRF) and the cyanoacrylates. Corfman et al.,[4] Omran and Hulka,[22] and Richart et al.[26] studied the effects of methyl and isobutyl cyanoacrylates in rabbits, monkeys, and pigs with varying results. The studies indicated the potential effectiveness of 2-methyl cyanoacrylate in producing tubal occlusion.

Davis et al. found that after uterotubal injections of aqueous 6 percent GRF, mice were more fertile than sham-operated controls that received aqueous injections.[8] The authors concluded that much higher doses of GRF would be required to produce occlusion.

These animal experiments led to the generalization that many toxic chemicals will produce necrosis, but occlusion will occur only after relatively prolonged contact, which leads to chronic injury and fibrosis. There is striking variation, however, in the usefulness of various animal models, and human trials may not parallel the animal experience.

Quinacrine A number of formulations have reached the clinical testing stage. These include quinacrine, silver nitrate in hydrophilic cream, and methyl cyanoacrylate. The agent most widely tested in humans is quinacrine in suspension. Zipper et al. tested two different concentrations of quinacrine introduced transcervically to the uterine fundus in two groups of patients by means of a biopsy cannula with an attached 10 ml syringe. The cannula was withdrawn one to two minutes after completion of the injection.[44] In Group A, 85 patients received a 2 ml suspension of 250 mg quinacrine a maximum of three times. In Group B, 37 patients received a maximum of two instillations of a 4 ml suspension containing 1 gm quinacrine. Occlusion was determined by tubal insufflation after each instillation of quinacrine. The results in 68 patients from Group A and all of the patients in Group B are shown in Table 18.1.

Zipper describes one complication in 250 instillations and no evidence of peritoneal irritation in any patient. Four patients whose tubes were patent after only one instillation became pregnant during the period of observation, an average of 7.3 months of exposure per woman.

Davidson and Wilkins studied changes in the Fallopian tubes of 10 women who had received a single injection of a 6 ml suspension containing 1 gm quinacrine transcervically into the uterine cavity via a flexible polyethylene cannula.[6] In patients with a large cervical os, a rubber stopper was used to prevent reflux of the quinacrine suspension, although some reflux into the vagina was seen in most cases after removal of the cannula. Pathological studies only were done in four women, two underwent clinical and pathological examination, and the rest were followed clinically from three weeks to seven months. Occlusion was demonstrated by Rubin tests except in patients who subsequently underwent vaginal hysterectomy and had histological examination of the tubes. The six patients followed clinically were found to have tubal occlusion when examined at least three weeks after the installa-

tion. Of the four patients who underwent hysterectomy within one week of instillation, one had bilateral epithelial necrosis in the intramural portion of the tubes, two had unilateral changes, and one had no change. The authors believe that they obtained higher intrauterine injection pressures than did Zipper and thus forced the quinacrine suspension through the tubal ostia. Since five patients were using an oral contraceptive during the entire course of the study, it may have exerted a potentiating effect.

Alvarado et al. studied the instillation of quinacrine at hysteroscopy in 30 women using 50 mg quinacrine in 0.25 cc saline introduced 5 mm into the intramural portion of the tubes by means of a catheter.[1] Occlusion was determined by hysterosalpingograms at three months in 16 patients as follows: (1) Bilateral occlusion occurred in six cases (37.5 percent); (2) unilateral occlusion occurred in six cases (37.5 percent); and (3) bilateral patency occurred in four cases (25 percent).

Quinones indicated early in 1974 that he had already performed 55 quinacrine instillations.[24] In the first group of 40 patients receiving 200 mg quinacrine per cc saline, only two patients (5 percent) had bilateral occlusion after one year. After 6 months, 13 had unilateral occlusion (32.5 percent), and 25 had bilateral patency (62.5 percent).

Richart et al. have had similarly poor results using a suspension of 800 mg quinacrine in 6 cc water. The suspension was administered using a Kahn cannula with a cervical olive in 64 patients. The injection was performed over a 30-second period and held in place for one minute. Hysterosalpingograms at three months showed bilateral closure rates of less than 50 percent.

Despite the simplicity of quinacrine lavage, the low rates of tubal occlusion that have been achieved even after repeated instillations suggest that the method in its present form is not clinically useful (see note, p. 187).

Silver nitrate Silver nitrate is another compound that has reached the clinical testing stage. Richart et al. introduced 0.2 ml of 10 percent silver nitrate in hydrophilic ointment into the isthmic and interstitial portions of the tube in 12 women via a polyethylene catheter, which was passed retrograde to the isthmus under culdoscopic control.[27] On hysterosalpingography at 8 to 12 weeks, bilateral cornual occlusion was observed in all patients.

Ringrose reported the results of a study using 10 percent and 15 percent silver nitrate paste delivered to the cornua through a cannula with a bulbous tip.[29] In his study, 106 women received the 10 percent concentration, and 54 received the 15 percent paste; the cases were tested for patency by hysterosalpingograms at three months with the results shown in Table 18.2.

Ringrose reported 4 percent amenorrhea and a gen-

Table 18.1 Occlusion after instillation of quinacrine

	Tubal Obstruction	
	Number	Percent
Group A		
After first instillation	24	35.2
Cumulative after 3 instillations	60	88.2
Group B		
After first instillation	24	64.8
Cumulative after 2 instillations	29	84.3

Table 18.2 Results of treatment with silver nitrate paste

	10% paste (106 women)	15% paste (54 women)
Bilateral occlusion	50%	70%
Unilateral occlusion	25%	24%
Bilateral patency	25%	6%

eral reduction in the amount of menstrual flow, as well as uterine cramps and spotting, but no major complications.[29] He also cites a subsequent study of a 20 percent silver nitrate paste in which 2 of 60 cases required hospitalization for peritoneal irritation. Although they are not reported in his paper, it is our understanding that a significant number of pregnancies occurred and that the complication rate may be higher than reported. Ringrose has subsequently added talc to his formula. This is an unacceptable additive because of its known effects in producing peritoneal granulomas.

Sodium morrhuate In 1966 Pitkin published a review of the hospital records of 371 patients sterilized during a 10-year period by injection of 5 percent sodium morrhuate in a ligature-isolated segment of Fallopian tube.[23] From follow-up questionnaires completed by 205 women, Pitkin found that 7.3 percent had conceived subsequent to the operation. Of 17 pregnancies in this group, seven carried full term, three resulted in early spontaneous abortions, one developed a tubal pregnancy, three had therapeutic abortions, and two were pregnant at the time of publication.

Tissue Adhesives

To date there have been few clinical experiences reported with tissue adhesives for sterilization, although interest in this method is increasing. Stevenson and Taylor observed the histological effects of methyl 2-cyanoacrylate in 12 patients who had a hysterectomy subsequent to MCA administration.[37] The MCA was injected through a polyethylene tube passed via a Foley catheter with a 5 ml balloon in the uterus. The tissue adhesive was administered 1 day, 2 days, and 1 (two patients), 2, 4, 6, 8, 10, 12, and 16 (two patients) weeks prior to hysterectomy. They found localized histotoxic effects confined to superficial layers of cells of the endometrium and Fallopian tube in the early cases and obliteration of the tube lumen after 12 weeks. The MCA was not identifiable histologically after 12 weeks and had presumably been eliminated from the genital tract.

Stevenson treated approximately 75 women, 50 percent of whom had both tubes blocked after a single application and 100 percent of whom showed tubal occlusion after two applications.[36]

Silastic Rubber

The direct delivery of rapidly polymerizing inert silicone rubber placed at the uterotubal junction has been advocated for sterilization. This procedure has the advantage of minimizing peritoneal irritation and decreasing any localized toxic effect, but it obviously requires a sophisticated delivery system.

In 1967 Hefnawi et al. studied the effects of silicone rubber plugs in rabbit uterine horns.[12] In their study 0.2–0.5 ml of Silastic and Elasticon rubber was injected in 64 rabbits. The rate of conception in the control horns was 79.4 percent, compared to 33.7 percent in horns with Silastic plugs occluding the oviduct and 19.6 percent in horns with Elasticon plugs. A number of intraperitoneal expulsions of the plugs were observed. The expulsions and lateral displacement rates of the Silastic plugs were higher than those recorded for Elasticon. After the removal of 12 intratubal plugs, the ovulation-implantation ratio reverted to 0.72, compared to a control ratio of 0.78.

Erb et al. felt that Hefnawi et al. had used a highly diluted, low-viscosity silicone system, which may have contributed to their high failure rate. Erb used 80 parts Dow Corning Silastic 382 Medical Elastomer and 20 parts 360 Medical Fluid with a 1 percent stannous octoate curing agent.[9] The material was introduced into the cornual region of the tubes of 20 rabbits at hysterotomy. An automatic dispenser controlled the rate of injection of the material through a catheter to a cannula with an obturator tip, which remains in the uterus after delivery of the plug. After 53 to 56 days, 38 of 40 plugs (95 percent) were in place. Pregnancy occurred subsequently in only one of the 38 occluded horns (5.3 percent of the animals), compared to a 73.7 percent pregnancy rate for sham-operated controls. The authors believe that the silicone plugs have the potential for reversibility, although this has not yet been demonstrated.

Rakshit carried out human trials of Dow Corning liquid silicone plastic mixed with 15 percent barium sulphate.[25] Silastic 521, 68-110, and 5392 were instilled in 47 cases, 37 transcervically and 10 at laparotomy. Some of the women underwent salpingectomy; the remainder were examined radiologically at unstated intervals to localize the radio-opaque silicone. Results are shown in Table 18.3.

Intratubal Devices and Plugs

It has been suggested that microporous plugs that adhere to the tubal epithelium might produce higher rates of occlusion than inert Silastics; however, the transcervical insertion of solid intratubal devices requires direct placement under visual control.

Table 18.3 Results of attempted sterilization with silicone and barium sulfate

Material	Installation Route	Satisfactory Block	Doubtful Block	Failure
S.521 and 68-110 (30 cases)	vaginal	21	6	3
S.5392 (7 cases)	vaginal	0	4	3
S.521 and 68-110 (10 cases)	abdominal (with ligation)	(no rejections up to 18 months; one pregnancy)		

Omran and Hulka evaluated Dacron felt intratubal devices in pigs, and reported a high incidence of infection and adhesions involving the uteri, tubes, and ovaries.[22] In a personal communication Meeker described his experiences with teflon plugs designed to be inserted through the fimbriated end of the tubes and secured by suture material at colpotomy.[18] Initial studies in baboons and rabbits give some indications of tubal blockage with minimal scar tissue formation and the possibility of patency after removal of the plugs. In current tests of plastic and metal alloy devices in monkeys and rabbits, however, Richart and Neuwirth's initial data indicate that permanent bonds do not form between the tissue and the plugs.[28] The occluding activity of the devices appears to be merely mechanical, in which case they would not be expected to be effective.

Hot Water

One of the more unusual methods currently under study is Moulding's work with steam and hot water as tubal occluding agents.[19] On the basis of his work with rabbits and human extirpated uteri, Moulding believes that steam, introduced at a low pressure by a catheter at hysteroscopy or using Thompson's balloon cannula, could destroy a longer portion of the oviduct than is possible with electrocauterization with a hysteroscope. These studies are preliminary, and no clinical trials are planned for the near future.

Hysterectomy

Methods that involve removal or incapacitation of the ovaries or uterus have not yet been mentioned. In this category oophorectomy and irradiation of the ovaries are of historical interest, although they are rarely advocated today. Elective vaginal and abdominal hysterectomy for sterilization are still endorsed by some on the grounds that, without a reproductive function, the uterus is a useless organ.[3] Opponents argue that elective hysterectomy involves unnecessary surgery and exposes the patient to a greater risk than does an abdominal tubal ligation procedure.

18.3 Delivery Systems

The choice of approach and delivery system for sterilization techniques depends upon many factors. The availability of financial support, skilled surgeons, anesthetists, operating rooms, electrical power, and repair facilities all play a role in determining which method will be employed. Training programs have also been an important factor, and their availability for teaching a particular approach often determines the method used in a particular hospital or country.

Patient motivation for sterilization is greatest immediately after delivery, a time at which the laparoscopic and hysteroscopic approaches are usually not employed because of technical problems. Hence the more traditional abdominal and vaginal tubal ligations are the most commonly practiced procedures and are usually performed within 48 hours postpartum, most often by the Pomeroy method. The demand for immediate postpartum sterilization has increased greatly over the past few years because of the obvious economic and motivational advantages of treating the puerperal woman, and emphasis has been placed on postpartum programs by international funding agencies. The Population Council has sponsored major postpartum family planning programs in Thailand, Venezuela, Colombia, and Indonesia, in which sterilization was an important component. In Table 18.4 postpartum program statistics from the Population Council show the numbers of total acceptors and percentage sterilized without regard to method since 1966.[33] Although the Population Council's postpartum program has been phased out, postpartum sterilization is an increasingly important component of family planning programs in many developing countries.

Postabortal patients are obviously equally good candidates for sterilization. The Joint Program for the Study of Abortion studied 72,988 legal abortion patients in the United States in 1970 and 1971 and found that 3.8 percent chose sterilization. Omran and Hulka have estimated that when sterilization is offered to women over age 30 with three or more children as part of postpartum care, 30 to 50 percent elect sterilization.[22] This number seems to be higher in countries other than the United States where data are available. All of the standard sterilization approaches have been combined with abortion, including hysterectomy, which has the highest associated morbidity rates.

As more experience has been gained with tubal ligation techniques, modifications have been made to simplify the operation and decrease the operating time. In

Table 18.4 Sterilizations in family planning programs

	1966	1967	1968	1969	1970	1971	1972
Total Acceptors	71,800	123,000	109,000	131,000	170,000	232,000	227,000
Percentage Sterilized	9.8%	9.3%	11.1%	9.2%	8.6%	8.8%	10.3%

Thailand, India, and Puerto Rico, for example, a mini-laparotomy approach has been used successfully, involving a small suprapubic incision and Pomeroy tubal ligation. The entire procedure can be done on an outpatient basis in 10 to 15 minutes, although general anesthesia is usually employed. The low morbidity and simplicity of the minilaparotomy make it competitive with newer, more experimental approaches.

Approaches that require only local anesthesia are advocated by many persons. Rapid, small-incision colpotomy techniques have been developed that have great cosmetic appeal and avoid the psychological trauma of abdominal surgery. The vaginal approach leaves less operative leeway, however, and usually requires greater technical skill on the part of the surgeon.

With the development of cold light sources and better distending media, endoscopic techniques previously used only for diagnostic purposes have been adapted for sterilization. Culdoscopy and laparoscopy have been used extensively in the past several years with good results. Cited advantages are increased visualization (and therefore less chance of error) and controlled bleeding. Disadvantages include the high cost of endoscopic equipment and the need for personnel with sophisticated training, good electrical power sources, and accessible repair centers.

In order to overcome the problems of training and cost involved in laparoscopy, the Agency for International Development sponsors an International Training Project at Johns Hopkins University, in which a team of two doctors and a nurse is sent to developing countries to deliver laparoscopic equipment and train local medical personnel in gynecological techniques. Thus far the project has reached about 39 clinics in 24 countries and has directly trained 110 physicians from countries other than the United States. Clifford Wheeless, the former director of the program, estimates a multiplier effect of approximately 2:1 in the training program, with the result that close to 250 doctors have been trained in laparoscopy.[39] Wheeless is also in the process of developing a "sterilization kit," to be sold for about $350, thereby radically reducing equipment costs.

The Association for Voluntary Sterilization has a similar training program, although emphasis is placed on the less complicated techniques, such as the modified suprapubic minilaparotomy used in Thailand. AVS-sponsored programs in laparoscopy and other methods have been carried out in Thailand, Colombia, and the Philippines.

Another attempt to make laparoscopy more adaptable to local conditions has been the development of the one-incision technique. Wheeless feels that the elimination of a second incision reduces operating time as well as the possibility of skin burns and visceral perforations, and it is easier to learn and teach.[40] The advantages of the one-incision technique are that it saves some operating time, is more cosmetically appealing, and avoids the bleeding risk of a second puncture. Disadvantages include less visual control due to the decreased optical field size and the need for smaller surgical instruments that require more manipulation to accomplish the procedure.

There is some debate over the use of laparoscopy for the puerperal patient. Although Steptoe and others feel that the procedure is contraindicated during the puerperium, Keith compared 167 puerperal and 70 nonpuerperal procedures and concluded that either period was acceptable.

The relative advantages and disadvantages of culdoscopy vis-à-vis colpotomy are similar to those of laparoscopy. Culdoscopy is sometimes cited as preferable to laparoscopy, since there is no abdominal incision and the instrumentation is somewhat simpler,[2] but, like laparoscopy, culdoscopic equipment is often prohibitively expensive and many gynecologists opt for direct location of the tubes at colpotomy. Advocates of culdoscopy mention the advantages of using only local anesthesia and the better visualization over an open vaginal approach. The complication rates of vaginal methods tend, however, to be higher than those of abdominal methods.

Hysteroscopy
Hysteroscopy is the most recent endoscopic technique to be used for sterilization procedures. There are obvious advantages to a nonsurgical approach, of which the foremost is the possibility of outpatient sterilization procedures; however, difficulties in occluding the interstitial portion of the Fallopian tubes have resulted in high failure rates for hysteroscopic sterilization. More serious than the failures, however, are recently reported complications associated with electrocoagulation at hysteroscopy. An estimated 500 cases of hysteroscopic sterilization reported to us included three cornual pregnancies and two small bowel perforations without evidence of uterine perforation, one of which resulted in

death from peritonitis and vascular collapse. In addition, a significant number of pregnancies have been reported in patients who had previously been thought to have tubal blockage. These reports are particularly disturbing when one realizes that increasing numbers of hysteroscopes are being marketed for sterilization as well as diagnostic use. Early Japanese publications suggesting considerable morbidity associated with hysteroscopic sterilization may be borne out by subsequent follow-up.

If hysteroscopy is to become an acceptable means of transcervical sterilization, there is an urgent need to develop superior occluding agents. The tissue adhesives such as GRF and MCA may be preferable to heat if the hysteroscopic delivery system can be improved. Semm believes that the dangers of high-frequency current can be avoided by his resistance-heating coagulation forceps or thermoprobes; however, in 42 cases Semm reports a 40 percent failure rate.[32]

Other Transcervical Approaches

Stevenson has reported the development of a microfocus miniature X-ray tube, which could provide an alternative to hysteroscopy.[36] His technique involves insertion of a disc applicator through the cervix with a cannula to conduct "hot" energy to produce a lesion at the uterotubal junction. Stevenson cites among the advantages of this method the possibility of using two X-ray tubes for a three-dimensional fused image, with a cheaper and faster technique than hysteroscopy. The potential of this approach is highly speculative, and no trials have been carried out.

With regard to the delivery of toxic agents, the problem revolves around the peritoneal cavity. Some agents, such as quinacrine, can be delivered using relatively simple systems, such as Zipper's cannula, because minimal peritoneal spill does not produce significant clinical side effects. The tube-occluding properties are not good, however, and even with three applications, there is a significant incidence of tubal patency. A chemical that is minimally epitheliotoxic in the peritoneum might be expected to exhibit similar properties in the tube, since the two epithelia are similar.

When a highly effective epitheliotoxic agent, such as silver nitrate, is used, peritoneal spillage must be avoided because the side effects are clinically unacceptable. In this case the system must be able to deliver the occluding agent to a 2–3 cm segment of interstitial and isthmic tube, while at the same time eliminating the potential for spilling the agent through the fimbria into the peritoneal cavity. Ideally, the whole procedure should be designed to be used by paramedical personnel and administered blindly on an outpatient basis.

Several balloon devices have been designed to meet these requirements for the delivery of relatively potent agents, in an attempt to achieve greater precision than is possible with simple catheters or cannulas. Corfman and Taylor devised a syringe mounted on a curved cannula to be placed at the uterine angle and guided to the cornua by a small balloon.[5] Thompson et al. produced an instrument for contrast-pressure delivery of sclerosing agents consisting of a small CO_2-filled balloon over a curved cannula to isolate the uterine cavity from the tubal ostia.[38] The occluding agent is forced into the tubal lumen through the cannula at a lesser pressure. The Thompson balloon has also been modified by the addition of a syringe device such as the Corfman and Taylor instrument described above. Stevenson used the same principle when he modified a Foley catheter by inserting a polyethylene tube through which he injected tissue adhesive.[37] In addition, Batelle Laboratories has developed a cannula with extendable arms designed to form a triangle that will assist in localizing the cornua and in placing the cannula tip at the tubal ostia.

Of all these designs, only the Stevenson balloon cannula has been successfully used in clinical trials, and his success may at least in part be ascribed to the polymerizing properties of MCA; however, his system produced occlusion in only 50 percent of the cases on one application and required two instillations for 100 percent success.

Reversibility

Despite much conjecture about the potential reversibility of some of the newer sterilization techniques, no procedures have yet been clinically proven to be consistently reversible. Reanastamosis procedures after tubal ligation have been notoriously unsuccessful when measured by number of live births. It remains to be seen whether it is possible to produce occlusion without necrosis with metal or polymer clips and plugs.

18.4 Prognosis: Research and Funding Needs

Great progress has been made in the dissemination of male sterilization procedures. The ease with which vasectomy techniques can be applied to large populations has been adequately demonstrated in a variety of countries and particularly in the vasectomy fairs held in India. Despite the desperate need for similar procedures for women, female sterilization has not been applied on a mass basis, largely because of the lack of a technique as simple as vasectomy.

In a sense our knowledge of human female sterilization has progressed little in the past 20 years. While cost-effectiveness studies and field tests are necessary for an objective assessment, a subjective appraisal indicates that the classical method of abdominal tubal ligation (albeit with the new modifications for miniprocedures) currently outweighs other approaches when compared for cost-effectiveness, including the necessary acquisition of technical skill and equipment, ease of teaching, and number of operations that can be done over the long term.

Despite the increased application of minilaparotomy and laparoscopic techniques, however, any procedure that invades the abdominal cavity requires a highly skilled surgeon and back-up anesthesiology. In addition, there are major complications from both simplified approaches, as shown by the bowel and vascular injuries reported on many occasions. Culdoscopy and colpotomy seem to be rapid procedures with cosmetic advantages, but the vaginal approach for sterilization has not been widely applied because most surgeons are more familiar with the abdominal approach to the uterus; both colpotomy and culdoscopic techniques require more specialized surgical skill.

Transcervical sterilization seems to hold the greatest promise for the future. Since transcervical techniques do not involve invasion of the peritoneal cavity, they eliminate the need for highly skilled surgeons and could be carried out by paramedical personnel in outpatient programs. The transcervical placement of intratubal plugs has been investigated as a potentially reversible procedure, but initial results do not seem promising. Even if the intratubal devices can be proved reversible in animals, it is difficult to conceive of a protocol for clinical testing because of the difficulties of locating large numbers of candidates for untested temporary sterilization procedures. The application of sclerosing agents seems more promising, although results of experiments using chemicals for transcervical tubal occlusion are as yet too tentative for widespread clinical use. Several agents have been identified that can effectively occlude the Fallopian tube. More research is needed on the development of an adequate delivery system as well as on the evaluation of the drugs for toxicity and safety.

Hysteroscopic visualization may be a means of providing precise delivery of caustic chemicals to the Fallopian tubes. The tubal ostia can be visualized with a hysteroscope, and a number of investigators have demonstrated that it is possible to deliver chemical injury to the cornual and interstitial portions of the tubes. Until modifications are introduced that preclude the complications and high failure rates developed in the early cautery series, however, hysteroscopy will not be widely applied. There is also a need for less expensive power supplies and light sources, to reduce the equipment costs. If these problems can be overcome, hysteroscopic sterilization seems to offer potential as a sterilization method.

The gaps in our knowledge of female sterilization techniques point to an urgent need for additional research. In the proceedings of the Battelle workshop in 1972, Speidel mentions that a perusal of the *Inventory of Federal Population Research* for that year revealed only two projects under the heading "Sterilization."[34] The FY 1973 *Inventory* presents only a slightly brighter picture. While the total number of projects listed in this category increased, the majority were vasectomy-related research awards.

The "ideal" procedure for female sterilization may never be identified, but simple procedures for large-scale outpatient programs can certainly be achieved within this decade if there is increased support for the development and refinement of existing technology. Most important is the creation of interdisciplinary teams—including sociologists, psychologists, chemists, and mechanical engineers—to study all aspects of sterilization and identify the most feasible combination of drug and delivery systems to ensure the mass fertility control that will be required if we are to deal effectively with current population growth rates.

References

1. Alvarado, A., R. Quinones, and R. Aznar. Tubal instillation of quinacrine under hysteroscopic control. In *Hysteroscopic sterilization*, ed. J. J. Sciarra. New York: Symposia Specialists, 1974.

2. Bank, A. H. Culdoscopic tubal sterilization. Fertil. Steril. 24(2):155, 1973.

3. Cali, R. W. Operations for sterilization of the female. Surg. Clin. N. Am. 53(2):495, 1973.

4. Corfman, P. A., R. M. Richart, and H. C. Taylor. Response of the rabbit oviduct to a tissue adhesive. Science 148(3675):1348, 1965.

5. Corfman, P. A., and H. C. Taylor. An instrument for transcervical treatment of the oviducts and uterine cornua. Obstet. Gynecol. 27:800, 1966.

6. Davidson, O. W., and C. Wilkins. Chemically induced tubal occlusion in the human female following a single instillation of quinacrine. Contraception 7(4):333, 1973.

7. Davis, H. C. Personal communication, May 3, 1974.

8. Davis, R. H., J. McDonald, G. Kyriazes, and H. Balin. Effect on fertility of intrauterotubal injection of gelatin. Obstet. Gynecol. 42(3):446, 1973.

9. Erb, R. A., R. H. Davis, G. Kyriazes, and H. Balin. Device and technique for blocking the Fallopian tubes. Contemp. Obstet. Gynecol.:92, February 1974.

10. Garcia, C. R. Oviduct anastomosis procedures. In *Human sterilization*, eds. R. M. Richart and D. J. Prager. Springfield, Ill.: Charles C Thomas, 1972.

11. Gutierrez-Najar, A. J. Culdoscopy as an aid to family planning. In *Female sterilization: Prognosis for simplified outpatient procedures*, eds. D. W. Duncan et al. New York: Academic Press, 1972.

12. Hefnawi, F., A-R. Fuchs, and K. A. Laurence. Control of fertility by temporary occlusion of the oviduct. Am J. Obstet. Gynecol. 99(3):421, 1967.

13. Hulka, J. F. Personal communication, April 23, 1974.

14. Hulka, J. F., and K. F. Omran. Comparative tubal occlusion rigid and spring-loaded clips. Fertil. Steril. 23(9):633, 1972.

15. Kroener, W. F., Jr. Surgical sterilization by fimbriectomy. Am. J. Obstet. Gynecol. 104:247, 1969.

16. Liston, W. A., W. Bradford, J. Downie, and M. G. Kerr. Female sterilisation by tubal electrocoagulation under laparoscopic control. Lancet:382, February 1970.

17. Martens, F. W. Attempted cryosurgical closure of the Fallopian tubes. In *Human sterilization*, eds. R. M. Richart and D. J. Prager. Springfield, Ill.: Charles C Thomas, 1972.

18. Meeker, C. Personal communication, May 17, 1974.

19. Moulding, T. S. Personal communication, April 25, 1974.

20. Neuwirth, R. S., S. Casthely, and Y.-H. Kim. Tubal pregnancy following application of tantalum clips at culdoscopy for sterilization. Am J. Obstet. Gynecol. 114(8):1066, 1972.

21. Neuwirth, R. S., R. M. Richart, and H. C. Taylor. Chemical induction of tubal blockade in the monkey. Obstet. Gynecol. 38(1):51, 1971.

22. Omran, K. F., and J. F. Hulka. Tubal occlusion: A comparative study. Int. J. Fertil. 15(4):226, 1970.

23. Pitkin, R. M. Sodium morrhuate for tubal sterilization. Obstet. Gynecol. 28(5):680, 1966.

24. Quinones, R. Personal communication, April 27, 1974.

25. Rakshit, B. Attempts at chemical blocking of the Fallopian tube for female sterilisation. J. Obstet. Gynecol. India 20:618, 1970.

26. Richart, R. M., R. S. Neuwirth, and H. C. Taylor. Experimental studies of fallopian tube occlusion. In *Human sterilization*, eds. R. M. Richart and D. J. Prager. Springfield, Ill.: Charles C Thomas, 1972.

27. Richart, R. M., A. J. Gutierrez, and R. S. Neuwirth. Transvaginal human sterilization: A preliminary report. Am. J. Obstet. Gynecol. 111:108, 1971.

28. Richart, R. M., and R. Neuwrith. *Current studies of Abcor and Battelle intratubal devices*. Sponsored by the World Health Organization.

29. Ringrose, C. A. Office tubal sterilization. Obstet. Gynecol. 42(1):151, 1973.

30. Salgado, C. Personal communication, May 17, 1974.

31. Salgado, C. Sterilisation induced by intra-uterine caustic injections. An. Brasil Genet.:503, June 1941.

32. Semm, K. Sterilisierung durch Thermokoagulation der Pars intramuralis tubae per hysteroscopiam. Endoscopy 5:218, 1973.

33. Sivin, I. Personal communication, April 1974.

34. Speidel, J. J. The role of human sterilization in family planning. In *Female sterilization: Prognosis for simplified outpatient procedures*, eds. D. W. Duncan et al. New York: Academic Press, 1972.

35. Steptoe, P. C. Recent advances in surgical methods of control of fertility and infertility. Br. Med. Bull. 26:60, 1970.

36. Stevenson, T. C. Personal communication, June 3, 1974.

37. Stevenson, T. C., and D. S. Taylor. The effect of methyl cyanoacrylate tissue adhesive on the human fallopian tube and endometrium. J. Obstet. Gynecol. 79:1028, 1972.

38. Thompson, H. E., C. A. Dafoe, T. S. Moulding, and L. E. Seitz. Evaluation of experimental methods of occluding the uterotubal junction. In *Female sterilization: Prognosis for simplified outpatient procedures*, eds. D. W. Duncan et al. New York: Academic Press, 1972.

39. Wheeless, C. R. Personal communication, April 1974.

40. Wheeless, C. R., and B. H. Thompson. Laparoscopic sterilization. Review of 3,600 cases. Obstet. Gynecol. 42(5):751, 1973.

41. Yoon, B. Personal communication, April 24, 1974.

42. Zipper, J., M. Medel, L. Pastene, and M. Rivera. Intrauterine instillation of chemical cytotoxic agents for tubal sterilization and treatment of functional metrorrhagias. Int. J. Fertil. 14(4):289, 1969.

43. Zipper, J., M. Medel, and R. Prager. Alterations in fertility induced by unilateral intrauterine instillation of cytotoxic compounds in rats. Am J. Obstet. Gynecol. 101(7):971, 1974.

44. Zipper, J., A. Stachetti, and M. Medel. Human fertility control by transvaginal application of quinacrine on the Fallopian tube. Fertil. Steril. 21(8):581, 1970.

Note added in proof: Central nervous system excitation has been reported following quinacrine lavage. It is our understanding that at least one death has occurred from this cause at the time of a quinacrine sterilization procedure.

19 Intrauterine Contraception   Howard J. Tatum

19.1 Introduction

The early history of intrauterine contraceptive devices (IUDs) is replete with reports of clinical trials employing foreign bodies made of metals, silkworm gut, and plastics. Medical prejudices of the late nineteenth and early twentieth centuries based upon the use of cervicouterine stem pessaries and perhaps coincident pelvic infections were severe impediments to serious studies of the IUD. The traditional conservatism (or fear of peer criticism) of the gynecologist resulted in delays in the presentation of clinical experiences with IUDs and in what may be described as surreptitious clinical experimentation.

The modern era of contraception with IUDs began with Oppenheimer's 1959 article in the *American Journal of Obstetrics and Gynecology*,[1] written at the request of Howard C. Taylor, who was then editor of the journal. This publication described the extremely favorable clinical experiences Oppenheimer had had with the Gräfenberg ring and the Tshihanra-Ota ring. As a result of these encouraging clinical data, from 1962 to 1964 a series of new IUDs appeared. These were developed and tested clinically by Margulies, Zipper and Sanhuerza, Lippes, Birnberg and Burnhill, Hall, and others.[2]

The disparity of results reported by these investigators pointed up the need for a uniform method of analysis whereby valid comparisons of clinical effectiveness and incidence of side effects could be made. This led to the establishment of the Cooperative Statistical Program (CSP) supported by the Population Council and under the direction of Christopher Tietze. The life table method of analysis was adapted from the life insurance actuary tables by Potter[3] for particular use for IUDs. This method was subsequently applied to other types of contraceptive methods. The most recent methodology for life table analyses was described in 1973 by Tietze and Lewit.[4]

The analyses that were carried out with this method were directed toward the principal side effects, which to a great extent determined the continuation rates, which in turn could be extrapolated to births averted. The side effects that resulted in closure of a segment or discontinuation of the method were: (1) pregnancy; (2) expulsion; (3) bleeding and/or pain; (4) other medical complications; (5) a planned pregnancy; or (6) oth-

er personal reasons. For comparative purposes, only first-segment data were initially considered. The first segment indicates the length of time the device has been used prior to the occurrence of an accidental pregnancy or prior to expulsion or removal for any purpose. Obviously, this is a somewhat artificial distinction since discontinuation of one method of contraception often leads to the adoption of another method. For this reason, consideration of multiple consecutive segments of contraception will give a more realistic measure of births averted than will data from a first or single segment. As a result of the CSP data, the Lippes loop came to be considered a standard with which corresponding results from other, less widely studied devices were compared.

Another and final component that influences the use-effectiveness of an IUD is related to the specific mechanism of contraceptive action. Investigations relevant to the mechanism of action will be considered separately.

19.2 Size and Shape of IUDs

Although Gräfenberg, Zipper, and Hall developed and tested IUDs that were relatively small in relation to the Lippes loop, not until 1968 did Tatum[5] propose the concept that in order to minimize the side effects, particularly pain, bleeding, and expulsion, an IUD should have a shape and size that conforms to the minimum size of the uterine cavity rather than obliging the cavity to conform to the size of the IUD (as in the Lippes loop and the Saf-T-Coil). He postulated that a reduction in shape and size and the related side effects would automatically increase the use-effectiveness of a device and therefore its continuation rate.

The T-Shaped IUD
Although the T shape of the uterine cavity was noted as early as 1858 by J. C. Guyon, no attempt was made to follow up on this lead until 1968 when Tatum independently considered the same anatomic configuration. The Tatum T IUD resulted from three separate lines of thought: (1) The uterine cavity is dynamic rather than static and is constantly undergoing changes in size and shape. (2) The minimum shape and dimensions of the uterine cavity that exist at the height of a

contraction resemble a T. (3) A T-shaped device offers relatively little mass to irritate the uterine musculature and thus encourage and enhance the expulsive forces of the myometrium.[2] These ideas led to a realization of the inadequacies of uterine cavity molds, which of necessity represent a single phase in the contraction pattern.

Although the arguments leading to the T were shown to be correct in that the device was associated with minimal pain and bleeding and a low expulsion rate, the contraceptive effect was unacceptably low —18 percent at one year. Presumably this low rate reflected the small surface area of the device (315 mm²). This demonstration set the stage for the use of a well-tolerated self-retaining intrauterine vehicle to carry a potent antifertility agent into the uterine cavity and provide long-term contraception.

19.3 Medicated IUDs

The idea of using an IUD as a vehicle or carrier for an active agent evolved from the development of the small self-retaining plain plastic T and the demonstration by Zipper and his associates[6] that metallic copper placed in the uterine cavity of the rabbit provided almost perfect contraception. The motivation for this latter development was Zipper's attempt to modify or inactivate the enzymatic environment of the endometrial cavity to the extent that nidation would be prevented. He was cognizant of certain enzyme systems' dependence upon and sensitivity to biologically active metals such as zinc, copper, silver, and iron. Of all the metals tested, zinc and copper proved to have the greatest influence upon implantation without at the same time manifesting severe maternal cytotoxic action (as seen with cadmium).

When the first clinical tests with the plain T proved disappointing with regard to contraceptive action, it seemed logical to Zipper and Tatum that a combination of copper and the T should complement each other. The first clinical test of this combination was performed in Santiago, Chile. Copper wire with a surface area of 30 mm² was wound around the upper end of the plastic T, and the device was introduced high in the uterine cavity. The pregnancy rate after one year of use was 5 per 100 women in contrast to 18 as obtained with the T without copper.[7]

Subsequent studies utilizing larger areas of metallic copper on the vertical arm of the T demonstrated a definite direct correlation between the surface area of copper and the contraceptive effectiveness. The reports and data that permitted this conclusion are summarized in a review by Tatum.[2] The addition of more than 200 mm² surface of copper on the vertical arm has been shown by Zipper and by Tatum[8] to contribute lit-

tle to the contraceptive effect. An important recent observation is that the placement of copper sleeves, 30 mm² in area, on each transverse arm of the T significantly increases the contraceptive efficiency of the TCu 200.

The logic behind this development was based upon two clinical observations. The first was the significant initial reduction in pregnancy rate achieved when only 30 mm² of copper was wound around the uppermost portion of the dependent arm of the T immediately below the crossbar (so that the copper was located in the superior aspect of the endometrial cavity). Subsequent additions of from 170 to 270 mm² of copper surface effected much more modest reductions in pregnancy rates. Thus the presence of copper high in the uterine cavity appears to be proportionately more effective in preventing pregnancy than when it is lower down. The second relevant clinical observation was an apparent decrease in contraceptive effectiveness when the Copper T was displaced downward as in partial or incomplete expulsion.

These observations led to the development of the TCu 380A, as reported in 1974 by Tatum.[9] A 1974 study by the Population Council confirmed that the position of copper within the uterine cavity and the exposed surface area of the copper are important in providing antifertility activity.[8] This concept will undoubtedly be reflected in the development of improved IUDs bearing adjunctive antifertility agents.

With the expanding use of the Copper T, the safety of the method became an important subject for investigation. The toxicity of copper was studied, particularly the effects of systemic absorption and its teratogenicity in case of accidental pregnancy.

Although some of the dissolved copper is known to enter the systemic circulation and to be distributed to many parts of the body (in rats), there is no evidence in humans that the small quantities of copper (10–50 μg/24 hr lost from the TCu 200) result in any toxic manifestations. It should be noted that 2,000–5,000 μg of copper are judged to be the minimum daily requirements of the adult human.

The presence of copper in the uterine cavity has not had any demonstrable effect upon the cervical epithelium, as judged by repetitive Papanicolaou smears over periods as long as six years. Reviews by Furst and Haro[10] and Gilman[11] provide convincing data indicating that metallic copper or copper salts do not have carcinogenic properties.

Detailed studies by Chang and Tatum[12] in three species of laboratory animals indicated that the copper wire did not produce any teratogenic effects upon developing fetuses. Gestation, parturition, and lactation were not affected by the copper. The subsequent development and fertility of the F_1 and F_2 generations were normal. At the time of this review, more than 500 accidental pregnancies have been recorded in women wearing Copper T IUDs. Of these, 172 elected to continue their pregnancy. None of the 500 pregnancies showed evidence of abnormal development or other indication of teratogenicity.

Mechanism of Contraceptive Action of Intrauterine Copper

The precise mechanism(s) whereby copper exerts its antifertility effect is not known. In most instances it does not prevent fertilization, although White,[13] Saito et al.,[14] and Loewit[15] have shown that copper salts as well as particulate copper are spermatodepressive and, in adequate concentrations, can be spermatocidal. Chang and Tatum[16] have shown that the contraceptive action of copper in the rat results in part from a local change in the endometrial environment, so that the blastocyst cannot implant. They also showed that the antifertility effect does not result from reduced estrogen uptake by the endometrium. All studies to date indicate clearly that the contraceptive action of copper is due to a local rather than a systemic effect. Although a number of endometrial enzyme systems have been reported to be influenced by the presence of metallic copper,[17,18] the significance of these changes in relation to nidation and fetal development is not known.

Leukocytic Infiltration

The propensity of copper to evoke an infiltration of leukocytes into the myometrium, the endometrium, and the uterine cavity was first reported by Zipper et al. in 1971.[19] These investigators stated that leukocytic infiltration had been found consistently in the endometria from women wearing the T or the TCu. They suggested that this mobilization may participate in the contraceptive action of the devices. Later, Cuadros and Hirsch[20] showed that metallic copper in the uterine cavity of monkeys caused a marked accumulation of leukocytes on the copper-bearing device and in the adjacent tissues. When a plain polyethylene device was used, only a scanty accumulation of leukocytes occurred. El Sahwi and Moyer[21] showed a direct relationship in the rabbit between fertility and the density of leukocytes within the uterine cavity. In their study, they used a relatively inert IUD made of Silastic. Thus the antifertility effect of most IUDs results at least in part from the propensity of the device to effect an accumulation of leukocytes within the cavity. We do not know yet precisely how these leukocytes, or products from them, make the intrauterine environment hostile to the blastocyst.

Special Clinical Attributes of the Copper T

Menstrual blood loss   The bleeding pattern associated with any contraceptive modality is very important, since major changes in either direction are apt to result in discontinuation of the method. Hefnawi et al.[22] and Israel et al.[23] observed that the Copper T was associated with less uterine bleeding than were the Lippes loop and the Dalkon shield; however, the menstrual bleeding of Copper-T wearers was somewhat greater than normal. These observations are supported by data of Tatum and Schmidt[24] derived from monkeys bearing diminutive plastic Ts with and without added metallic copper. The presence of metallic copper seems to cause a prolongation of the menstrual bleeding without effecting a change in the peripheral blood picture. The reduced blood loss caused by the Copper T in comparison with the Lippes loop may stem from the disparity in size of the devices.

Gravidity and parity   The small dimensions of the Copper T have permitted its successful use in nulligravid and nulliparous women. Although the pregnancy rate may be somewhat higher in nulligravid than in parous women, these differences are not so great as to preclude its use. Mishell et al.[25] studied the TCu 200 in nulliparous women and concluded that this device was a highly acceptable method for this group and provided an effective alternative to oral hormonal contraception.

19.4 Postpartum Insertion of IUDs

The need for an effective IUD for insertion during the puerperium has been apparent for many years. This interval in the reproductive life of the woman is psychologically and medically appropriate for the initiation of some form of fertility control. For many reasons, a systemically acting drug such as a steroid hormone is inadvisable, whereas a method that acts locally is preferable physiologically as well as pharmacologically. A principal shortcoming of IUD use during the immediate puerperium is the relatively high expulsion rate, presumably due to the spacious size of the endometrial cavity during this period of early involution. One must take into account the risk-benefit ratio, weighing the increased expulsion rate and the increased chance of uterine perforation that are associated with IUD insertions during the puerperium against the medical, psychological, and sociological advantages to the woman and her family of fertility control for some reasonable time following a delivery.

The ideal IUD for the first few months of the puerperium has not yet been developed. The conventional space-filling devices such as the Lippes loop and the Saf-T-Coil have been used with reasonable degrees of success. An expulsion rate of 15 to 25 or 30 percent within the first three months after delivery is to be expected. Although only limited data are yet available, the Copper T appears to be somewhat more effective than the larger IUDs. Tatum[9] reported an expulsion rate of 14.2 percent when the TCu 200 was introduced two to four weeks following delivery. This rate was reduced to 11.4 percent at five to eight weeks, and to 7 percent when the insertions were made 9 to 12 weeks after the delivery. At the latter interval, the rates for all events were comparable to interval insertions (not closer than three months to a full-term pregnancy termination).

19.5 Postabortion Insertion of IUDs

An effective contraceptive method immediately after an abortion is of utmost importance. Whether the abortion is spontaneous, elective, therapeutic, or illegally induced, the woman is usually psychologically and biologically receptive to some form of fertility control.

Traditionally the medical profession has disapproved of inserting a foreign body into the uterine cavity during the immediate puerperium (up to six days following termination of a pregnancy). This dictum was even more inviolate when the abortion was illegally induced, which implied potential if not actual uterine sepsis. These patients risk pregnancy the most and are least likely to seek good follow-up care.

A significant breakthrough occurred in 1972 when Tatum[2] reported a random comparison of two groups of potentially infected patients who were admitted for treatment of an induced illegal abortion. The treatment of both groups was identical except that Lippes loops were inserted in members of one group immediately after the surgical completion of the abortion, whereas the patients in the other group received their IUDs when they returned six to eight weeks later for postabortion checkup. The assignment to one or the other treatment group was made randomly. (Sealed identical envelopes containing a card that stated "Insert IUD" or "No IUD" were used.) The subsequent medical courses of the women in the two groups were compared with particular reference to: (1) number of days in the hospital; (2) highest temperature during hospital stay; and (3) complications arising during hospitalization and during the first four to six weeks after discharge from the hospital. Five clinical centers in several countries participated in this collaborative study; in all there were 2,388 patients. Of these, 1,179 did not immediately receive IUDs and 1,209 had IUDs inserted immediately after the curettage that completed the abortion. The only patients excluded from the study were those in septic shock or with fulminating peritonitis. Statistical evaluation of the histories of these patients yielded no evidence to suggest that the

insertion of an IUD immediately after completion of the potentially or actually infected abortion increased the chances of ensuing complications.

The data from this collaborative study suggest strongly that the traditional "hands-off" policy is now often unnecessary. The application of intrauterine contraception for this very-high-risk group of women seems to be not only warranted but medically feasible. These observations have been corroborated subsequently by a number of investigators.

Insertion of the Copper T immediately after a legal abortion has proved to be especially effective, as shown by Nygren and Johansson[26] and by Timonen and Luukkainen.[27] The incidence of subsequent complication was the same whether or not the IUD was inserted. Also, the contraceptive effectiveness and incidence of side effects, including expulsion, of the TCu 200 inserted at this point in the postabortion period were comparable to the results from routine insertions in family planning clinics.

19.6 Long-Lasting Copper T

The intrauterine environment causes a nonuniform dissolution of copper from the surface of copper wire. Microscopic and macroscopic cavitations in varying degrees result during the intrauterine life of the wire. The diameter of the wire diminishes irregularly, and flakes of copper oxide can occasionally be seen on and about the surface of the wire. Actual breaks or loss of continuity of the wire have been observed infrequently on TCu 200 devices removed from patients after intervals of intrauterine life ranging between eight months and three years. No signs or symptoms that could be attributed to corrosion or fragmentation of the wire were reported from more than 180,000 women bearing the wire-wound Copper T.

In spite of this absence of overt problems related to the dissolution of copper wire within the uterus, there is a theoretical limitation in duration of contraceptive effectiveness. Any IUD that has an effective life *in utero* of three years or less cannot be considered ideal in populations for which repetitive medical care is not readily available. From a demographic standpoint, an effective life *in utero* for an IUD should be more than three years and preferably at least five years. With this objective in mind, we applied copper to the T in the form of multiple sleeves instead of copper wires. This technique permits use of a thicker segment of copper, which will retain its integrity for considerably longer than can be expected for the 0.25-mm-diameter wire that is standard in the TCu 200. The multisleeved model, designated TCu 220C (C stands for "collars"), was first reported by Tatum in 1974.[9] Calculations based upon the dissolution rate of copper within the uterus and the wall thickness of the copper sleeves indicate that a life *in utero* of at least 25 years can be expected for this device. After one year of use the pregnancy rate obtained with the TCu 220C is about one-third that with the TCu 200. Although this difference is just short of being statistically significant, with additional time and a larger sample the differences may attain significance. The other clinical parameters such as expulsion, pain, and bleeding are almost identical for the two models.[8]

If the contraceptive effectiveness of the TCu 220C continues to be as favorable as it now appears, this device will become the method of choice because of its longer life. If further data confirm these optimistic figures, we will have overcome the disadvantages of a relatively short life span for the wire-wound T and will have made a major advance toward achieving satisfactory long-term, one-application contraception for the nulligravida and multipara alike. The demographic and economic implications of this advance could be enormous.

19.7 Other Copper-Bearing IUDs

With the demonstration that the addition of metallic copper increased the contraceptive effectiveness of the T-shaped IUD, this principle was applied to other IUDs. The Copper 7 developed by the G. D. Searle Company carries copper wire 0.20 mm in diameter and with a surface area of 200 mm². A number of clinical reports on the Cu 7 have appeared.[9,28] The most recent data derived from a random paired comparison of the TCu 200 and the Cu 7 by the Population Council were presented by Mishell in December 1974.[29] These data indicated that although the pregnancy rate achieved by the TCu 200 was about half that of the Cu 7, the difference was not statistically significant at the 95 percent confidence level. The expulsion rate for the Cu 7 was almost twice that of the TCu 200—a statistically significant difference. The other clinical parameters were essentially the same for both devices. The Copper 7 became the first copper-bearing IUD to be approved for commercial distribution in the United States by the FDA. Early approval of the Copper T is also expected.*

Two models of the Lippes loop bearing copper sleeves have been made and are being tested, one carrying a 135 mm² and the other a 200 mm² copper surface. One-year data from a comparison of the TCu 200 and Lippes loops A-135 and A-200 have been reported by Lippes et al.[30] According to Lippes, "The Copper T 200 performed better than either Copper Loop A-135 or Copper Loop A-200, in respect to closures for expulsion, removals for medical reasons, and continuation rates." This study corroborates the statement

made by Tatum: "Although the addition of metallic copper may cause a reduction in the rate of expulsion and the incidence and magnitude of uterine bleeding, it seems rather unlikely that side effects such as bleeding and pain which result from distension of the myometrium and compression of the endometrium will be altered significantly. It would be illogical, therefore, to assume that metallic copper will prove to be a panacea for the side effects of all shapes and sizes of IUDs!"[2] The addition of metallic copper to the Lippes loop is logical, however, since the loop will continue to provide acceptably low pregnancy rates even after the copper has been completely dissolved. On the other hand, the T without copper has an unacceptably low antifertility effect.

19.7 Other Metals on IUDs

Zipper et al.[31] have reported that both copper and zinc produce marked antifertility effects in the rabbit uterus but that silver, tin, and magnesium wires have little or no effect on implantations. Chang et al.[32] tested the anti-implantation effects of a series of metals in rat uteri: although less effective than copper, the metals zinc, cobalt, lead, nickel, and cadmium also produced marked reductions in implantations; the contraceptive properties of segments of silver, gold, and platinum were poor; and a combination of silver and platinum was also ineffective.

Intrauterine Zinc
As a result of these studies, Zipper et al.[33] placed 30 mm² each of copper and zinc wires on the vertical arm of the T IUD and tested this combination in women. The contraceptive effect of the Cu-Zn device after one year surpassed that of the T bearing 135 mm² of copper alone. Subsequent studies by Zipper and his associates[33] confirmed the efficient antifertility properties of intrauterine zinc but revealed at least two disadvantages of its use. At the end of one year they found a 35 percent decrease in the weight of the zinc wire, indicating a rather rapid dissolution rate. An even greater potential problem, reported by Cooper,[34] was the development of numerous areas of focal toxic degeneration in the endometrium of patients bearing the T that had pure zinc wire affixed to it. The endometrium reverted to its normal state after the zinc-bearing Ts were removed.

An apparently independent program by Anderson and the Ansell Rubber Company in Melbourne developed the Anderson-Ansell Latex Leaf IUD, which consists of silicone-rubber shield-shaped leaf impregnated with particles of metallic copper and metallic zinc. The preliminary clinical data presented by Anderson[35] in 1973 were exceptionally good; however, the problem of endometrial pathology has yet to be resolved.

19.8 Hormone-Releasing IUDs

The use of hormone-releasing IUDs was first reported by Doyle and Clewe in 1968.[36] Their preliminary studies applied the slow-release principle of progestins from silicone rubber to silicone elastomer rods impregnated with melengestrol acetate placed within the uteri of rats, rabbits, and monkeys. Their data demonstrated that steroids released from silicone elastomer rods within the uterine cavities increased the retention rate of the foreign body in rats and rabbits and produced typical secretory type of endometrium in estrogen-primed castrated monkeys.

In 1970 Croxatto et al.[37] were the first to show that a progestogen (megestrol acetate) within an intrauterine silicone elastomer capsule would prevent implantations in the experimental horn of a rabbit uterus, whereas normal implantations occurred in the contralateral control horn. Thus these investigators demonstrated that a progestogen acting locally was a contraceptive. The IUD as a vehicle for steroids to be released within the endometrial cavity was carried one step further by the 1970 studies of Scommegna and associates.[38] Silicone elastomer capsules containing progesterone were affixed to modified Lippes loops, which were then inserted into the uterine cavities of 34 human subjects. Endometrial changes were demonstrated that indicated localized absorption of progesterone. These investigators concluded from their short-term experiments that although the expulsion rate of the loop was not reduced by the presence of progesterone, histological changes in the endometrium presumably could interfere with the normal reproductive process.

More recently, Clewe and Doyle[39] have shown that silicone elastomer rods impregnated with melengestrol acetate suspended within one horn of a rat or rabbit uterus prevented implantations in that horn. Since implantations occurred normally in the contralateral control horn, their experiment demonstrated clearly that the antifertility effect of the exogenous progestin was local rather than systemic. The mechanism of this contraceptive action is not yet known. Preliminary clinical studies on women using a silicone elastomer Lippes loop impregnated with crystalline medroxyprogesterone were reported to be encouraging by Stryker and associates.[40]

Martinez Manautou et al.[41] reported on the results of 2,086 intrauterine progesterone-releasing systems studied during 11,500 woman-months. The individual systems in the form of a T were constructed to have delivery rates of 10, 25, 65, and 120 μg/day. General conclusions based upon these studies suggest that the contraceptive effectiveness of the 65 μg/day system is similar to that of the conventional hormonal contraceptives. Its advantage is in its local rather than systemic effects. Its principal side effect is intermenstrual bleeding, which diminishes when a second IUD is inserted after one year. The systems are structured to provide a constant release of progesterone for one full year. Biomembranes are expected to be developed in the near future, facilitating a two-year system. Although the precise mechanism(s) of contraceptive action is not known, the morphological and biochemical changes of the endometrium seem most important.

Investigations are under way in several different centers to evaluate the efficacy of using other potent synthetic progestins as IUD potentiators.

19.9 Nonmedicated IUDs

The Dalkon Shield

Davis and Israel[42] computed the average dimensions of the endometrial cavity at several levels from the intercornual plane downward toward the internal cervical os. Based upon these measurements and upon the premise postulated by Zipper and associates[7] that the antifertility effect of an "inert" IUD bears a direct relationship to the surface area of contact between the IUD and the endometrium, Davis[43] designed a device that he named the shield. This device is slightly pear-shaped, and its retention within the uterine cavity is enhanced by the presence of spicular projections along its lateral margins. Although the cephalocaudal and transverse dimensions of the shield are considerably smaller than those of Lippes loop "D", the total surface of the device is greater because a thin membrane partially covers the shield.

Preliminary clinical data collected by Davis[43] on the shield suggest that its antifertility effect is considerably better than the 18 percent pregnancy rate achieved by the plain T. The difference is probably related to the disparity in surface area between the two devices. It has been postulated that implantation may be jeopardized when normally opposing endometrial surfaces are separated by an inert membrane or barrier.

A random comparison of the Dalkon shield and the TCu 200 was undertaken by the Population Council. At the end of one year, the pregnancy rate for the TCu 200 was 1.4 per 100 women-years, while the rate for the Dalkon shield was 5.0. The expulsion rate for the shield was 3.0 and that for the T was 6.3. Removals for bleeding or pain were 11.6 for the TCu 200 and 14.2 for the shield.

Other investigators have reported clinical findings

differing from those of Davis, perhaps because Davis advised the use of contraceptive jelly in conjunction with the shield. While this adjunct was presumably to be used only for the first several months after the shield was inserted, some women may not have discontinued the practice.

Serious medical problems associated with the Dalkon shield appeared in late 1973 when the manufacturer began to receive reports of septic midtrimester spontaneous abortions in women using the shield. By May 1974 there had been four maternal deaths from sepsis and 36 septic abortions in women wearing the Dalkon shield. Sales were discontinued, and studies were undertaken to define the problem and to attempt to determine whether or not these clinical entities were generic to all IUDs or unique to the Dalkon shield. In an effort to clarify this issue, Tatum et al.[44] studied five currently used IUDs (Lippes loop, Saf-T-Coil, Copper T, Copper 7, and the Dalkon shield). All of these devices except the Dalkon shield utilized monofilament tails. The shield was equipped with a complex multifilament tail enclosed within a plastic sheath. This tail was shown to possess in vitro wicking properties for aqueous solutions and for live bacteria suspended in saline. Dalkon shields that had been electively removed from patients were studied bacteriologically and morphologically. The multifilament tails removed from patients were found to contain a wide variety of living bacteria. These bacteria were in the spaces between the 200 to 400 fibers within the plastic sheath and were clearly shown by transmission electron microscopy of the tails.

These studies showed conclusively that the tail of the Dalkon shield has physical characteristics that are completely different from those of the other IUDs currently in use in the United States. These data also demonstrated that this complex multifilament tail could under certain circumstances (such as pregnancy) contribute to the transmission of bacteria from the vagina and/or cervical canal into the uterine cavity and could provide a reservoir of microorganisms wherever the dependent end of the tail or a break in its sheath came into contact with an environment suitable for bacterial growth.

As a consequence of these studies, the A. H. Robins Company, in consultation with the FDA, withdrew all unused shields and indicated that new shields bearing a monofilament tail would be produced. At the time of this writing (January 1975), 14 deaths and 219 septic abortions have been reported among women wearing the Dalkon shield. Whether or not this clinical entity is limited to the shield and its complex tail has not yet been resolved. Perhaps time and a new monofilamented shield will clarify the question.

The Antigon F
The Antigon F IUD was developed by Paul Lebech and Mogens Osler in Copenhagen. It is constructed of high-density polyethylene and has a rather rigid frame covered by a plastic membrane. The tail is surgical suture consisting of six strands of synthetic fibers.

The Antigon F has been studied clinically in Denmark, Thailand, and the United States. While the preliminary data are encouraging, considerably more information from different clinics will be necessary before its relative efficacy will be known. The latest data on the Antigon were presented in December 1974 by Fuchs.[45, 46]

The Ypsilon
This is an ypsilon-shaped IUD consisting of a stainless steel spring foundation entirely covered with Silastic. It possesses a solid strand of Silastic as an appendage. The preliminary clinical data from the United States as reported by Soichet[47] are quite limited. The device has also been used in Brazil with encouraging results.[48] As with the Antigon F, much additional experience will be required with the Ypsilon before its true position is established with respect to the more widely used nonmedicated and medicated IUDs.

Fluid-Filled IUDs
The fluid-filled devices developed by Futoran and Kitrilakis[49] are semirigid, inflatable, and designed to fit most uterine cavities. The patient's subjective response determines the extent to which the device is inflated. It consists of a silicone polymer pouch reinforced with a Dacron mesh and is filled with saline through a fine Silastic tube, which, after being tied off when the appropriate volume of fluid is injected, serves as its appendage or tail.

19.10 Major Gaps in Our Knowledge

Mechanism of Action
While we as physicians and scientists should be concerned principally about safety and side effects, efficiency and reversibility, the precise mechanism(s) whereby the IUD effects contraception should be more or less academic. Since widespread implementation and acceptability of contraception is influenced to a considerable extent by religious and political pressures, however, it is necessary to attempt clarification of the mechanisms whereby any specific method prevents or limits conception.

The data currently available generally agree that the effect of the IUD is associated with a localized mobilization of leukocytes within the endometrial cavity. This sterile inflammatory response of the uterus to the

IUD is certainly one step in a chain of events that culminates in the prevention of a potential pregnancy. El Sahwi and Moyer[21] have shown that in the rabbit, implantation occurs in locations of the uterine cavity where the leukocytic infiltration effected by the IUD is minimal. An inverse relationship seems to exist between the number of implants and the number of leukocytes. Thus in experimental animals and in humans a common denominator in the mechanism of action of an IUD is most likely its propensity to evoke a mobilization of leukocytes to its vicinity.

The implications of this are not so obvious. A crucial question in many people's view is whether or not the egg has been fertilized prior to the action of the IUD. If fertilization has taken place, any subsequent interference with the zygote may be defined as an abortion. (A medically more acceptable definition is that abortion refers to premature disruption of an implanted or nidated embryo.) Of course, interference with the male (sperm) or female (ovum) gamete prior to their functional union cannot by any definition be classified as abortifacient.

Sagiroglu[50] has shown that the macrophages that have accumulated in the uterine cavity of women bearing nonmedicated IUDs phagocytize intact spermatozoa. He observed as many as 41 spermatozoa within a single macrophage. Based upon these observations, he concluded that this phagocytic attack on the spermatozoa constituted one mechanism for limiting conception. Hammerstein[51] has shown that metallic copper within a column of cervical mucus will limit sperm penetration and ascent through the mucus. Thus by these two examples, one with a nonmedicated IUD (Lippes loop) and the other with metallic copper (a potent antifertility agent), definite mechanisms are initiated by the IUD that affect only the male gamete.

Unpublished and very preliminary observations by Croxatto and his associates[52] suggest that metallic copper causes very rapid disintegration of human ova supended in Fallopian tube fluid. The presumption is that these ova are not fertilized at the time. The implication of these observations is extremely important, since they suggest that an ascending flow of copper-containing liquid from the uterine cavity into the Fallopian tube could effect the destruction of a prefertilized egg. Under no circumstances could this mechanism be considered abortifacient.

If further investigations (1) corroborate the spermatocidal and spermatodepressive action of both medicated (copper) and nonmedicated (Lippes loop) IUDs *and* (2) show conclusively that intrauterine copper can effect the destruction of unfertilized eggs within the Fallopian tube, the contraceptive action of these two types of IUDs cannot be considered abortifacient. A

major investigational effort should be made along these lines, since confirmation of the nonabortifacient mechanism of IUD contraception would overcome many of the present religious and political objections to this method.

These studies would very likely contribute much ancillary data on uterine and tubal motility, on the dynamics of active and passive fluid flow within the endometrial and tubal cavities, and on sperm, ovum, and zygote transport within the female genital tract. Additional information could also be expected in regard to phenomena contributing to and associated with the process of nidation or implantation of the blastocyst.

I anticipate that the studies that Horacio Croxatto and his group are undertaking will be most productive relevant to the basic physiology of nidation. These data will include interacting factors related to fertilization, to physiology of the blastocyst, to effects of zygote aging in regard to changes in the zona pellucida, to sperm penetration, and to sensitivity to exogenous substances that could interfere with these normal and essential stages in development.

Cuadros and his associates[53] have already shown by transmission and scanning electron microscopy that consistent morphological changes are produced in the human endometrium by the presence of nonmedicated and copper-containing IUDs. These changes relate to the accumulation of leukocytes, to the presence of a dense layer of mucopolysaccharides overlying the endometrial surface, and to a flattening of the endometrial cells in contact with the IUD. They have also shown that the IUD effects a deciliation of the surface epithelium. Although the functional significance of these morphological changes is not yet defined, these observations will add much to our basic knowledge of IUD function.

Although a number of endometrial enzyme systems have been reported to be influenced by the presence of the IUD, including copper,[54] the significance of these changes is not known.

Joshi and Sujan-Tejuja[55] carried out an exhaustive study in which they performed sequential analyses of the endometrium for total protein, acid-soluble nucleotide, ribonucleic acid (RNA), and both alkaline and acid phosphatases during five different phases of the menstrual cycle (days 6 to 8, 9 to 13, 16 to 20, 21 to 24, and 25 to 30) in control women and in women bearing the Lippes loop. They found no qualitative changes in the sequential shifts of any of these components except for the acid phosphatase. A marked increase in activity of the acid phosphatase was noted at midcycle in the IUD-bearing uterus, whereas little if any change was noted in the control endometria. On the other hand, significant quantitative increases occurred in all five analyzed biochemical parameters. They concluded from these studies that the IUD stimulates endometrial growth during the proliferative and early secretory phases of the cycle. Since the peak concentrations of total protein and of RNA occurred, on average, seven days earlier in the IUD-bearing uterus than in the control, they suggested that not only was the endometrial growth stimulated, but maturation was accelerated. They postulated that these changes, which are considered to reflect responses to endogenous ovarian hormones, indicated that the IUD might alter the sensitivity of the endometrium to these hormones.

19.11 Etiology of the Side Effects of IUDs

Since the use-effectiveness and continuation rates of IUDs are to a great extent predicated upon the types and frequency of side effects, it is essential to understand their etiology and to prevent or at least reduce their occurrence. The most important side effects (except for accidental pregnancy) that influence the acceptability of the IUD by a woman and her physician are (1) expulsion, (2) bleeding, (3) pain, and (4) other medical reasons. It is relevant here to comment briefly on each of these events with respect to possible etiological factors and preventive or curative measures.

Expulsion

As mentioned earlier in this paper, the uterus must be considered a dynamic rather than a static structure, the size and shape of the potential uterine cavity (there is no actual cavity until something distends the walls, such as pregnancy or an IUD) undergoing constant changes as a consequence of the rhythmic contractions of the myometrium. Any foreign body within the uterine cavity will tend to irritate the uterine musculature, causing it to oppose the distension and expel the foreign body. An important aspect of IUD design is therefore devising a shape and size that will cause a minimal degree of distension of the uterine cavity, and this was the logic behind the development of the T shape. We do not know whether contraceptive adjuncts to a nonmedicated IUD, such as copper or a progestin, can influence the retention rate of the device in the human.

A major gap in the IUD armamentarium is an IUD that will have an acceptably low expulsion rate when it is inserted during the early puerperium. Patient motivation for an effective contraceptive method is especially great at this time, and medical or paramedical personnel are usually available to initiate the method selected by the patient. An IUD that has been designed for this specific use is now being developed and

should be ready for clinical evaluation sometime in 1975.[56]

Proper insertion technique is of utmost importance in ensuring optimal retention of the IUD. The device must be placed high in the endometrial cavity, as close to the fundus of the uterus as is possible. The method whereby this correct placement is accomplished varies somewhat with the specific IUD being used. Devices such as the Copper T and the Saf-T-Coil are encased within an inserter tube until the fundus is reached. Then the inserter tube is withdrawn over a plunger, thus freeing the IUD within the cavity. Other devices such as the Lippes loop are freed from their enclosing inserter tube just above the internal cervical os. As more and more of the device is forced from the tube, the entire device moves toward the fundus (the so-called fundal-seeking process). Each type of device has specific characteristics that must be taken into consideration during the insertion procedure. The individual inserting the IUD must know these characteristics and must have determined the size and shape of the uterine cavity and the spacial relationship between the cervical canal and the endometrial cavity. If these details are neglected, the probability of uterine perforation and consequent intraperitoneal placement of the IUD is increased.

Bleeding

Most IUD removals for medical reasons result from abnormal uterine bleeding. Although the IUD does not alter the level or pattern of steroid hormones and gonadotropins during the menstrual cycle, it has local effects on the endometrium. Often these changes cause a 1–2 day premature onset of menstruation. An interesting hypothesis is that the endometrium reacts to the IUD by releasing prostaglandin. This in turn stimulates uterine contractions, which may prolong the interval of menstruation. The total measured blood loss during the menstrual cycle is increased over normal levels by the presence of an IUD. The blood loss during a normal period is about 35 ml, whereas it more than doubles when the woman is bearing a loop or a coil. Wearing a Copper T will often result in a 50 ml blood loss. Thus the amount of blood loss is less with a device that causes limited distortion of the endometrial cavity than with a larger device, which causes a greater degree of endometrial compression and myometrial distension. The reader is referred to the following treatises on uterine blood loss as a consequence of IUD use: Hefnawi et al.,[57] Liedholm et al.,[58] Israel et al.,[59] and Shaw and Moyer.[60]

A number of theories have been proposed to explain the precise cause of this increased bleeding. Morphological studies of the endometrium underlying IUDs have demonstrated areas of vascular erosion. Adjacent areas that are not in direct contact with the IUD show increased vascular permeability.

Shaw et al.[61,62] have shown in monkeys that the IUD is associated with greater fibrinolysis than in control uteri. Tatum and Schmidt[24] have demonstrated that in the monkey, the presence of a copper-wound IUD is associated with a significantly greater number of bleeding days than is the presence of the same IUD without copper wire. In spite of this bleeding tendency, which seems to be caused by the metallic copper, after two years no difference shows between the experimental and control monkey groups that can be detected by the total body hematological profile. No clinical evidence suggests chronic blood loss or anemia. In humans, Shaw and Moyer[60] have shown increases in fibrinolytic activator in endometrial cells underlying an IUD. Westrom and Bengtsson[63] have been able to reduce the menstrual blood loss effected by an IUD by the administration of the fibrinolytic inhibitor tranexamic acid. Hefnawi et al.[64] have shown that the fibrinolytic activity of menstrual blood from women bearing loops is significantly increased above normal, whereas the blood from Copper T users has fibrinolytic activity no different than that of control women.

Pelvic Infection

Although certain IUDs may, because of structural characteristics, predispose to ascending pelvic inflammatory disease,[65] no solid clinical data suggest that this problem is generic to all IUDs. Tietze and Lewitt[66] reviewed the data from the CSP of the Population Council and found that the incidence of salpingitis in IUD wearers was highest during the first two weeks following insertion. After one month the incidence steadily diminished. The conclusion is that salpingitis occurring one month or more after an IUD has been inserted (with the possible exception of the Dalkon shield with its multifilament tail) is more likely to be a result of venereal contact than of irritation by the IUD. A major problem that hinders clarification of the pelvic infection problem is that pelvic inflammatory disease (PID) is difficult to classify as to onset, extent, and causative agent. Seldom do two physicians agree on the definition of PID. It has become a "wastebasket" diagnosis for lower abdominal pain, vaginal discharge, and fever. Until more precise diagnostic criteria are agreed upon for PID, the normal incidence of this disease in any selected population sample will not be known, and hence changing incidences relevant to IUDs will be difficult if not impossible to verify.

Embedding

Almost any type of foreign body within the endometrial cavity may impinge some portion of its body on the endometrium with sufficient force to cause pressure necrosis of the underlying tissue. If the pressure is maintained, the foreign body will gradually sink deeper and deeper into the tissue, and epithelium will overgrow in an attempt to restore the continuity of the original surface. The reparative process may include fibroblastic as well as myometrial proliferation. While this type of embedding is usually asymptomatic, there are at least two potentially serious consequences: (1) The area of exposed surface of the IUD is reduced, which may result in a lessened contraceptive effect. (2) Removal of the IUD may become very difficult because of the embedding and overgrowth of uterine tissue. Nonreactile stainless steel IUDs seem to have a special propensity to become embedded in the uterine wall. Because of this problem the FDA forced the Majzlin spring IUD off the market and confiscated unsold supplies of the device—the first time that the FDA asserted its legal power in reference to an IUD. (The second time that FDA pressure resulted in the recall of an IUD was in 1974 with the Dalkon shield bearing the complex multifilament tail.) The Dalkon shield also has problems related to its removal, some of which may be caused by embedding of the lateral spicules within the epithelium and myometrium.

Uterine Perforation

Two types of uterine perforations may be encountered with most types of IUDs: cervical and fundal. Both types are usually asymptomatic but require different removal procedures.

Cervical perforations Any IUD that has a dependent protuberance, such as the Saf-T-Coil, Lippes loop, Copper 7, and Copper T, may impinge upon one of the endocervical ruga as a result of downward displacement or partial expulsion. Repetitive uterine contractions may force this protuberance to penetrate into and occasionally through the cervical tissue and erode through the vaginal epithelium over the cervix and become visible in the vagina. While this perforation is usually clinically silent, the device should be removed by upward pressure through the cervical canal, with the withdrawal being completed after the dependent portion has reentered the cervical canal. The principal reason for removing the perforated device is that by this downward descent it loses considerable contraceptive effect. The actual diameter of the dependent protuberance seems to have relatively little to do with the frequency with which it may perforate the cervix.

Fundal perforations Perforation of the wall of the fundus by an IUD occurs most frequently when the device is inserted after delivery and before the uterus has involuted completely. During this puerperal interval the entire uterine wall is soft and easily perforated. Occasionally a patient complains of sudden sharp pain at the time of the insertion, but more often there are no unusual symptoms at the time of insertion. Some perforations probably begin as deep penetrations and gradually continue their migration through the uterine wall and into the abdominal cavity.

Some of the total perforations remain extraperitoneal, whereas others are within the peritoneal cavity. Although not proved, it seems logical to assume that a device found within the peritoneal cavity was probably placed there at the time of insertion. From an anatomical point of view, a device that has passed through the entire uterine wall and has remained in an extraperitoneal location probably began its perforation at the time of insertion and then completed the perforation by gradual erosion through the remainder of the uterine wall.

In any event, certain complications result from extrauterine location of an IUD: (1) They no longer provide contraception. (2) If they have entered the peritoneal cavity and are closed devices (defined as having a hole encircled by the material of the device of sufficient diameter to permit entrance of a knuckle of bowel), they should be removed as soon as their presence has been diagnosed. (*Note*: Closed devices having these characteristics cannot by law be used in the United States because of the potential danger of bowel strangulation.)

The copper-bearing devices, such as the Copper 7 and the Copper T, should be removed from the peritoneal cavity as soon as is medically feasible. Because of the foreign body tissue response to the metallic copper, these devices are usually rather promptly enclosed by the omentum and remain fixed by adhesions.

A nonmedicated open IUD, such as the Lippes loop, is much less apt to evoke tissue reaction and adhesions than is a copper-bearing device. For this reason, many physicians believe that there is no medical necessity to remove them from the peritoneal cavity.

The Dalkon shield evokes much more foreign body reaction and adhesions than does the Lippes loop.[67] There are at least two possible explanations for this: (1) The Dalkon shield has both copper salts and small particles of metallic copper within its plastic matrix. Sufficient copper probably leaches out of the plastic to evoke a marked degree of tissue reaction. (2) If the multifilament tail of the device has been in contact with the vaginal bacterial flora long enough to have become impregnated with bacteria before the uterine perforation, bacteria housed within the interstices of the tail could provide a reservoir that could repetitively seed the peritoneal cavity, thus causing a localized

inflammatory process of bacterial origin. Because of this potential hazard, the Dalkon shield should be removed surgically as soon as its extrauterine location has been detected.

19.12 Effect of IUDs on Subsequent Pregnancy

Two major questions always in the minds of women who select IUDs for contraception and of physicians who are responsible for their care are: (1) Will the use of an IUD affect the woman's subsequent fertility should she wish to have additional pregnancies, will these pregnancies have a normal course, and will they terminate with the birth of a normal baby? (2) In case of a contraceptive failure with an IUD *in utero*, how is the pregnancy best handled? Is the hazard to the mother and/or the fetus increased? If the mother desires to continue the pregnancy, should an attempt be made to remove the IUD, or should it be left in place? Since the most solid data available are on the nonmedicated Lippes loop and on the Copper T, I limit my comments to them, and because of the timeliness of the issue a few relevant comments will be made about the Dalkon shield.

Reversibility of IUD Contraception
Tietze[68] did a review of the case records of women in the CSP study who used the Lippes loop for contraception and had it removed because they desired another pregnancy. Based upon life table analyses, the data indicated that for short-term users (1–3 years), normal fertility returned. The time of onset of pregnancy in relation to the removal of the loop was indistinguishable from the preloop data. There are as yet no meaningful data concerning the restoration of fertility after long-term use of the loop. The numbers available are very small, since most long-term wearers are terminators rather than spacers. In addition, since normal fertility diminishes with age, this factor must be accurately incorporated into the evaluation of the data.

A review of the reversibility of fertility among Copper-T wearers has been made by Tatum et al.[69] Some 710 women who had removals for a planned pregnancy were followed. Of these, 83 percent conceived within the normally expected time interval. Of those whose pregnancies had terminated at the data cutoff date, the distribution of live births (full term or premature), stillbirths, spontaneous abortions, induced abortions, and ectopic pregnancies were within normal rates. It should be noted that these data refer to short-term users only (up to three years of Copper T use). Thus it is safe to conclude that the use of the Copper T as a pregnancy spacer for this interval of time does not influence subsequent fertility.

Since each type of IUD may have unique properties

that influence the subsequent restoration of fertility, clinical data must be made available before predictions are justified. An example in point is the situation with the Dalkon shield. Because bacteria from the vagina have been shown by Tatum et al.[70] to migrate upward through the interfibrillar spaces within the sheath through the entire length of the tail, these bacteria could enter the endometrial cavity and thus produce a bacterial endometritis that could spread to include the Fallopian tubes and ovaries. If such a sequence of events takes place, fertility could be substantially reduced. A prospective study of former wearers of the Dalkon shield should be made, with special attention directed to the restoration of fertility.

Accidental Pregnancy with the IUD in Place
As with the question of restoration of fertility, the clinical course and recommended management of the accidental pregnancy with an IUD in place must be considered with respect to each specific IUD.

Lewit[71] reviewed the course of accidental pregnancies within the CSP studies. She concluded from information available on the Lippes loop that a pregnancy occurring with a loop in situ had about a 50 percent chance of terminating by a spontaneous abortion. Most clinicians have assumed that this figure is typical of most IUDs.

In a review of accidental pregnancies associated with the Copper T, Tatum and Schmidt[72, 73] provided data as to the outcome of these pregnancies if the IUD (1) is removed or expelled or (2) remains in place during the pregnancy. There were 704 accidental pregnancies, of which only 4 percent were lost to follow-up; 212 of these women elected to continue their pregnancy even though it had been unplanned. In 94 of these, the Copper T was either expelled or removed early in the pregnancy (Group A). In 118 women the IUD remained in place throughout the pregnancy (Group B). The pregnancies terminated in spontaneous abortions in 29 percent of Group A and 54 percent of Group B. This suggests that the continued presence of the IUD increases the likelihood that the pregnancy will terminate in an abortion. Live births resulted for 71 percent of Group A and 44 percent of Group B. Of these, 4 percent of Group A and 19 percent of Group B were premature. Based upon these data, we have concluded that removal of the Copper T early in pregnancy enhances the chance that the pregnancy will terminate in a live full-term birth, whereas if the device is left in place, there is better than 50 percent chance that the pregnancy will end in a spontaneous abortion, and if it does not abort, there is a 19 percent chance of premature birth.

These data are predicated upon an additional, very

significant condition: It is best if the IUD is removed early in pregnancy—*provided* this can be accomplished easily and with a minimum of force and trauma. If extraction is not readily accomplished or if the tails are not visible, no attempt should be made to force the extraction. Therefore the ease of extracting a specific IUD will govern, to a large extent, the rate of continuation of the associated pregnancy. I would hypothesize that removal of a Lippes loop or a Dalkon shield during early pregnancy would be more difficult and would produce more uterine trauma than would removal of a Copper T, and that this additional trauma would result in a higher rate of spontaneous abortion.

In any case of accidental pregnancy that coincides with use of an IUD or a steroidal contraceptive method, the question of teratogenic action must be considered. Chang and Tatum[12] have shown in three species of laboratory animals that metallic copper does not result in any demonstrable congenital defects. These studies were carried through three successive generations. No evidence of altered development or reproductive functions could be detected. In our human data, we have estimated that more than 200 pregnancies were allowed to progress spontaneously and terminated in a live birth. There has been no evidence of an unusual incidence of congenital abnormalities.

A similar negative effect has been ascertained in regard to the incidence of cervical neoplasia in Copper-T wearers.

19.13 Summary: The IUD as a Modern Contraceptive Method

Intrauterine contraception is the only contraceptive method in the female that has the following attributes:

1. Locally acting (nonsystemic)

2. Single introduction provides protection for prolonged periods of time

3. Not related to coitus

4. Reversible

5. Long-acting (years)

6. Inexpensive—can be mass-produced

7. Can be initiated by trained paramedic personnel

8. With the development of the Copper T, and later the Copper 7, effective IUDs have become available for the nulligravid and nulliparous woman. Although these two groups of women are not now of great importance from a demographic standpoint, they will become so throughout the world in time and with an increased awareness by women in the developing areas of the world of the advantages of child spacing and family planning.

The IUD method has the following disadvantages:

1. Need of pelvic manipulation by a physician or paramedic

2. Increased duration of menstrual bleeding per cycle

3. Traditional taboo against intrauterine placement of foreign body, which must be overcome by education.

References

1. Oppenheimer, W. Prevention of pregnancy by the Graefenberg Ring method. A re-evaluation after 28 years' experience. Am. J. Obstet. Gynecol. 78:446, 1959.

2. Tatum, H.J. Intrauterine contraception. Am J. Obstet. Gynecol. 112:1000, 1972.

3. Potter, R.G. Application of life table techniques to measurement of contraceptive effectiveness. Demography 3:297, 1966.

4. Tietze, C., and S. Lewit. Recommended procedures for the statistical evaluation of intrauterine contraception. Stud. Fam. Plann. 4:35, February 1973.

5. Tatum, H.J., and J.A. Zipper. The T intrauterine contraceptive device and recent advances in hormonal anticonceptional therapy. Proc. Sixth Northeast Obstetrics-Gynecology Congress, p. 78, Bahia, Brasil, October 4–9, 1968.

6. Zipper, J.A., M. Medel, and R. Prager. Toxic action of copper and zinc on implantation rates in rabbits. Abstracts, Sixth World Congress on Fertility and Sterility, p. 154, Tel Aviv, Israel, May 1968.

7. Zipper, J.A., H.J. Tatum, L. Pastene, M. Medel, and M. Rivera. Metallic copper as an intrauterine contraceptive adjunct to the T device. Am. J. Obstet. Gynecol. 105:1274, 1969.

8. Tatum, H.J. Comparative experience with newer models of the Copper T device in the U.S. In *Analysis of intrauterine conception,* eds. F. Hefnawi and S. Segal. Amsterdam: North-Holland, 1975.

9. Tatum, H.J. Copper-bearing intrauterine devices. Clin. Obstet. Gynecol. 17(1):93, March 1974.

10. Furst, A., and R.T. Haro. A survey of metal carcinogenesis. Prog. Exp. Tumor Res. 12:102, 1969.

11. Gilman, J.P.W. Metal carcinogenesis. II. A study on the carcinogenesis activity of cobalt, copper, iron and nickel compounds. Cancer Res. 22:158, 1962.

12. Chang, C.C., and H.J. Tatum. Absence of teratogenicity of intrauterine copper wire in rats, hamsters and rabbits. Contraception 7:413, 1973.

13. White, I.G. The toxicity of heavy metals to mammalian spermatozoa. Aust. J. Exp. Biol. 33:359, 1955.

14. Saito, S., I.M. Bush, F. Willet, and J. Whitmore. Effects of certain metals and chelating agents on rat and dog epididymal spermatozoan motility. Fertil. Steril. 18:517, 1967.

15. Loewit, K. Immobilization of human spermatozoa with iron: Basis for a new contraceptive? Contraception 3:219, 1971.

16. Chang, C.C., and H.J. Tatum. A study of the antifertility effect of intrauterine copper. Contraception 1:265, 1970.

17. Robles, F., E. Lopez de la Osa, U. Lerner, E. Johansson, P. Brenner, K. Hagenfeldt, and E. Diczfalusy. α-amylase, glycogen synthetase and phosphorylase in the human endometrium: Influence of the cycle and of the Copper T device. Contraception 6:373, 1972.

18. Chatterji, S., and K.R. Laumas. Effect of a copper wire as an IUD on some rat uterine enzymes. Contraception 9:65, 1974.

19. Zipper, J.A., H.J. Tatum, M. Medel, L. Pastene, and R. Rivera. Contraception through the use of intrauterine metals. I. Copper as an adjunct to the T device. Am. J. Obstet. Gynecol. 109:771, 1971.

20. Cuadros, A., and J.G. Hirsch. Copper on intrauterine devices stimulates leukocyte exudation. Science 175:175, 1972.

21. El Sahwi, S., and D.L. Moyer. The leukocytic response to an intrauterine foreign body in the rabbit. Fertil. Steril. 22:398, 1971.

22. Hefnawi, F., H. Askalani, and K. Zaki. Menstrual blood loss with copper intrauterine devices. Contraception 9:133, 1974.

23. Israel, R., S.T. Shaw, and M.A. Martin. Comparative quantitation of menstrual blood loss with the Lippes Loop, Dalkon Shield and Copper T intrauterine devices. Contraception 10:63, 1974.

24. Tatum, H.J., and F.H. Schmidt. Unpublished data, 1975.

25. Mishell, D.R., R. Israel, and N. Freid. A study of the Copper T intrauterine contraceptive device (TCu 200) in nulliparous women. Am. J. Obstet. Gynecol. 116:1092, 1973.

26. Nygren, K.G., and E.D.B. Johansson. Insertions of endouterine Copper T (TCu 200) immediately after first trimester legal abortion. Contraception 7:299, 1973.

27. Timonen, H., and T. Luukkainen. Immediate postabortion insertion of the Copper T (TCu 200) with 18 months follow-up. Contraception 9:153, 1974.

28. Bernstein, G.S., R. Israel, P. Seward, and D.R. Mishell. Clinical experience with the Copper 7 intrauterine device. Contraception 6:99, 1972.

29. Mishell, D.R., Jr. The clinic factor in evaluating intrauterine devices. Paper presented at the Third International Conference on Intrauterine Contraception, Cairo, Egypt, December 12–14, 1974.

30. Lippes, J., M. Zielezny, P.A. Ferro, and H. Sultz. Comparisons of two copper-bearing loops (size A) Copper T and loop D plain. Adv. Plan. Parent. 9:153, February 1974.

31. Zipper, J.A., M. Medel, and R. Prager. Suppression of fertility by intrauterine copper and zinc in rabbits. Am. J. Obstet. Gynecol. 105:529, 1969.

32. Chang, C.C., H.J. Tatum, and F.A. Kincl. The effect of intrauterine copper and other metals on implantation in rats and hamsters. Fertil. Steril. 21:274, 1970.

33. Zipper, J.A., M. Medel, L. Pastene, R. Rivera, and H.J. Tatum. Human fertility control through the use of endouterine metal antagonisms of trace elements (EMATE). Nobel Symposium No. 15, eds. E. Diczfalusy and U. Borell, p. 199. Stockholm, Sweden: Almqvist & Wiksell, 1970.

34. Copper, R.L. Personal communication reported in H.J.

Tatum, Intrauterine contraception, Am. J. Obstet. Gynecol. 112:1000, 1972.

35. Anderson, T. J. IUD Workshop (Battelle), Seattle, Washington, October 18–20, 1973.

36. Doyle, L. L., and T. H. Clewe. Preliminary studies on the effect of hormone-releasing intrauterine devices. Am. J. Obstet. Gynecol. 101:564, 1968.

37. Croxatto, H. B., R. Vera, and M. A. Parga. Estudio comparado de la accion del acetato de megestrol sobre la fertilidad. Proc. Fourth Annual Meeting of ALIRH, p. 77. Mexico, April 5–9, 1970.

38. Scommegna, A., G. N. Pandya, M. Christ, A. W. Lee, and M. R. Cohen. Intrauterine administration of progesterone by a slow releasing device. Fertil. Steril. 21:201, 1970.

39. Clewe, T. H., and L. L. Doyle. Personal communication reported in H. J. Tatum, Intrauterine contraception, Am. J. Obstet. Gynecol. 112:1000, 1972.

40. Stryker, J. C., L. L. Doyle, T. H. Clewe, and J. Lippes. Silastic Lippes loop with crystallin appeal. Proc. Ninth Annual Meeting, American Association of Planned Parenthood Physicians, Kansas City, Missouri, April 5–6, 1971.

41. Martinez Manautou, J., R. Aznar, and A. Rosado. Clinical experience with the intrauterine progesterone-releasing systems. Paper presented at the Third International Conference on Intrauterine Contraception, Cairo, Egypt, December 12–14, 1974.

42. Davis, H. J., and R. Israel. Uterine cavity measurements in relation to design of intrauterine contraceptive devices. In *Intrauterine contraception*, Amsterdam: Excerpta Medica Series 86:135, 1965.

43. Davis, H. J. The shield intrauterine device. Am. J. Obstet. Gynecol. 106:455, 1970.

44. Tatum, H. J., F. H. Schmidt, D. Phillips, M. McCarty, and W. M. O'Leary. The Dalkon Shield controversy: Structural and bacteriological studies on IUD tails. JAMA 231: 711, 1975.

45. Fuchs, F., and A. Risk. The Antigon-F, an improved intrauterine contraceptive device. Contraception 5:119, 1972.

46. Fuchs, F., L. L. Cederquist, S. Donovan, and N. H. Lauersen. Comparison of Antigon-F, Copper T and Ypsilon intrauterine contraceptive devices, Paper presented at the Third International Conference on Intrauterine Contraception, Cairo, Egypt, December 12–14, 1974.

47. Soichet, S. Ypsilon: A new silicone-covered stainless steel intrauterine contraceptive device. Am J. Obstet. Gynecol. 114:938, 1972.

48. Rodriquez, W. Paper presented at Tenth Brazilian Congress of Obstetricians and Gynecologists, Curitiba, Brazil, October 1972.

49. Futoran, J. M., and S. Kitrilakis. Experience with a fluid-filled intrauterine device. Obstet. Gynecol. 43:81, 1974.

50. Sagiroglu, N. Local effects of polyethylene intrauterine devices in women. Abstracts, Proc. Third International Conference on Intrauterine Contraception, p. 38, 1974.

51. Ullmann, G., and J. Hammerstein. Inhibition of sperm motility in vitro by copper wire. Contraception 6:71, 1972.

52. Croxatto, H. B. Personal communication, February 1975.

53. Cuadros, A., M. Bueno, E. Cobo, and J. Zuñiga. SEM of human endometrium under the effect of intrauterine devices. Abstracts, Proc. Third International Conference on Intrauterine Contraception, p. 25, 1974.

54. Robles, F., E. Lopez de la Osa, U. Lerner, E. Johansson, P. Brenner, K. Hagenfeldt, and E. Dczfalusy. α-amylase, glycogen synthetase and phosphorylase in the human endometrium: Influence of the cycle and of the Copper T device. Contraception 6:373, 1972.

55. Joshi, S. G., and S. Sujan-Tejuja. Biochemistry of the human endometrium in users of the intrauterine contraceptive device. Fertil. Steril. 20:98, 1969.

56. Tatum, H. J., T. Luukkainen, and A. Kosonen. Personal communication, January 1975.

57. Hefnawi, F., H. Askalani, and K. Zaki. Menstrual blood loss with copper intrauterine devices. Contraception 9:133, 1974.

58. Liedholm, P., N. O. Sjoberg, and B. Astedt. Increased menstrual blood loss and increased fibrinolytic activity of endometrium in women using copper intrauterine devices. Abstracts, Proc. Third International Conference on Intrauterine Contraception, p. 30, 1974.

59. Israel, R., S. T. Shaw, and M. A. Martin. Comparative quantitation of menstrual blood loss with the Lippes Loop, Dalkon Shield and Copper T intrauterine devices. Contraception 10:63, 1974.

60. Shaw, S. T., and D. L. Moyer. Problem bleeding with intrauterine devices. In *Intrauterine devices: Development, evaluation and program implementation*, eds. R. G. Wheeler, G. W. Duncan, and J. J. Speidel, p. 99. New York: Academic Press, 1974.

61. Shaw, S. T., R. W. Cihak, and D. L. Moyer. Fibrin proteolysis in the monkey uterine cavity: Variations with and without intrauterine device. Nature 228:1097, 1970.

62. Shaw, S. T., J. M. Jimenez, D. L. Moyer, and R. W. Cihak. Relationship of endometrial plasminogen activator to fibrin proteolysis in the uterine cavity of rhesus monkeys. Am. J. Obstet. Gynecol. 115:983, 1973.

63. Westrom, L., and L. P. Bengtsson. Effect of tranexamic acid (AMCA) in menorrhagia with intrauterine contraceptive devices. J. Reprod. Med. 5:154, 1970.

64. Hefnawi, F., A. A. Saleh, and O. Kandil. Intrauterine devices and blood loss. Abstracts, Proc. Third International Conference on Intrauterine Contraception, p. 28, 1974.

65. Tatum, H. J., F. H. Schmidt, D. Phillips, M. McCarty, and W. M. O'Leary. The Dalkon Shield controversy: Structural and bacteriological studies of IUD tails. JAMA 231: 711, 1975.

66. Tietze, C., and S. Lewit. Evaluation of intrauterine devices: Ninth progress report to the Cooperative Statistical Program. Stud. Fam. Plann. 55:1, 1970.

67. Whitson, L. G., R. Israel, and G. S. Bernstein. The extrauterine Dalkon Shield. Obstet. Gynecol. 44:418, 1974.

68. Tietze, C. Fertility after discontinuation of intrauterine and oral contraception, Proc. Sixth World Congress on Fertility and Sterilization, p. 237, Tel Aviv, Israel, 1968.

69. Tatum, H. J., F. H. Schmidt, and I. Sivin. Abstracts, Proc. Third International Conference on Intrauterine Contraception, p. 13, 1974.

70. Tatum, H. J., F. H. Schmidt, and D. Phillips. Morphological studies of Dalkon Shield tails removed from patients. Contraception 11:465, 1975.

71. Lewit, S. Outcome of pregnancy with intrauterine devices. Contraception 2:47, 1970.

72. Tatum, H. J., and F. H. Schmidt. Abstracts, Proc. Third International Conference on Intrauterine Contraception, p. 13, 1974.

Late Additions

Tatum, H. J., F. S. Schmidt, and A. K. Jain. Management and outcome of accidental pregnancies associated with copper T intrauterine devices. Am. J. Obstet. Gynecol. 126:869, 1976.

Tatum, H. J. Clinical aspects of intrauterine contraception: Circumspection 1976. Fertil. Steril. 28:3, 1977.

*Note added in proof: The Copper T model TCu-200B was approve by the USFDA on November 4, 1976.

20 The Morning-After Pill: A Report on Postcoital Contraception and Interception

John McLean Morris

20.1 Recent Developments

In 1963 postcoital contraception did not exist. The physician had nothing to offer the patient after exposure other than a douche or an abortion. But sufficient evidence had accumulated in rabbit studies and in the macaque monkey colony of van Wagenen that a notice appeared in the Yale–New Haven Hospital bulletin board:

VOLUNTEERS WANTED
Parous women—earn money each cycle
and help the wheels of science revolve

Three years later the first 100 successful midcycle exposures in women without pregnancy had been reported, and the term *morning-after pill* had been coined by the lay press. As estrogens do not interfere with fertilization and are therefore not contraceptives, the more scientifically correct term *interceptive* has been suggested for agents that interfere with implantation.

Historical Background

Interest at Yale in postcoital interception started in 1961 with the not-too-original idea that various alkaloids and antimetabolites used in treating gestational trophoblastic disease might interfere with implantation or development of the fertilized ovum and contribute to the development of postcoital conception control measures.

Based on observations made in rodents at this time by Segal and Nelson and subsequently by Chang, Blye, Greenwald, Duncan, and others, a group of nonsteroidal estrogen antagonists were added to the cytotoxic agents. While most of these agents proved effective in interrupting pregnancy in the rabbit, only one showed no evidence of teratogenicity and was found effective postcoitally in the macaque monkey. This compound, ORF-3858 (2-methyl-3-ethyl-4-phenyl-Δ-4 cyclohexenecarboxylic acid), described as an antiestrogen, led ultimately to a questioning of the use of such labels as antiestrogens, impeded estrogens, progestogen, antiprogestogen. Their definitions may be based on a special laboratory test, such as inhibition of the uterotropic activity of estradiol in the mouse or Clauberg, McPhail, or McGinty procedures in the rabbit, which may be somewhat misleading. All of the antiestrogens tested showed good uterotropic activity in the mouse, in general proportional to their effectiveness as postcoital agents and almost exactly proportional to their ability to compete with estradiol binding in the macromolecular fraction of human endometrium.

An Ortho Pharmaceutical report on ORF-3858 states that this compound is not estrogenic in the monkey. In terms of vaginal cornification, changes in the monkey's sex skin, and pattern of sexual behavior, it is highly estrogenic. These findings led to a study of steroidal and nonsteroidal estrogens.

As is often the case in scientific advance, we were unaware that the initial observations in this area had been made nearly 40 years previously and that it had taken this long to result in the clinical application of a laboratory observation.

Postovulatory Estrogen Interception

In 1926 Parkes and Bellerby in England and Smith at Johns Hopkins observed that crude ovarian extracts could interrupt pregnancy in the rat. In the subsequent three and a half decades very little was published on this matter. In 1963 Parkes noted "that there has been so far as I know, no determined effort to see whether the administration of estrogen during the third week of the human cycle would prevent any implantation that might otherwise take place." There were, however, some unpublished endeavors during this period that are perhaps worthy of note.

Throughout central Europe, particularly in Germany, efforts were made in the late 1940s to terminate early pregnancies with massive doses of stilbestrol. This method is unsuccessful when gonadotropin titers have reached certain levels. Van Wagenen and Dorfman administered large doses of theelin, diethylstilbestrol, and estradiol dipropionate to pregnant monkeys to observe the effect on the pregnancies. There was no interruption of pregnancy or any detectable effects on either mother or offspring. This work was not published.

In 1958 Eleanor Mears in London followed Parkes's suggestion more literally when she administered stilbestrol to women in the third week of the menstrual cycle. In eight cycles there were five pregnancies. This led her to the conclusion that estrogen would not interfere with implantation in women. The dosage used, however, was 3 to 10 mg per day. Although unpublished, these records were carefully kept and accompanied by temperature charts. Of interest is the fact that one of the patients did have the characteristic temperature drop with estrogen, but the pregnancy continued unaffected by the medication.

This work was unknown when a reasonably systematic study was undertaken at Yale of postcoital antifertility compounds in rabbits and subsequently in macaques and in humans. In essence the study showed that every compound that was uterotropic in the mouse was successful in preventing pregnancy in the rabbit, with the single exception of d-norgestrel. Other 19-norsteroids, androgens, stilbenes, triarylalkanes, diphenylindines, natural estrogens (conjugated, esterified, or unconjugated estrone, estradiol, estriol), and synthetic steroidal estrogens tested were, at various doses, effective interceptive agents. Some rather weak uterotropins such as testosterone, dihydrotestosterone, and estriol had a much higher ratio of antifertility effectiveness (rabbit) to uterotropic activity (mouse) than compounds such as estradiol. Digitalis, which will produce vaginal cornification but which is not uterotropic, was completely ineffective as an interceptive compound. Effective interceptive agents tested in the rabbit or in the macaque monkey include the following:

Estrone

Estradiol

Estriol

Ethinyl estradiol

Mestranol

Stilbestrol

Stilbestrol diphosphate

Clomid (MRL-41)

U11, 100A

U11, 555A

ORF-3858

RS-2874

RS-4574

Norethindrone

Conjugated estrogen (Premarin)

Esterified estrogen (Evex)

Sch-10015

Testosterone

Dihydrotestosterone

RS-2196

RS-2290

Dromostanolone

Oxymetholone

Chlorotrianisene (Tace)

Ethanoxytriphetol (Mer-25).

Emmens (1970) has reviewed the types and structures of compounds with postcoital antifertility activity. Certain cytotoxic agents and immunological techniques have also been effective in interrupting pregnancy.

In addition to requirements of effectiveness, interception involves the serious danger that at marginal doses or with incorrect timing a compound may prove teratogenic. This has not been observed with postcoital estrogens, but teratogenesis has been noted with a variety of other interceptive agents (Morris 1970).

Clinical effectiveness On the basis of continued success in the primate colony, it was felt that it would be safe to try interception as a contraceptive technique in women. This was first done in 1963. Volunteers were for the most part nurses, laboratory workers, and doctors' wives. Almost all were parous, had consorts of known fertility, and agreed to keep track of the time of intercourse. Huhner tests were done in almost all instances. (In general it has not been our policy to treat patients in the absence of a positive Huhner test.) The first 100 cycles were reported in 1966. There were no pregnancies in this series. The drugs originally used were stilbestrol, 25–50 mg/day; ethinyl estradiol, 0.5–2 mg/day; and in a few instances intravenous Premarin, 25 mg × 2. The latter was given usually because the patient came in on the third or fourth day following exposure. Subsequently the occurrence of pregnancies in the monkey at the 0.5 mg dose of ethinyl estradiol and one at the 1 mg dose caused us to abandon clinical use of this compound and substitute Premarin, 50 mg/day, although ethinyl estradiol has subsequently been shown by others to be effective.

The reason for the dosage and timing should be explained. There was no question from laboratory evidence that estrogen was an effective interceptive agent if given during the immediate postovulatory period. If x is the effective daily dose of an estrogen in the rabbit, the estrogen could be given as a single large dose ($5x$), but proved more effective if divided into three small doses ($3x$) during the preimplantation period. The dose of estrogen necessary to interrupt early established implantation was found to be approximately $30x$. The effectiveness, if any, of large doses of an estrogen in the preovulatory period appeared to be merely a reflection of sufficient estrogen levels persisting into the postovulatory period to the extent that implantation was prevented.

In terms of clinical effectiveness, estrogen must be considered a postovulatory rather than postcoital antifertility agent. If one used the commonly accepted three-day survival period for sperm in the female genital tract, and a postovulatory treatment period of three days was planned, then a five to six day period of administration might be required.

As the work progressed, it became evident that the effective survival time of sperm in the female genital tract was unknown. We have in a number of instances observed many motile sperm in cervical mucus five to seven days after exposure. Since these sperm are probably capable of fertilization, postcoital estrogen taken even after six days might be ingested prior to ovulation. Thus it would seem that any large series claiming 100 percent effectiveness with estrogen as an interceptive, unless all cases were single midcycle exposures, might be questioned in terms of accuracy of follow-up. Laboratory data and clinical experience suggest that the method itself is essentially 100 percent effective and that failures are probably related to timing or to failure to take a sufficient amount of estrogen.

Shortly after the initial report on postcoital estrogen in women was presented in 1966, other investigators confirmed the clinical observations, the largest series being those of Kuchera at the University of Michigan and McKinnon at UCLA with stilbestrol, and Haspels in Holland, using principally ethinyl estradiol. Effectiveness of estrogen interception in various reported and unreported series is summarized in Table 20.1.

Approximately 10 percent of the reported pregnancies have been ectopic. Side effects (principally nausea and vomiting) have been less with ethinyl estradiol, Premarin, or enteric-coated stilbestrol than with regular diethylstilbestrol or stilbestrol diphosphate. Cycle length has not been significantly altered. The stilbestrol induction of vaginal adenosis when given during organogenesis of the reproductive tract in the first trimester of pregnancy has been used quite erroneously to discourage the clinical use of estrogen interception.

Previllous implantation can be interrupted in some instances with very much higher doses of estrogen, but this is unsuccessful if gonadotropin (hCG) titers have reached significant levels.

Coital Progestogen Contraception

The interceptive action of estrogen as a postovulatory contraceptive must not be confused, as has been done by some, with the use of progestogens as coital contraceptives.

Some 19-norsteroids have been found to be weak interceptive agents. Nygren et al. (1972) in Sweden administered norethindrone 200 mg to 80 women at the end of the third week of the cycle, with 22 pregnancies in 301 cycles, resulting in a rather dismal Pearl index of 87.7. Lower doses (10–25 mg/day) given earlier on days 15–22, however, resulted in 17 pregnancies in 700 cycles, giving a much lower Pearl index of 29.2

In evaluating reports of the use of progestogens as

Table 20.1 Estrogen interception

Report	Estrogens Used[a]	No. of Cycles	Failures Related to: Timing/Dose	Method	Failure Rate Percent	Pearl Index
Morris and van Wagenen (1967)	DES, EE, CE	100	0	0	0	0
Kuchera (1971)	DES	1,000	0	0	0	0
Döring (1971)	EE, CE	32	0	0	0	0
Massey et al. (1971)	DES	247	4	0	1.6	19.2
Haspels (1972)	EE, DES, CE	2,000	14	0	0.7	8.4
Morris et al. (1973)	DES, EE, CE	750	7	1	1.1	13.2
McKinnon (1973)	DES	1,200	0	0	0	0
Schumacher (1973)	DES	257	0	0	0	0
Lehfeldt (1973)	EE	133	1	0	0.8	9.6
Kuchera (1973)	DES	298	6	0	3.0	36.0
Unreported series	DES, EE, CE	4,438[b]	6	3	0.2	1.2
Hall (1974)	DES	107	0	0	0	0
Total		10,462	38	4	0.4	4.8

[a] DES—diethylstilbestrol—(recommended dose 50 mg for 5 days); EE—ethinyl estradiol—(recommended dose 5 mg for 5 days); CE—conjugated estrogens—(recommended dose 50 mg for 5 days). [b] Approximate figure reported to author by various investigators.

postcoital contraceptives, it must be borne in mind that in animal studies progesterone itself is effective as a contraceptive only if taken in the preovulatory period (Morris 1973). The frequency of intercourse in some of the series, as reported in Table 20.2, was 7 to 11 times per cycle. Thus the midcycle exposure was probably protected not by the progestogen taken at that time but by the medication taken several days earlier.

Dosages in most instances are considerably larger than dosages contained in the daily minipill regimens, and in essence one may be taking pills throughout the cycle that prevent fertilization rather than acting as interceptives to prevent implantation. With an average of 10 exposures per cycle, the total dose per cycle would be 10 times that listed. Pregnancy rates were generally higher in the cycles with less frequent exposures. In some series it was felt that medication should precede the initial exposure by six hours, which is essentially the time required for a progestogen to change cervical mucus to the postovulatory pattern.

While these regimes appear to be effective, complications are essentially the same as those encountered with the use of the minipill, the principal one being bleeding or shortened cycles. But the medication was, in general, well accepted by the patient and effective at the higher dose levels.

There appears to be a very real place for coital con-traception (see Shearman 1973), but, as noted below, the differences between C-21 progestogens and most 19-norsteroids are sufficient that it may not be possible to use the two types of compounds interchangeably.

20.2 Basic Mechanisms and Gaps in Knowledge

Estrogens
Estrogens in the postovulatory period do not appear to have any direct effect on the blastocyst or to act on the basis of tubal transport. In the luteal phase they do alter the progestational endometrium and the uterine environment, as manifested by lowering of endometrial carbonic anhydrase. They also produce significant histological changes in the endometrium. The latter include stromal edema, hemorrhage, and loss of decidua. Glands show a persistence of basal vacuoles containing glycogen, persistence of cell membranes, and little or no secretion into the gland lumen. The histological picture prior to menstruation in treated women is sometimes similar to the Arias-Stella type of reaction. Histochemical staining shows a decreased alkaline phosphatase. With the electron microscope, destruction of the nucleolar channel system produced by progesterone can be demonstrated within 12 hours of estrogen administration.

Systemic manifestations of postovulatory estrogen

Table 20.2 Coital progestogen contraception

Report	Drug	Dose (mg)	No. of Cycles	No. of Pregnancies	Pearl Index
Rubio et al. (1970)	quingestanol	0.2	50	7	168
		0.3	100	3	36
		0.4	72	1	16.6
		0.5	927	5	6.5
		0.75	28	0	0
		0.8	1,004	0	0
Total			2,181	16	8.8
Kesserü et al. (1973)	d-norgestrel	0.15	239	9	45.2
		0.25	8,762	45	6.2
		0.3	4,085	23	6.8
		0.35	3,158	13	4.9
		0.4	25,558	75	3.5
Total			41,802	165	4.7
Zanartu et al. (1974)	retroprogestogen	40.0	783	3	4.5
	clogestone acetate	1.0	465	1	2.5
	norgestrieone	0.5	452	1	2.6
	ethynodiol diacetate	0.5	130	4	36.9
Total			1,830	9	5.9

include a lowering of serum progesterone levels (Johansson 1973) and of basal body temperature. The luteolytic effect has been demonstrated by a number of investigators including Johansson, Knobil, Auletta, Gore, and Board, but the mechanism has not been entirely explained. The administration of chorionic gonadotropin may bring progesterone values back to pretreatment levels, but the interceptive effect of estrogen cannot be reversed by concomitant progesterone administration.

There is evidence that progesterone alters carbohydrate pathways, increasing Krebs cycle activity and aerobic glycolysis with accumulation of high-energy phosphate bands. This appears to be reversed by estrogen back to the Emden-Myerhof pathway and hexose monophosphate shunt. Thus the blastocyst requirements for energy oxygen and conversion of CO_2 to bicarbonate in the previllous stage of implantation are no longer met after estrogen administration.

Progestogens

In defining progestogen it is important to point out the fundamental differences between the C-21 progestogens and the 19-norsteroids. In contrast to C-21 progestogens, 19-norsteroids in general:

1. will not maintain pregnancy in oophorectomized rodents

2. are uterotropic in high doses

3. will not produce nucleolar channel systems in human endometrium

4. may be virilizing in some instances, or have a virilizing effect on the fetus

5. have certain effects on carbohydrate and lipid metabolism

6. may lower the elevated endometrial carbonic anhydrase levels produced by progesterone.

The major contraceptive action of preovulatory progesterone appears to be on cervical mucus, causing interference with sperm transport. Effects demonstrated in the rabbit include interference with fertilization and increased ovum transport. Degenerating fertilized ova can be recovered, and the finding of fetal malformations after progesterone administration at the time of coitus in the rabbit suggests that the presence of increased progesterone immediately prior to ovulation could conceivably have a deleterious effect on the fetus.

Gaps in Our Knowledge

Unanswered questions concerning implantation relate both to the blastocyst and to the implantation site. What are the metabolic requirements of the blastocyst for preimplantation survival? Does the blastocyst depend on gonadotropin for prevention of immunological rejection? When does the fertilized ovum start to secrete gonadotropin? Is it present in the preimplantation blastocyst? Does the blastocyst have an angiogenesis factor to induce maternal blood supply? Why do rabbit blastocysts space evenly? What is the mechanism of ectopic pregnancy? Is it increased by estrogen? What is the role of the nucleolar channel system? What is decidua? What, if any, is the role of histamine? Are blastokinin or uterotropin related to carbonic anhydrase or other similar enzymes? What is the role of progesterone receptors? Can immunological means be used to prevent implantation? What is the role of carbonic anhydrase inhibitors? Why must the timing of fertilization, blastocyst development, implantation, and the hormonal environment be so exact?

Unanswered questions concerning ovarian hormones include the mechanism of their effect on basal body temperature and carbohydrate pathways. The role of prostaglandins in interception, if any, should be clarified. What is the mechanism of the nausea produced by estrogen? Is it related to effects on the liver or possibly even to prostaglandins? Further study should be applied to the effect of estrogen on müllerian duct development and on the fetal vagina, as well as to the possible role of preovulatory progesterone in fetal malformation.

Of more practical value is the possibility of effective estrogen-progesterone combination for midcycle protection against pregnancy. Would structural alterations in the steroid molecule or other estrogen or progestogen analogs yield an effective coital or postcoital pill? Would combinations of estrogens, 3-β-ol dehydrogenase inhibitors, carbonic anhydrase inhibitors, progesterone receptor binding agents, etc., prove more effective? Is there a practical role for hormones in contraception other than the prevention of ovulation?

20.3 Summary

There is no such thing as the ideal contraceptive that would fit every circumstance. Gynecological patients seek four types of fertility control.

The first are planners who come in before the fact seeking contraception. The best solution for them might be a symptom-free 100 percent effective device installed in the vagina, cervix, or uterus at a suitable time after puberty and removed only when the wearer consciously reaches the decision to have a child. An alternate ideal contraceptive would be an effective, nontoxic, and nonteratogenic pill or spermacide at the bedside table, taken at the time of exposure.

A second group of planners are those who have had

their family and wish sterilization. For this group a simple outpatient technique is needed for permanent sterilization or immunization against pregnancy.

There will always be those, however, who do not plan ahead. For the nonplanners coming in immediately after unprotected exposure, an interceptive technique is needed, assuming conception may have indeed already occurred.

And fourth, for those who have an implanted but unwanted pregnancy, a simple medical abortifacient is required.

Expressed in outline form, there are clinical requirements for:

A. Planners (before)
1. Contraception: IUD, pill, spermicide
2. Sterilization: glue, clip, immunization

B. Nonplanners (after)
3. Interception: postcoital pill
4. Abortion: medical abortifacient

The need for all four—contraception, sterilization, interception, and abortion—is evident. While planners probably outnumber nonplanners, the need for interception, particularly for those who are not having frequent intercourse or do not plan ahead, is borne out by a recent study from Johns Hopkins, which showed that of 2.4 million adolescent girls, less than half used any contraception at the time of their last intercourse.

If one assumes that a minimum of 1 percent of these unprotected exposures resulted in pregnancy and that an abortion would cost $200, postcoital pills might have saved $2.4 million in this group alone. Add to this the human anguish involved, and it becomes clear that research in interception is needed.

Contraception is not a take-it-or-leave-it matter. The future of mankind depends, not on the conquest of cancer or of space, but on the control of human reproduction.

References

Döring, G. K. Pille danach. Dtsch. Med. Wochenschr 97: 529, 1972.

Emmens, C. W. Postcoital contraception. Br. Med. Bull. 26: 45, 1970.

Hall, M. N. Use of the "morning-after-pill" in a college student health service. J. Am. Coll. Health Assoc. 22:395, 1974.

Haspels, A. A. Postcoital estrogen in large doses. IPPF Med. Bull. 6:3, 1972.

Johansson, E. D. B. Inhibition of the corpus luteum function in women taking large doses of diethylstilbestrol. Contraception 8:27, 1973.

Kesserü, E., A. Larrañaga, and J. Parada. Postcoital conception with d-norgestrel. Contraception 7:367, 1973.

Kuchera, L. K. Postcoital contraception with diethylstilbesterol. JAMA 218:562, 1971.

Kuchera, L. K. The morning-after pill. JAMA 224:1038, 1973.

Lehfeldt, H. Choice of ethinyl estradiol as a postcoital pill. Am. J. Obstet. Gynecol. 116:892, 1973.

Morris, J. McL., and G. van Wagenen. Compounds interfering with ovum implantation and development. III. The role of estrogens. Am. J. Obstet. Gynecol. 96:804, 1966.

Morris, J. McL., and G. van Wagenen. Postcoital oral contraception. Proc. Eighth Int. Conf. of IPPF, p. 256. Santiago, 1967.

Morris, J. McL. Postcoital antifertility agents and their teratogenic effect. Contraception 2:85, 1970.

Morris, J. McL., and G. van Wagenen. Interception: The use of postovulatory estrogens to prevent implantation. Am. J. Obstet. Gynecol. 115:101, 1973.

Morris, J. McL. Mechanisms involved in progesterone contraception and estrogen interception. Am. J. Obstet. Gynecol. 117:167, 1973.

Nygren, K-G., E. D. B. Johansson, and L. Wide. Postovulatory contraception in women with large doses of norethindrone. Contraception 5:445, 1972.

Rubio, B., E. Berman, A. Larrañaga, E. Guiloff, and J. J. Aguirre. A new postcoital oral contraception. Contraception 1:303, 1970.

Shearman, R. P. Postcoital contraception: A review. Contraception 7:459, 1973.

Zanartu, J. J., A. Dabancens, C. Oberti, R. Rodriquez-Bravo, and M. Garcia-Huidobro. Low-dosage oral progestogens to control fertility. Obstet. Gynecol. 43:87, 1974.

21 Injectable Contraceptive Preparations

Daniel R. Mishell, Jr.

The availability of a method of contraception that can be administered by injection at periodic intervals, varying from several months to a year or more, is an extremely important aspect of contraceptive development. There would be several advantages in developing such a method. These advantages include ease of administration by relatively untrained personnel and a probable high rate of acceptance by many people in developing countries who are accustomed to receiving injections for disease control. During the past decade a few injectable methods of contraception have been developed and used clinically. In addition, the use of prostaglandin injections as early abortifacients has undergone preliminary clinical trials. The injectable contraceptives developed thus far consist of long-acting progestogen preparations that are administered at intervals of one to six months.

21.1 Present Status

A total of four different injectable steroid formulations have undergone extensive clinical trials. One of these, depomedroxyprogesterone acetate (DMPA), a microcrystaline suspension of the progestogen, administered in a dosage of 150 mg every three months, is marketed in many countries throughout the world and has recently been released for restricted use as a contraceptive in the United States. Studies have also been undertaken with 300 mg of DMPA administered every six months, norethindrone enanthate, 200 mg every 12 weeks, and a combination of dihydroxyprogesterone acetofenide and estradiol enanthate monthly. This last preparation is reported to be widely used in Mexico, where many women request an injectable method of contraception. Clinical trials with norethindrone enanthate have involved 3,851 women for 39,712 cycles with an overall pregnancy rate of 0.66 per 100 woman-years.[1] Although there are relatively few published studies of clinical trials with this preparation, the 200 mg injection needs to be given exactly every 12 weeks, as this is the duration of the contraceptive effect. The pregnancy rate is increased when the injection is given at intervals of three months instead of 84 days.[2] Plans are now under way to expand clinical trials with various dosages of this agent, and WHO is planning to initiate trials in their network of Clinical Research

Centres to compare the effectiveness and bleeding patterns of norethindrone enanthate and DMPA.

DMPA, given in a dosage of 150 mg every three months, has been studied in more than 14,000 women for more than 150,000 woman-months of experience. As this formulation has been the most widely used injectable method of contraception, a considerable number of investigative reports have appeared concerning various aspects of its contraceptive use.

Use of DMPA injections provides a very effective method of contraception. Pregnancy rates from individual clinics with substantial numbers of patients vary from 0.0 to 0.5 per 100 woman-years. A clinical review in which the collective experience of 54 investigators with 3,857 women and a total of 72,215 woman-months' experience was published in 1973.[3] In this collaborative study, the drug failure (pregnancy) rate with the Pearl formula was 0.25 pregnancies per 100 woman-years, and with life table analysis, 0.31 pregnancies per 100 women at 12 months. Results of a similar collaborative study with DMPA, in doses of 300 mg every six months to 991 women for a total of 21,470 woman-months, were reported in 1972.[4] Using the Pearl formula, the pregnancy rate with this formulation was 1.73 per 100 woman-years; using life table analysis, the pregnancy rate at 12 months per 100 women was 2.28. As the contraceptive action of 150 mg usually lasts longer than three months, patients who delay receiving their next scheduled injection for a few weeks still remain protected against accidental pregnancy, and thus the effectiveness of this preparation is enhanced. It is advised that the drug be administered by deep intramuscular injection in the gluteal region without manual massage.

The drug acts in at least three different ways: First, it inhibits secretion of gonadotropins, especially the cyclic release of LH, and thus it inhibits ovulation; second, it increases the viscosity of cervical mucus, preventing the penetration of spermatozoa into the uterine cavity; and finally, it alters the endometrium in such a way as to diminish glandular proliferation and thus to impede nourishment of the blastocyst within the endometrial cavity.

A study using a radioimmunoassay method to measure blood levels of this drug showed relatively high fluctuating levels present for about the first three weeks after administration.[5] Thereafter the levels decreased with less fluctuation. The duration of pharmacologically effective serum levels has not been definitely established. In three women in whom serum gonadotropins were measured daily after a single injection of 150 mg DMPA, inhibition of the midcycle gonadotropin peak occurred for a variable period of time, from 110 to 155 days.[6] During treatment with DMPA, daily blood levels of both LH and FSH show some fluctuation, but the levels are generally similar to levels seen in the luteal phase of ovulatory cycles. After an injection of DMPA, daily measurement of serum progesterone revealed levels of this hormone to be persistently less than 1 ng/ml, indicating that ovulation is inhibited.[7]

Daily estradiol levels show only slight fluctuation and are usually in the range found in the early follicular phase of the normal menstrual cycle. Estradiol was measured in individual serum samples obtained from a group of women who had been receiving 150 mg injections of DMPA every three months for one to five years. Estradiol levels in these women were also mostly in the range of the early follicular phase of ovulatory cycles with mean levels about 40 μg/ml—significantly higher than estradiol levels in postmenopausal women.

When patients receiving the drug for long periods of time were examined, they were found to have a decreased uterine size, but no other signs or symptoms of de-estrogenization. There was no subjective decrease in breast size, and their vaginas remained moist and well rugated. Histological examination of the endometrium of patients at intervals during the first year of DMPA therapy showed no evidence of secretory endometrium.[8] The incidence of proliferative endometrium decreased rapidly after initiation of therapy with the majority of patients, showing either a low-lying quiescent type of endometrium with small, narrow, widely spaced glands and a pseudodecidual reaction in the stroma or an extremely scant atrophic type of endometrium. In contrast to the metabolic effects noted with the combination estrogen-progestogen oral contraceptives, no apparent changes in liver function, lipid metabolism, or blood pressure have been noted during DMPA treatment.[9] There is some evidence, however, that DMPA at a dosage of 150 mg every three months causes some deterioration of glucose tolerance and an increase in plasma insulin levels.[10] Although there is some evidence for a glucocorticoid effect of this steroid in animals, there is no consistent evidence of glucocorticoid activity in humans at the doses used in contraceptive formulation. Nearly all clinical studies demonstrate a significant gain in body weight during therapy, related to duration of usage.[3]

Beagle dogs treated with high doses of DMPA have an increased incidence of mammary cancer. Similar tumors in dogs have also been noted following administration of high doses of other related C-21 progestogens. Studies with DMPA in the monkey[11] as well as in humans have to date shown no increased incidence of mammary carcinoma, although adequate long-term epidemiological studies in the human have not been undertaken. The relevance of the carcinogenic effect of DMPA in the beagle to the development of breast cancer in humans is not known at the present time. Because high doses of the 19-nortestosterone type of progestogens are not associated with an increase in mammary tumors in beagles, the FDA decided that oral contraceptive preparations containing progestogens of the C-21 17-α-acetoxy type should be removed from the market, as these preparations have no advantages over compounds containing the 19-nortestosterone progestogens. Because the depot-injectable medroxyprogesterone acetate preparation is unique and has high efficacy as a contraceptive, however, the FDA decided that its benefit-risk ratio justified its use as a contraceptive in the United States for special patient populations.[12]

Patients receiving this drug show complete disruption of the normal menstrual cycle and a totally irregular bleeding pattern. During the three months after the first injection, the majority of patients bleed between 8 and 30 days of each 30-day time period.[8] Thereafter the incidence of increased bleeding gradually diminishes, and the majority of patients become completely amenorrheic after six months of therapy. Thereafter the incidence of amenorrhea continues to increase in direct proportion to the time in therapy, while the incidence of increased bleeding steadily diminishes. When bleeding does occur, it is usually not excessive and frequently is characterized as spotting. Menstrual bleeding can be regularized by the cyclic administration of oral estrogen,[13] and its use in conjunction with DMPA has been advocated by some to provide temporary regularization of excessive irregular bleeding.

At the end of one year, approximately 10 to 15 percent of women using this preparation discontinue because of irregular bleeding.[3,14] About 5 percent discontinue for other medical reasons, such as headache, nervousness, or weight gain. There is wide variation among clinical studies in the reported overall continuation rates at the end of one year. Studies using the life table method of data analysis report that only about 57 to 65 percent of the patients choosing this method of contraception continue using it after one year.[3,14] After discontinuing DMPA treatment, about half the patients resume a regular cyclic menstrual pattern within six months and about 75 percent have regular menses within one year.[14] When bleeding does resume after the effect of the last injection is dissipated, it is initially regular in about half the patients and irregular in the remainder.[15] In one study, some of the women were treated with hormonal steroids for a short time to induce regular menses.

McDaniel reported that of 226 Thai women who wished to conceive after discontinuing DMPA contraceptive therapy, about two-thirds had conceived at the end of nine months and three-fourths had conceived at the end of one year.[16] These data indicate that the cumulative pregnancy rate at the end of one year after stopping DMPA is less than that after discontinuing use of the IUD or conventional contraceptives. Because the patients in McDaniel's study received an estrogen supplement during a portion of each month, their incidence of resumption of fertility may have been higher than that of women treated with DMPA alone. The unpredictability of the time of onset of spontaneous ovulation after stopping DMPA therapy limits its use to women who are not at the time planning a future pregnancy.

21.2 Gaps in Our Knowledge

Despite the many published reports, there remain many gaps in our knowledge of the use of steroids and other possible injectable methods of contraception. We do not know whether the prolonged inhibition of ovulation caused by both DMPA and norethindrone enanthate occurs because of the inhibitory effect of the initial high blood levels of the drugs upon the hypothalamus or because of the prolonged duration of low blood levels—or a combination of both effects. For DMPA, we need to know whether the prolonged low levels of circulating estrogens are harmful to women and whether prolonged usage of the drug is carcinogenic in women as it is in beagles. Sociological studies also need to be undertaken to determine the acceptability of amenorrhea in various cultures. Much more needs to be known about the predictability of resumption of ovulation and fertility and whether use of long-acting steroids can cause irreversible sterility in some women. Furthermore, much more needs to be known about norethindrone enanthate. Information is not available concerning the effect on duration of effectiveness of varying the dosage as well as the concentration of the drug injected. Besides the lack of knowledge about norethindrone enanthate and DMPA, there is a great need to develop other types of injectable methods that will diminish the problems and improve the acceptability of currently available methods. The main problem that must be dealt with is the disruption of normal cyclic bleeding.

21.3 Potential Areas of Investigation

Potential new injectable methods for contraception may be categorized as follows:

1. Steroid formulations other than those currently available.
2. New vehicles for administering steroids that would allow a more constant rate of release from the injection site.
3. Agents that can be administered by intermittent injection and that would act in ways other than ovulation inhibition. This might include the development of luteolytic agents such as prostaglandin analogs and the development of immunological methods such as antisera to proteins produced exclusively by pregnancy.

The first two categories will be discussed in this section.

New Steroid Formulations
Several other progestogens that reportedly have prolonged activity have been synthesized by various pharmaceutical companies. Clinical testing of these agents, such as R-2323 and related drugs, needs to be initiated to determine their possible usefulness as injectable contraceptives. If these initial studies are promising, comparative clinical trials with DMPA and norethindrone enanthate need to be undertaken.

With these latter two agents, the frequency of undesirable side effects, mainly irregularity of bleeding, may be partially related to the rate of release from the injection site, the formation of a secondary depot, and the resultant variable blood level. As noted above, the amount of hormone released per day is initially high but decreases to a considerable extent thereafter. There is a resultant uneven time curve of the release of the compound from the depot.

A new approach to the development of long-acting contraceptive steroids has been suggested by Taubert and Kuhl. This approach involves linking steroid molecules by means of succinic acid to give dimeric and oligomeric steroid esters, which appear to be released at a slow and relatively even rate. They have succeeded in preparing steroid esters containing two (dimeric) and three (trimeric), and four (tetrameric) steroid molecules.

In preliminary experiments, a single injection of these compounds, derived from estradiol in oily solution, brought about an estrogenic effect of long duration. These short steroid chains, which are referred to as steroid oligomeres, are presumed to split in the organism into the hormonally active components at a rather slow rate. Synthesis of oligomeres of progestogens or derivatives of testosterone could produce a new type of injectable steroid that could be used as a contraceptive by both men and women.

In women, dimeric progestogens could be developed for use as injectable contraceptives. The main objective would be the development of a formulation that combines the advantage of a very long-lasting effect with an even rate of release from the secondary depot. This reduction of the dose released per day might reduce the incidence of undesirable side effects.

In men, dimeric or trimeric combinations of testosterone and ethynodiol or other easily esterifiable progestogens could be potentially useful as contraceptive agents. The acceptability and safety of such combinations would depend at least in part on finding the right dose-relationship between the two components. Both the progestogen and testosterone would be used to depress spermatogenesis via pituitary gonadotropin suppression. In addition, the testosterone component would prevent loss of libido and potency.

In addition to testing these agents in men, clinical testing of DMPA and other progestogens combined with a long-acting testosterone formulation, such as testosterone enanthate, should be undertaken.

Very little knowledge exists about another aspect of injectable contraception with progestogens in women, namely, the possible advantages of the addition of estrogenic agents to the formulation. Coutinho reported that in addition to excellent effectiveness, very good bleeding patterns were observed in two small series of patients treated with a combination of either DMPA and estradiol cyprionate or noregestrel and estradiol hexabenzonate. In addition to these long-acting estrogens, other types of long-acting estrogenic formulations have been developed. These include oily solutions of fatty acid esters such as estradiol 17-β enanthate, aqueous solutions of polyphosphate derivatives such as polyestriol phosphate, and ether derivatives such as quinesterol. This last compound is stored in adipose tissue and released at a slow rate. There is almost no factual knowledge as to whether the addition of any long-acting estrogens to the injectable formulation has an amenorrheic effect upon the bleeding pattern. Furthermore, as it is not known whether the low levels of circulating estradiol associated with DMPA have long-term harmful effects, such as premature development of osteoporosis, it has therefore not been determined whether the addition of an estrogen is necessary to prevent these effects. Finally, one must be concerned about possible increased carcinogenicity associated with the addition of long-acting estrogens to the injectable formulation.

New Vehicles
The injection of subdermal implants of Silastic cap-

sules containing progestogens is more a surgical procedure than a simple injection that can be performed by untrained personnel. Aside from that, much remains to be learned about biodegradable polymers that might be injected intramuscularly through a small gauge needle. It is believed that progestogens can be combined with these polymers in such a way that the steroids will be released at a relatively constant rate. The steroid can be either included or trapped in the matrix of the polymer or secreted with it to give a slow constant rate of release by hydrolysis. It has been suggested that these biodegradable polymers should be synthesized from small molecules of known toxicological properties and that the degradable products should be readily eliminated from the body. A few research organizations are initiating development of such polymers, but development costs are high and available resources for this important area of contraceptive development are extremely limited.

21.4 Summary: Funding Aspects

The available information indicates a great need for development of an effective and acceptable injectable contraceptive. The potential acceptability of such agents by different cultures has not been determined, however, and this must certainly be a part of the development procedure.

A relatively small amount of money has been made available by various agencies for the development of new injectable contraceptives and for studies to fill the many gaps in our knowledge. The Expanded Programme of Research, Development and Research Training of the World Health Organization has initiated a Task Force on Injectable Contraceptives as one of their 11 Task Forces. Studies funded by WHO include a comparative clinical trial of DMPA and norethindrone enanthate to determine differences in efficacy, bleeding patterns, and restoration of normal ovarian function, as well as projects for improving delivery systems by utilizing new polymers and preliminary synthesis of oligomeric steroids. The NIH Contraceptive Development Program has also expended a portion of its budget in this area. One project has been funded in which an injectable androgen is given once monthly and an oral steroid is given daily to act as a contraceptive in the male. Several projects involving the development of biodegradable synthetic polymer matrices have been funded. One contractor is preparing a system containing microcapsules together with progestins, and that system is undergoing preliminary clinical testing. Although contracts have been given to three other facilities to develop biodegradable polymers that produce a constant rate of release of the steroid, the CPR's *Report of Progress—1973* notes that development of such a system is quite complicated and "considerable research effort and time will be needed to reduce the concept to practice."

The ICCR of the Population Council is devoting a small portion of its effort to the development of injectable contraceptives. AID is not expending any funds in this area.

More funds must be expended in this branch of contraceptive research, especially since pharmaceutical companies are not now involved in developing an injectable contraceptive. Sociological studies to precisely determine the ultimate effect of injectable agents on contraceptive practice and fertility regulation might help in determining funding priorities. If, as suspected, the need proves great, efforts should be undertaken to provide additional funds or to allocate a greater percentage of available funds to this area of practical contraceptive development. These efforts will provide a very useful new means of contraception within a relatively short period of time.

References

1. Data on file with Schering, AG, D-1 Berlin 65, Postfach 65, 0311. Material on Noristerat/Depot contraceptive, 1973.

2. El-Mahgaub, S., and M. Karim. The long-term use of injectable norethisterone enanthate as a contraceptive. Contraception 5:21, 1972.

3. Schwallie, P. C., and J. R. Assenzo. Contraceptive use-efficacy study utilizing medroxyprogesterone acetate administered as an intramuscular injection once every 90 days. Fertil. Steril. 24:331, 1973.

4. Schwallie, P. C., and J. R. Assenzo. Contraceptive use-efficacy study utilizing Depo-Provera administered as an injection once every six months. Contraception 6:315, 1972.

5. Cornette, J. C., K. T. Kirton, and G. W. Duncan. Measurement of medroxyprogesterone acetate (Provera) by radioimmunoassay. J. Clin. Endocrinol. Metab. 33:459, 1971.

6. Mishell, D. R., Jr., M. Talas, A. F. Parlow, M. El-Habashy, and D. L. Moyer. In Proceedings of the Sixth World Congress on Fertility and Sterility, p. 203. Tel Aviv: The Israel Academy of Sciences and Humanities, 1968.

7. Mishell, D. R., Jr., K. M. Kharma, I. H. Thorneycroft, and R. M. Nakamura. Estrogenic activity in women receiving an injectable progestogen for contraception. Am. J. Obstet. Gynecol. 113:372, 1972.

8. Mishell, D. R., Jr., M. A. El-Habashy, R. G. Good, and D. L. Moyer. Contraception with an injectable progestin: A study of its use in postpartum women. Am. J. Obstet. Gynecol. 101:1046, 1968.

9. Mackay, E. V., S. K. Khoo, and R. R. Adam. Contraception with a six-monthly injection of progestogen. I. Effects on blood pressure, body weight and uterine bleeding pattern, side effects, efficacy and acceptability. Aust. N. Z. J. Obstet. Gynecol. 11:148, 1971.

10. Spellacy, W. N. Effects of oral contraceptives, estrogens and progestogens on protein, carbohydrate and lipid metabolism. In Human reproduction: Conception and contraception, eds. E. S. E. Hafez, and T. N. Evans. New York: Harper & Row, 1973.

11. Goldzieher, J. W., and D. C. Kraemer. The metabolism and effects of contraceptive steroids in primates. Acta Endocrinol. (Suppl: 166):389, 1972.

12. Berliner, V. R. U.S. Food and Drug Administration requirements for toxicity testing of contraceptive products: Meeting on pharmacological models to assess toxicity and side effects of fertility regulating agents. WHO Conference, Geneva, September 17–20, 1973.

13. El-Habashy, M. A., et al. Effect of supplementary oral estrogen on long-acting injectable progestogen contraception. J. Obstet. Gynecol. 35:51, 1970.

14. Scutchfield, P. D., W. N. Long, B. Corey, and C. W. Taylor, Jr. Medroxyprogesterone acetate as an injectable female contraceptive. Contraception 3:21, 1971.

15. Gardner, J. M., and D. R. Mishell, Jr. Study of patients upon discontinuation of injectable long-acting progestogen contraception. In Proc. Seventh Annual Meeting of Planned Parenthood Physicians, San Francisco, California, April 1969.

16. McDaniel, E. B., and T. Pardthaisong. Depo-medroxyprogesterone acetate as a contraceptive agent: Return of fertility after discontinuation of use. Contraception 8:407, 1973.

22 Bioengineering Aspects of Reproduction and Contraceptive Development

Thomas J. Lardner

22.1 Introduction

Bioengineering is the application of engineering and technology to problems of biology. It includes many diverse activities, among them:

Equipment and instrument development for clinical and research applications

Biomaterials compatibility studies

Engineering analyses of biological systems

Materials development.

Work in the field of bioengineering for reproductive biology and contraceptive technology started in 1969. The reason for this upsurge in activity has been a realization among engineers that technology may be able to contribute to a solution of the population problem. Another factor, no doubt, has been the awareness that research and development funds are available for work in reproductive biology and contraceptive technology. As a consequence, multidisciplinary bioengineering groups have been organized at a number of universities, at nonprofit research organizations, and at industrial firms. Many of these groups have concentrated on applying their engineering experience in such areas as biomaterials to developing and improving contraceptive devices, while other groups have participated in joint research efforts to develop sophisticated electronic sensing devices.

While bioengineering certainly has a role to play in helping to develop fertility regulation techniques and in helping to elucidate reproductive phenomena, it cannot play a *primary* role. Bioengineers can help in the development of hardware, in the quantification of parameters in different biological systems, and in the creation of new materials, but they must work with or be motivated by physicians, biological scientists, and clinicians who can identify problems of importance.

An outline of areas in which bioengineering might contribute is shown in Table 22.1. The efforts thus far in bioengineering can be classified into biomaterials studies, device and instrumentation development, and attempts to apply engineering methodology to the quantification of reproductive phenomena. Table 22.1 indicates the diverse areas in reproductive biology and contraceptive technology that require engineering input. Some of the recent contributions of engineering to contraceptive technology have been discussed in an excellent review article by Speidel and Ravenholt.[1]

The importance of a collaborative role for engineers in projects cannot be overstated. Important also is the realization that during a project the relative contribution of the engineer and the clinician will change. The engineer will be actively involved in hardware development after the clinical problem has been defined by collaboration between the clinician and the engineer. Once the hardware is in clinical testing, the engineer's role becomes less active, although the engineer must make an effort to understand the problems faced by the clinician.

Bioengineering activity in reproductive biology and contraceptive technology is at a watershed. Many of the organizations that entered the field of contraceptive device development in 1969 or 1970 have dropped out of programs or have failed to develop successful devices. The experience of these organizations has suggested the balance that is needed between the biological and the bioengineering sides. A few organizations have found that available funding is insufficient to develop and improve the contraceptive devices suggested by funding agencies. Some device development can be done cheaply but more often extensive and expensive programs are required.

Research efforts at universities have been reasonably successful at developing instrumentation for monitoring reproductive phenomena and for quantitative modeling of reproductive phenomena. But here, too, the long-term funding situation is unclear and the commitment of programs to reproductive biology is not assured.

22.2 Device and Instrument Development

Bioengineering work has been widely used in developing transducers and methods for detecting phenomena in reproductive biology and in developing devices for fertility regulation. Table 22.2 lists the activities in these areas.

Work on transducer design is proceeding at Stanford, at Case Western, with Blandau at the University of Washington, and with Fromm at Drexel, as a part of multidisciplinary research programs on either ovulation detection or on oviductal contractility.

In these programs the bioengineering group pro-

Table 22.1 Potential areas for bioengineering involvement in reproduction studies

	Instrument, Device, or Technique Development	Biomaterials Development	Quantification of Phenomena
Ovary	instrumentation to detect changes in ovarian temperature and blood flow		descriptions of processes of ovulation
Fertilization, Cell Cleavage			models of cell cleavage
Gamete Transport	instrumentation for measuring contractility, fluid secretions and fluid flow, ovum and sperm movement in the oviduct; instrumentation for detection of ciliary activity		models of effects of contractions and cilia on gamete transport
Uterus	instrumentation for studying contractile patterns; devices for measuring uterine size	materials for IUDs; polymer development for prescribed release of drugs in uterus, vagina	models of contractile patterns in the uterus
Uterotubal Junction and Cervix	device for visualization of the uterotubal junction; device for measurement of cervical mucus viscosity	materials for transcervical occlusion of the uterotubal junction	relation of viscosity to sperm transport in the cervix
Hormone Regulation of Reproductive Cycles			computer models and simulations of hormone interactions
Female Sterilization	techniques and devices	materials for clips and oviductal occlusive materials	
Abortion	simple and reliable instruments		
Male Tract	instruments for pressure and flow measurements; devices for reversible vasectomy	materials for vas valves, vas plugs, and stents	models of fluid flow in the tract and of blood flow to the tract
Sperm			analysis of sperm motility; relation of motility to energetics and morphology

vides the instrumentation and capability for data processing in order to help formulate hypotheses on the mechanisms of gamete transport and to suggest further experimentation. Miniaturized electronic and optical sensing and telemetry devices are being constructed to obtain data on in vivo oviductal contractile patterns and ovum movement; these data are unobtainable by other means.

These collaborative programs have been successful because the engineers have been willing to try to understand the physiologists' problems and to keep in mind the nature of the data needed, while the physiologists have been willing to work at understanding the kind of data the engineers can obtain without influencing normal physiological function.

The contribution of bioengineering efforts thus far to the development of new or improved contraceptive and fertility control devices is less clear. A group at Battelle Northwest, for example, has been investigating engineering aspects of the design of IUDs. A retrospective study of the correlation of the physical and material properties of IUDs with clinical performance has been made with the aim of identifying the properties that give improved performance. These studies have suggested modified designs. A conclusion reached by the Battelle group is that the performance of IUDs might be improved by an effort to measure the size of the uterine lumen before fitting an IUD. A device for determining the profile of the uterine lumen is presently undergoing preclinical study.

Methods and devices for female sterilization have been under active study.[2] One line of research in this area is aimed at developing methods and devices for fertility control at the uterotubal junction (UTJ). IITRI has constructed a hystereoscope to visualize the UTJ transcervically and to allow for the insertion of a plug or device. A similar instrument without the capability for visualization is being developed at the Franklin Institute for the delivery of occlusive material to the UTJ.

Table 22.2 Ongoing work in device and instrument development

Project Area	Active Groups
Instrumentation for Detection of Reproductive Events	
Detection of ovulation; changes in ovarian temperature and electrical impedence; changes in the vasculature of the vagina	University of Washington, Case Western Reserve University, University of Toronto
Ovum transport; optical detector for estimating the time of ovulation	University of Washington
Oviductal activity	University of Washington, University of Pennsylvania
Cervical mucus viscosity measurements	Technion
Forces associated with cervical dilation	University of North Carolina
Fertility Control Devices	
IUDs: Relation of physical characteristics to clinical performance; improved materials	Battelle, ALZA Corp., Franklin Institute, Techna Corp.
Uterine cavity measurement device	Battelle
Steerable hystereoscope cornuosalpingoguide	IITRI, Franklin Institute
Techniques for occluding the uterotubal junction	IITRI
Oviductal clips	University of North Carolina
Simplified equipment for pregnancy termination	Battelle
Reversible vasectomy devices	New York Medical College, Battelle, Abcor Corp., IITRI
Electrocoagulation of the Fallopian tubes	University of North Carolina

Improvement of simple and reliable equipment for uterine aspiration and for menstrual regulation was made at Battelle with the goal of providing equipment for developing countries.[3] The development of devices for reversible vasectomy is being investigated by a number of groups, each advocating a different technique. IITRI has developed a soft plastic device, Freund and his associates have developed a gold device, Abcor has developed a plug, and Battelle has developed a bypass concept.[4]

The success of programs in developing fertility control devices has been mixed. Some device programs have been very successful, such as the development of oviductal clips[5] and the upgrading of equipment for pregnancy termination. In both these programs, it should be noted, the task was clearly defined and the clinical needs were clearly identified. Furthermore, some hardware was already available, and clinical experience with that hardware could be used as a guide. Finally, there was a definite clinical need and encouragement from the clinicians to improve the existing devices and equipment.

Other programs have been less successful, such as the development of devices for reversible vasectomy. These programs have suffered from either too little engineering at the preliminary stages or too little clinical evaluation later in the program to evaluate potential problem areas. The final outcome of these programs is not clear.

22.3 Biomaterials Development

Material compatibility between a medical device and the tissue in which it is located is obviously important for the success of a device. Often it is necessary to ensure no tissue reaction; at other times the material should encourage a tissue reaction in order to develop good bonding between the device and the tissue. The quantification of the extent of tissue response with material properties is usually an integral part of biomaterials efforts. An enormous amount of literature has been generated on biomaterial compatibility.

Areas in contraceptive development for which biomaterial effort is needed are listed in Table 22.1. Programs involving biomaterials-related work are listed in Table 22.3. These efforts are part of programs aimed at developing contraceptive devices and techniques; no basic research work is presently underway on tissue response to different materials in the vas, uterus, and oviducts. The lack of this research data may be critical if the present product-device oriented programs do not lead to usable fertility control methods.

Additional discussion of biomaterials and of safety testing requirements for plastic devices, metal-releasing IUDs, and for hormone-releasing IUDs may be

Table 22.3 Ongoing work in biomaterials research

Project Area	Goal	Active Groups
Materials for improved "inert" IUDs	to relate material properties to the clinical performance of IUDs	Battelle Northwest, Franklin Institute, IITRI, Techna Corp., Abcor Corp.
Materials to allow controlled release of drugs	to relate material and drug properties and diffusion release rates to device performance	Battelle, ALZA Corp., Abcor Corp., Research Triangle Inst., Dynatech Co.
Materials for vasectomy valves, plugs, and stents	to find the best materials for fixing in place valves, plugs, and stents	New York Medical College (Freund), Abcor Corp., IITRI, Battelle Northwest
Materials for blockage of oviducts via a transcervical procedure	to find the best materials for blockage of oviducts	Franklin Institute, Battelle (Columbus), IITRI
Oviductal clips	to find the best material for occlusion of the oviduct	University of North Carolina (Hulka)

found in the proceedings of a meeting on pharmacological models in contraceptive development (WHO, 1973).

Work on the development of polymers and other substances for the controlled release of drugs is being performed by a number of firms and nonprofit research groups. The technology in this area is reasonably well established, and changes in material configurations are brought about by changes in the manufacturing processes. A large amount of this effort is presently in clinical stages, where the efficacy of the drug delivery systems can be established.

22.4 Engineering Methodology

Engineering methodology applied to reproductive biology attempts to describe quantitatively different reproductive phenomena and to assess the effects of different mechanisms. The phrase *biomechanics of reproductive biology* is often used to describe mathematical modeling of processes and events in reproductive biology. A list of some of the problems that have been investigated is given in Table 22.1. Much of this effort has been reasonably successful; the groups active in this area have been located at MIT and at the University of Illinois.

22.5 Conclusions and Recommendations

As can be seen from the preceding survey, a small amount of bioengineering activity has entered the fields of reproductive biology and contraceptive technology during the past seven years. This activity has been in the instrumentation for obtaining data on reproductive events, in developing devices for fertility regulation, and in applying engineering methodology to reproductive processes.

Research programs in which bioengineers contribute instrumentation and the capability for data processing and model building should be encouraged. In many cases, engineers can provide devices for physiological measurements that contribute to our understanding of reproductive events.

But the continued improvement of instrumentation should not become an end in itself. Often engineers develop equipment that is inappropriate for the measurements needed; often data are generated simply to allow engineers to computer-process them. These tendencies can be controlled in multidisciplinary programs once the bioengineer begins to understand the physiological processes involved. Examples of good programs using bioengineers are the programs at the University of Washington and the University of Pennsylvania. Investigators in ongoing biomedical programs in reproductive physiology should be encouraged to hire bioengineers to work with them. Engineers at the B.S. and M.S. levels are often able to make important contributions.

Many recent large-scale programs for the development of fertility control devices have been dominated by engineering considerations (e.g., the Battelle program on IUD development). These programs have not moved as quickly as they might, because clinical goals have been clouded by technological complexities whose importance is secondary to the goals. It is easier for engineers to focus on questions of design than it is for them to focus on clinical problems. For these reasons, action programs aimed at the improvement of specific fertility control methods should be modified. Programs to develop contraceptive technology should be clinically oriented; engineers should provide a service as part of these programs and work with results from clinical trials. Prototypes for specific hardware should be built with specific applications in mind. The advantages of a particular modification should be investigated and considered before clinical testing, but the motivation for the hardware should come from a clinical need.

Smaller programs involving physicians and engineers should be encouraged. Often these smaller collaborative efforts can yield immediate results (e.g., the work of Hulka and Clemens on the oviductal clip). Indeed, many small collaborative programs working on specific contraceptive devices are more likely to lead to something useful than large programs in which a major emphasis is on the engineering aspects.

Bioengineering activities in the past seven years have made contributions to fertility control methods and devices, to transducer development and instrumentation, and to the application of engineering methodology. In many cases, however, the potential contributions have been misdirected or have been inappropriate. More effort is needed to focus and direct the engineering work so it makes a contribution. Engineers respond well to goal-oriented research and development. Leadership is needed to help define goals for fertility control methods to which engineers can contribute.

References

1. Speidel, J., and R. Ravenholt. Needs for fertility control technology. In *Clinical Proceedings of the IPPF South East Asia and Oceania Congress*, 1974.

2. Duncan, G., R. Falb, and J. Speidel, eds. *Female sterilization*. New York: Academic Press, 1972.

3. *Pregnancy termination: Menstrual regulation update*. Population Report F-4, George Washington University, May 1974.

4. *Sterilization: Vasectomy, old and new techniques*. Population Report D-1, George Washington University, December 1973.

5. *Sterilization: Laparoscopic sterilization with clips*. Population Report C-4, George Washington University, March 1974.

23 The Role of Prostaglandins in Reproduction

Vivian J. Goldberg and
Peter W. Ramwell

Understanding of the humoral events in reproduction has advanced in three stages. First was the discovery and systematic study of the gonadal steroids. Subsequently, pituitary gonadotropic hormones and the hypothalamic releasing factors were discovered. In recent years much work has been done with a third major class of compounds, the prostaglandins (PGs). These compounds have a wide range of actions on reproductive processes, but in contrast to the previous two types of humoral agents, PGs are not localized in any particular tissue.

An analysis of the role of PGs in reproductive processes requires a separation of the possible physiological actions from the pharmacological effects of PGs. While the pharmacological effects are both dramatic and clinically significant, they may not reflect the true involvement, if any, of PGs in normal physiological processes. Furthermore, given to the whole animal, PGs may act at more than one site. Moreover, relatively few experimental protocols have been designed that attempt to isolate the site or sites of PG action. Other parameters are introduced by species differences in response to PG treatment that may further vary with reproductive state. A prominent feature of work done in this area is a lack of systematic experiments, which has resulted in a voluminous but superficial literature. The confusion and controversy surrounding the putative luteotropic versus luteolytic effects of PGs is a case in point.

The extensive, if not intensive, studies of PGs in recent years have been made possible by several important technical advances. First is the development of synthetic, high-purity PGs with reasonable stability and shelf life. A second development is the discovery that acetylenic fatty acids and nonsteroidal anti-inflammatory agents are potent inhibitors of PG synthetase. The use of these tools has allowed us to deduce a role of endogenous PG synthesis in response to hormonal stimulus. A third advance has been the development of radioimmunoassays for estimating the levels of endogenous PG. This method is more sensitive (by at least an order of magnitude) and less tedious than bioassay or gas chromatographic methods.

Reprinted from *Physiological reviews* 55 (1975), pp. 325–351, by permission of The American Physiological Society.

23.1 PGs and Gonadotropin Release

The first suggestion that PG may be involved in gonadotropin release was derived from experiments of Zor et al. (1970) in Field's laboratory. PGs, unlike a large number of putative neurotransmitters, were found to be specific in increasing anterior pituitary cAMP in vitro in male rats. Subsequently, Ratner et al. (1974) succeeded in showing that PGs stimulate the release of LH in hemipituitaries from male rats as well as increasing pituitary cAMP. Studies are now required of the effects of PGs on the pituitary or hypothalamus of female rats in various reproductive states.

The release of luteinizing hormone (LH) by PGs in vivo has been demonstrated. Carlson et al. (1973) observed an increase in serum LH following intracarotid infusion of $PGF_2\alpha$ (6 μg/hr) during the luteal phase in cycling ewes. Chamley and Christie (1973) failed to observe an LH elevation in the ewe, but the animals were either ovariectomized or anestrous. Labhsetwar (1973) observed an LH peak in hamsters 30 hours after $PGF_2\alpha$ injection on day 3 of pregnancy. A similar rise in serum LH was observed 10 minutes after intravenous injection of either PGE_1 (20 μg/rat) or $PGF_2\alpha$ (200 μg/rat) into the ovariectomized rat primed with progesterone and estrogen (Sato et al. 1974). Treatment of rats with pentobarbital on the morning of the proestrous day suppressed the LH surge and abolished ovulation, but infusion of PGE_1 (10 μg/rat) into the third ventricle of such animals on the afternoon of proestrus increased LH release and ovulation (Spies and Norman 1973). More PGE_2 (30 μg/rat) was required to reverse the pentobarbital effect; $PGF_2\alpha$ (10 μg/rat) was ineffective.

Exogenous PGs may act on the hypothalamus or higher centers to elicit LH release in the intact animal. Chatterjee (1973) has presented indirect evidence that, in rats, $PGF_2\alpha$ acts on the hypothalamus to release LH-releasing hormone (LH–RH). More convincing evidence from Lindner's (1973) laboratory is that LH–RH may be secreted by the hypothalamus in response to PGE_2. They found that antisera to LH–RH prevented the LH surge following PGE_2 administration (100 μg/rat), which normally doubled the LH levels in male and female rats.

To date, there is no direct evidence on the pharmacological effects of PG on FSH release either in vitro or in vivo.

The more difficult questions of the physiological role of PGs in the gonadal-hypothalamic-adenohypophysic axis have not been investigated directly. An early important finding was that ovulation was inhibited by administration of indomethacin (a commonly available PG-synthetase inhibitor) to rats primed with pregnant mare serum (PMS). This inhibition of ovulation induced by indomethacin could not be reversed by the subsequent administration of either synthetic LH–RH or LH (Behrman et al. 1972). Moreover, Tsafriri et al. (1973) found that indomethacin administration had no effect on the preovulatory LH surge in the rat and concluded that PGs probably do not have a physiological role in LH release in the rat.

In summary, the PGE compounds release LH in vitro and in vivo, and $PGF_2\alpha$ releases LH in vivo. Exogenous PGs may act on the hypothalamus or even higher centers, but there is no evidence that they have a physiological role.

23.2 Endogenous PG Synthesis in Ovulation

Although there is no evidence that PGs are required for gonadotropin release, data from several laboratories show PGs involved in ovum maturation and release. LH may stimulate ovarian PG synthesis. The addition of LH to either intact eight-day pregnant rats or to homogenates prepared from the ovaries of these rats increased the in vitro conversion of arachidonic acid to PG (Chasalow and Pharriss 1972). In addition, the secretion rate of ovary slices prepared from mature monkeys of unspecified reproductive state was increased by the addition of LH (100 ng/ml) to the medium; FSH and prolactin did not elicit this effect (Wilks et al. 1972).

The PG content of ovarian follicles increases as the follicles mature. Ovulation in estrous rabbits occurs 9 to 11 hours after the injection of human chorionic gonadotropin (hCG); and, five hours after the hCG injection, the PGE levels of the ovarian follicles are significantly higher than those observed at zero time (LeMaire et al. 1973). After nine hours the follicular levels of PGF as well as PGE were increased. These effects were eliminated when indomethacin was administered prior to the hCG injection (Yang et al. 1973). Similarly, the rise in follicular PGE and PGF, observed in rabbit ovaries 10 hours after mating, was abolished when indomethacin was administered immediately after coitus.

The finding (Grinwich et al. 1972; O'Grady et al. 1972) that indomethacin abolishes LH-induced ovulation is evidence that ovarian PG synthesis may be sig-

nificant. Tsafriri et al. (1973) hypothesized that the indomethacin acted on the ovary to suppress ovulation, since the LH levels of rats given indomethacin on the proestrous day were not depressed. Simultaneous treatment with PGE_2 (up to 750 μg/rat) partially overcame the indomethacin effect. In rabbits, the indomethacin block of follicle maturation and rupture could subsequently (12 hr after hCG injection) be reversed by infusing $PGF_2\alpha$ into the ovarian artery (Diaz-Infante et al. 1974).

The observation of unruptured luteinized follicles in the indomethacin-treated animals suggests that the endogenously produced PGs may be involved in the expulsion of the ovum from the ovary (Grinwich et al. 1972). In contrast, when Richman et al. (1974) infused the ovaries of hCG-treated rabbits, PGE_2 reduced the rate of follicle maturation and the number of ruptured follicles ($PGF_2\alpha$ had no effect). The addition of exogenous PGE may obscure the effects mediated by the endogenously synthesized PGE.

In summary, the evidence that PGs mediate ovulation is based on the ability of indomethacin in the rabbit to inhibit gonadotropin stimulation of both ovarian PG synthesis and ovulation. These studies clearly warrant further exploration of the role of PGs in these processes.

23.3 PG Mediation of LH Action on Granulosa Cells

One of the more controversial aspects of PG action is the possible role that PGs have in mediating or mimicking gonadotropin actions on granulosa and luteal cells. The effects of LH in stimulating PGE (and PGF) production by ovaries in vivo and in vitro have been discussed. The question at hand is whether PGs can replace LH in stimulating ovulation and luteinization.

Data obtained with rabbits argue against the involvement of PGs in LH-induced steroidogenesis. Although indomethacin treatment suppressed ovulation in LH-treated rabbits (Grinwich et al. 1972), the indomethacin-treated animals had luteinized follicles on day 8, and the progesterone 20-α-OH pregnen 4-en-zone levels were the same as controls.

Definitive work on the interrelationship of LH and PGs in the luteinization of monkey follicles has been performed in tissue culture by Channing et al. (1972a, b). The effects of PGE_1 and PGE_2 on morphological luteinization were similar to those of LH, but LH was more potent than PGE_2. LH was also more effective in promoting progestin secretion by luteinized granulosa cells than either PGE_2 or $PGF_2\alpha$. The progestin secretion of spontaneously luteinized cells was enhanced by the addition of PGE_2 and, to a lesser extent, of $PGF_2\alpha$. In view of these findings, it was surprising to observe that simultaneous additions of 0.1 μg/ml of hLH plus 10 μg/ml of any of the PGs resulted in an inhibition of progestin secretion to less than 30 percent of that observed with LH alone or less than 50 percent of that observed with PGE_2 alone. There was no effect on the spontaneous luteinization of granulosa cells from pre-ovulatory monkeys by 7-oxa-13-prostynoic acid (a PG inhibitor) at the doses tested, but hCG (0.1 μg/ml), LH (0.01 μg/ml), or PGE_2 effects on granulosa cells obtained from monkeys primed with PMS were inhibited at high concentrations of 7-oxa-13-prostynoic acid. The synthetase inhibitor eicosa-5,8,11,14-tetraynoic acid (at least 100 μg/ml) blocked the effects of hCG on the luteinization of cultured granulosa cells from PMS-treated monkeys. On the basis of these data, Channing concluded that PGs may mediate the action of LH in luteinization and the initiation of steroidogenesis.

In short-term incubations with freshly collected granulosa cells from pig ovaries, Kolena and Channing (1973) found a stimulation of cAMP content with LH and FSH. PGE_2 and PGE_1 were also capable of stimulating cAMP accumulation. The combination of LH and PGE_2 was a greater stimulant of cAMP production than either FSH plus PGE_2 or LH, FSH, or PGE_2 alone. (These experiments were the first demonstration of an FSH stimulation of ovarian adenylate cyclase.)

The results obtained with porcine granulosa cells are consistent with those obtained with rat Graafian follicle (Zor et al. 1972). In these studies, isolated follicles that were incubated with LH (5 μg/ml) for 18 hours were refractory to further stimulation by addition of LH (5 μg/ml), but the addition of PGE_2 resulted in an increase in the cAMP formed. These workers, like Kolena and Channing, were unable to demonstrate an inhibitory effect of 7-oxa-13-prostynoic acid on granulosa adenylate cyclase stimulated by LH or PGE_2.

The findings of additive effects of PGE_2 and LH on the porcine granulosa cell and rat follicle adenylate cyclase are inconsistent with the proposal of Kuehl et al. (1970) that there is a single gonadotropin-related site for PG action.

The temporal relationship among LH addition, PG synthesis, and cAMP formation suggests that PGs are not involved in the cAMP-mediated action of LH. Addition of LH to immature rat ovaries resulted in an increased accumulation of cAMP within 20 minutes (Lindner et al. 1974), while PGE levels did not rise significantly until the second hour of incubation. A delay in PG accumulation in the ovary following LH administration was observed in the rabbit by Yang et al. (1973) and also in the adult rat by Lindner et al. (1974). The cAMP-dependent effects observed when PGE was administered might be pharmacological. The ki-

netics of the LH-stimulated PG synthesis were such that the PGs appeared much later than the cAMP and could not be involved in the stimulation of adenylate cyclase observed within minutes of adding LH.

In summary, the initial work indicated a role for PGs in mediating the effects of LH because similar actions, including adenylate cyclase activation and steroidogenesis, were evoked with both agents. Subsequently it was found that PG antagonists and synthetase inhibitors did not consistently abolish LH action. Finally, the chronological sequence of LH and PG actions discount the possibility that PG mediates LH effects. Thus it appears that PGs are produced in the ovary in response to LH administration. Studies with PG-synthetase inhibitors indicate that ovarian PGs are necessary for follicle rupture but not for ovum maturation (Lindner et al. 1974) or luteinization of the granulosa cells (Grinwich et al. 1972). As described above, exogenous PGs can mimic many of the actions of LH on granulosa cells, including stimulation of cAMP formation, initiation of steroid production, and morphological transformation into luteinized cells. Since cAMP formation in response to LH stimulation occurred much earlier than PG synthesis in vivo and in vitro, a natural role for PG in cAMP-dependent processes may be ruled out.

23.4 Corpus Luteum Maintenance

PGs play a complicated role in the maintenance of the corpus luteum during pseudopregnancy and pregnancy. They may elicit different effects, depending on whether progestin production is studied in vivo or in vitro. In most of the species studied except primates, PGs administered in vivo promote luteolysis; in vitro, PGs promote steroidogenesis. The steroidogenic effect of $PGF_2\alpha$ on minced ovaries from pseudopregnant rats was first observed by Pharriss et al. (1968). Increased progesterone secretion by bovine corpora lutea was elicited by PGE_2 and PGE_1 (Speroff and Ramwell 1970), by PGA_1 and PGA_2 (Hansel et al. 1973), and possibly by $PGF_2\alpha$ (Hansel et al. 1973; Sellner and Wickersham 1970). Simultaneous incubation of luteal slices with LH and PGE_2 resulted in progestin secretion that was not greater than that with LH alone. The role of PGs in the developed corpus luteum may be similar to that postulated for granulosa cells; that is, PGs may mimic LH by stimulating adenylate cyclase (Marsh 1971) and promoting cAMP-dependent steroidogenic processes.

In view of the general steroidogenic effect of PGs in vitro, it is difficult to understand why these effects are not seen in vivo. The key to this problem is in the mechanism of luteal support. The secretory lifetime of the corpus luteum is determined by a number of endocrinological factors, which vary from species to species. PGs may interfere at different sites, depending on what these luteal-supporting factors are (e.g., LH in the ewe, estrogen in the rabbit, hCG in the human). PGs may act centrally on the hypothalamus or pituitary. Another site of action may be the steroid-secreting cells (Koering and Kirton 1973), where PGs would have lytic effects. Alternatively, they may promote the activity of an ovarian compartment, such as the developing follicle, to trigger (possibly through increased estrogen secretion) inappropriate ovulation. This possibility is suggested by the studies of Labhsetwar (1972a,b,c; 1973) on rats, hamsters, and mice, in which PGF$_2\alpha$ administration during the early days of pregnancy resulted in abrupt cessation of progesterone release and prompt ovulation. Finally, luteolysis may be a result of the vasoconstrictive action of PG on the ovarian vasculature.

The luteolytic effects of exogenous PGs are well established, and the literature has been reviewed by Labhsetwar (1974). Pharriss and Wyngarden (1969) were the first to report a luteolytic effect of PGF$_2\alpha$ on pseudopregnant rats. Intrauterine or intraventricular infusion of PGF$_2\alpha$ (1 mg/kg/day) resulted in a marked decrease in ovarian progesterone content and an increase in 20-α-hydroxyprogesterone. Morphological degeneration of the corpus luteum of guinea pigs following PGF$_2\alpha$ injection was observed by Blatchley and Donovan (1969). Since then similar data have been obtained for hamsters, rabbits, mice, cows, and ewes.

23.5 Luteolysis in Primates and Humans

Kirton et al. (1970) reported that injections of PGF$_2\alpha$ (30 mg/day) into mated rhesus monkeys for five days on postovulation days 7–11 did not result in premature menses or in lowered progestin levels. When PG was injected later in the cycle (postovulation days 11–15), lowered progestin levels and premature onset of menses resulted. The fertility rates for animals treated with PGF$_2\alpha$ were one of six compared with six of ten for untreated animals. Auletta et al. (1973) demonstrated that infusions of PGF$_2\alpha$ (50 mg/ml in 100 min) into the ovarian artery of postovulatory macaques resulted in a decrease of progesterone output to 10 percent of control values.

The effects of PGF$_2\alpha$ administration to humans were variable and depended on the age of the corpus luteum and the existence of pregnancy. Lehmann et al. (1972a,b) induced a fall in plasma progesterone and an early onset of menstruation in a woman infused with PGF$_2\alpha$ (25 mg in 5 hr) on postovulatory day 7. These findings were not confirmed in several other studies where women in the luteal phase of the cycle were in-

fused with similar doses of PGF$_2\alpha$. The progesterone levels did not decline and the menses were not induced, although there was staining and cramping in some subjects (LeMaire and Shapiro 1972; Jewelewicz et al. 1972). Vaginal bleeding (which was probably due to the effect of PGF$_2\alpha$ on the uterus) was not always accompanied by a fall in plasma progesterone (Bolognese and Corson 1973a).

The administration of large doses of PGF$_2\alpha$ (intravaginally or 24 mg intravenously) to early pregnant women (menses delayed 7–17 days) resulted in decrements in plasma progesterone, but successful abortion did not necessarily occur (Bolognese and Corson 1973b; Wentz and Jones 1973). Successful abortion was accompanied by a fall in hCG (and consequently a fall in plasma progesterone). Similarly, the fall in progesterone levels that may accompany the administration of progesterone to women in the late luteal phase could be reversed by the subsequent administration of hCG (Bolognese and Corson 1973a). These findings suggest that the primary site of PGF action in the termination of early pregnancy in humans may be the myometrium and not the corpus luteum.

Studies have been performed with monkeys to establish the relationship of plasma progesterone to PGF levels (Auletta et al. 1972). The fall in plasma progesterone that occurred four to five days before the onset of menses in normal cycling monkeys coincided with a rise in plasma PGF two to five days before the onset of menses. In monkeys treated with estrogen during the luteal phase, the plasma progesterone levels declined rapidly. Plasma PG rose while the progesterone declined in some of the estrogen-treated animals. Karsch et al. (1973) showed that the implantation of estrogen-containing capsules three days after the LH surge in monkeys caused decreases in plasma progesterone that were not accompanied by decrements in plasma LH levels. The luteolytic effects of estrogen have been observed before (see Knobil 1973 for review), but the mechanism of estrogen action has not been determined.

The factors that regulate the function of the primate corpus luteum are not completely known. Low levels of plasma LH are clearly required throughout the normal lifetime of the corpus luteum (see Knobil 1973 for review). The lifetime of the primate corpus luteum is not affected by the presence of the uterus. In other species, where PGs are known to be luteolytic, the uterus is a source of PGs and hysterectomy prolongs luteal function. It has been speculated that the primate corpus luteum has an intrinsically short functional life and that no other agents are required for its demise. The finding that increasing amounts of hCG are needed to elicit progesterone secretion by the corpus luteum during early pregnancy in the monkey supports this theory (Knobil 1973). The primate corpus luteum appears to become refractory to stimulation as it ages. Despite daily injections of hCG (50 IU/day beginning on postovulatory day 10), progesterone secretion eventually declined in the infertile monkey (Surve et al. 1973). More work is clearly needed to determine the regulation of luteal function in primates. Until these mechanisms are better understood, it will not be possible to identify the role of PGs.

Mechanisms of PG Action on Luteolysis

Specificity $PGF_2\alpha$ appears to be the most potent luteolytic PG. PGE_2 could terminate pregnancy in hamsters and rats, but much higher doses were required (Labhsetwar 1972d). High doses of PGE_1 terminated pregnancy in rats and hamsters (Labhsetwar 1974) but not in mice (Marley 1972). PGA_1 and PGA_2 and arachidonic acid were not luteolytic in hamsters and rats (Labhsetwar 1974).

Site of action The possible sites of action of PG in luteolysis include the hypothalamus and anterior pituitary, the lutein cells, and the ovarian vasculature. One possible mechanism of action is that PGs interfere with LH release and luteal function fails as a consequence of the withdrawal of pituitary support. There is no clear evidence that this situation occurs. Karsch et al. (1971) reported that continuous infusions of LH (begun as late as day 14 of the estrous cycle) could extend the lifetime of the corpus luteum in the intact cycling ewe; however, sheep with ovarian transplants, given concurrent infusions of LH and $PGF_2\alpha$, experienced a decline in progesterone secretion (Cerini et al. 1973) similar to that observed in animals infused with $PGF_2\alpha$ alone. These findings suggest that PG alone does not act by removing LH support of the corpus luteum; the findings also contrast with those of Chatterjee (1973), in whose studies $PGF_2\alpha$-induced luteolysis in the 10-day pregnant rat was prevented by the presence of a pituitary heterograft. These data suggest the possibility that the mechanisms of PG action vary among species. Since the endpoint of most experiments has been the termination of pregnancy or the decrease in progesterone secretion, these studies are difficult to evaluate. Unfortunately, gonadotropin levels have not been concurrently measured.

According to morphological, histochemical, and biochemical evidence, $PGF_2\alpha$ has a direct action on the lutein cell. Okamura et al. (1972) found degenerative changes in the corpora lutea of pregnant rats treated for four days with $PGF_2\alpha$ that included massive accumulations of lipid in the cytoplasm and lysosomelike granules. In a similar study with a different species, Koering and Kirton (1973) noted degenerative changes in the corpora lutea of $PGF_2\alpha$-treated rabbits as early as day 8 of pregnancy. The pathology observed after three days

of $PGF_2\alpha$ treatment (0.5 mg/kg/day) included autophagic vacuoles that contained lipid droplets. The corpora lutea of midpregnancy were more sensitive to $PGF_2\alpha$ treatment: animals that were given $PGF_2\alpha$ on days 11–13 and examined on day 14 exhibited more degeneration. Few luteal cells were recognizable, and only lytic cells remained. In each treated group, the serum progestin levels were markedly decreased in comparison with untreated controls.

In a histochemical study of the effects of PGE_2 or $PGF_2\alpha$ on pregnant rat corpora lutea (Fuchs and Mok 1974), the effects of $PGF_2\alpha$ treatment on 20-α-hydroxysteroid dehydrogenase (20-α-OH-SDH) activity appeared to be a function of gestational age. The production of 20-α-OH progesterone has been associated with luteolysis and is carried out by corpora lutea from earlier cycles during the first week of pregnancy and by all corpora lutea close to parturition. Administration of $PGF_2\alpha$ on days 4–6 had little effect on 20-α-OH-SDH activity when the animals were examined 48–72 hours after treatment, but rats infused with $PGF_2\alpha$ on days 9–12 or later in pregnancy exhibited intense 20-α-OH progesterone activity, which persisted for at least four days after the $PGF_2\alpha$ treatment. The effects of PGE_2 were similar, but much higher doses were required (which is consistent with Labhsetwar's observation that PGE_2 is luteolytic). The effects of $PGF_2\alpha$ infusion on day 10 on pregnancy termination could be reversed by the addition of progesterone, but the 20-α-OH-SDH activity was not inhibited. LH treatment—but not prolactin (2 mg/day) treatment—spared the pregnancy and prevented the activation of 20-α-OH-SDH (which supports Chatterjee's findings).

Using direct enzymatic assay, Strauss and Stambaugh (1974) measured luteal 20-α-OH-SDH levels in rats. $PGF_2\alpha$ induced this enzyme when pregnant rats were examined on day 10 or on day 16 after two days of $PGF_2\alpha$ treatment, which confirmed the histochemical findings. In these studies, LH, hCG, and prolactin (2 mg/day) maintained the pregnancy in the presence of $PGF_2\alpha$ and partially inhibited the induction of enzyme activity.

PG may exert its action through an effect on steroid synthesis. The activity of cholesterol ester synthetase and the tissue content of cholesterol ester were depressed in ovaries of gonadotropin-treated immature rats that had been given $PGF_2\alpha$ (Behrman et al. 1971). Ovarian slices from these animals also exhibited depressed progesterone synthesis.

Another possible mechanism of PG action on steroid synthesis may be the diversion of ovarian steroid production from progesterone synthesis to estrogen synthesis. Labhsetwar (1974) found that the ovarian estradiol output of pregnant hamsters (day 6) that had been treated with $PGF_2\alpha$ (250 μg) on day 5 was markedly increased over that of the control. Progesterone output by these animals was depressed. Thus PG may promote or mediate inappropriate estrogen secretion by the follicles.

$PGF_2\alpha$ contracts all four kinds of smooth muscle, and its venoconstrictive action may induce hypoxia in the ovary, which in turn may lead to luteolysis. There are data supporting and contradicting this explanation. Since PGE_2 is a vasodilator, the venoconstrictor hypothesis does not account for the luteolytic activity of this agent (Labhsetwar 1972d). $PGF_2\alpha$ was found to decrease ovarian blood flow in rats and rabbits (Pharriss et al. 1970; Gutknecht et al. 1971) in sheep (McCracken 1971), and in monkeys (Kirton et al. 1970). Other workers (Labhsetwar 1974) did not find a correlation between ovarian blood flow and a fall in the progesterone synthesis rate. The distribution of blood flow to various compartments of the ovary may change in response to PG without a change in the overall flow rate. Novy and Cook (1973) used the microsphere technique in pseudopregnant rabbits to measure blood flow following intravenous injection of a luteolytic dose of $PGF_2\alpha$. They found that blood flow significantly decreased to the corpus luteum and increased to the interstitial and follicular tissue, while overall ovarian blood flow remained unchanged. Ovarian blood flow accounts for 2 percent of the cardiac output, even though this organ constitutes only 0.1 percent of the animal's weight. The presence of a high flow rate in the ovary suggests that this organ may be sensitive to oxygen deprivation.

23.6 Endogenous PG Synthesis by the Uterus

The next question is whether the effects of exogenous PGs on progesterone synthesis are pharmacological or reflect processes that occur naturally. If PGs are natural luteolytic substances, PG levels in the ovarian artery, or in the ovary itself, should be elevated during the period of anticipated luteolysis. If PGs are indeed present during the late luteal stage, the site of synthesis, the control of synthesis, and the mechanism of action need to be uncovered.

The possibility that the uterus is the source of a luteolytic substance is supported by the observation—in guinea pigs, hamsters, rats, ewes, cows, and sows—that hysterectomy prolongs the functional life of the corpus luteum (for review, see Hilliard 1973; Hansel et al. 1973). McCracken et al. (1972) have presented evidence that $PGF_2\alpha$ produced in the uterus of sheep is the luteolytic agent in that species. Uterine venous blood from a donor animal, which was itself undergoing luteolysis (ovarian vein plasma levels of progesterone had fallen abruptly six hours earlier), was found to be capable of inducing a decrease in pro-

gesterone synthesis in a recipient ovary when the ovary was cross-circulated with the donor's blood. $PGF_2\alpha$ was identified and measured in the donor's uterine vein plasma. The same concentration of $PGF_2\alpha$ produced a rapid decline in the progesterone secretion rate, which was followed by an increase in estrogen secretion and a new LH peak when infused into the recipient's ovarian artery. Neither the luteolytic action nor a high $PGF_2\alpha$ concentration was observed in the uterine venous plasma taken from ewes that had recently ovulated and that had a functioning corpus luteum.

Other evidence in favor of $PGF_2\alpha$ as a natural luteolytic hormone includes the finding in guinea pigs (where $PGF_2\alpha$ is luteolytic) that intrauterine or subcutaneous administration of indomethacin after ovulation prolongs the functional lifetime of the corpora lutea (Horton and Poyser 1973).

The PGs carried by the uterine vein were thought to reach the ovarian artery by a countercurrent mechanism (the ovarian artery lies against the uterine vein in the sheep). Corpus luteum function was prolonged when the uterine vein and ovarian artery were separated (Hansel et al. 1973). McCracken et al. (1972) infused tritium-labeled $PGF_2\alpha$ (0.1 μCi/min; 10^{-11} M/min) into the uterine vein and observed labeled $PGF_2\alpha$ in the ovarian arterial blood 20 minutes later. At least 2 percent of the infused radioactivity was transferred. In separate experiments, Harrison et al. (1972) demonstrated that $PGF_2\alpha$-containing fluid accumulated in the uterus of ewes whose ovaries had been transplanted into the neck. The ovaries contained functional corpora lutea, even though several months had elapsed since the last observed estrus. These experiments appeared to indicate the need for a utero-ovarian transfer system that did not involve systemic circulation.

In contrast, Coudert et al. (1974a, b) have demonstrated that sheep have no direct anastomoses between the uterine-ovarian vein and the ovarian artery. Tritium-labeled $PGF_2\alpha$ was infused into the uterine vein at a similar rate and for a similar duration, as described by McCracken et al. (1972), but no transfer of $PGF_2\alpha$ was observed; therefore, the existence of a countercurrent mechanism for the distribution of PGs remains an open question.

23.7 Regulation of Uterine PG Production

Since the appearance of PGs in the uterine vein coincides with the onset of luteolysis, uterine PG synthesis may be regulated by the steroid hormones. For example, increased levels of $PGF_2\alpha$ were observed (Blatchley et al. 1971) in the utero-ovarian vein on day 7 of the guinea pig estrous cycle following three days of treatment (days 4–6) with estradiol (10 μg/day). Estrogen did not promote luteolysis in hysterectomized guinea pigs (Bland and Donovan 1970).

The effect of progesterone treatment on endometrial PG levels was studied in the cycling ewe (Wilson et al. 1972). Progesterone (40 mg/day) treatment on days 0 and 1 of the estrous cycle did not elevate endometrial concentrations of PGF$_2\alpha$ on days 5 and 9.

Chronically ovariectomized ewes were placed on various progesterone-estrogen regimens, and the effects on venous plasma PGF levels were observed (Caldwell et al. 1972). Administration of progesterone (20 mg/day) on days 1, 3, 5, 7, 9, and 11 (10 mg progesterone on day 11) and estradiol (50 μg on day 13) produced a pattern of PGF secretion similar to that observed in intact, normally cycling ewes. When estrogen antiserum was given simultaneously, the secretion of PGs was abolished. Treatment of the ovariectomized ewes with progesterone alone resulted in a diminution of PG secretion. Moreover, no detectable PG secretion occurred in ovariectomized and hysterectomized sheep following progesterone and estrogen treatment.

Ovariectomized mice were similar to ewes in their responses to sequential treatment with progesterone and estrogen (Saksena and Lau 1973). Uterine PGF content was higher in mice treated with progesterone (1 mg/day) for three days and estrogen (0.05 mg/day) for 3 days following progesterone than in mice receiving either no steroids or steroids in other combinations.

Estrogens were luteolytic in intact cows and ewes (Hansel et al. 1973) and could stimulate uterine PG synthesis in ewes and guinea pigs. The PGF$_2\alpha$ secretion rate has been measured in slices of endometrium prepared from mature monkeys of unknown reproductive states (Wilks et al. 1972); in all cases, the addition of progesterone or estrogen increased the PGF$_2\alpha$ secretion rate above controls.

PGs have been found in human menstrual fluid (Eglington et al. 1963). The hypothesis that the level of PGs in the human endometrium varies during the menstrual cycle (Pickles et al. 1965) has been confirmed by Downie et al. (1974). PGF$_2\alpha$ levels were elevated throughout the latter half of the luteal phase. PGE$_2$ levels peaked at onset of menstruation. Elevated plasma levels of 15-keto PGE$_2$ have been observed in the late luteal phase (Grieves et al. 1973).

Inappropriate uterine production of PGs has been postulated as the basis of dysmenorrhea in humans (Pickles et al. 1965). The administration of flufenamic acid (a PG-synthetase inhibitor) provided relief to patients whose symptoms were refractory to conventional treatments (Lindner et al. 1973); however, blood levels of PGF$_2\alpha$ in dysmenorrheic women were not dif-

ferent from those in normal women (Wilks et al. 1973).

The finding of an association between uterine PG content and cycle day in the various species studied suggests that uterine synthesis of PGs may be under hormonal control; this needs further study.

23.8 Tubal Contractility and Egg Transport

In all species studied, PGE inhibited the spontaneous contractions of the Fallopian tube, while PGF stimulated tubal contractility. This conclusion is based on in vivo and in vitro findings in rabbits (Horton et al. 1965; Spilman and Harper 1972; Aref et al. 1973), in sheep (Horton et al. 1965), and in humans (Coutinho and Maia 1971; Sandberg et al. 1965). An exception to the general rule that PGEs inhibit tubal contractility is the finding that tissue obtained from the distal (ovarian) segment of the human Fallopian tube is stimulated by PGE$_2$ and to a lesser extent by PGE$_1$ (Sandberg et al. 1965).

The effects of PG treatment on ova transport vary with species. In the rat, administration of high doses of PGE$_1$ during days 1–4 of pregnancy reduced the number of implantation sites, indicating tubal retention of ova. Administration of PGF$_2\alpha$ during the same period had no effects on the number of implantation sites (Labhsetwar 1972). In rabbits, the administration of PGE$_1$ or PGE$_2$ 13 hours after hCG-induced ovulation resulted in a slight acceleration of ova transport in the case of PGE$_1$ and a much greater acceleration in the case of PGF$_2\alpha$ (Ellinger and Kirton 1972; Aref et al. 1973; Chang and Hunt 1972). Ova of PGF$_2\alpha$-treated rabbits arrived in the uterus about 40 hours too early. Administration of PGE or PGF$_2\alpha$ four hours after ovulation resulted in premature loss of the cumulus cells from the ova (Ellinger and Kirton 1972).

Seminal fluid and PGs typically found in seminal fluid also have effects on Fallopian tubal contractility. Evidence has been obtained in the rabbit that PGs accelerate sperm transport in the female reproductive tract. Because rabbit semen contains low amounts of PGE$_1$ and because PGE$_1$ has similar effects on rabbit and human uterine motility, the rabbit was thought to be a good model for investigating the effects of added PG on tubal motility and sperm transport. Horton et al. (1965) found that the spontaneous contractions in the rabbit oviduct were inhibited within 10 minutes of the intravaginal administration of PGE$_1$. Significantly greater numbers of spermatozoa were found in rabbit oviducts two hours after insemination with semen samples containing an additional 75 μg of PGE$_1$ (Mandl 1972). These findings suggest that the high concentrations of PGE$_1$ present in human semen may accelerate sperm migration through the human female reproductive tract.

Evidence for a role of endogenous PG in normal tubal transport of ova comes from Chang's laboratory (Lau et al. 1973). Implantation was prevented by the administration of indomethacin (225 μg/animal) to mice on day 2 of pregnancy. This effect could be reversed by progesterone, PGE_2, or $PGF_2\alpha$. The timing of the indomethacin treatment was such that interference with ovulation was ruled out. Indomethacin may act on the Fallopian tube or on the uterus, or it may have a direct effect on the embryo.

Histoimmunological techniques have also been used to localize $PGF_2\alpha$ in the human Fallopian tube (Ogra et al. 1974). PG was found in the epithelium of tissue obtained during the proliferative phase and in the lamina propria of tissue obtained in the luteal phase. These findings suggest a role of PG in normal oviductal motility.

23.9 Uterine Contractility

The study of agents that affect uterine motility has usually been associated with processes that lead to the evacuation of uterine contents, as occurs in menstruation, abortion, and parturition. Changes in uterine motility may also affect transport of the egg and sperm and the implantation of the blastocysts. The potent smooth-muscle stimulating activity of PGs has led to the study of their effects on the pregnant and nonpregnant uterus.

In Vivo Effects on the Nonpregnant Uterus
PGs stimulate uterine contractions in women, especially around the time of ovulation. These effects have been observed with PGs extracted from seminal fluid (Karlson 1959; Eliasson and Posse 1960; for review see von Euler and Eliasson 1967). Introduction of PGs into the vagina resulted in contraction of the corpus and relaxation of the cervix (Karlson 1959). The contractile activity was thought to be due to an initial response to the mechanical irritation of the cervix or corpus when the fluid was injected. This stage was followed by a period of chemically induced contractions as the active agents directly affected the myometrium. In some cases, the activity changed to relaxation of the uterine muscle 20 to 40 minutes after intravaginal application of semen (Eliasson and Posse 1960).

These studies have been repeated with PGs in place of seminal fluid extracts. Intravenous administration of either PGE_2 or $PGF_2\alpha$ provoked uterine contractions (Coutinho and Maia 1971). Intravaginal application of PGE_2 during the luteal phase (days 20–22) resulted in uterine contractions that continued for several hours (Henzl et al. 1972).

In Vivo Effects on the Pregnant Human Uterus
Administration of PGE_1 and PGE_2 during midpregnancy results in an increase in tone and an increase in the amplitude of the contractions (Bygdeman et al. 1968). The use of PGs as midpregnancy abortifacients is discussed below.

In Vitro Effects
The in vitro effects of PGs on uterine contractility are generally excitatory. Bygdeman (1964) found, however, that PGs extracted from seminal fluid inhibited the contractile activity of myometrial strips from nonpregnant and pregnant women. In other studies, $PGF_2\alpha$ effected contraction in nonpregnant and pregnant myometrial strips (Sandberg et al. 1965). These contradictory observations have not been reconciled to date.

23.10 Abortion

PGs have been used to induce abortion in the first and second trimesters of pregnancy in women. PG use in the first trimester of pregnancy has been associated with a low success rate, a long induction-abortion interval, and deleterious side effects. While some of these problems have diminished with the intrauterine administration of a large dose of PG, vacuum aspiration remains the method of choice in early abortions.

PGs are proving to be more useful in second-trimester abortions. The previously used methods were hysterotomy and saline induction, both of which have serious drawbacks. The midpregnant uterus is refractory to oxytocin, and abortion cannot be induced with this compound. PGs, infused intravenously, intravaginally, intra-amniotically, or extra-amniotically, have been used to induce uterine contractions of sufficient vigor to evacuate the uterine contents. The experience with PGs in second-trimester abortions has been reviewed by Karim (1972a).

The first event in PG-induced abortion is the development of a high level of uterine contracture. The contracture may be the result of a direct action of PG, or it may be secondary to the ischemia resulting from PG-induced vasoconstriction. The stretch imparted to the noncontracting regions of the uterus may induce the release of endogenous PGs (Poyser et al. 1971). The stretch-induced release of PG could also raise the PG concentrations and reinforce the effect of administered PG.

A second mechanism that may be involved in PG-induced abortion is the withdrawal of the so-called progesterone block originally postulated by Csapo (1956). According to this hypothesis, the high levels of progesterone raise the threshold of electrical stimulation needed to produce contractions in the myometrium and make the myometrium refractory to contractile agents such as oxytocin and PG. Successful abortions were preceded by a decline in plasma progesterone levels (Csapo 1973), which indicates that a decrease in progesterone secretion is required.

The PG-induced contracture and vasoconstriction may compromise placental steroidogenesis. This decrease in progesterone output would help to reduce the progesterone block, and the effectiveness of the administered PGs would be enhanced.

23.11 Parturition

Some data indicate that PGs may be involved in normal parturition. The administration of PG-synthetase inhibitors such as aspirin or indomethacin to late-pregnant rats delayed parturition and resulted in a large proportion of stillborn pups (Aiken 1972; Chester et al. 1972; Waltman et al. 1973). Similar observations have been made with rabbits (O'Grady et al. 1972). The administration of $PGF_2\alpha$ antibody on day 17 of pregnancy resulted in delayed parturition in rats (Dunn et al. 1973). While no studies of the effects of indomethacin treatment on normal human labor have been performed, indomethacin treatment increased the induction-abortion interval in hypertonic saline-induced midtrimester abortion (Waltman et al. 1972).

$PGF_2\alpha$ (12 mg/day) could advance parturition when it was given to rats on days 17 and 18 of pregnancy. On day 20, all the treated rats delivered small fetuses, some of them alive (Deis 1971).

Plasma PG levels rise around the time of parturition in several species. In sheep the prepartum fall in progesterone is accompanied by a rise in estrogen. $PGF_2\alpha$ levels in the uterine vein rise rapidly in the 20 hours preceding parturition (Challis et al. 1972). The association of a circumnatal rise in estrogen with a surge of PG was confirmed by Thorburn et al. (1972a,b). The concentration of $PGF_2\alpha$ in the maternal cotyledons of the placenta and in the myometrium rose during labor (Liggins and Grieves 1971; Liggins et al. 1972).

The association of PGs with spontaneous labor in humans was demonstrated by Karim (1968) and Caldwell et al. (1971), who showed that the plasma $PGF_2\alpha$ levels were elevated during contractions and at delivery. Karim (1966) found $PGF_1\alpha$, $PGF_2\alpha$, PGE_1, and PGE_2 in amniotic fluid obtained during labor. $PGF_2\alpha$ was also found in the venous plasma of women during labor (Karim 1968). Until the onset of contractions, plasma $PGF_2\alpha$ levels of late-pregnant women were comparable to those of nonpregnant women (Brummer 1972b). $PGF_2\alpha$ and PGE_2 were also found in the amniotic fluid of women during spontaneous abortion (Karim 1972b) but were not apparent in the amniotic

fluid in women in term pregnancies who were not in labor (Karim and Devlin 1967). Decidual tissue obtained during labor contained higher levels of PGs than the corresponding amniotic fluid samples. The source of PGs that appear during labor may be the decidua, as suggested by Karim and Devlin (1967). The myometrium of the monkey has been shown to produce $PGF_2\alpha$ (Wilks et al. 1972), and human myometrial production of PGE can be increased by stretch (Kloeck and Jung 1973).

The role played by PGs in the coordination of spontaneous labor is obscure. In sheep the onset of labor is preceded by an increased level of estrogen, and Caldwell et al. (1972) have shown that estrogens provoke PG release from the sheep uterus. Estradiol infusion into pregnant women at term produced an increase in uterine activity that was not sufficient to achieve delivery (Larsen et al. 1973). There were no changes in the plasma levels of progesterone or PGF during the four-hour infusion.

PGs and oxytocin may have a physiological relationship. In the presence of PGs, ordinarily subthreshold doses of oxytocin may evoke contractions from human myometrial strips (Brummer 1972a). Vane and Williams (1973) have suggested that oxytocin may stimulate PG synthesis. The oxytocin-induced contractions of isolated nonpregnant rat uteri were abolished when indomethacin was added to the bathing fluid. The addition of indomethacin had no effect on the contractile activity of uteri stimulated with $PGF_2\alpha$. Indomethacin also reduced the PG output and abolished contractile activity of spontaneously contracting uteri from 17–22 day pregnant rats.

Further evidence for an interaction of PGs and oxytocin comes from the observation by Gillespie et al. (1972) that infusions of pregnant women at term with $PGF_2\alpha$ or PGE_2 were accompanied by a rise in oxytocin. Since infusion of PG into normal men also resulted in increased plasma levels of oxytocin, this effect is probably not mediated by the uterus.

When guinea pig myometrial strips were incubated in the presence of low concentrations of PGE_1, the dose-response curves for acetylcholine, vasopressin, and calcium were shifted to the left. The doses of these agents that produced half-maximal effects were reduced by a factor of two or more (Eagling et al., 1971, 1972). These findings suggest that PG mediates its effects at a site that is common to the spasmogens calcium, acetylcholine, and vasopressin. Support for this hypothesis comes from the observations of Carsten (1972, 1973) that PGE_2 and $PGF_2\alpha$ and oxytocin decrease ATP-dependent Ca^{++} binding by myometrial subcellular fractions prepared from pregnant and nonpregnant bovine uteri. PGs also increase the release of calcium from isolated sarcoplasmic reticulum prepared from bovine or human uteri (Carsten 1972, 1973).

Another possible site for oxytocin-PG interaction is the regulation of intracellular cyclic nucleotide levels. Oxytocin and $PGF_2\alpha$ promote the accumulation of cGMP in uterine tissue obtained from diethylstilbesterol-treated rats (Goldberg et al. 1973). Oxytocin and $PGF_2\alpha$ were able to inhibit up to 50 percent of the isoproterenol-stimulated cAMP accumulation in ovariectomized rat uteri (Bhalla et al. 1972). This effect conforms to the concept that cGMP and cAMP mediate opposing effects and that the contractile events in the uterus are subject to bidirectional control (Kolata 1973). It is not yet known how cAMP, whose formation is promoted by beta adrenergic agonists, such as isoproterenol, is coupled to smooth-muscle relaxation. Nor is it known what cGMP has to do with smooth-muscle contraction. Cyclic nucleotides may play a role in regulating calcium ion movements (Rasmussen 1970), which in turn affect contractility.

In summary, PGs recur repeatedly in the complex events of parturition. PGE and PGF may be produced by the decidua and PGE by the myometrium. The stimulus for PG production and release may be increased estrogen (as in the sheep), stretching of the tissue (as would occur during contractions), or the presence of oxytocin. The presence of PGs in the plasma may itself stimulate oxytocin release.

The actions of PGs in parturition are multiple. PGE and PGF can elicit muscle contractions in vivo in nonpregnant uteri and in vivo and in vitro in pregnant uteri of many species. (The early reports that PGs caused relaxation of nonpregnant uterine muscle in vitro are confusing and unexplained.) PGs may be involved in overcoming the progesterone block postulated by Csapo (1956). Progesterone synthesis by the placenta may be decreased by direct toxic effects of PGs or by ischemia resulting from the vasoconstricting properties of $PGF_2\alpha$ or from constriction of the vessels by the PG-stimulated contraction of the myometrium.

The role of PGs in the biochemical events leading to muscle contraction is not understood. PGs can modulate the cellular levels of the cyclic nucleotides either directly, since $PGF_2\alpha$ promotes cyclic GMP production, or indirectly, since $PGF_2\alpha$ and PGE_2 (in low concentrations) antagonize isoproterenol-stimulated cAMP accumulation. PGs may also be involved in calcium movements in the uterine muscle. To date, the relationship among these various biochemical events and the ultimate result of muscle contraction have not been explained.

23.12 The IUD

The intrauterine device (IUD) prevents implantation

and embryogenesis in many species. Chaudhuri (1971) suggested that PGs may mediate some of the observed effects of the IUD; subsequently he was able to measure an increase of PGE and PGF synthesis in the IUD-bearing horns of the rat uterus (Chaudhuri 1973). Increased uterine PG synthesis in the presence of the IUD has been observed in the sheep (Spilman and Duby 1972) and in the hamster (Saksena et al. 1974).

At least five explanations can be given for the antifertility effects of the IUD, and PGs could mediate any one of them. Changes in uterine contractility that impede sperm migration at the time of ovulation or that accelerate or retard ovum transport have been ruled out in humans. Sperm with good motility and morphology have been found in the oviducts of IUD-bearing women within 48 hours of coitus (Malkani and Sujan 1964; Morgenstern et al. 1966). Since fertilized ova have been recovered from the oviducts of IUD-bearing humans (Noyes et al. 1965) and monkeys (Kelly and Marston 1967), tubal contractility and tubal transport of ova are unaffected by the IUD.

Unusual patterns of uterine contractility have been observed in the IUD-bearing uterus and may account for the failure of implantation in the presence of an IUD (Bengtsson and Moawad 1966). The prelaborlike uterine contractions that were observed on day 25 of a 28-day menstrual cycle before the insertion of the IUD, occurred on day 19 of a 28-day cycle after the IUD was implanted. The laborlike contractions that accompanied the onset of menstruation in the normal cycle occurred as early as day 25 in the presence of the IUD. PGs have been shown to stimulate human uterine contractility; and although increased PG synthesis has not been measured in the IUD-bearing uterus in humans, PGs probably mediate this aspect of IUD action.

Leukocyte infiltration into the endometrium and uterine lumen characteristically follows IUD insertion, as was first observed by Greenwald et al. (1965) in the rat. The antifertility action of the IUD may be related to the leukocyte response, since increasing leukocyte counts in IUD-bearing rabbit uteri were associated with a decreasing number of implantation sites for corpora lutea (El Sahwi and Moyer 1971). The leukocyte infiltration is chronic (Moyer and Mishell 1971), with inflammatory cells persisting in the endometrium of humans for as long as three years after IUD insertion. The phagocytotic response appears to be enhanced in the IUD-bearing uterus in sheep (Hawk 1969) and in monkeys (Moyer et al. 1972). The increased phagocytotic activity may be directed against sperm as well as against bacteria, since polymorphonuclear leukocytes containing phagocytosed sperm were observed in the endometrium of IUD-bearing monkey uteri (Moyer et al. 1972). PGs may be involved in this aspect of IUD action, since PGE$_1$ is a leukotactic agent (Kaley and Weiner 1971) and PGE$_2$ can provoke leukocyte release (Kaley et al. 1972).

Another possible explanation for IUD action is that its presence stimulates the elaboration of an embryotoxic agent, but PGs themselves do not appear to be embryotoxic. PGF$_2\alpha$ (100 μg/ml) did not interfere with the development of mouse embryos in culture from the two-cell, four-cell, eight-cell, or morula stage into blastocysts. The subsequent development of the embryos in the uteri of foster mothers was unaffected by the PG treatment (Kirkpatrick 1974). In view of these findings, the unidentified embryotoxic agent is unlikely to be a PG.

Increased amounts of PG are synthesized in response to the uterine distension exerted by the IUD (Poyser et al. 1971); these amounts may cause premature luteolysis in the species that have luteolytic PGs. Decreases in luteal duration and luteal weight have been observed in sheep (Ginther et al. 1966; Stormshak et al. 1967). The luteolytic effects of the IUD could be reversed by administration of hCG (Stormshak et al. 1967). The IUD does not appear to affect cycle length in primates (Breed et al. 1972), and these data are compatible with the findings that PGs are not luteolytic in primates.

The presence of the IUD in humans has been associated with findings of abrasion, blisters with edema fluid, and ulcerations of the superficial endometrium (Bonney et al. 1966). These responses are characteristic of an inflammatory response. PGs are known to have many of the characteristics of a chemical mediator of inflammation (see Willis et al. 1972), including the leukotactic effect mentioned earlier. Whether these features make the endometrial surface unsuitable for implantation is not known.

No single action of the IUD has been shown to be responsible for the antifertility effects of the device. Likewise, no unequivocal role has been delineated for PGs.

23.13 Reproduction in the Male

Prostaglandins were so named because they were originally found in extracts of the human prostate gland, and much work has been done to characterize the PG content and secretion of the male reproductive tract. PGs in the male tract occupy a somewhat existential niche in biology: although everyone admits that they exist, no one is quite sure why. There are at least 13 PGs in seminal plasma (Hamberg and Samuelsson 1966; Samuelsson 1963), and PGs occur throughout the male reproductive tract (for review, see von Euler and Eliasson 1967).

Semen from normal human males contains PGE, PGF, PGA, and PGB compounds, with the PGE compounds predominating. The mean concentrations of the E series in normal men are PGE$_1$, 25μg/ml; PGE$_2$, 23 μg/ml; and PGE$_3$, 5.5 μg/ml. The concentrations of the F series are PGF$_1\alpha$, 3.6 μg/ml, and PGF$_2\alpha$, 4.4 ng/ml (Bygdeman and Samuelsson 1966). The combined concentrations of the A and B series were comparable to the concentrations of the E series. Seminal PGs appeared in the same fraction of semen (collected by the "split ejaculate" technique) as fructose; this occurrence indicated that PGs were synthesized in the seminal vesicles (Eliasson 1959). Collier and Flower (1971) found that aspirin administration resulted in a decrease in the PGE and PGF content of semen of humans. Furthermore, Bygdeman et al. (1970) found that in 40 percent of infertile men whose infertility could not be attributed to another cause, the PGE levels in the semen were significantly lower than in semen from fertile males. The therapeutic value of added PG to the semen of infertile men has not been evaluated.

The actions of PG in the elaboration of gonadal hormones and in gamete production may be surveyed in a manner analogous to the treatment of this subject in the female. PGs may stimulate interstitial-cell-stimulating hormone (ICSH) release from the pituitaries of male animals. Tissues from male rats were used in the studies done by Zor et al. (1970) and Ratner et al. (1974) on the effects of PG on the elaboration of gonadotropins by pituitary gland in vitro. Experiments with rats suggest that PGs may have an in vivo role in the elaboration of gonadotropins. Serum LH levels in male rats were doubled 15 minutes after injection of PGE$_2$, (100 μg/rat), and the simultaneous administration of PGE$_2$ and antiserum to LH-releasing hormone abolished the release of LH (Lindner et al. 1973).

The role of PGs in mediating FSH or LH effects in the male has not been investigated, nor are there any data on the involvement of PGs in spermatogenesis. Exogenous PGs may accelerate sperm transport. Hunt and Nicholson (1972) found that sperm labeled with tritiated thymidine appeared in the semen of chronically PGF$_2\alpha$-treated rabbits two days earlier than in vehicle-treated rabbits.

PGs present in the seminal fluid may promote the longevity or the motility of the sperm; however, this theory has been discounted by the finding of Eliasson et al. (1968) that PGE$_1$ has no effect on the oxygen uptake, fructose utilization, or lactate production of suspensions of washed human sperm.

Little is known about the physiological role of PGs in the male, but they may be involved in gonadotropin release and in sperm transit through the male ducts. These possibilities are suggestive and bear further investigation.

23.14 Conclusions

From the foregoing analysis of prostaglandin research in the reproductive field, it is clear that there have been three major discoveries: (1) PGs cause contractions of the human uterus during pregnancy; (2) PGs are luteolytic in many subprimate species, but not in humans; and (3) PG levels in the blood and amniotic fluid are elevated during labor in many species, including humans. These important findings have led to major advances in clinical medicine and animal husbandry and to a further understanding of some of the events in the reproductive cycle.

The finding by Bygdeman and Wiqvist that PGs cause a contraction of human smooth muscle was followed by the use of these agents in terminating pregnancy. Initially, PGs were used to induce labor at term (Karim; Anderson; Beazley). Later PGs were used to induce second-trimester abortions (Karim; Csapo; Anderson; Wiqvist; Embrey) and to terminate pregnancy in other conditions where oxytocin is ineffective (molar pregnancy, intrauterine death, and anencephaly). The use of $PGF_2\alpha$ to induce term labor has been associated with a significant risk of hypertonus and fetal distress. At present there are no clear advantages in inducing labor by $PGF_2\alpha$ rather than by oxytocin. Orally administered PGE_2 has recently been reintroduced for labor induction, but more tests are needed to establish the safety and efficacy of PGE_2 and its 15-methyl analog. Suction curettage remains the method of choice in first-trimester abortions, for which PGs have not proved to be useful. PGs are preferable to hysterotomy and saline induction in second-trimester abortions. Experimentation with dosage schedules and routes of administration are likely to establish procedures that have minimal induction-abortion intervals and diminished side effects.

Since PGs that contract the uterus have been found in the human endometrium (Pickles), inappropriate PG synthesis may be the pathology of dysmenorrhea. This hypothesis has been strengthened by the recent finding that PG-synthetase inhibitors are beneficial in this condition (Lindner).

The luteolytic actions of PGs were first noted by Pharriss; and Labhsetwar, McCracken, Inskeep, Horton, and Poyser have made substantial contributions to this field. The major advance, resulting from the original finding of the luteolytic action of PGs, is a better understanding of the regulation of this important steroidogenic gland. It is now known that $PGF_2\alpha$ is the authentic luteolysin in some species, while in others (e.g., cows), the uterine product may be a PG precursor.

PGs are used in veterinary practice to synchronize estrus in herds of sheep, cattle, pigs, and horses. PGs terminate the luteal phase, and the animals return to estrus within a few days (Louis et al. 1973; Inskeep 1973). This treatment simplifies breeding procedures and allows safe, early abortions before the animals are sent to market.

Many attempts have been made to demonstrate that PGs are luteolytic in humans, but it must be concluded that they are not. In monkeys, elevated plasma PG levels may occur during estrogen-induced luteolysis, but the source of these PGs is not known. The feasibility of further searches for a PG analog or precursor with luteolytic activity in humans remains to be seen. The real problem to be investigated is the mechanism of luteal regulation in humans.

Plasma PG levels are elevated during labor in sheep, goats (Thorburn), and humans (Karim; Caldwell). PG administration causes premature delivery in pregnant rats, and PG-synthetase inhibitors delay parturition in rats. These findings point to a possible role of PGs in circumnatal events.

No clinical applications have been made yet of these findings, but the use of synthetase inhibitors to prevent or curtail premature labor in humans should be investigated.

PGs play a possibly significant but not yet understood role in four areas: (1) Behrman initially demonstrated, and Ratner, Field, and Lindner have subsequently found, indications that PGs may be involved in the regulation of hypothalamic releasing factor release and the regulation of adenohypophyseal hormone secretion. There is no clear explanation of a PG role at these sites. (2) PGs are produced by follicles during ovulation (Caldwell; Armstrong; LeMaire; Lindner); however, the mechanisms of the regulation of ovarian PG synthesis and the actions of these agents are not known. (3) Although there is presently no direct evidence that PGs play a physiological role, circumstantial evidence suggests that they are involved in spermiogenesis and sperm maturation and transport. (4) The high concentration of PGs in the seminal fluid suggests their involvement in sperm transport in both the male and female reproductive tracts. These questions deserve further consideration.

Two subjects have not been extensively studied and were not discussed in the preceding analysis: (1) the possible teratogenic effects of PGs and of PG-synthetase inhibitors; and (2) the possible side effects in infants whose mothers have been treated with PG for labor induction. With the increasing use of PGs and with the possible use of synthetase inhibitors in the future, the immediate and long-range effect on the offspring of women treated with these agents should be examined.

References

Aiken, J. W. Aspirin and indomethacin prolong parturition in rats: Evidence that prostaglandins contribute to expulsion of foetus. Nature 240:21, 1972.

Aref, I., E. S. E. Hafez, and G. A. R. Kamar. Post-coital prostaglandins in vivo: Oviductal motility and egg transport in rabbits. Fertil. Steril. 24:671, 1973.

Auletta, F. J., B. V. Caldwell, G. van Wagenen, and J. M. Morris. Effects of postovulatory oestrogen on progesterone and prostaglandin F levels in the monkey. Contraception 6:411, 1972.

Auletta, F. J., L. Speroff, and B. V. Caldwell. PGF_2-alpha induced steroidogenesis and luteolysis in primate corpus luteum. J. Clin. Endocrinol. Metab. 36:405, 1973.

Behrman, H. R., A. J. MacDonald, and R. O. Greep. Regulation of ovarian cholesterol esters: Evidence for enzymatic sites of prostaglandin induced loss of corpus luteum function. Lipids 6:791, 1971.

Behrman, H. R., G. P. Orczyk, and R. O. Greep. Effect of synthetic gonadotropin-releasing hormone (Gn-RH) on ovulation blockade by aspirin and indomethacin. Prostaglandins 1:245, 1972.

Bengtsson, L. P., and A. H. Moawad. Lippes loop and myometrial activity. Lancet 1:146, 1966.

Bhalla, R. C., B. A. Sanborn, and S. G. Korenman. Hormonal interaction in the uterus: Inhibition of isoproternol-induced accumulation of adenosine $3':5'$-cyclic monophosphate by oxytocin and prostaglandins. Proc. Natl. Acad. Sci. USA 69:3761, 1972.

Bland, K. P., and B. T. Donovan. Oestrogen and progesterone and the function of the corpora lutea in the guinea pig. J. Endocrinol. 47:225, 1970.

Blatchley, F. R., and B. T. Donovan. Luteolytic effect of prostaglandin in guinea pig. Nature 221:1065, 1969.

Blatchley, F. R., B. T. Donovan, N. L. Poyser, E. W. Horton, C. J. Thompson, and M. Los. Identification of prostaglandin F_2-alpha in the utero-ovarian blood of guinea pig after treatment with oestrogen. Nature 230:243, 1971.

Bolognese, R. J., and S. L. Corson. The effect of vaginally administered prostaglandin F_2-alpha on corpus luteum function. Am. J. Obstet. Gynecol. 117:240, 1973a.

Bolognese, R. J., and S. L. Corson. Abortion of early pregnancy by the intravaginal administration of prostaglandin F_2-alpha. Am. J. Obstet. Gynecol. 117:246, 1973b.

Bonney, W. A., S. R. Glasser, T. H. Clewe, R. W. Noyes, and C. L. Cooper. Endometrial response to the intrauterine device. Am. J. Obstet. Gynecol. 96:101, 1966.

Breed, W. G., J. M. Stephenson, P. Eckstein, P. V. Peplow, and W. R. Butt. Effect of an intrauterine device on menstrual cyclicity and luteal function in the baboon. J. Reprod. Fertil. 28:249, 1972.

Brummer, H. C. Further studies on the interaction between prostaglandins and syntocinon on the isolated pregnant human myometrium. J. Obstet. Gynaecol. Br. Commonw. 79:526, 1972a.

Brummer, H. C. Serum PGF_2-alpha levels during late pregnancy, labour, and the puerperium. Prostaglandins 2:185, 1972b.

Bygdeman, M. The effect of different prostaglandins on human myometrium in vitro. Acta Physiol. Scand. (Suppl.242), 1964.

Bygdeman, M., and B. Samuelsson. Analyses of prostaglandins in human semen. Clin. Chim. Acta 132:465, 1966.

Bygdeman, M., S. U. Kwon, T. Mukherjee, and N. Wiqvist. Effect of intravenous infusion of prostaglandin E_1 and E_2 on motility of the pregnant human uterus. Am. J. Obstet. Gynecol. 102:317, 1968.

Bygdeman, M., B. Fredricsson, K. Svanborg, and B. Samuelsson. The relation between fertility and prostaglandin content of seminal fluid in man. Fertil. Steril. 21:622, 1970.

Caldwell, B. V., S. Burstein, W. A. Brock, and L. Speroff. Radio-immunoassay of the F prostaglandins. J. Clin. Endocrinol. 33:171, 1971.

Caldwell, B. V., A. S. Tillson, W. A. Brock, and L. Speroff. The effects of exogenous progesterone and estradiol on prostaglandin F levels in ovariectomized ewes. Prostaglandins 1:217, 1972.

Carlson, J. C., B. Barcikowski, and J. A. McCracken. PGF_2-alpha and the release of LH in sheep. J. Reprod. Fertil. 34:357, 1973.

Carsten, M. E. Prostaglandins' part in regulating uterine contraction by transport of calcium. In *Prostaglandins*, ed. E. M. Southern. Mount Kisco, N.Y.: Futura, 1972.

Carsten, M. E. Prostaglandins and cellular calcium transport in the pregnant human uterus. Am. J. Obstet. Gynecol. 117:824, 1973.

Cerini, M. E. D., W. A. Chamley, J. K. Findlay, and J. R. Goding. Luteolysis in sheep with ovarian autotransplants following concurrent infusions of luteinizing hormone and prostaglandin F_2-alpha into the ovarian artery. Prostaglandins 3:399, 1973.

Challis, J. R. G., F. A. Harrison, R. B. Heap, E. W. Horton, and N. L. Poyser. A possible role of oestrogens in the stimulation of prostaglandin F_2-alpha output at the time of parturition in a sheep. J. Reprod. Fertil. 30:485, 1972.

Chamley, W. A., and M. Christie. Failure of prostaglandin F_2-alpha to affect LH secretion in the ovariectomized ewe. Prostaglandins 3:405, 1973.

Chang, M. C., and D. M. Hunt. Effect of prostaglandin F_2-alpha on the early pregnancy of rabbits. Nature 236:120, 1972.

Channing, C. P. Stimulatory effects of prostaglandins upon luteinization of rhesus monkey granulosa cell cultures. Prostaglandins 2:331, 1972a.

Channing, C. P. Effects of prostaglandin inhibitors 7-oxa-13-prostynoic acid and eicosa-5,8,11,14-tetraynoic acid upon luteinization of rhesus monkey granulosa cells in culture. Prostaglandins 2:351, 1972b.

Chasalow, F. I., and B. B. Pharriss. Luteinizing hormone stimulation of ovarian prostaglandin biosynthesis. Prostaglandins 1:107, 1972.

Chatterjee, A. A possible mode of action of prostaglandins. VI. Failure of prostaglandin F_2-alpha in the interruption of pregnancy of rats having pituitary heterotransplant under the kidney capsule. Prostaglandins 4:915, 1973.

Chaudhuri, G. Intrauterine device: Possible role of prostaglandins. Lancet 1:480, 1971.

Chaudhuri, G. Release of prostaglandins by the I.U.D. Prostaglandins 3:773, 1973.

Chester, R., M. Dukes, S. R. Slater, and A. L. Walpole. Delay of parturition in the rat by anti-inflammatory agents which inhibit the biosynthesis of prostaglandins. Nature 240:37, 1972.

Collier, J. G., and R. J. Flower. Effect of aspirin on human seminal plasma prostaglandins. Lancet 2:852, 1971.

Coudert, S. P., G. D. Phillips, C. Faiman, W. Chernecki, and M. Palmer. A study of utero-ovarian circulation in sheep with reference to local transfer between venous and arterial blood. J. Reprod. Fertil. 36:319, 1974a.

Coudert, S. P., G. D. Phillips, C. Faiman, W. Chernecki, and M. Palmer. Infusion of tritiated PGF_2-alpha into the anterior uterine vein of the ewe: Absence of local venous-arterial transfer. J. Reprod. Fertil. 36:333, 1974b.

Coutinho, E. M., and H. S. Maia. The contractile response of the human uterus, Fallopian tubes, and ovary to prostaglandins in vivo. Fertil. Steril. 22:539, 1971.

Csapo, A. Progesterone "block." Am. J. Anat. 98:273, 1956.

Csapo, A. The prospects of prostaglandins in post-conceptional therapy. Prostaglandins 3:245, 1973.

Deis, R. P. Induction of lactogenesis and abortion by prostaglandin $F_2\alpha$ in pregnant rats. Nature 229:568, 1971.

Diaz-Infante, A., K. H. Wright, and E. E. Wallach. Effects of indomethacin and prostaglandin F_2-alpha on ovulation and ovarian contractility in the rabbit. Prostaglandins 5:567, 1974.

Downie, J., N. L. Poyser, and M. Wunderlich. Levels of prostaglandins in human endometrium during the normal menstrual cycle. J. Physiol. 236:465, 1974.

Dunn, M. V., N. G. Humphrey, G. R. Judkins, J. Z. Kendall, and G. W. Knight. The effect of PGF_2-alpha antibody on gestation length in the rat. N.Z. Med. J. 78:368, 1973.

Eagling, E. M., H. G. Lovell, and V. R. Pickles. Prostaglandins, myometrial "enhancement" and calcium. J. Physiol. 213:53P, 1971.

Eagling, E. M., H. G. Lovell, and V. R. Pickles. Interaction of prostaglandin E_1 and calcium in the guinea pig myometrium. Br. J. Pharmacol. 44:510, 1972.

Eglington, G., R. A. Raphael, G. N. Smith, W. J. Hall, and V. R. Pickles. Isolation and identification of two smooth muscle stimulants from menstrual fluid. Nature 200:960, 993, 1963.

Eliasson, R. Studies in prostaglandin. Acta Physiol. Scand. (Suppl. 158):1, 1959.

Eliasson, R., R. N. Murdock, and I. G. White. The metabolism of human spermatozoa in the presence of prostaglandin E_1. Acta Physiol. Scand. 73:379, 1968.

Eliasson, R., and N. Posse. The effect of prostaglandin on the non-pregnant human uterus in vivo. Acta Obstet. Gynecol. Scand. 39:112, 1960.

Ellinger, J. V., and K. T. Kirton. Ovum transport in rabbits injected with prostaglandins E_1 or F_2-alpha. J. Reprod. Biol. 7:106, 1972.

El Sahwi, S., and D. L. Moyer. The leukocytic response to an intrauterine foreign body in the rabbit. Fertil. Steril. 22:398, 1971.

Fuchs, A. R., and E. Mok. Histochemical study of the effects of prostaglandins F_2-alpha and E_2 on the corpus luteum of pregnant rats. Biol. Reprod. 10:24, 1974.

Gillespie, A., H. C. Brummer, and T. Chard. Oxytocin release by infused prostaglandin. Br. Med. J.:543, Feb. 26, 1972.

Ginther, O. J., A. L. Pope, and L. E. Casida. Local effects of an intrauterine plastic coil on the corpus luteum of the ewe. J. Anim. Sci. 25:472, 1966.

Goldberg, N. D., R. F. O'Dea, and M. K. Haddox. Cyclic GMP. In Advances in cyclic nucleotide research, vol. 3, eds. P. Greengard and G. A. Robison. New York: Raven Press, 1973.

Greenwald, G. S. Interruption of pregnancy in rats by uterine suture. J. Reprod. Fertil. 9:9, 1965.

Grieves, S. A., J. Z. Kendall, and J. C. Liggins. Measurement of PGF_2-alpha and its 15-keto metabolites in the human menstrual cycle. N.Z. Med. J. 78:367, 1973.

Grinwich, D. L., T. G. Kennedy, and D. T. Armstrong. Dissociation of ovulatory and steroidogenic actions of luteinizing hormone in rabbits with indomethacin, an inhibitor of prostaglandin synthesis. Prostaglandins 1:89, 1972.

Gutknecht, G. D., L. J. Wyngarden, and B. B. Pharriss. The effect of PGF_2-alpha on ovarian and plasma progesterone levels in the pregnant hamster. Proc. Soc. Exp. Biol. Med. 136:1151, 1971.

Hamberg, M., and B. Samuelsson. Prostaglandins in human seminal plasma. J. Biol. Chem. 241:257, 1966.

Hansel, W., P. W. Concannon, and J. H. Lukaszewska. Corpora lutea of the large domestic animals. Biol. Reprod. 8:222, 1973.

Harrison, F. A., R. B. Heap, E. W. Horton, and N. L. Poyser. Identification of prostaglandin F_2-alpha in uterine fluid from the nonpregnant sheep with autotransplanted ovary. J. Endocrinol. 53:215, 1972.

Hawk, H. W. Some effects of the IUD on reproductive function in the ewe. Fertil. Steril. 20:1, 1969.

Henzl, M. R., L. Noriega, R. Aznar, E. Ortega, and E. Segrea. The uterine effects of vaginally administered prostaglandin E_2. Prostaglandins 1:205, 1972.

Hilliard, J. Corpus luteum function in guinea pigs, hamsters, rats, mice, and rabbits. Biol. Reprod. 8:203, 1973.

Horton, E. W., I. H. M. Main, and C. J. Thompson. Effects of prostaglandins on the oviduct, studied in rabbits and ewes. J. Physiol. 180:514, 1965.

Horton, E. W., and N. L. Poyser. Elongation of the estrous cycle in the guinea pig following subcutaneous or intra-uterine administration of indomethacin. Br. J. Pharmacol. 49:98, 1973.

Hunt, W. L., and N. Nicholson. Studies on semen from rabbits injected with 3H-thymidine and treated with PGE_2 or PGF_2-alpha. Fertil. Steril. 23:763, 1972.

Inskeep, E. K. Potential uses of prostaglandins in control of reproductive cycles of domestic animals. J. Anim. Sci. 36: 1149, 1973.

Jewelewicz, R., B. Cantor, I. Dyrenfurth, M. P. Warren, and R. L. Vande Wiele. Intravenous infusion of prostaglandin F_2-alpha in the mid-luteal phase of the normal human menstrual cycle. Prostaglandins 1:443, 1972.

Kaley, G., and R. Weiner. Prostaglandin E_1: A potential mediator of the inflammatory response. Ann. N.Y. Acad. Sci. 180:338, 1971.

Kaley, G., E. J. Messina, and R. Weiner. The role of prostaglandin in microcirculatory regulation and inflammation. In *Prostaglandins in cellular biology*, eds. P. W. Ramwell and B. B. Pharriss. New York: Plenum Press, 1972.

Karim, S. M. M. Identification of prostaglandins in human amniotic fluid. J. Obstet. Gynaecol. Br. Commonw. 73:903, 1966.

Karim, S. M. M., and J. Devlin. Prostaglandin content of amniotic fluid during pregnancy and labour. J. Obstet. Gynaecol. Br. Commonw. 74:230, 1967.

Karim, S. M. M. Appearance of prostaglandin F_2-alpha in human blood during labour. Br. Med. J. 4:618, 1968.

Karim, S. M. M. Prostaglandins and human reproduction: Physiological roles and clinical uses of prostaglandins in relation to human reproduction. In *The prostaglandins: Progress in research*, ed. S. M. M. Karim. Oxford: Medical and Technical Publishing, 1972a.

Karim, S. M. M. Physiological role of prostaglandins in the control of parturition and menstruation. J. Reprod. Fertil. Suppl. 16:105, 1972b.

Karlson, S. The influence of seminal fluid on the motility of the nonpregnant human uterus. Acta Obstet. Gynecol. Scand. 38:503, 1959.

Karsch, F. J., J. F. Roche, J. W. Noveroske, D. L. Foster, H. W. Norton, and A. V. Nalbandov. Prolonged maintenance of the corpus luteum of the ewe by continuous infusion of luteinizing hormone. Biol. Reprod. 4:129, 1971.

Karsch, F. J., L. C. Krey, R. F. Weick, D. J. Dieshke, and E. Knobil. Functional luteolysis in the rhesus monkey. The role of estrogen. Endocrinology 92:1148, 1973.

Kelly, W. A., and J. H. Marston. Contraceptive action of intrauterine devices in the rhesus monkey. Nature 214:735, 1967.

Kirkpatrick, J. F. The absence of direct effects of PGF_2-alpha on preimplantation mouse embryos in vitro. Prostaglandins 5:107, 1974.

Kirton, K. T., B. B. Pharriss, and A. D. Forbes. Luteolytic effects of PGF_2-alpha in primates. Proc. Soc. Exp. Biol. Med. 133:314, 1970.

Kloeck, F. K., and H. Jung. In vitro release of prostaglandins from the human myometrium under the influence of stretching. Am. J. Obstet. Gynecol. 115:1066, 1973.

Knobil, E. On the regulation of the primate corpus luteum. Biol. Reprod. 8:246, 1973.

Koering, M. J., and K. T. Kirton. The effects of PGF_2-alpha on the structure and function of the rabbit ovary. Biol. Reprod. 9:226, 1973.

Kolata, G. B. Cyclic GMP: Cellular regulatory agent? Science 182:149, 1973.

Kolena, J., and C. P. Channing. Stimulatory effects of LH, FSH, and prostaglandins upon cyclic $3'5'$ AMP levels on porcine granulosa cells. Endocrinology 90:1543, 1972.

Kuehl, F. A., J. L. Humes, J. Tarnoff, V. J. Cirillo, and E. A. Ham. Prostaglandin receptor site: Evidence for an essential role in the action of luteinizing hormone. Science 169:883, 1970.

Labhsetwar, A. P. Effects of PGF_2-alpha on some reproductive processes of hamsters and rats. J. Endocrinol. 53:201, 1972a.

Labhsetwar, A. P. Prostaglandin E_2: Analysis of effects on pregnancy and corpus luteum in hamsters and rats. Acta Endocrinol. (Suppl. 170):1, 1972b.

Labhsetwar, A. P. Luteolytic and ovulation inducing properties of PGF_2-alpha in pregnant mice. J. Reprod. Fertil. 28:451, 1972c.

Labhsetwar, A. P. Prostaglandin E_2: Evidence for luteolytic effects. Prostaglandins 2:23, 1972d.

Labhsetwar, A. P. Neuroendocrine basis for ovulation in hamster treated with PGF_2-alpha. Endocrinology 92:606, 1973.

Labhsetwar, A. P. Prostaglandins and the reproductive cycle. Fed. Proc. 33:61, 1974.

Larsen, J. W., T. M. Hanson, B. V. Caldwell, and L. Speroff. The effect of estradiol infusion on uterine activity and peripheral levels of prostaglandin F and progesterone. Am. J. Obstet. Gynceol. 117:276, 1973.

Lau, I. F., S. K. Saksena, and M. C. Chang. Pregnancy biockade by indomethacin, an inhibitor of prostaglandin synthesis: Its reversal by prostaglandins and progesterone in mice. Prostaglandins 4:795, 1973.

Lehmann, F., F. Peters, M. Breckwoldt, and G. Bettendorf. Plasma-progestin during the infusion of prostaglandin F_2-alpha. Acta Endocrinol. (Suppl. 159):61, 1972a.

Lehmann, F., F. Peters, M. Breckwoldt, and G. Bettendorf. Plasma progesterone levels during the infusion of prostaglandin F_2-alpha in the human. Prostaglandins 1:269, 1972b.

LeMaire, W. J., and A. G. Shapiro. Prostaglandin F_2-alpha: Its effect on the corpus luteum of the menstrual cycle. Prostaglandins 1:259, 1972.

LeMaire, W. J., N. S. Yang, H. H. Behrman, and J. M. Marsh. Preovulatory changes in the concentration of prostaglandins in rabbit Graafian follicles. Prostaglandins 3:367, 1973.

Liggins, G. C., and S. Grieves. Possible role for prostaglandin F_2-alpha in parturition in sheep. Nature 232:629, 1971.

Liggins, G. C., S. A. Grieves, J. Z. Kendall, and B. S. Knox. The physiological roles of progesterone, oestradiol-17-beta and prostaglandin F_2-alpha in the control of ovine parturition. J. Reprod. Fertil. (Suppl.)16:85, 1972.

Lindner, H. R., U. Zor, S. Bauminger, A. Tsafriri, S. Lamprecht, Y. Koch, S. Antebi, and A. Schwartz. The use of prostaglandin synthetase inhibitors in the analysis of the role of prostaglandins in reproductive physiology. In *Prostaglandin synthesis inhibitors*, eds. H. J. Robinson and J. R. Vane. New York: Raven Press, 1974.

Louis, T. M., J. N. Spellflug, B. E. Sequin, and H. D. Hafs. Disappearance of injected $PGF_2\alpha$ in heifers. J. Anim. Sci. 37:319, 1973.

Malkani, P. K., and S. Sujan. Sperm migration in the female reproductive tract in the presence of intrauterine devices. Am. J. Obstet. Gynecol. 88:963, 1964.

Mandl, J. P. The effect of prostaglandin E_1 on rabbit sperm transport in vivo. J. Reprod. Fertil. 31:263, 1972.

Marley, B. P. Effect of prostaglandins F_2-alpha, E_2, and E_1 on fertility in mice. Nature New Biol. 235:213, 1972.

Marsh, J. The effect of prostaglandins on the adenyl cyclase of the bovine corpus luteum. Ann. N.Y. Acad. Sci. 180:416, 1971.

McCracken, J. Prostaglandin F_2-alpha and corpus luteum regression. Ann. N.Y. Acad. Sci. 180:456, 1971.

McCracken, J. A., J. C. Carlson, M. E. Glew, J. R. Goding, D. T. Baird, K. Green, and B. Samuelsson. Prostaglandin F_2-alpha identified as a luteolytic hormone in sheep. Nature New Biol. 238:129, 1972.

Morgenstern, L. L., M. C. Orgebin-Crist, T. H. Clewe, W. A. Bonney, and R. W. Noyes. Observations on spermatozoa in the human uterus and oviducts in the chronic presence of intrauterine devices. Am. J. Obstet. Gynecol. 96: 114, 1966.

Moyer, D. L., and D. R. Mishell. Reactions of human endometrium to the intrauterine foreign body. II. Long term effects on endometrial histology and cytology. Am. J. Obstet. Gynecol. 111:66, 1971.

Moyer, D. L., S. T. Shaw, N. Darwish, M. El Habashy, and S. El Sahwi. Investigations on intrauterine devices in *Macaca mulatta* monkeys. Acta Endocrinol. (Suppl. 166):381, 1972.

Novy, M. J., and M. J. Cook. Redistribution of blood flow by prostaglandin F_2-alpha in the rabbit ovary. Am. J. Obstet. Gynecol. 117:381, 1973.

Noyes, R. W., Z. Dickmann, T. H. Clewe, and W. A. Bonney. Pronuclear ovum from a patient using an intrauterine contraceptive device. 147:744, 1965.

Ogra, S. S., K. T. Kirton, T. B. Tomasi, and J. Lippes. Prostaglandins in the human Fallopian tube. Fertil. Steril. 25:250, 1974.

O'Grady, J. P., B. V. Caldwell, F. J. Auletta, and L. Speroff. The effects of an inhibitor of prostaglandin synthesis (indomethacin) on ovulation, pregnancy, and pseudopregnancy in the rabbit. Prostaglandins 1:97, 1972.

Okamura, H., S. L. Yang, K. H. Wright, and E. E. Wallach. The effect of prostaglandin F_2-alpha on the corpus luteum of the pregnant rat. An ultrastructural study. Fertil. Steril. 23: 475, 1972.

Pharriss, B. B., and L. J. Wyngarden. The effect of prostaglandin $F_2\alpha$ on the progestogen content of ovaries from pseudopregnant rats. Proc. Soc. Exp. Biol. Med. 130:92, 1969.

Pharriss, B. B., L. J. Wyngarden, and G. D. Gutknecht. Biological interaction between prostaglandins and luteotropins in the rat. In *Gonadotropins*, ed. E. Rosemberg. Los Altos: Geron-X, 1968.

Pharriss, B. B., J. C. Cornette, and G. D. Gutknecht. Vascular control of luteal steroidogenesis. J. Reprod. Fertil. Steril. Suppl. 10:97, 1970.

Pickles, V. R., W. J. Hall, F. A. Best, and G. N. Smith. Prostaglandins in endometrium and menstrual fluid from normal and dysmenorrheic subjects. J. Obstet. Gynaecol. Br. Commonw. 72:185, 1965.

Poyser, N. L., E. W. Horton, C. J. Thompson, and M. Los. Identification of prostaglandin F_2-alpha released by distension of guinea pig uterus in vitro. Nature 230:526, 1971.

Rasmussen, H. Cell communication, calcium ion, and cyclic adenosine monophosphate. Science 170:404, 1970.

Ratner, A., M. C. Wilson, L. Strivastava, and G. R. Peake. Stimulatory effects of PGE_1 on rat anterior pituitary cyclic AMP and luteinizing hormone release. Prostaglandins 5:165, 1974.

Richman, K. A., K. H. Wright, and E. E. Wallach. Local ovarian effects of prostaglandins E_2 and F_2-alpha on human chorionic hormone induced ovulation in the rabbit. Obstet. Gynecol. 43:203, 1974.

Saksena, S. K., and I. F. Lau. Effect of exogenous estradiol and progesterone on the uterine tissue levels of prostaglandin F_2-alpha in ovariectomized mice. Prostaglandins 3:317, 1973.

Saksena, S. K., I. F. Lau, and V. D. Castracane. Prostaglandin mediated action of IUDs. II. F-prostaglandins (PGF) in the uterine horn of pregnant rats and hamsters with intrauterine devices. Prostaglandins 5:97, 1974.

Samuelsson, B. Isolation and identification of prostaglandins from human seminal plasma. J. Biol. Chem. 238:3229, 1963.

Sandberg, F., A. Ingelman-Sundberg, and G. Ryden. The effect of prostaglandin F_1-alpha, F_1-beta, F_2-alpha, and F_2-beta on the human uterus and the Fallopian tubes in vitro. Acta Obstet. Gynecol. Scand. 44:585, 1965.

Sato, T., K. Taya, T. Jyujyo, M. Hirono, and M. Igarashi. The stimulatory effect of prostaglandins on luteinizing hormone release. Am. J. Obstet. Gynecol. 118:875, 1974.

Sellner, P. G., and E. W. Wickersham. Effects of prostaglandins on steroidogenesis. J. Anim. Sci. 31:230, 1970.

Speroff, L., and P. W. Ramwell. Prostaglandin stimulation of in vitro progesterone synthesis. J. Clin. Endocrinol. Metab. 30:345, 1970.

Spies, H. G., and R. L. Norman. Luteinizing hormone release and ovulation induced by the intraventricular infusion of prostaglandin E_1 into pentobarbitol blocked rats. Prostaglandins 4:131, 1973.

Spilman, E. H., and R. T. Duby. Prostaglandin mediated luteolytic effect of an intrauterine device in sheep. Prostaglandins 2:159, 1972.

Spilman, C. H., and M. J. K. Harper. Effect of prostaglandins on oviduct motility in conscious rabbits. J. Reprod. Biol. 7:106, 1972.

Stormshak, F., R. P. Lehman, and H. W. Hawk. Effect of intrauterine plastic spirals and hCG on the corpus luteum of the ewe. J. Reprod. Fertil. 14:373, 1967.

Strauss, J. F., and R. L. Stambaugh. Induction of 20-alpha hydroxy steroid dehydrogenase in rat corpora lutea of pregnancy by PGF₂-alpha. Prostaglandins 5:73, 1974.

Surve, A. H., F. E. Harrington, and R. L. Elton. Effect of hCG on the corpus luteum of the monkey. Proc. Soc. Exp. Biol. Med. 144:963, 1973.

Thorburn, G. D., R. I. Cox, W. B. Currie, B. J. Restall, and W. Schneider. Prostaglandin F concentration in the uteroovarian venous plasma of the ewe during the estrous cycle. J. Endocrinol. 53:325, 1972a.

Thorburn, G. D., D. H. Nicol, J. M. .Bassett, D. A. Shutt, and R. I. Cox. Parturition in the goat and sheep: Changes in corticosteroids, progesterone, oestrogens, and prostaglandin F. J. Reprod. Fertil. Suppl. 16:61, 1972b.

Tsafriri, A., Y. Koch, and H. R. Lindner. Ovulation rate and serum LH levels in rats treated with indomethacin or prostaglandin E₂. Prostaglandins 3:461, 1973.

Vane, J. R., and K. I. Williams. Prostaglandin production contributes to the contractions of rat isolated uterus. Br. J. Pharmacol. 45:146P, 1973.

von Euler, U. S., and R. Eliasson. *Prostaglandins*. New York: Academic Press, 1967.

Waltman, R., V. Tricomi, and A. Palav. Mid-trimester hypertonic saline-induced abortion: Effect of indomethacin on induction/abortion time. Am. J. Obstet. Gynecol. 114:829, 1972.

Waltman, R., V. Tricomi, E. H. Shabanah, and R. Arenas. The effect of anti-inflammatory drugs on parturition parameters in the rat. Prostaglandins 4:106, 1973.

Wentz, A. C., and G. S. Jones. Intravenous prostaglandin F₂-alpha for induction of menses. Fertil. Steril. 24:569, 1973.

Wilks, J. W., K. K. Forbes, and J. F. Norland. Synthesis of prostaglandin F₂-alpha by the ovary and uterus. J. Reprod. Med. 9:271, 1972.

Wilks, J. W., A. C. Wentz, and G. S. Jones. Prostaglandin alpha concentration in the blood of women during normal menstrual cycles and dysmenorrhea. J. Clin. Endocrinol. Metab. 37:469, 1973.

Willis, A. L., P. Davidson, P. W. Ramwell, W. F. Brocklehurst, and B. Smith. Release and actions of prostaglandins in inflammation and fever. Inhibition by antiinflammatory and antipyretic drugs. In *Prostaglandins in cellular biology*, eds. P. W. Ramwell and B. B. Pharriss. New York: Plenum Press, 1972.

Wilson, L., R. J. Cenedella, R. L. Butcher, and E. K. Inskeep. Levels of prostaglandins in the uterine endometrium during the ovine estrous cycle. J. Anim. Sci. 34:93, 1972.

Yang, N. S. T., J. M. Marsh, and W. J. LeMaire. Prostaglandin changes induced by ovulatory stimuli in rabbit Graafian follicles. The effect of indomethacin. Prostaglandins 4:395, 1973.

Zor, U., T. Kaneko, H. P. G. Schneider, S. M. McCann, and J. B. Field. Further studies on stimulation of anterior pituitary cyclic adenosine-3′,5′-monophosphate formation by hypothalamic extract and prostaglandins. J. Biol. Chem. 245:2883, 1970.

Zor, U., S. A. Lamprecht, T. Kaneko, H. P. G. Schneider, S. M. McCann, J. B. Field, A. Tsafriri, and H. R. Lindner. Functional relations between cyclic AMP, prostaglandins, and luteinizing hormone in rat pituitary and ovary. Adv. Cyclic Nucleotide Res. 1:503, 1972.

Bert W. O'Malley

24.1 Hormonal Regulation of Chromosome Structure and Function in Reproductive Tissues

The term *chromatin* was first used to describe the basic staining material of the cell nucleus, which was subsequently shown to consist of deoxyribonucleic acid (DNA) and proteins. Chromatin is currently defined as the diffuse, interface form of the chromosome of eukaryotic cells. It is a poorly defined mass of genetic material, composed primarily of DNA, histones, nonhistone proteins (acidic proteins), and RNA in a mass ratio of 1:1:2:0.05. The histones are composed basically of five main classes and are generally similar among all types of nucleated cells examined. In contrast, the nonhistone proteins are highly heterogeneous in terms of individual species, molecular weights, and immunological properties.

A major impetus to study this complex genetic species derived from the development of reproducible methodology by Zubay and Doty in 1959[1] and by Bonner.[2] Also in 1959, a major revelation was made by Weiss and Gladstone,[3] who described the association of a DNA-dependent RNA-synthesizing activity with chromatin; their work formed the basis for numerous subsequent studies on the enzymology of chromatin. This knowledge, coupled with revelations on the mechanism of regulation of RNA and DNA synthesis in bacteria and phage, has promoted a steady increase in our understanding of the structural and functional properties of the genetic material of nucleic cells. Still the structure and function of chromatin are far from completely elucidated and represent a major stumbling block to the development of theories for hormonal regulation of transcription or hormone-mediated differentiation and the development of eukaryotic cells.

Since 1959 the structure of native chromatin has been approached by almost every physical and chemical technique available. The eventual aim of such studies is to understand the structure of chromatin as related to its function properties in vivo. Unfortunately, the condition of chromatin in vivo differs markedly from the the state in which it is usually studied in vitro. Chromatin exists in the cell nucleus at a DNA concentration of about 10–50 mg/ml under conditions of ionic strength of about 0.15 M salt and in the presence of significant concentrations of divalent cation. In contrast, physical studies of chromatin have been for the most part performed at DNA concentrations of 0.01–0.5 mg/ml at very low ionic strength in the absence of calcium or magnesium. The solubility of the complex can differ under these in vitro conditions, and in many instances the complex exists as a precipitate at high ionic strength and a diffuse gel at low ionic strength in vitro. Functionally, the chromatin probably exists in a state in which it contains regions that are transcribable and regions that are totally repressed or nontranscribable. At this point, methods do not exist that would separate these active and inactive regions. Nevertheless, studies are being carried out on whole chromatin, even though we realize that only 5 to 10 percent of the total chromatin DNA is transcribed in most preparations.

An educated guess at the structure of chromatin at this time would be that the DNA is basically in the B-configuration and is highly supercoiled into a short thick particle. The proteins of chromatin are partially in the α-helical conformation and appear to interact with DNA for the most part by binding to the major groove. These proteins interact with DNA at the ends of the molecules and have a central helical nonbound region. The nonbound regions of the chromosome proteins may then interact in hydrophobic bonding with one another, providing at least a portion of the stabilizing energy for maintenance of the DNA in the supercoiled conformation.[4]

In the past six years, our knowledge of the composition and characteristics of mammalian RNA polymerase has blossomed under intense study from several laboratories. At present the consensus is that three distinct RNA polymerase forms exist in the eukaryotic nucleus: forms I, II, and III. Form I is primarily located in the nucleolus and is responsible for synthesis of ribosomal RNA. Forms II and III are located in the nucleoplasm. Polymerase II appears to be responsible for transcription of messenger RNA precursors, and type polymerase III synthesizes 4S and 5S RNA. Polymerase I is sensitive to α-amanitin, which represents a convenient test for this molecule.

Although many serious difficulties exist in work dealing with the structural composition and enzymology of chromatin, it is of basic importance that we understand this genetic complex. The number of workers in this area of research is rapidly increasing, but many more will be required to answer the questions of (1) what the mechanism of DNA replication is in normal cells and what the uncontrolled replication characteristics of neoplasia are; (2) how the chromosomal proteins relate to DNA replication; (3) how and why certain parts of the genome are expressed, while others are permanently repressed or temporarily repressed prior to induction with hormones; (4) how genes are induced to expression in an orderly fashion in response to differentiative stimuli and hormones; and (5) how specific gene restriction of the DNA by its chromosomal protein coat permits cell-specific expression of only the appropriate genes.

The histones seem to play an important supportive role in chromatin structure and gene repression, but they appear to not be involved in specific gene restriction or activation. The primary argument for this statement is that there are only five classes of histones, and these histones are similar in composition and quantity between different cells of the same organism and even between widely divergent organisms, for example, plants (peas) and mammals (calf thymus). The nonhistone or acidic chromosomal proteins appear to be more heavily implicated in specific gene restriction of transcription in chromatin. The evidence for this is (1) that nonhistone proteins are extremely heterogeneous as assessed by molecular weight estimation, charge separation, and immunochemical analysis; (2) that there are enough different species of nonhistones (hundreds to thousands) to account for specific gene interactions; (3) that the turnover of nonhistone proteins is much greater than that of histones; (4) that chemical modifications of nonhistones occur at a greater rate; (5) that the chromosomal concentration of nonhistone proteins is different for each tissue of the same organism, and in different species the composition is different; (6) that nonhistone proteins change in quantity and composition within the chromatin of hormone-stimulated or growing cells; (7) that the nonhistone proteins play an important role in the interaction of the steroid hormone receptor complex with target cell nuclei and chromatin; and (8) that certain fractions of the nonhistone proteins have been shown in a preliminary fashion to influence the rate of polymerase transcription of chromatin in vitro.

Paul and Gilmore[5,6] have provided perhaps the best original evidence implicating nonhistone proteins in specific restriction of transcription of chromatin. Early studies had demonstrated that the template activity of chromatin for bacterial polymerase was reduced to 5 to 10 percent of that of naked DNA, and the RNA transcribe from chromatin in vitro competed wholly with native RNA synthesized in vivo in the same tissue. Addition of histones to DNA abolished this activity as a template. Addition of either whole chromatin proteins to DNA under controlled conditions or of histones to dehistonized DNA led to template activity appropriate to the original chromatin and preserved the specificity of RNA synthesis characteristic of the original sample.

Important to a consideration of reproductive tissue development are the mechanisms active in spermiogenesis. In terms of chromatin, the most definitive studies have involved chromosomal protein-DNA interactions in Salmonid fish. At a particular stage in spermiogenesis, histones are removed from DNA and completely replaced by the even more basic protamines. The histones of trout spermatids are known to be acetylated and phosphorylated; in general these modifications occur in highly basic regions near the amino terminus of the molecule. Phosphorylation of these proteins occurs at about the time of histone replacement. Marushige and Dickson[7] have postulated that a local "unzipping" of the basic end of a modified histone molecule might sufficiently alter its overall binding to allow displacement by protamine. The subsequent appearance of small fragments of proteins, together with the presence of a protease activity in testis chromatin, have suggested that proteolysis may play a role in the removal of histones from DNA during maturation of spermatids.

Reproductive steroid hormones have previously been shown to have rather dramatic effects on the composition and structure of reproductive cell chromatin. Quantitative analysis of chromatin from various stages of reproductive tissue development has demonstrated that while the amounts of histone remained constant, the amounts of nonhistone increased during cell maturation and differentiation. Accompanying this increase in nonhistone proteins was a measurable increase in chromatin template capacity. Immunochemical studies using antibodies raised against DNA nonhistone protein complexes have revealed that the immunoreactive population of proteins changes during steroid hormone action on reproductive target tissue chromatins. During this period, structural analysis of chromosomal protein-DNA complexes, made by means of circular dichroism analysis, showed changes consistent with an increase in mean ellipticity that appear to represent an opening of the DNA, that is, removal of proteins from areas of the DNA.[8]

Incubation of tritiated estradiol directly with preparations of target tissue chromatin in vitro shows that very little of the tritiated steroid becomes bound to the chromatin; however, incubation of the preformed tritiated estradiol receptor complex from the uterus with uterine chromatin results in significant retention of the complex on the chromatin. Removal of histone (basic) proteins prior to the incubation exposes even more receptor-binding sites. Similar results with androgen receptor interactions with male target and nontarget tissues have been reported by researchers at three laboratories.[9,10]

The majority of studies on hormone-receptor interaction with target cell chromosomes appear to have been carried out in the chick oviduct system, using the tritiated progesterone receptor complex extracted and purified from oviduct cytosol.[11] Again it appears that tritiated progesterone requires the receptor to become associated with chromatin, and furthermore the receptor cannot bind to chromatin without first becoming complexed with the steroid hormone. The progesterone receptor complex appears to bind to oviduct chromatin to a much greater degree than to nontarget cell chromatin such as from the spleen, heart, lung, or hen erythrocyte. Experiments employing dissociation and reconstitution of chromosomal proteins to DNA to form hybrid chromatins have generally indicated that the histones play no significant role in the interaction of the hormone receptor complex with chromosomal DNA, but the nonhistones appear to play an important integral role. These studies have led to the generation of the "acceptor hypothesis" for target cell chromatin.[11] This hypothesis states that target cells contain nuclear chromosomal binding sites that are programmed to receive and bind the hormone-receptor complex upon its entry from the cytosol. This binding is specific, saturable, and high-affinity ($K_d \sim 10^{-8} \times 10^{-9}$ mol) in character.[12]

In summary, it can be speculated that after entry of the steroid-receptor complex into the nuclear compartment, the initial molecular interaction of the steroid receptor complex with chromatin may occur in two parts, a high-affinity reaction occurring with the hormone-receptor complex and the acceptor site, followed by a change in the chromatin that allows RNA polymerase to transcribe certain previously repressed gene sites.[12]

Considerable future research must center on the area of chromatin structure and function and the biochemistry of the hormone-receptor complex interaction with this species. The existence of the receptor and its translocation to the nucleus during the course of hormone action is now well substantiated. That steroid hormones can and do induce specific new mRNAs, which in turn code for new proteins to carry out new functions in reproductive cells, has also recently been proved. Research in the area of molecular biology and developmental biology of hormone action must now center on the nucleus. We must define the precise sequence of biochemical events that occurs following the binding of the hormone-receptor com-

plex onto the chromosome and the appearance of the first new mRNA molecules.[12]

24.2 Hormonal Regulation of Transcription in Reproductive Tissues

The elucidation of the molecular mechanisms by which reproductive hormones regulate gene transcription in their respective target tissues has been complicated by the enormous analytical complexity of eukaryotic DNA. Generally, advances in the field of reproductive hormone action have paralleled or followed technical advances in the field of molecular biology. The technical advances have provided the tools necessary to divide the transcriptional machinery into its component parts and have permitted the study of hormonal effects on RNA polymerase, chromatin template, and the types of RNA transcripts synthesized. While many of the early studies relied on indirect methods, such as blockage of the hormonal response by metabolic inhibitors, recent progress has allowed a more direct estimation of the hormonal induction of specific messenger RNAs. Two model systems that have provided the impetus for many of these advances in reproductive hormone action are the effect of estrogen in the castrate rat uterus and the effects of estrogen and progesterone in the immature chick oviduct. Results obtained in these systems have been quickly extended to studies of androgen action in the rat prostate and more recently to the effects of gonadotropins in their target tissues.[13,14]

Although hormonal effects on the labeling and accumulation of RNA had been demonstrated prior to the work of Ui and Mueller,[15] their studies using actinomycin D to block the stimulatory effect of estrogen on uterine RNA, protein, and lipid synthesis in ovariectomized rats suggested the primary importance of DNA-directed RNA synthesis in the early biosynthetic responses of the uterus to estrogen stimulation. Extending these studies to earlier times after estrogen stimulation, Hamilton,[16] Hamilton et al.,[17] and Means and Hamilton[18] demonstrated a rapid increase in the specific activity of pulse-labeled uterine nuclear RNA as soon as two minutes after estrogen administration in vivo to ovariectomized rats. This early effect could be abolished by actinomycin D but not by cycloheximide, again suggesting the primary importance of estrogen-stimulated RNA synthesis. In addition, these data also indicate that protein biosynthesis is not a necessary prerequisite for the early estrogen stimulation of nuclear RNA biosynthesis.

The ability to assay endogenous RNA polymerase activity in crudely isolated nuclei provided an additional method with which to study the early estrogen stimulation of uterine nuclear RNA synthesis. The initial experiments performed by Gorski[19] demonstrated that by one hour after the administration of estrogen to immature rats there was an increase in the activity of an endogenous nuclear RNA polymerase, which was later shown to synthesize predominantly ribosomal RNA (RNA polymerase I). Subsequent experiments by Hamilton et al.[17] indicated an increase also in the activity of RNA polymerase II, which synthesized more DNA-like RNA, but this occurred at much later times (e.g., at 6 to 12 hours). These workers also analyzed the base composition and nearest-neighbor dinucleotide frequency of the RNA products of polymerase I and polymerase II activities. Comparable studies were performed by Liao et al.[20] in the rat prostate after testosterone administration. Glasser et al.[21] reported that when endogenous RNA polymerase activities were assayed using conditions carefully designed to minimize ribonuclease degradation and to control for diurnal variations, a significant increase in polymerase II activity was observed as early as 15 minutes following estrogen treatment. This stimulation was biphasic with peaks at 30 minutes and 6 hours following hormone administration. Thus estrogen appeared to stimulate an initial peak of uterine polymerase II activity, which subsequently declined during the onset of polymerase I activity and then increased again at later times.

While these results correlated nicely with the previous studies describing the rapid synthesis of uterine nuclear RNA in response to estrogen, they did not distinguish between an increase in polymerase activity and an increased template availability. With the development of techniques to measure chromatin template capacity using exogenous, highly purified E. coli RNA polymerase, the response of the chromatin template to hormone administration could be measured. Barker and Warren[22] first showed a significant, tissue-specific elevation of uterine chromatin template capacity at two hours following in vivo administration of estrogen. These studies were extended by Teng and Hamilton,[23] who demonstrated an increased template capacity at 30 minutes as well as an increase in the specific activity of chromatin-associated RNA as early as 15 minutes after in vivo hormone administration. In somewhat earlier studies, Wilson and Loeb[24] had fractionated chromatin from the duck preen gland into presumptive euchromatin and heterochromatin and had localized both radioactive testosterone and newly synthesized RNA in the euchromatin fraction. Schwartz et al.[25] have demonstrated that the increase in chromatin template capacity seen in the chick oviduct following estrogen administration can be correlated with the number of initiation sites for RNA polymerase. These studies suggest that increased endogenous RNA polymerase activity results from a greater availability of

the chromatin template for polymerase molecules; however, Cox et al.[26] have shown that the greater amount of endogenous polymerase activity reflects an increase in the number of RNA polymerase molecules as well as in chromatin template capacity. Thus within 24 hours after estrogen administration to an immature chick, they were able to demonstrate a 400 percent increase in extractable polymerase I and a 100 percent increase in extractable polymerase II activities separated by DEAE-Sephadex chromatography.

In all of the previously mentioned studies, the effects on endogenous RNA polymerase activity were determined subsequent to in vivo administration of a hormone. Direct transcriptional effects of a hormone in vitro have been quite difficult to assess. Some progress in this area has been made by Raynaud-Jammet and Baulieu[27] and by Mohla et al.[28] These investigators reported the ability of the transformed estradiol-receptor complex to directly stimulate endogenous RNA polymerase I activity in isolated uterine nuclei. While this effect was somewhat variable, it did provide a basis for the future study of the direct effects of hormones in reconstituted cell-free systems.

In order to differentiate selective stimulatory effects of reproductive hormones on RNA synthesis from effects on total RNA synthesis, it was necessary to analyze carefully the types of RNA transcripts synthesized in response to hormone administration. Initial studies revealed that quantitative but not qualitative changes could be observed after hormone administration in target-tissue RNA populations when analysis was performed on sucrose gradients or by polyacrylamide gel electrophoresis. For example, Hamilton et al.[29] first reported that uterine, pulse-labeled nuclear RNA synthesized in response to estrogen consisted mostly of ribosomal RNA, as determined by base composition and sucrose-gradient analysis. Later studies by Knowler and Smellie[30] employed polyacrylamide gel electrophoresis to demonstrate an increased synthesis of pulse-labeled RNA greater than 45S (i.e., heterogeneous nuclear RNA). Finally, Luck and Hamilton[31] were able to demonstrate a stimulation of 45S ribosomal precursor processing during estrogen stimulation. Other more sensitive analytical techniques had to be employed, however, to determine whether hormone administration led to the synthesis of new types of RNA as well as an increased amount of RNA.

One of the first studies to indicate qualitative changes in hormonally induced RNA populations was performed by O'Malley and McGuire.[32] They utilized the techniques of nearest-neighbor dinucleotide frequency analysis and competitive DNA-RNA hybridization to demonstrate the appearance of new species of RNA in chick oviduct chromatin transcripts following estrogen administration. Church and McCarthy[33] performed similar hybridization experiments using the rabbit uterus. They were able to detect qualitative differences in nuclear RNA populations following estrogen treatment as well as an increased translocation of the percentage of the nuclear RNA molecules translocated to the cytoplasm. Under the conditions employed, however, only the rapidly hybridizing repetitive-sequence transcripts would have been detected, to the exclusion of the unique-sequence transcripts containing the majority of eukaryotic messenger RNA sequences. Liarakos et al.[34] have demonstrated an increased transcription of unique-sequence DNA in the chick oviduct after estrogen administration, but in these experiments qualitative changes were not determined. (Qualitative changes in a complex population of RNA transcripts, each present in a limited number of copies, are difficult to determine using the methods currently available.)

Another approach to this problem was the direct assessment of specific hormone-inducible messenger RNA levels in a target tissue by measuring the ability of an isolated mRNA fraction to support de novo synthesis of a specific protein in an in vitro translation system. Many indirect studies such as those performed by Liao and Williams-Ashman[35] had suggested hormonal effects on messenger RNA synthesis. In their experiments, the ability of prostatic ribosomes to respond to a synthetic messenger (poly AG) was measured. Not until the reports by Rosenfeld et al.[36] and Means et al.,[37] however, was an increase in a specific estrogen-inducible messenger RNA—ovalbumin mRNA— directly demonstrated by translation in the heterologous reticulocyte cell-free system.

More recently, with the availability of methods to purify specific messenger RNAs and the discovery that a complementary radioactive DNA copy of these messenger RNAs could be synthesized using viral reverse transcriptase, a powerful new hybridization probe for specific messenger RNA sequences has been developed. Using this probe, an increase in ovalbumin mRNA molecules could be correlated with the increased translation activity found after hormone administration.[38] This radioactive DNA probe was also utilized to determine the number of gene copies present in the chick genome that coded for ovalbumin mRNA.[39, 40] Since only a single gene copy could be detected using this technique, it appears that estrogen acts at the genome level to cause the repetitious transcription of a single ovalbumin gene that results in a high intracellular concentration of specific mRNA molecules of reasonably long half-life.[41] The availability of a high-specific-activity probe for a specific mRNA will also allow the detection of specific hormone-inducible mRNA sequences in reconstituted cell-free systems. This should provide a sensitive indi-

cator for assaying the effects of the hormone-receptor complex in vitro, and it should permit the identification of the chromatin-associated macromolecules responsible for hormonal induction of RNA synthesis. These new techniques may provide the impetus necessary to unravel the mechanism of reproductive hormone action at the transcriptional level.

24.3 Hormonal Regulation of Protein Synthesis in Reproductive Tissues

The initial studies on protein synthesis in reproductive tissue were carried out in Mueller's laboratory in the late 1950s.[42] They demonstrated that estrogen resulted in increased amino acid incorporation into protein in the rat uterus. Similar observations regarding effects of androgen on protein synthesis in prostate were made a few years later in Williams-Ashman's laboratory.[43] In 1962 Wilson[44] showed that testosterone increased the activity of ribonucleoprotein in prostate in vivo, and in the same year Liao and Williams-Ashman[45] made the initial observation that a hormone (testosterone) stimulated the activity of polyribosomes isolated from rat prostate and assayed in a cell-free system. These observations suggested that the rate-limiting step might be synthesis of RNA. Indeed, in 1963 Hamilton[46] and Ui and Mueller[15] provided evidence that stimulation of uterine protein synthesis by estrogen could be abolished by pretreatment with actinomycin D. Similar results were achieved in Williams-Ashman's laboratory[43] in the androgen-prostate model system.

One of the next major advances in our understanding of hormone-regulated protein synthesis was the theory of superinduction. Initial experiments on this phenomenon were obtained in the laboratories of Tomkins[47] and Kenny[48] in 1965. The theory says that actinomycin D results in increased levels of specific proteins. Although the reasons are not yet elucidated, the best bets are (1) decreased degradation of the protein in the absence of continued RNA synthesis, or (2) inhibition of the production of the mRNA by actinomycin D for a "repressor" molecule. Since these initial observations, superinduction has been reported to occur in reproductive target tissues in response to progesterone and estrogen.

Until 1966 no specific endpoint was available to investigate the action of estrogen on rat uterus. Notides and Gorski[49] showed in 1966 that estrogen stimulated the synthesis of a species of protein (IP for *induced protein*) within 30 minutes following administration to ovariectomized rats. The following year O'Malley and co-workers[50] introduced the chick oviduct as a unique model system for the study of the mechanism of action of both estrogen and progesterone. Estrogen induces the synthesis of specific oviduct proteins such as oval-bumin and lysozyme,[50] whereas progesterone controls the synthesis of avidin.[51] Evidence was also presented to suggest that both hormones acted at the level of gene transcription.

The first demonstration that gonadotropins stimulated protein synthesis in target tissues was provided in 1967 by Means's laboratory.[52] Here again the effects of FSH on the testis were manifest at the level of the polyribosome; moreover, inhibitor studies suggested that protein synthesis was controlled by previous effects of FSH on RNA synthesis. This model system remains the only one in which clear effects of a gonadotropin on RNA and protein synthesis have been demonstrated in detail.

The next advances that allowed development of the mechanism of protein synthesis in reproductive tissue were derived from studies with rabbit reticulocytes. These cells synthesize large quantities of globin. Lockard and Lingrel[53] demonstrated that treatment of polyribosomes with detergent resulted in the release of globin mRNA. This mRNA could be collected and could be translated in a lysate of reticulocytes. The second major contribution was made by Anderson and colleagues.[54] In a series of experiments they were able to isolate and partially purify four proteins that were required for the initiation of protein synthesis. These were the first successful studies to be reported in an eukaryotic system. Both of these contributions—the isolation and translation of specific mRNA and the isolation and purification of translation initiation factors—have proved very valuable in continuing studies to advance our understanding of the hormonal control of protein synthesis in reproductive tissues.

Means and O'Malley[55] demonstrated that the administration of estrogen to chicks caused a conversion of single ribosomes to polysomes in the oviduct. Moreover, these polysomes synthesized qualitatively different proteins both in vivo and in vitro. These data suggested that estrogen might cause the transcription of new species of mRNA. Stavnezer and Huang[56] were the first to demonstrate that the reticulocyte lysate was capable of translating mRNA from a heterologous system with fidelity. O'Malley and Means in 1972 utilized this system to translate ovalbumin[37] and avidin[57] mRNA from the oviduct. It was subsequently shown that estrogen regulated the intracellular concentration of mRNA of ovalbumin.[37] These experiments were confirmed by Schimke's laboratory.[58] O'Malley et al.[57] also showed that progesterone induced the mRNA for avidin. These were the first reports that sex steroid hormones induced the synthesis of mRNA for specific target tissue proteins. Finally, Palmiter[59] has revealed that the rates of mRNA translation for several specific oviduct proteins are con-

trolled differentially by sex steroids. Moreover, for optimal rates of protein synthesis in vivo, at least three steroid hormones (estrogen, progesterone, and testosterone) appear to be required.

24.4 Summary and Speculations on Future Applications of Basic Research to Contraceptive Development

Since reproductive tissue function is dependent on hormonal stimulation, blocking hormone action in certain target tissues would naturally lead to interruption of the reproductive process. The molecular information generated during the last decade on hormone action should provide some interesting new leads for contraceptives. When we consider the entire process of steroid hormone action as defined above, we should quickly realize that although blocking RNA or protein synthesis itself would inhibit the hormone response, the toxicity from such an approach would be unacceptable. It would be preferable to interfere with the earlier, more specific interactions such as the binding of steroid hormone to receptor, the amount of available cellular receptor, the activation of receptor, and the binding of hormone-receptor complex to the nuclear acceptor sites on chromatin. It seems quite conceivable to generate a new chemical agent that will competitively antagonize the binding of endogenous steroid hormone to receptor, irreversibly denature the steroid hormone receptor so that it cannot bind endogenous steroid hormone, or bind to the receptor in such a way that the receptor is not in the required conformation to carry out its physiological role, which is a consequence of binding to the nuclear acceptor sites.

The most specific, efficient, and nontoxic approach to chemical contraception would be the development of an agent to counteract the action of the pregnancy hormone, progesterone. Progesterone is obviously necessary for implantation and pregnancy, but with a couple of exceptions, it is not required for general cellular maintenance functions in other tissues in mammals. Thus elimination of the action of progesterone should have a specific effect on implantation in mammals. Furthermore, the best approach would seem to be initially blocking the action of this hormone rather than counteracting its effects by overdosage with other potent agents that produce side effects (e.g., estrogen). Toward this end, a precise understanding of the molecular sequence of events required for progesterone action in reproductive tissue should generate the insight required for designing new contraceptive agents. Possible approaches include:

1. Interference with the binding of progesterone to its target cell receptors. In this approach one could attempt to synthesize steroid derivatives that would bind covalently to a progesterone receptor and thus func-

tionally eliminate this binding molecule from the cell. The receptor binding capacity would then be totally absent until a new receptor is synthesized. During this period the steroid hormone, progesterone, would be unable to exert its actions in this cell.

2. Inactive analog binding to cell receptor molecules. This approach would involve synthesis of compounds that lack biological progestational activity but still bind to the target tissue receptor. This might be accomplished by minimum alterations in the A ring (the most critical area for binding specificity) rather than by altering the D, C, or B rings to cause biological inactivation. This method would "fool" the receptor into accepting and into binding and transporting an inactive steroid into the nucleus.

The most rewarding approach may be a combination of 1 and 2. In this approach one could covalently link an inactive steroid to the molecular receptor. This would require only a small dose of biologically inactive steroid and would provide maximum specificity and efficiency without any harmful side effects.

3. Destruction of the steroid hormone receptor so that it is unavailable to endogenous progesterone. This can be accomplished by: (a) synthesis of an inactive steroid that covalently binds the receptor, or by (b) hormone-induced destruction of receptor binding sites. Two interesting physiological experiments have recently shown that estrogen must first stimulate a progesterone-responsive cell to generate a sufficient concentration of progesterone receptor for subsequent physiological action, and a subsequent single large dose of progesterone somehow depletes the cell of available progesterone-binding sites. Future approaches may involve treatment with a large dose of weak estrogen, to prevent synthesis of progesterone receptor for about 25 days, or short-term treatment with a superphysiological dose of progesterone, to deplete the cell of progesterone receptor binding sites for about 5 days. If timed correctly during the cycle, administration of these hormones will effectively block progesterone binding to receptor, and in our laboratory they have been shown to block implantation and ensuing pregnancy. These compounds can be taken either orally or in a single injectable dose.

4. Prevention of receptor binding to nuclear acceptor sites. A short time ago some investigators felt this approach had no chance of success. Recently, however, evidence has accumulated that this mechanism is definitely feasible for new contraceptive development. This evidence is based on the fact that one of our safest and most efficient hormone analogs (spironolactone), which is a clinical, useful antagonist for aldosterone, has now been shown to work in this exact manner.[60] Spironolactone will bind to aldosterone receptor with the same affinity and with the same number of sites, but the spironolactone-receptor complex will not enter the nucleus in the whole cell, will not bind to nuclei in vitro, and will not bind to chromatin in vitro. It thus appears that this antagonist will bind to the receptor, but the receptor will not change to requisite conformation required for interaction with the nuclear acceptor sites. This phenomenon thus completely prevents the biological action of aldosterone in its target cells. I see no reason why we cannot generate hormone analogs that will interfere with progesterone action by the identical mechanism.

In summary, the past decade has provided numerous new revelations in the field of molecular biology. Our understanding of subcellular regulation has increased enormously. Only in the past few years has this information begun to be applied to cell and tissue physiology. If support continues for applied contraceptive research based on cellular and molecular biology, we will accomplish new and innovative mechanisms for the regulation of fertility.

References

1. Zubay, G., and P. Doty. The isolation and properties of deoxyribonucleo-protein particles containing single nucleic acid molecules. J. Mol. Biol. 1:1, 1959.

2. Bonner, J., G. R. Chalkley, M. Dahmus, D. Fambrough, F. Fujimara, R. C. Huang, J. Huberman, R. Jensen, K. Marushige, H. Ohlenbusch, B. Olivera, and J. Widholm. Isolation and characterization of chromosomal nucleoproteins. Meth. Enzymol. 12B:3, 1968.

3. Weiss, S. B., and L. Gladstone. A mammalian system for the incorporation of cytidine triphosphate into ribonucleic acid. J. Am. Chem. Soc. 81:4118, 1959.

4. Simpson, R. T. Structure and function of chromatin. Adv. Enzymol. 38:41, 1973.

5. Paul, J., and R. S. Gilmour. Template activity of DNA is restricted in chromatin. J. Mol. Biol. 16:242, 1966.

6. Paul, J., and R. S. Gilmour. Organ-specific restriction of transcription in mammalian chromatin. J. Mol. Biol. 34:305, 1968.

7. Marushige, K., and G. H. Dixon. Transformation of trout testis chromatin. J. Biol. Chem. 246:5799, 1971.

8. Spelsberg, T. C., W. Mitchell, F. C. Chytil, and B. W. O'Malley. Chromatin of the developing chick oviduct: Changes in the acidic proteins. Biochim. Biophys. Acta 312:765, 1973.

9. Liao, S., T. Liang, T. C. Shao, and J. L. Tymoczko. Androgen receptor cycling in prostate cells. In *Receptors for reproductive hormones*, eds. B. W. O'Malley and A. R. Means. N. Y.: Plenum Press, 1973.

10. Mainwaring, W. I. P., and B. M. Peterken. A reconstituted cell-free system for the specific transfer of steroid-receptor complexes into nuclear chromatin isolated from rat ventral prostate gland. Biochem. J. 125:285, 1971.

11. O'Malley, B. W., T. C. Spelsberg, W. T. Schrader, F. C. Chytil, and A. W. Steggles. Mechanisms of interaction of a hormone-receptor complex with the genome of a eukaryotic target cell. Nature (London) 235:141, 1972.

12. O'Malley, B. W., and A. R. Means. Female steroid hormones and target cell nuclei. Science 183:610, 1974.

13. Reel, J. R., and J. Gorski. Gonadotrophic regulation of precursor incorporation into ovarian RNA, protein and acid-soluble fractions. 1. Effects of pregnant mare serum gonadotrophin (PMSG), follicle-stimulating hormone (FSH), and luteinizing hormone (LH). Endocrinology 83:1083, 1968.

14. Jungmann, R. A., and J. S. Schweppe. Mechanism of action of gonadotropin. II. Control of ovarian nuclear ribonucleic acid polymerase activity and chromatin template capacity. J. Biol. Chem. 247:5543, 1972.

15. Ui, H., and G. C. Mueller. The role of RNA synthesis in early estrogen action. Proc. Natl. Acad. Sci. USA 50:256, 1963.

16. Hamilton, T. H. Sequences of RNA and protein synthesis during early estrogen action. Proc. Natl. Acad. Sci. USA 51:83, 1964.

17. Hamilton, T. H., C. C. Widnell, and J. R. Tata. Sequential stimulation by oestrogen of nuclear RNA synthesis and DNA-dependent RNA polymerase activities in rat uterus. Biochim. Biophys. Acta 108:168, 1965.

18. Means, A. R., and T. H. Hamilton. Evidence of depression of nuclear protein synthesis and concomitant stimulation of nuclear RNA synthesis during early estrogen action. Proc. Natl. Acad. Sci. USA 56:686, 1966.

19. Gorski, J. Early estrogen effects on the activity of uterine ribonucleic acid polymerase. J. Biol. Chem. 239:889, 1964.

20. Liao, S., K. Leininger, D. Sagher, and R. W. Barton. Rapid effect of testosterone on ribonucleic acid polymerase activity of rat ventral prostate. Endocrinology 77:763, 1965.

21. Glasser, S. R., F. C. Chytil, and T. C. Spelsberg. Early effects of oestradiol-17 on the chromatin and activity of the deoxyribonucleic acid-dependent ribonucleic acid polymerases (I & II) of the rat uterus. Biochem. J. 130:947, 1972.

22. Barker, K. L., and J. C. Warren. Template capacity of uterine chromatin control by estradiol. Proc. Natl. Acad. Sci. USA 56:1298, 1966.

23. Teng, C., and T. H. Hamilton. The role of chromatin in estrogen action in the uterus. I. The control of template capacity and chemical composition and the binding of H3-estradiol-17 beta. Proc. Natl. Acad. Sci. USA 60:1410, 1968.

24. Wilson, J. D., and P. M. Loeb. Estrogen and androgen control of cell biosynthesis in target organs. In Developmental and metabolic control mechanisms and neoplasia, Univ. of Texas M. D. Anderson Nineteenth Annual Symposium on Fundamental Cancer Research. Baltimore: Williams & Wilkins, 1975.

25. Schwartz, R. J., M.-J. Tsai, and B. W. O'Malley. Effect of estrogen on gene expression in the chick oviduct. V. Changes in the number of RNA polymerase binding and initiation sites in chromatin. J. Biol. Chem. 250:5175, 1975.

26. Cox, R. F., M. E. Haines, and N. H. Carey. Modification of the template capacity of chick-oviduct chromatin for form-B RNA polymerase by estradiol. Eur. J. Biochem. 32:513, 1973.

27. Raynaud-Jammet, M., and E.-E. Baulieu. Action de l'oestradiol in vitro: Augmentation de la biosynthèse de l'acide ribonucléique dans les noyaux utérins. C. R. Acad. Sci. (Paris) 268:3211, 1969.

28. Mohla, S., E. R. DeSombre, and E. V. Jensen. Tissue specific stimulation of RNA synthesis by transformed estradiol-receptor complex. Biochem. Biophys. Res. Commun. 46:661, 1972.

29. Hamilton, T. H., C. C. Widnell, and J. R. Tata. Synthesis of ribonucleic acid during early estrogen action. J. Biol. Chem. 243:408, 1968.

30. Knowler, J. T., and R. M. S. Smellie. The oestrogen-stimulated synthesis of heterogenous nuclear ribonucleic acid in the uterus of immature rats. Biochem. J. 131:689, 1973.

31. Luck, D. N., and T. H. Hamilton. Early estrogen action: Stimulation of the metabolism of high molecular weight and ribosomal (estradiol-17-RNA isolation-uterus-ribosomal RNA precursor-actinomycin D) RNAs. Proc. Natl. Acad. Sci. USA 69:157, 1972.

32. O'Malley, B. W., and W. L. McGuire. Studies on the mechanism of estrogen-mediated tissue differentiation: Regulation of nuclear transcription and induction of new RNA species. Proc. Natl. Acad. Sci. USA 60:1527, 1968.

33. Church, R. B., and B. W. McCarthy. Unstable nuclear RNA synthesis following estrogen stimulation. Biochim. Biophys. Acta 199:103, 1968.

34. Liarakos, C., J. M. Rosen, and B. W. O'Malley. Effect of estrogen on gene expression in the chick oviduct. II. Transcription of chick tritiated unique deoxyribonucleic acid as measured by hybridization in ribonucleic acid. Biochemistry 12:2809, 1973.

35. Liao, S., and H. G. Williams-Ashman. An effect of testosterone on amino acid incorporation by prostatic ribonucleoprotein particles. Proc. Natl. Acad. Sci. USA 48:1956, 1962.

36. Rosenfeld, G. C., J. P. Comstock, A. R. Means, and B. W. O'Malley. Estrogen-induced synthesis of ovalbumin messenger RNA and its translation in a cell-free system. Biochem. Biophys. Res. Commun. 46:1695, 1972.

37. Means, A. R., J. P. Comstock, G. C. Rosenfeld, and B. W. O'Malley. Ovalbumin messenger RNA of chick oviduct: Partial characterization, estrogen dependence and translation in vitro. Proc. Natl. Acad. Sci. USA 69:1146, 1972.

38. Harris, S. E., J. M. Rosen, A. R. Means, and B. W. O'Malley. Use of a specific probe for ovalbumin messenger RNA to quantitate estrogen-induced gene transcripts. Biochemistry 14:2072, 1975.

39. Harris, S. E., A. R. Means, W. M. Mitchell, and B. W. O'Malley. Synthesis of [³H]DNA complementary to ovalbumin messenger RNA: Evidence for limited copies of the ovalbumin gene in chick oviduct. Proc. Natl. Acad. Sci. USA 70:3776, 1973.

40. Sullivan, D., R. Palacios, J. Stavnezer, J. M. Taylor, A. J. Faras, M. L. Kiley, N. Summers, J. M. Bishop, and R. T. Schimke. Synthesis of a deoxyribonucleic acid sequence complementary to ovalbumin messenger ribonucleic acid and quantification of ovalbumin genes. J. Biol. Chem. 248:7530, 1973.

243   Hormonal Control of Gene Expression

41. Palmiter, R. D. Rate of ovalbumin messenger ribonucleic acid synthesis in the oviduct of estrogen-primed chicks. J. Biol. Chem. 248:8260, 1973.

42. Mueller, G. C., A. Herranen, and K. Jervell. Studies on the mechanism of action of estrogen. Recent Prog. Horm. Res. 8:95, 1958.

43. Williams-Ashman, H. G., S. Liao, R. L. Hancock, L. Jurkowitz, and D. A. Silverman. Testicular hormone and the synthesis of ribonucleic acids and proteins in the prostate gland. Recent Prog. Horm. Res. 20:247, 1964.

44. Wilson, J. D. Localization of the biochemical site of action of testosterone on protein synthesis in the seminal vesicle of the rat. J. Clin. Invest. 41:153, 1962.

45. Liao, S., and H. G. Williams-Ashman. An effect of testosterone on amino acid incorporation by prostatic ribonucleoprotein particles. Proc. Natl. Acad. Sci. USA 48:1956, 1962.

46. Hamilton, T. H. Isotopic studies on estrogen-induced accelerations of ribonucleic acid and protein synthesis. Proc. Natl. Acad. Sci. USA 49:373.

47. Tomkins, G. M., L. D. Garren, R. R. Howell, and B. Peterkofsky. The regulation of enzyme synthesis by steroid hormones: The role of translation. J. Cell. Comp. Physiol. 66:137, 1965.

48. Kenney, F. T., W. D. Wicks, and D. L. Greenman. Hydrocortisone stimulation of RNA synthesis in induction of hepatic enzymes. J. Cell. Comp. Physiol. 66 (Suppl.I):125, 1965.

49. Notides, A., and J. Gorski. Estrogen-induced synthesis of a specific uterine protein. Proc. Natl. Acad. Sci. USA 56:230, 1966.

50. O'Malley, B. W., and P. O. Kohler. Studies on steroid regulation of synthesis of a specific oviduct protein in a new monolayer culture system. Proc. Natl. Acad. Sci. USA 58:2359, 1967.

51. O'Malley, B. W. In vitro hormonal induction of a specific protein (avidin) in chick oviduct. Biochemistry 6:2546, 1967.

52. Means, A. R., and P. F. Hall. Effect of FSH on protein biosynthesis in testes of the immature rat. Endocrinology 81:1151, 1967.

53. Lockard, R. E., and J. B. Lingrel. The synthesis of mouse hemoglobin beta-chains in a rabbit reticulocyte cell-free system programmed with mouse reticulocyte 9S RNA. Biochem. Biophys. Res. Commun. 37:204, 1969.

54. Prichard, P. M., J. M. Gilbert, D. A. Shafritz, and W. F. Anderson. Factors for the initiation of hemoglobin synthesis by rabbit reticulocyte ribosome. Nature 226:511, 1970.

55. Means, A. R., I. B. Abrass, and B. W. O'Malley. Protein biosynthesis on chick oviduct polyribosomes. I. Changes during estrogen-mediated tissue differentiation. Biochemistry 10:1561, 1971.

56. Stavnezer, J., and R. C. Huang. Synthesis of a mouse immunoglobulin light chain in a rabbit reticulocyte cell-free system. Nature 230:172, 1971.

57. O'Malley, B. W., G. C. Rosenfeld, J. P. Comstock, and A. R. Means. Steroid hormone induction of a specific translatable messenger RNA. Nature New Biol. 240:2031, 1973.

58. Rhoads, R. E., G. S. McKnight, and R. T. Schimke. Quantitative measurement of ovalbumin messenger ribonucleic acid activity. Localization in polysomes, induction by estrogen, and effect of actinomycin D. J. Biol. Chem. 248:2031, 1973.

59. Palmiter, R. D. Regulation of protein synthesis in chick oviduct. I. Independent regulation of ovalbumin, conalbumin, ovimucoid and lysozyme induction. J. Biol. Chem. 247:6450, 1972.

60. Marver, D., J. Stewart, J. W. Funder, D. Feldman, and I. S. Edelman. Renal aldosterone receptors: Studies with ^{3}H aldosterone and the antimineralocorticoid ^{3}H spirolactone (SC-26304). Proc. Natl. Acad. Sci. USA 71:1431, 1974.

25 Hormone-Receptor Interaction in the Mechanism of Reproductive Hormone Action

E. V. Jensen, K. J. Catt, J. Gorski, and H. G. Williams-Ashman

25.1 Introduction

The molecular basis for the control of reproduction has long been a subject of fascination and challenge for chemists and biologists alike. During the first half of this century, a variety of humoral factors associated with mammalian reproduction were identified, and their physiological functions, chemical nature, and metabolic pathways of synthesis and degradation were elucidated. With the availability of information on what the sex hormones are and what they do, the question of how they do it began to receive investigative attention. The past sesquidecade has seen a rapid expansion of knowledge providing insight into the biochemical mechanisms by which steroid and protein hormones exert their regulatory effects on reproductive processes.

Progress in the understanding of hormone mechanisms has been enhanced by a number of concurrent developments in biomedical science. The tremendous explosion of knowledge in the field of molecular biology, establishing a chemical basis for the control of cell growth and function by information coded in the genome, permitted a rational search for biochemical processes that might be sensitive to hormonal modulation in cells of endocrine-responsive tissues. The availability of radioactive hormones and substrates of high specific activity and the introduction of automated instrumentation for the detection and measurement of radioisotopes in biological materials, as well as the development of sensitive techniques for the separation and identification of minute amounts of steroids and of macromolecular substances, have facilitated the tracking of the hormone molecule within the target cell and the delineation of early biochemical response. The concept of a cyclic nucleotide serving as a "second messenger" to deliver the regulatory signal to the appropriate intracellular effector site has provided a unifying pattern for the action of peptide hormones whose primary interaction is at the plasma membrane, while the discovery of intracellular receptor proteins for steroid hormones has led to recognition of the entity that actually interacts with the genome to elicit a biological response.

Aided by the foregoing developments, investigations of the mechanisms of reproductive hormone action have followed two general lines of attack.

Attempting to establish the temporal sequence of biochemical events leading to eventual stimulation of growth or function, the first approach involves a search for biochemical processes in responsive tissues in which changes can be detected especially early after exposure to hormone. The second approach determines the fate of the hormone itself during its pathway of interaction with receptor substances in the target cell. Both types of experiment have yielded fundamental data that are mutually complementary. In the past few years the two lines of investigation have begun to converge to yield a rational pattern for hormone action.

This essay is a discussion of the second of these investigative approaches. It summarizes the most significant stages in the development of our understanding of receptor substances for steroid sex hormones and for gonadotropins in their respective target cells and the implications of hormone-receptor interaction in the control of fertility. The large body of information concerning response of biochemical processes to hormonal stimulation is discussed only to the extent that involvement of hormone-receptor complexes has been demonstrated. We make no attempt here to provide complete documentation of primary literature reports; detailed reference to the abundance of excellent work from numerous laboratories is provided by the many review articles and monographs that are available. A few such reviews are listed at the end of this article, along with selected papers that have contributed to novel concepts or experimental directions.

25.2 Steroid Hormone Receptors

Estrogens
Estrogen binding in reproductive tissues The fact that tissues of the reproductive tract contain characteristic hormone-binding components or receptors was first recognized in 1958 and 1959 after two technical achievements: the synthesis, in Reading and Chicago respectively, of hexestrol and estradiol labeled with carrier-free tritium and the development of an analytical technique (since supplanted by more efficient methods) for the routine determination of tritium in animal tissues. Early studies of the fate of tritiated hexestrol in young goats and sheep (Glascock and Hoekstra) and of estradiol in immature rats (Jensen

245 Hormone-Receptor Interaction

and Jacobson) demonstrated a striking uptake and retention of radioactive hormone by such reproductive tissues as uterus, vagina, and anterior pituitary. Estradiol was found to bind in the immature rat uterus and to evoke biological response without itself undergoing chemical change, suggesting that the action of the hormone involves its interaction with macromolecules rather than its participation in chemical reactions of steroid metabolism as had been previously considered. After micromethods were developed for the conversion of tritiated estradiol into other steroidal estrogens, it was demonstrated that 17α-methylestradiol, 17α-ethynylestradiol, and estriol, as well as hexestrol, resemble estradiol in being taken up and bound in the rat uterus and vagina without chemical change. In contrast, after the administration of estrone or mestranol, the target tissues were found to accumulate estradiol and 17α-ethynylestradiol, respectively, indicating that these steroids with only one free hydroxyl group can serve as metabolic precursors of the dihydroxy substances that bind preferentially to the receptors.

The antiestrogen ethamoxytriphetol and later the related compounds nafoxidine, clomiphene, and Parke-Davis CI-628 were shown to prevent the specific uptake and retention of estradiol by target tissue receptors in vivo. The observed correlation between the reduction in hormone incorporation and the inhibition of uterine growth when different amounts of nafoxidine are administered provided the first evidence that binding of hormone to receptor actually is involved in its biological action. In contrast, actinomycin-D and puromycin, substances previously found by Mueller to block the uterotropic action of estradiol in the rat, show no inhibition of the characteristic uptake and retention of hormone by uterine tissue, suggesting that the binding of estradiol to receptor is an early step in the uterotropic process, apparently initiating a sequence of biochemical events that can be blocked at later stages by these inhibitors of RNA and protein synthesis.

In the early 1960s estradiol and other estrogenic steroids labeled with tritium of high specific activity became available commercially, and an increasing number of investigators began to undertake receptor studies. Important early observations concerning the interaction of estrogens with target tissues in vivo were reported from many laboratories, in particular those of Stone, Gorski, King, Talwar, Terenius, Eisenfeld, and Baulieu. Using cell fractionation techniques, several investigators found that administered estradiol is localized in two regions of uterine cells, the nucleus and the high-speed supernatant or cytosol fraction. Although at first investigators disagreed about the relative distribution of hormone between the two binding sites, the contention of Gorski and of Jensen that the overwhelming majority of the uterine estradiol is localized in the nucleus became generally accepted after its confirmation by the valuable drymount autoradiographic technique developed by Stumpf and Roth. Both by serial sectioning and by autoradiography estradiol was found to bind in both endometrium and myometrium, with a somewhat higher concentration observed in endometrium. The autoradiographic technique of Stumpf proved extremely useful in demonstrating the specific binding of estrogens in hypothalamus and other neurological tissues where the proportion of receptor-containing cells is small but real, as first shown by biochemical experiments of Eisenfeld and of Kato and Villee.

In the mid-1960s reports from the laboratories of Stone, Jensen, and Terenius first described simple in vitro systems in which one could demonstrate an interaction of estrogens with excised uterine tissue that showed the characteristics observed in vivo, including nuclear localization, sensitivity to antiestrogens of the ethamoxytriphetol type, and, as found later, formation of the same nuclear and extranuclear hormone-receptor complexes. The uptake and binding of estradiol by uterine tissue in vitro was found to be highly sensitive to sulfhydryl-blocking reagents, suggesting that sulfhydryl-containing substances are involved in the binding phenomenon. By carrying out in vitro experiments at different temperatures, Gorski and Jensen showed that nuclear localization of the hormone is much more temperature-dependent than is extranuclear binding and that warming of uteri first exposed to estradiol in the cold results in a shift of extranuclear hormone into the nucleus. This observation was important in the development of current concepts of the interaction pathway of steroid hormones in target cells. An ingenious superfusion technique for studying the interaction of estrogens with reproductive tissues under steady-state conditions was later devised by Gurpide.

Estrogen-receptor complexes Talwar demonstrated that the radioactive estradiol in uterine cytosol exists in combination with a macromolecule, and Jungblut in the Chicago group devised a salt extraction procedure, later improved by Puca and Bresciana, for solubilizing the nuclear hormone as a macromolecular complex. Then in 1966 the field of receptor studies entered a new phase when Toft and Gorski applied the technique of sucrose gradient ultracentrifugation for the detection and characterization of estrogen-receptor complexes. They found that the complex of uterine cytosol sediments as a discrete entity, with a coefficient now known to be about 8S, and that the receptor is predominantly protein in nature, inasmuch as the sedimentation peak is destroyed by the action of proteases but not nucleases. Using the sedimentation technique, the laboratories of Erdos, of Korenman, and of Baulieu made the important observation that in the presence of salt the 8S cytosol complex is dissociated into a steroid-binding subunit, which the Jensen group demonstrated to be different from the binding unit of the nuclear complex in that the former sediments at about 4S in salt-containing sucrose gradients, as compared with the value of 5S they had previously observed for the nuclear complex. Although the estrogen receptor in uterine cytosol of immature rats or calves exists entirely in the 8S form under conditions of low ionic strength, King and Notides found that part of the receptor in cytosol from adult rat and human uteri sediments as the unaggregated subunit, even in low-salt sucrose gradients, a phenomenon demonstrated by Notides to result from the action of a proteolytic enzyme present in the uteri of mature animals that destroys the ability of the receptor unit to form the 8S complex. It was further shown by Erdos, by Rochefort, and by W. L. McGuire that in sucrose gradients containing 0.15 M salt the estrogen-receptor complex of immature rat uterine cytosol can exist in an intermediate state of aggregation, sedimenting at about 6S.

The elucidation of relation between the cytosol and nuclear forms of the estrogen-receptor complex represents a major advance in receptor research, inasmuch as the two-step pathway proposed for estradiol in uterine cells has provided a general model for the interaction of all classes of steroid hormones with their respective target tissues (Figure 25.1). A relation between cytosol and nuclear binding was first indicated by early in vivo studies by Jensen in which varying doses of the antiestrogen nafoxidine were found to reduce nuclear and extranuclear binding of estradiol proportionately. Experiments with increasing doses of tritiated estradiol demonstrated that the interaction with the uterus in vivo consists of two phenomena: an uptake process, which is not saturable even with hyperphysiological amounts of hormone, and a retention process, which becomes saturated as physiological levels of hormone are exceeded. After Gorski and Jensen observed that the 8S extranuclear complex is formed in vitro simply by adding estradiol to uterine cytosol and that a physiological dose of estradiol in vivo utilizes only a small fraction of the total cytosol-binding capacity, Jensen proposed in 1966 that the 8S extranuclear receptor protein, present in excess amounts, might serve as an uptake receptor, bringing the hormone to the nucleus, where it is retained by nuclear receptors.

During the following year a considerable body of mutually consistent evidence accumulated to indicate that the estradiol-receptor complex of the nucleus is actually derived from the initially formed extranuclear complex by a temperature-dependent, hormone-induced translocation. In Wotiz's laboratory more

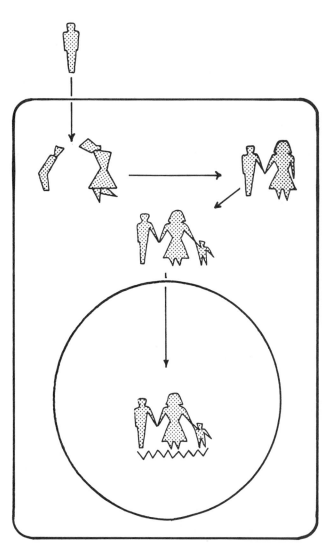

Figure 25.1 Schematic representation of the interaction of steroid hormones with receptors in target cells. The hormone binds to an extranuclear receptor protein, inducing its transformation to an activated form, which, for the estrogen receptor, appears to involve the addition of a macromolecular species. The activated steroid-receptor family is translocated to the nucleus where it binds in the chromatin. In the O'Malley modification, based on the properties of the progesterone receptor of chick oviduct, the receptor complex consists of two protein chains, each bearing steroid, with one couple of the mixed foursome binding to DNA and the other to acidic proteins of the chromatin.

radioactivity was found to be bound to uterine nuclei when they are incubated with tritiated estradiol in uterine cytosol than when in buffer alone. Both the Gorski and Jensen groups observed the previously mentioned shift of uterine radioactivity from an extranuclear 8S form to a nuclear 5S form when tissues that had been exposed to tritiated estradiol in the cold were warmed to physiological temperature. Especially compelling was the finding in these two laboratories that, unlike the 8S extranuclear complex, which can be formed by direct addition of estradiol to uterine cytosol, the 5S complex is not produced by treatment of uterine nuclei or nuclear extract with estradiol alone, but is readily obtained if the nuclei are incubated with estradiol in uterine cytosol containing the 8S receptor. The Jensen group showed, and Gorski confirmed, that the administration of estradiol in vivo depletes the receptor content of rat uterine cytosol, compatible with the movement of the receptor complex to the nucleus. On the basis of this variety of evidence, Gorski and Jensen proposed independently in 1967 a rudimentary form of the currently accepted two-step interaction mechanism in which the 8S cytosol complex (then called 9.5S) undergoes temperature-dependent translocation to produce the 5S nuclear complex.

After it was established in 1968 that the 8S cytosol complex contains a binding subunit, Jensen recognized that the conversion of this unit from a 4S to a 5S form accompanies the translocation process. At first this change was believed to take place in the nucleus, but in 1970 Brecher in the Jensen laboratory reported that the conversion of the receptor subunit from its native (4S) form to the nuclear (5S) modification does not require nuclei but may be effected by warming uterine cytosol in the presence but not the absence of estradiol, a finding soon confirmed by Hamilton. The Jensen group showed that during 4S to 5S transformation the extranuclear estradiol-receptor complex acquires a striking ability to bind to isolated nuclei, and W. L. McGuire reported a similar affinity of transformed complex for chromatin, suggesting that the temperature-dependent process associated with translocation is the estrogen-induced conversion of the receptor to an active form that can bind in the genome. The ability of the transformed complex to bind not only to chromatin and to DNA but also to a variety of polyanions was subsequently reported by Baulieu, who suggested the term *acidophilic activation* for the transformation process.

The molecular basis for estrogen-induced transformation or activation of the receptor protein is not completely understood, but careful studies in the laboratories of Notides, of Alberts, and of Jungblut indicate that this phenomenon probably involves more than a change in receptor conformation. On the basis

of kinetic evidence for a second-order reaction and the elution properties of native as compared to transformed complex on Sephadex columns, it appears that receptor transformation involves the addition of a macromolecular component or possibly a dimerization of the 4S unit.

The presence of a similar receptor system in which estradiol reacts with an extranuclear protein to form a complex that is translocated to the nucleus was later demonstrated for anterior pituitary in the laboratories of Notides, of Leavitt, of Eisenfeld, and of Clark, and for rat mammary tumor by W. L. McGuire, by Wittliff, and by Kyser in the Jensen group. Siiteri, Notides, and Hähnel have characterized the receptor system of human uterus. Irvine and associates demonstrated in 1961 that hormone-dependent human breast cancers incorporate more tritiated hexestrol in vivo than do autonomous cancers. Jensen in 1970 initially reported that the estrogen-receptor content of excised specimens of human breast cancers can be used to predict response to endocrine ablation in patients with advanced breast cancer. Since then, studies of estrogen receptors and more recently of androgen and progestin receptors in human breast cancers have been carried out in many laboratories.

The precise fate of the transformed estradiol-receptor complex in the target cell nucleus and the nature of the intranuclear acceptor site to which it binds in vivo have been the subjects of considerable investigation and speculation, but little is known with certainty. Early studies from the laboratories of King, of Chalkley, and of Hamilton demonstrated an association with chromatin, and Stumpf showed by autoradiography that the complex probably is not localized in the nucleolus. Under proper conditions Liao could extract the estradiol-receptor complex from uterine nuclei in combination with ribonucleoprotein particles, while a recent report by Puca describes the isolation of a basic protein from calf uterine nuclei that shows many of the properties characteristic of the nuclear acceptor substance. As described below, the finding by O'Malley that the progesterone receptor of chick oviduct appears to consist of two steroid-binding proteins, one of which interacts with DNA and the other with certain nonhistone proteins of the chromatin, raises the interesting possibility that a similar phenomenon may be involved in the interaction of estrogen-receptor complex with target cell chromatin.

Controversial attempts have been made to distinguish specific, saturable interaction of the estradiol-receptor complex in isolated target cell nuclei from the binding shown by transformed complex with nuclei from all tissues; however, the early saturation experiments of Jensen and the more precise studies of Clark, using his valuable exchange technique for determining the actual amount of receptor present in the nucleus, show the limited capacity of uterine nuclei to retain translocated complex in vivo. According to Clark, a physiological dose of estradiol in the immature rat leads on the average to the appearance of about 6,000 receptor molecules in each uterine nucleus, whereas Jensen estimated from depletion studies that at least 14,000 receptor molecules, representing approximately half the original extranuclear binding capacity, disappear from the cytosol at the nadir four hours after hormone injection. These results indicate that, under physiological conditions. a substantial number of estrogen-receptor complexes are translocated to the nucleus for interaction with chromatin. Recent studies by Clark and Gorski have demonstrated that full biological response requires the presence of estrogen-receptor complex in the nucleus for a prolonged period of time, suggesting that the complex does not simply trigger an initial event but participates in nuclear processes on a continuing basis.

Most experimental findings concerning the action of estrogens and other steroid hormones are consistent with the two-step translocation mechanism involving interaction of the transformed hormone-receptor complex with the RNA-synthesizing system in the genome. A few observations, however, are difficult to reconcile with this interaction pathway: Sonnenschein reports that, in contrast to the situation in uterus, the nuclei of pituitary tumor cells contain a substantial amount of unoccupied estrogen receptors before exposure to hormone. Liao has found that the nucleus and not the cytoplasm of vaginal epithelium cells contains a specific receptor for androst-5-ene-3β,17β-diol, a C_{19} steroid that elicits an estrogenlike effect in this tissue, and Baulieu has made similar observations of the presence of an estrogen receptor in chick liver nuclei. Both Rochefort and Ruh have reported that dihydrotestosterone and testosterone can effect the translocation of extranuclear estrogen receptor to the nucleus in surviving uterine tissue, even though these androgenic hormones are alleged not to bind to the receptor protein. As first reported for androgens in prostate, Liao has observed an extremely rapid, estrogen-induced stimulation of a reaction involved in the initiation of protein synthesis in uterine tissue by a process that appears to be independent of any interaction in the nucleus. The significance of these phenomena in the overall picture of steroid hormone action remains to be evaluated.

Effect of receptor complex on RNA synthesis Although transformed estradiol-receptor complex binds strongly with isolated nuclei from many if not all tissues, the biochemical result of this binding appears to be highly tissue-specific. Only with nuclei of hormone-dependent tissues can this interaction in vitro be shown to exert an influence on RNA polymerase reactions. While the numerous investigations of biochemical response of cell components to estrogenic stimulation in vivo, including the elegant work of O'Malley and of Schimke on induction of ovalbumin mRNA synthesis in chick oviduct and that of Gorski on mRNA for "induced protein" in rat uterus, are outside the scope of this discussion, studies on the RNA polymerase activity of isolated uterine nuclei are relevant because of its sensitivity to the action of estrogen-receptor complexes in vitro.

Following the pioneer experiments of Mueller, much evidence has been obtained to indicate that enhanced synthesis of all types of RNA is an early response of the rat uterus to estrogenic stimulation in vivo. Gorski showed further that administration of estradiol to immature rats doubles the RNA polymerase activity of their uterine nuclei but not of their liver nuclei, as determined by an in vitro assay now known to measure the nucleolar enzyme, polymerase I. More recently, Glasser and associates demonstrated that RNA polymerase II activity is also elevated in uterine nuclei isolated from estrogen-treated animals, though at an earlier time than polymerase I. After attempts to stimulate the RNA polymerase system of uterine nuclei by direct treatment with estradiol proved unsuccessful, Baulieu made the important observation that incubation of nuclei from heifer endometrium with the estrogen-receptor complex of endometrial cytosol causes an enhancement of RNA polymerase I activity comparable to that observed in rat uterine nuclei after hormone administration in vivo; Mousseron-Canet found similar stimulation when estrogen-receptor complex was added directly to the polymerase assay system. Mohla in the Jensen laboratory then showed that to elicit this stimulatory action the estradiol-receptor complex must be in the transformed state and that the sensitivity to stimulation by estrogen-receptor complex is a specific characteristic of nuclei from hormone-dependent tissues. Using the binding of tritiated actinomycin D as an indicator of chromatin template activity, Leclercq and Heuson found similarly that exposure to transformed estradiol-receptor complex results in increased capacity for actinomycin D incorporation in uterine but not in diaphragm nuclei. In recent studies with induced rat mammary tumors, DeSombre found that incubation with estrogen-receptor complex enhances RNA polymerase activity in nuclei from hormone-dependent but not from autonomous tumors.

So far, stimulation of isolated nuclei by estrogen-receptor complexes has been observed only for RNA polymerase I and not for polymerase II, although augmentation of both enzymatic activities results from the action of the hormone in vivo. Because of evidence suggesting that the enhancement of polymerase I by estradiol in vivo may require the prior stimulation of polymerase II as well as the synthesis of protein, reservations have been expressed about the physiological significance of the effect of estrogen-receptor complexes on RNA polymerase in isolated nuclei. The specificity of this phenomenon for nuclei of hormone-dependent tissues and tumors, however, and the fact that prior administration of estradiol in vivo eliminates the susceptibility of uterine nuclei to further stimulation in vitro, suggests that the transformed estradiol-receptor complex exerts an effect on the RNA-synthesizing system in target cell nuclei similar to that resulting from the action of the hormone in vivo. The susceptibility of its nuclei to stimulation in vitro appears to be a convenient criterion of hormone dependency of a tissue; it also provides a simple means of testing the biological activity of receptor preparations during various stages of purification.

Receptor levels Detailed information is lacking about the control of the biosynthesis of the receptor protein in target cells. Jensen has reported that all examined rat tissues contain small amounts of 8S receptor protein in their cytosols, but that target tissues contain much higher levels than do nontarget tissues. During differentiation, the nuclei of hormone-dependent tissues appear to acquire the need for hormonal stimulation, accompanied by an increased level of the receptor protein required for the hormone's action. Recently DeSombre has found that carcinogen-induced rat mammary tumors that regress on ovariectomy show substantial levels of cytosol receptor and possess nuclei with RNA polymerase systems susceptible to stimulation by estrogen-receptor complex, whereas autonomous tumors, with nuclei insensitive to stimulation by receptor complex, generally show low receptor levels. Some autonomous tumors with insensitive nuclei still possess substantial receptor levels, however, indicating that the loss of hormone-dependency by the nucleus is not always accompanied by a reduced production of receptor. Similarly, Shyamala has described autonomous mouse mammary tumors, which contain cytoplasmic estrogen receptor that does not undergo hormone-induced translocation to the nucleus on incubation of tumor slices with estradiol at 37°C. A clue to the origin of the cytoplasmic receptor is provided by the studies of Jungblut, who extracted from the microsomal fraction of young pig uteri two nonaggregating forms of an estrogen-binding protein that appear to be precursors of the aggregating receptor protein of the cytoplasm.

Observations have been made by Jacobson, by Kellie, and by de Hertogh of the variation of cytoplasmic receptor level in rat uterus with the ovarian cycle and by Hughes in the Chicago group of the gradual decline in uterine receptor content of mature rats following ovariectomy; all these observations point to an ovarian contribution to the control of receptor biosynthesis, even though the highest receptor levels are found in the uterus of the immature rat. Similar cyclic changes in the estrogen-binding capacity of monkey oviduct were described by Brenner. Jensen, Gorski, and, more recently, Muldoon showed that the depletion of cytoplasmic receptor induced by the administration of estradiol is a stimulus to receptor resynthesis. In contrast, Clark has found that the nuclear translocation of receptor induced by nafoxidine is for some reason not followed by receptor replenishment, providing an explanation for the weak estrogenic but strong antiestrogenic properties of this class of substance.

Receptor purification Because of their instability and tendency to aggregate, purification of the different forms of the estrogen-receptor protein—to provide material in amounts sufficient for analysis, structure determination, and production of specific antibodies—has encountered considerable difficulty. While in the Chicago laboratory, Puca found that the addition of calcium ions to calf uterine cytosol in the presence of 0.4 M salt yields a stabilized form of the cytosol receptor, sedimenting at 4.5S in either high- or low-salt sucrose gradients, which is resistant to aggregation during purification procedures. Later, in Naples, he showed that this stabilization is due to a proteolytic factor present in uterine cytosol that is activated by calcium ions to act on the receptor protein to reduce or eliminate its tendency to aggregate. Mueller and Jensen further observed that the nuclear estradiol-receptor complex loses its tendency to aggregate on aging or on further purification, during which its sedimentation properties change from 5.2S to 4.8S. By a combination of salt precipitation, gel filtration, ion-exchange chromatography, and acrylamide gel electrophoresis, the Jensen group has purified these nonaggregating forms of the cytosol and nuclear estradiol-receptor complexes to apparent homogeneity and determined the amino acid composition of the nuclear protein (MW 66,000; pI 5.8). The yields of the final products have been low, however, and firm criteria of purity have not as yet been established. The physiological significance of these stabilized forms of the hormone-receptor complex is not clear, although partially purified preparations of both the 4.5S cytosol and 4.8S nuclear complexes are found to stimulate the RNA polymerase activity of isolated uterine nuclei.

The use of affinity chromatography for purification of estrogen receptors has had only limited success. Early attempts by Jungblut in 1966 and by Mueller in 1969 to employ estradiol affinity columns encountered remarkable difficulty in eluting the adsorbed receptor protein in an undenatured form. In 1973 the laboratories of Cuatrecasas and of Baulieu each reported that affinity columns in which the estradiol is attached to the supporting matrix by a long chain of amino acid polymer are suitable for the efficient purification of the calcium-stabilized (4.5S) form of the cytosol complex. In spite of these exciting indications, estrogen-receptor purification in tangible quantity has not as yet been achieved.

Progestins

Progesterone receptors in mammalian tissues Although modest retention of radioactive progesterone in the uterus of the ovariectomized rat was first reported by Laumas in 1966, most early attempts to demonstrate selective uptake and binding of progesterone by mammalian reproductive tissues in vivo proved unsuccessful until it was recognized that the presence of progesterone receptors in target cells depends strongly on prestimulation by estrogen. In 1968 Katzman observed that the retention of locally administered progesterone by the ovariectomized mouse vagina is markedly increased in animals pretreated with estrogen for 48 hours, and in 1970 Bardin reported that the accumulation of progesterone in the uteri of ovariectomized guinea pigs is increased sevenfold by the prior administration of estrogen. Selective binding of progesterone, dependent on estrogen pretreatment, was demonstrated for the rabbit uterus by Wiest and for the hamster uterus and other reproductive tissues by Lisk and by Leavitt.

Because of the interaction pattern already established for the estrogenic hormones, studies of progesterone receptors moved rapidly to the use of broken cell systems and the search for receptor proteins in the cytosol fraction of target cells. Between 1970 and 1973 there appeared several reports describing specific progesterone-receptor complexes in the cytosol fraction of uterine homogenates from guinea pig (Baulieu, Bardin, Vihko, Stavely), rabbit (Wiest, J. L. McGuire, Ryan, Stavely), mouse (O'Malley), and human (Wiest, Laumas, King), after either administration of tritiated progesterone to the animal or addition of hormone directly to the cytosol. Because it was found to react with glucocorticoids as well as progesterone, some uncertainty arose regarding the significance of the binding protein first detected by Reel and by Baulieu in rat uterine cytosol, but later studies by O'Malley, by Terenius, by Ryan, and by Stavely confirmed the presence of specific progesterone receptors in this system.

In many of the above investigations, the level of progesterone receptor in the cytosol is markedly increased by pretreatment of the animal with estrogen. In the ovariectomized guinea pig, Baulieu detected an increase in progesterone receptor within six hours after estrogen administration, with a maximum eightfold increase observed at 24 hours. In addition, the nature of the receptor protein appears to be changed as a result of the estrogen administration. In low-salt sucrose gradients, values of between 4S and 5S are reported for the progesterone-receptor complex of uterine cytosol from unstimulated animals, but after estrogen treatment the complex is found to sediment, either wholly or in part, as a larger entity, with reported coefficients ranging from 6.5S to 8S. As with the estrogen receptor, the 6.5–8S cytosol complex is dissociated to a 4S subunit in the presence of salt.

Although the results of cell fractionation have not always been consistent, autoradiographic studies by Stumpf clearly demonstrated a selective nuclear concentration of radioactive steroid in oviduct, uterus, and vagina but not in diaphragm or liver of the estrogen-primed, castrate guinea pig receiving tritiated progesterone. Progesterone-induced translocation of receptor protein to the uterine nucleus in the estrogen-primed, ovariectomized rat was demonstrated by Clark, using his exchange technique to estimate total nuclear receptor. From the uterine nuclei of rabbits receiving tritiated progesterone in vivo, Wiest has extracted a progesterone-receptor complex, sedimenting at about 4S.

As might be expected, the progesterone receptor content of reproductive tissues varies considerably with the ovarian cycle and throughout pregnancy. Milgrom in the Baulieu group has shown that in cytosol from guinea pig uterus, the receptor concentration ranges from a maximum of about 40,000 progesterone-binding sites per cell at proestrus to a minimum of 2,500 at diestrus. At proestrus the 6.7S form of the receptor predominates, as compared to the 4.5S form at diestrus and a mixture of both at postestrus. Similar results for rat uterus were reported by the O'Malley group. Luukkainen and associates observed a higher concentration of cytosol receptor in hyperplastic human endometrium than in endometrium during the proliferative or secretory phases. They have also reported progesterone-binding components in pregnant rat uterine microsomes that are different from the cytosol receptors, which, in analogy with the observations of Jungblut on estrogen-binding components of pig uterine microsomes, may represent precursors of the actual cytoplasmic progesterone receptors. In both the rat and the rabbit, Ryan found that the concentration of progesterone receptors in the myometrial cytosol decreases after midpregnancy to about half its former level, rising again just prior to parturition.

Progesterone receptors in the chick oviduct By far the most extensive studies, providing the bulk of present information concerning progesterone receptors and their significance in hormone action, have been carried out by O'Malley and his associates with a nonmammalian system, the chick oviduct. After preliminary stimulation with estrogen, this tissue responds to the further action of estrogen by synthesizing ovalbumin, whereas progesterone treatment induces the production of avidin. In 1969 the O'Malley group reported the binding of radioactive steroid in both the cytosol and nuclear fractions of oviduct from estrogen-prestimulated chicks receiving tritiated progesterone in vivo, and in 1970, in collaboration with Sherman, they described cytoplasmic and nuclear progesterone-receptor complexes obtained both in vivo and in vitro that are readily distinguishable from binding to transcortin (CBG) by gel filtration through Agarose. Pretreatment of the chick with estrogen was found to cause a 20-fold increase in the level of progesterone receptor in the oviduct. The cytoplasmic complex, produced either by administration of tritiated progesterone in vivo or by direct addition of the hormone to oviduct cytosol, was found to sediment as a single 3.8S peak in salt-containing sucrose gradients but as a mixture of 5S and 8S entities in low-salt gradients. The complex extracted by 0.3 M KCl from oviduct nuclei, either after hormone treatment in vivo or on incubation of excised tissue with tritiated progesterone at 37°C in vitro, sediments in salt-containing gradients at 4S, indistinguishable by this criterion from the cytosol complex. The protein nature of the cytoplasmic receptor is indicated by the destruction of the 3.8S complex by incubation with pronase but not with ribonuclease or deoxyribonuclease. The steroid bound in the complexes was shown to be unchanged progesterone.

Except for the lack of detectable difference in sedimentation rate between the nuclear and cytoplasmic complexes, the interaction of progesterone with receptor proteins in chick oviduct was shown to resemble closely that previously described for estradiol in rat uterus. In 1970 and 1971 the O'Malley group reported evidence that the nuclear progesterone-receptor complex is derived from an initial cytosol complex by a temperature-dependent translocation process. Not only does incubation of excised oviduct tissue with progesterone at 2°C give rise almost exclusively to extranuclear binding, shifting to nuclear complex as the tissues are warmed to 37°C, but in oviduct tissue incubated with progesterone in vitro at 37°C, the progressive increase in the amount of nuclear complex is accompanied by a corresponding depletion of cytoplasmic-receptor capacity. No nuclear-receptor protein can be extracted from nuclei of oviduct tissue that has not been exposed previously to progesterone either in vivo or in vitro. Although earlier experiments suffered from the instability of the cytoplasmic receptor at 37°C, in 1975 O'Malley reported incubation experiments carried out at 25°C that clearly demon-

strated the dependence on cytosol receptor for the binding of progesterone in isolated oviduct nuclei and the importance of hormone-induced, temperature-dependent conversion of the native cytoplasmic complex to an active form that can bind in the nucleus. In contrast to the transformed estrogen-receptor complex, which binds strongly to isolated nuclei or chromatin from many tissues, the temperature-activated progesterone-receptor complex of oviduct cytosol was found to possess a remarkable specific affinity for oviduct nuclei, compared with spleen or heart nuclei.

O'Malley has carried out detailed investigations on the nature of the acceptor site with which the translocated progesterone-receptor complex associates in the oviduct nucleus. The striking preference of the complex for oviduct nuclei was shown to depend on components of the nonhistone (acidic) proteins of the oviduct chromatin. In an ingenious set of "exchange" experiments, in which chromatins from oviduct, heart, and erythrocytes were separated into DNA, histone, and acidic protein components that were variously recombined to produce reconstituted hybrid chromatins, O'Malley demonstrated that the specificity of nuclear binding resides in the AP_3 subfraction of the acidic nuclear proteins. Not only does deletion of the AP_3 fraction result in a marked loss in binding ability in the reconstituted oviduct chromatin, but hybrid chromatin containing heart or erythrocyte DNA combined with oviduct proteins resembles oviduct chromatin in its affinity for receptor complex, whereas oviduct DNA combined with heart or erythrocyte proteins shows little binding of the complex. After separation of the receptor protein into two 4S progesterone-binding subunits, which are incorporated equally into oviduct nuclei on hormone treatment in vivo or in vitro, O'Malley demonstrated that component A binds nonspecifically to DNA but not to chromatin, whereas component B binds to chromatin and shows a specific affinity for chromatin from oviduct as compared to spleen. Without detracting from the elegance of these experiments, it should be recognized that evidence that the tissue specificity of nuclear binding resides in the AP_3 fraction of the oviduct chromatin proteins and in the B component of the receptor has been obtained with what probably is the native or nonactivated form of the receptor. In view of O'Malley's recent finding that temperature-dependent receptor activation is as important in the progesterone system as it is for estrogens and other classes of steroid hormones, the significance of the tissue specificity will be even more compelling when it has been demonstrated with the activated form of the progesterone-receptor complex, which undoubtedly is the entity that interacts with the nucleus in vivo.

On the basis of the foregoing observations, O'Malley has proposed a modified version of the translocation mechanism for the progesterone-receptor complex in the oviduct in which there is binding both with DNA and with acidic proteins, with the latter association, involving the B component of the receptor, responsible for the tissue specificity of the phenomenon. This interaction is postulated to enhance template activity of the chromatin by making initiation sites available for the synthesis of mRNA for avidin and other oviduct proteins. The concept of a double receptor-component interaction is of considerable interest in its potential extension to the other classes of steroid hormones.

Purification of progesterone receptors In 1972, using conventional techniques of hydroxylapatite chromatography and gel filtration through Sephadex G-200, Vihko and associates achieved a 200-fold purification of the progesterone receptor of guinea pig uterine cytosol. By a sequence of ammonium sulfate precipitation, gel filtration through Agarose, and DEAE-cellulose chromatography, Schrader in the O'Malley group separated the 8S cytoplasmic progesterone receptor into two 4S components (called A and B) with purification of 800- and 3,000-fold, respectively. Recently the O'Malley group has developed an affinity chromatography system, involving deoxycorticosterone coupled to albumin-Sepharose, that can effect a 2,000-fold purification of cytoplasmic progesterone receptor complex that has been subjected to preliminary purification by precipitation with ammonium sulfate. Subsequent ion-exchange chromatography on DEAE-Sephadex separates the partially purified complex into its A and B components, each of which shows a single band on SDS-gel electrophoresis, corresponding to molecular weights of 110,000 and 117,000, respectively. Originally it was found that, once separated, the two components did not recombine to regenerate the 8S entity, but Schrader has devised conditions under which the two chains associate to form a 6S dimer.

Androgens
Androgen-binding in reproductive tissues In promoting the growth and maintenance of genital and accessory sex tissues, androgenic hormones perform a function in the male that is analogous to that of estrogens in the female. In mammals, but not in all classes of vertebrates, androgen action exhibits a number of special features that are fundamentally different from the action of estrogens or progestins. Androgenic steroids, secreted by the immature testis during restricted and critical periods of fetal and/or neonatal life, are mandatory for the initial and irreversible morphogenesis or organization of certain tissues that in adulthood are responsive to testosterone and related hormones; these tissues include male genital glands and ducts, external

male genital structures, and the regions of the hypothalamus that are normally responsible for adult male modes of gonadotropin release by the anterior hypophysis, as well as masculine modalities of sexual behavior. Moreover, mutants exist of certain mammalian species that are partially or completely resistant to the biological action of endogenous or exogenous androgens, a phenomenon not as yet observed with estrogens or progestins. Finally, the metabolic transformation of circulating testosterone in various tissues yields many different steroid products, some of which have little or no androgenic activities but others of which may either represent active androgenic forms of testosterone or may even exert qualitatively different types of biological responses (e.g., etiocholanolone, formed in liver, which is nonandrogenic but pyrogenic and may also affect erythropoiesis). It must also be remembered that, in addition to the classical male secondary sexual organs and parts of the hypothalamo-hypophyseal axis, the germinal epithelium of the testis also represents a target for androgenic hormones.

Most studies of the binding of androgens to receptor substances have been concerned with ventral prostate and seminal vesicle. Early attempts to demonstrate selective uptake and retention of androgenic steroids in male accessory sex tissues in vivo did not reveal any dramatic accumulation. Using testosterone labeled with ^{14}C, a small tendency for selective uptake by the rat prostate and seminal vesicle was reported by Greer in 1959, Butenandt in 1960, Samuels in 1962, Mosebach in 1964, and Lawrence in 1965. This occurs especially if only unconjugated steroid is considered, and Pearlman in 1961 noted a small concentration of radioactivity in the ventral prostate of rats receiving a constant infusion of androstenedione labeled with tritium of low specific activity. In most of these experiments the greatest amount of radioactive steroid was found in the liver and kidney.

After testosterone and other androgens labeled with tritium of high specific activity became available commercially, a significant in vivo affinity of androgens for their target tissues could be demonstrated. In 1967 Resko reported the selective accumulation of a testosterone metabolite, chromatographically similar to androstenedione, by prostate and seminal vesicle of castrated guinea pigs receiving tritiated testosterone in vivo. In 1968 and 1969 the laboratories of Tveter, of Wilson, of Liao, and of Eisenfeld reported similar binding of radioactive androgen in rat target tissues; Migeon observed uptake by dog prostate. In contrast to the dog prostate, where microsomal binding appears to predominate, cell fractionation experiments of Mangan, of Wilson, of Liao, and of Mainwaring demonstrated that the accumulation of steroid in the rat prostate results from its retention in the nucleus, a finding confirmed by the autoradiographic studies of Tveter and of Stumpf. Uptake and nuclear localization of radioactive androgen in the mouse prostate was described by Thomas. In 1970 and 1971 Blaquier, Tveter, and French and associates found that the rat epididymis also concentrates androgenic steroids in vivo with predominantly nuclear localization. Similar nuclear accumulation of androgens in rat pituitary was demonstrated by a number of investigators, including Whalen, Eisenfeld, McEwen, Beyer, and Jouan, as well as by the autoradiographic experiments of Stumpf. Pfaff, Whalen, McEwen, Eisenfeld, and Lindner have observed less pronounced but significant steroid concentration in the hypothalamus and other regions of the brain.

Certain antiandrogenic compounds, such as cyproterone, cyproterone acetate, and flutamide, were shown by Liao, by Eisenfeld, by Voigt, and by Peets to block the incorporation of radioactive steroid in the rat prostate, seminal vesicles, and anterior pituitary and to prevent the formation of specific androgen-receptor complexes.

Androgen-receptor complexes A major advance in the understanding of the interaction of androgenic hormones with male accessory sex tissues came in 1968 when, following earlier metabolic studies of Shimazaki and of Farnsworth, Liao and Wilson established that after the administration of tritiated testosterone to castrated rats, the radioactive steroid that binds with receptors in the prostate, seminal vesicle, and preputial gland is not testosterone but dihydrotestosterone (17β-hydroxy-5α-androstan-3-one). Liao found similar results when incubating minced prostatic tissue with testosterone in vitro. Although reduction of testosterone to dihydrotestosterone can take place in the liver and other organs, this conversion was demonstrated to occur readily in whole prostatic tissue and also in isolated prostatic nuclei if a NADPH-generating system is present.

Recognition that dihydrotestosterone is the proximate androgenic species in the prostate nucleus opened the way for detailed studies of androgen receptors by a large number of investigators. In earlier experiments the dihydrotestosterone-receptor complexes detected were produced by the reduction of tritiated testosterone in the tissue, but after tritiated dihydrotestosterone of high specific radioactivity became available, it was possible to demonstrate its direct reaction with intracellular receptors in a manner similar to that previously employed with estradiol in female reproductive tissues.

Wilson, Liao, and Mainwaring first showed that the dihydrotestosterone bound in the prostatic nuclei of testosterone-treated castrated rats is extracted by exposure to KCl solutions to yield a macromolecular complex, which Liao showed to sediment at 3.0S in salt-containing sucrose gradients. The cytosol fraction of prostate homogenates from similar rats was found to contain a dihydrotestosterone-receptor complex, reported by Unhjem to sediment at 9.5S, and by Mainwaring at 8S, in low-salt sucrose gradients. Similar nuclear and cytosol complexes were obtained by Liao and by Mainwaring, respectively, on incubation of excised prostatic tissue with tritiated testosterone in vitro, while direct addition of labeled dihydrotestosterone, but not testosterone, to prostatic cytosol was found to produce a complex reported by Mainwaring and by Baulieu to sediment in low-salt gradients at 8S. In the presence of salt this complex dissociates into a subunit, described by Baulieu as 4–5S and by Liao as 3.5S (a value later revised to 3.8S on the basis of more precise sedimentation experiments carried out in glycerol-containing sucrose gradients). Voigt has identified the cytosol complex by means of agar-gel electrophoresis, and Bruchovsky has characterized both the cytosol and nuclear complexes by chromatography on cellulose phosphate. Liao, Baulieu, and Voigt all found that the binding of dihydrotestosterone to the receptor protein in prostatic cytosol is abolished in the presence of cyproterone or cyproterone acetate, and Liao and Peets described similar inhibition with flutamide.

In analogy to the case of estrogens and progestins, the dihydrotestosterone complex found in prostatic nuclei appears to be derived from the extranuclear complex by a hormone-induced translocation, involving a temperature-dependent and hormone-dependent transformation of the receptor protein. Mainwaring, Liao, and Stumpf each found that incubation of surviving prostatic tissue with tritiated dihydrotestosterone at 2°C results in little nuclear accumulation of labeled steroid, in contrast to 37°C, where nuclear accumulation resembling that in vivo is seen by either biochemical or autoradiographic methods. Liao has shown that prostatic nuclei from castrated rats do not contain any significant amount of androgen-binding proteins and that exposure of such nuclei to dihydrotestosterone alone does not produce nuclear complex. In the absence of dihydrotestosterone, little cytosol receptor binds to isolated prostate nuclei. As described by Liao, by Baulieu, and by Mainwaring, incubation of prostate nuclei with a dihydrotestosterone-cytosol mixture at 20°, 25°, or 37°, but not at 2°C, results in substantial nuclear binding and the formation of salt-extractable 3.0S complex. Under the same conditions that dihydrotestosterone produces nuclear complex, testosterone, which binds only weakly to the cytosol receptor, does not induce its nuclear translocation. Mainwaring later reported similar findings in regard to binding with isolated chromatin. Recently Liao has shown that incubation of prostate cytosol with dihydrotestosterone at 20° but not at 0°C causes the transformation of the hormone-receptor complex from its native (3.8S) form to the nuclear (3.0S) form, as determined by sedimentation in salt-containing sucrose gradients, and Mainwaring has concluded that warming to 30°C produces a change in the cytoplasmic androgen-receptor complex necessary for its binding with chromatin.

Similar cytoplasmic and nuclear binding with the formation of an 8S cytoplasmic complex was observed by Mainwaring in normal human prostate and in some but not all specimens of benign prostatic hyperplasia. Cyproterone-sensitive binding of dihydrotestosterone to receptors in rat epididymis was described by Blaquier and by French and associates, giving rise, both in vivo and in vitro, to cytoplasmic and nuclear complexes reported by Blaquier to sediment at 8.4S and 3.5S, respectively. Evidence has been presented to indicate that the nuclear complex is produced by the temperature-dependent translocation of the extranuclear complex. The cytoplasmic complex is distinguished from the cyproterone-insensitive binding to a 4S protein, called androgen-binding protein (ABP), that French has demonstrated to be present in epididymis; this substance apparently is produced in the testis and is carried to the epididymis, where it binds with both testosterone and dihydrotestosterone but is not incorporated in the nucleus. In addition to ABP, French and Steinberger demonstrated the presence in rat testis tubules of an androgen-receptor system that, after in vivo administration of tritiated testosterone, gives rise to cytoplasmic and nuclear complexes similar to those observed in prostate and epididymis. Whether these receptors are present in Sertoli cells or in germinal epithelium and whether they play a role in an effect of androgen on spermatogenesis remains to be established. Blaquier has shown spermatozoa to be devoid of androgen receptors.

Although the exact nature of the nuclear component that binds the androgen-receptor complex is not clearly understood, a number of experimental observations provide some information about this acceptor site. Early experiments of Wilson with the duck preen gland and of Mangan with the rat prostate indicated that labeled androgen administered in vivo becomes associated with chromatin, particularly euchromatin. Prostatic chromatin appears to have a special affinity for androgen-receptor complex. Both Liao and Mainwaring have observed that, during an incubation at 20° or 37°C with the cytosol complex obtained from prostate, significantly more radioactivity (shown by Liao to be 3S complex) is bound to prostatic nuclei than to nuclei from such tissues as liver, kidney, brain, thymus, and diaphragm. Mainwaring has also demonstrat-

ed that, on incubation at 4°C with either nuclear or cytoplasmic dihydrotestosterone-receptor complex, chromatin from rat prostate or seminal vesicle binds more radioactivity than does chromatin from liver, kidney, and spleen, and the O'Malley group has made similar observations concerning prostate and testis chromatin as compared to that from spleen, liver, or lung. In these in vitro experiments the capacity of nuclei or of chromatin to bind receptor complex is saturable at levels equal to or less than the binding capacity in vivo. Liao has also demonstrated specific binding of androgen-receptor complex with deoxyribonucleoprotein complexes reconstructed from purified DNA and salt-extractable proteins of prostate nuclei.

Liao and associates found that the dihydrotestosterone-receptor complex but not the receptor protein itself can bind strongly to ribonucleoprotein (RNP) particles from prostate nuclei but not from nuclei of liver thymus or uterus. Analogous preferential binding of the estrogen-receptor complex of uterine cytosol to RNP particles from uterine nuclei was also observed. On the basis of these findings, Liao has suggested that specific RNP may constitute at least a portion of the acceptor site in target tissue and that steroid-receptor complex, translocated to the nucleus, may participate in the processing of newly synthesized nuclear RNA, being translocated with RNP particles to the ribosome, where receptor is released for participation in a new reaction cycle with another molecule of hormone.

Recently Liao has described an extremely rapid stimulation by administered dihydrotestosterone of a reaction involved in the initiation of protein synthesis in ribosomal particles in the ventral prostate of the castrated rat. The factor affected appears to be a cytosol protein that binds methionyl-$tRNA_f$. Because the stimulatory action is blocked by cyproterone, which prevents binding of hormone to the cytoplasmic receptor, this effect appears to involve the hormone-receptor complex in an action that is independent of its translocation to the nucleus.

Thus the interaction pathway of androgenic hormones in many target cells involves conversion of testosterone to dihydrotestosterone, which binds to cytoplasmic receptors and is transferred to the nucleus. This recognition provided a potential explanation for certain phenomena of inherited androgen resistance in rats (Stanley and Gumbreck), mice (Lyon and Hawkes), and humans (testicular feminizing syndrome). Androgen resistance in so-called Tfm mutants was first considered to be associated with a defect in the conversion of testosterone to dihydrotestosterone; however, studies from the laboratories of Bardin, of Tomkins, and of Wilson demonstrated that androgen-sensitive tissues such as preputial gland, kidney, submandibular gland, and fetal anlage of Tfm rats and mice exhibit normal conversion of testosterone to dihydrotestosterone, but these tissues have difficulty concentrating androgen, especially in the nuclei. Later Bardin showed that cytosols from preputial gland of the Tfm rat and from kidney of the Tfm mouse lack the 8S receptor protein normally found in these tissues. These findings, along with observations that Tfm animals are resistant to exogenous dihydrotestosterone as well as testosterone, indicate that the genetic defect is in the receptor system rather than in the enzymes of reduction.

Whether the testicular feminization syndrome in humans results from a similar defect in androgen receptors is difficult to ascertain because of the lack of a suitable target organ for study. Imperato-McGinley and associates have reported a deficiency in the overall conversion of testosterone to dihydrotestosterone, as indicated by plasma and urinary steroid levels, and Wilson has described two types of familial male pseudohermaphroditism, one that appears to involve abnormal dihydrotestosterone synthesis and the other a defect in androgen action. The animal models and the fact that patients with testicular feminizing syndrome are generally resistant to administered dihydrotestosterone as well as to testosterone suggest that a defective receptor system is probably involved in the etiology of this condition in humans.

Effect of receptor complexes on RNA synthesis

Williams-Ashman reported in 1962 that an early response of target cells to the action of androgenic hormones is enhanced synthesis of nuclear RNA and also that prostatic nuclei isolated from testosterone-treated rats show increased RNA polymerase activity. These findings were confirmed by Liao, who also showed that the base composition of the RNA synthesized by the isolated nuclei is altered, as indicated by nearest-neighbor frequency determination. Mainwaring has found that the activity of the solubilized RNA polymerase I from rat prostate nuclei and especially from nucleoli is significantly increased within one hour after androgen treatment.

Although Villee has reported stimulation of RNA polymerase in prostatic nuclei by treatment with dihydrotestosterone in the absence of receptor, this observation has not been confirmed by others. In 1972 and 1973 Griffiths and associates reported that incubation of prostatic nuclei or nucleoli with either dihydrotestosterone or receptor alone did not influence RNA polymerase activity of isolated prostatic nuclei or nucleoli, but that incubation with either the cytoplasmic or nuclear dihydrotestosterone-receptor complex resulted in a 50 to 100 percent increase in RNA polymerase I activity. Greater stimulation is observed when prostatic chromatin rather than liver chromatin or calf thymus DNA is used as template. In contrast to the experience thus far with estrogen-receptor complexes and isolated uterine nuclei, small but significant stimulation of polymerase II is also observed, especially under the most recently described experimental conditions. The tissue specificity of this stimulatory effect of receptor complex on isolated nuclei and nucleoli remains to be established.

Although many of the actions of testosterone in the rodent prostate and seminal vesicle appear to be mediated through its conversion to dihydrotestosterone, which interacts with the receptor, in certain tissues this compound may not be the proximate androgen. Testosterone itself may be the active androgen in rat uterus and levator ani and in mouse kidney, whereas 5α androstanediols appear to be active in dog prostate. The influence of testosterone on reproductive behavior appears to result from its conversion in the brain to dihydrotestosterone and estradiol, the latter through an aromatization process described by Ryan.

Receptor purification

Because of its instability and tendency to lose bound steroid during purification procedures, the isolation of androgen-receptor protein has proved difficult. Several investigators have employed an ammonium sulfate precipitation to concentrate the prostatic cytosol receptor and remove a substantial amount of contaminating proteins, including a substance (α protein) demonstrated by Liao to bind dihydrotestosterone without further interaction with the nucleus. Recently the Mainwaring group has described the use of DNA-cellulose chromatography followed by isoelectric focusing to provide a preparation of cytoplasmic receptor purified some 2,300-fold.

25.3 Gonadotropin Receptors

Receptors for LH were originally defined in the testis and ovary by in vivo and in vitro binding studies with radioiodinated LH and hCG. In early studies performed by Lunenfeld and Eshkol, Espeland et al., and DeKretser et al., the labeled hormone was localized by autoradiography to the anticipated target sites—the Leydig cells of the testis and the luteinized cells of the ovary. In addition, studies by Mancini et al. on the cellular distribution within the testis of gonadotropins localized by immunohistochemical methods showed that FSH was confined to the Sertoli cells, and LH was confined to the Leydig cells and peritubular cells. The location and properties of LH/hCG receptors have been analyzed and described by several groups, including Mougdal et al., Catt and Dufau, Reichert et al., Rajaneimi et al., Lee and Ryan, Kammerman, Channing et al., and Midgley et al. More recently, in vitro binding studies with labeled gonadotropins have been performed with slices, cell suspensions, and homogenates of the testis and ovary. Whereas the LH/hCG receptors have been subjected to fairly extensive study since 1971, observations upon receptors for FSH and prolactin have been more recently described by Means, Rabinowitz, Reichert, Friesen, and their colleagues.

Preparation of Labeled Gonadotropins

Gonadotropin-binding studies have been most frequently performed with radioiodinated hormones, usually prepared by labeling the glycoprotein with ^{125}I; a relatively small number of studies have been prepared with tritium-labeled gonadotropins, usually of rather low specific activity. The conditions employed for iodination of gonadotropins as radioimmunoassay tracer are usually unsuitable for the preparation of labeled hormones for receptor binding sites. Also the approximate calculations of specific activity applied to radioimmunoassay tracers are too inaccurate to use in quantitative binding studies. The various gonadotropins exhibit marked differences in susceptibility to damage during the radioiodination procedure, and differential loss of biological activity and immunoreactivity is frequently observed.

FSH and prolactin are more readily inactivated than LH or hCG during iodination, predominantly by the reagents employed rather than by the addition of iodine per se. For receptor studies, the degree of iodination should not exceed one atom per molecule, and iodination conditions should be chosen to minimize oxidative tracer damage. Modifications of the chloramine T procedure have been applied to iodination of several peptide hormones for receptor binding studies, including ACTH, insulin, growth hormone, LH, hCG, and FSH. For hLH and hCG, satisfactory tracer has been prepared by iodination in the presence of low concentrations of chloramine T, for short time periods and at low temperature. Purification of the labeled hormone has been performed by gel filtration, cellulose adsorption, chromatography on Sepharose–Concanavalin A, and occasionally by electrophoresis. LH is more readily damaged than hCG during iodination, and labeled hCG has been more widely used for binding studies on LH receptors of the testis and ovary. The preparation of biologically active iodinated FSH and prolactin has been more difficult to achieve, and several reports have indicated that the lactoperoxidase iodination procedure is a more suitable method for labeling these hormones for binding studies.

The availability of suitable tracer has been a relatively greater problem in studies on peptide hormone receptors than in those concerned with steroid hormones. The hormones must be obtained in highly purified and active forms, the labeling procedure should not lead to significant loss of biological activity, and the labeled peptide should exhibit satisfactory stability during binding studies and storage. Most gonadotropin preparations employed for labeling are not of maximum attainable biological activity (e.g., the biological potency of most highly purified hCG is 15,000–18,000 IU/mg, whereas the activity of the usually available hCG preparations is in the range of 10,000–12,000 IU/mg). The iodinated derivatives of such hormones must therefore contain a portion of labeled inactive molecules, for which correction should be made during calculation of binding constants derived from equilibrium or kinetic data. To this end, the labeled peptide hormone should be characterized by the following procedures prior to use in quantitative binding studies.

Determination of specific activity This should be performed by bioassay or radioligand-receptor assay; in the latter procedure the labeled hormone is assayed by self-displacement by addition of increasing concentrations of tracer to the radioreceptor assay. Measurement of specific activity can also be performed by self-displacement in a specific radioimmunoassay system for the gonadotropin, but the values obtained may be less biologically relevant than those derived by radioligand-receptor assay. Bioassay by conventional procedures is not usually practical for labeled gonadotropins but can be more readily performed in vitro by employing the steroidogenic response of testicular or ovarian target cells (e.g., testosterone production by dispersed Leydig cells). Such methods are much more sensitive than in vivo bioassays and are much more convenient for the assay of radioiodinated gonadotropins that stimulate steroidogenesis.

Determination of the proportion of radioactive hormone that can be bound by an excess of receptor sites This value indicates the content of active hormone in the labeled preparation and can provide a correction factor for calculation of binding constants (e.g., if only 30 percent of the tracer is bound by excess receptors, then 70 percent of the total radioactivity will always be present as inactive tracer in the "free" fraction, which should be corrected accordingly). Such correction factors are usually approximate, since exposure to high concentrations of cell membranes or homogenates may increase hormone degradation and give too low a value for the content of biologically active hormone.

Evaluation of the physicochemical properties of the iodinated gonadotropin The labeled hormone must retain its original physicochemical properties, at least to the extent of its migration on gel filtration and in an appropriate electrophoresis system. These tests should be performed first to evaluate the labeling procedure and then intermittently as quality-control measures.

A particular feature of labeled peptide hormones is their tendency to exhibit nonspecific adsorption to a variety of tissue preparations and physical surfaces. This is minimized by the use of relatively undamaged tracer and by the inclusion of carrier proteins in incubation media during binding studies. The nonspecific bound radioactivity is usually measured as that which is not displaced from binding sites by incubation from time zero with an excess of the unlabeled hormone.

Location of Gonadotropin Receptors

Receptors for LH and hCG have been demonstrated by DeKretser, Catt, Dufau, and others in the Leydig cells of the testis, but not in other tissues of the male. No binding sites for LH are demonstrable in the seminiferous tubule, and the tubule does not respond to LH with cAMP or steroid formation. In the ovary, autoradiographic studies by Midgley and colleagues showed that LH receptors are present in the interstitial tissue and theca cells of the developing follicle. These investigators also showed that LH receptors begin to appear in the granulosa cells of the maturing follicles of the rat ovary at the time of antrum formation. Channing and Kammerman have demonstrated receptors for LH in the granulosa cells of maturing ovarian follicles of the pig ovary. Although LH receptors are clearly present in the maturing granulosa cells, Lindner and colleagues showed injected gonadotropins to be localized mainly in the theca cells, and it is uncertain when the LH receptors of the granulosa cell become occupied by endogenous LH. In addition, LH receptors have been demonstrated in the corpus luteum of man, rhesus monkey, pig, cow, and rat.

Receptors for FSH have been more difficult to demonstrate, particularly in the testis. The studies by Mancini's group and by Means and colleagues, however, have provided good evidence that FSH receptors are present in the Sertoli cells of the testis. Ovarian receptors for FSH have been identified in the granulosa cells of immature animals by the Ann Arbor group. In the rat, FSH receptors are present in small follicles prior to the development of LH receptors; in this species, treatment with FSH has been shown by Zeleznik in Midgley's laboratory to be followed by the appearance of LH receptors in the granulosa cells.

Catt and Dufau have localized receptors for LH and hCG to the plasma membrane of the Leydig cell, and Rajaneimi, Midgley, and colleagues have localized them to the cells of the corpus luteum by autoradiographic and cell fractionation. No electron microscopy data are available concerning the subcellular localization of labeled FSH, but immunohistochemical studies by Mancini's group and binding analysis with testis fractions by Means and colleagues have indicated that the receptor sites are associated with the plasma membrane of the tubule cells, specifically of the Sertoli cell.

Prolactin receptors have also been relatively difficult to demonstrate, but Friesen and colleagues have recently showed them to occur in the lactating mammary gland as well as in other tissues, including the liver, kidney, and adrenal gland.

Gonadotropin-Binding Studies In Vitro

In vitro studies upon gonadotropin receptors have been performed with intact testes and ovarian slices or sections; with cell dispersions from ovarian follicles, corpus luteum, and testis interstitium; and with homogenates of the testis and ovary. Such preparations have been employed for localization of the receptors, for characterization of the receptor population, for quantitative binding studies to determine affinity and rate constants, and for development of radioligand-receptor systems to use in quantitation of gonadotropins and in structure-function studies with modified gonadotropins.

Quantitative binding studies have shown that the receptor-gonadotropin interaction is characterized by high association constant ($\sim 10^{10}$ M^{-1}) and low binding capacity (~ 1 pmole/g). Rate constants for association and dissociation are temperature-dependent, with relatively slow dissociation at lower temperatures. At body temperature more rapid dissociation occurs, but quantitative studies are complicated by accompanying degradation of receptors and hormone. In general, the interaction between hCG and testis receptors follows the behavior predicted for a simple bimolecular chemical reaction.

Testis and ovarian homogenates have been employed for specific radioligand-receptor assays, most extensively for LH/hCG and more recently for FSH. In contrast to the LH/hCG assays the initial assays for FSH have displayed relatively low tracer binding, usually only a few percent of the labeled hormone. The radioligand-receptor assays for gonadotropins developed by Catt and Dufau, Reichert et al., Lee and Ryan, and Saxena et al. possess the virtues of biological specificity, relatively high precision and accuracy, rapidity, and considerably greater convenience than conventional bioassays. They are, in general, less sensitive than radioimmunoassay and about 100-fold more sensitive than conventional bioassay. The LH/hCG radioligand-receptor assay is responsive to LH from a wide variety of species—including humans, primates, sheep, cows, pigs, and rats—and to the placental gonadotropins of humans, monkeys, and horses. In most radioligand-receptor assays, relatively simple homogenates of the appropriate target tissue—testis, ovary, seminiferous tubules, or mammary gland—have been incubated with ^{125}I-labeled tracer hormone and appropriate standards. In some cases partially purified preparations of cell membrane have been employed. The sensitivity of such assays has not been sufficiently high to measure peripheral hormone levels in nonpregnant animals, but the methods are applicable to the measurement of CG during pregnancy in man and monkey and of prolactin during pregnancy in the rat. Recently measurements of plasma gonadotropins in postmenopausal women and in cycling women at the time of the LH peak have been performed by radioligand-receptor assay.

An important aspect of the measurement of gonadotropins is the divergence in apparent potency that can be observed between various classical in vivo bioassays, radioimmunoassays, and in vitro assays such as the radioligand-receptor method. This is partly attributable to the differences between pituitary and urinary LH in man and the varying efficacies of these and other forms of LH in the individual bioassay procedures —largely due to the differing half-lives of the individual forms of LH and hCG and the uncertainty whether plasma LH should be assayed against pituitary or urinary standards. Variations in plasma half-life between LH and hCG preparations are partly dependent on the degree of sialylation of the glycoprotein molecules; those with the most abundant sialic acid residues show the longest half-life and often the greatest biological activity. Since in vitro assays are not responsive to factors that influence metabolism in vivo, they would be expected to provide generally higher potency values than those obtained with in vivo bioassays; this is frequently confirmed.

Gonadotropin-binding systems have also been of value for the study of structure-function relations in components and derivatives of the gonadotropic hormones in vitro. Removal of sialic acid from LH and hCG causes a major loss of biological activity measured by conventional in vivo bioassays. Dufau and colleagues demonstrated, however, that the binding activity of the desialylated hormones is not reduced and is usually slightly enhanced. These investigators also showed that removal of the adjacent galactose residue from the hCG molecule had no effect on binding activity, indicating that neither of the major terminal carbohydrate residues is essential for interaction of the hormone with the receptor site. The in vitro activities of the modified glycoproteins, in terms of stimulation of cAMP and testosterone production, are significantly reduced, however. The steroidogenic activities of the asialo-hCG and asialo-agalacto-hCG preparations are about 50 percent and 15 percent, respectively, of that of the native hormone. The hCG derivatives that retain binding activity and show reduced agonist activity are potential competitive antagonists and may prove to be of considerable value as inhibitors of gonadotropin activity in vitro. Further studies on the role of sugar residues in gonadotropin binding and activity have been described by Bahl, Moyle, and colleagues.

Ward, Papkoff, and others have showed that a variety of chemical modifications of the protein portion of the LH or hCG molecule interfere with binding to the receptor site. These include reduction of disulfide bonds, performic acid oxidation, and succinylation. Progressive nitration of tyrosine residues leads to serial loss of binding activity of ovine LH, the susceptible residues being probably in the α subunit. In iodinated LH and hCG the labeled tyrosine residues have also been shown to be situated in the α subunit.

In addition to studies on the role of carbohydrate residues in receptor binding and activation, in vitro systems have been used to evaluate the biological activity of subunits of LH, hCG, FSH, and TSH. The existence of a common α subunit and specific β subunits in these glycoprotein hormones had suggested that the α subunit could be responsible for a common function of the various hormones, such as activation of adenylate cyclase, while the β subunit appears more likely to be responsible for the specific recognition of the hormone by the receptor site. Initial reports on the biological properties of glycoprotein hormone subunits by Gospodarowicz, Papkoff, and others suggested that the isolated subunits may exhibit specific biological activities, most clearly the lipolysis in isolated fat cells. Evidence of specific actions in the testis or ovary was less convincing, and a number of studies were performed to determine the true activity, if any, of the isolated subunits. Application of the radioligand-receptor assay to a variety of α and β subunits of LH and hCG by Catt and colleagues showed that the intrinsic activity of the subunits was equivalent only to that seen by conventional bioassays; identical values were also obtained by a sensitive in vitro bioassay based upon testosterone formation by isolated rat testes, indicating that the apparent activity of certain subunit preparations was entirely attributable to contamination with intact hormone. No enhancement of specific functions, such as receptor binding and target cell activation, was detectable in either of the subunits. The absence of biological activity in hCG subunits was also demonstrated by the neutralization studies with specific antisera, followed by bioassay. Reichert has shown that subunits of FSH also exhibit minimal binding-inhibition activity in FSH radioligand-receptor assays, to an extent commensurate with the degree of contamination with undissociated hormone.

Reichert has used radioligand-receptor assay to evaluate the recombination of homologous and heterologous pairs of gonadotropin subunits; this assay provides a rapid and convenient system for kinetic studies of subunit combination and dissociation. The characteristic slopes of the human and nonhuman LH preparations in the rat testis/hCG radioligand assay are determined by the respective β subunits of these hormones. Also, the β subunit of hCG confers higher binding affinity upon recombinations with α subunits of LH, reflecting the generally higher binding potency of hCG in receptor assay systems.

Gonadotropin Binding and Target Cell Activation

Catt, Dufau, and colleagues have examined the relationship between hormone binding and target cell activation during uptake of labeled hCG by the rat testis. Increased binding of hormone to receptor sites is evident over a wide range of hCG concentration, greatly exceeding that necessary to induce maximum steroidogenesis, and is accompanied by a correspondingly large rise in cAMP formation. Such an effect suggests that the testis contains a large proportion, possibly as high as 99 percent, of "spare" receptors; most of these receptors are coupled to adenylate cyclase. Such spare receptors are obviously not redundant in the thermodynamic sense, since they would operate to enhance the rate of association between hormone and target cell and may thus increase the sensitivity of the cell to activation by a given level of trophic hormone.

The association between hormone binding and cAMP formation has also been demonstrated by Means for FSH in the tubules of the testis and by Clark and Menon for hCG in the granulosa cells of the ovary. At low levels of hCG, however, Catt, Moyle, Menon, and their colleagues have observed a dissociation between steroidogenesis and cAMP formation. Cyclic AMP levels do not begin to rise until testosterone production in testis tissue or dispersed Leydig cells is almost maximal. This suggests that cAMP may not be involved in the steroidogenic response to physiological levels of LH, or that only an extremely small rise or translocation of cAMP in a critical intracellular compartment may occur during the initial phase of steroidogenesis. The latter possibility is supported by the finding that phosphodiesterase inhibitors consistently enhance the testosterone response induced by submaximal concentrations of hCG. The production of testosterone by dispersed Leydig cells in the presence of theophylline or methylisobutylxanthine (MIX) has been applied by Dufau and colleagues to the development of an in vitro bioassay of sensitivity comparable to that of radioimmunoassay, with the capacity to bioassay circulating levels of LH and hCG.

Induction of Receptors

Measurement of binding sites in the ovary has been a fruitful source of information about the induction of LH receptors during follicle development. Female rats show minimal response in ovarian weight to exogenous gonadotropins in the first week of life, and Weizmann's group showed that stimulation of cAMP by LH in the ovarian follicles of the newborn rat cannot be demonstrated at a time when prostaglandins can activate cAMP formation. Such results suggest that LH receptor sites are not present or are not coupled to adenylate cyclase in the newborn animal. Development of gonadotropin responsiveness seems to require secretion of endogenous estrogen during the first few days of life, probably formed locally in the theca interna cells. Ross's group has shown that administration of estrogen enhances ovarian uptake of labeled FSH in immature hypophysectomized female rats. Estrogen probably causes the induction of FSH receptors in the granulosa cell during the first week or so of postnatal life. In slightly older female rats (21 days), Zeleznik and colleagues showed that LH receptors could be induced in the granulosa cells of ovarian follicles by treatment with FSH for two days. Channing has reported that comparable changes can be produced in vitro by incubation of porcine granulosa cells with FSH. Thus the development of LH receptors in the granulosa cell appears to depend upon the action of FSH and normally occurs around the time of antrum formation. The above studies, and those of Ericson, Ryan, and colleagues, suggest that a relationship exists between the appearance of LH receptor sites, the development of gap junctions between granulosa cells at the time of antrum formation, and the acquisition of responsiveness to gonadotropins.

Kammerman and Channing showed that the granulosa cells of large follicles contain many more LH receptors than those of small follicles and give a much larger cAMP response to stimulation by LH in vitro; however, the degree to which these are occupied by endogenous LH in vivo is not known. The access of circulating gonadotropins to granulosa cells is probably limited, and many of the receptors may remain unoccupied until the time of ovulation. The ability of cultured granulosa cells to undergo luteinization in vitro suggests that LH is bound to a proportion of the receptor sites but is presumably unable to initiate luteinization until the cells are removed from proximity to the ovum or antral fluid. Receptors for LH have also been demonstrated in the theca cells of large ovarian follicles, a finding consistent with the responsiveness of the tissue to LH during its effect upon ovulation.

In the testis of the newborn rat, Frowein and Engel observed binding of gonadotropins to receptors at a time when the Leydig cells are said to be relatively insensitive to the actions of LH. In older animals, FSH has been shown by Odell and colleagues to induce sensitivity to LH, and it may play a role in the onset of sexual maturation. Such a role would presumably involve the induction of LH receptors in the Leydig cell, a mechanism that has not yet been demonstrated by hormone-binding studies. But the induction of LH receptors by FSH probably takes place in both sexes, during follicle maturation in the female and during maturation of the testis in the male.

Solubilization of Gonadotropin Receptors

Dufau and colleagues have extracted receptors for LH from particulate binding fractions of the testis and ovary, using nonionic detergents, including Triton X-100 and Lubrol. The Triton-solubilized receptors have a molecular weight in the region of 200,000 and behave as asymmetric molecules with Stokes radium of 64 Å. The free receptor migrates as a 6.5S species on sucrose density gradient ultracentrifugation, and the receptor-hormone complex migrates as a 7.5S species. The hormonal specificity of the detergent-solubilized receptors is retained, and their binding affinity is slightly reduced. The soluble receptors lose binding activity after exposure to trypsin, indicating that protein forms a major component of the binding site. Treatment with phospholipase A also destroys binding activity, suggesting that phospholipid could be a functionally important part of the binding complex. Recently the LH-hCG receptors of rat testis have been isolated by Dufau and colleagues in highly purified form by affinity chromatography of detergent-solubilized receptors on Agarose gel coupled to hCG. Purification of gonadotropin receptors by affinity chromatography appears to have considerable potential for isolating the receptors in a homogeneous form and in a quantity suitable for structural analysis.

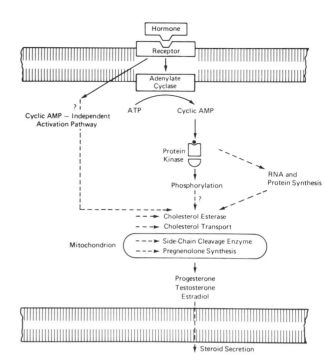

Figure 25.2 Action of gonadotropins on steroidogenic target cells of testis and ovary. Protein hormone interacts with receptor in the plasma membrane, inducing the formation of a second messenger that serves as the intracellular effector of processes that lead to enhanced steroidogenesis.

Reviews

Baulieu, E. E. A 1972 survey of the mode of action of steroid hormones. *Proc. Fourth International Congress on Endocrinology*, p. 30. Amsterdam: Excerpta Medica, 1973.

Channing, C. R., and S. Kammerman. Binding of gonadotropins to ovarian cells. Biol. Reprod. 10:179, 1974.

Dufau, M. L., and A. R. Means. *Hormone binding and target cell activation in the testis*. New York: Plenum Press, 1974.

Gorski, J., D. Toft, G. Shyamala, D. Smith, and A. Notides. Hormone receptors: Studies on the interaction of estrogen with the uterus. Recent Prog. Horm. Res. 24:45, 1968.

Jensen, E. V., and E. R. DeSombre. Mechanism of action of the female sex hormones. Ann. Rev. Biochem. 41:203, 1972.

Jensen, E. V., S. Mohla, T. A. Gorell, and E. R. DeSombre. The role of estrophilin in estrogen action. Vitam. Horm. 32:89, 1974.

King, R. J. B., and W. I. P. Mainwaring. *Steroid-cell interactions*. Baltimore: University Park Press, 1974.

Liao, S. Cellular receptors and mechanism of action of steroid hormones. Int. Rev. Cytol. 41:87, 1975.

Liao, S., and S. Fang. Receptor proteins for androgens and the mode of action of androgens on gene transcription in ventral prostate. Vitam. Horm. 27:17, 1970.

O'Malley, B. W., and A. R. Means. *Receptors for reproductive hormones*. New York: Plenum Press, 1973.

O'Malley, B. W., and A. R. Means. Female steroid hormones and target cell nuclei. Science 183:610, 1974.

Raspe, G., ed. *Advances in the biosciences*, Vol. 7: *Schering workshop on steroid hormone receptors*. New York: Pergamon Press, 1971.

Williams-Ashman, H. G., and A. H. Reddi. Actions of vertebrate sex hormones. Ann. Rev. Physiol. 33:31, 1971.

Selected References

Anderson, J. N., J. H. Clark, and E. J. Peck, Jr. Oestrogen and nuclear binding sites: Determination of specific sites by ^{3}H-estradiol exchange. Biochem. J. 126, 1972.

Anderson, K. M., and S. Liao. Selective retention of dihydrotestosterone by prostatic nuclei. Nature 219:277, 1968.

Anderson, J. N., E. J. Peck, Jr., and J. H. Clark. Nuclear receptor-estrogen complex: Relationship between concentration and early uterotropic responses. Endocrinology 92: 1488, 1973.

Bardin, C. W., and L. P. Bullock. Testicular feminization: Studies of the molecular basis of a genetic defect. J. Invest. Dermatol. 63:75, 1974.

Baulieu, E. E., and I. Jung. A prostatic cytosol receptor. Biochem. Biophys. Res. Commun. 38:599, 1970.

Bruchovsky, N., and J. D. Wilson. Evidence that dihydrotestosterone is the active form of testosterone. Clin. Res. 14:74, 1968.

Bruchovsky, N., and J. D. Wilson. The intranuclear binding of testosterone and 5α-androstan-17β-ol-3-one by rat prostate. J. Biol. Chem. 243:5953, 1968.

Buller, R. E., D. O. Toft, W. T. Schrader, and B. W. O'Malley. Progesterone-binding components of chick oviduct. VIII. Receptor activation and hormone-dependent binding to purified nuclei. J. Biol. Chem. 250:801, 1975.

Castro, A. E., A. Alonso, and R. E. Mancini. Localization of follicle stimulating and luteinizing hormones in the rat testes using immunohistochemical methods. J. Endocrinol. 52:129, 1972.

Catt, K. J., and M. L. Dufau. Spare gonadotropin receptors in rat testis. Nature New Biol. 244:219, 1973.

Catt, K. J., M. L. Dufau, and T. Tsuruhara. Radioligand-receptor assay of luteinizing hormone and chorionic gonadotropin. J. Clin. Endocrinol. Metab. 34:123, 1972.

Catt, K. J., T. Tsuruhara, and M. L. Dufau. Gonadotropin binding sites of the rat testis. Biochem. Biophys. Acta 279: 194, 1972.

Clark, J. H., J. N. Anderson, and E. J. Peck, Jr. Estrogen receptor–anti-estrogen complex: Atypical binding by uterine nuclei and effects on uterine growth. Steroids 22:707, 1973.

Dufau, M. L., E. H. Charreau, and K. J. Catt. Characteristics of a soluble gonadotropin receptor from the rat testis. J. Biol. Chem. 248:6973, 1973.

Dufau, M. L., K. Watanabe, and K. J. Catt. Stimulation of cyclic AMP production by the rat testis during incubation with hCG in vitro. Endocrinology 92:6, 1973.

Dorrington, J. H., and I. B. Fritz. Effects of gonadotropins on cyclic AMP production by isolated seminiferous tubule and interstitial cell preparations. Endocrinology 94:395, 1974.

Davies, P., and K. Griffiths. Further studies on the stimulation of prostatic ribonucleic acid polymerase by 5α-dihydrotestosterone complexes. J. Endocrinol. 62:385, 1974.

Erdos, T. Properties of a uterine oestradiol receptor. Biochem. Biophys. Res. Commun. 32:338, 1968.

Falk, R. J., and C. W. Bardin. Uptake of tritiated progesterone by the uterus of the ovariectomized guinea pig. Endocrinology 86:1059, 1970.

Fang, S., K. M. Anderson, and S. Liao. Receptor proteins for androgens: On the role of specific proteins in selective retention of 17β-hydroxy-5α-androstan-3-one by rat ventral prostate in vivo and in vitro. J. Biol. Chem. 244:6584, 1969.

Feil, P. D., S. R. Glasser, D. O. Toft, and B. W. O'Malley. Progesterone binding in the mouse and rat uterus. Endocrinology 91:738, 1972.

Glascock, R. F., and W. G. Hoekstra. Selective accumulation of tritium-labelled hexoestrol by the reproductive organs of immature female goats and sheep. Biochem. J. 72: 673, 1959.

Gospodarowicz, D. Properties of the luteinizing hormone receptor of isolated bovine corpus luteum plasma membranes. J. Biol. Chem. 248:5042, 1973.

Irving, R., and W. I. P. Mainwaring. Partial purification of steroid-receptor complexes by DNA-cellulose chromatography and isoelectric focusing. J. Steroid Biochem. 5:711, 1974.

Jensen, E. V., and H. I. Jacobson. Basic guides to the mechanism of estrogen action. Recent Prog. Horm. Res. 18: 381, 1962.

Jensen, E. V., and H. I. Jacobson. Fate of steroid estrogens in target tissues. In *Biological activities of steroids in relation to cancer*, eds. G. Pincus and E. P. Vollmer, p. 161. New York: Academic Press, 1960.

Jensen, E. V., T. Suzuki, T. Kawashima, W. E. Stumpf, P. W. Jungblut, and E. R. DeSombre. A two step mechanism for the interaction of estradiol with rat uterus. Proc. Natl. Acad. Sci. USA 59:632, 1968.

Jensen, E. V., T. Suzuki, M. Numata, S. Smith, and E. R. DeSombre. Estrogen-binding substances of target tissues. Steroids 13:417, 1969.

Kammerman, S., and R. E. Canfield. The inhibition of binding of iodinated human chorionic gonadotropin to mouse ovary in vivo. Endocrinology 90:384, 1972.

Korenman, S. G., and B. R. Rao. Reversible disaggregation of the cytosol-estrogen binding protein of uterine cytosol. Proc. Natl. Acad. Sci. USA 61:1028, 1968.

Kuhn, R. W., W. T. Schrader, R. G. Smith, and B. W. O'Malley. Progesterone binding components of chick oviduct. X. Purification by affinity chromatography. J. Biol. Chem. 250:4220, 1975.

Lee, C. Y., and R. J. Ryan. Luteinizing hormone receptors: Specific binding of human luteinizing hormone to homogenates of luteinized rat ovaries. Proc. Natl. Acad. Sci. USA 69:3520, 1972.

Lee, C. Y., and R. J. Ryan. Interaction of ovarian receptors with human luteinizing hormone and human chorionic gonadotropin. Biochemistry 12:4609, 1973.

Liang, T., and S. Liao. A very rapid effect of androgen on initiation of protein synthesis in prostate. Proc. Natl. Acad. Sci. USA 72:706, 1975.

Liao, S., T. Liang, and J. L. Tymoczko. Ribonucleoprotein binding of steroid-"receptor" complexes. Nature New Biol. 241:211, 1973.

Little, M., G. C. Rosenfeld, and P. W. Jungblut. Cytoplasmic estradiol "receptors" associated with the microsomal fraction of pig uterus. Hoppe-Seyler's Z. Physiol. Chem. 353:231, 1972.

Mainwaring, W. I. P. A soluble androgen receptor in the cytoplasm of rat prostate. J. Endocrinol. 45:531, 1969.

Mainwaring, W. I. P., and B. M. Peterken. A reconstituted cell-free system for specific transfer of steroid-receptor complexes into nuclear chromatin isolated from rat ventral prostate gland. Biochem. J. 125:285, 1971.

Means, A. R. Specific interaction of ^{3}H-FSH in rat testis binding sites. In *Receptors for reproductive hormones*, eds. B. W. O'Malley and A. R. Means, p. 431. New York: Plenum Press, 1973.

Milgrom, E., M. Atger, and E. E. Baulieu. Progesterone in uterus and plasma. IV. Progesterone receptors in guinea pig uterus cytosol. Steroids 16:741, 1970.

Milgrom, E., M. Atger, M. Perrot, and E. E. Baulieu. Progesterone in uterus and plasma. VI. Uterine progesterone receptors during the estrus cycle and implantation in the guinea pig. Endocrinology 90:1071, 1972.

Mougdal, N. R., W. R. Moyle, and R. O. Greep. Specific binding of luteinizing hormone to Leydig tumor cells. J. Biol. Chem. 246:4983, 1971.

Notides, A. C., D. E. Hamilton, and J. H. Rudolph. Action of a human uterine protease on the estrogen receptor. Endocrinology 93:210, 1973.

Notides, A. C., and S. Nielsen. The molecular mechanism of the in vitro 4S and 5S transformation of the uterine estrogen receptor. J. Biol. Chem. 249:1866, 1974.

O'Malley, B. W., M. R. Sherman, and D. O. Toft. Progesterone "receptors" in the cytoplasm and nucleus of chick oviduct target tissue. Proc. Natl. Acad. Sci. USA 67:501, 1970.

Podratz, K. C., and P. A. Katzman. Effect of estradiol on uptake and retention of progesterone by the vagina of the ovariectomized mouse. Fed. Proc. 27:497, 1968.

Puca, G. A., E. Nola, V. Sica, and F. Bresciani. Estrogen-binding proteins of calf uterus. Interrelationship between various forms and identification of receptor-transforming factor. Biochemistry 11:4157, 1972.

Puca, G. A., V. Sica, and E. Nola. Identification of a high affinity nuclear acceptor site for estrogen receptor of calf uterus. Proc. Natl. Acad. Sci. USA 71:979, 1974.

Rajaniemi, M., and T. Vanha-Pertulla. Attachment to the luteal plasma membranes. An early event in the action of luteinizing hormone. J. Endocrinol. 57:199, 1973.

Raynaud-Jammet, C., and E. E. Baulieu. Action de l'oestradiol in vitro: Augmentation de la biosynthèse d'acide ribonucléique dans les noyaux utérine. C. R. Acad. Sci. (Paris) 268D:3211, 1969.

Reichert, L. E., and V. K. Bhalia. Development of a radioligand tissue receptor assay for human follicle-stimulating hormone. Endocrinology 94:483, 1974.

Reichert, L. E., G. M. Lawson, F. L. Leidenberger, and C. G. Trowbridge. Influence of α and β subunits on the kinetics of formation and activity of native and hybrid molecules of LH and hCG. Endocrinology 93:938, 1973.

Ritzen, E. M., L. Hagenas, V. Hansson, F. S. French, and S. N. Nayfeh. Androgen binding proteins in different testis compartments. J. Steroid Biochem. 5:849, 1974.

Rochefort, H., F. Lignon, and F. Capony. Formation of estrogen nuclear receptor in uterus: Effect of androgens, estrone and nafoxidine. Biochem. Biophys. Res. Commun. 47:662, 1972.

Sar, M., S. Liao, and W. E. Stumpf. Nuclear concentration of androgens in rat seminal vesicles and prostate demonstrated by dry-mount autoradiography. Endocrinology 86:1108, 1970.

Schrader, W. T., D. O. Toft, and B. W. O'Malley. Progesterone-binding protein of chick oviduct. VI. Interaction of purified progesterone-receptor components with nuclear constituents. J. Biol. Chem. 247:2401, 1972.

Shiu, R. P. C., P. A. Kelly, and H. G. Friesen. Radioreceptor assay for prolactin and other lactogenic hormones. Science 180:968, 1973.

Shyamala, G., and J. Gorski. Estrogen receptors in the rat uterus. Studies on the interaction of cytosol and nuclear binding sites. J. Biol. Chem. 244:1097, 1969.

Spelsberg, T. C., A. W. Steggles, F. Chytil, and B. W. O'Malley. Progesterone-binding components of chick oviduct. V. Exchange of progesterone-binding capacity from target to non-target tissue chromatins. J. Biol. Chem. 247:1368, 1972.

Stumpf, W. E., and L. J. Roth. High resolution autoradiography with dry-mounted, freeze-dried frozen sections. J. Histochem. Cytochem. 14:274, 1966.

Toft, D., and J. Gorski. A receptor molecule for estrogens: Isolation from rat uterus and preliminary characterization. Proc. Natl. Acad. Sci. USA 55:1574, 1966.

Tsuruhara, T., M. L. Dufau, J. Hickman, and K. J. Catt. Biological properties of hCG after removal of terminal sialic acid and galactose residues. Endocrinology 91:296, 1972.

Tveter, K. J., and A. Attramadal. Selective uptake of radioactivity in rat ventral prostate following administration of testosterone-1,2-^{3}H. Acta Endocrinol. 59:218, 1968.

Wiest, W. G., and B. R. Rao. Progesterone binding proteins in rabbit uterus and human endometrium. Adv. Biosci. 7:251, 1971.

26 The Control of Testicular Function

Emil Steinberger,
Ronald S. Swerdloff, and
Richard Horton

Scientific progress in reproductive endocrinology has moved rapidly in the past fifteen years. At the beginning of this period we knew (1) that the testes produced sex hormones and sperm; (2) that the pituitary controlled both of these processes; and (3) that the testicles exercised feedback influences on the secretion of hormones from the pituitary gland. Progress was hampered by difficulties in the measurement of pituitary and gonadal hormones and by primitive notions of how the brain was involved in the control of reproductive functions.

Much of the progress in reproductive medicine in the past decade has been a result of the development of techniques allowing accurate measurement of extremely small amounts of pituitary and gonadal hormones in biological fluids. These methodological advances permitted studies of the dynamics of hormonal secretion in animal models, normal human subjects, and patients with reproductive problems. As a result, we have gained considerable understanding of the physiological processes responsible for normal sexual maturation, maintenance of male hormone secretion and spermatogenesis in the normal adult, and the decline in reproductive function in the aged. We also gained new insight into the biochemical processes involved in the synthesis of male sex hormones and the control of sperm production and hormone synthesis by the hypothalamus and pituitary gland. These studies were logically followed by investigations of the effects of gonadal hormones on peripheral tissues.

Information gleaned from normal physiology was soon applied to pathological states, making possible quantitative diagnosis of the underfunctioning testes. Physicians are now readily able to diagnose gonadal insufficiency and to localize the anatomical level of the defect. In this way gonadal inadequacy due to defects in the brain and pituitary can be separated from that originating in the testis. This has resulted in the rational treatment of patients with abnormal gonadal function; specific therapy is determined by the functional and anatomical site of the defect. The practical importance of this knowledge is its potential for early detection of central nervous system lesions and thus institution of life-saving therapy. Not only has progress occurred in the treatment of adult patients with underfunctioning testes, but treatment of children with delayed and premature puberty can now be logically approached.

There are many practical problems in need of attention, such as:

1. Development of effective and safe male contraceptive agents. The information gained in the past fifteen years has given us the background to attack this problem from several directions.

2. Understanding of infertility due to abnormalities in sperm production. Future studies must be directed toward gaining a better understanding of the complex process of sperm maturation and the defects responsible for isolated failure of this process.

3. Clarification of the effects of male sex hormones on other organs such as the prostate, and on bone and vascular systems. For example, we must learn more about the effects of male sex hormones on the prostate gland and their relation to the development of both malignant and benign growth of prostatic tissue. The role of gonadal hormones in the development and modification of atherosclerosis needs to be clarified. The effect of gonadal hormones on intellectual processes and affect requires a great deal of study. Methodological advances have placed into the hands of clinical investigators the tools with which to approach these problems rationally.

26.1 The Hypothalamic-Pituitary-Gonadal Axis

Historical Introduction

The reproductive axis in men includes the extrahypothalamic central nervous system, the hypothalamus, the pituitary gland, and the testes. Before 1962, indirect evidence led to the development of the physiological concept of a closed-loop feedback system that embodied the following elements: (1) the hypothalamus stimulates the pituitary to secrete gonadotropins; (2) LH and FSH regulate the testicular production of gonadal steroids and spermatozoa; and (3) the gonadal hormones in turn inhibit the secretion of LH and FSH (for review, see Paulsen 1974). Experimental work in the past decade has focused on obtaining direct evidence to clarify the complex interactions responsible for these events and to define the hormones and the sites of control of the reproductive axis. The hypothalamus is the integrative center of the reproductive axis. At this level both neural messages from the central nervous system and at least part of the humoral messages from the testes act to modulate the secretion of hypothalamic gonadotropin-releasing hormone and thereby gonadotropin secretion. The concept that hypothalamic releasing hormones capable of modulating pituitary function are released from the hypothalamus into the capillaries of the median eminence and are delivered via this portal system to the pituitary gland was formulated by Green and Harris in 1947. The experimental work leading to the isolation and synthesis of these substances, including gonadotropin-releasing hormone (GnRH) or luteinizing-hormone-releasing factor (LRF), was conducted primarily in the laboratories of Schally and his associates (1971).

The early work on the hypothalamic-pituitary-gonadal relationships and on the gonadopituitary feedback mechanisms was seriously hampered by lack of sufficiently sensitive techniques for the measurement of gonadotropins in the blood. Most of the experimental studies had to be based on information obtained from the measurement of gonadotropins by bioassay in either animal pituitary glands or human urine. The bioassays are relatively difficult to carry out, require a large number of animals, and, as mentioned above, are quite insensitive. In spite of the recent development of more sensitive techniques (radioimmunoassays), the bioassays remain an important tool in the endocrine laboratory for the verification of radioimmunoassay systems and for determining the biological activity of an immunologically identifiable hormone. The sensitivity, specificity, and time requirements of various gonadotropin bioassay systems have been reviewed by Swerdloff and Odell (1968a). It is worth recalling that as late as 1962, investigators debated about whether there were separate gonadotropin hormones or multiple biological effects of a single hormone (Paulsen 1974).

An extremely important methodological advance in hormone measurement occurred in 1960 when Yalow and Berson described the technique for radioimmunoassay of plasma insulin. With this report endocrinology entered a new era in which hormones could be measured easily in small amounts of blood. This technique was soon adapted for the measurement of other hormones, including gonadotropins. In 1962 Wide described a hemagglutination immunoassay for hLH based on the cross-reaction of hLH with antibodies directed against hCG. In 1964 Paul and Odell described a radioimmunoassay for hCG. By 1965–1966 purified preparations of hLH suitable for iodination had become available, and a number of investigators described radioimmunoassays for hLH (Rizkallah et al.

1965; Bagshawe et al. 1966; Midgley 1966; Odell et al. 1966).

In 1966–1967, radioimmunoassays for hFSH were developed (Faiman and Ryan 1967; Rocca and Albert 1967). Radioimmunoassays for rat LH and FSH soon followed (Monroe et al. 1968; Niswender et al. 1968), as did LH and FSH assay systems for many other species. These techniques allowed LH and FSH to be measured in small amounts of serum and launched physiological studies in humans and experimental animals.

The role of gonadal steroids in controlling the release of gonadotropins has been recognized since the important parabiotic studies of Moore and Price in 1932 demonstrated an inhibitory effect of estrogens on pituitary gonadotropins. Greep and Jones (1950) then showed a similar effect of testosterone on pituitary LH in castrated male rats, and later Greep (1961) proposed that androgens also have an inhibitory effect on gonadotropin secretion.

The nature of feedback control of pituitary FSH production remained an enigma for decades. The problem was investigated by evaluating the effect of castration and subsequent administration of gonadal hormones on pituitary gonadotropins. Unfortunately the reports on the effect of castration were conflicting, suggesting either an increase, no change, or a decrease in pituitary levels of FSH (Hellbaum and Greep 1943; Paesi et al. 1955; Bogdanove et al. 1964; Hafiez et al. 1972). This mystery was clarified in 1966 when Steinberger and Duckett demonstrated that following castration the pituitary FSH content initially drops below normal, subsequently returns to normal, and ultimately reaches elevated levels.

Gonadotropin Secretion by the Pituitary Gland

Plasma levels of gonadotropins Soon after the development of adequate radioimmunoassay techniques for hLH and hFSH, levels of these hormones in normal men were reported by a number of investigators (Odell et al. 1966; Schlaff et al. 1968; Odell et al. 1968; Ryan and Faiman 1968). Some reports suggested the presence of a diurnal (circadian) rhythm while others failed to confirm this finding (Faiman and Winter 1971; Boyar et al. 1972a; Swerdloff et al. 1972a; Saxena et al. 1972). One of the reasons for this confusion may have been the failure to recognize that both LH and FSH are secreted in pulses (Nankin and Troen 1971; Boyar et al. 1972a; Boon et al. 1972; Rubin et al. 1972; Krieger et al. 1972; Naftolin et al. 1972a; Santen and Bardin 1973; Alford et al. 1973; Smith et al. 1974). Multiple frequent sampling (Nankin and Troen 1971, 1972; Boyar et al. 1972a; Boon et al. 1972; Rubin et al. 1972; Krieger et al. 1972; Naftolin et al. 1972a, 1973;

Alford et al. 1973; Santen and Bardin 1973; Leymarie et al. 1974) and particularly sampling every two minutes for eight hours (Smith et al. 1974) clearly established the pulsatile nature of pituitary and gonadal hormone secretion. It remains unclear how the classic concept of a gonadopituitary feedback mechanism accords with the observations on the oscillatory behavior of plasma levels of both pituitary and gonadal hormones. Although some investigators have demonstrated a relationship between the secretory patterns of gonadotropins and the hormone responses of the gonad, the correlations are weak and do not indicate a one-to-one relationship (Naftolin et al. 1973). Perhaps synergistic effects of pituitary hormones are important in stimulation of secretion of gonadal steroids (Johnson and Ewing 1971; Hafiez et al. 1972; Odell et al. 1973). Alternatively, the poor correlation between the testosterone and LH spikes could indicate that the moment-to-moment pulsatory gonadotropin secretion is independent of gonadal feedback. Further studies will be essential to provide greater insight into the exact relationship between pulsatile patterns of gonadotropin and gonadal steroid secretion.

Although the understanding of the pulsatile character of the hormone levels is incomplete, these findings have had an important impact on clinical studies and investigative work. Santen and Bardin (1973) demonstrated that fluctuations in serum levels are so great that a single measurement of LH in a normal man has confidence limits of ±50 percent. FSH variations apparently are of lesser magnitude. These authors recommended measurement of LH over a three hour period either by multiple sampling or by continuous integrated collection, thereby reducing the confidence limits to ±18 percent. Similarly, studies on techniques for best sampling of testosterone levels revealed that three samples obtained within a one hour period provide for adequate reduction of the error of estimate due to the oscillating nature of plasma testosterone levels (Goldzieher et al., 1976).

Metabolic clearance rates of gonadotropins The availability of purified LH and FSH for administration to humans and the development of sensitive hormonal measurement systems have allowed us to determine the metabolic clearance rates and production rates of LH in men (Kohler et al. 1968; Marshall et al. 1973) and of LH and FSH in women (Cable et al. 1969). These studies indicate that the gonadal status of the subject does not influence the disappearance rate of LH or FSH. Metabolic clearance rates of FSH in women are less than those of LH, with the half-life of LH approximately half that of FSH. Metabolic clearance rates of FSH in men have not been determined. These studies demonstrate that a large portion of the pituitary content of gonadotropins is turned over each day and indicate that gonadotropin synthesis by the pituitary is an active process.

Regulation of gonadotropin secretion: LH production
Despite the considerable body of knowledge accumulated prior to the 1960s, a great deal of confusion existed concerning the specific role of testicular hormones in regulating LH production, particularly regarding the quantitative nature of these interrelationships and the site of the inhibitory activity within the hypothalamic-pituitary complex. Studies using the pituitary content of LH and FSH as an indicator of secretory state were difficult to interpret. In 1959 Gans reported that testosterone administration caused reduction of plasma LH levels in castrated male rats. Subsequently Ramirez and McCann demonstrated an increase in serum LH levels following castration of rats (1963a) and prevention of this rise by administration of testosterone (1963b; 1965). These results were promptly confirmed (Parlow 1964). Following the development of radioimmunoassay techniques, dose-response relationships were established in experimental animals, and these showed a fall in serum LH with increasing levels of testosterone (Gay and Dever 1971; Swerdloff et al. 1972a; Swerdloff and Walsh 1973). It became apparent that the duration of the castrated state influenced the responsiveness of the hypothalamic-pituitary axis to the inhibitory action of testosterone (Gay and Dever 1971; Swerdloff and Walsh 1973) and that androgenic activity of steroid compounds correlated well with their ability to inhibit gonadotropins (Swerdloff et al. 1973).

By the mid-1960s androgen administration was demonstrated to suppress LH levels in eugonadal men (Swerdloff and Odell 1968b; Franchimont 1968; Alder et al. 1968; Peterson et al. 1968). Estradiol had also been shown to be more potent than testosterone in inhibiting LH secretion in both men and experimental animals (Swerdloff and Odell 1968b; Gay and Dever 1971; Swerdloff and Walsh 1973; Walsh et al. 1973a). Since estradiol was known to circulate in eugonadal men, the possibility existed that estradiol was the primary inhibitor of LH secretion. Naftolin et al. (1972b) had actually proposed that all effects of testosterone on the central nervous system might be due to brain tissue aromatization of testosterone to estrogens, but a number of studies were promptly performed which demonstrated that androgens that cannot be metabolized to estrogens (because of their biochemical structure) will inhibit gonadotropin secretion in both man and lower animals (Naftolin and Feder 1973; Swerdloff et al. 1972b; Stewart-Bentley et al. 1974).

These studies were conducted with pharmacological doses of steroids and were followed by attempts to infuse steroids in amounts that would come close to simulating physiological concentrations of the hormones in blood (Stewart-Bentley et al. 1974; Sherins and Loriaux 1973). They demonstrated suppression of serum LH levels by physiological levels of both testosterone and estradiol. Thus at the present time the roles of testosterone and estradiol in LH inhibition remain unclear. While it is possible that synergistic effects of the two hormones are responsible for physiological control of LH, data from experimental animals fail to show such synergism (Gay and Dever 1971; Swerdloff and Walsh 1973). It is of interest that patients with congenital and organ resistance to testosterone and elevated serum estradiol levels (testicular feminization) have high blood LH concentrations (Judd et al. 1972).

Regulation of gonadotropin secretion: FSH production
Castration of both men and experimental animals ultimately results in elevated serum FSH levels (Gay and Dever 1971; Odell and Swerdloff 1968; Swerdloff et al. 1971; Walsh et al. 1973b), thus confirming the important role of the testes in feedback control of FSH secretion. At one time, most investigators believed that this inhibitory activity of the testes on FSH secretion was the result of gonadal hormones feeding back on the hypothalamus and pituitary. An alternate hypothesis, the "utilization theory," held that the testes normally metabolize gonadotropins, thereby preventing their excretion in the urine in a biologically active form; thus in the absence of the testes the urinary concentration of gonadotropins rises (Heller and Nelson 1948; Howard et al. 1950; Paulsen 1974). This concept gradually fell into disrepute and was finally refuted by the observation that the metabolic clearance rate for LH was not changed significantly by castration.

Throughout this period investigators continued their attempt to discover which testicular hormones controlled FSH secretion. After some initial uncertainty (Swerdloff and Odell 1968b; Franchimont 1968; Peterson et al. 1968), it became apparent that administration of pharmacological amounts of testosterone will suppress FSH as well as LH secretion (Steinberger and Duckett 1968; Swerdloff et al. 1972b; Walsh et al. 1973b). A number of other steroids including estradiol have similar effects. Estradiol is known to be secreted by the testes, and estradiol receptors have been identified in the hypothalamus and pituitary (Reichlin 1974). Studies in experimental animals have failed to demonstrate, however, that estradiol administration produces preferential FSH-inhibiting activities (Gay and Dever 1971; Swerdloff and Walsh 1973). Attempts have been made to determine the effect of physiological amounts of testosterone and estradiol on LH and FSH in man (Stewart-Bentley et al. 1974). One study suggests that physiological amounts of testosterone and estradiol suppress LH but not FSH; in another study using higher doses of the steroids, suppres-

sion of both LH and FSH was observed (Sherins and Loriaux 1973).

There is considerable evidence that a seminiferous tubule factor may also be important in the feedback regulation of FSH. This concept dates back to the work of McCullagh and Walsh (1935), who suggested that a substance originating in the germinal epithelium inhibits pituitary FSH production. They named this substance *inhibin*. The suggestion was based to a great extent on the observations that serum FSH is elevated in conditions where the germinal epithelium is selectively injured, but both serum and urinary LH and testosterone are normal. Circumstances supporting this group of findings include testes irradiation (Paulsen 1968); antispermatogenic agents (Van Thiel et al. 1972); early cryptorchidism in rats (Steinberger and Duckett 1966; Swerdloff et al. 1971; Steinberger and Chowdhury 1974); some patients with severe oligospermia or azoospermia (Rosen and Weintraub 1971; deKretser et al. 1972; Leonard et al. 1972); and patients with the "Sertoli cell only" syndrome (Ryan et al. 1970). Howard et al. (1950) suggested that inhibin is secreted by the Sertoli cells, and Johnsen (1964) proposed that it is a lipid substance found in the residual bodies of spermatogenic tissue. Two recent reports have indicated that a peptide substance with selective FSH-inhibiting activity has been isolated from both the semen and testes of experimental animals (Franchimont and Chari 1974; Baker et al. 1976). These findings are of considerable practical importance, since a selective FSH inhibitor might be considered as a potential male contraceptive.

Age and the Pituitary-Gonadal Axis
Aging It has been known for many years that gonadotropin levels are elevated in postmenopausal women. Similarly, increased plasma LH levels were found in aged men (Schalch et al. 1968; Evans et al. 1971; Schiavi et al. 1974), though data showing elevation in circulating levels of FSH in elderly males have been inconsistent. Rubens et al. (1974) observed elevations in FSH in males over the age of 65, while Nieschlag et al. (1973) were not able to confirm this finding. A suggestion was made that two populations of elderly men exist, one with increased serum LH and the other with low levels of both hormones. The elevations in serum gonadotropins in elderly men are associated with lower total and free levels of serum testosterone (Vermeulen et al. 1972; Rubens et al. 1974), suggesting a primary testicular abnormality. This conclusion is supported by the finding of impaired testosterone response to hCG stimulation in elderly men (Ryan and Faiman 1968; Vermeulen et al. 1972; Longcope 1973; Stearns et al. 1973; Nieschlag et al. 1973; Rubens et al.

1974). Walsh et al. (1973b) reported a correlation between serum FSH levels in elderly men and the degree of damage to spermatogenic tubules. This suggests the possibility that the gonadotropin changes are related to a decrease in an inhibiting factor (inhibin) production by the testes with advancing age. The mechanism for these age-related changes is unknown, but the histological changes in the testes of these elderly men show a pattern suggesting alterations in blood supply that might accompany atherosclerosis (Sasano and Ichijo 1969).

Puberty Until the last decade it was generally believed that no gonadotropins were secreted prior to puberty and that puberty was initiated by the onset of LH and FSH secretion. This was proven to be incorrect by the demonstration that LH is present in the serum (Odell et al. 1967) and urine (Rifkind et al. 1967) of prepubertal children. High levels of FSH have been found in the serum of the fetus, the levels decreasing as term approaches (Grumbach and Kaplan 1973). Both plasma LH and FSH are detectable at birth and rise during sexual maturation, FSH increasing to a greater degree than LH in the early stages of puberty. The pulsatile pattern of LH secretion is first detectable at about stage III of puberty, manifested as a sleep-associated rise in gonadotropins that is not present in either the prepubertal child or the adult (Boyar et al. 1972b). The physiological mechanisms that produce increasing mean blood LH and FSH during maturation of children are not completely understood. Several possibilities exist: (1) the hypothalamus develops an increasing capacity to secrete LRH and/or a decreased sensitivity to the inhibitory influences of gonadal steroids on LRH secretion; (2) the pituitary becomes more responsive to the effects of LRH and secretes increasing amounts of gonadotropins; or (3) areas of the central nervous system outside the hypothalamus mediate the changes listed in the first possibility above.

In the prepubertal human, the gonads function as a part of a dynamic feedback system. Thus serum LH and FSH levels are elevated in agonadal children prior to the time that puberty would normally have occurred (Winter and Faiman 1972a), but for unknown reasons levels found in castrated adults are not reached until the individual attains the chronological age associated with normal pubertal development. This may be due to inherent hypothalamic maturation or to changing pituitary sensitivity to secreted GnRH.

Once it had been demonstrated that the gonads exerted an inhibitory influence on the hypothalamic-pituitary axis prior to puberty, the question arose of why the normal immature child with low circulating gonadal steroids did not have high serum gonadotropins. Data presented for experimental animals (Byrnes and Meyer 1951; Ramirez and McCann 1965) and to a limited extent for humans (Kelch et al. 1973) indicate that the immature hypothalamus is more sensitive to the inhibitory effects of gonadal steroids than the mature hypothalamus. One theory of sexual maturation states that the primary initiating event in pubertal development is an increase in the hypothalamic threshold for negative feedback; with increasing age, the "gonadotat" becomes progressively less sensitive to the inhibitory effects of sex steroids, resulting in increasing secretion of LH and FSH. While at the present time this effect on the secretion of LH and FSH is presumed to occur at the hypothalamic level, adequate techniques are not yet available for measuring serum GnRH during sexual maturation.

The role of the pituitary gland in the maturation process has been investigated in both humans and experimental animals. In human studies, synthetic GnRH has been administered in different doses to prepubertal, pubertal, and adult subjects. Roth et al. (1973) have demonstrated that an increasing pituitary response to GnRH might be a factor responsible for sexual maturation in boys. The increment in serum FSH above baseline was not influenced by age, but the increment in LH increased with age. Thus their study and that of Job et al. (1972) showed that prepubertal boys have a higher serum FSH to LH ratio after GnRH administration than does the adult male.

Role of the gonads in the maturation process Until recently the gonad was generally believed to play a rather passive role in sexual maturation, hormonal secretion of the gonad being entirely determined by the amount of gonadotropic hormone to which it was exposed. In the past several years evidence has accumulated indicating that the gonad (at least in the male) also undergoes maturational changes, becoming progressively more sensitive to gonadotropin during the process of pubertal development. The immature in contrast to the adult male rat is not responsive to the effects of administered LH five days after hypophysectomy (Swerdloff et al. 1973; Odell et al. 1974). This suggested that the immature gonad of intact animals might be intrinsically less capable of responding to the stimulatory effects of pituitary hormones.

In subsequent studies in intact male animals, the same investigators demonstrated that immature animals secrete much less testosterone after a bolus dose of LH than do adults. With increasing age, this response to LH gradually increased to adult levels (Odell et al. 1974). The mechanism of increasing testis response to LH with age was unclear, but the observation that FSH administration tends to normalize the response to LH in hypophysectomized immature rats (Odell et al. 1974) suggested that exposure of the normal immature male to FSH might result in increasing testosterone levels. More recent studies have demonstrated that treatment of immature intact male rats with FSH will result in increased serum testosterone levels (reflected by increased ventral prostate weight) and will significantly augment the testosterone secretion in response to exogenous LH (Swerdloff et al. 1972a; Odell et al. 1974). Data in the human appear to support this concept of gonadal maturation. Diminished responsiveness of the prepubertal testis to hCG has been demonstrated (Saez and Bertrand 1968; Frasier et al. 1969; Winter and Faiman 1972b) with the magnitude of testosterone responses in boys increasing with age (Winter and Faiman 1972b). While Winter and Faiman (1972b) found the testosterone response to hCG correlated with both basal LH and FSH levels, Sizonenko et al. (1973) reported that the magnitude of response to hCG correlated best with basal serum FSH concentration.

The observation that serum FSH rises in boys earlier in puberty than serum LH and that elevations of both gonadotropins precede the steep increase in serum testosterone suggests a possible etiological relationship of these events. The marked progress that has been made in the past fifteen years toward understanding the physiological events leading to sexual maturation is reflected in the studies described above. This information is of critical importance in dealing with the clinical problems of precocious and delayed puberty.

Influence of Nonreproductive Factors on Gonadotropin Secretion

It is well known that factors outside the classical hypothalamic-pituitary-end organ system may influence the secretion of other pituitary hormones; however, physical exercise, changes in blood sugar, infusions of arginine, and injection of vasopressin have been shown to have little or no effect on serum LH and FSH levels (Swerdloff and Odell 1968a; Guevara et al. 1970).

Studies in experimental animals indicate that the sensory systems such as olfaction and light perception have important roles as modifiers of reproductive and nonreproductive function in female rodents; for example, odors from an animal of the opposite sex have important effects on the cyclicity and sexual behavior of more primitive species than humans. The role of such pheromones in the human is unclear.

Light has long been known to influence the reproductive function of female animals of many species (Fiske 1941; Everett et al. 1949). Blind girls have early menarche (Zacharias and Wurtman 1964), while constant light results in precocious puberty in female rats. Similar studies have not been done in blind boys, but blind men do not appear to have abnormal night-day patterns of blood LH, FSH, or gonadal steroid levels (Bodenheimer et al. 1973). Additional study is warranted on the influence of light and smell on reproductive functions of both sexes.

Evidence that higher cortical function may influence the reproductive axis includes the frequent occurrence of menstrual abnormalities in emotionally stressed women and the demonstration of depressed serum testosterone levels in mentally stressed men (Kreuz et al. 1972).

Nutritional factors influence reproductive function in both males and females. In immature male rats and bulls, caloric restriction has been shown to delay testicular growth, spermatogenesis, and seminal vesicle growth (Davies et al. 1957; Leathem 1961). Undernourished adult animals also demonstrate atrophy of the testes, seminal vesicles, and prostate (Mason 1933; Mulinos and Pomerantz 1941; Pazos and Huggins 1945; Reid 1949). Similar abnormalities can be seen in protein deficiency (Leathem 1961; Guilbert and Goss 1932; Leathem 1954; Aschkenasy 1954; Leathem and DeFeo 1952; Svajgr et al. 1972). Human data have indicated that adequate protein and calorie intake is required for normal reproductive function in women. Amenorrhea is common in victims of concentration camps and in underdeveloped countries (Klebanow 1949; Keys 1950; Zubirán and Gómez-Mont 1953; Holmberg and Nylander 1971). Impaired reproductive function also appears to occur in undernourished men (Mont 1964; McLaren 1969). The pathogenesis of these abnormalities of reproductive function in situations of altered nutrition is unclear, although many people believe that the alterations occur at the hypothalamic-pituitary level rather than at the periphery. Not all the data support this contention, however. Studies in undernourished experimental animals have demonstrated either increased, decreased, or unchanged pituitary content of gonadotropins (Marrian and Parkes 1929; Mason and Wolfe 1930; Werner 1939; Pomerantz and Mulinos 1939; Maddock and Heller 1947; Meites and Reed 1949; Rinaldini 1949; Vanderlinde and Westerfeld 1950; Blivaiss et al. 1954; Perloff et al. 1954). Urinary gonadotropin levels in humans have been found to be decreased in starvation (Bliss and Migeon 1957; Mont 1964; Daughaday 1968; Ney 1969; McLaren 1969; Suryanarayana et al. 1969). A study by Root and Russ (1972) reported a blunted rise in serum and pituitary gonadotropins in starved male rats. Most older studies indicated normal testicular responsiveness to exogenous gonadotropins in undernourished animals (Mulinos and Pomerantz 1941; Maddock and Heller 1947; Rinaldini 1949). In contrast, recent reports have suggested that undernourished men have a primary testicular defect with low serum testosterone and increased serum LH levels.

Recent studies by Wurtman and Fernstrom (1974)

have demonstrated that tryptophan-deficient diets lower brain neurotransmitter concentrations. Administration of norepinephrine, epinephrine, and dopamine (all neurotransmitters) has been shown to affect LRH, LH, and FSH secretion. Nutrition and its influence on hormonal function deserve further investigation.

26.2 Testicular Steroids

Androgen Synthesis

Historical introduction The rapid acquisition of knowledge during the past fifteen years has been based on a number of fundamental discoveries made in the distant past. Probably the first observation pointing toward the concept of a humoral messenger system related to testicular function dates back to antiquity in Annon's description of somatic changes in castrated men. Berthold's observation (1849) that postcastration cockscomb atrophy can be prevented by testicular implants provided the first experimental evidence that testes may produce a substance that is capable of influencing other tissues. The description of the Leydig cells (Leydig 1857) and the discovery of lipids in the Leydig cells (Loisel 1903) suggested that this substance is produced by a specific cell type in the testis and that it may be lipid in nature. Preparation of an androgenically potent lipid extract from bull testes (McGee 1927) placed androgens in the class of lipids. The isolation of the first androgen, androsterone, from human urine (Butenandt 1932) and crystalline testosterone from bull testes (David et al. 1935) settled the question of the testicular site of androgen production and its exact chemical structure. The demonstration of the in vitro synthesis of testosterone from cholesterol (Butenandt and Hanisch 1935) pointed toward the identity of the major chemical precursor of androgens. In summary, these investigations established the endocrine function of the testis and demonstrated that C19 steroids, particularly testosterone, are biologically potent androgens.

Studies of androgen biogenesis and its control were heralded by the in vitro demonstration that testicular tissue incorporates acetate into steroids (Srere et al. 1950) and that it can utilize acetate for testosterone synthesis (Brady 1951). Subsequently, human testes were demonstrated to synthesize testosterone from acetate and to secrete the de novo formed testosterone into the testicular venous system (Savard et al. 1952; Lucas et al. 1957).

The 1960s were marked by the elucidation of androgen biogenetic pathways and the hormonal control of androgen synthesis. By the late 1960s and early 1970s, the molecular mechanisms underlying gonadotropic hormone action in the testes became the major topics of investigation.

Biogenesis of cholesterol David et al. (1935) suggested that testosterone was probably the major androgen produced by mammalian testes. Comparative studies conducted in various mammalian species, including man, confirmed this suggestion and revealed many species similarities in the androgen biogenetic process and in the identity of its major end products.

These studies also demonstrated the pivotal role of cholesterol as the precursor of androgens and posed the question whether the testis is capable of utilizing extragonadally formed cholesterol or whether it must rely totally on de novo synthesis of the cholesterol in the testis. The available evidence points to the capacity for de novo cholesterol synthesis in most steroid-forming tissues, including the testis (Morris and Chaikoff 1959; Gerson et al. 1964). The capacity for the utilization of extragonadally formed cholesterol has also been demonstrated in a number of mammalian species, however.

In the 1960s the details of pathways leading to the formation of cholesterol were greatly elucidated. The major cholesterol precursor, squalene, was demonstrated to form from acetate, most likely via the mevalonic acid→farnesyl→merolidyl pathway, similar to that found in the microorganisms and in the liver. The details of the conversion of squalene to cholesterol are not entirely clear. Lanosterol is most likely a pivotal intermediate. Whether it is converted to cholesterol via the Δ^8-cholesterol, Δ^7-dihydrocholesterol pathway or via a zymosterol→desmosterol pathway remains to be established. For reviews, see Danielsson and Tchen (1968) and Eik-Nes (1970).

Conversion of cholesterol to pregnenolone The process of conversion of cholesterol to pregnenolone has received considerable attention, particularly since it may play an important role as the rate-limiting step in androgen biogenesis (Forchielli et al. 1969). Similar to studies concerned with cholesterol biosynthesis, extensive investigations have been conducted on the conversion of cholesterol to pregnenolone in tissues other than the testis. The fundamental steps observed in other tissues have been demonstrated to occur also in the testis. Staple et al. (1956) suggested that the key step in this transformation involved the splitting of the carbon-carbon bond of the cholesterol side chain with the release of a 6-carbon fragment (isocaproic acid).

The conversion of cholesterol to pregnenolone takes place in mitochondria and requires both TPNH and oxygen (Halkerston et al. 1961). The first step in this transformation probably involves the formation of 20α cholesterol. Some investigators consider this to be the rate-limiting step (Hall 1970). Others, however, suggest that hydroxylation at C22 precedes the 20α hydroxylation (Shimizu et al. 1962). Formation of a $20\alpha,20R$-dihydrocholesterol intermediate has been established firmly (Shimizu et al. 1962). The cleavage of the (20–22) bond in this dihydroxy intermediate most likely does not require oxygen.

The biochemical details of the cleavage process still are not clearly understood. It appears that the 6-carbon chain cleaved from cholesterol is isocapralaldehyde, which subsequently is oxidized to isocaproic acid (Satoh et al. 1966). For detailed reviews of this topic see Forchielli et al. (1969) and Hall (1970).

Formation of androgens from pregnenolone The pathways leading to the formation of androgens from pregnenolone have been the topic of numerous studies in several mammalian species. The most commonly utilized has been the rat; however, a considerable body of literature has also accumulated dealing with steroid metabolism in the testes of rabbits, dogs, monkeys, and men.

The transformation of pregnenolone to testosterone can occur via precursors with a double bond either in the C5 (Δ^5 pathway) or the C4 (Δ^4 pathway) positions. The *preferred* pathway has not been entirely clarified, and there is some evidence that in different species, different pathways may be preferred. While the mechanisms or reasons for the selection of one pathway over another are entirely unknown, depending upon whether pregnenolone is acted upon first by the Δ^5-3β-hydroxy steroid dehydrogenase and isomerase or by 17α-hydroxylase, the formation of either progesterone or 17α hydroxypregnenolone results. Thus either the Δ^4 or the Δ^5 pathway will prevail.

Kinetic studies suggest that in the rat, guinea pig, and other rodents, the Δ^4 pathway (pregnenolone →progesterone →17α-hydroxyprogesterone→androstenedione →testosterone) is preferred, while in other species, such as the canine and possibly the human, the Δ^5 pathway (pregnenolone →17α-hydroxypregnenolone→dehydroepiandrosterone→Δ^5-androstene-3β,17β-diol) is preferred.

The physiological significance of the selection between the two pathways remains to be determined. Theoretically, at any point in the Δ^5 pathway the precursor can enter the Δ^4 pathway. The Δ^5-3β-hydroxysteroid dehydrogenase and the Δ^5–Δ^4 isomerase may not be substrate-specific. The same enzyme may therefore be capable of converting any of the intermediates in the Δ^5 pathway to the respective intermediate of the Δ^4 pathway.

The crucial step in the biogenetic process leading to the formation of androgens is the cleavage of the two carbon side chains of 17α hydroxyprogesterone or 17α hydroxypregnenolone. This is an irreversible reaction leading directly to the formation of "weak" androgens (androstenedione and DHEA, respectively). The conversion of androstenedione to testosterone is ac-

complished by an oxidoreductase and is a reversible reaction. Under normal physiological conditions this reaction is driven toward the C17 reduced product, testosterone. Although testosterone is apparently converted at the site of its action in the target organ, tissue, or cell to a 5α-reduced androgen, the evidence strongly suggests that the androgen-secreting cells produce and secrete principally testosterone as the major circulating androgen.

Enzymes involved in steroidogenesis Steroid enzymology has trailed behind many other areas of enzymology (e.g., that concerned with energy metabolism); however, the enzymatic activities necessary for the major conversion steps in the steroid biogenetic pathways have been investigated to a certain extent.

Most studies concerned with the conversion of cholesterol to pregnenolone were done initially on adrenal gland tissue rather than on the testis, but it was subsequently demonstrated that similar reactions occurred in testicular tissue. This series of conversions is accomplished primarily by the action of three enzymes: cholesterol-20α-hydroxylase, cholesterol-22R-hydroxylase, and cholesterol-C20-C22-lyase. The two-step hydroxylation that must precede the cholesterol side-chain cleavage appears to require both reduced TPN$^+$ and molecular oxygen. The details of these reactions are not entirely clear. Since TPNH and molecular oxygen are characteristic requirements for hydroxylation reactions of steroids, however, side-chain cleavage probably involves at least one hydroxylation.

TPNH is assumed to donate electrons to a transport system in which cytochrome P-450 activates oxygen. Numerous studies suggest that the side-chain cleavage involves "mixed function" (Mason 1957) oxidation, in which one atom of oxygen is retained by the steroid while the other is reduced to water. The question of the supply of the reducing equivalents (NADPH) for side-chain cleavage has not been clarified. Hall (1970) suggests that "side-chain cleavage has its own pool of reduced TPN$^+$, generated via reversed electron transport at the expense of high-energy compounds synthesized in conjunction with the oxidation of succinate." (See two excellent reviews dealing with this question: Forchielli et al. 1969; Hall 1970.)

The formation of progesterone from pregnenolone requires the action of two enzymes: Δ^5–Δ^4 isomerase and Δ^5-3β-hydroxysteroid dehydrogenase. The reaction requires the presence of NAD and NADH. Hydroxylation of progesterone is accomplished by 17α-hydroxylase, and the reaction requires NADPH as cofactor and molecular oxygen. The C17-C20-lyase accomplishes the side-chain cleavage of 17α-hydroxyprogesterone and has the same oxygen and cofactor requirements as the hydroxylation reaction. The C19 steroid formed, androstenedione, is a weak androgen and serves as the immediate precursor to testosterone. The conversion of androstenedione to testosterone is accomplished by 17α-hydroxysteroid dehydrogenase in the presence of NADPH. This enzyme probably is not substrate-specific, and it may also reduce DHEA to androstenediol.

The requirements for molecular oxygen for steroid hydroxylation have been reevaluated and confirmed in a series of elegant experiments utilizing double-isotope-tracer techniques in which the stable isotope of oxygen (^{18}O) was employed as the tracer for molecular oxygen and mass spectrometry was used for analysis of the products (Tamaoki et al. 1969).

Cellular localization of androgen synthesis and secretion in the testes The Leydig cells were believed to be the site of androgen production in the testis as early as the turn of the twentieth century. This belief has been supported by evidence gained from physiomorphological and cytochemical studies. Direct evidence did not arise, however, until the demonstration of in vitro androgen biogenesis in Leydig cells separated mechanically from the seminiferous tubules (Christensen and Mason 1965) and in Leydig cell cultures used to demonstrate steroid conversions (Steinberger et al. 1967). While these studies established the Leydig cell as the site of androgen production in the testis, they did not eliminate the possibility of androgen synthesis in cells associated with the seminiferous tubules (Lacy and Pettitt 1970). Evidence has surfaced that the seminiferous tubules are most likely not involved in the de novo androgen synthesis, but they may be active in the metabolism of androgens and possibly of other steroids.

The relationship of various intracellular organelles to the androgen biogenetic pathway has been investigated extensively (for review, see Christensen and Gillim 1969). Electron-microscopic and cell fractionation studies of the steroid-producing cells, coupled with examination of steroid-biogenetic potential of the various subcellular organelles, provided a considerable amount of anatomical information concerning the subcellular sites of androgen synthesis. Using this information, deductions were made concerning the route of the intermediates through the various organelles during the steroidogenic process.

Cholesterol, either synthesized in the smooth endoplasmic reticulum or derived from extracellular pools, is thought to be brought into the mitochondria, where the side-chain cleavage takes place and pregnenolone is formed. Pregnenolone is translocated to the smooth endoplasmic reticulum, where the enzymes involved in its conversion to testosterone are localized. Testosterone, formed in the smooth endoplasmic reticulum, is transferred to the cytoplasm and secreted by the cell.

Mechanisms involved in the intracellular transport of the intermediates and secretion of the steroids remain essentially unexplored. Studies of mitochondrial enzymes of the adrenal cortical cells suggest that the hydroxylating enzymes are most likely located in the inner membrane of the mitochondria (Yago and Ichii 1969; Dodge et al. 1970). Samuels et al. (1974) have attempted to investigate the details of secretion mechanisms and patterns of migration of androgen precursors from cytosol to the microsomes. Their study suggests that pregnenolone is specifically concentrated on and bound to the outer surface of the microsomes. There it is converted to progesterone, which interacts with the cytochrome P-450 complex within the membrane matrix. The cytochrome catalyzes the "mixed function" oxidase reactions, forming androstenedione. This C19 steroid diffuses toward cytosol and is partly reduced at 17α position to testosterone at the outer surface of the microsome.

This fascinating study suggests that the capacity for specific differential binding of androgen precursors to intracellular membranes may be the basic mechanism responsible for the intracellular flow of precursors. The possibility that the trophic hormones may influence the specific binding by the membranes should be seriously considered.

Differentiation of steroid biosynthetic pathways in developing testes Physiological studies suggested that fetal testes must be producing an androgen (Price and Pannabecker 1956). In vitro studies of incubates of fetal testicular tissue demonstrated the capacity of the tissue to convert suitable precursors to testosterone (Noumura et al. 1966). This has been demonstrated to occur in a number of mammalian species (Lipsett and Tullner 1965; Bloch 1967), including man (Acevedo et al. 1961; Bloch 1964; Serra et al. 1970).

The application of sensitive radioimmunoassay techniques permitted measurement of endogenous testosterone levels to confirm the physiological and the in vitro observations regarding the capacity of fetal testicular tissue to produce testosterone. During the perinatal period rat testicular tissue converts appropriate precursors to testosterone in vitro at rates similar to or higher than the mature testis (Steinberger and Ficher 1968) and shows an extremely high endogenous concentration of testosterone (Tcholakian 1974). As the animal develops, the capacity of testicular tissue for in vitro testosterone production diminishes. Instead, the tissue acquires the capacity to form considerable amounts of 5α-androstanediol and androsterone. The peak of this activity occurs between postnatal days 20 and 25 and coincides with the nadir in the capacity to produce testosterone. With further development of the testis, the biosynthetic pattern gradually reverses, and the capacity to form in vitro testosterone, rather than 5α-reduced androgens, becomes more prominent

(Steinberger and Ficher 1968; Ficher and Steinberger 1968; Steinberger and Ficher 1969). The mechanisms controlling this pattern of differentiation of the steroid biogenetic pathways in the developing testis are unknown. Some evidence suggests that gonadotropins are most likely not involved in this process (Steinberger and Ficher 1969).

Recent studies (Rivarola et al. 1972; Lloret and Weisz 1974) suggest that the seminiferous tubules are capable of reducing testosterone to 5α-androstanediol, particularly during the fourth week after birth; these studies indicate that changes in the biogenetic pattern may involve the participation of the seminiferous tubules in the 5α-reduction process. This possibility is interesting because it may be related to the role of androgens in the initiation of spermatogenesis (see below). Additional information is required, however, before this possibility can be considered seriously. It should be noted that morphological and cytochemical studies of developing Leydig cells in the past led a number of investigators to the hypothesis that the developing Leydig cells may be undergoing changes reflected by changes in their androgen biogenetic capacity (Roosen-Runge and Anderson 1959).

Intratesticular testosterone The extragonadal role of testosterone was the first to be recognized because removal of the source of testosterone production, the testes, resulted in morphologically, physiologically, and psychologically discernible extragonadal changes associated with the drastically diminished circulating testosterone levels. The possibility of an intratesticular role for testosterone in the growth of seminiferous tubules and in the process of spermatogenesis was not raised until later, and not until the past few years has this question been clarified. The problem in demonstrating the effect of testosterone on the testes arose from the inability of testosterone replacement therapy to affect spermatogenesis at a dose that stimulates growth of sex accessories beyond normal. To produce an effect on seminiferous tubules, testosterone had to be administered at doses resulting in pharmacological circulating levels. Recent investigations have revealed that testosterone concentration in human testicular tissue is many times greater than its concentration in blood (E. Steinberger et al. 1974b). This creates a steep testes-blood gradient. It had been suggested that testes do not store testosterone, as the pituitary stores gonadotropins. This suggestion was confirmed in studies where testosterone synthesis was blocked in vivo, and it was demonstrated that both plasma and testicular concentrations of testosterone declined to very low levels within three to six hours (Tcholakian et al. 1974). The data do not prove, however, that there is no short-term storage of testosterone in the testes and that there is no mechanism concerned with its release. The stor-

age may be accomplished by binding the steroid to an androgen-binding protein (Hansson et al. 1973a; Steinberger et al. 1974a) or by other not yet explored mechanisms. The possiblity of an important physiological role of this mechanism in the action of testosterone on spermatogenesis should not be neglected.

Androgen Secretion by the Testes
Historical introduction Until the early 1960s the study of gonadal function in vivo depended upon crude bioassay techniques for gonadotropins; the only sex steroids measurable were the ketosteroids in urine, which were thought to originate primarily from the gonads; however, castration was known to only partially lower ketosteroids. One of the major advances during this period was the demonstration that the ketosteroids were derived from both adrenal and gonadal C19 steroids, which were interconvertible in the body (Vande Wiele et al. 1963; Tait 1963).

The modern studies on the origins and metabolism of ketosteroids by the Columbia University group soon led to a burst of interest in measuring testosterone, which was known to be synthesized by testicular tissue and to be a very potent androgen. The introduction of chromatographic techniques with isotopic tracer steroids and classical colorimetric tests led quickly in the early 1960s to reports of testosterone in testicular vein blood (West et al. 1952), urine (Camacho and Migeon 1963; Horton et al. 1963), and finally peripheral blood (Finkelstein et al. 1961; Riondel et al. 1963). Other potential androgens such as dehydroisoandrosterone and androstenedione were also quantitated in human peripheral blood.

Development of modern techniques The decade 1963 to 1973 witnessed an amazing revolution and sophistication in hormone methodology. The ability to measure steroids, particularly the sex steroids, progressed from the classical approaches of organic chemistry (colorimetric and gravimetric), useful for substances in the milligram and microgram range, to highly specific and sensitive assays useful in the nanogram and picogram range. In this short time a number of techniques were developed and declined as more satisfactory approaches were introduced.

These techniques include double isotope derivative or dilution assays (Hudson et al. 1963), gas liquid chromatography (Brownie et al. 1964), competitive protein binding (Murphy 1968; Mayes and Nugent 1968), and most recently radioimmunoassay (RIA) (Midgley et al. 1971). With the RIA approach, large molecules such as proteins can be utilized as antigenic carriers to yield antibodies that are useful as reagents to quantitate unknown biological samples. Steroids can also be rendered antigenic by chemical conjugation to proteins or polymers. These approaches use chemically pure reference compounds for comparison with the unknown sample to compete with high-specific-activity labeled tracer in the bound-free relationship that leads to the typical RIA standard curve. The ease of performing RIAs has resulted in the widespread availability of steroid and protein hormone assays in large medical centers and also in commercial reference laboratories, available locally to all practicing physicians. With adequate training in reproduction, the practicing internist, pediatrician, or gynecologist has laboratory endocrine tools found until recently only in a handful of research laboratories.

Steroid secretion by the testes Considerable dynamic understanding is now available about the sex hormone secretions from the testis during the human life span. This interest extends down to function, control, and secretion of the fetal testis since sexual development and critical imprinting of the higher brain and basal structures (hypothalamus) play a key role in male development (Jost 1951). Although the fetal testis is capable of function, only minimal data currently exist on human and subhuman fetal testicular function, although a number of groups are studying subhuman species (Lipsett and Tullner 1965; Siiteri and Wilson 1974). At birth there are measurable levels of male hormones, although controversies rage on differences in levels between the sexes and on the function of these hormones in the neonatal period (Lindner 1961; Noumura et al. 1966). During childhood and adolescence, marked changes that have been related to changes in gonadotropin levels and feedback sensitivity occur in testicular hormonal function (Frasier et al. 1969). In the adult, in addition to wide variations in androgen levels between individuals, there are diurnal variations and short-term episodic secretions of male hormones and even suggestions of longer periods of cyclicity. In lower mammals, the male responds to visual and olfactory stimuli by heightened pituitary secretion of gonadotropin and marked increases in testosterone secretion and mating behavior (Saginor and Horton 1968; Vermeulen et al. 1972). The primate does not demonstrate this dramatic neuroendocrine response, but other more subtle behavioral and neuroendocrine events (Michael 1974) may be uncovered that bear on human personality patterns and reproductive behavior (Pincus 1956; Lunde and Hamburg 1972). In aging men, testosterone levels fall only slightly up to the age of sixty (Ruben and Vermeulen, in press); however, the actual secretion of testosterone declines (Kent and Acone 1966), levels of gonadotropins rise, and recent evidence suggests some resistance of the Leydig cells to gonadotropin stimulation (Ruben and Vermeulen, in press). This suggests that the human male has some analog, although much less dramatic, to the female

menopause. The biochemical and behavioral effects of these changes are unclear.

The human testis also secretes 17α-hydroxyprogesterone, androstenedione, and estradiol-17β (Resko and Eik-Nes 1966; Strott and Lipsett 1968). The first two are weak progestational and androgenic compounds. The last is a potent steroid, the major estrogen of the female. About 10–15 µg per day of estradiol-17β are thought to be secreted by the adult testes; the remainder of blood estradiol is derived from peripheral conversion of testosterone (Korenman et al. 1963; Horton and Tait 1966; Kelch et al. 1972; Baird et al. 1973). Although low in magnitude, levels of estradiol in men are not markedly different from levels observed in prepubertal girls, or in adult women during the follicular phase of the menstrual cycle, and they exceed levels in postmenopausal women (MacDonald et al. 1967; Baird et al. 1968). The physiological role of 17α-hydroxyprogesterone (1–2 mg per day) and estradiol in males is a mystery.

One of the most interesting developments in the last decade has been the demonstration that a number of sex steroids are derived both by direct secretion and by peripheral conversion of precursors (prehormones) secreted from the gonad and/or adrenal cortex. This phenomenon of peripheral conversion accounts for the source of testosterone in the prepubertal male and adult woman (from androstenedione) (Korenman et al. 1963; Horton and Tait 1966; Kelch et al. 1972; Baird et al. 1968; Longcope et al. 1968) and of dihydrotestosterone (Ito and Horton 1971) and androstan-3α,17β-diol (from testosterone) (Kinouchi and Horton 1974) in male blood. In the adult human male, testosterone secretion by the Leydig cell (4–9 mg per day) is many times greater than testicular and adrenal androstenedione (1–2 mg), so that less than 10 percent of blood testosterone is derived from peripheral conversion of precursors. The secretion of prehormones with minimal biological activity and peripheral conversion to potent hormones may represent a higher level of hormone control influenced by peripheral target and non-target tissue. Dihydrotestosterone is now thought to be a peripheral conversion product of testosterone with significant levels in male and female blood. Interconversion studies suggest that androgen target tissues such as prostate may be the source (Eik-Nes 1964, 1970), and thus measurements of dihydrotestosterone in vivo may reflect, at least in part, target tissue events (Kinouchi and Horton 1974).

The study of gonadotropin control of the Leydig cell has indicated the presence of a dynamic feedback between androgens (and estrogen) and the CNS secretion of gonadotropins (Hooker 1948). LH acts almost instantaneously early in the steroid biosynthetic pathway, perhaps via the adenyl cyclase–cAMP system to increase testosterone synthesis and secretion (Hall and Eik-Nes 1962; Dorrington and Fritz 1974). Animal models (in vivo) and perfusion studies (in vitro) form the mainstay of our current knowledge (VanDemark and Ewing 1963; Eik-Nes 1971). The sympathetic nervous system also plays a role in Leydig cell function since β adrenergic stimulation increases testosterone secretion. Since LH appears to be the Leydig cell regulator, hCG probably causes Leydig cell activity during fetal development, and evidence of Leydig cell activity is observed in the fetal testes (Eik-Nes 1971). LH may also play a role in peripheral testosterone action, since recent work suggests that testosterone-to-dihydrotestosterone conversion is enhanced in seminiferous tubules by gonadotropins. The role of other trophic hormones such as FSH and prolactin appears minimal, although the importance of the interaction between LH and FSH for Leydig cell secretion and metabolism remains unclear. Other factors, such as substances in plasma and the prostaglandins, may also play some supporting role (Eik-Nes 1971). This subject requires further elucidation.

The modern clinical approach to gonadal disorders is clearly based upon methodology and concepts of neuroendocrine control that have developed primarily in the period since 1960. Clinical approaches allow classification of disorders at the central (secondary) or gonadal (primary) level (Paulsen et al. 1968). This is now accomplished by comparing blood levels of testosterone with levels of gonadotropins (FSH and LH) using RIA techniques. Currently available probes can be used to define hypothalamic disease (clomiphene—Lipsett et al. 1966; Odell et al. 1967), pituitary disease (response to GnRH—Kastin et al. 1971), or gonadal disease (hCG stimulation). The availability of long-acting preparations of testosterone and parenteral gonadotropin (FSH-like and LH-like) allow substitution therapy and/or treatment of male infertility.

In contrast to disorders of the thyroid and adrenal glands, various social and methodological influences delayed research into gonadal function until the late 1950s, so no distinct biosynthetic disorders of the gonad were known. This has been partially remedied, and disorders of most biosynthetic steps leading to testosterone synthesis by the Leydig cell have now been described in patients. These disorders include problems in enzyme steps of the cholesterol side-chain cleavage (desmolase—Zachmann et al. 1972), 3β-ol dehydrogenase (Zachmann et al. 1970), 17α-hydroxylase (Biglieri et al. 1966; Horton and Frasier 1967), and 17β-hydroxysteroid dehydrogenase (Saez et al. 1971). Although understanding of Leydig cell steroidogenesis in Klinefelter's syndrome, a common disorder, has increased, the pathophysiology and ontogeny of this chromosomal disorder have not been clarified (Paul-

sen et al. 1968). In the rare testicular feminization syndrome, in which testosterone is inactive on target tissues, recent knowledge about peripheral conversion of testosterone to dihydrotestosterone and the importance of cytoplasmic and nuclear receptors provides new insight and new understanding about hormone action (Wilson and Walker 1969; Northcutt et al. 1969; Bardin et al. 1973).

Studies of the metabolism of C19 steroids provided the impetus for many of the developments subsequently made in this field. The availability of ^{3}H- and ^{14}C-labeled steroids stimulated many studies of the metabolic rate and excretion patterns of steroids (Korenman and Lipsett 1964). Early studies indicated that only small amounts of testosterone appeared unchanged in urine (glucuronides and sulfates—Camacho and Migeon 1963; Horton et al. 1963). Most of it, as well as some C19 steroids of adrenal origin, are metabolized to a series of C19 O$_2$ ketosteroids such as androsterone and etiocholanolone, which have minimal androgenicity. Measurements of testosterone glucuronide provided considerable insight into androgen physiology, however (Korenman and Lipsett 1964; Kirschner and Bardin 1972), and determinations of testosterone secretion were possible in the male, but urine testosterone in the female was subsequently shown to be derived from multiple sources, the major one being androstenedione (Korenman et al. 1963; Horton and Tait 1966; Baird et al. 1968; Kelch et al. 1972; Baird et al. 1973). Studies of testosterone production rates in the male, using either blood or urine measurements, yield values of 4–10 mg per day. Disappearance times and studies of metabolic clearance rates following single injections or constant infusion of radioactive steroid indicated that testosterone was cleared principally by the liver and that its clearance rate (1,000 liters per day) was intermediate between that of cortisol and that of aldosterone. This finding was subsequently explained by the discovery of testosterone binding to plasma globulin.

The discovery that testosterone and estradiol are bound to a specific β globulin—TBG or SHBG (Pearlman et al. 1967)— has led to a concept that the unbound (free and albumin-bound) androgen or estrogen is biologically important. The levels of both SHBG and circulating sex steroids bound to it are increased in pregnancy or with oral contraceptive use, whereas the freely diffusible unbound steroid fraction remains unaltered. Because of this relationship, work in this field is tending to focus on measurement of total and free hormone concentrations (Vermeulen et al. 1969).

The sex steroid binding protein has affinity for both testosterone-dihydrotestosterone and estradiol. The importance of interactions between androgens, estrogens, and SHBG in conditions such as gynecomastia is unclear at this time.

Subsequent work has uncovered alterations in production rates and metabolic clearance of androgens and estrogens in hyper- and hypothyroidism (Southren et al. 1968) and enhanced clearance of androgens in hirsutism and virilization states (Bardin and Lipsett 1967). This appears to represent both alterations in free hormone levels and induction of hepatic enzymes by secreted testosterone itself. An area of great research interest involves studies of steroid kinetics in women with disorders of excess androgen production and metabolism. The liver possesses most of the enzymes that metabolize testosterone and estrogen, including Δ^4-reductase, 3α-, 3β-, and 17β- hydroxysteroid reductases as well as sulfotransferases and glucuronyl transferases. Many drugs and thyroxin markedly affect the activity of these enzymes (Berliner and Dougherty 1960; Stylianou et al. 1961; Baulieu et al. 1965).

Metabolic studies in the androgen field have recently shifted from examining the degradative role of the liver and kidney to looking at the activity of target tissues (McGuire and Tomkins 1959; Yates and Urquhart 1962; Schriefers 1967; Naftolin et al. 1972b). Steroid hormones are bound to specific cytoplasmic receptors, after which they are transported to the nucleus and interact principally at the level of nuclear transcription. Testosterone follows this general pattern, but it is converted to DHT in the cytoplasm and possibly in the nucleus (Bruchovsky and Wilson 1968; Haltmeyer and Eik-Nes 1972). DHT appears to be the androgenic messenger in sexual target tissues, suggesting that it may have a role in cancerous states and in prostatic hyperplasia and neoplasia. The prostate may even play a role as an active endocrine organ rather than a passive receptor for sex hormones from the gonad (Siiteri and Wilson 1970; Wilson 1972).

In summary, with respect to Leydig cell secretion in the male, the major advances since 1960 are:

1. Development and general availability of methodology for steroid analysis. This is vital for basic and applied research as well as for clinical diagnosis and management of disease.

2. Increased understanding of the complexity of Leydig cell secretions and control from conception throughout life.

3. The development of new, more complex concepts of gonadal-CNS feedback and suggestions of many behavioral effects of reproductive hormones.

Hormonal Control of Steroidogenesis
Historical introduction Testosterone has been shown to be a secretory product of the testis of all mammalian species that have been investigated. Physiological studies provided indirect evidence that administration of a gonadotropin with ICSH activity (ICSH, hCG, PMS) will stimulate androgen production by the testes (for review, see Steinberger and Steinberger 1972).

In vivo studies In the past fifteen years abundant direct evidence has been presented for the stimulatory action of ICSH on testosterone secretion by the testes. Some of the most extensive studies have been conducted in Eik-Nes's laboratory, utilizing an in vitro dog testis perfusion system. The relation of temperature, rate of blood flow, and concentration of the gonadotropic hormone to the rate of testosterone secretion has been documented, and the remarkable rapidity of the secretory response (a 400 percent change in 10 minutes) has been demonstrated (for review, see Eik-Nes 1970). Clinical studies (Kirschner et al. 1965) demonstrated a profound stimulatory effect of hCG on plasma testosterone levels and production rates in male humans.

In vitro studies Recently a series of in vitro experiments were performed to demonstrate the stimulatory effect of ICSH on testosterone production by testicular tissue and isolated Leydig cells. The sensitivity and precision of the system were sufficient to make it suitable as an in vitro bioassay technique capable of detecting ICSH activity in human serum (Catt et al. 1974).

In vitro biogenetic studies were in agreement with the in vivo and in vitro secretory studies, which showed that ICSH promotes incorporation of ^{14}C-acetate into ^{14}C-testosterone and conversion of ^{3}H-cholesterol to ^{3}H-testosterone in testicular incubations (Hall and Eik-Nes 1962; Dorfman and Ungar 1965).

The biochemical site of ICSH action on the androgen biosynthetic pathway in the testes has been studied in considerable detail. Halkerston et al. (1961) and Koritz (1962) suggested that ICSH stimulates steroidogenesis at some step(s) beyond cholesterol and before pregnenolone. This was subsequently supported by work from Hall's and Dorfman's laboratories (for reviews, see Hall 1970; Forchielli et al. 1969; Steinberger and Steinberger 1972). Actually, many of the ideas concerning the mechanism and site of action of ICSH have been postulated by analogy from work on the effect of ACTH on adrenal steroidogenesis or LH on corpus luteum. Fortunately, data obtained in most studies dealing directly with the effect of ICSH on testicular steroidogenesis are in agreement with data derived from the other two systems. Evidence has been presented in support of the concept that ICSH has a profound effect on the side-chain cleavage of cholesterol (Dorfman et al. 1967; Forchielli et al. 1969). The specific point at which ICSH acts in the series of reactions related to the cleavage process is not entirely clear. Hall and Young's (1968) suggestion that ICSH "accelerates steroidogenesis by specifically stimulating the 20α-hydroxylation of cholesterol" has been supported by studies of other investigators and is generally accepted, but the mechanism by which ICSH produces this effect has so far eluded clarification. In an attempt to develop an experimental approach to this problem, an analogy was drawn with the adrenal gland. It is generally accepted that TPNH and molecular oxygen are characteristic requirements for hydroxylation reactions of the steroids. It has been suggested that ICSH makes TPNH available, and numerous studies testing this idea have been conducted in the ovary and the adrenal gland. In the testes, stimulation of cAMP by ICSH has been demonstrated and cAMP has been termed a "second messenger" (Catt et al. 1974).

It is tempting to accept the hypothesis that the principal action of ICSH on steroidogenesis is confined to cAMP stimulation, resulting in increased levels of TPNH. Recent studies in the adrenal gland suggest that ACTH stimulates steroidogenesis via a cell-membrane-bound process involving activation of adenyl cyclase stimulation of cAMP synthesis and activation of protein kinase, the latter modulating synthesis of a specific protein(s) involved in the cholesterol side-chain cleavage. Although ICSH has been shown to stimulate protein synthesis in the testes, the role of the de novo synthesized protein in regulation of cholesterol side-chain cleavage is unclear. In experiments utilizing mitochondrial preparations, the increase of ^{14}C-amino acid incorporation into protein did not appear to correlate with stimulation of steroid synthesis, and studies utilizing puromycin to block protein synthesis failed to support the hypothesis that de novo protein synthesis is obligatory for the occurrence of cholesterol side-chain cleavage (Forchielli et al. 1969). These experiments, however, were conducted under specific in vitro conditions, which may not reflect a physiological in vivo state. Further studies will be required to clarify the relationship between protein synthesis and steroidogenesis.

Most of the studies discussed so far deal primarily with acute experiments, primarily short-term in vitro incubations, short-term organ perfusions, or short-term (a few days) administration of the hormone to experimental subjects. Changes occurring subsequent to chronic stimulation with ICSH may involve more than cholesterol side-chain cleavage. As far back as 1956, Samuels and Helmreich observed a progressive increase in the activity of Δ^5-3β-hydroxysteroid dehydrogenase in testes of hypophysectomized rats injected daily with hCG for a long period. Increased activities of C17-C20-lyase, Δ^4-5α-reductase, and 17α-hydroxlyase have been reported in testes of immature animals treated chronically with hCG. These findings

suggest that ICSH may affect the androgen production by the testes by mechanisms other than regulation of cholesterol side-chain cleavage, perhaps influencing all enzymes related to conversion of cholesterol to testosterone and its 5α-reduced metabolites. It remains to be discovered whether an effect on enzymes other than those involved in cholesterol side-chain cleavage is a specific function of ICSH or whether it is merely a reflection of a general, complex "trophic" response of the cell to ICSH. Furthermore, in the studies suggesting an effect of ICSH on enzymes other than those involved with cleavage of cholesterol side chain, some of the experiments produce conflicting results.

A possible role of FSH in testicular steroidogenesis has been suggested by a number of reports, although the classic hypothesis ascribes no steroidogenic function to FSH. Johnson and Ewing (1971) reported potentiation by FSH of the ICSH effect on testicular testosterone production in vivo. Differences between the effects of ICSH and PMS (a gonadotropin with both FSH and ICSH activity) on the biosynthetic pathways in posthypophysectomy regressed testes have been noted (Steinberger and Ficher 1973). So far, however, no conclusive evidence has been mustered to support directly the possibility that FSH has an important physiological role in testicular androgen production.

Product inhibition may play an important role in controlling the rates of androgen synthesis. In vitro, pregnenolone inhibits cholesterol side-chain cleavage. Progesterone shares in this effect but is less potent, and other C21 steroids are ineffective. Similarly, the side-chain cleavage of 17α-hydroxypregnenolone is inhibited by a number of C21 steroids. Recently in vivo administration of 17β-estradiol to adult male rats has been demonstrated to stop testosterone production within several hours. This may also be an example of a product-inhibition phenomenon, since neither pituitary nor plasma LH levels were affected at the time when testosterone synthesis was suppressed (Tcholakian et al. 1974). Similar observations were made in humans following administration of fluoxymesterone (Jones et al. 1974).

Application of In Vitro Biosynthesis Techniques for Study of Pathology in Human Testes
Utilization of radiolabeled precursors has been a useful approach for the in vitro investigations of normal testicular steroid biosynthetic pathways. Application of similar techniques to studies of steroid biosynthesis in testicular tissue from men with defective testicular function has yielded interesting and important information concerning the pathophysiology of certain testicular lesions. Routine testicular biopsy provides a sufficient amount of tissue for in vitro study of the androgen biosynthetic pathways, and study of steroid

biosynthetic pathways in testicular tissue incubates from reproductively and endocrinologically normal males provides the necessary baseline for interpretation of data obtained from men with testicular abnormalities (E. Steinberger et al. 1970b; A. Steinberger et al. 1970).

Characteristic patterns of androgen biosynthesis were demonstrated in testicular tissue from men with well-defined testicular abnormalities, such as hypogonadotropic hypogonadism, Klinefelter's syndrome, or testicular feminization (E. Steinberger et al. 1974b). Of particular interest is the observation of extremely active synthesis of testosterone in vitro in incubates of testicular tissue from patients with Klinefelter's syndrome (E. Steinberger et al. 1974b) casting doubt on the assumption that testes of Klinefelter patients have defective Leydig cells. The reduced plasma levels of testosterone and particularly the diminished response to an hCG stimulation test may be due to an actual decrease in the total mass of Leydig cells, resulting in lower total testosterone production under conditions of normal or increased stimulation. This hypothesis is corroborated by the observation of a high testicular vein level of testosterone in patients with Klinefelter's syndrome (E. Steinberger et al. 1974b).

Similarly, the capacity of the testicular tissue of patients with testicular feminization to form testosterone in vitro is great, providing direct evidence that the testes of these patients are indeed capable of testosterone synthesis at a rate at least as high as normal testes (E. Steinberger et al. 1970b).

Several exciting reports have shown specific enzyme defects in vitro in the testicular tissue from patients with oligospermia and infertility. Diagnosis of the specific defect enabled the physician to treat the condition satisfactorily (Steinberger et al. 1974c).

26.3 Hormonal Control of Spermatogenesis

Historical Introduction
During the past two decades a series of discoveries have firmly identified the central nervous system (specifically the hypothalamus) as the primary control site of gonadal growth and functions. Clinical observations at the turn of the century led a number of investigators to suggest that certain structures in the brain are responsible for inducing and maintaining testicular function. In the 1920s the effects of the pituitary and its gonadotropic secretions on gonadal function were demonstrated. Until the 1950s the pituitary gland reigned as the primary "controller" of gonadal function, and then evidence began to accumulate suggesting that the hypothalamus may be producing a substance that in turn stimulates the pituitary gland to secrete gonadotropins. This substance, LRF, has been purified and synthesized, and it was shown to stimulate secretion of both LH and FSH.

Role of Hormones in Initiation and Maintenance of Spermatogenesis
Subsequent to the demonstration that removal of the pituitary gland prevents development of immature testes and causes regression of seminiferous epithelium and Leydig cell function in adult testes, Greep et al. (1936) suggested that the two gonadotropic substances, LH and FSH, affect Leydig cells and seminiferous epithelium, respectively. The evidence leading to this conclusion was based, however, on experiments conducted with relatively impure hormones, and the testicular response was judged in a qualitative fashion. Furthermore, most of the work was conducted either with hypophysectomized animals or with immature males. Recently it has become abundantly clear that in many instances hypophysectomized animals may retain residual pituitary tissue capable of a low degree of gonadotropin production (Lostroh et al. 1963), while immature animals produce varying amounts of gonadotropins throughout the maturation process. Because of the difficulty of obtaining an experimental model totally devoid of gonadotropins and because of the cross-contamination of the two gonadotropins used in experiments calling for replacement therapy, the results obtained were either difficult to interpret or contradictory. Furthermore, the lack of a quantitative approach for the assessment of the response of the germinal epithelium to the various experimental manipulations led to additional difficulties.

The role of ICSH in Leydig cell function has now been clearly established, but its possible direct role in the growth and function of the seminiferous tubules still remains unresolved. In the 1960s the possibility of a synergism between ICSH and FSH was proposed. It has been suggested that both hormones are necessary for "complete spermatogenesis" (Woods and Simpson 1961; Lostroh 1963). In these studies, however, incomplete hypophysectomy (Lostroh et al. 1963), impure gonadotropins, and nonquantitative evaluation of spermatogenesis remained significant problems.

In an attempt to clarify and systematize some of the difficulties encountered in resolving the question of hormonal control of the seminiferous tubule function, Steinberger and Steinberger (1969) suggested that the hormonal requirements for initiation of spermatogenesis in immature testes and its reinitiation subsequent to posthypophysectomy regression may differ from those required for its maintenance. Furthermore, they suggested that quantitatively normal spermatogenesis may require a different hormonal milieu from that required for qualitative progression of the spermatogenic process.

It has been generally accepted, on the basis of numerous early experiments, that hypophysectomy induces an arrest of spermatogenesis at the stage of primary spermatocytes. In other words, lack of gonadotropins prevents completion of the meiotic division and formation of the haploid cells, the spermatids. This conclusion was based on qualitative microscopic observations of histological sections of the testes. Utilizing a quantitative technique for the analysis of seminiferous epithelium, Clermont and Morgentaler (1955) demonstrated that hypophysectomy causes specifically a partial loss of type A spermatogonia. Whether this is due to an increased rate of spontaneous degeneration or a decrease in mitotic activity is not clear. The remaining type A spermatogonia form type B spermatogonia, which in turn form primary spermatocytes without further loss. In addition to changes in spermatogonia, a substantial attrition of primary spermatocytes occurs during the lengthy meiotic prophase; however, some of the spermatocytes apparently do complete the meiotic division and form spermatids, but these degenerate spontaneously during early stages of development so that no mature spermatids are formed. These studies suggest that lack of gonadotropins (and lack of testosterone, since the latter should not be formed in absence of ICSH) affects type A spermatogonia and primary spermatocytes, causing relative diminution in cell numbers rather than an absolute block at a certain stage of germ cell development. Quantitative evaluation of seminiferous epithelium in hypophysectomized animals treated with ICSH or FSH led to the conclusion that FSH may have no role in spermatogenesis: "As far as FSH is concerned, it may be suggested that this hormone did not exert an influence per se (on seminiferous epithelium), but influenced the Leydig cells through its ICSH contaminant" (Clermont and Harvey 1967). These authors observed no difference in maintenance of spermatogenesis when either ICSH, FSH, or testosterone was used for replacement therapy.

Utilizing both in vitro (tissue culture) and in vivo (estrogen-blocked rats) approaches, Steinberger reevaluated the role of testosterone in spermatogenesis and proposed the concept of "consecutive" action of hormones on the germinal epithelium (for review, see Steinberger 1971). This concept assumes that different hormones may be required at different stages of germ cell development, particularly during the initial wave of spermatogenesis at puberty. High intratesticular concentration of testosterone is required for meiosis to undergo completion. In other words, the late meiotic prophase and metaphase appear to be testosterone-dependent. The initiation of the spermatogenic process in prepubertal testes, i.e., the induction of spermatogonial divisions leading to formation of more mature germ cells, may also be under the control of testosterone. The evidence for this, however, is only indirect (Steinberger 1974).

In summary, recent studies provide evidence pointing toward an important role for testosterone at two crucial stages of the spermatogenic process, its initiation and the completion of the meiotic division. The role of testosterone in remaining segments of the spermatogenic process is still unclear; however, evidence is accumulating that testosterone may also play a role in the quantitative expression of spermiogenesis.

Subsequent to Greep's suggestion that FSH is the hormone responsible for stimulation of spermatogenesis, numerous studies were conducted to confirm his findings and to clarify with greater precision the site in the spermatogenic process where FSH may exhibit its effect. Early attempts to define FSH action on spermatogenesis met with failure. Simpson et al. (1944) and Randolph et al. (1959) suggested that ICSH is the primary gonadotropin involved in seminiferous tubule function. Subsequently Woods and Simpson (1961), using highly purified gonadotropins (by 1961 standards), demonstrated that ICSH even at a "very low" dose maintains spermatogenesis, while FSH at doses showing no ICSH contamination produces "only slight effect on testicular weight and development." At higher doses, FSH maintained spermatogenesis, but the sex accessories were also stimulated, suggesting ICSH contamination. Although accepting the possibility of a synergistic effect of the two hormones, Woods and Simpson also concluded that ICSH is the primary spermatogenic hormone. Similar conclusions were reached by Lostroh (1963) and by von Berswordt-Wallrabe and Neumann (1968). Von Berswordt-Wallrabe et al. (1968) utilized an androgen antagonist (cyproterone acetate) to eliminate androgenic activity resulting from possible ICSH contamination of their FSH preparation. On the basis of these experiments, they concluded: "FSH by itself does not exert any detectable effects in the testes of hypophysectomized mature rats. Neither the hypothesis that formation of type A stem cells may be under direct pituitary control, nor the observation that FSH may produce a secretory hypertrophy of the Sertoli cells was found to be substantiated. It is concluded that FSH alone has no influence on testicular events in hypophysectomized rats." As mentioned above, Clermont and Harvey (1967), utilizing qualitative techniques for evaluation of the spermatogenic process, arrived at a similar conclusion.

In animals with estrogen-blocked pituitary gonadotropins, treatment with testosterone from birth has been shown to allow spermatogenesis to proceed through meiosis and to form spermatids up to steps 14 to 15 of spermiogenesis; however, completion of spermiogenesis and formation of spermatozoa did not occur until an FSH-like substance was also administered. Consequently, FSH appears to be necessary for completion of spermiogenesis. Whether FSH affects the spermatids directly or creates a condition that permits testosterone to influence the completion of spermiogenesis cannot be stated with certainty at this point (for review, see Steinberger and Steinberger 1969).

To summarize, it appears that spermatogenesis can be maintained in hypophysectomized males by testosterone in the absence of gonadotropins, but its initiation at puberty requires the presence of FSH. Recently, an extensive series of experiments has also demonstrated that reinitiation of spermatogenesis subsequent to posthypophysectomy regression of the testes also requires the presence of an FSH-like hormonal activity (von Berswordt-Wallrabe and Neumann 1968).

In the early 1940s a number of investigators (Selye and Friedman 1941; Ruzicka and Prelog 1943; Leathem and Brent 1943; Masson 1945; and others) reported maintenance of spermatogenesis in hypophysectomized animals treated with various "weak" androgens. They concluded that sufficiently high doses of "weak" androgens will elicit a spermatogenic response. In light of recent observations that the "active" androgen, at least at extragonadal target tissues, is a 5α-reduced androgen, dihydrotestosterone, and in view of the fact that developing testes are capable of preferential synthesis of 5α-reduced androgens, particularly 5α-androstane-3α,17β-diol during development, the question of the effect of C19 steroids other than testosterone on spermatogenesis has been reevaluated. That certain "weak" androgens such as DHEA, androstenedione, or androstenediol can maintain spermatogenesis can be explained by their intratesticular conversion to testosterone. Study of the 5α-reduced androgens revealed that a number of them (DHT, 5α-androstanediol, and androsterone) compare with testosterone in ability to maintain spermatogenesis in hypophysectomized rats. Their ability to initiate spermatogenesis in newborn estrogen-blocked rats varies, however. Some, such as androstanediol, had an effect equal to testosterone; others, such as androsterone, were barely capable of supporting early stages of germinal epithelium development (Chowdhury and Steinberger 1973).

There has also been a recent reevaluation of the suggestion that pregnenolone may act like a "gonadotropin" on spermatogenesis (Selye and Friedman 1941). A series of C21 steroids (pregnenolone, progesterone,

17α-hydroxyprogesterone, and 17α-hydroxypregnenolone) were shown to maintain spermatogenesis in hypophysectomized rats despite the atrophy of sex accessories equal to that of untreated hypophysectomized animals, suggesting the presence of very low, if any, circulating levels of androgens (Steinberger and Chowdhury 1973). Whether these steroids affect spermatogenesis directly or have to be converted to androgens in the testes is unclear at this time. Harris and Bartke (1974) observed relatively high levels of testosterone in the rete testis fluid of hypophysectomized pregnenolone-treated rats in spite of markedly depressed (to hypophysectomy levels) circulating testosterone. E. Steinberger et al. (1975) demonstrated conversion in the testes of radiolabeled pregnenolone tracer administered in vivo to testosterone. The rate of conversion was, however, extremely low. Undoubtedly, more extensive studies are needed to establish the mode of action of the C21 steroids on seminiferous epithelium.

In summary, solid evidence has accumulated in the past decade implicating androgens as the crucial hormones required for spermatogenesis. Whether testosterone, its 5α-reduced metabolites, or both are the active steroids remains to be elucidated. It has been firmly established that some of the 5α-reduced androgens can produce the same effect on spermatogenesis as testosterone. The early suggestion that pregnenolone can maintain spermatogenesis in hypophysectomized animals has been confirmed and shown to hold true for a number of other C21 steroids. Their mode of action (via conversion to androgens?) remains to be determined.

Application of tissue culture techniques to the study of spermatogenesis has provided a number of important observations. The in vivo study of mechanisms involved in control of spermatogenesis is complicated by the interaction of the entire organism with the testes and by the influence of the various feedback mechanisms. An in vitro organ culture provides a simplified experimental model in which the environment can be more rigidly controlled and the direct effect of various agents can be investigated. Investigators utilizing these techniques have demonstrated that the meiotic prophase can proceed until the late stages of pachytene spermatocytes in the absence of hormones in a chemically defined medium; however, glutamine appears to be essential for this process. It is of interest that glutamine is essential for differentiation of other tissues, such as the retina.

Studies with organ cultures have also demonstrated the hormonal independence of the transformation of type A to type B spermatogonia and the transformation of the latter to resting spermatocytes. This finding has confirmed the results obtained in vivo in estrogen-blocked newborn rats, where formation of type B spermatogonia and resting spermatocytes could be observed for months after initiation of estrogen treatment in the absence of gonadotropins and testosterone. In addition, studies of testicular organ cultures showed that the germinal stem cells can divide in the absence of hormones for an indefinite period of time. Under the in vitro conditions, they fail to evolve into more advanced types of germinal epithelium cells; however, they retain the capacity to enter spermatogenesis and form spermatozoa when transplanted into testes of adult rats (for review of the in vitro studies, see E. Steinberger et al. 1970a).

Molecular Mechanisms Concerned with the Effect of Hormones on Seminiferous Tubules and the Role of the Sertoli Cell in Spermatogenesis

That Sertoli cells may be concerned with the economy of the germinal cells had been mentioned by Sertoli (1865). He called them "nurse" cells and suggested that they perform a "nutritive" function for the germ cells. Subsequently it has been suggested that they are also phagocytic (for review, see Vilar et al. 1967). On the basis of rather limited histochemical studies, Lacy (1962) speculated that the Sertoli cell may respond to hormonal stimulation and also be a source of a "nonandrogenic" testicular hormone, although later (1967) he suggested that this hormone may in fact be an androgenic steroid.

The first direct evidence for an effect of FSH on the morphology of the Sertoli cells was obtained in studies of organ cultures of immature rat testes (E. Steinberger et al. 1964). This observation was subsequently confirmed by Murphy (1965) in vivo. She also made cell counts in histological sections of the testes and suggested that FSH stimulates replication of Sertoli cells in testes of adult animals. Utilizing ^{3}H-thymidine labeling and radioautographic techniques, Steinberger and Steinberger (1971) were unable to confirm this suggestion either in vivo or in organ cultures utilizing testes from immature or adult rats.

The observation that FSH may produce a morphological change in the Sertoli cells led to a concerted effort to investigate the possibility that the Sertoli cell may indeed be the target cell for FSH action. Labeled FSH was shown by bright-light microscopy to localize in the seminiferous tubules (Mancini et al. 1967, 1968), and electron-microscopic studies suggested that it localizes in the cytoplasm of the Sertoli cells (Castro et al. 1970, 1972). The preferential localization of FSH in Sertoli cells was compatible with the idea that the cells may be the site of its biological activity, or at least the site where it is modified or stored prior to exerting its effect on other cell types in the seminiferous tubule.

Specific binding of ^{3}H-FSH to testicular tissue, and more specifically to the seminiferous tubules in vitro, was demonstrated by Means and Vaitukaitis (1972) and later confirmed with ^{125}I-labeled FSH by Bhalla and Reichert (1974) and A. Steinberger et al. (1974a). Utilizing a combination of mechanical, enzymic, and tissue culture techniques, A. Steinberger et al. (1974a, b) demonstrated that interstitial cells, peritubular cells, and germinal cells do not bind ^{125}I-labeled FSH, while seminiferous tubules depleted of germ cells show the same degree of specific binding as whole seminiferous tubules, suggesting that the Sertoli cells may be the primary site of specific FSH binding. This suggestion has recently been supported by direct evidence from experiments showing specific binding of radiolabeled FSH to isolated and culture-grown Sertoli cells. The binding was demonstrated to occur in cultures grown for 11 days in the absence of hormones, suggesting that the receptors are not hormone-dependent (A. Steinberger et al. 1975).

Localization of FSH in Sertoli cells using light and electron microscopy and studies on FSH binding provide a significant body of evidence in support of the hypothesis that at least one of the targets of biological action of FSH in the testis is the Sertoli cell. A series of recent biochemical observations provided further support for this idea and served as the starting point for investigations of the details of the molecular mechanisms responsible for FSH action in the Sertoli cells. Three almost parallel lines of biochemical evidence have evolved for the effect of FSH on the seminiferous tubules.

Means and Hall (1968) demonstrated an increase of protein synthesis in testes of immature rats treated with FSH. This effect was limited to a specific age during maturation. Similarly, FSH-induced RNA synthesis was restricted to testes from animals approximately 20 days of age (Means 1971). The stimulation of protein synthesis was probably secondary to the increase in RNA synthesis.

The second line of evidence deals with in vitro stimulation of adenyl cyclase activity by FSH. Sutherland and Rall (1962) were first to demonstrate the presence of adenyl cyclase in testicular tissue, and Murad et al. (1969) were first to demonstrate in vitro stimulation of adenyl cyclase by addition of FSH to testicular homogenates. This observation was subsequently confirmed by Kuehl et al. (1970), who showed a similar effect of FSH on isolated seminiferous tubules. Subsequently Dorrington et al. (1972) showed increased cAMP levels in isolated seminiferous tubules incubated with FSH. These studies provided evidence for localization of an FSH-responsive cAMP system within seminiferous tubules. The cell types of the seminiferous tubule in which the FSH-dependent process takes place remain to be determined. Utilizing a combination of mechanical, enzymic, and tissue culture techniques, Heindel et al. (1975) separated the peritubular cells, Sertoli cells, and germ cells. Only fractions containing Sertoli cells responded to FSH with increased production of cAMP. Sertoli cells maintained in culture for up to 11 days retained the capacity to respond to FSH with increased cAMP production (A. Steinberger et al. 1975). These studies provided the first direct evidence that Sertoli cells are the exclusive site of FSH stimulation of cAMP and provided a new approach to in vitro study of the molecular mechanisms associated with FSH action on the testes.

The demonstration of cAMP-dependent protein kinase in testicular tissue (Reddi et al. 1971) suggested the possibility that the link between stimulation of adenyl cyclase by FSH and the ultimate increase in protein synthesis could be mediated via a cAMP-dependent protein kinase. Indeed, an increase in protein kinase was observed in isolated seminiferous tubules incubated with FSH. The greatest response was noted in testes of 16-day-old rats, and no stimulation was observed in animals older than 30 days (Means et al. 1974).

Although the FSH-induced increases in adenyl cyclase and cAMP show a temporal relationship, suggesting that FSH controls the cAMP levels in the testes primarily by affecting its synthesis, the presence of a phosphodiesterase in the testes (Kuehl et al. 1970) suggests that the regulatory mechanism may also involve activation of this enzyme, particularly since a testis-specific phosphodiesterase isoenzyme has been demonstrated (Christiansen and Desautel 1973).

The third line of evidence deals with demonstration of an androgen-binding protein (ABP) and an androgen receptor in the testicular tissue. In 1972 and 1973 several groups of investigators reported the presence of a specific ABP (Vernon et al. 1972; Ritzen et al. 1973; Hansson et al. 1973a; E. Steinberger et al. 1974a) in the rete testes, efferent duct fluid (French and Ritzen 1973), and the epididymis (Ritzen et al. 1971).

Subsequent to the demonstration of ABP, considerable effort has been expended in defining its physiochemical properties (Hansson et al. 1973; Sanborn et al. 1974). As reported previously for the epididymal ABP (Ritzen et al. 1971), the testicular protein showed high-affinity androgen-binding activity ($K_a \approx 5 \times 10^8$ M^{-1} for testosterone) and a rapid dissociation constant ($t_{1/2} = 3$ min, 0°C, 30% glycerol buffer).

Physiological studies of ABP revealed its dependence on pituitary gonadotropins. Hypophysectomy resulted in a slow progressive loss of this protein from the testes (Vernon et al. 1973; E. Steinberger et al. 1974a; Hansson et al. 1974a), and FSH treatment of hypophysectomized rats maintained and, in posthypophysectomy-regressed animals, partly restored its lev-

els (E. Steinberger et al. 1974a; Hansson et al. 1974a; Sanborn et al. 1975a). Hansson et al. (1973b) and E. Steinberger et al. (1974a) suggested that ABP is probably produced by the Sertoli cells. This suggestion has been supported by subsequent studies with isolated Sertoli cells cultured in vitro (Fritz et al. 1974; A. Steinberger et al. 1975).

On the basis of the studies discussed in this section, E. Steinberger et al. (1974a) suggested the following hypothesis for the molecular events concerned with hormonal control of spermatogenesis: (1) FSH is bound specifically to the Sertoli cells; there it stimulates cAMP production. (2) Cyclic AMP activates a protein kinase that mediates processes leading to the synthesis of proteins, one of which is the ABP. (3) Testosterone enters the Sertoli cells from the interstitial area and is bound to the specific binding protein. (4) The androgen-protein complex influences spermatogenesis.

This series of events could explain the FSH dependence of the initiation of the spermatogenic process. Also, the maintenance of spermatogenesis in hypophysectomized males by testosterone could be explained if it is assumed that one of the effects of the androgen-protein complex is to assure continuous formation of more ABP. This hypothesis would explain the difficulty in reinitiating spermatogenesis in posthypophysectomy-regressed testes with testosterone (Nelson and Gallagher 1936).

This suggestion may not hold true, however, in light of a recent demonstration of induction of ABP with testosterone in posthypophysectomy-regressed rat testes (Elkington et al. 1975).

Recently a cytoplasmic testosterone receptor, distinct from ABP and similar to testosterone receptors in the epididymis and ventral prostate, has been demonstrated in the testes (Hansson et al. 1974b). The possibility has to be considered that ABP is involved primarily in transport of androgens in the testes, analogous to the steroid-binding proteins in blood, and that the androgen receptor mediates the molecular mechanisms involved in the effects of testosterone on germ cells. Undoubtedly, the details of these molecular mechanisms will require considerable study before they are clearly elucidated; however, the presence of these mechanisms and their importance in mediation of hormonal effects in the testes have been definitely demonstrated in the past two to three years.

References

Acevedo, H. F., L. R. Axelrod, E. Ishikawa, and F. Takaki. Steroidogenesis in the human fetal testis: The conversion of pregnenolone-7α-H³ to dehydroepiandrosterone, testosterone and 4-androstene-3,17-dione. J. Clin. Endocrinol. Metab. 21:1611, 1961.

Alder, A., H. Burger. J. Davis, A. Dulmanis, B. Hudson, G. Sarfaty, and W. Straffon. Carcinoma of prostate: Response of plasma luteinizing hormone and testosterone to oestrogen therapy. Br. Med. J. 1:28, 1968.

Alford, F. P., H. W. G. Baker, H. G. Burger, D. M. de-Kretser, B. Hudson, M. W. Johns, J. P. Masterson, Y. C. Patel, and G. C. Rennie. Temporal patterns of integrated plasma hormone levels during sleep and wakefulness. II. Follicle-stimulating hormone, luteinizing hormone, testosterone and estradiol. J. Clin. Endocrinol. Metab. 37:848, 1973.

Aschkenasy, A. Action de la testostérone, de la thyroxine et de la cortisone sur l'évolution de l'anémie et de la leucopénie protéiprivés. Sang 25:15, 1954.

Bagshawe, K. D., C. E. Wilde, and A. H. Orr. Radioimmunoassay for human chorionic gonadotrophin and luteinising hormone. Lancet 1:1118, 1966.

Baird, D., R. Horton, C. Longcope, and J. F. Tait. Steroid prehormones. Perspect. Biol. Med. 11:384, 1968.

Baird, D. T., A. Galbraith, I. S. Fraser, and J. E. Newsam. The concentration of oestrone and oestradiol-17β in spermatic venous blood in man. J. Endocrinol. 57:285, 1973.

Baker, H. W. G., H. G. Burger, D. M. deKretser, A. Dulmanis, L. W. Eddie, B. Hudson, E. J. Keogh, V. W. K. Lee, and G. C. Rennie. Clinical and basic studies in male reproductive endocrinology. Recent Prog. Horm. Res. 32:429, 1976.

Bardin, C. W., and M. B. Lipsett. Testosterone and androstenedione blood production rates in normal women and women with idiopathic hirsutism or polycystic ovaries. J. Clin. Invest. 46:891, 1967.

Bardin, C. W., L. P. Bullock, R. J. Sherins, I. Mowszowicz, and W. R. Blackburn. Androgen metabolism and mechanism of action in male pseudohermaphroditism: A study of testicular feminization. Recent Prog. Horm. Res. 29:65, 1973.

Baulieu, E-E., C. Corpéchot, F. Dray, R. Emiliozzi, M. C. Lebeau, P. Mauvais-Jarvis, and P. Robel. An adrenal secreted "androgen": Dehydroisoandrosterone sulfate. Its metabolism and a tentative generalization on the metabolism of other steroid conjugates in man. Recent Prog. Horm. Res. 21:411, 1965.

Berliner, D. L., and T. F. Dougherty. Influence of reticuloendothelial and other cells on the metabolic fate of steroids. Ann. NY Acad. Sci 88:14, 1960.

Berthold, A. A. Transplantation der Hoden. Arch. Anat. Physiol. 16:42, 1849.

Bhalla, V. K., and L. E. Reichert, Jr. FSH receptors in rat testes: Chemical properties and solubilization studies. In Hormone binding and cell regulation in the testis, ed. M. L. Dufau, and A. R. Means, p. 201. New York: Plenum Press, 1974.

Biglieri, E. G., M. A. Herron, and N. Brust. 17-hydroxylation deficiency in man. J. Clin. Invest. 45:1946, 1966.

Bliss, E. L., and C. J. Migeon. Endocrinology of anorexia nervosa. J. Clin. Endocrinol. Metab. 17:766, 1957.

Blivaiss, B. B., R. O. Hanson, R. E. Rosenzweig, and K. McNeil. Sexual development in female rats treated with cortisone. Proc. Soc. Exp. Biol. Med. 86:678, 1954.

Bloch, E. Metabolism of 4-14C-progesterone by human fetal testis and ovaries. Endocrinology 74:833, 1964.

Bloch, E. The conversion of 7-3H-pregnenolone and 4-14C-progesterone to testosterone and androstenedione by mammalian fetal testes in vitro. Steroids 9:415, 1967.

Bodenheimer, S., J. S. D. Winter, and C. Faiman. Diurnal rhythms of serum gonadotropins, testosterone, estradiol and cortisol in blind men. J. Clin. Endocrinol. Metab. 37:472, 1973.

Bogdanove, E. M., A. F. Parlow, J. N. Bogdanove, I. Bhargava, and E. V. Crabill. Specific LH and FSH bio-assays in rats with hypothalamic lesions and accessory sex gland hypertrophy. Endocrinology 74:114, 1964.

Boon, D. A., R. E. Keenan, and W. R. Slaunwhite, Jr. Plasma testosterone in men: Variation, but not circadian rhythm. Steroids 20:269, 1972.

Boyar, R., M. Perlow, L. Hellman, S. Kapen, and E. Weitzman. Twenty-four hour pattern of luteinizing hormone secretion in normal men with sleep stage recording. J. Clin. Endocrinol. Metab. 35:73, 1972a.

Boyar, R., J. Finkelstein, H. Roffwarg, S. Kapen, E. Weitzman, and L. Hellman. Synchronization of LH secretion with sleep during puberty. N. Engl. J. Med. 287:582, 1972b.

Brady, R. O. Biosynthesis of radioactive testosterone in vitro. J. Biol. Chem. 193:145, 1951.

Brownie, A., H. J. van der Molen, E. E. Nishizawa, and K. B. Eik-Nes. Determination of testosterone in human peripheral blood using gas-liquid chromatography with electron capture detection. J. Clin. Endocrinol. Metab. 24:1091, 1964.

Bruchovsky, N., and J. D. Wilson. Conversion of testosterone to 5α-androstan-17β-ol-3-one by rat prostate in vivo and in vitro. J. Biol. Chem. 243:2012, 1968.

Butenandt, A. Über die Chemie der Sexualhormon. Z. Angew. Chem. 45:655, 1932.

Butenandt, A., and G. Hanisch. Über Testosteron. Umwandlung des Dehydrosterons im Androstendiol und Testosterone: Ein Weg zur Darstellung des Testosterons aus Cholesterin. Z. Physiol. Chem. 237:89, 1935.

Byrnes, W. W., and R. K. Meyer. The inhibition of gonadotrophic hormone secretion by physiological doses of estrogen. Endocrinology 48:133, 1951.

Cable, Y. D., P. O. Kohler, C. M. Cargille, and G. T. Ross. Production rates and metabolic clearance rates of human follicle-stimulating hormone in premenopausal and postmenopausal women. J. Clin. Invest. 48:359, 1969.

Camacho, A., and C. J. Migeon. Isolation, identification and quantitation of testosterone in the urine of normal adults and in patients with endocrine disorders. J. Clin. Endocrinol. Metab. 23:301, 1963.

Castro, A. E., A. C. Seiguer, and R. E. Mancini. Electron microscopic study on the localization of labeled gonadotropins in the Sertoli and Leydig cells of the rat testis. Proc. Soc. Exp. Biol. Med. 133:582, 1970.

Castro, A. E., A. Alonso, and R. E. Mancini. Localization of follicle-stimulating and luteinizing hormones in the rat testis using immunohistological tests. J. Endocrinol. 52:129, 1972.

Catt, K. J., T. Tsuruhara, C. Mendelson, J. M. Ketelslegers, and M. L. Dufau. Gonadotropin binding and activation of the interstitial cells of the testis. In *Hormone binding and target cell activation in the testis*, ed. M.L. Dufau and A.R. Means, p. 1. New York: Plenum Press, 1974.

Chowdhury, A. K., and E. Steinberger. Effect of 5α reduced androgens on initiation and maintenance of spermatogenesis. Biol. Reprod. 9:62, 1973.

Christensen, A. K., and S. W. Gillim. The correlation of fine structure and function in steroid-secreting cells, with emphasis on those of the gonads. In *The gonads*, ed. K.W. McKerns, p. 415. New York: Appleton-Century-Crofts, 1969.

Christensen, A. K., and N. R. Mason. Comparative ability of seminiferous tubules and interstitial tissue of rat testes to synthesize androgens from progesterone-4¹⁴C in vitro. Endocrinology 76:646, 1965.

Christiansen, R. O., and M. Desautel. Induction of highly specific testicular isozyme of cyclic nucleotide phosphodiesterase by interstitial cell stimulating hormone (ICSH) and FSH. Clin. Res. 21:289, 1973.

Clermont, Y., and S. C. Harvey. Effects of hormones on spermatogenesis of the rat. In *Endocrinology of the testis*, Ciba Foundation Colloquia on Endocrinology, Vol. 16, eds. G. E. W. Wolstenholme and M. O'Connor, p. 173. Boston: Little, Brown, 1967.

Clermont, Y., and H. Morgentaler. Quantitative study of spermatogenesis in the hypophysectomized rat. Endocrinology 57:369, 1955.

Danielsson, H., and T. Tchen. Steroid metabolism. In *Metabolic pathways*, Vol. 2, 3rd ed., ed. D. N. Greenberg, p. 117. New York: Academic Press, 1968.

Daughaday, W. H. The adenohypophysis. In *Textbook of endocrinology*, 4th ed., ed. R. J. Williams, p. 27. Philadelphia: W. B. Saunders Co., 1968.

David, K., E. Dingemanse, J. Freud, and E. Laqueur. Über Krystallinisches männliches Hormon aus Hoden (Testosteron), wirksamer als aus Harn oder aus Cholesterin bereitetes Androsteron. Z. Physiol. Chem. 233:281, 1935.

Davies, D. V., T. Mann, and L. E. A. Rowson. Effect of nutrition on the onset of male sex hormone activity and sperm formation in monozygous bull-calves. Proc. R. Soc. Lond. [Biol.] 147:332, 1957.

deKretser, D. M., H. G. Burger, D. Fortune, B. Hudson, A. R. Long, C. A. Paulsen, and H. P. Taft. Hormonal, histological and chromosomal studies in adult males with testicular disorders. J. Clin. Endocrinol. Metab. 35:392, 1972.

Dodge, A. H., A. K. Christensen, and R. B. Clayton. Localization of a steroid 11β-hydroxylase in the inner membrane subfraction of rat adrenal mitochondria. Endocrinology 87: 254, 1970.

Dorfman, R. I., and F. Ungar. *Metabolism of steroid hormones*. New York: Academic Press, 1965.

Dorfman, R. I., K. M. J. Menon, D. C. Sharma, S. Joshi, and E. Forchielli. Steroid hormone biosynthesis in rat, rabbit, and capuchine testis. In *Endocrinology of the Testis*, Ciba

Foundation Colloquia on Endocrinology, Vol. 16, eds. G. E. W. Wolstenholme and M. O'Connor, p. 91. Boston: Little, Brown, 1967.

Dorrington, J. H., and I. B. Fritz. Effects of gonadotropins on cyclic AMP production by isolated seminiferous tubule and interstitial cell preparations. Endocrinology 94:395, 1974.

Dorrington, J. H., R. G. Vernon, and I. B. Fritz. The effect of gonadotrophins on the 3′,5′-AMP levels of seminiferous tubules. Biochem. Biophys. Res. Commun. 46:1523, 1972.

Eik-Nes, K. B. Effects of gonadotrophins on secretion of steroids by the testis and ovary. Physiol. Rev. 44:609, 1964.

Eik-Nes, K. B. Synthesis and secretion of androstenedione and testosterone. In *The androgens of the testis*, ed. K. B. Eik-Nes, p. 1. New York: Marcel Dekker, 1970.

Eik-Nes, K. B. Production and secretion of testicular steroids. Recent Prog. Horm. Res. 27:517, 1971.

Elkington, J. S. H., B. M. Sanborn, and E. Steinberger. The effect of testosterone propionate on the concentration of testicular and epididymal androgen binding activity in the hypophysectomized rat. Mol. Cell. Endocrinol. 2:151, 1975.

Evans, J. I., A. W. MacLean, A. A. A. Ismail, and D. Love. Concentrations of plasma testosterone in normal men during sleep. Nature 229:261, 1971.

Everett, J. W., C. H. Sawyer, and J. E. Markee. A neurogenic timing factor in control of the ovulatory discharge of luteinizing hormone in the cyclic rat. Endocrinology 44:234, 1949.

Faiman, C., and R. J. Ryan. Radioimmunoassay for human follicle stimulating hormone. J. Clin. Endocrinol. Metab. 27: 444, 1967.

Faiman, C., and J. S. D. Winter. Diurnal cycles in plasma FSH, testosterone and cortisol in men. J. Clin. Endocrinol. Metab. 33:186, 1971.

Ficher, M., and E. Steinberger. Conversion of progesterone to androsterone by testicular tissue at different stages of maturation. Steroids 12:491, 1968.

Finkelstein, M., E. Forchielli, and R. I. Dorfman. Estimation of testosterone in human plasma. J. Clin. Endocrinol. Metab. 21:98, 1961.

Fiske, V. M. Effect of light on sexual maturation, estrous cycles, and anterior pituitary of the rat. Endocrinology 29:187, 1941.

Forchielli, E., K. M. J. Menon, and R. I. Dorfman. Control of testicular steroid biosynthesis. In *The gonads*, ed. K. W. McKerns, p. 519. New York: Appleton-Century-Crofts, 1969.

Franchimont, P. Le dosage radio-immunologique des gonadotrophines. Ann. Endocrinol. 29:403, 1968.

Franchimont, P., and S. Chari. Personal communication, 1974.

Frasier, S. D., F. Gafford, and R. Horton. Plasma androgens in childhood and adolescence. J. Clin. Endocrinol. Metab. 29:1404, 1969.

French, F. S., and E. M. Ritzen. A high-affinity androgen-binding protein (ABP) in rat testis: Evidence for secretion into efferent duct fluid and absorption by epididymis. Endocrinology 93:88, 1973.

Fritz, I. B., B. Kopec, K. Lam, and R. G. Vernon. Effects of FSH on levels of androgen binding protein in the testis. In *Hormone binding and target cell activation in the testis*, eds. M. L. Dufau and A. R. Means, p. 311. New York: Plenum Press, 1974.

Gans, E. The ICSH content of serum of intact and gonadectomized rats and of rats treated with sex hormones. Acta Endocrinol. (Kbh.) 32:373, 1959.

Gay, V. L., and N. W. Dever. Effects of testosterone propionate and estradiol benzoate—alone or in combination—on serum LH and FSH in orchidectomized rats. Endocrinology 89:161, 1971.

Gerson, T., F. B. Shorland, and G. G. Dunckley. Effect of β-sitosterol on cholesterol and lipid metabolism in the rat. Nature 200:579, 1964.

Goldzieher, J. M., T. S. Dozier, K. S. Smith, and E. Steinberger. Improving the diagnostic reliability of rapidly fluctuating plasma hormone levels by optimized multiple-sampling techniques. J. Clin. Endocrinol. Metab. 43:824, 1976.

Green, J. D., and G. W. Harris. The neurovascular link between the neurohypophysis and adenohypophysis. J. Endocrinol. 5:136, 1947.

Greep, R. O. Physiology of the anterior hypophysis in relation to reproduction. In *Sex and internal secretions*, Vol. 1, ed. W. C. Young, p. 240. Baltimore: Williams & Wilkins, 1961.

Greep, R. O., and I. C. Jones. Steroid control of pituitary function. Recent Prog. Horm. Res. 5:197, 1950.

Greep, R. O., H. L. Fevold, and F. L. Hisaw. Effects of two hypophyseal gonadotropic hormones on the reproductive system of the male rat. Anat. Rec. 65:261, 1936.

Grumbach, M. M., and S. L. Kaplan. Ontogenesis of growth hormone, insulin, prolactin, and gonadotropin secretion in the human foetus. In *Proceedings of Sir Joseph Barkoft Centenary Symposium*, p. 462. London: Cambridge University Press, 1973.

Guevara, A., M. H. Luria, and R. G. Wieland. Serum gonadotropin levels during medical stress (myocardial infarction). Metabolism 19:79, 1970.

Guilbert, H. R., and H. Goss. Some effects of restricted protein intake on estrous cycle and gestation in rat. J. Nutr. 5:251, 1932.

Hafiez, A. A., C. W. Lloyd, and A. Bartke. The role of prolactin in the regulation of testis function: The effects of prolactin and luteinizing hormone on the plasma levels of testosterone and androstenedione in hypophysectomized rats. J. Endocrinol. 52:327, 1972.

Halkerston, I. D., J. Eichhorn, and O. Hechter. A requirement for reduced triphosphopyridine nucleotide for cholesterol side-chain cleavage by mitochondrial fractions of bovine adrenal cortex. J. Biol. Chem. 236:374, 1961.

Hall, P. F. Gonadotrophic regulation of testicular function. In *The androgens of the testis*, ed. K. B. Eik-Nes, p. 73. New York: Marcel Dekker, 1970.

Hall, P. F., and K. B. Eik-Nes. The action of gonadotropic hormones upon rabbit testis in vitro. Biochim. Biophys. Acta 63:411, 1962.

Hall, P. F., and D. G. Young. Site of action of trophic hormones upon the biosynthetic pathways to steroid hormones. Endocrinology 82:559, 1968.

Haltmeyer, G. C., and K. B. Eik-Nes. Production and secretion of 5α-dihydrotestosterone by the canine prostate. Acta Endocrinol. (Kbh.) 69:394, 1972.

Hansson, V., O. Djoseland, E. Reusch, A. Attramadal, and O. Torgersen. An androgen binding protein in the testis cytosol fraction of adult rats. Comparison with the androgen binding protein in the epididymis. Steroids 21:457, 1973a.

Hansson, V., F. S. French, S. C. Weddington, W. S, McLean, D. J. Tindall, A. A. Smith, and S. N. Nayfeh. Androgen transport mechanisms in the testis and epididymis. IRCS Med. Sci. (73-111) 3-10-33, 1973b.

Hansson, V., F. S. French, S. Weddington, S. N. Nayfeh, and E. M. Ritzen. FSH stimulation of testicular androgen binding protein (ABP). In *Hormone binding and target cell activation in the testis*, eds. M. L. Dufau and A. R. Means, p. 287. New York: Plenum Press, 1974a.

Hansson, V., W. S. McLean, A. A. Smith, D. J. Tindall, S C. Weddington, S. N. Nayfeh, F. S. French, and E. M. Ritzen. Androgen receptors in rat testis. Steroids 23:823, 1974b.

Harris, M. E., and A. Bartke. Maintenance of rete testis fluid testosterone and dihydrotestosterone levels by pregnenolone and other C-21 steroids in hypophysectomized rats. Eighth Annual Meeting of the Society for the Study of Reproduction, Abstract No. 145. Ottawa, Canada, August 1974.

Heindel, J. J., R. Rothenberg, G. A. Robison, and A. Steinberger. LH and FSH stimulation of cyclic AMP in specific cell types isolated from the testes. J. Cyclic Nucleotide Res. 1:69, 1975.

Hellbaum, A. A., and R. O. Greep. Qualitative changes induced in gonadotropic complex of pituitary by testosterone propionate. Endocrinology 32:33, 1943.

Heller, C. G., and W. O. Nelson. The testis-pituitary relationship in man. Recent Prog. Horm. Res. 3:229, 1948.

Holmberg, N. G., and I. Nylander. Weight loss in secondary amenorrhea. A gynecologic, endocrinologic and psychiatric investigation of 54 consecutive clinic cases. Acta Obstet. Gynecol. Scand. 50:241, 1971.

Hooker, C. W. Biology of the interstitial cells of the testis. Recent Prog. Horm. Res. 3:173, 1948.

Horton, R., and S. D. Frasier. Androstenedione and its conversion to plasma testosterone in congenital adrenal hyperplasia. J. Clin. Invest. 46:1003, 1967.

Horton, R., and J. F. Tait. Androstenedione production and inter-conversion rates measured in peripheral blood and studies on the possible site of its conversion to testosterone. J. Clin. Invest. 45:301, 1966.

Horton, R., J. M. Rosner, and P. H. Forsham. Urinary excretion pattern of injected H[3]-testosterone. Proc. Soc. Exp. Biol. Med. 114:400, 1963.

Howard, R. P., R. C. Sniffen, F. A. Simmons, and F. Albright. Testicular deficiency: A clinical and pathologic study. J. Clin. Endocrinol. Metab. 10:121, 1950.

Hudson, B., J. Coghlan, A. Dulmanis, M. Wintour, and I. Ekkel. The estimation of testosterone in biological fluids. 1. Testosterone in plasma. Aust. J. Exp. Biol. 41:235, 1963.

Ito, T., and R. Horton. The source of plasma dihydrotestosterone in man. J. Clin. Invest. 50:1621, 1971.

Job, J. C., P. E. Garnier, J. L. Chaussain, and G. Milhaud. Elevation of serum gonadotropins (LH and FSH) after releasing hormone (LH-RH) injection in normal children and in patients with disorders of puberty. J. Clin. Endocrinol. Metab. 35:473, 1972.

Johnsen, S. G. Studies on the testicular-hypophyseal feedback mechanism in man. Acta Endocrinol. (Kbh.) 45 (Suppl. 90):99, 1964.

Johnson, B. H., and L. L. Ewing. Follicle-stimulating hormone and the regulation of testosterone secretion in rabbit testes. Science 173:635, 1971.

Jones, T. M., R. L. Landau, and V. S. Fang. Effects of administration of synthetic oral androgens on testicular function in young adult men. Fifty-Sixth Annual Meeting of the Endocrine Society, Abstract No. 186. Atlanta, Georgia, June 1974.

Jost, A. La physiologie de l'hypophyse foetale. Biol. Med. (Paris) 40:205, 1951.

Judd, H. L., C. R. Hamilton, J. J. Barlow, S. S. C. Yen, and B. Kliman. Androgen and gonadotropin dynamics in testicular feminization syndrome. J. Clin. Endocrinol. Metab. 34:229, 1972.

Kastin, A. J., A. V. Schally, C. Gual, A. R. Midgley, Jr., A. Arimura, M. C. Miller III, and A. Cabeza. Administration of LH-releasing hormone of human origin to man. J. Clin. Endocrinol. Metab. 32:287, 1971.

Kelch, R. P., M. R. Jenner, R. Weinstein, S. L. Kaplan, and M. M. Grumbach. Estradiol and testosterone secretion by human, simian, and canine testes, in males with hypogonadism and in male pseudohermaphrodites with the feminizing testes syndrome. J. Clin. Invest. 51:824, 1972

Kelch, R. P., S. L. Kaplan, and M. M. Grumbach. Suppression of urinary and plasma follicle-stimulating hormone by exogenous estrogens in prepubertal and pubertal children. J. Clin. Invest. 52:1122, 1973.

Kent, J. R., and A. B. Acone. Plasma testosterone levels and aging in males. In Androgens in normal and pathological conditions, ed. A. Vermeulen, p. 31. Amsterdam: Excerpta Medica, 1966.

Keys, A. Biology of Human Starvation. Minneapolis: University of Minnesota Press, 1950.

Kinouchi, T., and R. Horton. 3α-androstanediol kinetics in man. J. Clin. Endocrinol. Metab. 38:262, 1974.

Kirschner, M. A., and C. W. Bardin. Androgen production and metabolism in normal and virilized women. Metabolism 21:667, 1972.

Kirschner, M. A., M. B. Lipsett, and D. R. Collins. Plasma ketosteroids and testosterone in man: A study of the pituitary-testicular axis. J. Clin. Invest. 44:657, 1965.

Klebanow, D. Fertilitätsstörungen als Spätfolge chronischen Hungers und schwere seelischer Traumen. Geburtshilfe Frauenheilkd. 9:420, 1949.

Kohler, P. O., G. T. Ross, and W. D. Odell. Metabolic clearance and production rates of human luteinizing hormone in pre- and postmenopausal women. J. Clin. Invest. 47:38, 1968.

Korenman, S. G., and M. B. Lipsett. Is testosterone glucuronoside uniquely derived from plasma testosterone? J. Clin. Invest. 43:2125, 1964.

Korenman, S. G., H. Wilson, and M. Lipsett. Testosterone production rates in normal adults. J. Clin. Invest. 42:1753, 1963.

Koritz, S. B. The effect of calcium ions and freezing on the in vitro synthesis of pregnenolone by rat adrenal preparations. Biochim. Biophys. Acta 56:63, 1962.

Kreuz, L. E., R. M. Rose, and J. R. Jennings. Suppression of plasma testosterone levels and psychological stress. Arch. Gen. Psychiatry 26:479, 1972.

Krieger, D. T., R. Ossowski, M. Fogel, and W. Allen. Lack of circadian periodicity of human serum FSH and LH levels. J. Clin. Endocrinol. Metab. 35:619, 1972.

Kuehl, F. A., Jr., D. J. Patanelli, J. Tarnoff, and J. L. Humes. Testicular adenyl cyclase: Stimulation by the pituitary gonadotrophins. Biol. Reprod. 2:154, 1970.

Lacy, D. Certain aspects of testis structure and function. Br. Med. Bull. 18:205, 1962.

Lacy, D. Seminiferous tubule in mammals. Endeavour 26:101, 1967.

Lacy, D., and A. J. Pettitt. Sites of hormone production in the mammalian testis, and their significance in the control of male fertility. Br. Med. Bull. 26:87, 1970.

Leathem, J. H. Hormonal and nutritional influences on the male reproductive system. Anat. Rec. 118:323, 1954.

Leathem, J. H. Nutritional effects on endocrine secretions. In Sex and internal secretions, Vol. 1, ed. W. C. Young, p. 666. Baltimore: Williams & Wilkins, 1961.

Leathem, J. H., and B. J. Brent. Influence of pregneninolone and pregnenolone on spermatogenesis in hypophysectomized adult rats. Proc. Soc. Exp. Biol. Med. 52:341, 1943.

Leathem, J. H., and V. J. DeFeo. Response of mouse gonad to equine pituitary gonadotrophins as influenced by dietary protein restriction. Anat. Rec. 112:356, 1952.

Leonard, J. M., R. B. Leach, M. Couture, and C. A. Paulsen. Plasma and urinary follicle-stimulating hormone levels in oligospermia. J. Clin. Endocrinol. Metab. 34:209, 1972.

Leydig, F. von. Lehrbuch der Histologie des Menschen und der Thiere, Frankfurt am M., 1857.

Leymarie, P., M. Roger, M. Castanier, and R. Scholler. Circadian variations of plasma testosterone and estrogens in normal men. A study by frequent sampling. J. Ster. Biochem. 5:167, 1974.

Lindner, H. Androgens and related compounds in the spermatic vein blood of domestic animals. I. Neutral steroids secreted by the bull testis. J. Endocrinol. 23:139, 1961.

Lipsett, M. B., and W. W. Tullner. Testosterone synthesis by the fetal rabbit gonad. Endocrinology 77:273, 1965.

Lipsett, M. B., H. Wilson, M. A. Kirschner, S. G. Korenman, L. M. Fishman, G. A. Sarfaty, and C. W. Bardin. Studies on Leydig cell physiology and pathology: Secretion and metabolism of testosterone. Recent Prog. Horm. Res. 22: 245, 1966.

Lloret, A. P., and J. Weisz. Metabolism of testosterone and 5α-dihydrotestosterone in vitro by the seminiferous tubules of the mature rat. Endocrinology 95:1306, 1974.

Loisel, G. Les graisses du testicule chez quelques mammifères. C. R. Soc. Biol. (Paris) 55:1009, 1903.

Longcope, C. The effect of human chorionic gonadotropin on plasma steroid levels in young and old men. Steroids 21:583, 1973.

Longcope, C., D. S. Layne, and J. F. Tait. Metabolic clearance rates and interconversions of estrone and 17β-estradiol in normal males and females. J. Clin. Invest. 47:93, 1968.

Lostroh, A. J. Effect of follicle-stimulating hormone and interstitial cell stimulating hormone on spermatogenesis in Long-Evans rats hypophysectomized for six months. Acta Endocrinol. (Kbh.) 43:592, 1963.

Lostroh, A. J., R. Johnson, and C. W. Jordan, Jr. Effect of ovine gonadotrophins and antiserum to interstitial cell-stimulating hormone on the testis of the hypophysectomized rat. Acta Endocrinol. (Kbh.) 44:536, 1963.

Lucas, W. M., W. F. Whitmore, and C. D. West. Identification of testosterone in human spermatic vein blood. J. Clin. Endocrinol. Metab. 17:465, 1957.

Lunde, D. T., and D. A. Hamburg. Techniques for assessing the effects of sex hormones on affect, arousal, and aggression in humans. Recent Prog. Horm. Res. 28:627, 1972.

McCullagh, D. R., and E. L. Walsh. Experimental hypertrophy and atrophy of the prostate gland. Endocrinology 19: 466, 1935.

McGee, L. C. Effect of injection of lipoid fraction of bull testicle in capons. Proc. Inst. Med. Chicago 6:242, 1927.

McGuire, J. S., Jr., and G. M. Tomkins. The effects of thryoxin administration on the enzymic reduction of Δ^4-3-ketosteroids. J. Biol. Chem. 234:791, 1959.

McLaren, D. S. Undernutrition. In Diseases of metabolism, 6th ed., ed. P. K. Bondy, p. 1245. Philadelphia: W. B. Saunders, 1969.

MacDonald, P. C., R. P. Rombaut, and P. K. Siiteri. Plasma precursors of estrogen. I. Extent of conversion of plasma Δ^4-androstenedione to estrone in normal males and nonpregnant normal, castrate and adrenalectomized females. J. Clin. Endocrinol. Metab. 27:1103, 1967.

Maddock, W. O., and C. G. Heller. Dichotomy between hypophyseal content and amount of circulating gonadotrophins during starvation. Proc. Soc. Exp. Biol. Med. 66:595, 1947.

Mancini, R. E., A. Castro, and A. C. Seiguer. Histologic localization of follicle-stimulating and luteinizing hormones in the rat testis. J. Histochem. Cytochem. 15:516, 1967.

Mancini, R. E., A. C. Seiguer, and A. P. Lloret. The effect of gonadotropins in the testis of hypophysectomized patients. In Gonadotropins, ed. E. Rosemberg, p. 503. Los Altos, Calif.: Geron-X, 1968.

Marrian, G. F., and A. S. Parkes. The effect of anterior pituitary preparations administered during dietary anoestrus. Proc. Roy. Soc. Lond. [Biol.] 105:248, 1929.

Marshall, J. C., D. C. Anderson, T. R. Fraser, and P. Harsoulis. Human luteinizing hormone in man: Studies of metabolism and biological action. J. Endocrinol. 56:431, 1973.

Mason, H. F. Mechanisms of oxygen metabolism. Science 125:1185, 1957.

Mason, K. E. Differences in testis injury and repair after vitamin A deficiency, vitamin E deficiency, and inanition. Am. J. Anat. 52:153, 1933.

Mason, K. E., and J. M. Wolfe. The physiological activity of the hypophysis of rats under various experimental conditions. Anat. Rec. 45:232, 1930.

Masson, G. Spermatogenic activity of various steroids. Am. J. Med. Sci. 209:324, 1945.

Mayes, D., and C. A. Nugent. Determination of plasma testosterone by the use of competitive protein binding. J. Clin. Endocrinol. Metab. 28:1169, 1968.

Means, A. R. Concerning the mechanism of FSH action: Rapid stimulation of testicular synthesis of nuclear RNA. Endocrinology 89:981, 1971.

Means, A. R., and P. F. Hall. Protein biosynthesis in the testis: I. Comparison between stimulation by FSH and glucose. Endocrinology 82:597, 1968.

Means, A. R., and J. Vaitukaitis. Peptide hormone "receptors": Specific binding of ^{3}H-FSH to testis. Endocrinology 90:39, 1972.

Means, A. R., E. MacDougall, T. R. Soderling, and J. D. Corbin. Testicular adenosine 3':5'-monophosphate-dependent protein kinase. Regulation by follicle-stimulating hormone. J. Biol. Chem. 249:1231, 1974.

Meites, J., and J. O. Reed. Effect of restricted feed intake in intact and ovariectomized rats on pituitary lactogen and gonadotrophin. Proc. Soc. Exp. Biol. Med. 70:513, 1949.

Michael, R. P. Steroids, sex attractiveness and sex behavior in primates. Fourth International Congress on Hormonal Steroids, Mexico City, 1974.

Midgley, A. R., Jr. Radioimmunoassay: A method for human chorionic gonadotropin and human luteinizing hormone. Endocrinology 79:10, 1966.

Midgley, A. R., Jr., G. D. Niswender, V. L. Gay, and L. E. Reichert, Jr. Use of antibodies for characterization of gonadotropins and steroids. Recent Prog. Horm. Res. 27:235, 1971.

Monroe, S. E., A. F. Parlow, and A. R. Midgley, Jr. Radioimmunoassay for rat luteinizing hormone. Endocrinology 83:1004, 1968.

Mont, F. G. Undernutrition. In Modern nutrition in health and disease, 4th ed., eds. M. G. Wohl and R. S. Goodhart, p. 984. Philadelphia: Lea & Febiger, 1964.

Moore, C. R., and D. Price. Gonad hormone functions and the reciprocal influence between gonads and hypophysis with its bearing on the problem of sex hormone antagonism. Am. J. Anat. 50:13, 1932.

Morris, M. D., and I. L. Chaikoff. The origin of cholesterol in liver, small intestine, adrenal gland, and testis of the rat: Dietary versus endogenous contributions. J. Biol. Chem. 234:1095, 1959.

Mulinos, M. G., and L. Pomerantz. The reproductive organs in malnutrition. Effects of chorionic gonadotropin upon atrophic genitalia of underfed male rats. Endocrinology 29: 267, 1941.

Murad, F., S. Strauch, and M. Vaughan. The effect of gonadotropins on testicular adenyl cyclase. Biochim. Biophys. Acta 177:591, 1969.

Murphy, B. E. P. Binding of testosterone and estradiol in plasma. Can. J. Biochem. 46:299, 1968.

Murphy, H. D. Sertoli cell stimulation following intratesticular injections of FSH in the hypophysectomized rat. Proc. Soc. Exp. Biol. Med. 118:1202, 1965.

Naftolin, F., and H. H. Feder. Suppression of luteinizing hormone secretion in male rats by 5α-androstan-17β-ol-3-one (dihydrotestosterone) propionate. J. Endocrinol. 56:155, 1973.

Naftolin, F., S. S. C. Yen, and C. C. Tsai. Gonadotrophins —Rapid cycling of plasma in normal men. Nature New Biol. 236:92, 1972a.

Naftolin, F., K. J. Ryan, and Z. Petro. Aromatization of androstenedione by the anterior hypothalamus of adult male and female rats. Endocrinology 90:295, 1972b.

Naftolin, F., H. L. Judd, and S. S. C. Yen. Pulsatile patterns of gonadotropins and testosterone in man: The effects of clomiphene with and without testosterone. J. Clin. Endocrinol. Metab. 36:285, 1973.

Nankin, H. R., and P. Troen. Repetitive luteinizing hormone elevations in serum of normal men. J. Clin. Endocrinol. Metab. 33:558, 1971.

Nankin, H. R., and P. Troen. Overnight patterns of serum luteinizing hormone in normal men. J. Clin. Endocrinol. Metab. 35:705, 1972.

Nelson, W. O., and T. F. Gallagher. Some effects of androgenic substances in the rat. Science 84:230, 1936.

Ney, R. L. The anterior pituitary gland. In Diseases of metabolism, 6th ed., ed. P. K. Bondy, p. 718. Philadephia: W. B. Saunders, 1969.

Nieschlag, E., K. H. Kley, and W. Wiegelmann. Age dependence of the endocrine testicular function in adult men. Acta Endocrinol. (Kbh.) Suppl. 177:122, 1973.

Niswender, G. D., A. R. Midgley, Jr., S. E. Monroe, and L. E. Reichert, Jr. Radioimmunoassay for rat luteinizing hormone with antiovine LH serum and ovine LH-131I. Proc. Soc. Exp. Biol. Med. 128:807, 1968.

Northcutt, R. C., D. P. Island, and G. W. Liddle. An explanation for the target organ unresponsiveness to testosterone in the testicular feminization syndrome. J. Clin. Endocrinol. Metab. 29:422, 1969.

Noumura, T., J. Weisz, and C. W. Lloyd. In vitro conversion of 7-3H-progesterone to androgens by the rat testis during the second half of fetal life. Endocrinology 78:245, 1966.

Odell, W. D., and R. S. Swerdloff. Radioimmunoassay of luteinizing and follicle-stimulating hormones in human serum. In Radioisotopes in medicine: In vitro studies, eds. R. L. Hayes, F. A. Goswitz, and B. E. P. Murphy, p. 165. A.E.C. Symposium Series, No. 13, 1968.

Odell, W. D., G. T. Ross, and P. L. Rayford. Radioimmuno-assay for human luteinizing hormone. Metabolism 15:287, 1966.

Odell, W. D., G. T. Ross, and P. L. Rayford. Radioimmuno-assay for LH in human plasma or serum: Physiological studies. J. Clin. Invest. 46:248, 1967.

Odell, W. D., A. F. Parlow, C. M. Cargille, and G. T. Ross. Radioimmunoassay for human follicle-stimulating hormone: Physiological studies. J. Clin. Invest. 47:2551, 1968.

Odell, W. D., R. S. Swerdloff, H. S. Jacobs, and M. A. Hescox. FSH induction of sensitivity to LH: One cause of sexual maturation in the male rat. Endocrinology 92:160, 1973.

Odell, W. D., R. S. Swerdloff, J. Bain, F. Wollesen, and P. K. Grover. The effect of sexual maturation on testicular response to LH stimulation of testosterone secretion in the intact rat. Endocrinology 95:1380, 1974.

Paesi, F. J. A., S. E. deJongh, M. J. Hoogstra, and A. Engelbregt. The follicle-stimulating hormone-content of the hypophysis of the rat as influenced by gonadectomy and oestrogen treatment. Acta Endocrinol. (Kbh.) 19:49, 1955.

Parlow, A. F. Differential action of small doses of estradiol on gonadotrophins in the rat. Endocrinology 75:1, 1964.

Paul, W. E., and W. D. Odell. Radiation inactivation of the immunological and biological activities of human chorionic gonadotropin. Nature 203:979, 1964.

Paulsen, C. A. Effect of human chorionic gonadotrophin and human menopausal gonadotrophin therapy on testicular function. In Gonadotropins, ed. E. Rosemberg, p. 491. Los Altos, Calif.: Geron-X, 1968.

Paulsen, C. A., D. L. Gordon, R. W. Carpenter, H. M. Gandy, and W. D. Drucker. Klinefelter's syndrome and its variants: A hormonal and chromosomal study. Recent Prog. Horm. Res. 24:321, 1968.

Paulsen, C. A. The testes. In Textbook of endocrinology, 5th ed., ed. R. H. Williams, p. 323. Philadelphia: W. B. Saunders, 1974.

Pazos, R., Jr., and C. Huggins. Effect of androgen on the prostate in starvation. Endocrinology 36:416, 1945.

Pearlman, W. H., O. Crépy, and M. Murphy. Testosterone-binding levels in the serum of women during the normal menstrual cycle, pregnancy, and the postpartum period. J. Clin. Endocrinol. Metab. 27:1012, 1967.

Perloff, W. H., E. M. Lasché, J. H. Nodine, N. G. Schneeberg, and C. B. Vieillard. The starvation state and functional hypopituitarism. JAMA 155:1307, 1954.

Peterson, N. T., Jr., A. R. Midgley, Jr., and R. B. Jaffe. Regulation of human gonadotropins. III. Luteinizing hormone and follicle stimulating hormone in sera from adult males. J. Clin. Endocrinol. Metab. 28:1473, 1968.

Pincus, G. Aging and urinary steroid excretion. In Hormones and the aging process, eds. E. T. Engle and G. Pincus, p. 1. New York: Academic Press, 1956.

Pomerantz, L., and M. G. Mulinos. Pseudo-hypophysectomy produced by inanition. Am. J. Physiol. 126:P601, 1939.

Price, D., and R. Pannabecker. Organ culture studies of foetal rat reproductive tracts. Ciba Foundation Colloquia on Aging 2:3, 1956.

Ramirez, V. D., and S. M. McCann. Comparison of the regulation of luteinizing hormone (LH) secretion in immature and adult rats. Endocrinology 72:452, 1963a.

Ramirez, V. D., and S. M. McCann. Increased sensitivity of immature male rats to negative feedback of testosterone on luteinizing hormone secretion. Forty-fifth Annual Meeting of the Endocrine Society, Abstract No. 155, Atlantic City, N.J., June 1963b.

Ramirez, V. D., and S. M. McCann. Inhibition effect of testosterone on luteinizing hormone secretion in immature and adult rats. Endocrinology 76:412, 1965.

Randolph, P. W., A. J. Lostroh, R. Grattarola, P. G. Squire, and P. H. Li. Effect of ovine interstitial cell-stimulating hormone on spermatogenesis in the hypophysectomized mouse. Endocrinology 65:433, 1959.

Reddi, A. H., L. L. Ewing, and H. G. Williams-Ashman. Protein phosphokinase reactions in mammalian testis. Stimulatory effects of adenosine $3':5'$-cyclic monophosphate on the phosphorylation of basic proteins. Biochem. J. 122:333, 1971.

Reichlin, S. Neuroendocrinology. In Textbook of endocrinology, 5th ed., ed. R. H. Williams, p. 774. Philadelphia: W. B. Saunders, 1974.

Reid, J. T. Relationship of nutrition to fertility in animals. J. Am. Vet. Med. Assoc. 114:158, 1949.

Resko, J. A., and K. B. Eik-Nes. Diurnal testosterone levels in peripheral plasma of human male subjects. J. Clin. Endocrinol. Metab. 26:573, 1966.

Rifkind, A. B., H. E. Kulin, and G. T. Ross. Follicle-stimulating hormone (FSH) and luteinizing hormone (LH) in the urine of prepubertal children. J. Clin. Invest. 46:1925, 1967.

Rinaldini, L. M. Effect of chronic inanition on the gonadotrophic content of the pituitary gland. J. Endocrinol. 6:54, 1949.

Riondel, A., J. F. Tait, M. Gut, S. A. S. Tait, E. Joachim, and B. Little. Estimation of testosterone in human peripheral blood using S^{35}-thiosemicarbazide. J. Clin. Endocrinol. Metab. 23:620, 1963.

Ritzen, E. M., S. N. Nayfeh, F. S. French, and M. C. Dobbins. Demonstration of androgen binding components of rat epididymis cytosol and comparison with binding components in prostate and other tissues. Endocrinology 89:143, 1971.

Ritzen, E. M., M. C. Dobbins, D. J. Tindall, F. S. French, and S. N. Nayfeh. Characterization of an androgen binding protein in rat testis and epididymis. Steroids 21:593, 1973.

Rivarola, M. A., E. J. Podesta, and H. E. Chemes. In vitro testosterone-^{14}C metabolism by rat seminiferous tubules at different stages of development: Formation of 5α-androstandiol at meiosis. Endocrinology 91:537, 1972.

Rizkallah, T., M. L. Taymor, M. Park, and R. Batt. An immunoassay method for human luteinizing hormone of pituitary origin. J. Clin. Endocrinol. Metab. 25:943, 1965.

Rocca, D., and A. Albert. Daily urinary excretion of follicle-stimulating hormone during the menstrual cycle. Mayo Clin. Proc. 42:536, 1967.

Roosen-Runge, E. C., and D. Anderson. The development of the interstitial cells in the testis of the albino rat. Acta Anat. (Basel) 37:125, 1959.

Root, A. W., and R. D. Russ. Short-term effects of castration and starvation upon pituitary and serum levels of luteinizing hormone and follicle stimulating hormone in male rats. Acta Endocrinol. (Kbh.) 70:665, 1972.

Rosen, S. W., and B. D. Weintraub. Monotropic increase of serum FSH correlated with low sperm count in young men with idiopathic oligospermia and aspermia. J. Clin. Endocrinol. Metab. 32:410, 1971.

Roth, J. C., M. M. Grumbach, and S. L. Kaplan. Effect of synthetic luteinizing hormone-releasing factor on serum testosterone and gonadotropins in prepubertal, pubertal and adult males. J. Clin. Endocrinol. Metab. 37:680, 1973.

Ruben, G., and A. Vermeulen. J. Clin. Endocrinol. Metab., in press.

Rubens, R., M. Dhont, and A. Vermeulen. Further studies on Leydig cell function in old age. J. Clin. Endocrinol. Metab. 39:40, 1974.

Rubin, R. T., A. Kales, R. Adler, T. Fagan, and W. D. Odell. Gonadotropin secretion during sleep in normal adult men. Science 175:196, 1972.

Ruzicka, L., and V. Prelog. Untersuchungen von Extrakten aus Testes. (1. Mitteilung). Zur Kenntnis der Lipoide aus Schweinetestes. Helv. Chim. Acta 26:975, 1943.

Ryan, R. J., and C. Faiman. Radioimmunoassay of FSH and LH in human serum: The effects of age, and infusion of several polyamines in males. In Gonadotropins, ed. E. Rosemberg, p. 333. Los Altos, Calif.: Geron-X, 1968.

Ryan, R. J., M. D. Cloutier, A. B. Hayles, J. Paris, and R. V. Randall. The clinical utility of radioimmunoassays for serum follicle-stimulating hormone (FSH) and luteinizing hormone (LH). Med. Clin. North Am. 54:1049, 1970.

Saez, J. M., and J. Bertrand. Studies on testicular function in children: Plasma concentrations of testosterone, dihydroepiandrosterone and its sulfate before and after stimulation with human chorionic gonadotrophin (1). Steroids 12:749, 1968.

Saez, J. M., E. de Peretti, A. M. Morera, M. David, and J. Bertrand. Familial male pseudohermaphroditism with gynecomastia due to a testicular 17-ketosteroid reductase defect. I. Studies in vivo. J. Clin. Endocrinol. Metab. 32:604, 1971.

Saginor, M., and R. Horton. Reflex release of gonadotropin and increased plasma testosterone concentration in male rabbits during copulation. Endocrinology 82:627, 1968.

Samuels, L. T., and H. Helmreich. The influence of chorionic gonadotropin on the 3β-ol dehydrogenase activity of testes and adrenals. Endocrinology 58:435, 1956.

Samuels, L. T., L. Bussmann, K. Matsumoto, and R. A. Huseby. Organization of androgen biosynthesis in the testis. Fourth International Congress on Hormonal Steroids, Mexico City, September 1974.

Sanborn, B. M., J. S. H. Elkington, A. K. Chowdhury, R. K. Tcholakian, and E. Steinberger. Hormonal influences on the level of testicular androgen binding activity: Effect of FSH following hypophysectomy. Endocrinology 96:304, 1975a.

Sanborn, B. M., J. S. H. Elkington, A. Steinberger, E. Steinberger, and M. L. Meistrich. Androgen binding in the testis: In vitro production of androgen binding protein by Sertoli cell cultures and measurement of nuclear bound androgen by a nuclear exchange assay. In *Hormonal regulation of spermatogenesis*, eds. F. S. French, V. Hansson, E. M. Ritzen, and S. N. Nayfeh, p. 293. New York: Plenum Press, 1975b.

Sanborn, B. M., J. S. H. Elkington, and E. Steinberger. Properties of rat testicular androgen binding proteins. In *Hormone binding and target cell activation in the testis*, eds. M. L. Dufau and A. R. Means, p. 291. New York: Plenum Press, 1974.

Santen, R. J., and C. W. Bardin. Episodic luteinizing hormone secretion in man. Pulse analysis, clinical interpretation, physiologic mechanisms. J. Clin. Invest. 52:2617, 1973.

Sasano, N., and S. Ichijo. Vascular patterns of the human testis with special reference to its senile changes. Tohoku J. Exp. Med. 99:269, 1969.

Satoh, P., G. Constantopoulos, and T. T. Tchen. Cleavage of cholesterol side chain by adrenal cortex. IV. Effect of phosphate and various nucleotides on a soluble enzyme system. Biochemistry 5:1646, 1966.

Savard, K., R. K. Dorfman, and E. Poutasse. Biogenesis of androgens in the human testis. J. Clin. Endocrinol. Metab. 12:935, 1952.

Saxena, B. B., R. Malva, G. Leyendecker, and H. M. Gandy. Further characterization of the radioimmunoassay of human pituitary FSH. In *Gonadotropins*, eds. B. Saxena, C. G. Beling, and H. M. Gandy, p. 399. New York: Wiley-Interscience, 1972.

Schalch, D. S., A. F. Parlow, R. C. Boon, and S. Reichlin. Measurement of human LH in plasma by radioimmunoassay. J. Clin. Invest. 47:665, 1968.

Schally, A. V., R. M. G. Nair, T. W. Redding, and A. Arimura. Isolation of the luteinizing hormone and follicle-stimulating hormone-releasing hormone from porcine hypothalami. J. Biol. Chem. 246:7230, 1971.

Schiavi, R. C., D. M. Davis. D. White, A. Edwards, G. Igel, and C. Fisher. Plasma testosterone during nocturnal sleep in normal men. Steroids 24:191, 1974.

Schlaff, S., S. W. Rosen, and J. Roth. Antibody to human follicle-stimulating hormone: Cross-reactivity with three other hormones. J. Clin. Invest. 47:1722, 1968.

Schriefers, H. Factors regulating the metabolism of steroids. Vitam. Horm. 25:271, 1967.

Selye, H., and S. Friedman. The action of various steroid hormones on the testis. Endocrinology 28:129, 1941.

Serra, B. G., G. Perez-Palacios, and R. B. Jaffe. De novo testosterone biosynthesis in the human fetal testis. J. Clin. Endocrinol. Metab. 30:141, 1970.

Sertoli, E. Dell'esistenza di particolari cellule ramificati nei canalicoli seminiferi del testicolo umano. Il Morgagni 7:31, 1865.

Sherins, R. J., and D. L. Loriaux. Studies on the role of sex steroids in the feedback control of FSH concentrations in men. J. Clin. Endocrinol. Metab. 36:886, 1973.

Shimizu, K., M. Gut, and R. I. Dorfman. 20, 22α-dihydroxy-cholesterol, and intermediate in the biosynthesis of pregnenolone (3β-hydroxypregn-5-en-20-one) from cholesterol. J. Biol. Chem. 237:699, 1962.

Siiteri, P., and J. D. Wilson. Dihydrotestosterone in prostatic hypertrophy. I. The formation and content of dihydrotestosterone in the hypertrophic prostate of man. J. Clin. Invest. 49:1737, 1970.

Siiteri, P., and J. D. Wilson. Testosterone formation and metabolism during male sexual differentiation in the human embryo. J. Clin. Endocrinol. Metab. 38:113, 1974.

Simpson, M. E., C. H. Li, and H. M. Evans. Sensitivity of reproductive system of hypophysectomized 40 day male rats to gonadotropic substances. Endocrinology 35:96, 1944.

Sizonenko, P. C., A. Cuendet, and L. Paunier. FSH. I. Evidence for its mediating role on testosterone secretion in cryptorchidism. J. Clin. Endocrinol. Metab. 37:68, 1973.

Smith, K. D., R. K. Tcholakian, M. Chowdhury, and E. Steinberger. Rapid oscillations in plasma levels of testosterone, LH and FSH in man. Fertil. Steril. 25:965, 1974.

Southren, A. K., G. G. Gordon, and S. Tochimoto. Further study of factors affecting the metabolic clearance rate of testosterone in man. J. Clin. Endocrinol. Metab. 28:1105, 1968.

Srere, P. A., I. L. Chaikoff, S. S. Treitman, and L. S. Burstein. The extra-hepatic synthesis of cholesterol. J. Biol. Chem. 182:629, 1950.

Staple, E., W. S. Lynn, Jr., and S. Gurin. An enzymatic cleavage of the cholesterol side chain. J. Biol. Chem. 219:845, 1956.

Stearns, E. L., J. S. D. Winter, and C. Faiman. Effects of aging on serum testosterone, free testosterone and serum gonadotropin levels in men. Fifty-fifth Annual Meeting of the Endocrine Society, Abstract No. 96. Chicago, Ill., 1973.

Steinberger, A., and E. Steinberger. Replication pattern of Sertoli cells in maturing rat testis in vivo and in organ culture. Biol. Reprod. 4:84, 1971.

Steinberger, A., M. Ficher, and E. Steinberger. Studies of spermatogenesis and steroid metabolism in cultures of human testicular tissue. In *The human testis*, eds. E. Rosemberg and C. A. Paulsen, p. 333. New York: Plenum Press, 1970.

Steinberger, A., K. H. Thanki, and B. Siegal. FSH binding in rat testes during maturation and following hypophysectomy. Cellular localization of FSH receptors. In *Hormone binding and target cell activation in the testis*, eds. M. L. Dufau and A. R. Means, p. 177. New York: Plenum Press, 1974a.

Steinberger, A., K. H. Thanki, and B. Siegal. Sertoli cells—primary site of FSH activity in the testes. Seventh Annual Meeting of the Society for the Study of Reproduction, Abstract No. 21. Ottawa, Canada, August 1974b.

Steinberger, A., J. J. Heindel, J. N. Lindsey, J. S. H. Elkington, B. M. Sanborn, and E. Steinberger. Isolation and culture of FSH responsive Sertoli cells. Endocrinol. Res. Commun. 2:261, 1975.

Steinberger, E. Hormonal control of mammalian spermatogenesis. Physiol. Rev. 51:1, 1971.

Steinberger, E. Maturation of male germinal epithelium. In *Control of onset of puberty*, eds. M. M. Grumbach, G. D.

Grave, and F. E. Mayer, p. 386. New York: John Wiley & Sons, 1974.

Steinberger, E., and A. Chowdhury. Effect of C_{21} steroids on spermatogenesis in hypophysectomized rats. Fifty-fifth Annual Meeting of the Endocrine Society, Abstract No. 98. Chicago, Ill., 1973.

Steinberger, E., and M. Chowdhury. Control of pituitary FSH in male rats. Acta Endocrinol. (Kbh.) 76:235, 1974.

Steinberger, E., and G. E. Duckett. Pituitary "total" gonadotropins: FSH and LH in orchiectomized or cryptorchid rats. Endocrinology 79:912, 1966.

Steinberger, E., and G. E. Duckett. Effect of testosterone on the release of FSH from the pituitary gland. Acta Endocrinol. (Kbh.) 57:289, 1968.

Steinberger, E., and M. Ficher. Conversion of progesterone to testosterone by testicular tissue at different stages of maturation. Steroids 11:351, 1968.

Steinberger, E., and M. Ficher. Differentiation of steroid biosynthetic pathways in developing testes. Biol. Reprod. 1 (Suppl. 1):119, 1969.

Steinberger, E., amd M. Ficher. Effect of hypophysectomy and gonadotropin treatment on metabolism of ^{3}H-progesterone by rat testicular tissue. Steroids 22:425, 1973.

Steinberger, E., and A. Steinberger. The spermatogenic function of the testes. In *The gonads*, ed. K. W. McKerns, p. 715. New York: Appleton-Century-Crofts, 1969.

Steinberger, E., A. Steinberger, and W. H. Perloff. Initiation of spermatogenesis in vitro. Endocrinology 74:788, 1964.

Steinberger, E., A. Steinberger, O. Vilar, I. I. Salamon, and B. N. Sud. Microscopy, cytochemistry and steroid biosynthetic activity of Leydig cells in culture. In *Endocrinology of the testis*, Ciba Foundation Colloquia on Endocrinology 16, eds. G. E. W. Wolstenholme and M. O'Connor, p. 56. Boston: Little, Brown, 1967.

Steinberger, E., A. Steinberger, and M. Ficher. Study of spermatogenesis and steroid metabolism in cultures of mammalian testes. Recent Prog. Horm. Res. 26:547, 1970a.

Steinberger, E., M. Ficher, and K. D. Smith. Relation of in vitro metabolism of steroids in human testicular tissue to histologic and clinical findings. In *The human testis*, eds. E. Rosemberg and C. A. Paulsen, p. 439. New York: Plenum Press, 1970b.

Steinberger, E., A. Root, M. Ficher, and K. D. Smith. The role of androgens in the initiation of spermatogenesis in man. J. Clin. Endocrinol. Metab. 37:746, 1973.

Steinberger, E., A. Steinberger, and B. Sanborn. Endocrine control of spermatogenesis. In *Physiology and genetics of reproduction, Part A*, eds. E. M. Coutinho and F. Fuchs, p. 163. New York: Plenum Press, 1974a.

Steinberger, E., K. D. Smith, R. K. Tcholakian, A. K. Chowdhury, A. Steinberger, M. Ficher, and C. A. Paulsen. Steroidogenesis in human testes. In *Male fertility and sterility*, Proceedings of the Serono Symposia, Vol. 5, eds. R. E. Mancini and L. Martini, p. 149. New York: Academic Press, 1974b.

Steinberger, E., M. Ficher, and K. D. Smith. An enzymatic defect in androgen biosynthesis in human testis: A case report and response to therapy. Andrologia 6:59, 1974c.

Steinberger, E., A. K. Chowdhury, R. K. Tcholakian, and H. Roll. Effect of C_{21} steroids on sex accessory organs and testes of mature hypophysectomized rats. Endocrinology 96: 1319, 1975.

Stewart-Bentley, M., W. D. Odell, and R. Horton. The feedback control of luteinizing hormone in normal adult men. J. Clin. Endocrinol. Metab. 38:545, 1974.

Strott, C. A., and M. B. Lipsett. Measurement of 17-hydroxyprogesterone in human plasma. J. Clin. Endocrinol. Metab. 28:1426, 1968.

Stylianou, M., E. Forchielli, M. Tummillo, and R. I. Dorfman. Metabolism in vitro of 4-C^{14} testosterone by a human liver homogenate. J. Biol. Chem. 236:692, 1961.

Suryanarayana, B. V., J. R. Kent, L. Meister, and A. F. Parlow. Pituitary-gonadal axis during prolonged total starvation in obese men. Am. J. Clin. Nutr. 22:767, 1969.

Sutherland, E. W., and T. W. Rall. Formation of a cyclic adenine ribonucleotide by tissue particles. J. Biol. Chem. 232:1077, 1962.

Svagr, A. J., D. L. Hammell, M. J. Degeeter, V. W. Hays, G. L. Cromwell, and R. H. Dutt. Reproductive performance of sows on a protein-restricted diet. J. Reprod. Fertil. 30: 455, 1972.

Swerdloff, R. S., and W. D. Odell. Gonadotropins: Present concepts in the human. Calif. Med. 109:467, 1968a.

Swerdloff, R. S., and W. D. Odell. Feedback control of LH and FSH secretion. Lancet 2:683, 1968b.

Swerdloff, R. S., and P. C. Walsh. Testosterone and estradiol suppression of LH and FSH in adult male rats: Duration of castration, duration of treatment and combined treatment. Acta Endocrinol. (Kbh.) 73:11, 1973.

Swerdloff, R. S., P. C. Walsh, H. S. Jacobs, and W. D. Odell. Serum LH and FSH during sexual maturation in the male rat: Effect of castration and cryptorchidism. Endocrinology 88:120, 1971.

Swerdloff, R. S., H. S. Jacobs, and W. D. Odell. Hypothalamic-pituitary-gonadal interrelations in the rat during sexual maturation. In *Gonadotropins*, eds. B. B. Saxena, C. C. Beling, and H. M. Gandy, p. 546. New York: Wiley-Interscience, 1972a.

Swerdloff, R. S., P. C. Walsh, and W. C. Odell. Control of LH and FSH secretion in the male: Evidence that aromatization of androgens to estradiol is not required for inhibition of gonadotropin secretion. Steroids 20:13, 1972b.

Swerdloff, R. S., P. K. Grover, H. S. Jacobs, and J. Bain. Search for a substance which selectively inhibits FSH— Effects of steroids and prostaglandins on serum FSH and LH levels. Steroids 21:703, 1973.

Tait, J. F. Review: The use of isotopic steroids for the measurement of production rates in vivo. J. Clin. Endocrinol. Metab. 23:1285, 1963.

Tamaoki, B.-I., H. Inano, and H. Nakano. In vitro synthesis and conversion of androgens in testicular tissue. In *The gonads*, ed. K. W. McKerns, p. 547. New York: Appleton-Century-Crofts, 1969.

Tcholakian, R. K. Relationship of levels of testicular and plasma testosterone and sex accessory weights in 1 to 120 day old rats. Seventh Annual Meeting of the Society for the

Study of Reproduction, Abstract No. 140. Ottawa, Canada, August 1974.

Tcholakian, R. K., M. Chowdhury, and E. Steinberger. Time of action of 17β-oestradiol on luteinizing hormone and testosterone. J. Endocrinol. 63:411, 1974.

VanDemark, N. L., and L. L. Ewing. Factors affecting testicular metabolism and function. I. A simplified perfusion technique for short-term maintenance of rabbit testis. J. Reprod. Fertil. 6:1, 1963.

Vanderlinde, R. E., and W. W. Westerfeld. The inactivation of estrone by rats in relation to dietary effects on the liver. Endocrinology 47:265, 1950.

Vande Wiele, R. L., P. C. MacDonald, E. Gurpide, and S. Lieberman. Studies on the secretion and interconversion of the androgens. Recent Prog. Horm. Res. 19:275, 1963.

Van Thiel, D. H., R. J. Sherins, G. H. Myers, Jr., and V. T. DeVita, Jr. Evidence for a specific seminiferous tubular factor affecting follicle-stimulating hormone secretion in man. J. Clin. Invest. 51:1009, 1972.

Vermeulen, A., L. Verdonck, M. van der Straeten, and N. Orie. Capacity of the testosterone-binding globulin in human plasma and influence of specific binding of testosterone on its metabolic clearance rate. J. Clin. Endocrinol. Metab. 29:1470, 1969.

Vermeulen, A., R. Rubens, and L. Verdonck. Testosterone secretion and metabolism in male senescence. J. Clin. Endocrinol. Metab. 34:730, 1972.

Vernon, R. G., J. H. Dorrington, and I. B. Fritz. Testosterone binding by rat testicular seminiferous tubules. Fourth International Congress of Endocrinology, Washington, D.C., June 1972.

Vernon, R. G., B. Kopec, and I. B. Fritz. Studies on the distribution of the high-affinity testosterone-binding protein in rat seminiferous tubules. J. Endocrinol. 57:ii, 1973.

Vilar, O., A. Steinberger, and E. Steinberger. An electron microscopic study of cultured rat testicular fragments. Z. Zellforsch. 78:221, 1967.

von Berswordt-Wallrabe, R., and F. Neumann. Successful reinitiation and restoration of spermatogenesis in hypophysectomized rats with pregnant mare's serum after a long-term regression period. Experientia 24:499, 1968.

von Berswordt-Wallrabe, R., H. Steinbeck, and F. Neumann. Effect of FSH on the testicular structure of rats. Endokrinologie 53:35, 1968.

Walsh, P. C., R. S. Swerdloff, and W. D. Odell. Feedback control of FSH in the male: Role of estrogen. Acta Endocrinol. (Kbh.) 74:449, 1973a.

Walsh, P. C., R. S. Swerdloff, and W. D. Odell. Feedback regulation of gonadotropin secretion in men. J. Urol. 110:84, 1973b.

Werner, S. C. Failure of gonadotropic function of the rat hypophysis during chronic inanition. Proc. Soc. Exp. Biol. Med. 41:101, 1939.

West, C. D., V. P. Hollander, T. H. Kritchevsky, and K. Dobriner. The isolation and identification of testosterone, Δ⁴-androstenedione-3,17, and 7-ketocholesterol from spermatic vein blood. J. Clin. Endocrinol. Metab. 12:915, 1952.

Wide, L. An immunological method for the assay of human chorionic gonadotrophin. Acta Endocrinol. (Kbh.) Suppl. 70, 1962.

Wilson, J. D. Recent studies on the mechanism of action of testosterone. N. Engl. J. Med. 287:1284, 1972.

Wilson, J. D., and J. D. Walker. The conversion of testosterone to 5α-androstan-17β-ol-3-one (dihydrotestosterone) by skin slices of man. J. Clin. Invest. 48:371, 1969.

Winter, J. S. D., and C. Faiman. Serum gonadotropin concentrations in agonadal children and adults. J. Clin. Endocrinol. Metab. 35:561, 1972a.

Winter, J. S. D., and C. Faiman. Pituitary-gonadal relations in male children and adolescents. Pediatr. Res. 6:126, 1972b.

Woods, M. C., and M. E. Simpson. Pituitary control of the testis of the hypophysectomized rat. Endocrinology 69:91, 1961.

Wurtman, R. J., and J. D. Fernstrom. Effects of the diet on brain neurotransmitters. Nutr. Rev. 32:193, 1974.

Yago, N., and S. Ichii. Submitochondrial distribution of components of the steroid 11β-hydroxylase and cholesterol sidechain-cleaving enzyme systems in hog adrenal cortex. J. Biochem. 65:215, 1969.

Yalow, R. S., and S. A. Berson. Immunoassay of endogenous plasma insulin in man. J. Clin. Invest. 39:1157, 1960.

Yates, F. E., and J. Urquhart. Control of plasma concentrations of adreno-cortical hormones. Physiol. Rev. 42:359, 1962.

Zacharias, L., and R. J. Wurtman. Blindness: Its relation to age of menarche. Science 144:1154, 1964.

Zachmann, M., J. A. Vollmin, G. Mürset, H.-Ch. Curtius, and A. Prader. Unusual type of congenital adrenal hyperplasia probably due to deficiency of 3β-hydroxysteroid dehydrogenase. Case report of a surviving girl and steroid studies. J. Clin. Endocrinol. Metab. 30:719, 1970.

Zachmann, M., A. Vollmin, W. Hamilton, and A. Prader. Steroid 17, 20-desmolase deficiency: A new cause of male pseudohermaphroditism. Clin. Endocrinol. (Oxford) 1:369, 1972.

Zubirán, S., and F. Gómez-Mont. Endocrine disturbances in chronic human malnutrition. Vitam. Horm. 11:97, 1953.

27 Spermatogenesis

Yves Clermont

27.1 Mammalian Spermatogenesis

Spermatogenesis is the elaborate cytological process by which a spermatogonial stem cell produces the spermatozoa. This process of cell differentiation lasts five to eight weeks, depending on the animal species, and takes place within the delicate seminiferous tubules forming the bulk of the testis. The elaboration of spermatozoa by the seminiferous epithelium is so intricate that its analysis at the biochemical level has been initiated only recently. Less work is being done at present on the formation of the spermatozoon than on the biochemical composition and modification of the fully formed spermatozoon as it travels through the male and female reproductive tract; however, numerous microscopists have studied the morphological or structural aspects of the spermatogenic process.

Spermatogenesis can be divided into three phases, each presenting well-characterized and distinctive cytological features. The first phase concerns the youngest cells of the germ cell line, the spermatogonia; most of these cells proliferate to give rise to spermatocytes, while the remainder maintain their own number by renewing themselves. The second phase involves the primary and secondary spermatocytes that go through a process of reductional or meiotic divisions leading to the formation of haploid cells, the spermatids. The third phase concerns the spermatids, each of which goes through a complex metamorphosis leading to the production of a highly differentiated motile cell, the spermatozoon.

Spermatogonial Proliferation, Differentiation, and Renewal

During the past decade a good deal of attention has been given to the behavior of spermatogonia (5, 32). The continuous production of spermatozoa by the seminiferous epithelium, resulting in the maintenance of male fertility, depends on the active proliferation of spermatogonia, which must yield large numbers of differentiating cells, the spermatocytes as well as cells of their own kind, to serve as future stem cells. The importance of this phase of spermatogenesis in terms of the biology of fertility is therefore obvious, since a depletion of the stem cell population results in temporary or permanent sterility.

At the end of the last century the French histologist

Claude Regaud (31), in his classical studies on the rat seminiferous epithelium, made a clear distinction, in terms of morphological appearance and function, between two main categories of spermatogonia: the dustlike spermatogonia, now called the type A spermatogonia, and the crustlike spermatogonia, now referred to as type B spermatogonia. The former show an interphasic nucleus containing a finely granulated dustlike chromatin; they are considered to be nondifferentiated or noncommitted cells, and "stem cells" are to be found among them. The latter show an interphasic nucleus with distinct flakes or crusts of deeply stained chromatin attached to the nuclear membrane; these cells are committed to the production of spermatocytes and are therefore termed differentiating spermatogonia. This classification of spermatogonia was initially devised for the rat but was later found to be applicable to all mammals, including humans (5). Obviously there are some differences in the nuclear characteristics of the spermatogonia among species; however, type A and type B spermatogonia can be easily identified in all species.

As a result of more recent investigations, done mainly in rats, mice, and monkeys, each one of these two categories of spermatogonia can now be subdivided into subtypes (5). The differences between rodents and primates are important enough for each to be separately reviewed.

The spermatogonial population of the rat has been extensively studied in both radioautographs of testicular sections and dissected tubules from animals injected with ^{3}H-thymidine. Observations on such material led to the conclusion that among the type A spermatogonia were two classes of stem cells that could be distinguished on the basis of their morphological characteristics and proliferative behavior. The first class was called "reserve type A" or "type A_0" spermatogonia. Isolated or paired along the tubular limiting membrane, these cells were found to be generally quiescent (i.e., they did not actively divide), as indicated by their low mitotic index and their negligible labeling index after ^{3}H-thymidine administration. The second class was called the "renewing type A" spermatogonia. These cells were arranged in groups of four or more cells along the tubular wall. They proliferated actively and in a quasisynchronous manner. In the rat or mouse, four successive generations of these cells (types A_1–A_4) appear along the tubular limiting membrane. Thus type A_1 cells give rise to type A_2 cells, which in turn yield type A_3 cells, which finally produce type A_4 cells. As a result of the divisions of the type A_4 spermatogonia, two categories of cells are formed along the tubular wall: new type A_1 cells and the so-called intermediate-type spermatogonia (in fact, these cells belong to the general type B category, and they are committed to produce spermatocytes). The intermediate spermatogonia divide to give rise to type B spermatogonia, which in turn produce a generation of primary spermatocytes. This scheme of spermatogonial renewal in rodents, which proposes the existence of two classes of spermatogonial stem cells, was questioned by some authors (22, 28), but recent observations on the rat (20) indicate that the scheme is valid.

Several studies on various species of monkeys also supported the existence of two classes of spermatogonial stem cells (4, 6). In monkeys as well as in man (3), type A spermatogonia can be classified on the basis of their nuclear characteristics into two distinct classes: the dark and the pale type A spermatogonia. The dark type A cells have a nucleus containing a finely granulated but deeply stained chromatin, while the pale type A cells have a nucleus showing a finely granulated but pale stained chromatin. The dark type A spermatogonia form the nonproliferative elements of the spermatogonial population, since they do not incorporate ^{3}H-thymidine and thus can be considered reserve stem cells. The pale type A spermatogonia periodically divide, and as a result of these mitoses, new pale type A spermatogonia are produced that can serve as stem cells, and type B spermatogonia are produced that are destined to become spermatocytes. The pale type A cells can thus be considered as renewing stem cells. In monkeys four consecutive generations of type B (B_1–B_4) cells appear along the tubular limiting membrane, the last generation (type B_4) being the progenitors of primary spermatocytes. In men there are also dark and pale type A as well as type B spermatogonia, but their exact proliferative behavior remains to be clarified.

Why emphasize the spermatogonial stem cells? First, since the proliferative activity and continuous renewal of this class of germ cells explain the continuous production of differentiating germ cells and thus of spermatozoa throughout the adult life of animals, including man, the spermatogonial stem cells are directly related to the maintenance of male fertility. The proliferative activity of spermatogonia may be modified to a certain extent in animals with sexual cycles resulting in periods of fertility or sterility. Second, an abnormally low population of stem cells may result in oligospermia and sterility. The causes of such deple-

tion or malfunctioning of stem cells remain to be understood. Third, the existence of two classes of stem cells (reserve and renewing) provides an explanation for the regenerative capacity of the seminiferous epithelium following the partial destruction of the spermatogonia by various physical agents or chemical substances, in particular those having a deleterious effect on dividing cells.

The reserve nature of some type A spermatogonia (type A_0) was demonstrated in an analysis of the behavior of the spermatogonial stem cells following X-irradiation (10). On days 12 to 14 following irradiation (300 r) of the rat testis, the renewing type A spermatogonia disappeared from the seminiferous tubules, while the reserve type A stem cell population was only partly affected. The surviving type A_0 cells became proliferative, as indicated by their capacity to incorporate ^{3}H-thymidine, and quantitatively restored the stem cell population (A_1–A_4). Once this population of cells was restored, some type A_0 spermatogonia returned to a reserve stem cell condition. These observations on X-irradiated testes demonstrated the reserve function of some type A spermatogonia and their role in the repair of the seminiferous epithelium following its partial destruction. In addition, these observations suggested the following interaction between the two classes of stem cells: The renewing stem cells, through the action of a mitotic inhibitory substance, would normally prevent the reserve type A spermatogonia from undergoing mitosis. Following destruction through X-irradiation of type A_1–A_4 cells, the mitotic inhibition would disappear and the reserve type A_0 spermatogonia would begin to initiate the series of divisions that would reconstitute the population of type A_1–A_4 cells. As the number of the latter cells returned to normal, their inhibitory action on some type A_0 cells would reexert itself, and these spermatogonia would once again reenter a state of dormancy and become reserve stem cells.

These data suggested the possible existence of a mitotic inhibitor falling within the category of "chalones." A chalone is defined as an "internal secretion produced by a tissue for the purpose of controlling by inhibition the mitotic activity of that same tissue" (2). Experimental evidence for the existence of a spermatogonial chalone has come from studies in which an extract of normal testis was administered to animals several days after their testes were irradiated. The extract inhibited the incorporation of ^{3}H-thymidine and mitosis in the type A spermatogonia (presumably type A_0) that were in the process of repopulating the seminiferous epithelium with new type A spermatogonia (8). The demonstration of such a spermatogonial chalone, a substance that also appears to regulate growth of the seminiferous tubules (9), throws some light on one of the complex mechanisms that intervenes during this first phase of spermatogenesis.

The renewal of stem cells is still not well understood. Thus, for example, we do not know what factors determine the fate of the progeny of dividing stem cells (i.e., whether they remain stem cells or take the path of differentiation into spermatocytes). It is not clear also what really happens in terms of cell differentiation during the successive divisions of the differentiating type B spermatogonia. Do these successive divisions (2–4) only increase numerically the precursors of spermatocytes, or is there some stepwise modification of the chromosomes or chromosomal activity that prepares, at the molecular level, the next phase of the differentiation of germ cells into spermatozoa?

The following additional features related to the first phase of spermatogenesis have been disclosed by various experimental approaches:

The renewing type A_1 spermatogonia initiate spermatogenesis with the regularity of a clock, at fixed intervals (e.g., every 12 days in the rat, every 16 days in man), and no factors (hormonal or other) appear to influence this parameter. Once engaged in spermatogenesis, the evolution of spermatogonia progresses at a given and fixed pace.

The spermatogonia that form groups along the limiting membrane are connected to each other by delicate open intercellular bridges (12). This unique feature may partly explain the synchronous or quasisynchronous evolution of clusters of germ cells.

The proliferative spermatogonia (i.e., the renewing types A_1–A_4) as well as the differentiating type B spermatogonia, have remarkably long DNA-synthetic phases, compared to somatic cells, which tend to lengthen with differentiation (21). The significance of this in terms of cell differentiation remains to be clarified.

In the seminiferous tubules of normal animals, though varying with the species, spermatogonia are often seen to degenerate. This is not a haphazard, accidental, or insignificant phenomenon, since the incidence of cell death is constant for a given animal species. The reasons for such a well-regulated elimination of a given fraction of the spermatogonial population are not understood (33).

The spermatogonia are located within the so-called basal compartment of the seminiferous epithelium, a compartment that is delimited by the limiting membrane of the seminiferous tubules and on the luminal side by tightly attached processes of Sertoli cells. This basal compartment, which can be permeated with large-size molecules, constitutes a milieu that is different from that of the adluminal compartment in which spermatocytes and spermatids develop (11, 16).

Spermatogonial renewal and development have been said to be influenced by hormones (androgens, FSH), but the exact nature of such a trophic stimulation remains to be elucidated.

Meiosis

The spermatocytes, produced by divisions of the last generation of type B spermatogonia, pursue their differentiation into spermatozoa by undergoing meiosis—two successive divisions leading to the production of haploid cells, the spermatids. These two divisions, sometimes referred to as reduction divisions, are strikingly different morphologically from that of a standard cell division or mitosis. This explains the peculiar terminology accompanying the steps of the prophase of the first of the two divisions of maturation. Another interesting feature is that the cytological appearance of meiotic cells is remarkably similar from one species to another or from one genus to another, and thus what follows can be applied to all mammalian species.

Although discoveries concerning the structure of DNA, and in particular its replication during mitosis, throw some light on the mechanism of meiosis, the peculiar behavior of chromosomes during the reduction divisions are far from explained.

Soon after their formation, the spermatocytes, which closely resemble the parent type B cells, enter a long DNA-synthetic phase, during which most of their DNA is replicated. If observations performed on meiotic cells of plants can be applied to animal tissues, some 99.7 percent of the DNA is synthesized during the preleptotene stage, but some residual DNA synthesis (0.3 percent) takes place later during the meiotic prophase. In meiotic cells this delayed DNA synthesis may play a role in the pairing of the homologous chromosomes that takes place later (29, 30).

Following the preleptotene stage, the spermatocytes enter the first step of the prophase of the first meiotic division, called leptotene. Here the chromatin takes a fine filamentous texture, which is the first sign of the formation of chromosomes at the light-microscopic level. This is followed by the so-called zygotene stage, during which homologous chromosomes pair. The paired chromosomes assume the shape of delicate loops attached by their extremity to one area of the nuclear envelope. Here they are said to take the characteristic "bouquet" configuration. In the nuclei of these cells, electron-microscopic studies revealed the presence of a spirally arranged tripartite structure composed of two lateral elements flanking a third central element, the whole system called a synaptinemal complex. This peculiar structure appears to be the site of attachment or binding of homologous chromosomes observed during the zygotene and the next step of the meiotic prophase, called the pachytene step. The origin, nature, and function of the synaptinemal complex have been extensively studied by a few authors (26, 27, 34) but still remain mysterious.

Following the zygotene stage, the cell enters the so-called pachytene condition. As the nuclear volume progressively increases, the pachytene chromosomes, which are bivalents (i.e., a pair of homologous chromosomes), shorten and become more compact. This stage lasts 8 to 9 days in mice, 10 to 12 days in rats and monkeys, and 16 days in humans. One may thus refer to these spermatocytes as being in the early, mid, or late pachytene stage. Accompanying an increase in nuclear volume is a corresponding increase in cytoplasmic volume.

In the cytoplasm there is a well-demarcated spheroidal Golgi apparatus with a pair of centrioles in proximity. In addition to small mitochondria and cisternae of endoplasmic reticulum there is a newly acquired chromophilic mass called the chromatoid body. This pleomorphic organelle, spongy in appearance, is composed of granulofilamentous material frequently associated with the smooth-surfaced vesicles of the endoplasmic reticulum. The origin and composition of this cytoplasmic structure remain obscure (15). During this long stage in which the homologous chromosomes are closely coupled, portions of homologous chromosomes are exchanged (crossing over). This presupposes a breakage of DNA chains, followed by recombination of the loose ends of the DNA molecules on the DNA chains of the opposite chromosomes. This phenomenon contributes to an exchange of genetic information between chromosomes of maternal and of paternal origin and therefore to a mixing of parental genetic characteristics. The sex chromosomes—the large X and the small Y chromosomes—also pair in the so-called sex vesicle, a chromophilic mass attached to the nuclear envelope. There is no morphological sign at the light- and electron-microscopic level of the exchange of chromosomal segments during the pachytene stage; it becomes apparent during the following step of the meiotic prophase, called the diplotene stage. This stage features a partial separation of the homologous chromosomes, which remain attached at certain points—chiasmata—along the chromosomes.

Following the diplotene stage, the chromosome contracts even more and becomes very deeply stained (diakinesis). Following dissolution of the nuclear envelope and formation of the spindle, the chromosomes align at the equatorial plate to form a typical metaphase plate. During anaphase the chromosomes disentangle, separate, and move toward their respective poles. No centromere split is necessary, since the homologs maintain their individual centromere. The random distribution of the homologs to the two new nuclei also contributes to further mixing of the parental genetic material. Following telophase, two new cells are formed—the secondary spermatocytes. The latter cells contain a haploid number of chromosomes; some contain the X chromosome in addition to the autosomes, and others contain the Y chromosome. Each of these chromosomes is already composed of two double helices of DNA or two chromatids. These secondary spermatocytes have a relatively short interphase during which no DNA synthesis takes place. Their spherical nuclei show some granulated or globular chromatin masses. In the cytoplasm is a spheroidal Golgi zone next to the nucleus, a chromatoid body, as well as the usual cytoplasmic organelles. These cells soon enter the second maturation division, during which the short and thick chromosomes first form a metaphase plate; then, following a splitting of the centromere, each chromatid is carried to the two poles of the spindle in a manner identical to that seen in an ordinary mitosis. It should be remembered, however, that the total number of metaphase chromosomes is half that seen in a division of a somatic cell. Similarly, the daughter cells (spermatids) that receive the chromosomal halves or chromatids also contain a haploid number of chromosomes.

Such a remarkable piece of cytological engineering does not take place without hazards; faults are frequent, possibly more frequent than usually believed. These anomalies, which result in the degeneration of a fair percentage of spermatocytes during meiotic divisions, can also be morphologically detected by analysis of the karyotypes. Chromosomal anomalies originating during meiosis can also be found in the offspring and will result in well-characterized genetic disorders and diseases accompanied frequently by sterility (trisomy (21), Klinefelter's syndrome, etc.).

Other features of meiosis, disclosed in recent years, merit brief mention. During the long prophase of the first meiotic division, the chromosomes (in contrast to the mitotic chromosomes) are not inactive in terms of RNA synthesis. Appreciable RNA synthesis takes place in the nucleus, principally during mid or late pachytene. This RNA is accompanied by nuclear protein synthesis. The newly synthesized RNA remains inside the nucleus and associated with the chromosomes and is released into the cytoplasm of the spermatocytes during diakinesis. This RNA is eventually seen in the cytoplasm of the spermatids, and since there is relatively little RNA synthesis in spermatids, the "meiotic" RNA must contain a good deal of the genetic information necessary to proceed with the differentiation taking place during spermiogenesis (19, 24, 25). In relation to the spermatocytes, an endonuclease has been isolated from meiotic cells in plants that appears to have a specific action on meiotic chromosomes and to play a significant role in the crossing-over phenomenon (30).

Spermatocytes originating from a group or cluster of renewing stem cells evolve through meiosis at a fixed pace—always the same for a given species—and in a quasisynchronous manner. This quasisynchronous evolution may be related to the existence of open intercellular bridges that exist between the spermatocytes (12).

Soon after their formation, the spermatocytes are pushed up from the basal compartment into the adluminal compartment created by the Sertoli cells. This takes place through the active participation of the cytoplasmic processes of the Sertoli cells, which slide on the basement membrane under the spermatocytes and push the spermatocytes upward. The spermatocytes as well as the spermatids will therefore pursue their differentiation in a new milieu conditioned by the Sertoli cells.

Although spermatocytes appear to require the presence of hormones to progress through meiosis, the exact nature of this frequently discussed trophic action remains totally obscure.

Spermiogenesis
The newly formed spermatid soon undertakes an extraordinarily complex series of changes that constitute a true metamorphosis, leading to the production of the highly differentiated motile cell, the spermatozoon. This exceptional example of cell differentiation has attracted the attention of innumerable light and electron microscopists over the past 20 years. Probably because of the complexity of the topic and the amplitude of the descriptive task, no one has yet attempted to write a comprehensive review on this topic, even limited to mammalian species. The analyses of mammalian spermiogenesis at the ultrastructural level, initiated by Fawcett and collaborators in the early 1950s and pursued actively since then by the Harvard group and others, have brought to light cytological features that have clearly shown the intricacies of the evolutionary changes taking place in the nucleus and cytoplasm of spermatids during spermiogenesis. Considering that these morphological changes constitute the expression of even more complex phenomena at the molecular level, one wonders how and when these mechanisms of spermatid differentiation will ever be elucidated.

The newly formed spermatid is a rather modest-looking cell with a small spherical nucleus showing a granulated chromatin and a rather pale stained cytoplasm. The usual array of organelles are present: a spheroidal and compact Golgi apparatus next to the nucleus, a pair of centrioles proximal to but outside the Golgi zone, mitochondria with a peculiar arrangement of their cristae due to the dilatation of the intercristal space, some free clusters of ribosomes, and an endoplasmic reticulum mainly composed of interconnected cisternae with occasional ribosomes attached to them. A chromatoid body is also clearly visible, floating in the cytoplasm.

During the first phase of spermiogenesis (corresponding to the Golgi and cap phases (7, 23)), the most important changes take place in the Golgi apparatus and the centrioles. The Golgi apparatus soon starts to elaborate secretorylike granules rich in glycoproteins, as shown by the periodic acid-Schiff or acid-silver techniques. These granules apparently fuse into a single granule (the acrosomic granule) that becomes closely apposed to the nuclear surface. The granule continues to grow by the addition of material, elaborated by the stacks of Golgi saccules. As a result, the acrosomic granule spreads over the surface of the nucleus, forming a caplike covering. The nucleus underlying this acrosome cap does not remain indifferent, since the nuclear envelope loses nuclear pores and cisternal space and undergoes condensation of chromatin on its inner aspect. Between the nuclear envelope and the inner acrosomal membrane (i.e., the membrane delimiting the acrosomic system that faces the nucleus), a granulofilamentous and possibly binding material forms, which is particularly evident at the margin of the acrosome cap. As the acrosomic system develops at one pole of the nucleus, the centrioles establish contact with the nuclear envelope at the other pole. The proximal centriole lies sideways on the nuclear surface, while the distal centriole is perpendicular to the surface of the nucleus and soon starts to grow a typical flagellum (with the characteristic nine peripheral pairs plus one central pair of microtubules). The proximal centriole attaches strongly to the nuclear envelope at the level of the electron-dense basal plate (a layer of dense material seen at the surface of the nuclear envelope). During this first phase of spermiogenesis the mitochondria do not undergo any significant modification while the chromatoid body slowly migrates toward the centriolar pole of the nucleus.

During the middle third of spermiogenesis (called the acrosome phase (23)), the morphological appearance of the spermatid goes through a number of rather dramatic modifications. The nucleus, which had been located in the central portion of the cytoplasm, rotates and moves toward the periphery of the cell, with the acrosomic system coming in contact with the cytoplasmic membrane. As a result, the cell becomes elongated, with the nucleus at one pole and the bulk of cytoplasm at the other. Thereafter the nucleus itself starts to change in shape because of the rearrangement and condensation of the chromatin. This packaging of DNA proteins appears to be very well programmed and genetically controlled, since at the termination of the condensation the nucleus has a size and shape that is characteristic for each given animal species. With some exceptions, the nuclei of mammalian spermatids generally assume either a spatulate or a falciform shape, and in each category the shapes remain morphologically distinctive. Thus, for example, among spatulate spermatozoa, the nuclei of human spermatozoa have a distinctive flattened apical extremity and a globular caudal portion, giving them a pyriform shape when viewed from the side (13, 14).

The relatively rapid condensation of the nuclear chromatin, for which no biochemical mechanisms have as yet been proposed, results in the formation of a superfluous nuclear envelope, which will eventually be resorbed so that the envelope will finally tightly fit the condensed chromatin. At the apical extremity of the nucleus where the acrosomic system stops growing, the Golgi apparatus, which had been contributing material to its content, detaches from the nucleus and floats freely in the cytoplasm. The content of the acrosomic system condenses while it readjusts (at times with profound structural modifications, particularly in falciform spermatozoa) to the transforming apical portion of the nucleus.

Between the inner acrosomal membrane and the nuclear membrane there is now a distinct gap called the subacrosomal space, which is filled with some granulofilamentous material. At the basal or caudal extremity of the nucleus, a new delicate fibrillar structure appears—the caudal tube or manchette. This is a veil-like structure that inserts on a ring surrounding the nucleus close to the margin of the acrosome cap and extends caudally along the flagellum for a short distance. It is made up of numerous microtubules. The exact function of this caudal tube remains unknown, but it may contribute to orienting the flow of cytoplasm that may exist in these cells. Closely applied to the basal portion of the nucleus, the centriolar apparatus undergoes complex modifications accompanied by transformation of the proximal centriole and addition of reinforcing electron-dense, cross-striated longitudinal columns around the two centrioles. The end result is the formation of a strong collar or connecting piece (17).

Toward the end of the acrosome phase nine coarse fibers form along the flagellum, each fiber facing a pair of microtubules of the axonemal complex. The exact nature and role of these coarse fibers remains to be studied. The chromatoid body that floats around the forming connecting piece contributes some of its substance toward the formation of the annulus, a delicate ringlike structure that surrounds the flagellum next to the centrioles.

During the third and last phase of spermiogenesis (referred to as the maturation phase (23)) many additional subtle changes take place. The chromatin in the nucleus of maturing spermatids undergoes a further and final condensation and assumes a paracrystalline state. The nucleus thus takes its definitive shape. This modification of the chromatin is accompanied by a modification of the acidic proteins associated with the DNA. The content of the acrosomic system also undergoes a further condensation (although not final, since further changes and condensations may take place in the acrosomic system of epididymal spermatozoa) and readjustment at the surface of the nucleus (particularly striking in falciform spermatids). In the subacrosomal space material accumulates, densifies, and forms an apparently rigid capsule that tightly covers a good part of the apical portion of the nucleus. In rodents this material takes the shape of a rigid pointed and angular structure called the perforatorium. The composition and role of this structure remain to be discovered.

At the caudal extremity of the cell the following changes are taking place: Early during the maturation phase the annulus slides down the flagellum over a given and fixed distance; as if this were a signal, the mitochondria (which up to now were dispersed in the cytoplasm) migrate, possibly carried by some circular streaming of the cytoplasm, toward the flagellum, along which they line up side by side. These mitochondria subsequently condense as a result of a loss of their intercristal fluid and take the shape of slightly curved rodlets. They adhere tightly to the now fully developed coarse fibers that are seen along the flagellum and are arranged side by side and tip to tip in a very regular manner, following a spiral generating line (1). They will occupy the portion of the flagellum seen between the neck piece and the annulus that is referred to as the middle piece of the tail. After this is done, the caudal tube abruptly disappears. Distal to the middle piece of the tail, a striated fibrous sheath appears and forms a girdle around the coarse fibers of the flagellum.

Now that the cell has almost completed its transformation into a spermatozoon, it must get rid of the long droplet of superfluous cytoplasm that can be seen along the flagellum. This cytoplasmic body contains, in addition to lipid droplets, an abundance of free ribosomes, a few cisternae of endoplasmic reticulum, residual mitochondria, and fragments of the chromatoid body. These cytoplasmic droplets flow toward the nuclear or head portion of the cell, and most of its cytoplasmic mass is detached through the effective action of cytoplasmic processes of the Sertoli cells. These processes, acting like pseudopods, virtually cut off this so-called residual cytoplasm and simultaneously release the spermatozoon from the seminiferous epithelium, a phenomenon called spermiation (18).

The durations of spermiogenesis and of each of the various steps are fixed and constant for a given animal species. Spermatids, like spermatogonia and spermatocytes, evolve synchronously in groups, and the elements of the groups are connected by open intercellular bridges. These persist until the very end of spermiogenesis when the spermatids cast off their residual cytoplasm.

Spermiogenesis is a delicate and intricate process and thus sensitive to adverse conditions (hormonal or nutritional deficiencies, noxious substances, chromosomal defects acquired during meiosis, etc.). In such instances abnormalities are frequent and tend to take place during the acrosome phase, the time of the most elaborate morphological changes of the nucleus and cytoplasmic organelles.

The differentiation of spermatids takes place in close association with the Sertoli cells and in the environment they create. This aspect of spermatogenesis has received a good deal of attention with the development of the concept of the blood-testis barrier (11, 16). The close association of acrosome and maturation phase spermatids with Sertoli cells was clearly indicated in the early light-microscopic descriptions of the seminiferous epithelium, in which the spermatids were seen to be inserted head first in the apical Sertoli cytoplasm. Electron-microscopic studies have reemphasized this by demonstrating modifications of the cytoplasmic structures of the Sertoli cells (cisternae of the ribosomal endoplasmic reticulum running parallel to the cell membrane; presence of bundles of filaments) adjacent to the acrosome-covered nucleus of spermatids. Thus on the one hand spermiogenesis cannot be dissociated from the Sertoli cell structure and function, but on the other hand the exact nature of the interaction between Sertoli cells and spermatids remains to be elucidated. Sertoli cells have been considered recently as producers, under FSH stimulation, of androgen-binding proteins and as a means of concentrating such androgen-protein complexes around spermatids. Whether spermatids constitute a target for androgens remains to be proved, however.

A number of cytochemical studies have been performed on spermatids, but these analyses remain fragmentary. The most extensive studies concern the evolution of nucleoproteins (19, 24).

The Cycle of the Seminiferous Epithelium
Germ cells at various steps of spermatogenesis are not arranged at random within the seminiferous epithelium but tend to form cellular associations of fixed composition. Owing to the precise and regular timing of the steps of spermatogenesis, spermatids at given steps of spermiogenesis are associated with spermatocytes and spermatogonia at given steps of their respective development. These characteristic cellular groupings, which reappar at regular intervals in segments of tubules, represent stages of a cycle of the seminiferous epithelium that may be defined as "a complete series of the successive cellular associations appearing in any one given area of the seminiferous epithelium" (23). The number of stages composing the cycle varies with the species and the criteria used to characterize them. This histological feature of the seminiferous epithelium and, in particular, the detailed classification into stages of the cycle have been useful in the study of the various aspects of spermatogenesis, especially the mode of proliferation and renewal of spermatogonia and spermiogenesis. They have also been useful in the determination, by means of radioautography, of the exact duration of spermatogenesis and of its parts (5).

27.2 Goals for Research on Spermatogenesis

Knowledge of the various aspects of spermatogenesis is considerably greater now than it was around 1950. The progress made during the last 25 years arose mainly from the development of new methods of investigation, such as the use of radioactive tracers combined with radioautography, or the use of the electron microscope. As a result of the extensive electron-microscopic studies, the morphological aspects of the cytological events taking place during the differentiation of germ cells into spermatozoa have been widely studied. The ultrastructural complexities of the changes taking place, particularly in spermatids, lent themselves beautifully to this descriptive analysis. With recent technological advances in microscopy, such as freeze fracture or freeze etching techniques, scanning electron microscopy, high-voltage electron microscopy, EM radioautography, and cytochemistry, many more studies on germ cells and Sertoli cells will rapidly add masses of valuable information to what is already known. These morphological studies are absolutely essential to gain some understanding of spermatogenesis; without such "visualization," this process of cell differentiation would remain vague and its analysis at the molecular level would remain difficult, incomplete, and imprecise.

While the morphological aspects of spermatogenesis have received a good deal of attention, many other fundamental facets of the spermatogenic process have been touched only superficially. A few characteristic examples are (a) in relation to spermatogonia, the mechanisms that control the differentiation of stem cells into either new stem cells or differentiating type B spermatogonia; (b) in relation to spermatocytes, the molecular processes that lead to the synapsis of homologous chromosomes and crossing over; (c) in relation to spermatids, most of the controlling molecular mechanisms involved in the structural modifications of the nucleus or cytoplasmic organelles during spermiogenesis. In terms of the extracellular factors that influence spermatogenesis, the current speculation should be buttressed with more solid information. Thus, for example, the influence of hormones (gonadotropins and androgens) on spermatogenesis has been discussed for years, but although it is clear that spermatogenesis requires the presence of gametogenic hormones to undergo completion, it is not known whether hormones act directly on germ cells or indirectly through their action on Sertoli cells. Therefore the direct and positive role of hormones on the mechanism of germ cell differentiation remains to be demonstrated. Another feature that retains the attention of many investigators is the relationship between Sertoli cells and germ cells, for while the morphological aspects of this association have been well analyzed, the functional aspects remain mysterious and the exact role of Sertoli cells in conditioning the differentiation of spermatids awaits further studies. In summary, while a good many of the phenomena taking place during spermatogenesis have been extensively studied at the structural level, most if not all of these phenomena remain to be analyzed and clarified at the molecular level. Controlling mechanisms are obscure and also need to be systematically studied.

References

1. André, J. Contribution à la connaissance du chondriome: Étude de ses modifications ultrastructurales pendant la spermatogenèse. J. Ultrastruct. Res. Suppl. 3:1962.

2. Bullough, W. S. *The evolution of differentiation*. New York: Academic Press, 1967.

3. Clermont, Y. Renewal of spermatogonia in man. Am. J. Anat. 118:509, 1966.

4. Clermont, Y. Two classes of spermatogonial stem cells in the monkey (*Cercopithecus aethiops*). Am. J. Anat. 126:57, 1969.

5. Clermont, Y. Kinetics of spermatognesis in mammals: Seminiferous epithelium cycle and spermatogonial renewal. Physiol. Rev. 52:198, 1972.

6. Clermont, Y., and M. Antar. Duration of the cycle of the seminiferous epithelium and the spermatogonial renewal in the monkey *Macaca arctoides*. Am. J. Anat. 136:153, 1973.

7. Clermont, Y., and C. P. Leblond. Spermiogenesis of man, monkey, ram and other mammals as shown by the "periodic acid-Schiff" technique. Am. J. Anat. 96:229, 1955.

8. Clermont, Y., and A. Mauger. Existence of a spermatogonial chalone in the rat testis. Cell Tissue Kinet. 7:171, 1974.

9. Clermont, Y., and A. Mauger. Effect of a spermatogonial chalone on the growing rat testis. Anat. Rec. 178:330 (Abstract), 1974.

10. Dym, M., and Y. Clermont. Role of spermatogonia in the repair of the seminiferous epithelium following X-irradiation of the rat testis. Am. J. Anat. 128:265, 1970.

11. Dym, M., and D. W. Fawcett. The blood testis barrier in the rat and the physiological compartmentation of the seminiferous epithelium. Biol. Reprod. 3:308, 1970.

12. Dym, M., and D. W. Fawcett. Further observations on the number of spermatogonia, spermatocytes and spermatids connected by intercellular bridges in the mammalian testis. Biol. Reprod. 4:195, 1971.

13. Fawcett, D. W. The structure of the mammalian spermatozoon. Int. Rev. Cytol. 7:195, 1958.

14. Fawcett, D. W. A comparative view of sperm ultrastructure. Biol. Reprod. 2:90, 1970.

15. Fawcett, D. W., E. M. Eddy, and D. M. Phillips. Observation on the fine structure and relationships of the chromatoid body in mammalian spermatogenesis. Biol. Reprod. 2:129, 1970.

16. Fawcett, D. W., L. V. Leak, and P. M. Heidger. Electron microscopic observations on the structural components of the blood-testis barrier. J. Reprod. Fertil. Suppl. 10:105, 1970.

17. Fawcett, D. W., and D. M. Phillips. The fine structure and development of the neck region of the mammalian spermatozoon. Anat. Rec. 165:153, 1969.

18. Fawcett, D. W., and D. M. Phillips. Observation on the release of spermatozoa and on changes in the head during passage through the epididymis. J. Reprod. Fertil. Suppl. 6:405, 1969.

19. Gledhill, B. L. Nucleic acids of the testis. In *The testis*, Vol. 2, eds. A. D. Johnson, W. R. Gomes, and N. L. Van Demark, p. 307. New York: Academic Press, 1970.

20. Hermo, L. The existence of two classes of spermatogonial stem cells in the rat testis. Anat. Rec. 175:343 (Abstract), 1973.

21. Huckins, C. Kinetic profiles of spermatogonia in testes of adult Sprague-Dawley rats. Cell Tissue Kinet. 4:139, 1971.

22. Huckins, C. The spermatogonial stem cell population in adult rats. I. Their morphology, proliferation and maturation. Anat. Rec. 169:533, 1971.

23. Leblond, C. P., and Y. Clermont. Spermiogenesis of rat, mouse, hamster and guinea pig as revealed by the "periodic acid-fuchsin sulfurous acid" technique. Am. J. Anat. 90:167, 1952.

24. Monesi, V. Synthetic activities during spermatogenesis in the mouse. Exp. Cell Res. 39:197, 1965.

25. Monesi, V. Chromosome activities during meiosis and spermiogenesis. J. Reprod. Fertil. Suppl. 13:1, 1971.

26. Moses, M. J. Structural patterns and the functional organization of chromosomes. In *The role of chromosomes in development*, p. 11. New York: Academic Press, 1964.

27. Moses, M. J. Synaptinemal complex. Ann. Rev. Genet. 2:363, 1968.

28. Oakberg, E. F. Spermatogonial stem cell renewal in the mouse. Anat. Rec. 169:515, 1971.

29. Ohno, S. Morphological aspects of meiosis and their genetical significance. In *Advances in experimental medicine and biology*, Vol. 10: *The human testis*, eds. E. Rosemberg and C. A. Paulsen, p. 115. New York: Plenum Press, 1970.

30. Pearson, P. L. The behavior of chromosomes. In *Advances in the biosciences*, Vol. 10: *Schering Workshop on Contraception: The masculine gender*, ed. G. Raspé, p. 15. New York: Pergamon Press, 1973.

31. Regaud, C. Etude sur la structure des tubes séminifères et sur la spermatogenèse chez les mammifères. Arch. Anat. Microsc. 4:101, 231, 1901.

32. Roosen-Runge, E. C. The process of spermatogenesis in mammals. Biol. Rev. 37:343, 1962.

33. Roosen-Runge, E. C. Germinal cell loss in normal metazoan spermatogenesis. J. Reprod. Fertil. 35:339, 1973.

34. Solari, A. J., and L. L. Tres. Ultrastructure and histochemistry of the nucleus during male meiotic prophase. In *Advances in experimental medicine and biology*, Vol. 10: *The human testis*, eds. E. Rosemberg and C. A. Paulsen, p. 127. New York: Plenum Press, 1970.

28 The Ultrastructure and Functions of the Sertoli Cell

Don W. Fawcett

More than a century has passed since Sertoli described the supporting cells of the seminiferous epithelium that bear his name (70). Without the benefit of the microtome, he demonstrated by maceration techniques that the supporting cells were basically columnar in form but with ramifying processes that extend toward the lumen to envelope-associated clusters of germ cells. The clusters of synchronously developing spermatids and the expanded apical portion of the Sertoli cell in which they are embedded were recognized in 1871 as a functional unit by von Ebner, who is credited with introducing the concept of a symbiotic relationship between the developing germ cells and the Sertoli cells (21, 22). This interpretation, based solely upon the topographical relations between the two populations of cells, persists to the present, even though there is still very little solid evidence bearing upon the nature or degree of their physiological interdependence.

The application since 1960 of the electron microscope to studies of the testis has led to a much clearer understanding of the organization of the seminiferous epithelium, including the ultrastructural characteristics of the Sertoli cells, their role in the maintenance of the blood-testis permeability barrier, and their participation in sperm release. The biochemistry of these cells has lagged behind morphological studies for lack of a satisfactory means of dissociating them from germ cells and interstitial cells. Significant progress is now being made, however, in assessing their responses to hormonal stimulation and identifying their secretory products.

28.1 Organization of the Seminiferous Epithelium

The seminiferous epithelium has a number of characteristics that make it unique among epithelia. It is made up of two distinct categories of cells—a postmitotic population of Sertoli cells and a proliferating population of germ cells in various stages of their differentiation into spermatozoa. The Sertoli cells extend from base to free surface and are provided with an elaborate array of lateral processes that extend into the interstices between the associated spermatogonia, spermatocytes, and spermatids (Figures 28.1, 28.2). The Sertoli cells are long-lived and cease to proliferate before puberty, whereas the germ cells are a constantly renewing population, with their stem cells at the

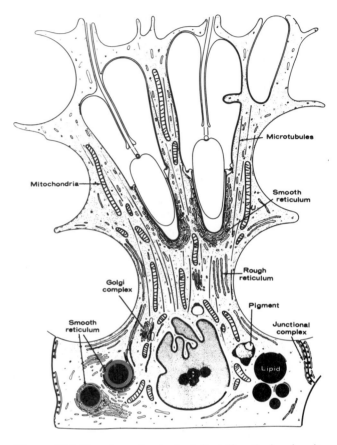

Figure 28.1 Drawing of a typical Sertoli cell showing its shape and relationships to the germ cells as well as the form and distribution of its principal organelles and inclusions.

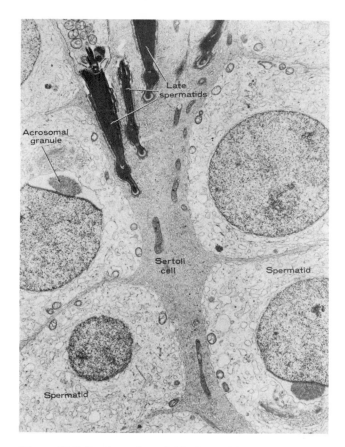

Figure 28.2 Section of seminiferous epithelium from chinchilla testis illustrating the Sertoli cell–germ cell relationships. Columnar portion of supporting cell sends thin laminar processes between spermatids arranged in vertical rows along its sides. Another set of more advanced spermatids occupies deep recesses in its apical cytoplasm.

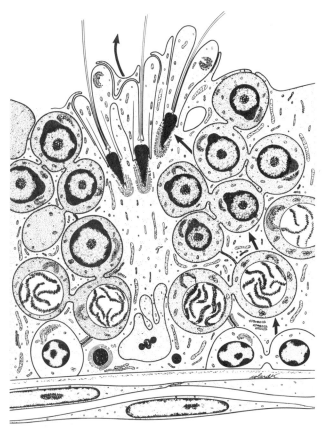

Figure 28.3 A drawing of the cellular relationships in the seminiferous epithelium. A sessile population of columnar Sertoli cells is surrounded by a mobile population differentiating germ cells moving upward along the sides of the supporting cell. After elongation the spermatids establish a new relationship occupying deep recesses in the apex of the Sertoli cell.

base and more advanced stages at successively higher levels in the epithelium. The germ cells slowly move upward along the sides of the supporting cells as they differentiate. When the spermatids approach the surface, they elongate and establish a new relationship to the supporting cells, occupying deep recesses in their apical cytoplasm (Figure 28.3). The occurrence of two populations, one fixed and the other constantly moving upward, is a feature peculiar to the seminiferous epithelium. The continually changing relationships between the germ cells and the supporting cells create some problems of cell coherence and cell communication that may have important implications for the control and maintenance of spermatogenesis (25).

In other columnar epithelia the cells have on their lateral surfaces of contact local specializations of the cell membranes that maintain cohesion and communication between cells. The mechanical function of assuring cell attachment is subserved by beltlike *zonulae adherentes* that encircle their apical ends and by *desmosomes* scattered over their lateral surfaces. The

communication between cells, which is essential for physiological integration of the entire epithelium, is maintained through *nexuses* or *gap junctions*—specialized sites of close membrane apposition that permit passage of ions and small molecules from cell to cell. In addition to providing low-resistance electrical coupling of cells, the gap junctions are also sites of very firm attachment of opposing membranes. In the seminiferous epithelium, on the other hand, neither desmosomes, zonulae adherentes, nor gap junctions are found on the interfaces between Sertoli cells and germ cells.

The absence of gap junctions is especially surprising, for if one considers the highly integrated nature of the spermatogenic cycle in mammals and the precise timing of events in germ-cell differentiation, one would expect to find abundant specializations for cell-to-cell communication. But the presence of such firm attachments on the interface between germ cells and supporting cells would prevent their movement relative to one another. Thus it seems that in the seminiferous epithelium upward mobility of the germ cells is maintained at the sacrifice of one of the commonest and most efficient mechanisms for communication among epithelial cells (25). In the absence of such membrane specializations it seems reasonable to conclude that whatever influence the Sertoli cells have on differentiation of the germ cells is probably mediated indirectly by alterations in the extracellular fluid environment in which the germ cells develop or by release of molecules to which the germ cell membranes are freely permeable.

In secretory and absorbing epithelia in general, the intercellular spaces are closed by juxtaluminal *zonulae occludentes*—circumferential bands of fusion of the opposing membranes. These deny access of water-soluble substances to the intercellular clefts from the lumen but permit free access of blood-borne metabolites to the cells through the base of the epithelium. In the seminiferous epithelium there are no juxtaluminal occluding junctions; such a tight closure would prevent ascent of the germ cells, which, in effect, develop in expanded intercellular clefts between neighboring Sertoli cells. There are, however, occluding junctions between adjacent Sertoli cells near the base of the epithelium (Figure 28.4). These are of a type unique to Sertoli cells. They tend to be located just above the spermatogonia and therefore partition the epithelium into two compartments—a basal compartment containing the spermatogonia and preleptotene spermatocytes and an adluminal compartment containing the more advanced stages of germ cells (20, 33). Any diffusible substances in the perivascular spaces of the interstitial tissue have access to the stem cells in the basal compartment; however, the occluding junctions between the overarching processes of the Sertoli cells constitute a permeability barrier that isolates the differentiating germ cells from the general extracellular fluid compartment of the testis. The existence of this permeability barrier is probably necessary for the secretory function of the epithelium (*vide infra*). It may also enable the Sertoli cells to create in the adluminal compartment a special microenvironment essential for meiosis and further differentiation of the germ cells.

A number of investigators have emphasized the probable importance of the Sertoli cells as "bridge cells" between the bloodstream and the germ cells (81). This concept has been strengthened by the discovery that the occluding junctions between these cells are the morphological basis of the blood-testis permeability barrier. Since extracellular diffusion into the epithelium is barred, any substances reaching the germ cells in the adluminal compartment must traverse the Sertoli cells and are subject to modification in passage.

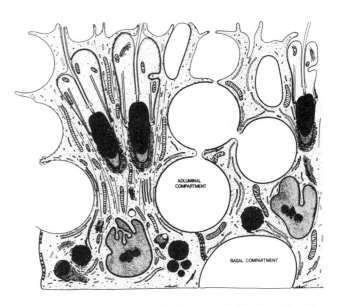

Figure 28.4 Drawing illustrating how occluding junctions between adjacent Sertoli cells mar their base, divide the epithelium into a basal compartment containing spermatogonia and preleptolene spermatocytes and an adluminal compartment containing meiotic and postmeiotic stages of the germ cells.

28.2 Ultrastructure

The Nucleus

The nucleus was usually described by classical cytologists as irregularly oval or pyramidal, with its long axis perpendicular to the lamina propria. It is now evident that the nuclear shape is far more irregular than was appreciated by light microscopy. In most of the species studied to date the nucleus is deeply invaginated (Figure 28.1), but the lobules demarcated are so closely apposed and superimposed in the thicker sections viewed with the light microscope that they may present a relatively simple outline (6, 18). The nucleoplasm is of a fine fibrogranular texture and remarkably homogeneous, being generally devoid of the karyosomes and peripheral clumps of coarse chromatin that characterize most somatic cell nuclei. Thus it seems to have an unusually high proportion of euchromatin, a feature not uncommon in exceptionally active cells.

The limited amount of heterochromatin in the Sertoli cells of laboratory rodents is concentrated in two spheroidal masses on either side of the nucleolus, forming a tripartite complex that is highly characteristic of this cell type (Figure 28.5). These juxtanucleolar bodies were first observed before the turn of the century, but only recently have they been recognized by Feulgen staining as nucleolus-associated heterochromatin. The nucleolus proper is made up of the usual anastomosing strands of fine filaments and particles of ribonucleoprotein. There is still no satisfactory expla-

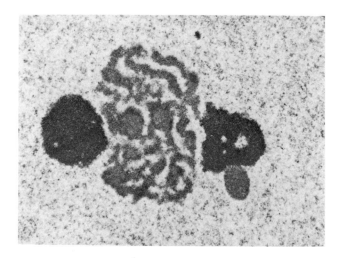

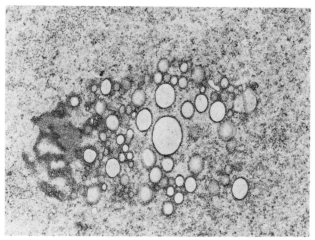

Figure 28.5 Nucleolus of a Sertoli cell from the Chinese hamster *Cricetulus griseus*. Similar nucleolar complexes are found in mice, rats, and several other laboratory rodents. Central portion is composed of a typical nucleolonema and represents the nucleolus proper. The two dense masses of heterochromatin regularly found in close association with it are called satellite karyosomes.

Figure 28.6 Sertoli cell nucleolus from the domestic bull. Lower left, anastomosing strands' granular and fibrillar material of the nucleolonema. Bulk of nucleolus is composed of vesicles of varying size bearing minute ribosomelike granules on their outer surfaces. Significance of these membrane-limited components of the nucleolus is not known. They are found in bull (*Box taurus*), ram (*Ovis aries*), African buffalo (*Syncerus coffer*), gerenuk (*Litocranius walleri*), and probably in many other ruminants.

nation for the occurrence, in these species, of two discrete satellite karyosomes in symmetrical relationship to the nucleolus. Hybridization with labeled nucleic acids has shown that the satellite DNA, which is usually associated with the centromeric regions of chromosomes, binds to the juxtanucleolar bodies of Sertoli cells (62). This would indicate that the centromeres are all closely associated in the heterochromatin adjacent to the nucleolus. No explanation for this unusual nuclear organization has been offered. It is not found in all species.

In bulls, rams, and other ruminants, an unusual differentiation of the nucleolus is of particular interest to cell biologists. Within the strands of the nucleolonema are membrane-limited tubules and vesicles of varying size (Figure 28.6). Similar vesicles are clustered in the meshes of and outside of the nucleolonema (61). Adhering to the outer surfaces of the vesicles are small dense particles apparently identical to the granular component of the nucleolus. The association of these particles with the membranes of intranuclear vesicles is reminiscent of the association of ribosomes with the membranes of the endoplasmic reticulum in the cytoplasm. Small clusters of granule-studded vesicles are occasionally encountered at the periphery of the nucleus, but there is no evidence that they discharge their content into the perinuclear cistern or through the pores into the cytoplasm. Their significance is unknown. The only nucleolar differentiation at all comparable is the so-called nucleolar channel system

found in the human endometrial epithelium in the secretory phase of the cycle (16, 80). The membrane-limited tubules are transient structures confined to one phase of the cycle, whereas the nucleolar vesicles of Sertoli cells are enduring structures with no known cyclic changes. Neither of these structures has attracted the investigative attention it deserves because reproductive biologists in general have yet to develop a strong interest in morphological changes at the subcellular level.

The nuclear envelope is abundantly provided with pores, which are most evident in freeze-cleaving preparations that present extensive views of the nuclear surface. The distribution of pores is more uniform than in many other cell types, possibly because of the absence of peripheral masses of chromatin.

Cytoplasmic Organelles

Interest of reproductive biologists in the cytoplasmic organelles of Sertoli cells has centered upon two questions: (1) Is there cytological evidence of protein synthetic activity? (2) Do these cells have the ultrastructural characteristics commonly associated with the synthesis of steroids? Cells actively engaged in synthesis of large amounts of protein-rich secretory product usually contain a well-developed system of tubular or cisternal elements of the endoplasmic reticulum with many associated ribosomes. Such cells also tend to be

305   Ultrastructure and Functions of the Sertoli Cell

clearly polarized with a well-developed supranuclear Golgi apparatus, often containing secretory granules in various stages of condensation. The Sertoli cells have only a limited amount of granular endoplasmic reticulum. Although predominately tubular in form, parallel arrays of a few cisternae are occasionally encountered, especially in the basal portion of the cell. Instead of a single Golgi complex consistent in location, there are multiple small Golgi complexes, each consisting of a few short parallel saccules and associated small vesicles. No condensing vacuoles or dense secretory granules are observed in the vicinity of the Golgi complexes or elsewhere in the cytoplasm. Thus on the basis of ultrastructural criteria one may say that the Sertoli cell has a degree of development of the granular endoplasmic reticulum consistent with appreciable protein synthesis, but there is no evidence of concentration of a product in the Golgi complex or of formation and release of secretory granules.

The cytological features typically found in steroid-secreting cells include an elaborate development of the smooth endoplasmic reticulum, a prominent Golgi complex, and abundant mitochondria, which are often unusually variable in size and may have tubular instead of lamellar cristae (27). The smooth endoplasmic reticulum is well represented in Sertoli cell cytoplasm and in some species is more extensively developed than the granular reticulum. The ram, for example, has conspicuous aggregations of tubular and cisternal elements of smooth reticulum in the basal cytoplasm (Figure 28.7). The cisternae are often arranged in multilayered concentric systems around lipid droplets, a configuration also commonly seen in steroid-secreting cells. The mitochondria, however, do not conform to the expectations of steroid-secreting cells. Most are long and slender with foliate cristae, but some are cup-shaped (12). The Golgi apparatus, as already described, consists of multiple small units dispersed in the cytoplasm, and none of these has the appearance of being especially active in synthesis or concentration of secretory product. Thus the only cytological characteristic of Seroli cells that is suggestive of steroidogenesis is its well-developed smooth endoplasmic reticulum, clearly associated with lipid droplets (Figure 28.7). This finding alone is not sufficient to warrant the conclusion that Sertoli cells are engaged in the biosynthesis of estrogens or androgens. In other cell types with a well-developed smooth reticulum, the enzymes of this versatile organelle are involved in a variety of physiological activities other than metabolism of steroids—cholesterol and triglyceride synthesis, calcium sequestration, and metabolism of various lipid-soluble drugs, to name only a few.

The smooth reticulum in properly fixed Sertoli cells

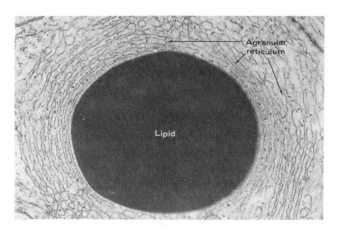

Figure 28.7 Smooth reticulum in the form of fenestrated cisternae arranged concentrically around lipid droplets, a frequent occurrence in the ram Sertoli cell.

is generally in a tubular or cisternal configuration, but in certain stages of the rodent spermatogenic cycle, especially those immediately following spermiation, the endoplasmic reticulum is reported to become distended so that it appears vesicular or vacuolar (43). The coexistence in neighboring seminiferous tubules of supporting cells with distended reticulum and others with tubules of more orthodox form has led some workers to distinguish two types of Sertoli cells (39, 46), but probably these appearances merely reflect different phases of physiological activity of a single cell type.

Especially striking are dense accumulations of smooth reticulum localized adjacent to the membrane that lines recesses in the apical cytoplasm occupied by advanced spermatids. In electron micrographs these sharply circumscribed masses of reticulum appear to form a cap over the developing acrosome of each of the spermatids (Figure 28.8). The mobilization of Sertoli cell reticulum in this close topographical relationship to developing acrosomes on the associated spermatids is one of the few morphological indications of significant interaction between the supporting cells and the germ cells (23, 25). Just what function the reticulum may have in differentiation of the acrosome remains an intriguing problem. It has been pointed out that the Sertoli cells extending the full thickness of the epithelium may have to provide for the differing needs of two or more generations of germ cells located at different levels in the epithelium. The accumulations of reticulum just described suggest that this may be accomplished by local mobilization of organelles in different proportions or configurations in different regions of the cytoplasm.

The Sertoli cell cytoplasm contains a variety of membrane-limited dense bodies that are all believed

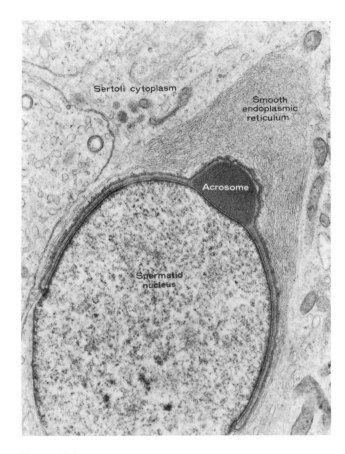

Figure 28.8 Ram spermatid at stage shortly before onset of nuclear condensation. Smooth endoplasmic reticulum of the Sertoli cell forms a conspicuous caplike aggregation of membrane precisely localized over the acrosomal cap of each developing spermatid. Similar localization of smooth reticulum is seen in many other species.

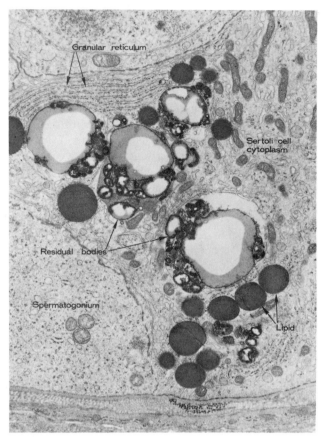

Figure 28.9 Electron micrograph of the base of a monkey Sertoli cell showing several heterophagic vacuoles or residual bodies in an advanced state of degradation. A number of droplets of lipid are also present. (Micrograph by M. Dym.)

to be part of a well-developed intracellular digestive system. (63). Small spherical bodies with a homogeneous content are considered to be primary lysosomes. Larger masses, irregular in outline and heterogeneous in their fine structure and density, are interpreted as heterophagic vacuoles containing substances in the process of degradation (Figure 28.9). Extremely dense irregular masses are identified as lipofuscin pigment deposits and interpreted as the undigestible residues of lysosomal activity (18). The majority of these bodies are found near the base of the cell.

Crystalline cytoplasmic inclusions are normally found in the Sertoli cells of humans but not in the testes of other species (2, 20, 24, 54, 58). These are of two kinds. The large Charcot-Böttcher crystalloids (8–15 μ long and 2–3 μ thick) appear in electron micrographs as bundles of 150 Å filaments or tubules. The filaments are less well ordered than the subunits of true crystals. The bundles may bifurcate, and they may have central defects occupied by the ground substance of the cyto-

plasm. The smaller crystals of Spangaro (1–5 μ long and 1 μ thick) described by light microscopists (76) do not seem to have been identified in electron micrographs. No functional significance has been attributed to these cyrstalline or paracrystalline inclusions. Since they are limited to the humans, they are probably not essential to Sertoli cell function.

The Cytoplasmic Matrix
The principal components of cytoplasmic matrix that resist extraction during specimen preparation for electron microscopy are microfilaments and microtubules. These are of interest because of their involvement in movements of organelles within the cytoplasm and in determination of cell shape. In general, the shape changes associated with cell motility are attributed to contractility of an ectoplasmic zone of cytoplasm rich in 60–70 Å filaments that have been identified as actin. A second category of 100 Å filaments that have not been chemically characterized seems to have a sup-

porting or cytoskeletal function. Microtubules 250 Å in diameter participate in the maintenance of cell shape and have an important role in determining the direction of cytoplasmic flow and the movements of organelles and inclusions within the cytoplasm. Microtubules and both categories of filaments are present in Sertoli cell cytoplasm, but their distribution and relative abundance varies in different stages of the cycle.

The thicker filaments occur in bundles associated with the special occluding junctions between neighboring Sertoli cells near the base of epithelium. The bundles of filaments are interposed between the cell membrane and a subsurface cistern of the endoplasmic reticulum. They are circumferentially oriented and course-parallel to each other and to the cell base. Similar junctional specializations line the recesses in the apical cytoplasm occupied by the heads of elongated spermatids. Filaments of this character (100 Å) are seldom found elsewhere in the cytoplasm, but they may rarely be observed in regularly spaced bundles between cisternae of the reticulum in the infranuclear region. An exception to this general statement is found in the testis of the macaque at the transitional zone near the junction of the seminiferous tubules with the *tubuli recti*, where 100 Å filaments are the predominant component of the cytoplasm (19). These Sertoli cells have an appearance very different from those elsewhere in the tubules. Their cytoplasm in histological sections is pale-staining and poor in organelles. In electron micrographs the pale areas are found to be filled with closely packed filaments. Such a high concentration of filaments has not been reported for other species; however, the transitional segment has been neglected in ultrastructural studies, and its filament concentration may be found more commonly when it is studied in other species.

The other category of thinner filaments (60–70 Å) is of general occurrence but is relatively inconspicuous, being found as randomly oriented individual filaments or occasionally assembled in small bundles parallel to the long axis in the columnar portion of the cell.

Cytoplasmic microtubules are present at all stages, but they are most obvious and most consistent in their orientation in cells supporting advanced spermatids deeply recessed in the cell apex (11). They are found throughout the columnar portion of such cells, oriented parallel to the cell axis. In sections transverse to this axis at the level of the condensed nuclei of advanced spermatids, circular cross sections of microtubules are numerous and remarkably uniform in their spacing (Figure 28.10). They have usually been interpreted as cytoskeletal elements providing internal support for the columnar portion of the Sertoli cell, but this may not be their only function. Their uniform spacing and parallel orientation is reminiscent of the

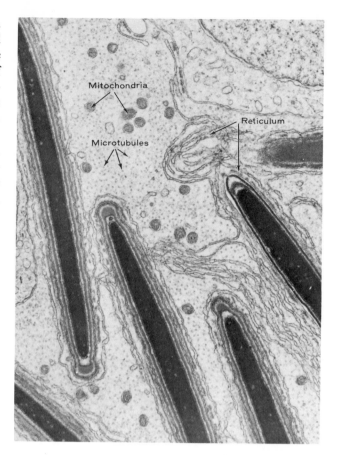

Figure 28.10 Apical region of a ram Sertoli cell section parallel to the basal lamina. Transverse sections of condensed heads of several late spermatids are surrounded by cisternal profiles of smooth endoplasmic reticulum. Punctate profiles of numerous microtubules are evenly distributed throughout Sertoli cell cytoplasm. Small round sections of mitochondria also appear. Both microtubules and mitochondria present circular profiles, because they are oriented parallel to the vertical cell axis and therefore in this horizontal section are cut transversely.

arrangement of microtubules in nerve axons. There is abundant evidence that the neurotubules are involved in axoplasmic flow or in the more rapid movement of vesicles and other particulate cytoplasmic constituents along the axon. By analogy it seems likely that the microtubules of Sertoli cells are involved in the flow of cytoplasm associated with movement of late spermatids upward and downward in the epithelium at different stages of spermiogenesis.

28.3 Participation in Sperm Release

In classical accounts of spermiogenesis, the spermatids were considered to develop as individual cells and were thought to be released into the lumen with a flask-shaped lobule of excess cytoplasm still attached to them. This tab of cytoplasm was said to be cast off by a process of active constriction, and the spherical residual bodies thus formed were believed to be phagocytized by the Sertoli cells while the spermatozoa were transported along the tubules to the rete testis and ductuli efferentes. One of the major contributions of electron-microscopic studies of the seminiferous epithelium has been a clarification of the mechanism of sperm release and the demonstration of a complex and active role of the Sertoli cells in this process (29). Ultrastructural studies of spermiation in several species are in substantial agreement on the following sequence of events.

Active elongation of the spermatids results in adluminal displacement of the bulk of their cytoplasm, which comes to surround the base of the flagellum that projects into the lumen (7). Their condensed nucleus and acrosome occupy deep conforming recesses in the apical surface of the Sertoli cells (Figure 28.11A). At this stage the spermatids appear to be drawn deeper into the epithelium, so their nuclei are at or near the level of the Sertoli cell nuclei. These movements require the coordinated action of a number of Sertoli cells, since the large syncytial clusters of spermatids joined by intercellular bridges span several supporting cells and must be moved as a unit. Concurrently with this deeper penetration of the germ cells, the Sertoli cells extend multiple studlike processes into each lobe of spermatid cytoplasm (66, 67, 68). They are expanded at their tips and appear in thin sections as round profiles bounded by two membranes. These processes are interpreted as hold-fast devices of the Sertoli cells grasping the spermatid cytoplasm. In addition, thin laminar processes of the free surface of the supporting cells envelop the rounded lobes of spermatid cytoplasm projecting into the lumen. The intercrescent processes of the Sertoli cells, their overarching laminar processes, and the persisting intercellular bridges connecting the spermatids all serve to fix the lobules of

excess cytoplasm in the epithelium. As the process of spermiation progresses, the nucleus, base of flagellum, and other axial components of the spermatids are displaced toward the lumen, while their eccentric lobules of residual cytoplasm remain fixed (Figure 28.11B). This adluminal shift of the head, neck, and flagellum is attributed to active movements of the apical cytoplasm of the Sertoli cells.

The progressive extrusion of the axial components of the spermatid, while the cytoplasmic lobule is held immobile, results in a gradual reversal of the relative positions of these two parts of the spermatid. The neck region, which at an earlier stage was deep in the epithelium and some distance rostral to the residual cytoplasm, is later situated in the lumen and is connected to the residual cytoplasm by a slender stalk that runs rostrally along the side of the spermatid nucleus (Figure 28.11C). With further adluminal displacement of the head, this cytoplasmic stalk becomes extremely attenuated and finally gives way. Its proximal portion then retracts to the neck region of the free spermatozoan to form its cytoplasmic droplet. The distal portion of the stalk retracts into the residual cytoplasm, which rounds up near the surface of the epithelium (Figure 28.11D). In this way individual free spermatozoa are separated from syncytial cell bodies that remain in the epithelium, partially or completely enveloped by slender Sertoli cell processes. Thus, contrary to the classical interpretation, the residual bodies are not normally cast off into the lumen with

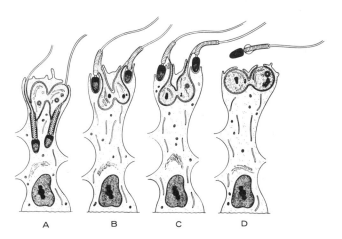

Figure 28.11 Successive stages in sperm release. A: Elongated spermatids deeply embedded in the Sertoli cell with cytoplasm caudal to the middle piece. B: Extrusion of axial components of spermatids while lobules of cytoplasm are held in the epithelium. C: Continued extrusion of sperm head resulting in attenuation of slender stalk connecting cytoplasm to neck region. D: Breaking of stalk with retraction of its proximal portion to neck region, forming the cytoplasmic droplet and leaving behind rounded residual bodies still held in the epithelium.

the spermatozoa but are retained within the epithelium throughout spermiogenesis and spermiation; however, agents that damage or interfere with the normal physiology of Sertoli cells may result in intraluminal residual bodies. The traditional observations of unreduced spermatids and free residual bodies in the lumen were almost certainly artifacts due to a combination of mechanical damage in excising the tissue and shrinkage attributable to the harsher fixation and embedding procedures used for light microscopy.

A much simpler mechanism of spermiation has been proposed for amphibian testes (8). Evidence from studies on the toad shows that luteinizing hormone (LH) causes the Sertoli cells to imbibe water, and the resulting swelling of their apical cytoplasm effaces the niches occupied by the maturing spermatids, thus expelling them into the lumen. Some investigators have endeavored to extend this interpretation to the mammal (9, 82), but their evidence for Sertoli cell swelling in response to LH has gone unconfirmed where adequate fixation was achieved through perfusion. Moreover, passive swelling would be expected to release residual bodies as well as spermatozoa, and this is not supported by ultrastructural studies. Spermiation in the mammal appears to involve complex active movements of the apical region of the Sertoli cell. These movements probably depend upon the actinlike category of small cytoplasmic filaments and possibly upon cytoplasmic flow directed along microtubules.

28.4 Phagocytic Function

The disposal of the residual bodies and of the considerable number of germ cells that normally degenerate during spermatogenesis is generally attributed to phagocytosis and intracellular digestion by Sertoli cells (64, 4). Phagocytosis is not a common property of epithelia, and the few that exhibit this behavior are characterized by a highly heterogeneous cytoplasm with an abundance of lysosomes. It has been possible to demonstrate phagocytic potential of Sertoli cells by injecting dyes or carbon particles into the rete testis and observing their uptake from the lumen of the distal ends of the seminiferous tubules (15). But they do not show the voracity that would seem to be required to rapidly dispose of the large volume of residual cytoplasm discarded in the course of normal spermatogenesis. The number of primary lysosomes found in their apical cytoplasm also seems quite inadequate for a task of this magnitude.

Examination of the epithelium by electron microscopy immediately after spermiation suggests that separation of spermatozoa from spermatid cytoplasm may initiate autophagy in the latter. There is evidence of early dissolution of the membrane of the residual body

and beginning degradation of its organelles and inclusions while it is still extracellular with respect to the Sertoli cell. Thus the initial phases of disposal of residual bodies and degenerating germ cells probably depend upon activation of their own lysosomal system and autophagic dissolution of many of their constituents. There seems to be no doubt, however, that later stages of their degradation do take place within the Sertoli cell. Dense masses of lipofuscin pigment found in the basal cytoplasm are assumed to be indigestible end products of this heterophagic activity of Sertoli cells.

Considering the enormous numbers of residual bodies formed in each spermatogenic cycle and the number of cycles in a reproductive lifetime, it is remarkable that more lipochrome pigment does not accumulate in these cells. They would seem to have a burden of protoplasmic disposal many times greater than that of tissue macrophages or fixed elements of the reticuloendothelial system. Several tissues such as cardiac muscle, ovary, and adrenal, which are not involved in heterophagic activity, accumulate far more pigment than do Sertoli cells. One must conclude that the mechanisms of the latter for disposal of residual cytoplasm are remarkably efficient. This subject deserves more study than it has yet had. The degree to which the small molecular products of residual body degradation are reutilized by the Sertoli cells or the developing germ cells is unknown.

28.5 Maintenance of the Blood-Testis Permeability Barrier

In the past decade a number of physiological studies have shown that when vital dyes (17) and a broad spectrum of other compounds having widely differing molecular weights are introduced into the bloodstream, they rapidly appear in the testicular lymph but not in the fluid collected from the rete testis. These observations have clearly established the presence of a blood-testis permeability barrier located somewhere immediately around or within the wall of the seminiferous tubules (48, 49, 73, 84).

A more precise localization of the barrier has been achieved by morphological investigations using electron-opaque particulate tracers such as carbon, colloidal thorium dioxide, ferritin, lanthanum nitrate, or the enzyme peroxidase, which can be localized histochemically by its dense reaction product with diaminobenzidine (26, 20, 1). When these substances are injected intravascularly or interstitially they rapidly diffuse throughout the intertubular tissue. The larger particulates are usually excluded from the tubules by the layer of peritubular myoid cells, but they are able to traverse certain intercellular clefts not closed by occluding cell-to-cell junctions. This adventitial layer therefore constitutes a significant impediment to diffusion of large molecules into the tubules, but it is ineffective against the smaller tracers, peroxidase and lanthanum, which readily traverse many of the intercellular clefts between myoid cells and reach the base of the seminiferous epithelium. They also enter the intercellular clefts surrounding spermatogonia and may penetrate a short distance into the interspace between the overarching processes of the supporting cells. There the tracer is stopped abruptly by occluding junctional complexes between adjacent Sertoli cells (Figure 28.12). These are confined to the basal third of the epithelium and constitute the most effective component of the blood-testis permeability barrier.

The occluding junctions consist of symmetrical specializations of the neighboring Sertoli cells (Figure 28.13), each having subsurface cisternae of endoplasmic reticulum separated from the opposing cell membranes by parallel bundles of filaments (30, 60, 20). The membranes in the junctional region are generally 150–200 Å apart, but in limited areas they approach to within 20 Å of one another and have the appearance of small gap junctions or nexuses. In addition, there are multiple sites, spaced at more or less regular intervals along the junctional complex, where the outer leaflets of the opposing membranes come into contact and appear to be fused (Figure 28.14), as they are in the juxtaluminal tight junctions of other epithelia. Studies on thin sections alone could not ascertain whether these focal tight junctions were punctate attachments or long lines of membrane fusion running circumferentially around the cell parallel to its base. In experiments involving the use of lanthanum as an extracellular tracer, however, the lanthanum may under certain conditions penetrate far enough into the junction to distribute dense contrast medium on both sides of one or more of the sites of membrane fusion (59). In oblique views these then appeared in negative image as thin white lines transversing the dense background of lanthanum. Such images suggested that the membrane fusions were linear and of considerable extent.

This inference has now been substantiated by the technique of freeze-cleaving, which provides extensive *en face* views of the interior of the Sertoli cell membranes (25, 33). Replicas of planes of cleavage through the junctional specializations show on the inwardly directed outer half-membrane (B face) many long parallel rows of 65–110 Å particles (Figure 28.15). The spacing of the rows varies from 40 to 300 nm, and they are not interconnected as are the A face rods or ridges of typical *zonulae occludentes*. The outwardly directed inner half-membrane (A face) is characterized by a series of shallow grooves that complement the

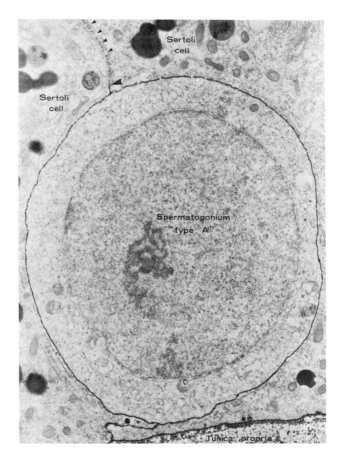

Figure 28.12 Electron micrograph of seminiferous epithelium from monkey testes in which peroxidase was used as a probe of the extracellular space. The dense tracer has penetrated the base of the epithelium and surrounds a spermatogonium. It extends a short distance into the interspace between two Sertoli cells and is stopped abruptly (large arrow) by an occluding junctional complex. These complexes are the morphological basis of the blood-testis barrier. (Micrograph by M. Dym.)

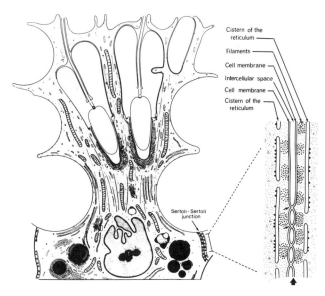

Figure 28.13 Diagrammatic representation of the location and fine structural components of the junctional specializations between Sertoli cells. The opposing membranes are fused at multiple sites. Under the opposing membrane are bundles of filaments parallel to the surface, and deep to the filaments are cisternae of the endoplasmic reticulum. The fusion of membranes closes the intercellular spaces. The significance of the associated filaments and reticulum is not known.

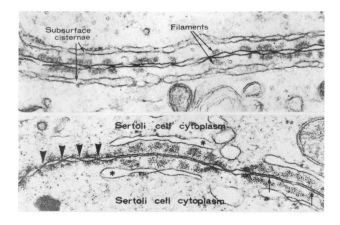

Figure 28.14 Electron micrographs illustrating Sertoli junctions of ram and rat testis. The components shown here were presented diagrammatically in Figure 28.13.

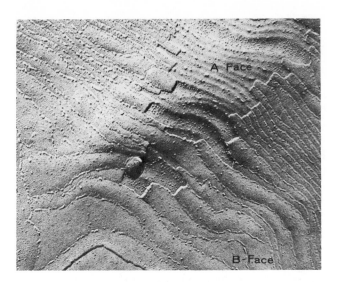

Figure 28.15 Freeze-cleaving preparation of the junctional region of the interface between two Sertoli cells showing representative areas of both the A and B faces of the membranes. The rows of membrane intercalated particles are mainly associated with the B face. (Micrograph by N. B. Gilula and D. W. Fawcett)

rows of particles on the B face. Discontinuities in the linear particle aggregates of the B face are usually represented by groups or short rows of particles that have adhered to the grooves on the A face.

These parallel linear arrays of particles seen within the plane of the membrane correspond to the focal contacts and lines of membrane fusion seen in thin sections of the Sertoli junctions. The extensive views presented in the freeze-cleaving technique make it quite clear that the circumferential lines of membrane fusion extend for long distances around the base of the cell parallel to the basal lamina.

The nonjunctional areas of the A face contain many randomly distributed intramembranous particles of varying size. In addition, between the successive rows of the occluding junction, one occasionally observes on the A face particles of uniform size (70 Å) closely packed in rows with a center-to-center spacing of 100 Å (Figure 28.16). These aggregates may form single rows of limited length or several rows in close proximity. They appear to represent an unusual form of gap junction and correspond to the areas of close membrane apposition recognized in thin sections of Sertoli junctions. They are, no doubt, the basis for the electrical coupling (77) and communication between Sertoli cells that enables them to coordinate their activities.

The Sertoli junctions differ from other occluding junctions (a) in their location near the base of the epithelium, (b) in the linear aggregation of membrane-intercalated particles of varying size associated with

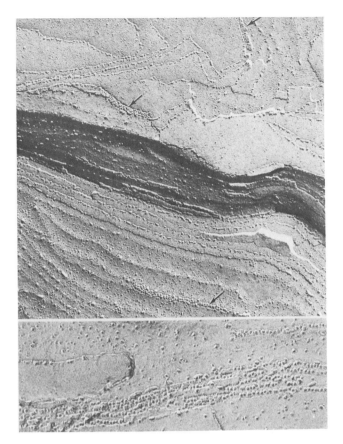

Figure 28.16 Additional examples of Sertoli cell junctional complexes as revealed by freeze fracturing. Small aggregations of closely packed particles on the A face represent small nexuses or gap junctions and are believed to be for electrical coupling of Sertoli cells and integration of their physiological activities. (Micrograph by N. B. Gilula and D. W. Fawcett.)

the B face, (c) in the lack of anastomoses between the linear particle arrays, and, (d) in the very large number of parallel lines of membrane fusion (20–35) arranged in series. Probably none of these is a complete seal, since blind endings of lines of fusion can be seen both in tracer studies and in freeze-fracture preparations. But aggregately these multiple rows constitute a highly effective barrier against penetration of the intercellular spaces from the base of the epithelium.

In a comparative study of the juxtaluminal occluding junctions of a wide range of epithelia, a positive correlation has been found between the number of rows of membrane-intercalated rods in freeze-fracture images and the "tightness" of the permeability barrier as measured by transepithelial electrical resistance (14). Although no data are available on the resistance across the seminiferous epithelium, the exceptionally large number of parallel rows of membrane fusion in the Sertoli junctions suggests that this is one of the "tight

est" epithelial permeability barriers in the body. It is also exceptionally resistant to hypertonic lithium chloride or urea, agents that very rapidly uncouple liver cells and that open up the occluding endothelial junctions of the cerebral capillaries that constitute the blood-brain permeability barrier.

In newborn rats the occluding Sertoli junctions are not present and there is no blood-testis barrier. They develop concurrently with the acquisition of a lumen by the seminiferous cords and the onset of spermatogenesis. Their differentiation does not seem to be directly hormone-dependent since suppression of gonadotropin release by clomiphene or estrogen administration delays, but does not prevent, their development (83).

The compartmentation of the epithelium by occluding Sertoli cell junctions obviously cannot be permanent. At any given time there must be certain segments of seminiferous tubules, representing particular stages of the cycle, where the junctional specializations break down transiently to permit syncytial groups of preleptotene spermatocytes to move up from the basal compartment into the abluminal compartment. As yet, no adequate explanation exists for how this is accomplished or what its local control is. There is no experimental evidence for the existence of segments of tubule that lack a barrier and where tracers can penetrate to the lumen. A progressive dissolution of the junctions on the adluminal side of the ascending germ cells may be accompanied by the simultaneous formation of a new occluding junction on their abluminal side so that at no time is the barrier open. This phenomenon deserves further study, even though it presents serious technical difficulties.

28.6 Secretory Function

Both endocrine and exocrine secretory functions have been attributed to the Sertoli cells, but in all cases the physiological evidence is incomplete and the morphological evidence is ambiguous. Certainly they do not have the cytological characteristics of typical secretory cells.

Abundant experimental evidence shows that the fetal testes are responsible for inhibition of development of the müllerian ducts as well as for maintenance of the wolffian ducts and virilization of the external genitalia (40). Androgens produced by the fetal interstitial Leydig cells stimulate the wolffian ducts and cause male differentiation of the genitalia. The müllerian ducts, on the other hand, are unaffected by androgens. But when juxtaposed in vitro to isolated seminiferous cords, a diffusible product, called antimüllerian substance or antimüllerian hormone, causes their regression. Ingenious experiments involving segregation of seminiferous cords from Leydig cells, elimination of germ cells from the seminiferous cords, and establishment of monolayer cultures of fetal Sertoli cells have demonstrated that the so-called antimüllerian hormone originates in the Sertoli cells (41, 42, 5). Its chemical nature has not been determined, nor is it known whether its production is limited to a particular period of fetal development.

A very significant recent advance has been the discovery of an androgen-binding protein (ABP) with a high affinity for testosterone and dihydrotestosterone. This is synthesized in the seminiferous tubules and released into the lumen (32, 35, 36). The synthesis of ABP is stimulated by FSH, and evidence points to the Sertoli cell as its site of origin. The production of ABP may help to achieve the high intratubular concentrations of androgen required for maintenance of spermatogenesis. Added to the tubular fluid, it results in accumulation of androgen in rete testis fluid in concentrations 10 to 15 times those found in the peripheral blood (37). There is reason to believe that these high intraluminal concentrations of androgen are necessary to maintain the cytological differentiation and normal function of the initial segments of *ductus epididymidis* (28). Incontestable biochemical evidence shows that FSH administration results in increased protein synthesis in seminiferous tubules of immature animals (55, 56). There is also physiological evidence for production and release of ABP in the adult in response to FSH stimulation. Moreover ^{125}I-labeled FSH has been found to bind specifically to Sertoli cells and not to other cell types in the seminiferous epithelium. Thus the Sertoli cells seem to represent the primary site of FSH action in the testes (78).

Cytological evidence of exocrine secretory activity by Sertoli cells is largely lacking. They are endowed with an amount of granular endoplasmic reticulum consistent with fairly active protein synthesis, but no product is visible within the cisternae of this organelle; no secretory granules have been identified in association with the Golgi apparatus; and no images suggestive of release of a secretory product by exocytosis have thus far been reported by electron microscopists.

The intimate intermingling of interstitial tissue and seminiferous tubules has made it difficult to distinguish their respective biochemical functions. The suggestion that the tubules, as well as the Leydig cells, have a capacity for biosynthesis of steroids has been advanced repeatedly but remains a subject of controversy (6, 58). The idea has been strongly supported by the finding that canine testicular tumors that are believed to originate from Sertoli cells secrete estrogens (38). Analysis of lipid extracted from testes of irradiated animals, together with results of histochemical

and ultrastructural investigations, led to the speculation that the stimulus initiating progressive differentiation of spermatogonia might be a steroid elaborated by the Sertoli cell in response to the ingestion of residual bodies from the previous cycle of spermatogenesis (50, 51, 52, 53). The evidence supporting this interesting thesis was rather tenuous, and it has not been widely accepted.

In recent years it has been shown that in some rodent species the seminiferous tubules can be separated from the interstitial tissue by taking advantage of a natural plane of cleavage provided by the lumen of extensive peritubular lymphatic sinusoids (13). This seemed to offer, for the first time, the possibility of direct analysis of the respective contributions of the two components to testicular steroidogenesis. When the two fractions were incubated with ^{14}C-progesterone, both converted the labeled compound to testosterone in vitro, but the specific activity of the interstitial tissue was 40 to 140 times greater than that of the tubules (13). In other studies using these two tissue fractions, significant qualitative differences in the steroid intermediates were reported, and it was concluded that the tubules have a steroidogenic function utilizing the same precursors but following a biosynthetic pathway involving intermediates that are not formed in significant amounts by isolated interstitial tissue (3). In these studies the amount of androgen produced by the tubules was so small that it was difficult to exclude the possibility of minor contamination by Leydig cells.

Other investigators, using a different approach, conclude that the interstitial cells are certainly the major and probably the only source of testicular androgens (34). Thus the question of steroidogenesis by Sertoli cells remains unresolved by biochemical methods. Morphological studies affirm that they possess some but not all of the characteristics of steroidogenic cells. The abundance of smooth endoplasmic reticulum, often closely associated with lipid droplets, is strongly reminiscent of similar associations in known steroidogenic cells, but the extensive smooth membranes of Sertoli cells and their constituent hydroxylases and other enzymes could equally well be interpreted as differentiations for conversion of steroids of interstitial cell origin to specific metabolites required for spermatogenesis. An interesting recent finding is that the high concentrations of androgens normally found in the rete testis can be maintained in hypophysectomized rats by administration of pregnenolone and other C21 steroids (37). This seems to indicate that the maintenance of spermatogenesis in hypophysectomized rats by these compounds (37) is due to their conversion to testosterone in the testis—very likely in the Sertoli cells.

The seminiferous epithelium can secrete fluid against an osmotic pressure gradient. In rams testicu-

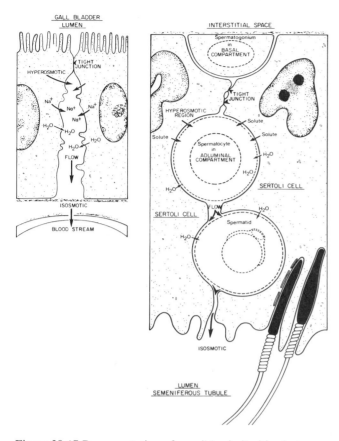

Figure 28.17 Representation of possible similarities between mechanism of absorption of water in gallbladder epithelium (A) and fluid secretion by the seminiferous epithelium (B). In gallbladder epithelium a standing osmotic gradient is thought to be created by active pumping of solute into the intercellular clefts below juxtaluminal tight junctions. Water then follows, and fluid essentially isosmotic with blood emerges from base of the epithelium. Similar morphological relations exist if one inverts the seminiferous epithelium (B). Tight junctions near base prevent direct access to adluminal intercellular clefts from base of the epithelium. Possibly if solute were pumped into clefts around the germ cells a standing gradient might be created in adluminal compartment that would move water from base to lumen. Schema at present is purely conjectural.

lar fluid is formed at a rate of 0.5 to 1.0 ml per 100 gm testis per hour, and the composition of that fluid differs significantly from that of blood plasma or lymph. It contains relatively little protein but has higher concentrations of chloride and potassium than plasma and is rich in inositol and glutamate (72). The formation of this fluid begins before the germ cells have reached an advanced stage of differentiation, and it persists after elimination of germ cells. The Sertoli cells are therefore believed to be mainly responsible for elaboration of the testicular fluid and for maintenance of its unusual composition.

It has been proposed that the standing gradient hypothesis of fluid transport, which is generally accepted with certain modifications for gallbladder epithelium, might also account for the secretion of fluid by the seminiferous epithelium (71, 72). The gallbladder epithelium has occluding cell-to-cell junctions near its luminal surface and moves water from lumen to base by actively pumping sodium ions across the lateral cell membranes into the intercellular clefts, creating an hypertonic region immediately below the junctions (Figure 28.17). Water follows, diluting the sodium so that the fluid emerging at the base of the epithelium is isosmotic with the blood. An extracellular osmotic gradient is thus maintained that moves water from lumen to base, concentrating the contents of the gallbladder.

The seminiferous epithelium, on the other hand, moves water from its base to the tubule lumen. The row of occluding Sertoli junctions near the base of the epithelium may be considered analogous to the juxtaluminal tight junctions of gallbladder epithelium. With the intercellular clefts closed at the base and open to the lumen, the polarity of the system would be reversed. It is speculated that active pumping of some solute into the intercellular clefts above the Sertoli junctions may create a standing gradient in the adluminal compartment that would move water from base to lumen (Figure 28.17). In the case of the seminiferous epithelium, the solute pumped is not sodium, for the rate of secretion is not diminished by ouabain. It is altered by carbonic anhydrase inhibitors, however, which may effect active chloride transport. The fluid secreted is also rich in potassium (71).

While the applicability of the standing gradient hypothesis to the seminiferous epithelium has not yet been established beyond doubt, it seems to offer a plausible mechanism for secretion of tubule fluid. Moreover, since the lumen does not appear in the seminiferous cords and fluid secretion by the epithelium does not begin until about the time of differentiation of the Sertoli junctions (83), fluid secretion by the tubules may well be dependent upon development of the necessary morphological relations for creation of a standing gradient in the adluminal compartment.

28.7 Response to Injury

The shape of the Sertoli cell is so elaborate and its relationship to the germ cells is so complex that it is difficult in routine histological preparations even to define cell limits because of extensive interdigitation and superimposition. The cytological characteristics of Sertoli cells were thus studied relatively little in the past. Investigations of human male infertility and experimental studies on the effects of antispermatogenic agents focused almost exclusively upon changes in the germ cells. The ability of Sertoli cells to survive injury by ionizing radiation, to tolerate elevated temperature in cryptorchidism, and to persist after elimination of germ cells by pharmacological agents has fostered the belief that these cells are extraordinarily resistant to damage.

In the past decade improved fixation, plastic embedding, and the cutting of sections one-fifth to one-tenth the thickness of routine paraffin sections have made it possible to exploit more fully the resolving power of the light microscope. As a result of these technical advances, together with the wider use of the electron microscope, it has become apparent that the Sertoli cells are actually responsive to a variety of agents and may prove to be very sensitive indicators of testicular damage.

Their repertoire of cytological reactions to injury seems to be rather restricted. The most common response is the development of many clear, cytoplasmic vacuoles of varying size (Figure 28.18). In electron micrographs, each of these is found to be limited by a membrane but usually appears entirely empty. The virtual absence of material precipitated by the fixative implies that the content of these vacuoles in the living state is aqueous and includes little or no protein. They are usually spherical but may become very large and may be so closely packed that they assume polygonal profiles by mutual deformation. This change in the Sertoli cells has been observed in a wide variety of seemingly unrelated forms of experimental insult to the seminiferous epithelium, including exposure to the hypoxia of simulated high altitude (10), deficiency of vitamin A (74), induction of allergic orchitis, and administration of the antifertility agents bis dichloroacetyl diamine (WIN 18446) (31) and the alkylating agent 2,3,5 tris ethylene iminobenzyquinone (Trenimon) (44). It is also observed in certain male sterile mutants of the mouse and in many cases of human infertility of unknown provenance.

Thus the accumulation of watery vacuoles seems to be a nonspecific response of Sertoli cells to a wide variety of injuries. Whether these vacuoles arise by dilation and rounding up of cisternae of the endoplasmic reticulum or by endocytosis of droplets of fluid has not

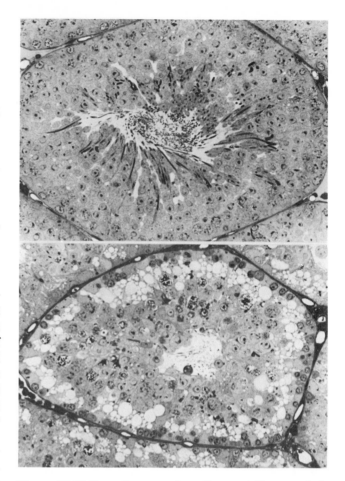

Figure 28.18 Top: Cross section of a seminiferous tubule from a normal hamster. Bottom: Comparable section from an animal subjected to simulated high altitude. The Sertoli cell show extensive vacuolation. This seems to be a nonspecific reaction of Sertoli cells to injury. It is seen after a wide variety of agents that affect spermatogenesis. (Photomicrographs courtesy of R. Yates.)

been clearly established. It is conceivable that this intracellular accumulation of fluid results from damage to a secretory process or a transcellular transport mechanism. That it often appears before there is obvious damage to germ cells suggests that many changes hitherto attributed to a direct action upon the germ cells may actually be secondary to interference with Sertoli cell function. These findings serve to reemphasize the need for further study of the physiology and biochemistry of this remarkable and poorly understood cell type.

28.8 Landmark Advances of the Past Two Decades

1. The definitive demonstration, by electron microscopy, that the Sertoli cells are individual and not syncytial.

2. Description of the fine structural features of the cell that were beyond the reach of the light microscope.

3. Description of the complex active role of the Sertoli cell in sperm release, and residual body retention.

4. Identification of the occluding junctional complexes between Sertoli cells as the structural basis of the blood-testis permeability barrier.

5. Recognition that the Sertoli junctions achieve a compartmentation of the seminiferous epithelium into a basal compartment containing the spermatogonia and an adluminal compartment containing more advanced stages of germ cells. Realization of possible implications of this arrangement for control of spermatogenesis and as a safeguard against autoimmunization against sperm antigens.

6. The demonstration by the freeze-cleaving technique of the unique nature of the Sertoli cell occluding junctions and the identification of atypical gap junctions that are believed to be the basis for electrical coupling and coordination of the activities of the supporting cells.

7. Discovery of a factor in the fetal testis that inhibits the müllerian duct, and accumulation of evidence for its production by the Sertoli cells.

8. Recognition that the Sertoli cells are probably the primary site of FSH activity in the testis (based upon selective binding of labeled gonadotropin and demonstration of increased protein synthesis in response to FSH administration).

9. Identification of ABP and demonstration that it is produced by the Sertoli cells in response to FSH stimulation.

10. Discovery that high levels of androgen in the rete testis fluid can be maintained in hypophysectomized rats by administration of C_{21} steroids. This can best be explained by conversion of these compounds to testosterone and dihydrotestosterone in the testis —probably by the Sertoli cells.

11. Recognition that the Sertoli cells are highly sensitive to a wide variety of agents and exhibit a nonspecific response to injury consisting of accumulation of large numbers of watery vacuoles in the cytoplasm.

28.9 Gaps in Our Knowledge

1. Although the Sertoli cells have long been regarded as "nurse cells" or "sustentacular cells," we still do not know what they contribute to the germ cells or how essential this is for their development.

2. Recent evidence suggests that Sertoli cells in hypophysectomized animals can produce androgens from C_{21} steroids. Still unknown is the degree to which this mechanism operates in intact animals, as well as the degree to which normal spermatogenesis depends upon steroids or steroid metabolites produced by Sertoli cells.

3. Sertoli cells are believed to produce ABP. It remains to be established whether the principal function of ABP is to maintain a steep gradient tending to facilitate diffusion of androgen into the seminiferous epithelium or whether its principal function is the transport of androgen in high concentration to maintain normal cytological differentiation and function of the head of the epididymis.

4. Morphological studies of spermiation indicate that the germ cells are relatively passive. The concurrent movement of sperm into the lumen and the retention of residual bodies depend upon complex motor activities of the Sertoli cells. This would seem to be a vulnerable step in spermatogenesis that deserves more intensive study. Certain antifertility agents appear to interfere with sperm release; others appear to cause premature release of immature forms. Either effect has potential for contraception in the male.

5. There is evidence for production by the seminiferous tubules of a factor (inhibin) that exerts a negative feedback on FSH release by the pituitary. Other evidence suggests a local feedback from the tubules to the Leydig cells. Further research is needed to determine whether these factors originate in the germ cells or the supporting cells; efforts are needed to isolate and characterize them.

6. The occluding junctions between Sertoli cells near the base of the seminiferous epithelium constitute a tight permeability barrier that isolates meiotic and postmeiotic germ cells from the general extracellular fluid compartment of the testis. Further study is needed to discover the mechanism controlling the opening and closing of this barrier and to determine whether the barrier is indeed essential for fluid secretion and germ cell differentiation.

References

1. Aoki, A., and D. W. Fawcett. Impermeability of Sertoli cell junctions to prolonged exposure to peroxidase. Andrologie 7:63, 1975.

2. Bawa, S. R. The fine structure of the Sertoli cell of the human testes. J. Ultrastruct. Res. 9:459, 1963.

3. Bell, J. B. C., C. D. Vinson, and D. Lacy. Studies on the structure and function of the mammalian testis. III. In vitro steroidogenesis by the seminiferous tubules of rat testis. Proc. R. Soc. Lond. [B] 176:433, 1971.

4. Black, V. H. Gonocytes in fetal guinea-pig testes: Phagocytosis of degenerating gonocytes by Sertoli cells. Am. J. Anat. 131:415, 1971.

5. Blanchard, M. G., and N. Josso. Source of the anti-Müllerian hormone synthesized by the fetal testis. II. Müllerian inhibiting activity of fetal bovine Sertoli cells in tissue culture. Pediatr. Res., 1974.

6. Brökelmann, J. Fine structure of germ cells and Sertoli cells during the cycle of the seminiferous epithelium in the rat. Z. Zellforsch, Mikrosk. Anat. 59:820, 1963.

7. Burgos, N. H., and D. W. Fawcett. Studies on the fine structure of the mammalian testis. I. Differentiation of the spermatids in the cat. J. Biophys. Biochem. Cytol. 1:287, 1955.

8. Burgos, M. H., and R. Vitale-Calpe. The mechanism of spermiation in the toad. Am. J. Anat. 120:227, 1967.

9. Burgos, M. H., and R. Vitale-Calpe. Gonadotropic control of spermiation. In Progress in endocrinology, ed. C. Gual, p. 1030. Amsterdam: Excerpta Medica, 1969.

10. Chen, I-Li, and R. D. Yates. Effects of simulated high altitude on hamster testes. Anat. Rec. 178 (Abstract), 1974.

11. Christensen, A. K. Microtubules in Sertoli cells of guinea pig testis. Anat. Rec. 151 (Abstract), 1965.

12. Christensen, A. K., and G. B. Chapman. Cup-shaped mitochondria in interstitial cells of the albino rat testis. Exp. Cell Res. 18:576, 1959.

13. Christensen, A. K., and N. R. Mason. Comparative ability of seminiferous tubules and interstitial tissue of rat testes to synthesize androgens from progesteron-4-^{14}C in vitro. Endocrinology 76:646, 1965.

14. Claude, P., and D. A. Goodenough. The ultrastructure of the zonula occludens in freeze-fractured material from tight and leaky epithelia. J. Cell Biol. 53:390, 1973.

15. Clegg, E. J., and E. W. MacMillan. The uptake of vital dyes and particulate matter by the Sertoli cells of the rat testis. J. Anat. 99:219, 1965.

16. Clyman, M. J. A new structure observed in the nucleolus of the human endometrial epithelial cell. Am. J. Obstet. Gynecol. 86:430, 1963.

17. Debruyn, P. P. H., R. C. Robertson, and R. S. Farr. In vivo affinity of deaminocridine dyes for nuclei. Anat. Rec. 108:279, 1950.

18. Dym, M. The fine structure of the monkey Sertoli cell and its role in maintaining the blood-testis barrier. Anat. Rec. 175:639, 1973.

19. Dym, M. The fine structure of monkey Sertoli cells in the transitional zone at the junction of the seminiferous tubules with the tubuli recti. Am. J. Anat. 140:1, 1974.

20. Dym, M., and D. W. Fawcett. Observations on the blood-testis barrier of the rat and on the physiological compartmentation of the seminiferous epithelium. Biol. Reprod. 3:308, 1970.

21. Ebner, V. von. Untersuchungen uber den Bau der samenkanalchen und die enwickelung der Spermatozoiden bei den Saugethieren und Menschen. Untersuchungen aus dem Institut fur Physiologie und Histologie im Graz (Liepzig) 2: 200, 1871.

22. Ebner, V. von. Zur Spermatogenese bei den Saugethieren. Arch. Mikrobiol. Anat. 31:236, 1898.

23. Fawcett, D. W. Interrelations of cell types within the seminiferous epithelium and their implications for control of spermatogenesis. In Regulation of mammalian reproduction, ed. S. Segal. Springfield, Ill.: Charles C Thomas, 1973.

24. Fawcett, D. W., and M. H. Burgos. The fine structure of Sertoli cells in the human testes. Anat. Rec. 124:401 (Abstract), 1956.

25. Fawcett, D. W. Interactions between Sertoli cells and germ cells. In Male fertility and sterility, eds. R. E. Mancini and L. Martini, p. 13. New York: Academic Press, 1974.

26. Fawcett, D. W., L. V. Leak, and P. N. Heidger. Electron microscopic observations on the structural components of the blood-testis barrier. J. Reprod. Fertil. Suppl. 10:105, 1970.

27. Fawcett, D. W., J. A. Long, and A. L. Jones. The ultrastructure of the endocrine glands. Recent Prog. Horm. Res. 25:315, 1969.

28. Fawcett, D. W., and A. Hoffer. Dependence of the initial segment of the rat epididymal duct upon substances in the testicular fluid. In Proceedings of the 14th Conference of the Anatomical Society of Australia and New Zealand, p. 51, 1976.

29. Fawcett, D. W., and D. M. Phillips. Observations on the release of spermatozoa and on the changes in the head during passage through the epididymis. J. Reprod. Fertil. Suppl. 6:418, 1969.

30. Flickinger, C., and D. W. Fawcett. Junctional specializations of the Sertoli cells in the seminiferous epithelium. Anat. Rec. 158:207, 1967.

31. Flores, M., and D. W. Fawcett. Ultrastructural effects of the antispermatogenic compound, WIN 18446 (bis dichloroacetyl diamine). Anat. Rec. 172:319, 1972.

32. French, F. S., and E. M. Ritzen. Androgen binding protein in efferent duct fluid of rat testis. J. Reprod. Fertil. 32:479, 1973.

33. Gilula, N. B., D. W. Fawcett, and A. Aoki. Ultrastructural and experimental observations on the Sertoli cell junctions of the mammalian testis. Dev. Biol. 50:142, 1976.

34. Hall, P. F., D. C. Irby, and D. M. deKretser. Conversion of cholesterol to androgens by rat testes: Comparison of interstitial cells and seminiferous tubules. Endocrinology 84: 488, 1969.

35. Hansson, V., O. Trygstad, F. S. French, W. S. McLean, A. A. Smith, D. J. Tindall, S. C. Weddington, P. Petrusz, S. N. Nahfeh, and E. M. Ritzen. Androgen transport and receptor mechanisms in the testis and epididymis (in press).

36. Hansson, V., F. S. French, S. C. Weddington, W. S. McLean, D. J. Tindall, A. A. Smith, S. N. Nahfeh, and E. M. Ritzen. Androgen transport mechanisms in the testis and epididymis. Int. Res. Commun. Syst. November 1973.

37. Harris, M. E., and A. Bartke. Maintenance of rete testis fluid testosterone and dihydrotestosterone levels by pregnenolone and other C-21 steroids in hypophysectomized rats. Proc. Soc. Study Reprod. (Abstract 145), 1974.

38. Huggins, C., and P. V. Moulder. Estrogen production by Sertoli cell tumors of the testes. Cancer Res. 5:510, 1945.

39. Johnson, S. G. Two types of Sertoli cells in man. Acta Endocrinol. 61:111, 1969.

40. Jost, A. Hormonal factors in the sex differentiation of the mammalian fetus. Phil Trans. R. Soc. Lond. [B] 259:119, 1970.

41. Josso, N. Permeability of membranes to Müllerian inhibiting substance synthesized by the human fetal testis in vitro: A clue to its biochemical nature. J. Clin. Endocrinol. 34:265, 1972.

42. Josso, N. In vitro synthesis of Müllerian-inhibiting hormone by seminiferous tubules isolated from the calf fetal testis. Endocrinology 93:829, 1973.

43. Kerr, J. B., and D. Dekretzer. Fine structure of the Sertoli cell throughout the cycle of the seminiferous epithelium in the normal and cryptorchid rat. In Electron microscopy, Vol. 2, eds. J. V. Sanders and D. J. Goodchild, p. 428. Canberra: Australian Acad. Sci., 1974.

44. Kierszenbaum, A. L. Effect of Trenimon on the ultrastructure of Sertoli cells in the mouse. Virchows Arch. [Zellpathol.] 5:1, 1970.

45. Kierszenbaum, A. L., and R. E. Mancini. Structural changes manifested by Sertoli cells during experimental allergic orchitis in guinea pigs. J. Reprod. Fertil. 33:119, 1973.

46. Kierszenbaum, A. L. RNA synthetic activity of Sertoli cells in mouse testis. Biol. Reprod. 11:365, 1974.

47. Kingsley-Smith, B. V., and D. Lacy. Residual bodies of seminiferous tubules of the rat. Nature 184:249, 1959.

48. Kormano, M. Dye permeability and alkaline phosphatase activity of testicular capillaries in the postnatal rat. Histochemie 9:327, 1967.

49. Kormano, M. Penetration of intravenous trypan blue into the rat testis and epididymis. Acta Histochem. 30:133, 1968.

50. Lacy, D. Certain aspects of testis structure and function. Br. Med. Bull. 18:205, 1962.

51. Lacy, D. The seminiferous tubules in mammals. Endeavour 26:101, 1967.

52. Lacy, D., and B. Lofts. The use of ionizing radiation and estrogen treatment in the detection of hormone synthesis by the Sertoli cell. J. Physiol. (London) 161:23, 1961.

53. Lacy, D., and A. J. Pettitt. Sites of hormone production in the mammalian testis and their significance in the control of male fertility. Br. Med. Bull. 26:87, 1970.

54. Lubarsch, O. Uber das Vorkommen kristallinischer und krystalloider Bilderungen in den Zellen des Menschlichen Hodens. Arch. Pathol. Anat. Physiol. 145:316, 1886.

55. Means, A. R. Concerning the mechanism of FSH action. Rapid stimulation of testicular synthesis of nuclear RNA. Endocrinology 89:981, 1971.

56. Means, A. R. Concerning the testicular action of FSH on cells of the seminiferous epithelium. In Biology of reproduction, Proc. Symp. Pan American Congress of Anatomy, p. 368. New Orleans, 1972.

57. Nagano, T. Some observations on the structure of interstitial cells and Sertoli cells of the human testes. Gunma Symp. Endocrinol. 2:19, 1965.

58. Nagano, T. Some observations on the fine structure of the Sertoli cells in the human testes. Z. Zellforsch Mikrosk. Anat. 73:89, 1966.

59. Neaves, W. B. Permeability of Sertoli cell tight junctions to lanthanum after ligation of ductus deferens and ductuli efferentes. J. Cell Biol. 59:559, 1973.

60. Nicander, L. An electron microscopical study of cell contacts in the seminiferous tubules of some mammals. Z. Zellforsch. Mikros. Anat. 83:375, 1967.

61. Nicander, L., M. Abdul-Raouf, and B. Crabo. On the ultrastructure of seminiferous tubules in bull calves. Acta Morphol. Neerl. Scand. 4:127, 1961.

62. Pardue, M. L., and L. G. Gall. Chromosomal localization of mouse satellite DNA. Science 168:1356, 1970.

63. Reddy, K. J., and D. J. Svoboda. Lysosomal activity in Sertoli cells of normal and degenerating germinal epithelial cells of rat testis. Am. J. Pathol. 51:1, 1967.

64. Régaud, C. Etudes sur la structure des tubes seminifères et sur la spermatogénèse chez les mammifères. Arch. Anat. Microsc. Morphol. Exp. 4:101, 331, 1901.

65. Sapsford, C. S. The development of the Sertoli cell of the rat and mouse: its existence as a mononucleate unit. J. Anat. 97:225, 1963.

66. Sapsford, C. S., and C. A. Rae. Sertoli cell–spermatid relationships ultrastructural studies of the movements of mature spermatids into the lumen of the seminiferous tubule. J. Anat. 103:215, 1968.

67. Sapsford, C. S., C. A. Rae, and K. W. Cleland. Ultrastructural studies on spermatids and Sertoli cells during early spermiogenesis in the bandocoot Perameles nasuta Geoffroy (Marsupalia). Aust. J. Zool. 15:881, 1967.

68. Sapsford, C. S., C. A. Rae, and K. W. Cleland. Ultrastructural studies on maturing spermatids and on Sertoli cells in the bandicoot (Permaeles nasuta). Aust. J. Zool. 17:195, 1969.

69. Sapsford, C. S., C. A. Rae, and K. W. Cleland. The fate of residual bodies and degenerating germ cells and the lipid cycle in Sertoli cells in the bandicoot Perameles nasuta. Aust. J. Zool. 17:729, 1969.

70. Sertoli, E. De l'esistenza di particulari cellule ramificate nei canaliculi seminiferi dell testicolo umano. Morgagni 7: 31, 1865.

71. Setchell, B. P. Testicular blood supply, lymphatic drainage, and secretion of fluid. In The testis, Vol. 1, eds. A. D. Johnson, W. R. Gomes, and N. L. Vandemark, p. 101. New York: Academic Press, 1970.

72. Setchell, B. P. Fluid secretion by the testis. J. Reprod. Fertil. 14:347, 1967.

73. Setchell, B. P., T. W. Scott, J. R. Voglmayer, and G. M. Waites. Characteristics of testicular spermatozoa and the fluid which transports them into the epididymis. Biol. Reprod. Suppl. 1:40, 1969.

74. Sherins, R. J. Increased FSH and compensated Leydig cell failure in men with disorders of spermatogenesis. Biol. Reprod. (in press).

75. Sohval, A. R., Y. Suzuki, J. L. Gabrilove, and J. Churg. Ultrastructure of crystalloids in spermatogonia and Sertoli cells of normal human testis. J. Ultrastruct. Res. 34:83, 1971.

76. Spangaro, S. Uber die histologischen Veranderungen des Hodens, Nebenhodens, und Samenleiters von Geburt an biz zum Griesalter, mit besonderer Berucksichtigung der Hodenatrophie, des elastischen Gewebes und des Vorkommens von Krystallen im Hoden. Anat. Rec. 18:593, 1902.

77. Spitzer, N. C. Low resistance junctions in male germinal tissues of the lily and the rat. Ph.D. thesis, Division of Medical Sciences, Graduate School of Arts and Sciences, Harvard University, 1969.

78. Steinberger, A., K. H. Thanki, and B. Siegal. Sertoli cells—primary site of FSH activity in the testes. Proc. Soc. Study Reprod. 21 (Abstract), 1974.

79. Suzuki, F., and T. Nagano. The postnatal development of the junctional complexes of mouse Sertoli cells as revealed by freeze-fracture. Anat. Rec. 185:403, 1976.

80. Tersakis, J. A. The nucleolar channel system in the human endometrium. J. Cell Biol. 27:293, 1965.

81. Vilar, O., M. I. Perez Del Cerro, and R. E. Manami. The Sertoli cell as a "bridge-cell" between the basal membrane and the germ cells. Exp. Cell Res. 27:158, 1962.

82. Vitale-Calpe, R., and M. H. Burgos. The mechanism of spermiation in the hamster. I. Ultrastructure of spontaneous spermiation. J. Ultrastruct. Res. 31:394, 1970.

83. Vitale-Calpe, R., D. W. Fawcett, and M. Dym. The normal development of the blood-testis barrier and the effects of clomiphene and estrogen treatment. Anat. Rec. 176:333, 1973.

84. Waites, G. M. H., and B. P. Setchell. Some physiological aspects of the function of the testis. In *The gonads*, ed. W. W. McKerns, p. 649. New York: Appleton-Century-Crofts, 1969.

29 Leydig Cells

William B. Neaves

29.1 Significant Recent Developments

In the last 10 years many lines of evidence strengthened the identification of Leydig cells as the major source of testicular androgen. At the same time, the traditional role of Leydig cells in the maintenance of extratesticular aspects of maleness was expanded to include an important intratesticular role in support of spermatogenesis. The outstanding effects of Leydig cell function, both in the testis and elsewhere, were increasingly attributed to the action of testosterone on target tissues.

Basic research in morphology, biochemistry, and physiology elucidated many details of testosterone production by Leydig cells. Electron microscopy revealed the subcellular structure of the Leydig cell, thereby providing the background for correlation of cellular ultrastructure with the synthesis and secretion of steroid hormones. Biochemical analysis of testicular cell fractions permitted the assignment of specific steroidogenic functions to various Leydig cell organelles. Metabolic studies identified the rate-limiting step in testosterone synthesis and demonstrated the ability of luteinizing hormone (LH) to influence this step. New methods for measuring plasma levels of testosterone and LH confirmed the traditional roles of these hormones in feedback control of Leydig cell function.

The importance of Leydig cells to the gametogenic function of the testis has been underscored by numerous experiments showing that maintenance of spermatogenesis after hypophysectomy can be achieved either by specific restoration of Leydig cell function or by administration of large doses of testosterone. It has become apparent that the action of LH on spermatogenesis is mediated by the secretion of testosterone by Leydig cells. Realization that the Leydig cells played a major role in supporting spermatogenesis has been accompanied by the development of a contraceptive strategy based on the suppression of Leydig cell function. In its most promising form, this strategy relies on administration of progestin to block pituitary secretion of LH, combined with testosterone replacement therapy to maintain extratesticular aspects of maleness. As a result of these recent developments, the relevance of Leydig cells to fertility control has been firmly established.

Cellular Origin of Testicular Androgens

Since the beginning of this century, Leydig cells have been considered the probable source of testicular androgens (1). During the last decade, crucial support for this view has come from a variety of sources. Christensen and Mason (2) showed that separated interstitial tissue, containing the Leydig cells of the testis, metabolized progesterone to testosterone much more efficiently than did the seminiferous tubules. Van der Molen and co-workers (3) demonstrated that synthesis of testosterone from endogenous precursors occurs in isolated interstitial tissue but not in isolated seminiferous tubules. They also found the highest concentrations of endogenous testosterone in the interstitial tissue of the testis (4). Histochemists have repeatedly shown that Leydig cells contain 3β-hydroxysteroid dehydrogenase, an essential enzyme in the conversion of pregnenolone to testosterone (5). Using fluorescent antibodies against steroid-protein conjugates, Woods and Domm (6) found that Leydig cells were the principal source of testicular steroids. Steinberger and co-workers (7) have employed tissue culture techniques to provide direct demonstration of steroid biogenesis in Leydig cells. While none of these studies eliminates Sertoli cells of the seminiferous tubules as a possible source of some androgens, they make it highly unlikely that their contribution is significant compared to Leydig cells. Although attempts have been made to link androgen synthesis with Sertoli cells (8), as yet no evidence exists that Sertoli cells are capable of de novo steroid biosynthesis (3).

Biological Significance

Over 50 years passed between Leydig's (9) discovery of the testicular interstitial cells that now bear his name and generation of the hypothesis that these cells are the source of a testicular hormone important in the development of secondary sex characteristics and sexual instincts (1). In subsequent years, Leydig cells have become increasingly associated with the development and maintenance of extratesticular aspects of maleness, a role that hinges on their secretion of the male hormone, testosterone. Perhaps because they were initially linked with extratesticular (secondary) sexual attributes, relatively little attention was directed to the possibility that Leydig cells might play an important role inside the testis. This neglect may also have been encouraged by the growing realization that hormones, by traveling through the blood, generally act on target tissues some distance from their cells of origin. Evidence that androgens could also stimulate spermatogenesis, although available by the late 1930s, was slow to influence the concept of Leydig cell function. While recognition of the androgen dependency of spermatogenesis developed, thought gradually turned to the significance of the location of Leydig cells in close proximity to the germinal epithelium. Only recently has it become apparent that the primary function of Leydig cells may be provision of the androgen stimulus required for maintenance of spermatogenesis in the germinal epithelium.

Role in spermatogenesis The androgen dependency of spermatogenesis has become a generally accepted concept during the last decade. Numerous experiments have suggested that LH, a major pituitary factor affecting spermatogenesis, exerts its influence on the germinal epithelium through stimulation of androgen secretion by the Leydig cells (10). Hence the primary function of Leydig cells may be secretion of the testosterone required to sustain spermatogenesis.

Several lines of evidence suggest that the germinal epithelium has a higher testosterone requirement than other androgen target tissues. The maintenance of spermatogenesis in hypophysectomized rats by testosterone administration requires relatively massive doses (11), so that plasma testosterone levels far in excess of those necessary for maintenance of accessory sex organs must be obtained. The administration of physiological doses of testosterone to hypophysectomized mammals maintains accessory sex organs but fails to restore spermatogenesis. On the other hand, administration of physiological doses of testosterone to intact mammals actually suppresses spermatogenesis. Morse and Heller (12) have shown that this effect is associated with a modest elevation of plasma testosterone levels and a striking reduction in plasma LH levels and in testicular testosterone concentration.

Presumably, the exogenous testosterone suppresses plasma LH while maintaining somewhat elevated plasma testosterone levels. The virtual absence of plasma LH leads to inactivation of the Leydig cells, decline in testicular testosterone concentration, and failure of spermatogenesis, which requires more testosterone than is provided by the levels of exogenous testosterone in testicular arterial blood. The seminiferous tubules are normally surrounded by lymph containing up to 10 times as much testosterone per unit volume as the arterial blood entering the testis (13). Highest concentrations of endogenous testosterone occur in the testicular interstitial tissue, a finding that favors the hypothesis that testosterone is synthesized by the

Leydig cells and transported to the seminiferous tubules (4).

It appears that the intimate association of Leydig cells with seminiferous tubules (Figure 29.1) has great physiological significance in terms of the dependency of spermatogenesis on high local concentrations of testosterone. This view is further supported by experiments performed almost 30 years ago (14). Spermatogenesis was maintained in hypophysectomized rats by intratesticular pellets of testosterone, whereas the same pellets administered subcutaneously were relatively ineffective. In similar experiments with hypophysectomized monkeys, seminiferous tubules nearest the testosterone pellet underwent complete spermatogenesis, while those more distant remained degenerate (15). The ability of testosterone to substitute for functioning Leydig cells in these and in more recent hypophysectomy experiments by Clermont and Harvey (16) indicates that Leydig cells influence spermatogenesis principally through their secretion of testosterone.

Leydig cells and masculinity The androgen-dependency of masculine traits, including the characteristic development of accessory sex organs, was firmly established in the first half of this century (17). Circulating androgen levels are generally believed to control the development of accessory sex organs, even though these levels may fluctuate from moment to moment, so that single measurements of plasma testosterone show no correlation with accessory organ weight (18). Circulating androgens in the male are thought to originate in the testis. Conclusive confirmation of the testicular origin of androgens in blood has come from the recent demonstration that plasma testosterone drops to undetectable levels soon after castration (19).

Other roles of Leydig cells Unexplained variation in the quantity and organization of interstitial tissue in different mammalian species may serve as a warning

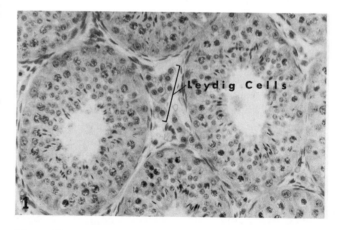

Figure 29.1 Leydig cells (× 600), showing their close association with seminiferous tubules.

that our list of Leydig cell functions is incomplete. The great quantity of Leydig cells in some species may reflect their role in processes other than testosterone production. The unusual abundance of Leydig cells in domestic boars and stallions may be related to the fact that both secrete large amounts of estrogen, the purpose of which remains obscure (20). In addition, the boar testis produces Δ^{16}-androstenone, which is thought to serve as a pheromone (21). Recent analysis shows that the boar testis contains 10 times as much Δ^{16}-androstenone as testosterone (22). Fawcett and co-workers (20) have speculated that the characteristic abundance of Leydig cells in many fossorial mammals may be related to the production of steroid olfactory signals more suited to their environment than conventional visual signals of reproductive status.

Whether the modest quantities of Leydig cells present in most mammals, including humans, serve functions in addition to androgen secretion remains to be determined. Human Leydig cells may secrete estrogen. The human testes normally secrete about $50\,\mu$g of estradiol per day (23). The fact that chorionic gonadotropin (CG) stimulates testicular estrogen production suggests that Leydig cells may be the source of this hormone (24). This issue remains controversial, however, since other indirect evidence suggests that estrogens are secreted by Sertoli cells.

Fundamental Morphological Advances

Significant advances in Leydig cell morphology during the last decade have been achieved at the subcellular level. By opening the cytoplasm of Leydig cells to fine structural analysis, high-resolution electron microscopy provided the necessary morphological background for functional correlations in the areas of cellular biochemistry and physiology. These largely descriptive studies cleared the way for increasingly experimental approaches to the relationship of structure to function in Leydig cells.

The availability of excellent reviews of recent advances in Leydig cell ultrastructure (25,26) make detailed coverage of the subject unnecessary in this discussion. Accordingly, consideration of subcellular structure (Figure 29.2) is limited to major organelles and inclusions for which functional correlations are available.

Endoplasmic reticulum The endoplasmic reticulum is a membranous organelle that extends throughout the cytoplasm as a closed system of tubules and flattened sacs. Smooth reticulum is that portion of the organelle with no ribosomes on its outer surface. The striking abundance of smooth endoplasmic reticulum in Leydig cells of the opossum encouraged Christensen and Fawcett (27) to speculate that this organelle might play a major role in the synthesis of hormonal steroids.

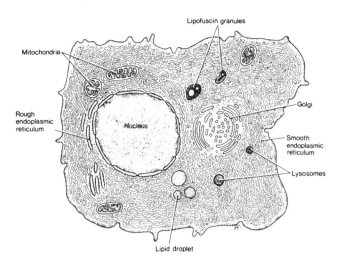

Figure 29.2 Morphology of the Leydig cell.

Since then the occurrence of large amounts of smooth reticulum has been widely recognized as the most distinctive cytoplasmic characteristic of Leydig cells from a great variety of species. Christensen (28) correlated morphological and biochemical evidence suggesting that the relative abundance of smooth reticulum in various species reflects the extent to which the Leydig cells rely on internally synthesized cholesterol for conversion to steroid hormones. His correlations, which imply that the smooth reticulum is involved in cholesterol synthesis, have been supported by localization of many cholesterol biosynthetic enzymes in the microsome (endoplasmic reticulum) fraction of testicular homogenates.

The microsome fraction of testicular homogenates also contains enzymes in the pathway from pregnenolone to testosterone, suggesting that the endoplasmic reticulum can convert precursor steroids to testosterone. Murota and co-workers (29) have strengthened this suggestion by electron-microscopic verification of poorly developed endoplasmic reticulum in Leydig cells of patients whose testicular microsomal fractions exhibited decreased conversion of progesterone to testosterone. Chronic stimulation of immature Leydig cells with CG has been shown to increase activities of several enzymes in the pathway from pregnenolone to testosterone (30) and to increase the quantities of smooth endoplasmic reticulum seen in electron micrographs (31). Morphological correlations such as these support the role of the smooth reticulum in testosterone synthesis.

Considerable structural variation has been described in the smooth reticulum. It is generally agreed that tubular and cisternal profiles more accurately reflect the form of the smooth reticulum in living cells (25) than do vesicular conformations. The functional distinction between tubular and cisternal forms is problematical, especially since the two may be freely interconvertible (28). An indication that the tubular form may be more active than the cisternal form in hormone synthesis has come from the association of exclusively tubular smooth reticulum with elevated plasma testosterone levels in seasonally breeding mammals (32).

The relationship of smooth reticulum to other organelles and inclusions may have functional significance. Christensen and Fawcett (33) noted the tendency for smooth reticulum to be segregated from other organelles in the peripheral cytoplasm of adult Leydig cells. Ichihara (34) subsequently described the development of this phenomenon in Leydig cells just prior to puberty. Neaves (35) showed that proliferation and peripheral segregation of smooth reticulum could be induced in poorly differentiated Leydig tumor cells by treatment with CG. These findings, plus the association of a segregated smooth reticulum with high plasma testosterone levels (32), suggest that the functional activity of Leydig cells may in some cases be inferred from the disposition of their smooth reticulum.

Mitochondria The mitochondrion is a discrete organelle composed of two membranous sacs, one within the other. The inner sac forms infoldings or invaginations (cristae) and encloses an amorphous matrix. In addition to their common role in cellular respiration and adenosine triphosphate production, mitochondria of Leydig cells have been associated with conversion of cholesterol to pregnenolone, a crucial step in the biosynthesis of testosterone (36). Apart from the occurrence of tubular cristae in some species, Leydig cell mitochondria are not structurally distinctive, in spite of their specific role in steroidogenesis.

Administration of exogenous gonadotropin promotes subtle changes in the fine structure of Leydig cell mitochondria. They become more pleomorphic (31), cristae increase (37), and the intracristal spaces widen (38). Similar changes occur in mitochondria of Leydig tumor cells after gonadotropin treatment (35). It is suspected that gonadotropin-induced alteration of mitochondrial structure may be related to the reactions in steroidogenesis that are thought to be located inside the mitochondrion.

Lipid droplets Lipid droplets are homogeneous, dense inclusions not bounded by a unit membrane and usually spherical in conformation. Lipid droplets in steroid-producing cells contain detectable quantities of cholesterol by the Schultz test and probably represent stores of esterified cholesterol that may be converted to steroid hormones when the proper stimulus occurs (25). The proper stimulus seems to be pituitary gonadotropin or its analogs. LH promotes a decrease in the content of esterified cholesterol in normal testes and in Leydig cell tumors (39). Morphological correlates of gonadotropin-induced cholesterol ester depletion may be found in the dramatic reduction of lipid droplets described in immature Leydig cells treated with CG (31, 40).

The depletion of lipid droplets in pubertal Leydig cells of rats coincides with the phase of maximum accessory sex organ growth (41). In seasonally breeding mammals, depletion of Leydig cell lipid droplets parallels elevation of plasma testosterone levels (32). These recent findings support the view that lipid droplets contain androgen precursor and suggest that their depletion may be a morphological indication of increased functional activity in the Leydig cell.

Golgi complex The Golgi complex, consisting of several stacks of closely packed cisternae and associated vesicles, has been implicated in the secretion of some steroid hormones (42). There is striking disparity, however, between the morphological correlates of Golgi function in protein-secreting cells and in steroid-secreting cells (26). Notably absent in the latter cells are prominent secretory vesicles. Coated vesicles associated with the Golgi complex have been suggested to function in progesterone secretion (43), but they have been discounted as major agents in steroid function because of their scarcity (44). Convincing demonstration of a relationship between the Golgi complex and the specific function of Leydig cells has yet to appear. An indication that the Golgi complex may not play a major role in testosterone secretion in some species has come from a report that this organelle is scarce and poorly developed during periods of maximal Leydig cell activity in hyrax (32).

Microbodies, lysosomes, and lipofuscin granules Microbodies and lysosomes are membrane-bound cytoplasmic vesicles containing catalase and acid hydrolase activities, respectively. The moderately dense, amorphous matrix is similar in the two organelles, so that cytochemical tests are necessary to identify them specifically. Whether microbodies have a distinctive role in Leydig cell function is not yet known (45). Neither is it evident that lysosomes are directly involved in steroid synthesis or secretion.

Lipofuscin granules are membrane-bound bodies, often irregular in profile, containing a very dense, heterogeneous matrix, which usually shows some acid hydrolase activity. The biochemistry of lipofuscin is poorly understood, but it is thought to consist primarily of indigestible products of lysosomal oxidation of lipids (37). In Leydig cells of guinea pigs (40) and humans (37), lipofuscin granules increase in response to gonadotropin administration. The significance of this observation is obscure, although it may be explained by accelerated lysosomal destruction of exhausted steroidogenic organelles.

Fundamental Biochemical Advances

Widespread interest in the biosynthesis of androgens by Leydig cells is reflected in a voluminous record of experimental investigations during the last decade. Much of the published data is based on the study of crude slices or homogenates of whole testes and therefore may not accurately reflect biochemical events within Leydig cells. In spite of this, cautious interpretation of these findings has provided an invaluable framework for our growing understanding of androgen biosynthesis in Leydig cells.

Extension of biochemical studies directly to Leydig cells has been inhibited by the difficulty of separating these cells from other testicular cells. As early as 1965, Christensen and Mason (2) demonstrated the feasibility of separating interstitial tissue from seminiferous tubules for use in steroid metabolism experiments. Their successful utilization of isolated interstitial tissue resulted in direct confirmation of the primary role of Leydig cells in testosterone synthesis; however, the necessarily laborious dissection of individual testes, coupled with relatively low yields of Leydig cells, has apparently discouraged widespread adoption of such preparations in biochemical studies of androgenesis. Recently Moyle and co-workers have obtained a transplantable Leydig cell tumor that exhibits many features expected in normal Leydig cells, including testosterone secretion and responsiveness to LH (46). As they demonstrated in the case of hormonally induced depletion of cholesterol (39), the large mass and relative cellular homogeneity of the tumor enable study of aspects of Leydig cell biochemistry that are obscured in ordinary testicular preparations.

Investigation of relatively pure Leydig cell populations, whether they come from tumor models or from improved testicular fractionation techniques, is a desirable alternative to the study of heterogeneous testicular preparations. For the moment, however, many facets of Leydig cell biochemistry must be inferred from work done on the whole testis or, in a few cases, on other steroidogenic tissues.

In several instances, research on steroid biochemistry in the testis has been preceded by similar work in hepatic, adrenal, or ovarian tissues. In this sense, a substantial amount of research on testicular steroidogenesis cannot be considered innovative. One should not, however, depreciate the practical value of establishing for the testis the validity of common principles of steroid biosynthesis discovered first in other tissues. If credit for some innovative discoveries in steroid biosynthesis seems to be either misplaced or neglected in the following paragraphs, it may be because this survey is largely confined to findings made specifically with testicular material.

Synthesis and storage of cholesterol The search for obligatory precursors of steroid hormones has focused on cholesterol, with careful experiments by Hall (47) strongly favoring cholesterol as the source of all testicular androgens. The origin of this cholesterol seems to be within the testis itself, since studies by Morris and Chaikoff (48) and Gerson and co-workers (49) indicate in situ formation of most testicular cholesterol. Testicular biosynthesis of cholesterol has been intensively studied by Gaylor and co-workers, who have demonstrated the formation of squalene and lanosterol from acetate (50) as well as the conversion of lanosterol to cholesterol and other C27 sterols (51). Most enzymatic steps in the synthesis of cholesterol from acetate were localized in the microsome fraction of testicular homogenates (Figure 29.3). Although the control of testicular cholesterol synthesis is still poorly understood, there is suggestive evidence that testosterone produced in the Leydig cell may regulate cholesterol synthesis through a feedback control system (51).

Findings on testicular cholesterol synthesis tend to be quickly incorporated into the store of information concerning Leydig cell biochemistry. The potential hazard of this tendency is indicated by Hall's (47) demonstration that the pool of testicular cholesterol involved in biosynthesis of androgens is small. This fact is not surprising in view of the small portion of the testis composed of Leydig cells. Indeed, even in the case of the Leydig cell cholesterol pool, Moyle's (52) data suggest that only a small fraction is involved in steroidogenesis.

The cholesterol in the metabolically active androgen precursor pool of Leydig cell tumors is derived from esterified cholesterol, synthesized in advance and stored until required for conversion to steroids (52). Retrieval of stored cholesterol for conversion of tes-

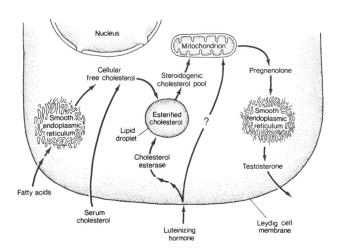

Figure 29.3 Diagram showing the synthesis and storage of cholesterol, conversion of cholesterol to pregnenolone, and conversion of pregnenolone to testosterone by the Leydig cell.

tosterone requires hydrolysis of the ester, a step that is stimulated by LH. Moyle (52) has shown that the steroids synthesized in the first two hours after stimulation of Leydig tumor with LH are derived from stored cholesterol rather than from cholesterol in the medium or from cholesterol newly synthesized within the cell. The factors influencing cholesterol storage in Leydig cells are still obscure, although experiments with prolactin suggest that this hormone may favor intracellular accumulation of cholesterol esters.

Conversion of cholesterol to pregnenolone The conversion of cholesterol to steroid hormones begins with cholesterol side-chain cleavage, a series of enzymatic steps leading to pregnenolone. Toren and co-workers (53) associated cholesterol side-chain cleavage with the mitochondrial fraction of testicular homogenates. Moyle (52) extended this association to the mitochondria of Leydig cell tumors while further demonstrating the probable localization of cholesterol side-chain cleavage in the inner mitochondrial membrane. Hall and Eik-Nes, studying metabolism of testis slices in vitro, produced convincing evidence that LH stimulates testicular steroidogenesis by accelerating cholesterol side-chain cleavage (47, 54, 55). They also showed that the rate-limiting step in androgen synthesis is the first event in side-chain cleavage, namely 20α-hydroxylation of cholesterol (56).

The mechanism whereby LH stimulates side-chain cleavage is still unsettled. Substrate availability could be the crucial factor, in which case LH may simply enhance hydrolysis of cholesterol esters, thereby releasing metabolically active cholesterol (52). In addition to its demonstrable ability to increase substrate availability, LH could conceivably influence other factors in 20α-hydroxylation, such as production of TPNH, activation of oxygen, or removal of pregnenolone inhibition. Several lines of evidence indicate that the stimulatory effect of LH on steroidogenesis may involve cAMP. Like LH, cAMP stimulates steroid synthesis in the testis (57) and in Leydig cell tumors (58). LH encourages formation of cAMP, apparently by increasing the activity of an adenyl cyclase (59) associated with the cell membrane. Hence LH binds to the Leydig cell surface (60), where it promotes intracellular accumulation of cAMP, which in turn activates a series of kinases by binding with an inhibiting subunit of a protein kinase (61). Release of the active kinase somehow stimulates hydrolysis of cholesterol esters and may also exert other influences on mitochondrial cleavage of the cholesterol side chain.

Conversion of pregnenolone to testosterone There are conflicting views regarding the preferred pathway from pregnenolone to testosterone in the Leydig cell. This is probably attributable to the many difficulties and pitfalls involved in the interpretation of results de-

rived from analysis of intermediate steroids present in the testis or from recovery of labeled steroids following incubation of testicular preparations with labeled intermediates. It is also possible that some degree of species variation has contributed to the diversity of opinion regarding steroidogenic pathways.

Although other pathways may be involved, the bulk of available evidence favors testicular androgen formation via either progesterone or 17α-hydroxypregnenolone (10). General support seems to exist for the concept of progression from pregnenolone through progesterone to testosterone (62). The first step, conversion of pregnenolone to progesterone, is catalyzed by the 3β-hydroxysteroid dehydrogenase complex. Next, the enzyme 17α-hydroxylase reduces progesterone to 17α-hydroxyprogesterone, which is converted to androstenedione by C17-C20 lyase. Finally, testosterone is produced from the reduction of androstenedione by 17β-hydroxysteroid dehydrogenase. Tamaoki and co-workers have localized all these enzymes in the microsome fraction of testicular homogenates from a variety of species, including humans (29). Detailed discussion of testicular conversion of pregnenolone to testosterone is presented in a review by Tamaoki and co-workers (63).

Steroid secretion The cellular biochemistry of steroid synthesis has been studied intensively during the last decade, and many significant facts have been revealed. The biochemistry of steroid secretion, on the other hand, has been seriously neglected. Hardly more has been achieved to date than the identification of certain steroid secretory products in testicular venous blood. On the basis of their relative abundance in testicular venous versus arterial blood, the human testis has been found to secrete testosterone (64), testosterone sulfate (65), and pregnenolone sulfate (66). While all intermediates in steroid biosynthesis may escape the biosynthetic process and thereby be excreted by the testis, to date there is no evidence that the human testis secretes any steroids other than testosterone in amounts sufficient for significant biological effects (67).

Since Leydig cells are considered to be the principal steroid-producing cells of the testis, the presence of testosterone and its precursors in testicular venous blood has been attributed to the secretory activity of Leydig cells. The mechanisms are unknown whereby steroids, either free or conjugated, leave the Leydig cell and enter testicular venous blood.

Fundamental Physiological Advances
Effects of LH on Leydig cells Eik-Nes, Hall, and others have shown repeatedly that gonadotropins with LH activity (LH, hCG, PMS) increase the secretion of testicular testosterone in vivo and increase the synthe-

sis of testosterone by testicular slices in vitro (68). LH apparently stimulates testosterone biosynthesis by accelerating the first step in cholesterol side-chain cleavage (56). Acceleration of this rate-limiting step may be a consequence of increased substrate availability caused by the effect of LH on cholesterol ester hydrolysis (52). Increased secretion of testosterone under the influence of LH seems to be merely the result of increased biosynthesis; there is no evidence that significant quantities of testosterone can be stored inside Leydig cells for secretion at a later time. In short, testosterone is probably secreted as soon as it is synthesized, so that acute effects of LH on testicular secretion of testosterone can be explained solely by stimulation of cholesterol side-chain cleavage. Increased testosterone secretion following LH administration is evident within 15 minutes, both in vivo (57) and in vitro (46).

Working with separated interstitial tissue and seminiferous tubules from rat testes, van der Molen and co-workers (69) found that LH specifically increased levels of cAMP in interstitial tissue but not in seminiferous tubules. LH also stimulated testosterone production in the isolated interstitial tissue. This evidence strongly suggests that the steroidogenic action of LH is confined to testicular Leydig cells.

Prolonged treatment with LH (actually hCG) in vivo has effects beyond the side-chain cleavage of cholesterol. When hCG is administered to immature or hypophysectomized adult rats for a few days, several enzymes in the pathway from pregnenolone through progesterone to testosterone show increased activity (30, 70). After two to five days of hCG administration, normal Leydig cells from immature mice (31) and Leydig cells from a murine testicular tumor (35) both show increased quantities of smooth endoplasmic reticulum. Although no increase has been found in the wet weight or protein content of the microsome fraction from testes of animals chronically stimulated with hCG (30, 70), this may not be inconsistent with proliferation of Leydig cell smooth endoplasmic reticulum. It is likely that an increase in Leydig cell microsomes (smooth endoplasmic reticulum) would be obscured by the sheer bulk of testicular microsomes in the preparations studied.

Some reservations have been expressed regarding the ability of Leydig cells from intact adult mammals to exhibit a microsomal response to chronically administered LH. For example, Shikita and Hall (70) could not demonstrate an increase in microsomal enzyme activity from testes of intact adult rats after repeated daily injections of CG. Their finding has been attributed to the possibility that Leydig cells in adult mammals are maximally stimulated by endogenous gonadotropin and hence cannot respond to additional exogenous gonadotropin.

Other evidence supports the ability of adult Leydig cells to increase their steroidogenic capacity under continuing treatment with exogenous gonadotropin. Van der Molen and co-workers (69) have shown that testosterone secretion by the adult rat testis in response to intravenous administration of hCG is increased fourfold by repeated daily subcutaneous injections of the same hormone. DeKretser (37) found that prolonged CG therapy in men with initially normal plasma testosterone levels resulted in elevation of these levels and in proliferation of smooth endoplasmic reticulum in their Leydig cells. Increased quantities of smooth endoplasmic reticulum have also been reported in Leydig cells of adult rats repeatedly treated with CG (71). These observations suggest that adult Leydig cells are not maximally stimulated by exogenous gonadotropin.

It is important to realize that LH probably does more than merely increase testosterone synthesis. The rapid disappearance of testosterone from the testis after hypophysectomy (72) indicates the importance of LH and possibly other pituitary factors in supporting even minimal levels of testosterone production by Leydig cells. Indeed, LH seems necessary to maintain the differentiated state of Leydig cells. The regression and redifferentiation of Leydig cells that occurs after hypophysectomy can be reversed by administration of LH (73). As Aoki (31) has shown, the differentiation of Leydig cells normally occurring just prior to puberty can be prematurely induced by administration of CG.

The key role played by LH in the development and functioning of Leydig cells suggests that its impact on cellular metabolism may be more extensive than has yet been recognized. For example, LH can influence the oxygen metabolism of Leydig cells. Hamberger and Steward (74) found a rapid rise in oxygen uptake by isolated Leydig cells following addition of LH to the incubation medium. The response was specific for Leydig cells, since neither seminiferous tubules nor nerve cells increased their oxygen consumption in the presence of LH.

Effects of FSH on Leydig cells Almost 40 years have passed since Greep and co-workers suggested that Leydig cells of the interstitial tissue are the testicular target of LH and that FSH acts on the seminiferous tubules (Figure 29.4). This view has never been seriously challenged, in spite of occasional reports that FSH may act synergistically with LH in stimulating androgen production by Leydig cells (75, 76, 77). Continuing support for Greep's hypotheses has come from a variety of experiments during the last decade.

FSH is unable to influence oxygen uptake by Leydig

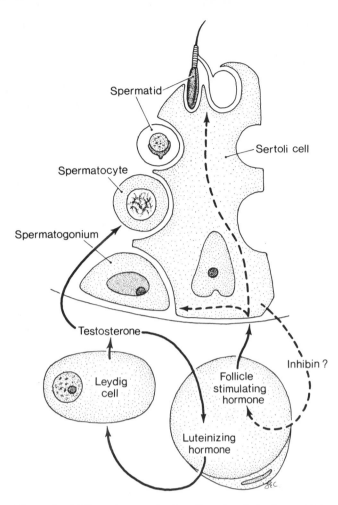

Figure 29.4 LH action on the Leydig cells of the interstitial tissue and FSH action on the seminiferous tubules.

cells; LH stimulates oxygen consumption by these cells (74). FSH increases levels of cAMP in the seminiferous tubules but not in interstitial tissue, while LH does just the opposite (69, 78). Furthermore, FSH does not act synergistically with LH to elevate cAMP levels in isolated Leydig cells (78). The secretion of testosterone by the testes of intact rats is not influenced by in vivo administration of FSH (69). FSH binds specifically to the seminiferous tubules (79). These findings tend to minimize the possibility that FSH exerts significant control over the function of Leydig cells. However, recent studies by Catt and others suggest that FSH may stimulate development of LH binding sites on the Leydig cell surface.

Feedback control of Leydig cell function Simultaneous study of circulating androgens and gonadotropins in male subjects by sensitive radioimmunoassay techniques has demonstrated the influence of androgens (particularly testosterone) on the secretion of LH and vice versa (80). These findings support the classical view that testosterone secreted by Leydig cells into

the general circulation governs blood levels of LH, which in turn control the production of testosterone by Leydig cells.

Since the extratesticular effects of Leydig cell function are mediated by blood levels of testosterone, it is logical that blood levels of testosterone should be involved in the feedback control of Leydig cells. Inside the testis, however, local testosterone concentrations probably mediate the effect of Leydig cells on spermatogenesis. To the extent that blood levels of testosterone reflect testicular testosterone concentrations, the classical feedback loop may be adequate for governing the role of Leydig cells in spermatogenesis. Whether spermatogenesis involves other feedback control of the Leydig cells is an open question. Spermatogenesis does influence the secretion of FSH by a route as yet unidentified (80), but FSH appears to have little or no influence on Leydig cell function. The possibility of a direct feedback link between the seminiferous epithelium and Leydig cells is raised by the discovery of a specific estradiol receptor in Leydig cells (3). This is a particularly interesting finding in view of previous suggestions that the seminiferous epithelium produces an estrogen that functions in feedback control of spermatogenesis (81).

The possibility that spermatogenesis may exert significant feedback control on Leydig cells, either directly or indirectly, is a very serious issue in the development of male contraceptives. Certain contraceptive strategies strive for specific inhibition or interruption of spermatogenesis while tacitly assuming that the endocrine function of the testis will remain normal. It is already apparent that this assumption may be unjustified, since several different antispermatogenic agents appear to promote Leydig cell hyperplasia (82), perhaps by interfering with the balance of pituitary gonadotropins through their common effect on spermatogenesis. Depending on the degree to which spermatogenic feedback influences the Leydig cells, antispermatogenic contraceptive strategies may threaten normal Leydig cell function.

29.2 Unsolved Problems in Leydig Cell Biology

Biological Significance of Leydig Cell Function
The role of Leydig cells in the maintenance of extratesticular aspects of maleness is firmly established. In the last decade it has become increasingly apparent that Leydig cells may also be involved in the support of spermatogenesis. Much evidence has suggested that the androgen needed for spermatogenesis is provided by Leydig cells. There is still some concern, however, that Sertoli cells may play a role in meeting the androgen requirements of the germinal epithelium. Clarification of the relative roles of Leydig cells and Sertoli

cells in the support and regulation of spermatogenesis is urgently needed.

The apparent roles of Leydig cells, both inside and outside the testis, seem to hinge on their secretion of testosterone. It would be premature, however, to assume that Leydig cells produce no other important secretions or have no other biological roles. Comparative studies have raised the possibility that Leydig cells may produce functional steroids other than testosterone. This possibility poses problems for contraceptive strategies that rely on suppression of normal Leydig cell secretion. These strategies hope to substitute exogenous steroid for normally functioning Leydig cells, an endeavor that will demand exhaustive knowledge of the identity and significance of all Leydig cell products. Although it appears likely that testosterone is the only essential secretion of the human Leydig cell, rigorous proof of this is needed.

Morphology

Outstanding unsolved problems in Leydig cell morphology center around the functional significance of structural variation in the organelles and inclusions that are involved in steroidogenesis. The meaning of various structural forms of the smooth endoplasmic reticulum is still obscure in most species. The importance of subtle structural alterations in Leydig cell mitochondria has not been explained. The ultrastructural correlates of cholesterol storage and utilization in steroid hormone synthesis are largely unexplored. Fine structural manifestations of steroid secretion have not been detected.

Progress in these areas will require close correlation of fine structural observations with appropriate biochemical and physiological parameters. Apart from its fundamental contribution to Leydig cell biology, the resulting information will enhance the yield of functional inference that can be obtained from ultrastructural analysis of testicular biopsies. Improved interpretation of testicular biopsies should prove particularly valuable in monitoring the success of contraceptive strategies that hope to preserve normally functioning Leydig cells.

A previously neglected aspect of Leydig cell morphology is the physical relationship of Leydig cells to the seminiferous tubules. A recent comparative survey of the organization of interstitial tissue in the mammalian testis has revealed great variation in the association between Leydig cells and other testicular elements (20). Since this variation cannot be explained phylogenetically, it probably reflects currently unknown physiological variables. Exploration of the physiological correlates of morphological variation in the testicular interstitial tissue will yield new insight

into the microenvironmental requirements of spermatogenesis.

Cytochemistry

Very little progress has occurred in Leydig cell cytochemistry during the last decade, in spite of its great potential for refining the correlation of morphological and biochemical information at the subcellular level. Due to technical difficulties, successful visualization of steroidogenic enzyme activity at the electron-microscopic level has still not been achieved. Neither has it been possible to immobilize labeled steroids within the cell. New technical approaches to these problems, such as preparation of frozen thin sections for high-resolution autoradiography, are being explored (25). Success in this area would permit detailed localization of steroid biosynthetic steps within the organelles of individual Leydig cells.

Biochemistry

Many details of cholesterol biosynthesis in the testis have been established in the last decade, but certain steps remain equivocal. For example, it is still uncertain whether the pathway from lanosterol to cholesterol leads through Δ^7-dehydrocholesterol or desmosterol. Resolution of this problem is particularly important to the interpretation of experimental results derived from pharmacological blockage of the terminal steps of cholesterol synthesis. The factors controlling cholesterol biosynthesis in the testis are poorly understood. The relative roles of pituitary factors such as LH and prolactin require further investigation. Stored cholesterol, especially cholesterol ester, seems to be the immediate precursor for testicular steroidogenesis. The size of the precursor pool within Leydig cells has not been established, however. Investigation of reasonably pure Leydig cell preparations might be expected to improve understanding of the precursor pool.

The mechanism whereby LH stimulates cholesterol side-chain cleavage requires clarification. LH is known to increase substrate availability for this reaction, but whether it also exerts a direct influence on enzymatic events inside the mitochondrion remains to be determined. It is also necessary to explore the possibility that LH may have an additional effect on the transport of pregnenolone out of the mitochondrion.

The preferred pathway from pregnenolone to testosterone is not established firmly. There are several pitfalls responsible for persistent uncertainty in this area. Interpretation of results from incubations of labeled intermediates of the various pathways with testis slices is complicated by the possibility of differential permeability of the Leydig cells to different intermediates and by the lack of information about various pool sizes. Interpretation of isolated intermediates between pregnenolone and testosterone is equivocal since abundance of an intermediate may only mean that it is slowly metabolized, not that it is part of a predominant pathway. Eik-Nes (62) has emphasized the possibility that intracellular architecture may be the controlling factor in the selection of pathways from pregnenolone to testosterone. If this is the case, demonstration of the preferred pathway may be achieved by innovative cytochemical techniques rather than by traditional biochemical analysis of cell homogenates.

While the synthesis of testicular steroids has been studied intensively, less attention has been directed to in vivo secretion of steroids. As mentioned earlier, an exhaustive list of Leydig cell secretory products is not available. Comparison of the chemical compositions of testicular arterial and venous blood has already suggested that human Leydig cells secrete steroids other than testosterone. Rigorous application of this approach is required to complete the list.

Physiology

LH is clearly the principal regulator of Leydig cell function in vivo. FSH alone does not influence Leydig cell function, but there are conflicting reports that it may be able to synergize with LH in stimulating Leydig cells. The possibility that the ratio of the two hormones may be a significant factor in controlling Leydig cells is reflected in the popular explanation of Leydig cell hypertrophy following pharmacological interference with spermatogenesis. Changes in the Leydig cell population after exposure to antispermatogenic agents have been attributed to disturbance in the balance of pituitary gonadotropins. Because of its importance to male contraceptive strategy, the possibility that FSH acts synergistically with LH on Leydig cells in vivo must be thoroughly investigated. At the same time, the role of other pituitary factors in Leydig cell biology requires exploration. An example is prolactin, which is suspected to stimulate cholesterol synthesis and storage in Leydig cells.

An outstanding issue in Leydig cell physiology is the possible spermatogenic feedback on testosterone secretion. If FSH can act synergistically on Leydig cells, then the ability of spermatogenesis to influence pituitary secretion of FSH may secondarily affect testosterone secretion. Whether direct feedback occurs between the germinal epithelium and Leydig cells is an open question. The suspected secretion of estrogen by Sertoli cells coupled with recent discovery of an estrogen receptor in Leydig cells should encourage further research in this area.

29.3 Relevance of Leydig Cells to Fertility Control

Leydig cells are the major source of androgen in the male. Their principal function is synthesis and secretion of testosterone, the hormone that promotes the development and maintenance of maleness. Leydig cells can be considered to exert at least two effects in adult males, each dependent on testosterone as the mediating agent. Their primary effect is in support of spermatogenesis. As noted previously, spermatogenesis appears to require high concentrations of testosterone in the immediate vicinity of the seminiferous tubules. This requirement may be fulfilled by the location of Leydig cells in the intertubular spaces and by their secretion of testosterone into the interstitial fluid surrounding the tubules. The secondary effect of Leydig cells encompasses all extratesticular actions of testosterone, particularly the maintenance of androgen target organs and masculine traits. These actions are mediated by modest amounts of testosterone acquired by the blood during its passage through the interstitial tissue of the testis.

It is apparent that the acceptability of any male contraceptive technique will depend on the degree to which the attributes of maleness are affected. Willing sacrifice of masculine physical characteristics, libido, or potency for the sake of birth control cannot be expected. Hence a major concern in the development of a male contraceptive will be the extent to which secondary effects of Leydig cell function are preserved. Whether these effects are preserved by retention of normally functioning Leydig cells or by administration of exogenous androgen may prove to be relatively unimportant to the maintenance of overt masculinity.

The fact that certain aspects of Leydig cell function appear to be duplicated by administration of exogenous testosterone may be extremely important to the development of male contraceptives. As will be seen, some of the most promising approaches to male contraception depend on the premise that exogenous testosterone can substitute adequately for the secondary effects of Leydig cell function.

Based on these considerations, male contraceptive strategies, both current and hypothetical, can be divided into two categories. In the first category are strategies that hope to preserve normally functioning Leydig cells. These include contraception by pharmacological interference with spermatogenesis and sperm maturation and by vasectomy. The second category is reserved for strategies that rely on exogenous testosterone to achieve the secondary effects of Leydig cell function. These include contraception by suppression of normal Leydig cell function and by castration.

Preservation of Normally Functioning Leydig Cells
Pharmacological interference with spermatogenesis A popular approach to the interruption of spermatogenesis has been the search for cytotoxic agents that selectively attack developing germ cells. The bis(dichloroacetyl) diamines at first seemed promising in this regard. The earliest effects of this agent are seen in advanced spermatids, where there is gross distortion of the acrosome (83). Unfortunately, the effects are not limited to the germinal epithelium. Reddy and Svoboda (82) have reported true hyperplasia of Leydig cells in rats treated with bis(dichloroacetyl) diamines. Workers using other antispermatogenic agents have also reported Leydig cell hyperplasia (84), suggesting that the interstitial effects of these agents may not be caused by direct action on the Leydig cells. Most workers have attributed changes in the Leydig cell population to a disturbance in the balance of pituitary hormones resulting from interruption of spermatogenesis (82). If this interpretation is correct, it holds a significant threat to all contraceptive strategies that hope to preserve normal Leydig cell functions after selective interference with spermatogenesis. For this reason, contraception by obstruction of epididymal sperm maturation may prove a more promising strategy.

Pharmacological interference with sperm maturation To become fully functional, sperm must undergo a period of maturation in the epididymis. Although the contribution of the epididymis to sperm maturation is not clearly understood, it is known to be androgen-dependent. Hence one strategy for interfering with sperm maturation involves specific blockage of androgen action on the epididymis. An encouraging development for this strategy was recently reported by Prasad (85). Small amounts of an androgen antagonist —cyproterone acetate—implanted subcutaneously in rats seem to inhibit potential motility of epididymal sperm without affecting the testes, accessory glands, or libido. This finding suggests that dissection of the extratesticular effects of Leydig cell function can be achieved in a way that is contraceptively useful.

Vasectomy The fact that many vasectomized men develop antibodies to sperm antigens (86) has generated fears that vasectomy may indirectly threaten Leydig cell function by predisposing the testis to autoimmune disease. It is difficult to judge the seriousness of this threat, since the relationship of vasectomy to the development of orchitis is only beginning to be investigated in animal models (87). There is some reason for concern that allergic orchitis might impair Leydig cell function. Testicular tissue damaged by the autoimmune process exhibits diminished capacity to convert progesterone to testosterone (88), but it remains to be seen whether this effect is due to immune factors directed at Leydig cells or to other causes, such as gonadotropin imbalance following interruption of spermatogenesis (89). The basis for autoimmune attack on Leydig cells has been established by the demonstration of steroid-secreting cell antibodies in some human diseases (90). Apart from encouraging the development of autoimmunity, vasectomy might affect the testis in other ways. Some of these, including vascular impairment and thermoregulatory interference, have been discussed in a recent review of the biological aspects of vasectomy (91).

Considering the extensive use of vasectomy to achieve birth control, it should come as a surprise to find that its effect on Leydig cell function is still controversial. Animal model studies are particularly troublesome, with postvasectomy reports of reduced urinary excretion of 17-ketosteroids (92) and diminished testicular metabolism of androgen precursors (93) continuing to appear. Since animal models provide a means of predicting long-term effects of vasectomy in men, resolution of conflict over the consequences of vasectomy in these species is sorely needed.

Meanwhile, data from studies of vasectomized men remain unduly scarce. The little evidence available suggests that blood levels of testosterone are normal in the first three months after vasectomy (94, 95) and that Leydig cells show no morphological change (96, 97). These findings are in agreement with extensive clinical experience showing no association of vasectomy with sudden or overt pathological changes in the Leydig cells. The possibility remains, however, that vasectomy might induce subtle degeneration of Leydig cell function over a period of years. This possibility should stimulate efforts to extend follow-up studies of vasectomized men so that evidence from longer postoperative intervals can be obtained.

Substitution of Exogenous Androgen
Suppression of normal Leydig cell function One of the most promising approaches to male contraception is based on the ability of certain exogenous steroids to depress plasma levels of LH, thereby depriving Leydig cells of their functional stimulus (11). In the absence of testosterone secretion by the Leydig cells, testicular testosterone levels fall below the requirements of spermatogenesis, and sterility is achieved (12). Cessation of Leydig cell function, however, demands that exogenous testosterone be administered to maintain the extragonadal attributes of maleness. Since the extragonadal effects of testosterone can be obtained with far smaller doses than are required to support spermatogenesis, maintenance of secondary sexual characteristics does not interfere with the achievement of sterility.

Administration of exogenous testosterone is very effective in depressing plasma levels of LH. In adult men, daily doses (50 mg) of testosterone propionate have been shown to reduce plasma LH to undetectable levels while maintaining plasma testosterone at twice the normal level (12). This regimen produces spermatogenic arrest while supporting secondary sexual characteristics and appears to be reversible after suspension of treatment. Objections to this very attractive contraceptive approach center around two concerns. First, there is some evidence that testosterone conjugates may effect liver function (98) and later serum lipoproteins (99). Second, the necessity of maintaining somewhat elevated plasma testosterone levels to suppress plasma LH raises the possibility that hyperstimulation of accessory sex organs may occur. Considering the incidence and complications of prostatic hypertrophy among adult men, the potential consequences of chronically elevated plasma testosterone must be carefully investigated.

The first objection may be met by administration of free testosterone in subcutaneous Silastic implants. Frick (100) has noted essentially normal liver function and blood chemistry in men with Silastic implants containing unconjugated testosterone. The objection to elevated plasma testosterone may call for a different steroid for suppression of plasma LH. Since various progestins are effective in preventing release of LH from the pituitary into the blood, a regimen could probably be developed that would rely on progestin to suppress plasma LH with administration of just enough testosterone to maintain normal plasma testosterone levels. Such a plan should eliminate the possibility of accessory organ hypertrophy. A program coordinated by the Population Council seems to have achieved this goal. As reported by Frick (100), oral administration of progestin combined with subcutaneous testosterone implants achieved cessation of spermatogenesis without elevation of plasma testosterone in an encouraging number of adult men representing a wide range of ages.

An outstanding advantage of male contraception by steroid therapy is its great potential for reversibility (101). Steroid contraception, especially in its most acceptable form, has the disadvantage of requiring considerable attention by the patient, with daily ingestion of progestin being combined with periodic replacement of testosterone implants. This is further complicated by the fact that the testosterone dosage required to achieve normal plasma testosterone levels must be adjusted to the individual patient (100).

Castration Although there is historical precedence for its use in humans, birth control by castration appears ridiculous from our current perspective, and there is scant reason to expect that its status will improve in the near future. Nevertheless, it should be emphasized that the practical difference between contraception by suppression of Leydig cell function and contraception by castration is probably restricted to the irreversibility of the latter. Both dispense entirely with normal testicular functions, endocrine and exocrine, and both rely on androgen replacement therapy to maintain secondary sexual characteristics.

Contraception by castration is included in this discussion primarily to provoke consideration of the extent to which Leydig cell function can be replaced by administration of a single exogenous steroid, testosterone. It has been noted that testosterone is the primary secretory product of Leydig cells in most mammals, but it is highly likely that Leydig cells in certain species, such as the boar, secrete large quantities of other steroids. Even in humans, Leydig cells secrete small quantities of testosterone precursors and metabolites. That these or any other currently unknown products of Leydig cell activity exert biologically significant effects elsewhere in the organism seems unlikely on the basis of existing evidence. In spite of this, continuing investigation of contraceptive techniques involving suppression of Leydig cell function must focus not only on the potential side effects of administered steroids but also on the possibility that replacement therapy may be deficient.

If Leydig cell function is really as simple as available evidence suggests, castration coupled with testosterone replacement therapy may be a relatively acceptable means of achieving permanent sterility. On the other hand, should Leydig cell function prove more complex, then contraception by Leydig cell suppression is surely less promising than it now appears.

Cosmetic Considerations
From the preceding discussion and its emphasis on the role of Leydig cells in maintaining the male habitus, it is apparent that acceptable contraceptive strategies must strive to preserve the physical appearance of those who elect to use them. In this respect, it becomes important to consider the effect of various contraceptives on the size of the testes and hence on the appearance of the scrotum.

The size of the testis is closely correlated with the diameter of the seminiferous tubules. Accordingly, a contraceptive that involves destruction of the seminiferous tubules should have a relatively devastating effect on testicular size. It is also clear that the diameter of the seminiferous tubules is related to spermatogenic activity. Complete suppression of spermatogenesis should therefore reduce seminiferous tubule diameter to such an extent that the size of the testis approaches that seen prior to puberty. Further clinical trials of steroid contraceptives involving suppression of spermatogenesis will test this expectation.

Should severe testicular shrinkage be a concomitant of suppressed spermatogenesis, testosterone replacement therapy cannot be expected to restore normal scrotal morphology. Depending on the importance of normal scrotal morphology to the individual, some form of testicular prosthesis may be indicated. If this seems impractical, other contraceptive methods must be considered. The availability of adequate testicular prosthesis is not a problem, since Silastic testes are currently used in clinical situations demanding total castration. Considering the successful utilization of subcutaneous Silastic capsules for long-term administration of steroid hormones, it may not be entirely fanciful to suggest that cosmetic and therapeutic requirements could be met simultaneously by scrotal implantation of Silastic testes designed to contain a lifetime supply of hormonal steroids and engineered to release them at physiological rates.

29.3 Potential Value of Future Research

By playing crucial roles in gametogenesis and in the expression of masculinity, Leydig cells occupy a central position in male reproductive biology. From the practical viewpoint of fertility control, the dual role of the Leydig cell presents opportunities and at the same time poses problems. Opportunity is manifest in the dependency of spermatogenesis on normal Leydig cell function; suppression of Leydig cell function has been shown to inhibit sperm production and hence fertility. Problems are evident in the tendency of masculinity to deteriorate following impairment of Leydig cell function; interference with testosterone production will threaten libido, potency, and male physique. Some contraceptive strategies may choose to exploit the opportunities inherent in Leydig cell function, but all must seek to avoid the problems.

In the future, three areas of Leydig cell research will be especially significant for fertility control. These areas are (1) the physiological relationship between Leydig cells and seminiferous epithelium, (2) the effects of various contraceptive methods on Leydig cell function, and (3) the ability of exogenous steroids to substitute for normal Leydig cell function.

Continuing investigation of the relationship between Leydig cells and the seminiferous epithelium will be necessary to refine our understanding of the role that Leydig cells play in gametogenesis. Improved understanding of this role may open new approaches to contraception while allowing perfection of existing strategies. It will also permit increasingly complete explanation of spermatogenic inhibition following suppression of Leydig cell function. The ability to explain the mechanisms behind such a contraceptive strategy will be important in promoting its acceptance by an increasingly sophisticated public.

The relationship between Leydig cells and the seminiferous epithelium is particularly crucial to contraceptive strategies that hope to retain normal Leydig cell function while inhibiting spermatogenesis by other means. Future research must determine whether interrupted spermatogenesis is compatible with persistence of normal Leydig cell function. The issue hinges on possible involvement of Leydig cells in the feedback control of spermatogenesis. This is one of many examples in which a fundamental aspect of Leydig cell physiology has great significance for fertility control.

Spermatogenic inhibition is only one contraceptive strategy that may threaten Leydig cell function. Even strategies with no immediate effect on the testis (e.g., vasectomy) may eventually alter Leydig cells. Hence it is important that researchers monitor the effects of various contraceptives on Leydig cells, both in animal models and in human patients. In humans, combined study of plasma hormone levels and ultrastructural analysis of testicular biopsies should yield informative correlations. Proper interpretation of testicular biopsies will benefit from additional progress in understanding the fundamental relationship between the fine structure of Leydig cells and synthesis of steroids.

In some respects, such as maintenance of most masculine traits, impairment of normal Leydig cell function appears to be countered by administration of exogenous testosterone. Hence the ability of exogenous steroid to substitute for normal Leydig cell function is a major practical consideration limiting contraceptive exploitation of the Leydig cell's gametogenic role. Rigorous demonstration of the essential components of steroid replacement therapy will be an important contribution to fertility control, even if it does no more than indicate necessity for testosterone alone. To be able to state with complete confidence that exogenous testosterone replaces all extratesticular effects of Leydig cell function should enhance public acceptance of any contraceptive method that interferes with Leydig cell function.

Although the areas of Leydig cell research that have been mentioned appear to be among those particularly relevant to current problems in fertility control, they have emerged from a broad front of basic research that should not be allowed to lapse in the future. As existing problems are solved, new ones tend to arise in their place, and the ability to cope with them may well entail research efforts that would appear frivolous by present standards. This concern is not expressed to discourage the concept of directed research based on rational predictions. Instead it is forwarded in recognition of the fact that perspectives often change through time, so that yesterday's prognostications often seem myopic in retrospect.

29.5 Summary

During the last decade convincing evidence from a variety of investigations has reinforced the view that Leydig cells are the principal source of the male hormone, testosterone. Through their secretion of testosterone, Leydig cells promote the development and maintenance of extratesticular aspects of maleness. In recent years Leydig cells have been shown to play a major role inside the testis, where they mediate the effects of LH on spermatogenesis. Spermatogenesis requires high local concentrations of testosterone, a condition that appears to be met by the location of Leydig cells near the seminiferous tubules and by their secretion of testosterone in response to stimulation by LH. Because of their crucial role in the production of sperm as well as in the expression of masculinity, Leydig cells occupy a central position in male reproductive biology.

Outstanding fundamental advances in all areas of Leydig cell biology have been achieved in the last 10 years. Basic research in morphology, biochemistry, and physiology have elucidated many details of testosterone production by Leydig cells. Electron microscopy has revealed the internal architecture of the Leydig cell and established the structural background for our understanding of subcellular function. Biochemical analysis of cell fractions has demonstrated the roles of various Leydig cell organelles in testosterone biosynthesis. Metabolic studies have clarified details of the stimulation of Leydig cells by LH. New techniques for measuring blood levels of testosterone and LH have confirmed the suspected importance of these hormones in feedback control of Leydig cell function.

Although great progress has been made, major gaps still remain in our knowledge of Leydig cell biology. Clarification is urgently needed of the relative roles of Leydig cells and Sertoli cells in the support and regulation of spermatogenesis. The possibility that spermatogenesis exerts feedback control on Leydig cells requires exploration. A complete list of Leydig cell secretions, a prerequisite of definitive replacement therapy, is still missing. Correlation of subcellular structure and function needs refinement to be clinically useful. Leydig cell cytochemistry has been seriously neglected, and many biochemical details of steroid biosynthesis have not been established.

In spite of these gaps, the dual role of Leydig cells in support of both masculinity and spermatogenesis has firmly established their relevance to fertility control. Since the acceptability of any contraceptive will require that masculinity be unaffected, all birth control strategies must strive to preserve the extratesticular effects of Leydig cell function. Some strategies seek to exploit the role of Leydig cells in spermatogenesis by suppressing their function and hence stopping sperm production. These strategies must rely on steroid-replacement therapy to maintain the extratesticular aspects of maleness.

Future research in Leydig cell biology should include areas of special significance to fertility control. The promise shown by contraceptives that suppress Leydig cell function demands thorough definition of the physiological relationship between Leydig cells and seminiferous epithelium. Acceptance of Leydig cell suppression also requires rigorous demonstration of the adequacy of steroid replacement therapy. The effects of other contraceptives on Leydig cell structure and function must be carefully monitored in animal models and in human patients.

Selected Reviews

Morphology
Christensen, A. K. Leydig cells. In *Handbook of physiology*; Section 7: Endocrinology; Vol. 5: *Male reproductive system*, p. 57. Baltimore: Williams & Wilkins, 1975.

Christensen, A. K., and S. W. Gillim. The correlation of fine structure and function in steroid-secreting cells, with emphasis on those of the gonads. In *The gonads*, ed. K. W. McKerns, p. 415. New York: Appleton-Century-Crofts, 1969.

Fawcett, D. W., J. A. Long, and A. L. Jones. The ultrastructure of endocrine glands. Recent Prog. Horm. Res. 25:314, 1969.

Biochemistry
Eik-Nes, K. B. Synthesis and secretion of androstenedione and testosterone. In *The androgens of the testis*, ed. K. B. Eik-Nes, p. 1. New York: M. Dekker, 1970.

Hall, P. F. Gonadotrophic regulation of testicular function. In *The androgens of the testis*, ed. K. B. Eik-Nes, p. 73. New York: M. Dekker, 1970.

Tamaoki, B. Steroidogenesis and cell structure: Biochemical pursuit of sites of steroid biosynthesis. J. Steroid Biochem. 4:89, 1973.

Physiology
Hall, P. F. Endocrinology of the testis. In *The testis*, Vol. 2, eds. A. D. Johnson, W. R. Gomes, and N. L. Van Demark, p. 1. New York: Academic Press, 1970.

Parkes, A. S. The internal secretions of the testis. In *Marshall's physiology of reproduction*, Vol. 3, ed. A. S. Parkes, p. 412. London: Longmans, Green, 1966.

Steinberger, A., and E. Steinberger. Hormonal control of spermatogenesis. In *The regulation of mammalian reproduc-*

tion, eds. S. J. Segal, R. Crozier, P. A. Corfman, and P. G. Condliffe, p. 139. Springfield, Ill.: C. C Thomas, 1973.

Steinberger, E., and A. Steinberger. Testis: Basic and clinical aspects. In *Reproductive biology*, eds. H. Balin and S. Glasser, p. 144. Amsterdam: Excerpta Medica, 1972.

References

1. Bouin, P., and P. Ancel. Recherches sur les cellules interstitielles du testicule des mammifères. Arch. Zool. Exp. Genet. (Ser. IV) 1:437, 1903.

2. Christensen, A. K., and N. R. Mason. The comparative ability of seminiferous tubules and interstitial tissue of rat testis to synthesize androgens from progesterone-4-^{14}C in vitro. Endocrinology 76:646, 1965.

3. van der Molen, H. J., H. de Bruijn, B. Cooke, and F. de Jong. In *The endocrine function of the human testis*, eds. V. James, M. Serio, and L. Martini, p. 533. New York: Academic Press, 1973.

4. Cooke, B. A., F. H. deJong, H. J. van der Molen, and F. F. G. Rommerts. Endogenous testosterone concentrations in rat testis interstitial tissue and seminiferous tubules during in vitro incubation. Nature New Biol. 237:255, 1972.

5. Baille, A. H., M. M. Ferguson, and D. M. Hart. *Developments in steroid histochemistry*, New York: Academic Press, 1966.

6. Woods, J. E., and L. V. Domm. Histochemical identification of the androgen-producing cells in the gonads of domestic fowl and albino rat. Gen. Comp. Endocrinol. 7:559, 1966.

7. Steinberger, E., A. Steinberger, and M. Fischer. Study of spermatogenesis and steroid metabolism in cultures of mammalian testis. Rec. Prog. Horm. Res. 26:547, 1970.

8. Lacy, D., In *The endocrine function of the human testis*, Vol. 1, eds. V. James, M. Serio, and L. Martini, p. 493. New York: Academic Press, 1973.

9. Leydig, F. Zur Anatomie de männlichen Geschlechtsorgane und Analdrusen der Saugetiere. Z. Wiss. Zool. 2:1, 1850.

10. Steinberger, A., and E. Steinberger. In *The regulation of mammalian reproduction*, eds. S. J. Segal, R. Crozier, P. A. Corfman, and P. G. Condliffe, p. 139. Springfield, Ill.: C. C Thomas, 1973.

11. Heller, C. G., H. C. Morse, M. Su, and M. J. Rowley. In *The human testis*, eds. E. Rosemberg and C. A. Paulsen, p. 249. New York: Plenum Press, 1970.

12. Morse, H. C., and C. G. Heller. Testosterone concentrations in testis of normal men: Effects of testosterone propionate administration. Biol. Reprod. 9:102, 1973.

13. Lindner, H. R. Partition of androgen between the lymph and venous blood of the testis in the ram. J. Endocrinol. 25:483, 1963.

14. Dvoskin, S. Reinitiation of spermatogenesis by pellets of testosterone and its esters in hypophysectomized rats. Anat. Rec. 99:329, 1947.

15. Smith, P. E. Maintenance and restoration of spermatogenesis in hypophysectomized rhesus monkeys by androgen administration. Yale J. Biol. Med. 17:281, 1944.

16. Clermont, Y., and S. C. Harvey. In *Endocrinology of the testis*, eds. G. Wolstenholme and M. O'Connor, p. 173. Boston: Little, Brown, 1967.

17. Parkes, A. S. In *Marshall's physiology of reproduction*, Vol. 3, ed. A. S. Parkes, p. 412. London: Longmans, Green, 1966.

18. Neaves, W. B., and P. S. Bramley. Relationship between blood levels of testosterone and accessory sex gland weight in impala, *Aepyceros melampus*. Comp. Biochem. Physiol. 24A:983, 1972.

19. Coyotupa, J., A. Parlow, and N. Kovasic. Serum testosterone and dihydrotestosterone levels following orchiectomy in the adult rat. Endocrinology 92:1579, 1973.

20. Fawcett, D. W., W. Neaves, and M. Flores. Comparative observations on intertubular lymphatics and the organization of the interstitial tissue of the mammalian testis. Biol. Reprod. 9:500, 1973.

21. Sink, H. D. Theoretical aspects of sex odor in swine. J. Theor. Biol. 17:174, 1967.

22. Claus, R., B. Hoffman, and H. Karg. Determination of 5a-androst-16-en-3-one, a boar taint steroid in pigs, with reference to relationships to testosterone. J. Anim. Sci. 33:1293, 1971.

23. Fishman, L. M., G. Sarfaty, H. Wilson, and M. Lipsett. In *The endocrinology of the testis*, eds. G. Wolstenholme and M. O'Connor, p. 156. Boston: Little, Brown, 1967.

24. Maddock, W. O., and W. O. Nelson. The effects of chorionic gonadotropin in adult men: Increased estrogen and 17-ketosteroid excretion, gynecomastia, Leydig cell stimulation and seminiferous tubule damage. J. Clin. Endocrinol. Metab. 12:985, 1952.

25. Christensen, A. K., and S. W. Gillim. In *The gonads*, ed. K. W. McKerns, p. 415. New York: Appleton-Century-Crofts, 1969.

26. Fawcett, D. W., J. A. Long, and A. L. Jones. The ultrastructure of endocrine glands. Recent Prog. Horm. Res. 25:315, 1969.

27. Christensen, A. K., and D. W. Fawcett. The normal fine structure of opossum testicular interstitial cells. J. Biophys. Biochem. Cytol. 9:653, 1961.

28. Christensen, A. K. The fine structure of testicular interstitial cells in guinea pigs. J. Cell Biol. 26:911, 1965.

29. Murota, S., M. Shikita, and B. Tamaoki. Androgen formation in the testicular tissue of patients with prostatic carcinoma. Biochem. Biophys. Acta 117:241, 1966.

30. Shikita, M., and P. F. Hall. The action of human chorionic gonadotropin in vivo upon microsomal enzymes of immature rat testis. Biochem. Biophys. Acta 136:484, 1967.

31. Aoki, A. Hormonal control of Leydig cell differentiation. Protoplasma 71:209, 1970.

32. Neaves, W. B. Changes in testicular Leydig cells and in plasma testosterone levels among seasonally breeding rock hyrax. Biol. Reprod. 8:451, 1973.

33. Christensen, A. K., and D. W. Fawcett. The fine structure of testicular interstitial cells in mice. Am. J. Anat. 118:551, 1966.

34. Ichihara, I. The fine structure of testicular interstitial cells in mice during postnatal development. Z. Zellforsch. 108:475, 1970.

35. Neaves, W. B. Ultrastructural transformation of a murine Leydig cell tumor after gonadotropin administration. J. Natl. Cancer Inst. 50:1069, 1973.

36. Hall, P. F. In *The androgens of the testis*, ed. K. B. Eik-Nes, p. 73. New York: M. Dekker, 1970.

37. de Kretser, D. M. Changes in the fine structure of the human testicular interstitial cells after treatment with human gonadotropins. Z. Zellforsch. 83:344, 1967.

38. Russo, J., and F. L. Sacerdote. Ultrastructural changes induced by HCG in the Leydig cell of the adult mouse testis. Z. Zellforsch. 112:363, 1971.

39. Pokel, J. D., W. R. Moyle, and R. O. Greep. Depletion of esterified cholesterol in mouse testis and Leydig cell tumors by luteinizing hormone. Endocrinology 91:323, 1972.

40. Merkow, L., H. F. Acevedo, M. Slifkin, and B. J. Caito. Studies on the interstitial cells of the testis. 1. The ultrastructure in the immature guinea pig and the effect of stimulation with human chorionic gonadotropin. Am. J. Pathol. 53:47, 1968.

41. Clegg, E. J. Further studies on artificial cryptorchidism: Quantitative changes in the interstitial cells of the rat testis. J. Endocrinol. 21:433, 1961.

42. Long, J. A., and A. L. Jones. The fine structure of the zona glomerulosa and zona fasciculata of the adrenal cortex of the opossum. Am. J. Anat. 120:463, 1967.

43. Cavazos, L. F., L. L. Anderson, W. D. Belt, D. M. Hendricks, R. R. Kraeling, and R. M. Melampy. Fine structure and progesterone levels in the corpus luteum of the pig during the estrous cycle. Biol. Reprod. 1:83, 1969.

44. Gillim, S. W., A. K. Christensen, and C. E. McLennan. Fine structure of the human menstrual corpus luteum at its stage of maximum secretory activity. Am. J. Anat. 126:409, 1969.

45. Reddy, J., and D. Svoboda. Microbodies (peroxisomes) identification in interstitial cells of the testis. J. Histochem. Cytochem. 20:140, 1972.

46. Moyle, W. R., and D. T. Armstrong. Stimulation of testosterone biosynthesis by luteinizing hormone in transplantable moose Leydig cell tumors. Steroids 15:681, 1970.

47. Hall, P. F. The effect of interstitial cell stimulating hormone on the biosynthesis of testicular cholesterol from acetate-1-C^{14}. Biochemistry 2:1232, 1963.

48. Morris, M. D., and I. L. Chaikoff. The origin of cholesterol in liver, small intestine, adrenal gland and testis of the rat: Dietary versus endogenous contributions. J. Biol. Chem. 234:1095, 1959.

49. Gerson, T., F. Shortland, and G. Dunckley. The effect of β-sitosterol on the metabolism of cholesterol and lipids in rats on a diet low in fat. Biochem. J. 93:385, 1964.

50. Tsai, S. C., B. P. Ying, and J. Gaylor. Testicular sterols. 1. Incorporation of mevolonate and acetate into sterols by testicular tissue from rats. Arch. Biochem. Biophys. 105:329, 1964.

51. Gaylor, J. L., Y. Chang, M. Nightingale, E. Recio, and B. Ying. Testicular sterols. IV. End-product steroid inhibition of lanosterol demethylation. Biochemistry 4:1114, 1965.

52. Moyle, W. R. The action of luteinizing hormone on steroidogenesis in transplantable mouse testes tumors. Ph.D. thesis, Harvard University, Cambridge, Massachusetts, 1970.

53. Toren, D., K. M. Menon, E. Forchielli, and R. I. Dorfman. In vitro enzymatic cleavage of the cholesterol side chain in rat testis preparations. Steroids 3:381, 1964.

54. Hall, P. F. On the stimulation of testicular steroidogenesis in the rabbit by interstitial cell–stimulating hormone. Endocrinology 78:690, 1966.

55. Hall, P. F., and K. B. Eik-Nes. The effect of interstitial cell–stimulating hormone on the production of pregnenolone by rabbit testis in the presence of an inhibitor of 17α-hydrolase. Biochem. Biophys. Acta 86:604, 1964.

56. Hall, P. F., and D. G. Young. Site of action of trophic hormones upon the biosynthetic pathways to steroid hormones. Endocrinology 82:559, 1968.

57. Eik-Nes, K. B. In *Endocrinology of the testis*, eds. G. Wolstenholme and M. O'Connor, p. 1200. Boston: Little, Brown, 1967.

58. Moyle, W. R., N. R. Moudgal, and R. O. Greep. Cessation of steroidogenesis in Leydig cell tumors after removal of luteinizing hormone and adenosine cyclic 3',5'-monophosphate. J. Biol. Chem. 246:4978, 1971.

59. Murad, F., B. S. Strauch, and M. Vaughan. The effect of gonadotropins on testicular adenyl cyclase. Biochem. Biophys. Acta 177:591, 1969.

60. Moudgal, N. R., W. R. Moyle, and R. O. Greep. Specific binding of luteinizing hormone to Leydig cell tumor cells. J. Biol. Chem. 246:4983, 1971.

61. Garren, L. D., G. N. Gill, H. Masui, and G. M. Walton. On the mechanism of action of ACTH. Recent Prog. Horm. Res. 27:433, 1971.

62. Eik-Nes, K. B. In *The androgens of the testis*, ed. K. B. Eik-Nes, p. 1. New York: M. Dekker, 1970.

63. Tamaoki, B. I., H. Inano, and H. Nakano. In *The gonads*, ed. K. W. McKerns, p. 547. New York: Appleton-Century-Crofts, 1969.

64. Hollander, N., and V. P. Hollander. The microdetermination of testosterone in human spermatic vein blood. J. Clin. Endocrinol. Metab. 18:966, 1958.

65. Saez, J. M., S. Saez, and C. Migeon. Identification and measurement of testosterone in the sulfate fraction of plasma of normal subjects and patients with gonadal and adrenal disorders. Steroids 9:1, 1967.

66. Laatikainen, T., E. A. Laitinen, and R. Viho. Secretion of neutral steroid sulfates by the human testis. J. Clin. Endocrinol. Metab. 29:219, 1969.

67. Lipsett, M. B. In *The human testis*, eds. E. Rosemberg and C. A. Paulsen, p. 407. New York: Plenum Press, 1970.

68. Hall, P. F., and K. B. Eik-Nes. The action of gonadotrophic hormones upon rabbit testis in vitro. Biochem. Biophys. Acta 63:411, 1962.

69. van der Molen, H. J., H. W. A. de Bruijn, B. A. Cooke, F. H. de Jong, and F. F. G. Rommerts. In *The endocrine*

function of the human testis, Vol. 1, eds. V. James, M. Serio, and L. Martini, p. 459. New York: Academic Press, 1973.

70. Shikita, M., and P. F. Hall. Action of human chorionic gonadotropin in vivo upon microsomal enzymes in testes of hypophysectomized rats. Biochem. Biophys. Acta 141:433, 1967.

71. Schwarz, W., and H. J. Merkerm. Die Hodenzwischenzellen der Ratte nach Hypophysektomie und nach Behandlung mit Choriongonadotropin und Amphenon B. Z. Zellforsch. 65:272, 1965.

72. Fariss, B. L., T. J. Hurley III, S. Hane, and P. H. Forsham. Testicular testosterone response to human chorionic gonadotropin in the rat. Proc. Soc. Exp. Biol. Med. 130:864, 1969.

73. Woods, M. C., and M. E. Simpson. Pituitary control of the testis of the hypophysectomized rat. Endocrinology 69:91, 1961.

74. Hamberger, L. A., and V. W. Steward. Action of gonadotropins in vitro on the respiration of isolated interstitial cells from the testis of the rat. Endocrinology 83:855, 1968.

75. Johnson, B. H., and L. L. Ewing. Follicle-stimulating hormone and the regulation of testosterone secretion in rabbit testis. Science 173:635, 1971.

76. Parlow, A. F., and L. E Reichert. Influence of follicle-stimulating hormone on the prostate assay of luteinizing hormone. Endocrinology 73:377, 1963.

77. Sizonenko, P. C., A. Cuendet, and L. Paunier. FSH. I. Evidence for its mediating role on testosterone secretion in cryptorchidism. J. Clin. Endocrinol. Metab. 37:68, 1973.

78. Dorrington, J. H., and I. B. Fritz. Effects of gonadotropins on cyclic AMP production by isolated seminiferous tubule and interstitial cell preparations. Endocrinology 94:395, 1974.

79. Means, A. R., and J. Vaitukaitis. Peptide hormone "receptors": Specific binding of ^{3}H-FSH to testis. Endocrinology 90:39, 1972.

80. Franchimont, P. In *The endocrine function of the human testis*, Vol. 1, eds. V. James, M. Serio, and L. Martini, p. 439. New York: Academic Press, 1973.

81. Hall, P. F. In *The testis*, Vol. 2, eds. A. D. Johnson, W. R. Gomes, and N. L. Van Demark, p. 1. New York: Academic Press, 1970.

82. Reddy, K. J., and D. J. Svoboda. Alterations in rat testis due to an antispermatogenic agent. Arch. Pathol. 84:376, 1967.

83. Flores, M., and D. W. Fawcett. Ultrastructural effects of the antispermatogenic compound WIN-18446 (bis dichloracetyl diamine). Anat. Rec. 172:310, 1972.

84. Benson, W. R., and F. S. Clare. Regenerative changes and spermatic granulomas in the rat testis after treatment with dl-ethionine. Am. J. Pathol. 49:981, 1966.

85. Prasad, M. R. N. Limiting male fertility by selectively depriving the epididymis of androgen. Res. Reprod. 5:3, 1973.

86. Ansbacher, R. Vasectomy: Sperm antibodies. Fertil. Steril. 24:788, 1973.

87. Alexander, N. J. Autoimmune hypospermatogenesis in vasectomized guinea pigs. Contraception 8:147, 1973.

88. Becker, W. G., C. A. Snipes, and C. J. Migeon. Progesterone-4-^{14}C metabolism to androgens by testes of normal and isoimmune aspermatogenic guinea pigs. Endocrinology 78:737, 1966.

89. Katsh, S., and G. W. Duncan. Pituitary gonadotropin content of aspermatogenic guinea pigs. Proc. Soc. Exp. Biol. Med. 127:470, 1968.

90. Anderson, J. R., R. B. Goudie, K. Gray, and D. A. Stuart-Smith, Immunological features of idiopathic Addison's disease: An antibody to cells producing steroid hormones. Clin. Exp. Immunol. 3:107, 1968.

91. Neaves, W. B. In *Handbook of physiology*; Section 7: Endocrinology; Vol. 5: *Male reproductive system*, p. 303. Baltimore: Williams & Wilkins, 1975.

92. Sackler, A. M., A. S. Weltman, V. Pandhi, and R. Schwartz. Gonadal effects of vasectomy and vasoligation. Science 179:293, 1973.

93. Collins, P. M., J. B. G. Bell, and W. N. Tsang. The effect of vasectomy on steroid metabolism by the seminiferous tubules and interstitial tissue of the rat testis: A comparison with the effects of aging. J. Endocrinol. 55:18, 1972.

94. Bunge, R. G. Plasma testosterone levels in man after vasectomy. Invest. Urol. 10:9, 1972.

95. Wieland, R. G., M. C. Hallberg, E. M. Zorn, D. E. Klein, and S. S. Luria. Pituitary-gonadal function before and after vasectomy. Fertil. Steril. 23:779, 1972.

96. Kubota, R. Electron microscopic studies of the testis after vasectomy in rats and men. Jap. J. Urol. 60:373, 1969.

97. Nelson, W. O. In *Studies on testis and ovary, eggs and sperm*, ed. E. T. Engle, p. 3. Springfield Ill.: C. C Thomas, 1952.

98. Foss, G. C., and S. L. Simpson. Oral methyltestosterone and jaundice. Br. Med. J. 1:259, 1959.

99. Furman, R. H., R. P. Howard, L. N. Norcia, and E. C. Keaty. The influence of androgens, estrogens, and related steroids on serum lipids and lipoproteins. Am. J. Med. 24:80, 1958.

100. Frick, J. Control of spermatogenesis in men by combined administration of progestin and androgen. Contraception 8:191, 1973.

101. MacLeod, J. In *Fertility disturbances in men and women*, ed. C. A. Joel, p. 265. Basel: S. Karger, 1971.

30 The Blood-Testis Barrier
B. P. Setchell

The term *blood-testis barrier* is somewhat misleading. The testis consists of two major components, the seminiferous tubules and the interstitial tissue, and there is a more effective barrier between the bloodstream and the contents of the tubules than between the blood and the interstitial tissue. Since the tubules comprise an overwhelming majority of the testis in most species, however, it seems appropriate to continue using the simple term *blood-testis barrier* which was coined by analogy with the blood-brain barrier. The same experiments—vital staining with injected dyes—that revealed the existence of the blood-brain barrier more than 50 years ago showed that the cells inside the seminiferous tubules, like the brain, remained free of dye. No particular importance was attached to this observation, however, or to later observations with other dyes or radioactive compounds, until Kormano noticed in 1967 that the exclusion of dyes from the seminiferous tubules was not seen in animals before puberty. Independently of these studies Waites and I noticed that the amounts of radioactive rubidium ions in the testis one minute after injection (expressed as the ratio of cpm/g tissue to cpm/g body weight) was about half the value for iodoantipyrine, whereas in other tissues, with the notable exception of the brain, the two markers gave similar results. Rubidium is virtually excluded from the brain by the blood-brain barrier, and therefore the differences found in the testis also suggested a barrier to free entry there. This barrier was also apparently located in the seminiferous tubules, because when normal tubular function was destroyed by injecting the animals with cadmium salts, the difference between the rubidium and iodoantipyrine values disappeared.

The final convincing proof of a barrier within the testis came when we compared the composition of fluids collected from various sites in the testis and then studied the rate at which marker substances passed from one fluid to another. The site of the barrier was localized within the testis by electron microscopy with electron-opaque markers by Fawcett and his colleagues.

30.1 Composition of Fluids Within The Testis

These studies depended on the development of techniques for collecting fluid from within the seminiferous tubules and from between the tubules. In the testis are a number of tubules that are usually two-ended; both ends open into the rete testis, from which the efferent ducts carry the spermatozoa, still suspended in fluid, into the epididymis (Figure 30.1). The spaces between the blood capillaries and the tubules are thought to drain into lymphatic vessels in the interstitial spaces and in the septa of the testis and thence into lymphatic ducts on the outside of the spermatic cord. The lymphatic ducts are comparatively easy to cannulate in large domestic mammals such as rams and boars.

Lymph from the spermatic cord, except for the absence of erythrocytes, is quite similar to blood plasma. The high concentrations of testosterone and protein are noteworthy. The concentration of testosterone is about two-thirds that in blood from the internal spermatic vein, i.e., much higher than the concentration in arterial blood. This ratio persists after gonadotropin stimulation. Thus the seminiferous tubules are normally exposed to a much higher concentration of testosterone than are other tissues of the body, a point that is often overlooked in studies on the effects of steroids on spermatogenesis. The concentration of protein in testicular lymph is higher than in lymph elsewhere in the body except in the liver, and this high concentra-

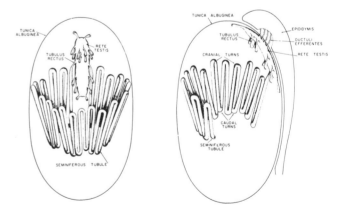

Figure 30.1 Diagrams illustrating the arrangement of the rete testis and seminiferous tubules in the rat. The basic arrangement is probably similar in other species except for the location of the rete, which extends along the epididymal margin of the testis in man and is centrally placed along the long axis of the testis in rams and in many other species. From Clermont and Huckins (1961).

tion persists even when the flow of lymph is increased by heating the testis or by raising venous pressure. In other tissues, increasing lymph flow lowers its protein concentration to a value thought to be that of filtered fluid, and therefore we can probably conclude that the filtered fluid in the testis is unusually rich in protein.

By contrast, the composition of fluid from within the seminiferous tubules or rete testis is quite different from either blood plasma or testicular lymph (Figure 30.2). Fluid has been collected for analysis in four ways. First, the rete testis has been cannulated in a number of species, and long-lasting chronic preparations have proved possible in some of these. Fluid collected in this way is referred to as rete testis fluid (RTF). Second, fluid has been removed directly from the seminiferous tubules of rats by micropuncture techniques; this fluid is called free-flow seminiferous tubule fluid. Third, if a column of oil is injected into a tubule and left there, continued secretion of aqueous fluid by the wall of the tubule breaks up the oil column into droplets, and this so-called primary fluid can then be removed by micropuncture for analysis. Fourth, the fluid secreted inside the tubules and rete can be retained there for 15 hours by ligating the efferent ducts. Then the difference between the two testes in their content of any substance is equal to the amount of this substance in the retained secreted fluid. If this amount is divided by the volume of retained fluid (estimated by the difference in weight between the ligated and unligated testes), a concentration can be calculated. These values are referred to as concentrations in total secreted fluid. This technique can be modified by decapuslating the testis (thereby removing the rete testis), dispersing the tubular cells, and removing the cellular debris by centrifugation. The supernatant fluid is largely from the lumina of the tubules but is contaminated by some lymph and cellular contents. A correction can be made, however, by treating the contralateral, unligated testis of the same animal in the same way and assuming that the fluid from the unligated testis contains the same amount of lymph and cellular contents. The concentration of a substance in the additional tubular fluid is given by a similar calculation: [(amount of substance in fluid from ligated testis) − (amount in fluid from unligated testis)] / [(volume of fluid from ligated testis) − (volume of fluid from unligated testis)]. All the fluids are quite different from blood plasma or testicular lymph, and though different results were obtained for the different fluids, these differences suggest where fluid is secreted in the testis and how it moves.

Fluid from catheters in the rete testis is opalescent and colorless; it is an uncontaminated, homogeneous suspension of living testicular spermatozoa of normal

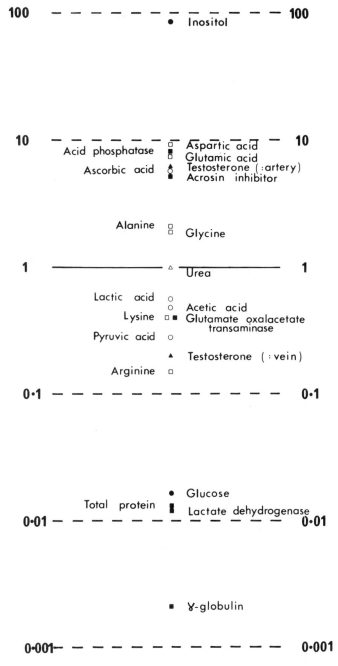

Figure 30.2 Ratios of the concentrations of various organic substances in rete testis fluid of rams to their concentrations in blood plasma (log plot). Two values are plotted for testosterone because of the different concentrations of this substance in arterial and testicular venous blood. ■ = proteins; □ = amino acids; ● = carbohydrates; ○ = organic acids; △ = urea; ▲ = testosterone.

morphology, and it represents a good source of material for in vitro studies.

Spermatozoa

The concentration of spermatozoa in RTF (30 to 100 × 10^6 per ml) is much less than that in ejaculated semen in all species so far studied. But the spermatocrit (percentage by volume of the fluid occupied by spermatozoa after centrifugation) of fluid collected from the seminiferous tubules is greater than that of RTF, and the calculated concentration of spermatozoa in the total secreted fluid is also higher than that in RTF.

The spermatozoa in RTF are apparently infertile and relatively immotile, sometimes exhibiting vibratory circular movements that appear to be nonpropulsive. They usually possess the clear cytoplasmic droplet of immature epididymal spermatozoa and are different from epididymal or ejaculated spermatozoa in a number of ways.

Ions

The potassium concentration in RTF is about three times higher than in blood plasma; sodium and chloride concentrations show smaller but consistent differences, and these differences persist even when the concentration of spermatozoa is drastically reduced by locally heating the testis. The concentration of potassium is higher in free-flow micropuncture fluid than in RTF and even higher in primary fluid. The concentrations of sodium and chloride are highest in RTF and least in primary fluid. All fluids are isosmotic with plasma. Primary and free-flow fluids are probably commensurately higher in bicarbonate than RTF. The calculated concentration of potassium in total secreted fluid lies between that of RTF and that of free-flow tubular fluid, suggesting that the retained secretion is a mixture of these two fluids. The ionic composition of additional tubular fluid (ATF) is very similar to that of free-flow tubular fluid (Figure 30.3).

The concentration of calcium and magnesium in RTF is about half that in blood plasma, but this may be because about half the Ca and Mg in blood plasma is protein-bound, and the protein concentration of RTF is very low. The inorganic phosphate concentration of RTF is only a fraction of that of blood plasma.

Carbohydrates

RTF contains practically no glucose or fructose but does contain high concentrations of inositol in all species so far examined, except in the wallaby. No other carbohydrates could be detected in RTF by gas-liquid chromatography of the trimethylsilane derivatives, except in galactose-fed rats when galactitol was present with increased concentrations of inositol.

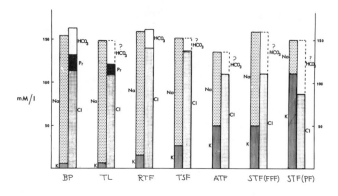

Figure 30.3 Concentrations of ions and protein in various fluids from the rat testis. BP = blood plasma; TL = testicular lymph; RTF = rete testis fluid; TSF = total secreted fluid; ATF = additional tubular fluid; STF (FFF) = tubular free-flow fluid; STF (PF) = tubular primary fluid.

Amino Acids

RTF contains less of most of the free amino acids than does blood plasma or testicular lymph, but certain of them are present in very much higher concentrations. These acids include glutamic, aspartic, alanine, and glycine in the ram, bull, boar, and wallaby. In the rat there is more lysine in RTF than in plasma and proline substitutes for glutamic acid.

Proteins

RTF is markedly different from blood plasma and testicular lymph both in the concentration of total protein and in the nature of proteins present. Initially, all the plasma proteins were thought to be present, but in lower concentrations and, except for α_2 macroglobulin, with greater differences in the concentrations of larger proteins, particularly γ globulin. Subsequently, with more sophisticated techniques for separation, a number of specific proteins have been demonstrated in RTF, and many of the individual plasma proteins do not appear in RTF. Tubular fluid contains even less of the plasma proteins and more specific proteins than RTF contains.

The activity per unit total protein of certain enzymes in RTF is appreciably higher than in blood plasma. Furthermore, when certain enzymes (malic dehydrogenase—EC 1.1.1.3.7—and glutamate oxalacetate transaminase—EC 2.6.1.1) are separated into their isoenzymes, one isoenzyme present in RTF is found in testis tissue but not in blood plasma. With lactic dehydrogenase (EC 1.1.1.27), the isoenzyme present in RTF is isoenzyme I, which is found in many tissues including testis and blood plasma, and not isoenzyme x, which is specific to the testis, particularly the germinal cells.

Ram RTF contains concentrations of LH that have been determined by radioimmunoassay to be comparable to those in blood plasma, but neither rat RTF collected by catheter nor the supernatant obtained by centrifuging homogenized EDL contains any detectable LH. RTF from rats, rabbits, and rams contains appreciable concentrations of a testosterone-binding protein, which also binds 5α dihydrotestosterone. In rats this protein is not found in blood or lymph but only in RTF, into which it is secreted by the Sertoli cells under the influence of FSH. In rabbits and rams a similar protein is also found in blood plasma and testicular lymph, but this protein is from a different source and its production is under different control.

Ram RTF also contains an appreciable concentration of an inhibitor of acrosin and trypsin; this is a peptide with a molecular weight of about 6,000 daltons. There is also a protein with a molecular weight of about 25,000 daltons, which may be the long-sought-for inhibin, the feedback from the seminiferous epithelium to the pituitary that controls FSH production.

Steroids
The concentration of testosterone and certain other steroids in RTF has been shown to be appreciably higher than that in peripheral plasma in the ram, bull, rat, and rhesus monkey. In the ram the ratio of RTF to plasma concentrations of testosterone from the interstitial spermatic vein is 0.2, whereas in the rat it is 0.9. There are also high concentrations of estrogens in boar RTF, but they are not as high in RTF as in testicular lymph or plasma from the internal spermatic vein. Cholesterol is present in RTF in low concentrations.

The concentration of testosterone in rat RTF was decreased by hypophysectomy or the parenteral administration of small doses of testosterone propionate and increased by injections of hCG. Testosterone concentration in the RTF of hypophysectomised rats could be restored to normal by repeated injections of pregnenolone, which had comparatively little effect on the concentration of testosterone in testicular venous plasma.

Conclusions
The differences in composition between the fluid inside the seminiferous tubules and that in the excurrent ducts of the testis and blood plasma or testicular lymph lead to the conclusion that substances do not diffuse freely into and out of the tubules; otherwise the concentrations would equalize. It is therefore relevant to consider just how substances do penetrate into the tubules. The simplest route would be through the walls of the tubules, but the differences in sperm concentration and ion and protein composition between seminiferous tubular fluid and RTF suggest that two distinct secretions occur in the testis, one in the tubules and the other in the rete testis or *tubuli recti*. To explain

the differences between primary fluid and free-flow fluid, it is necessary to postulate that a potassium-rich fluid is secreted in the tubules and that this secretion is diluted by a sodium- and chloride-rich secretion from the rete testis that is drawn into the tubules and mixed there by the peristaltic action of the tubules.

If this is so, then there is an alternative route for compounds to reach the cells lining the seminiferous tubules, namely through the rete testis epithelium and then down the lumina of the seminiferous tubules.

30.2 Functional Evidence for a Blood-Testis Barrier

Experiments to study the function of the blood-testis barrier have depended largely on the study of the passage of radioactive and other markers from the blood into testicular lymph and into fluid from inside the tubular system. The rate of passage into the lymph gives a measure of the permeability of the capillaries; the rate of entry into fluid from inside the tubular system measures the rate of penetration into the seminiferous tubules.

Substances introduced into the bloodstream come quite rapidly into equilibrium with testicular lymph. This is so for proteins such as albumin and large water-soluble molecules such as inulin and ^{51}Cr-EDTA as well as for ions. These results suggest a high capillary permeability, but apparently it is not high enough to produce unusually high volumes of distribution of ^{131}I-labeled human serum albumin in the rat testis. Furthermore the curves of the venous concentrations of ^{51}Cr-labeled red blood cells and ^{125}I-albumin, after the intra-arterial injection of a mixture of these markers, do not differ appreciably as they should do if capillary permeability is very high.

The transport of glucose through the testicular capillaries is passive, not carrier-mediated, because the rate of entry of ^{14}C-L-glucose into testicular lymph from blood plasma is equal to that of ^{3}H-D-glucose. For a comparison it may be recalled that D-glucose passes out of the brain capillaries much more readily than L-glucose, because D-glucose is transported by a specific carrier in the brain. Also, when the concentration of glucose in blood plasma is suddenly raised, the ratio of testicular lymph to plasma concentrations rises (after an initial temporary fall) from control values of 0.8 toward unity. The low values at normal glucose concentrations are probably due to utilization of glucose by the tubules, and this becomes less significant as the concentration rises. By contrast, the ratio of the concentration of glucose in cerebrospinal fluid (CSF) to that in plasma (which is about 0.6 at normal plasma glucose concentrations) falls at high glucose concentrations because of the characteristics of the carrier in the brain capillaries or the cells surrounding them. It would therefore appear that transport across testicular capillaries is by comparatively unrestricted passive diffusion.

Three methods have been used to study the rate of penetration of substances into the seminiferous tubules. The simplest and most direct, but least physiological, is to isolate seminiferous tubules and use them to study the rate at which substances enter, either with the cut ends of the tubules occluded using a special chamber or with the cut ends free.

The volumes of distribution (i.e., the ratio of cpm/g tissue to cpm/ml medium or plasma) for sucrose in these preparations were considerably greater than those in vivo and moreover could be reduced by cooling the testis during isolation of the tubules and incorporating 6.3 percent bovine serum albumin into the media in which the tubules were isolated and incubated. Therefore, unless special precautions are taken, the permeability of isolated tubules appears to be abnormally high.

The second technique was based on similar techniques used for studying the rate of passage of substances into CSF. The plasma concentration of the substance under investigation is raised and then ideally held constant while RTF and lymph are collected (Figure 30.4). So far, no one has collected sufficient tubular fluid to be able to analyze it for anything but ions and proteins, but it is tempting to believe that fluid from the rete testis reflects the relative concentrations inside the tubules, if not their absolute values. As discussed earlier, RTF and tubular fluid are not identical, and this technique may give biased results if the substance under investigation penetrates the epithelium of the rete testis more readily than it does the wall of the seminiferous tubule. Alternatively, the concentration of the marker in blood plasma can be compared with the concentration of the seminiferous tubular fluid or ATF calculated by the difference technique.

The third technique is somewhat indirect and requires measurement in vivo of the volume of distribution of the test substances, defined in μl/g as (cpm/g testis)/(cpm/μl plasma). The volume can be compared with simultaneous measurements of the volume of distribution for substances whose distribution in the testis is known.

30.3 Entry of Individual Substances

Water, Ions, and Small Organic Molecules
If tritiated water is infused intravenously, the radioactivity in RTF reaches the same level as in blood plasma during the first half hour. The entry rates of ethanol, urea, glycerol, and bicarbonate into RTF are only slightly slower. Creatinine enters RTF much more slowly, but p-aminohippurate and ^{51}Cr-EDTA do not

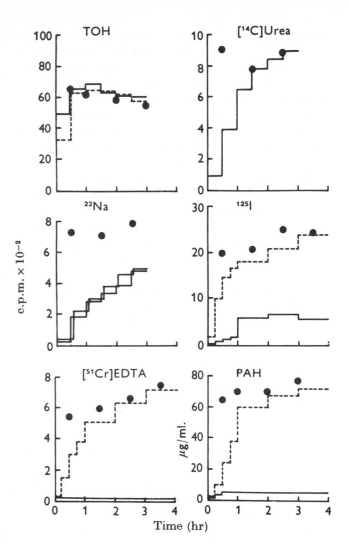

Figure 30.4 Concentrations of various substances in blood plasma (filled circles), rete testis fluid (solid lines), and testicular lymph (dashed lines) from rams during intravenous infusion, in most instances after a priming dose, of a number of marker substances. The two lines for ^{22}Na apply to the two testes of the same animal. From Setchell et al. (1969).

appear in RTF at all, even in experiments lasting up to six hours (Figure 30.4). Except for bicarbonate, all the other ions studied (Na⁺, K⁺, Pb⁺, Cl⁻, I⁻, CSN⁻, acetate, propionate, butyrate) entered RTF slowly and were still significantly lower than in blood plasma after three hours. When using radioactive rubidium as a marker for radioactive potassium, taking advantage of its more convenient radiochemical properties and assuming that the two ions probably behave similarly, equilibrium between plasma and RTF in the amount of radioactive rubidium per unit of nonradioactive potassium was reached only between 48 and 72 hours.

When radioactive rubidium was injected intraperitoneally into rats, the rubidium in the testes increased progressively, but did not reach equilibrium with plasma even after six hours, unlike other organs such as liver, kidney, and muscle. A similar time-course was seen in isolated tubules with their ends occluded and incubated in media containing radioactive rubidium, and the exchange was drastically reduced by the addition of ouabain, suggesting that Na-K activated adenosine triphosphatase (ATPase) is involved. It was not possible, however, to detect any ouabain-sensitive ATPase activity in homogenates of whole testes or tubules, probably because of the high concentrations of other ATPases present in the testis.

The concentration of radioactive rubidium in total secreted fluid was negligible up to six hours after injection. Radioactive sodium and potassium did enter RTF and ATF (both fluids were studied in the same rats). The rate of entry, measured as (cpm/μl fluid)/(cpm/μl plasma), was higher for potassium into ATF than into RTF and for sodium into RTF than into ATF, but when transfer constants (k_{out}) were calculated and when allowance was made for the different concentrations in the two fluids, the rete testis appeared to be more permeable to potassium ($k_{out} = 0.0046$ min⁻¹) than to sodium ($k_{out} = 0.0015$ min⁻¹) and more permeable than the tubules to either potassium ($k_{out} = 0.0010$ min⁻¹) or sodium ($k_{out} = 0.0020$ min⁻¹).

Carbohydrates

The entry of glucose cannot be studied directly because of its high rate of metabolism, but it is possible to use the closely related analog 3-0-methylglucose (30MG), which in other tissues is transported like glucose but not metabolized. This substance, when infused intravenously, appears quickly in ram RTF and reaches equilibrium within several hours. In rats its volume of distribution in the testis is appreciably greater in the EDL than in the unligated testis. The calculated concentration in the accumulated fluid was 56 percent of that in plasma after three hours. The volume of distribution of 30MG in vivo is reduced to only slightly more than that for sucrose by increasing the

concentration of glucose in the plasma, either by injecting glucose or by making the rats diabetic (Figure 30.5).

In isolated seminiferous tubules, 30MG is distributed rapidly into about 60 percent of the tissue water. This volume of distribution is reduced by including glucose or mannose in the incubating medium, slightly reduced by including galactose, and unaffected by including fructose, sucrose, or inositol; 30MG already in the tubules can be driven out by the addition of glucose to the medium, a phenomenon known as counterflow. The entry of 30MG is unaffected by inhibitors such as phloridzin, 2:4 dinitrophenol, or ouabain, by sodium-free medium, or by the presence or absence of insulin.

This evidence indicates that glucose enters the tubules by a mobile carrier-facilitated diffusion, not by active transport or by simple diffusion; the carrier system is not sensitive to insulin; that is, it is similar to that in erythrocytes but not to that in muscle cells. The K_m of the carrier in the rat has been calculated to be about 11mM in vitro and 8mM in vivo, which would suggest that the uptake of glucose by the testis should depend on its plasma concentration. It has not been possible to obtain evidence in the rat, but there appears to be no relation between glucose uptake and concentration in the ram; the characteristics of the carrier may be different in this species.

Radioactive inositol enters RTF from blood very slowly, and more radioactivity is found in RTF inositol after infusion of ¹⁴C-glucose than after ³H-inositol. The rate of increase in the specific radioactivity is still slow, however, suggesting that in the testis a large pool of inositol exchanges comparatively slowly.

Sucrose, sodium, and inulin rapidly occupy a volume of about 10 to 15 percent of the rat testis in vivo. This volume is probably equivalent to the interstitial extracellular fluid and lymph spaces. After the first hour the volumes of distribution of these markers do not increase further and are no greater in the EDL than in the unligated testes; in fact, the volume of distribution in the ligated testis is often slightly less, presumably because of a slight compression of the interstitial spaces by the distended tubules.

Amino Acids

The entry of only a small number of amino acids into the seminiferous tubules has been measured. Glutamate enters ram RTF very slowly; glycine enters slightly more rapidly, but more radioactivity appears in most of the amino acids that are present in high concentrations in RTF after an infusion of radioactive glucose than after an infusion of either glutamate or glycine.

Somewhat more rapid entry into rat RTF has been

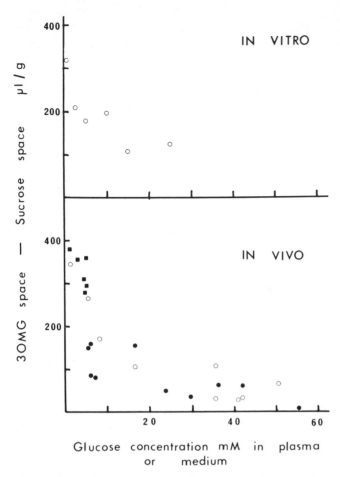

Figure 30.5 Relationship of the concentration of glucose in the plasma or medium to the amount of 30MG entering the seminiferous tubules, expressed as the volume of distribution for 30MG less the volume of distribution for sucrose, which is known to be excluded from tubules. ○ = normal rats; ■ = alloxan diabetic rats; ● = streptozotocin diabetic rats. Rats were injected with insulin or infused with glucose to give the lowered or raised plasma glucose concentrations shown. From A. Middleton and B. P. Setchell (unpublished data).

demonstrated for a number of amino acids, but this has not been substantiated by measuring the volumes of distribution for the EDL and unligated testes. These volumes are only slightly greater than those for sucrose, and the concentrations in the total secreted fluid were only a fraction of that in plasma.

Proteins

Little radioactivity appeared in the RTF when [125]I- or ^{131}I-labeled human serum albumin was infused into the bloodstream of rams or rats. Even when the counts precipitable with 5 percent trichloracetic acid (TCA) are expressed per unit of total protein present, RTF does not come into equilibrium with blood plasma in the ram for about four days. The situation is similar with ovine prolactin in the ram, but equilibrium is reached with smaller proteins like insulin in about 24 hours. With FSH, LH, and growth hormone, the radioactivity per unit total protein in RTF exceeds that in blood from four hours after the beginning of the infusion, but the exact significance of this finding must await precise estimates of the amounts of these hormones present in RTF.

Radioactively labeled sheep and rat FSH and rat LH appear to enter the fluid accumulating in the rat testis after EDL more rapidly than human serum albumin does. Much of the radioactivity in the testis fluid is not protein-bound, however, and much of the protein-bound activity is not immunoreactive FSH or LH. Therefore the entry of unchanged FSH and LH may be slower than at first appears. These hormones certainly do not pass through the walls of the tubules readily, but this is compatible with their present suggested sites of action—LH on the interstitial cells and FSH on the Sertoli cells.

Steroids

Initial experiments involved injection of radioactively labeled steroids into the animal and then autoradiography of the testis or separation of the testis into tubules and interstitial tissue. The results of these studies were rather confusing, probably due to artifacts in some of the techniques.

More recently, a study has been made of the penetration of some labeled steroids from blood into RTF. Testosterone and dehydroepiandrosterone appeared to be readily transferred from blood to RTF, whereas cholesterol was excluded. Between these extremes, the appearance of radioactivity in RTF suggested the following order of entry rates: testosterone > progesterone > pregnenolone > 5α-reduced androgens > estrogens > corticosteroids. This study made the important and unjustified assumptions that the radioactive steroids in arterial blood reflected the steroids bathing the walls of the seminiferous tubules and that

RTF was representative of the fluid inside the seminiferous tubules.

To remedy these shortcomings, a further experiment was done in which radioactive steroids (testosterone, dihydrotestosterone, 5α-androstane-3α,17β-diol, or androstenedione) were infused intravenously into rats whose efferent ducts on one testis had been ligated 24 hours previously. After 30 or 60 minutes of infusion of arterial and testicular venous blood, RTF and ATF were collected, and radioactivity was measured and separated by thin layer chromatography. These observations confirmed that testosterone penetrated readily into RTF and that the 5α-reduced androgens penetrated poorly. The penetration into tubular fluid was similar (Figure 30.6). There was little radioactive androstenedione in the testicular fluids or in testicular venous blood. Apparently the radioactive androstenedione in arterial blood was converted in the interstitial tissue into testosterone, which was then penetrating through the walls of the seminiferous tubules and rete. The absence of major differences in rates of appearance of the various steroids in RTF and ATF suggests similarity in the permeability of the two epithelia to steroids.

When labeled progesterone was infused into one testicular artery of a boar, some radioactivity appeared in the RTF but most of it had been transformed into highly polar compounds, which were also present in higher concentrations in plasma from the internal spermatic vein. When labeled pregnenolone was infused, much less radioactivity appeared in the RTF, but again a high proportion was present as polar compounds.

Drugs
The penetration of a number of established antifertility compounds into RTF has been studied in rats. The esters of methanesulphonic acid all entered the RTF to reach 20 to 25 percent of blood levels within three hours. When the compounds were injected 11 to 15 hours before collection of RTF, the amount of radioactivity in RTF usually exceeded that in blood. The radioactivity was usually present as the compound injected, except that ^{35}S-methylene dimethanesulphonate was entirely broken down after penetration into the tubule into methanesulphonic acid, which itself did not enter the tubules readily. α Chlorohydrin penetrated into RTF in rats almost as quickly as tritiated water does, attaining blood levels within 40 minutes.

A study has also been made of the entry of series of barbiturates, sulphonamides, and salicylic acid into RTF. The transfer constants were highly correlated with the lipid solubilities of these drugs, but they bore little relation to molecular size, the percentage ionized or the pKa (Figure 30.7).

Conclusions
Functional evidence has revealed that the blood-testis barrier represents a wide range of permeability, from total exclusion from the tubules to almost free transfer into the tubules. It is not yet possible to suggest a chemical basis to account for the variations in rate of penetration observed to date. An outstanding problem is to define the source of the compounds found in seminiferous tubule and RTF, whether they are derived from the blood, synthesized in the interstitium, or synthesized inside the barrier in the germinal epithelium.

30.4 Structure of the Blood-Testis Barrier

Capillaries
The capillary wall represents the first barrier that substances must cross in order to leave the bloodstream. The testicular arterioles and capillaries of eutherian

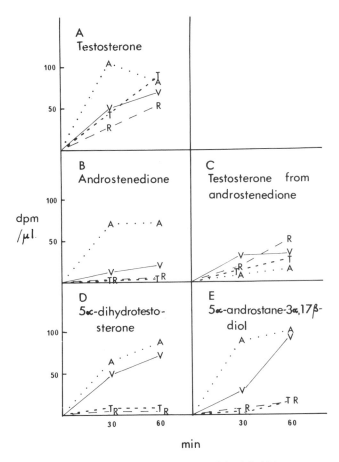

Figure 30.6 Radioactivity in dpm/μl original fluid in areas on Silica gel thin-layer chromatograms corresponding to the steroid infused (Panels A, B, D, and E) or in the area corresponding to testosterone when androstenedione was infused (Panel C). The fluids are arterial blood (A), testicular venous blood (V), rete testis fluid (RTF), and additional tubular fluid (T). Each point is the mean of two rats.

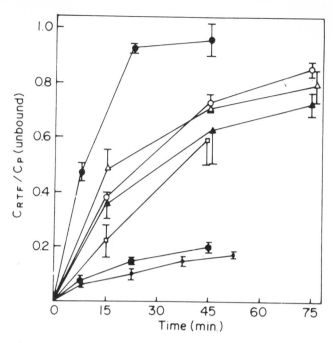

Figure 30.7 Ratios of the concentrations of various substances in rete testis fluid (C_{RTF}) to their concentration in blood plasma (C_P) during intravenous infusions. ● = thiopental, PC (partition coefficient chloroform: phosphate buffer pH 7.4) = 102; ○ = pentobarbital, PC = 21; ▲ = barbital, PC = 2.0; △ = sulfamethoxypyridazine, PC = 1.6; □ = sulfanilamide, PC = 0.027; ⬟ = sulfaguanidine, PC = 0.0018; ■ = salicylic acid, PC = 0.0003. Each point represents the mean ± SD of three to five experiments. From Okumura et al. (1975).

mammals with scrotal testes are supplied by an elongated, coiling artery, which is surrounded by the multiple veins of the pampiniform plexus. This arrangement, and the analogous arterial and venous retia in marsupials, acts as a countercurrent heat exchanger and almost eliminates the difference between systolic and diastolic blood pressure. The capillaries of the testis seem to be orientated either parallel to the tubules and larger vessels in the interstitial spaces or at right angles to the tubules. This organization develops only at puberty, but so far there is no explanation why the capillaries are arranged in this way. The Leydig cells lie near intertubular capillaries, and the capillary arrangement might have the effect of carrying the testosterone from the Leydig cells first around the tubular walls through the extracellular, intertubular fluid.

The pressure in the vessels in the interstitial spaces near the Leydig cells might be such that filtration of a protein-rich fluid from blood to tissue occurs there, whereas the capillaries around the tubules may be at a lower pressure so that they resorb fluid. These differences in capillary pressure would seem to be supported by the observation that changes in venous pressure cause greater changes in the diameter of the peritubu-

lar capillaries, compared with the intertubular capillaries, and the lumina of the peritubular capillaries disappear when intratesticular pressure is raised after ligation of the efferent ducts and accumulation of fluid in the testis. Whether or not the two types of capillary act in this way, they seem to have a similar ultrastructure, namely an unfenestrated endothelium with no spaces between adjacent cells and with a definite basement membrane, but with no pericytes. The endothelium of the small blood vessels of the testis has an unusual appearance because of a large number of microvillous processes.

It is usual to describe the interstitial tissue as a loose connective tissue containing blood and lymph vessels and islands of Leydig cells, but there are marked species differences in the actual arrangement of these structures. In the guinea pig the Leydig cells lie in clusters around the blood vessels, with the greater part of the interstitium occupied by peritubular lymphatic sinusoids of irregular outline. These are bounded by an attenuated endothelial lining, which covers the vessels and their associated Leydig cell clusters and also forms the outermost layer of the peritubular boundary tissue. The anatomy in the rat is very similar except that there are gaps in the endothelial covering of the Leydig cells and blood vessels. In the larger mammals, such as the bull, ram, elephant, monkey, and human, the Leydig cells are not as closely associated with the blood vessels. Instead, they are found in clusters of varying size scattered in loose connective tissue, which is drained by a conspicuous lymphatic vessel located either centrally or eccentrically in each intertubular area. Finally, in the boar, the warthog, the zebra, and the naked mole rat, there are larger areas (up to 60 percent of the space) filled with closely packed epitheloid Leydig cells with very little interstitial connective tissue and a few small lymphatic vessels.

Seminiferous Tubules

The seminiferous tubules in most species are surrounded by four concentric layers: an inner noncellular layer, which is well developed in species such as the ram into a multilamellated structure; an inner cellular layer, which in most species is formed by myoid cells that are probably responsible for the contractile activity of the tubules; an outer noncellular layer, mainly collagen; and an outer cellular layer, which may be the cells lining the peritubular lymphatic spaces.

The myoid cells are dependent on a normal hormonal environment for their development. Inside the tubules the only cells abutting on the boundary tissue are spermatogonia and Sertoli cells. All the other germinal cells, spermatocytes, spermatids, and developing spermatozoa are sandwiched between pairs of Sertoli cells or embedded in their luminal surfaces. Pairs of

Sertoli cells are joined above the spermatogonia but below the spermatocytes by specialized junctions, and it has been suggested that these junctions divide the intercellular spaces into a basal compartment around the spermatogonia and between them and Sertoli cells and an adluminal compartment between the Sertoli cells and the other germinal cells (Figure 30.8).

The sites of restricted permeability have been defined by examining the testes of animals injected or perfused with various electron-opaque markers. In the rat and guinea pig the larger markers such as carbon, thorium, and ferritin spread throughout the interstitial tissue but do not pass the myoid cells, which form tight end-to-end junctions with one another. Smaller markers, such as peroxidase and lanthanum, are also stopped at the narrow junctions between pairs of myoid cells at most sites. In certain areas of the tubule these markers get past the myoid cells and then penetrate between the spermatogonia and the Sertoli cells and between adjacent Sertoli cells as far as their specialized junctions. There the markers stop. The penetration of markers through the myoid layer seems to be random and is not associated with any particular stage of the spermatogenic cycle.

In primates the situation is rather different. In humans and monkeys the myoid cells do not form tight junctions with one another, and therefore in monkeys offer little or no resistance to the entry of the markers. The Sertoli-Sertoli cell junctions in monkeys act as the only barrier to penetration, but it appears to be just as effective as the dual barrier in rodents. Similar results have been reported in fowls.

It has recently been shown that the integrity of the Sertoli-Sertoli cell junction appears to be beginning to break down 24 hours after ligation of the efferent ducts, presumably because of pressure due to the accumulated fluid. Later the pressure decreases. Presumably the junctions then allow the fluid to pass readily from the tubules into the interstitial spaces.

30.5 Disturbances of the Blood-Testis Barrier

Temperature
The testes of most mammals are contained in a scrotum maintained at a temperature lower than the rest of the body. Therefore temperature may affect the blood-testis barrier, but structural and functional evidence exists for a barrier that is also effective in birds, in which the testis is normally at a temperature of 41°C or higher.

The evidence on the effect of temperature on the blood-testis barrier in mammals is rather confusing. The entry of ^{131}I-iodoantipyrine into the rat testis during the first minute after intravenous injection increased sharply as the temperature of the testis was

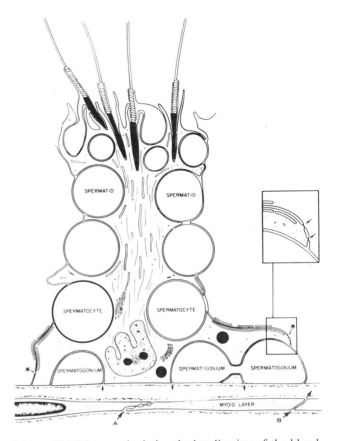

Figure 30.8 Diagram depicting the localization of the blood-testis barrier and the compartmentalization of the germinal epithelium by tight junctions between adjacent Sertoli cells. Note the germ cells and their relationship to a columnar Sertoli cell. The primary barrier in rodents to substances penetrating from the interstitium is the myoid layer. The majority of cell junctions in this layer are closed by a tight apposition of membranes (at A). Over a small fraction of the tubule surface, myoid junctions exhibit an interspace 200 Å in width and are therefore open (at B). Material gaining access to the base of the epithelium by passing through open junctions in the myoid layer is free to enter the intercellular gap between the spermatogonia and the Sertoli cells. Deeper penetration is prevented by occluding junctions (stars) on the Sertoli-Sertoli boundaries. These tight junctions constitute a second and more effective component of the blood-testis barrier. In effect, the Sertoli cells and their tight junctions delimit a basal compartment in the germinal epithelium, containing the spermatogonia and early preleptotene spermatocytes, and an adluminal compartment, containing the spermatocytes and spermatids. Substances traversing open junctions in the myoid cell layer have direct access to cells in the basal compartment, but to reach the cells in the adluminal compartment, substances must pass through the Sertoli cells or enter via the lumen from the rete testis. From Dym and Fawcett (1970).

raised to 43°C or 45°C, suggesting that blood flow was substantially increased. The entry of ^{86}Rb at the same time, however, increased only marginally, suggesting that the permeability to rubidium was less at the higher temperature. Furthermore the permeability of isolated tubules to ^{86}Rb was greatest at 33°C and decreased at higher temperatures. These findings conflict with direct observations on the passage of rubidium from blood to RTF in the rat, in which after 30 minutes the entry of rubidium into the testis at 41°C was 90 percent greater than into the control testis at 33°C. Conversely, entry of radioactivity during androstenedione infusion was correspondingly decreased at 41°C, although the entry rates of radioactivity associated with testosterone were unchanged by this amount of heat.

Effect of Cadmium
An early effect of cadmium in the rat appears to be an increase in permeability of the testicular capillaries to a variety of markers, including ^{131}I-labeled human serum albumin. Even earlier changes can be detected in the amount of ^{86}Rb entering the tubules, however, and perhaps cadmium also damages the integrity of the tubular barrier. Lanthanum freely penetrates the myoid layer of guinea pig seminiferous tubules a few hours after cadmium administration. Increased staining of the tubular contents of the guinea pig after the parenteral injection of dyes was seen 24 hours after cadmium injections, but tubular staining was normal 5 and 12 hours after cadmium injection. There was no increased entry of serum albumin or γ globulin into the tubules until 72 hours after cadmium injection. Blood flow was drastically reduced in the rat 6 hours after injection of cadmium, so these changes after 24 hours and longer may have been secondary to the fall in blood flow that would probably have occurred in the guinea pig by then.

Cadmium may increase the permeability of the rete rather than that of the tubules, as abnormal amounts of serum proteins can be detected in rat RTF as early as 15 minutes after the injection of cadmium whereas there is no change in the proteins of the fluid from the seminiferous tubules.

Effect of Immunization of the Animal to Testis-Specific Antigens
There is some suggestion that acriflavine and γ globulin enter the seminiferous tubule more readily in the guinea pig if it has been immunized with testis homogenate and Freund's complete adjuvant. In addition, when adjuvant alone was injected into guinea pigs, peroxidase got past myoid cells more readily but was still stopped at the junctions between Sertoli cells. This treatment caused collagen fibers to disappear

from the peritubular spaces and peroxidase to appear in some Sertoli cells and type B spermatogonia.

The significance of these observations is uncertain, because the normal rete is apparently more permeable to dyes and protein than are the tubules, and the immunological reaction seems to begin at the rete testis and spread from there along the tubules. Mature spermatozoa were affected before early spermatids, and in young guinea pigs with spermatids in the testis but no sperm in the excurrent ducts, there was no damage when they were immunized with testis homogenate. Therefore it would appear that an antigen-antibody reaction must occur in the rete before the permeability of the blood-testis barrier elsewhere in the testis increases, or alternatively, antibodies entering at the rete are carried into the lumina of the tubules and act on the germinal cells from the lumen. The action of the adjuvant may be to increase the permeability of the rete rather than that of the tubules themselves.

Immunological damage cannot be produced by the passive transfer of antibodies, however, although injected antibodies do produce a reaction in the rete. Furthermore, when lymph node cells from an actively immunized animal are injected into the testis of a nonimmunized recipient, there is a cellular reaction in the interstitial tissue. But when macrophages collected from the peritoneal cavity are used instead of the lymph node cells, the reaction in the testis occurs more rapidly and begins in the rete.

30.6 Consequences of the Blood-Testis Barrier

Spermatogenesis
Since a restriction on the entry of dyes and other markers into the tubules does not develop until after postnatal day 15 in rats, it must be assumed that the primary function of the blood-testis barrier is to create stable and favorable conditions for the main function of the testis, the production of spermatozoa. It is obvious from the unusual composition of the fluid inside the tubules that rather special conditions are created there, but we do not yet know how these conditions favor spermatogenesis. Indeed, ATF and RTF are far enough away from the critical steps in spermatogenesis that we are uncertain whether their composition reflects the special conditions needed for the critical steps or whether they represent what is left over after the cells have taken what they need. It may be like trying to find out what a family eats by analyzing its kitchen waste.

Some of the substances present in high concentration in the fluid such as glycine, glutamine, and aspartic acid may be important in the synthesis of purine and pyrimidine bases, but it is not even known whether the testis synthesizes most of its own bases or extracts them as such from the blood. It is well known that ^{3}H-thymidine is taken up from the blood and incorporated in DNA in the dividing germ cells, but the quantitative importance of this process has not been evaluated. Glutamic acid is one of the amino acids found necessary for the normal development of duck and chicken gonads in tissue culture, and glutamine has been shown to stimulate the differentiation of testicular cells in chemically defined media.

In view of the relatively high concentration of α_2 macroglobulin in RTF, it is interesting to recall that α_2 macroglobulin will stimulate DNA synthesis by bone marrow cells after X-irradiation and that these or similar proteins are present in elevated concentrations in blood plasma during periods of rapid cell division; α_2 macroglobulin has also been shown to bind and inhibit a number of proteinases.

Another clue to a possible functional significance of the barrier may lie in the separation of the spermatogonia and the other germinal cells inside the basal and adluminal compartments, respectively. The spermatogonia are diploid cells dividing mitotically like stem cells elsewhere in the body, the only difference being that the spermatogonial divisions are synchronized along appreciable lengths of the tubules. This synchrony may result at least in part from the persistence of cellular linkages after the cells have divided or from other factors associated with the spermatogenic cycle. The spermatocytes, on the other hand, enter the long prophase of the meiotic division at about the same time that they move from the basal to the adluminal compartment and lose contact with the boundary tissue. The exact timing of this separation is difficult to establish, but it may be argued that the Sertoli cells commit the spermatocytes to enter into meiosis by removing them from the basal compartment, whereas the cells remaining in the basal compartment continue to divide mitotically.

A meiosis-inducing effect by the Sertoli cells could be mediated through the fluid microenvironment of the germinal cells, which is probably secreted by the Sertoli cells. Efforts have not been successful in demonstrating RTF activity stimulating cultured testicular cells to complete meiosis or stimulating starfish oocytes to divide meiotically, as 1-methyladenine does.

The blood-testis barrier will have to be considered in evaluating the recently described spermatogonial chalone. If this chalone is produced by the dividing spermatogonia, it would probably remain in the basal compartment to repress mitosis in the type A_0 spermatogonia. If it is produced by the later stages, however, its access to the dividing spermatogonia would have to

be indirect, probably via the Sertoli cells. Similarly, if mitotic activity in the seminiferous tubules is dependent on a mitotic stimulator secreted by the underlying mesenchymal tissue, as in the epidermis, this is likely to have its major effect on the spermatogonia in the basal compartment.

Endocrinological Consequences
The suggestion that gonadotropins may not gain access to the seminiferous tubules has not been supported by subsequent evidence; however, even though these hormones seem to enter the tubules more quickly than other proteins, their entry is still slow compared with smaller molecules. The slow entry of gonadotropins would serve to shield the germinal epithelium from any sudden fluctuations in the concentrations of gonadotropins in the plasma (e.g., those caused by periodic release of these hormones from the pituitary). It has recently been demonstrated, however, that there are specific receptors for LH in the Leydig cells, and it has also been suggested that FSH acts on the Sertoli cells. Therefore it may not be necessary for either of these hormones to pass beyond the blood-testis barrier.

The ready entry of some steroids, particularly testosterone, makes it unlikely that in normal testes the de novo synthesis of steroids from cholesterol inside the tubules is of any consequence. Although cholesterol itself has been shown not to enter the tubules, considerable amounts are present, probably synthesized there from acetate. This conclusion is based on experiments in which radioactivity was incorporated from acetate into cholesterol, but none of the radioactivity appeared in testosterone. The majority of the cholesterol in the testis is inside the tubules, which suggests that this cholesterol is probably not involved in the synthesis of testosterone.

Nevertheless, transformation of one steroid into another certainly appears to occur inside the tubules, as it does in many other tissues of the body such as skin and hair. Evidently the transformation of one steroid into another is a much more common phenomenon than de novo synthesis. If a permeant steroid is transformed inside the tubules into a nonpermeant one (e.g., testosterone into 5α-androstane-3α 17β, diol) a concentration gradient would build up without any expenditure of energy. So far no steroid has been found in the fluid inside the tubules in higher concentrations than in lymph or blood from the internal spermatic vein, but a comprehensive search has not been made.

The barrier could also be important in retaining any substance of endocrinological significance formed inside the tubule, so that it leaves the testis in RTF to be reabsorbed in the caput epididymidis. Such a substance, inhibin, has been postulated as the basis of a feedback mechanism to the pituitary on the rate of spermatogenesis and has been found in RTF. Inhibin appears to be a protein with a molecular weight of at least 20,000 daltons, and the balance of evidence suggests that it is probably produced by the Sertoli cells in response to the numbers of cells in the later stages of spermatogenesis. It cannot be predicted whether it would be secreted on the tubular or blood side of the barrier, or on both sides, but obviously the blood-testis barrier will be important in determining its pathway to the pituitary.

Immunological Consequences

Once a cell becomes haploid, it becomes foreign to the immunological system of the body. Therefore an animal can be immunized against its own spermatozoa or testis cells. This does not happen naturally, because the haploid cells are isolated immunologically by the blood-testis barrier from the rest of the body. Likewise, the barrier excludes from the tubules naturally occurring antibodies reacting with spermatozoa and antibodies induced by injecting just spermatozoa or testis. If the injections include Freund's complete adjuvant, however, the testis shows immunological damage, and this has been shown to result at least in part from a breakdown in the normal function of the barrier.

Effects on Spermatozoa

The blood-testis barrier maintains the peculiar composition of the fluid inside the tubules and rete testis, and this may have important effects on the spermatozoa the fluid normally contains. One obvious function of the fluid is to transport the spermatozoa out of the testis into the epididymis, but this could be done by a fluid of any reasonable composition. Two other functions are probably served by the fluid. First, it may supply the spermatozoa with exogenous substrate and help control their endogenous metabolism. Second, it may inhibit the motility of the spermatozoa. RTF certainly stimulates the oxygen uptake of ram and boar testicular spermatozoa, compared with an ionic mixture with the same composition, and at the same time it also preserves their lipid reserves, which normally decrease during incubation. Testicular spermatozoa do not show much motility under any of the conditions so far tested, but they have the necessary apparatus and no one has yet explained why they are not motile. Indeed, no one has convincingly shown why epididymal spermatozoa, as they develop the capacity for movement, are normally held immotile. The two phenomena may be linked. The high potassium content of RTF, which becomes even higher in the epididymis, may be involved. The other possibility is that the peculiar

amino acid composition of the fluid may have some significance. Some amino acids inhibit sea urchin spermatozoa, and poly-L-glutamic acid, which is normally present in the reproductive tract of the hen, has an inhibitory but life-extending action on cock spermatozoa, although elimination of this substance from the oviducts by an immunological method had no effect on the fertility of the hens. The epididymal seminal plasma of mammals may act in a manner similar to that of the spermatophore fluid of the squid or the spermathecal fluid in bees. Inhibition of spermatozoal metabolism in the epididymis would have the effect of conserving their reserves until after ejaculation, when the inhibitors would be diluted by the accessory fluid. A knowledge of the exact role of testicular fluid in sperm survival in the epididymis could be vital to understanding how better to preserve spermatozoa outside the body.

Another important consequence of the barrier is that it enables a high concentration to be maintained in the fluid of the polypeptide that selectively inhibits the acrosomal proteinase or acrosin, which enables the spermatozoa to penetrate the ovum at the moment of fertilization. This enzyme also allows spermatozoa to penetrate other cells, and it is therefore not surprising that the inhibitory peptide is present when the spermatozoa leave the germinal epithelium and is not just added to the semen at the moment of ejaculation, as was previously believed. Its action is probably reinforced by the action of α_2 macroglobulin, which also combines with and inhibits proteinases. This latter inhibition is more pronounced for large substrate molecules, and proteinases bound to α_2 macroglobulin can be further inhibited by small inhibitor molecules. The α_2 macroglobulin and the peptide inhibitor together may thus be important in dealing with any proteinases that leak out of acrosome.

It will also be important to see whether the macroglobulin molecules attach themselves to the sperm surface. If they do, their removal may be a part of capacitation. The small peptide inhibitor from RTF can block fertilization in vitro, has a molecular weight of about 6,000 daltons, and would probably be lost from the fluid into the bloodstream if the barrier did not exist.

30.7 Summary

The blood-testis barrier prevents many substances from passing readily into or out of the seminiferous tubules of the testis, where the spermatozoa are formed. Inside the tubules are the cells that give rise to the spermatozoa and also the Sertoli cells; the barrier is formed by special junctions between adjacent pairs of Sertoli cells. The barrier is probably important in providing the right conditions for the special type of cell division necessary for the formation of the spermatozoa from the stem cells, and it probably enables fluids quite different from blood plasma to circulate in the tubules and carry the sperm into the epididymis to become mature and fertile. It also enables the spermatozoa to develop, although they are immunologically foreign to the rest of the body. Reduction in effectiveness of the barrier may be a possible way of controlling sperm production and fertility in men, and maintenance of the barrier may be important in minimizing the production of mutations due to the effects of drugs.

Key References

Clermont, Y., and C. Huckins. Microscopic anatomy of the sex cords and seminiferous tubules in growing and adult male albino rats. Am. J. Anat. 108:79, 1961.

Cooper, T. G., and G. M. H. Waites. Testosterone in rete testis fluid and blood of rams and rats. J. Endocrinol. 62:619, 1974.

Cooper, T. G., and G. M. H. Waites. Steroids entry into rete testis fluid and the blood-testis barrier. J. Endocrinol. 65:195, 1975.

Dym, M. The fine structure of the monkey (*Macaca*) Sertoli cell and its role in maintaining the blood-testis barrier. Anat. Rec. 175:639, 1973.

Dym, M., and D. W. Fawcett. The blood testis barrier in the rat and the physiological compartmentation of the seminiferous epithelium. Biol. Reprod. 3:308, 1970.

Evans, R. W. The lipid metabolism of the mammalian spermatozoa. Ph.D. thesis. Council for National Academic Awards, England, 1975.

Fawcett, D. W. The architecture of the interstitial tissue of the testis and of the cell junctions in the seminiferous tubules. Adv. Biosci. 10:83, 1973.

Fawcett, D. W. Interactions between Sertoli cells and germ cells. In *Male fertility and sterility*, eds. R. E. Mancini and L. Martini, p. 13. New York: Academic Press, 1974.

Fawcett, D. W. Ultrastructure and function of the Sertoli cell. In *Handbook of Physiology*, Section 7: Endocrinology, Vol. 5: *Male reproductive system*, eds. D. W. Hamilton and R. O. Greep, p. 21. Baltimore: Williams & Wilkins, 1975.

Fawcett, D. W., L. V. Leak, and P. M. Heidger. Electron microscopic observations on the structural components of the blood-testis barrier. J. Reprod. Fertil. Suppl. 10:105, 1970.

Fawcett, D. W., W. B. Neaves, and M. N. Flores. Comparative observations on intertubular lymphatics and the organization of the interstitial tissue of the mammalian testis. Biol. Reprod. 9:500, 1973.

French, F. S., and R. M. Ritzen. A high affinity androgen-binding protein (APB) in rat testis: Evidence for secretion into efferent duct fluid and absorption by the epididymis. Endocrinology 93:88, 1973.

Hansson, V., E. M. Ritzen, F. S. French, and S. N. Nayfeh. Androgen transport and receptor mechanisms in testis and epididymis. In *Handbook of Physiology*, Section 7: Endocrinology, Vol. 5: *Male reproductive system*, eds. D. W. Hamilton and R. O. Greep, p. 173. Baltimore: Williams & Wilkins, 1975.

Harris, M. E., and A. Bartke. Concentration of testosterone in testis fluid of the rat. Endocrinology 95:701, 1974.

Harris, M. E., and A. Bartke. Maintenance of rete testis fluid testosterone and dihydrotestosterone levels by pregnenolone and other C_{21} steroids in hypophysectomized rats. Endocrinology 96:1396, 1975.

Kormano, M. Dye permeability and alkaline phosphatase activity of testicular capillaries in the post-natal rat. Histochemie 9:327, 1967.

Koskimies, A. I., and M. Kormano. The proteins in fluids from the seminiferous tubules and rete testis of the rat. J. Reprod. Fertil. 34:433, 1972.

Main, S. J. The blood-testis barrier and temperature. Ph.D. thesis, University of Reading, England, 1975.

Okumura, E., I. P. Lee, and R. L. Dixon. Permeability of selected drugs and chemicals across the blood testis barrier of the rat. J. Pharmacol. Exp. Ther. 194:89, 1975.

Setchell, B. P. The blood–testicular fluid barrier in sheep. J. Physiol. 189:63P, 1967.

Setchell, B. P. Testicular blood supply, lymphatic drainage and secretion of fluid. In *The testis*, Vol. 1, eds. A. D. Johnson, N. L. Van Demark, and W. R. Gomes, p. 101. New York: Academic Press, 1970.

Setchell, B. P. The entry of substances into the seminiferous tubules. In *Male fertility and sterility*, eds. R. E. Mancini and L. Martini, p. 37. New York: Academic Press, 1974.

Setchell, B. P., R. V. Davies, and S. J. Main. Inhibin. In *The testis*, Vol. 4, eds. A. D. Johnson, W. R. Gomes, and N. L. Van Demark. New York: Academic Press, 1976.

Setchell, B. P., B. T. Hinton, F. Jacks, and R. V. Davies. The restricted penetration of iodinated rat FSH and LH into the seminiferous tubules of the rat testis. Med. Cell. Endocrinol. 6:59.

Setchell, B. P., and S. J. Main. Inhibin. Biobliog. Reprod. 24:245, 361, 1974.

Setchell, B. P., and S. J. Main. The blood-testis barrier and steroids. In *Hormonal regulation of spermatogenesis*, eds. F. S. French et al. New York: Plenum Press, 1975.

Setchell, B. P., T. W. Scott, J. K. Voglmayr, and G. M. H. Waites. Characteristics of testicular spermatozoa and the fluid which transports them into the epididymis. Biol. Reprod. Suppl. 1:40, 1969.

Setchell, B. P., J. K. Voglmayr, and G. M. H. Waites. A blood-testis barrier restricting passage from blood into rete testis fluid but not into lymph. J. Physiol. (London) 200:73, 1969.

Setchell, B. P., and G. M. H. Waites. The blood testis barrier. In *Handbook of Physiology*, Section 7: Endocrinology, Vol. 5: *Male reproductive system*, eds. D. W. Hamilton and R. O. Greep, p. 143. Baltimore: Williams & Wilkins, 1975.

Tindall, D. J., R. Vitale, and A. R. Means. Androgen binding protein as a biochemical marker of formation of the blood-testis barrier. Endocrinology 97:636, 1975.

Tuck, R. R., B. P. Setchell, G. M. H. Waites, and J. A. Young. The composition of fluid collected by micropuncture and catheterization from the seminiferous tubules and rete testis of rats. Pfluegers Arch. Ges. Physiol. 318:225, 1970.

Vitale, R., D. W. Fawcett, and M. Dym. The normal development of the blood-testis barrier and the effects of clomiphene and estrogen treatment. Anat. Rec. 176:333, 1973.

Voglmayr, J. K. Metabolic changes in spermatozoa during epididymal transit. In *Handbook of physiology*, Section 7: Endocrinology, Vol. 5: *Male reproductive system*, eds. D. W. Hamilton and R. O. Greep, p. 437. Baltimore: Williams & Wilkins, 1975.

Waites, G. M. H., A. R. Jones, S. J. Main, and T. G. Cooper. The entry of anti-fertility and other compounds into the testis. Adv. Biosci. 10:101, 1973.

Waites, G. M. H., and B. P. Setchell. Changes in blood flow and vascular permeability of the testis, epididymis and accessory reproductive organs of the rat after the administration of cadmium chloride. J. Endocrinol. 32:329, 1966.

Willson, J. T., N. A. Jones, S. Katsch, and S. W. Smith. Penetration of the testicular-tubular barrier by horse radish peroxidase induced by adjuvant. Anat. Rec. 176:85, 1973.

31 The Structure of the Spermatozoon

Don W. Fawcett

31.1 Introduction

Three hundred years have passed since the discovery of the spermatozoon (1677), and thus it is timely to review what we know of the structure of this fascinating cell. The pace of accumulation of this knowledge provides a good example of the slow beginnings of science and the rapid recent acceleration in the rate of discovery, due mainly to advances in instrumentation. Using a microscope with a highly convex lens, von Leeuwenhoek was able to observe the general form of spermatozoa and the character of their swimming movements well enough to write a description that would be difficult to improve upon today:

Their bodies were rounded, but blunt in front and running to a point behind, and furnished with a long thin tail about five or six times as long as the body, and very transparent, and with a thickness about one twenty-fifth that of the body . . . [they] moved forward with a snake-like motion of the tail, as eels do when swimming in water. (27)

The introduction of the compound microscope and the progressive improvement of its resolving power sharpened the images of the surface contours of the spermatozoon but contributed little to our understanding of its internal structure. Indeed, most of what was observed from 1677 to 1950 can be displayed in a very simple drawing (Figure 31.1).

The development in the 1950s of the electron microscope and of microtomes capable of cutting ultrathin sections (4×10^{-6} in. thick) initiated an exciting and remarkably fruitful period of exploration of biological structure at magnifications up to half a million times and resolutions now down to 5 Å. The sperm tail, which previously appeared to be devoid of substructure, was soon found to have a remarkably complex internal organization (Figures 31.2–31.4). In the past decade the transmission electron microscope has provided the structural basis for a sliding filament theory of sperm motility; it has clarified the nature of the acrosome reaction and demonstrated the events of sperm penetration and gamete fusion. With the recent development of the freeze-cleaving technique it is now possible to split the sperm cell membrane (4×10^{-7} in. thick) in half and to examine regional specializations within the plane of the membrane—specializations

Reprinted with permission from *Developmental Biology* 44: 394–436, 1975.

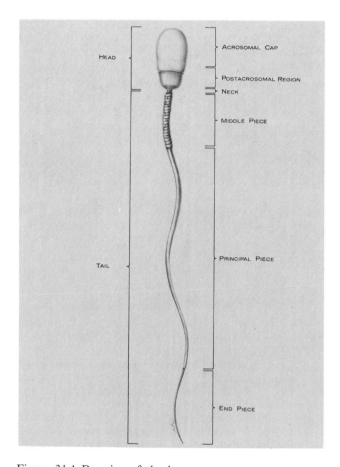

Figure 31.1 Drawing of the human spermatozoon as seen with the light microscope.

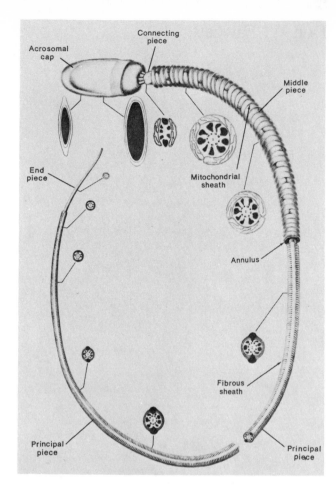

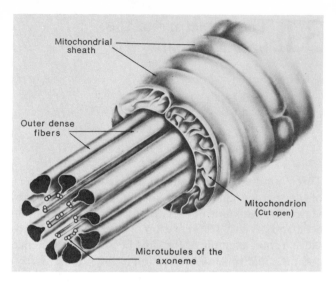

Figure 31.3 The middle piece of a typical mammalian spermatozoon, showing the close proximity of the mitochondrial sheath to the outer dense fibers and the relationship of the latter to the doublets of the axoneme.

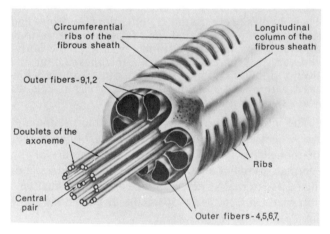

Figure 31.4 A segment from the principal piece of a spermatozoon illustrating one of the two longitudinal columns of the fibrous sheath and the associated ribs. Inward prolongation of the longitudinal columns attaching to doublets 3 and 8 divide the tail into two unequal compartments, one containing three and the other four outer fibers.

Figure 31.2 A schematic representation of a typical mammalian spermatozoon as it would appear with the cell membrane removed to reveal the underlying structural components. An acrosomal cap covers the anterior two thirds of the nucleus. The connecting piece is inserted in an implantation fossa in the posterior aspect of the nucleus.

The internal structure of the sperm flagellum is best understood from the study of cross sections at various levels. Running through the axis of the sperm tail for its entire length is the axoneme, a longitudinal bundle of microtubules similar to that found in cilia and flagella in general. Outside of the axoneme is a row of nine longitudinally oriented outer dense fibers that are not found in other flagella. Three segments of the sperm tail are defined by the nature of the sheaths that envelope the core complex of microtubules and dense fibers. The middle piece is characterized by a sheath of circumferentially oriented mitochondria. A dense annulus marks the caudal end of the middle piece. In the long principal piece, the core complex is enclosed in a fibrous sheath of circumferential dense fibers. The end piece is the portion beyond the termination of the fibrous sheath, consisting only of the axoneme. The plasma membrane invests all of the structures shown.

that may well be involved in gamete recognition and fusion, which are the essential features of fertilization.

Since it is the gamete that is transferred between the sexes, the spermatozoon is a logical target of efforts at conception control. An obvious and early approach was the interposition of mechanical barriers to sperm transfer (condom or diaphragm). The realization that successful fertilization in the mammal depends upon sperm motility made it reasonable to take advantage of their accessibility during transfer, to destroy motility by intravaginally administered surface-active or cytotoxic agents (spermicidal creams or jellies). These simple direct approaches remain the only widely used means of reversible fertility control in the male.

The development of more acceptable oral or injectable antifertility agents that will achieve a temporal separation of the contraceptive act from coitus will require a detailed understanding of the morphological and chemical basis of sperm motility, the control of spermatogenesis, the mechanism of sperm release, and the nature of sperm maturation and activation. Because research on the reproductive biology of the male has attracted less attention and support than that of the female, serious gaps remain in our knowledge—gaps that must be filled if we are to identify vulnerable steps in these processes that would lend themselves to pharmacological suppression. The simple things have already been done and further progress now becomes increasingly costly, requiring expensive instrumentation and a high degree of sophistication both in the methods employed and in the training of the scientists who will pursue these problems.

The structural analysis of the spermatozoon has probably been carried further than has that of any other differentiated cell type, yet the essential molecular mechanisms of motility, activation, zona penetration, and syngamy still elude us.

The remarkably productive decade of scientific discovery just past has not produced a safe and effective new male contraceptive, but this should not surprise or discourage either the scientists or those who support them. There have been other unexpected benefits. Studies of spermatozoa and methods for their long-term preservation have already been of inestimable value to animal breeding for the production of food and fiber for an expanding population. No less impressive have been their contributions to cell biology in general. Highly specialized though they are, spermatozoa have a number of components and properties in common with all cells. Their ready availability and their occurrence as suspensions of free-swmming cells make them ideal material for many investigations that cannot be carried out on the cells of organized tissues. The pioneering studies on nucleic acids, which were to lead to the revolutionary recent advances in molecular biology, were carried out on spermatozoa. Our present understanding of the interactions of histones with DNA is firmly based on studies of sperm nuclei. Studies of the genesis of sperm tails have clarified the role of centrioles as organizers in cell differentiation. Our knowledge of the chemistry of microtubules and of their assembly from molecular subunits is also based upon such studies. Investigations of the surface of the spermatozoon are shedding new light upon the distribution of binding sites, regional specializations, and stability of cell membranes. The basic understanding of cell organelles that has been gained from research on spermatozoa has significance for all of biology and medicine, and these returns must be taken into account in any assessment of the societal benefits of research in reproductive biology.

31.2 The Sperm Head

The Nucleus

In the development of the spermatozoon, its nucleus acquires a shape characteristic of each species. This shaping of the nucleus takes place while its chromatin is undergoing a remarkable condensation that renders it metabolically inert and highly resistant to digestion. Associated with this morphological transformation of the nucleus is a progressive stabilization of the chromatin through establishment of disulfide bonds (22, 14). This is accompanied by a progressive decrease in the binding of tritiated actinomycin D by DNA as its binding sites are obliterated by cross-linking (26).

These changes in the physical state of the chromatin have been interpreted as a stratagem of nature to protect the genome from damage on the perilous journey to the site of fertilization and to diminish nuclear volume in order to streamline the cell and facilitate motility. Light microscopists anticipated that if higher magnification could be achieved, it would be possible to see in the condensed nucleus a precise arrangement of closely packed chromosomes, but this expectation has not been borne out by electron-microscopic studies. The chromatin of the mature mammalian spermatozoon usually appears uniformly dense with no indication of chromosomal boundaries and no other resolvable organization. The homogeneous, dense chromatin is interrupted only by randomly distributed small clear areas that seem to represent random defects in the condensation process.

Polarization microscopy (59, 60) and X-ray diffraction (118) have demonstrated a highly ordered substructure in the sperm heads of invertebrates. This has fostered the belief that a comparable degree of organization probably exists in mammalian sperm nuclei but is obscured by the close packing and intense staining of condensed chromatin in electron micrographs.

Some support for this view has come from recent studies with the freeze-cleaving technique that have revealed a lamellar substructure in the nuclei of mature spermatozoa from several different species (62, 63, 46).

In the majority of species the uniformity of the spermatozoa is quite remarkable; hundreds of millions are produced each day with very little variation in head shape and with a surprisingly small percentage of developmental anomalies. Human spermatozoa are exceptional in this regard: they exhibit considerable variability in head shape and have a surprising frequency of sizable irregular cavities in the condensed chromatin. These are usually called *nuclear vacuoles*—although they are unlike other vacuoles in not being limited by a membrane. As a rule, they appear empty in electron micrographs or contain a sparse granular precipitate. They may be single or multiple, and some are large enough to distort the shape of the sperm head. Whether these anomalies of nuclear condensation have an effect upon fertilizing capacity is not known and will be difficult to ascertain without a comparable animal model.

In addition to these relatively gross defects visible at low magnification, electron micrographs disclose a marked variation in the degree of chromatin condensation. Whereas in other species this progresses to a dense homogeneous state in nearly all sperm, a significant proportion of the spermatozoa in human ejaculates have nuclei that still display the coarse granular pattern characteristic of the penultimate stage of condensation. When exposed to agents that break disulfide bonds, these nuclei decondense more rapidly than do those with dense homogeneous chromatin (15). This heterogeneity in nuclear ultrastructure in the human ejaculate suggests that the process of chromatin condensation does not proceed to completion in all members of the sperm population. Here again it is not clear whether incomplete condensation is correlated with diminished fertilizing capacity. Comparative studies suggest that this is probably not the case, for in at least one rodent species (*Citellus*) none of the sperm heads become fully condensed and there is no evidence of low fertility.

The discovery that the human Y chromosome can be selectively stained with fluorescent quinacrin dyes (86) has made it possible to identify with some confidence the male-determining spermatozoa by the presence of a brightly fluorescent spot in the nucleus (8). It was expected that selective staining of the Y chromosome would provide evidence for or against a consistent arrangement of the chromosomes within the sperm nucleus. Unfortunately it has not done so. The bright yellow spot is usually situated in the anterior half of the nucleus, but a precisely reproducible local-ization has not been demonstrated. This cannot be interpreted as conclusive evidence one way or the other, however, because a consistent pattern of chromosomal arrangement might be considerably distorted by the occurrence of intranuclear vacuoles of the kind described above. Enumeration of sperm with two fluorescent spots, in which diploidy can be ruled out by comparative measurement of DNA content, has made it possible to estimate the frequency of nondisjunction in the second meiotic division, which is the only other way in which a YY sperm can arise (33). Examination of ejaculates by this relatively new technique may yield other useful genetic information.

Acrosome

Cytologists using the light microscope were not able to clearly resolve the limits of the acrosome or membranous investments of the sperm head. The frequent artifactual loosening and separation of the plasmalemma and underlying acrosomal membrane (18) led to descriptions by light microscopists of a *galea capitis* or head cap, which they envisioned as a separate structure overlying the acrosome. The early electron-microscopic studies eliminated confusion on this point by clearly showing that the acrosome is not confined to the tip of the sperm head but is actually a membrane-limited, caplike structure closely applied to the tapering anterior portion of the nucleus (34, 36). The cell membrane directly invests it (Figure 31.5). Thus there is no structure conforming to traditional descriptions of the *galea capitis,* and this term has now been abandoned.

The outer acrosomal membrane immediately beneath the cell membrane is continuous at the posterior margin of the cap with the inner acrosomal membrane, which is closely applied to the nuclear envelope. The two acrosomal membranes run parallel throughout most of their extent and enclose a narrow cavity occupied by an acrosomal content of low electron density.

In the human spermatozoon the acrosome is relatively small and does not extend anteriorly much beyond the leading edge of the nucleus (34, 89). In many other mammalian species, however, a conspicuous thickening of the acrosomal cap extends anteriorly well beyond the nucleus. This region, designated the *apical segment* of the acrosome, often has a shape characteristic of the species (36). The part of the cap that extends back over the anterior portion of the nucleus is referred to as the *principal segment*. A narrower caudal portion of the cap is called the *equatorial segment* (78, 36). In the human spermatozoon a linear differentiation within this segment gives its limiting membrane a pentalaminar appearance (89). In freeze-cleaving preparations of guinea pig spermatozoa a differentiation of the content of the equatorial segment

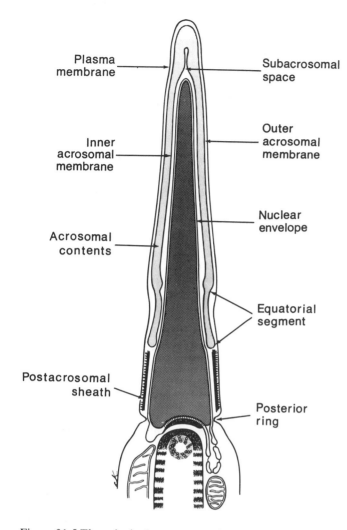

Plasma membrane

Inner acrosomal membrane

Acrosomal contents

Postacrosomal sheath

Subacrosomal space

Outer acrosomal membrane

Nuclear envelope

Equatorial segment

Posterior ring

Figure 31.5 The principal components in a sagittal section of a primate sperm head. The posterior ring marks the junction of the head and neck. The fusion of the cell membrane with the underlying nuclear envelope in this circumferential groove isolates the interstitial spaces of the head from the remainder of the sperm.

results in a palisade formation of parallel ridges running obliquely forward from the caudal margin of the cap (46). No functional significance has been assigned to these structural details, but interest in this region runs high because its fate during fertilization is different from that of the other segments of the acrosome. It persists after the more anterior regions have been lost in the acrosome reaction (13, 123).

Cytochemical studies of the acrosome have shown its contents to be rich in carbohydrate (65), and chemical analyses have established the presence of galactose, mannose, fucose, galactosamine, glucosamine, and sialic acid (24, 57). In earlier electron-microscopic studies the acrosomal contents were described as homogeneous, but later studies have consistently identified areas of differing density (35, 37, 42). These are most evident in the apical segment and especially after glycolmethacrylate-embedding (42). There is often a pale outer zone around an inner zone of greater density. In the rabbit spermatozoon, discrete dense bodies with ill-defined boundaries are described in this region of the acrosome. In electron micrographs these exhibit a fine periodic structure interpreted as a crystal lattice (42). In the rat a highly ordered substructure with a periodicity of 42 Å has also been observed in a cortical zone on the convex portion of the curved acrosome (93), and a similar periodicity has been described in the acrosome of the human sperm (87, 88, 89).

In the presence of a recently ovulated egg, capacitated sperm undergo the acrosome reaction (9, 45, 123). The outer membrane over the apical and principal segments of the acrosome fuses at multiple sites with the overlying cell membrane, creating openings through which the enzyme-rich contents of the acrosome are released (Figure 31.6). This process of membrane fusion and vesiculation progresses until the major part of the outer acrosomal membrane and the overlying cell membrane are lost, leaving the anterior half of the sperm head invested only by the inner acrosomal membrane (9, 12, 13). The equatorial segment does not seem to participate in the acrosome reaction but remains intact. The free edge of its outer membrane left by dissolution of the anterior regions of the acrosome becomes continuous with the margin of the cell membrane interrupted in the same process.

Penetration of the egg envelope was originally attributed to a mechanical function of the acrosome, but some 30 years ago the localization of hyaluronidase activity in this portion of the spermatozoon directed attention to the probable role of lytic enzymes (99, 5). This interpretation has gained general acceptance in the period of heightened interest in hydrolytic enzymes that followed the identification of lysosomes as cell organelles of widespread occurrence. Several acid hydrolases have since been identified in acrosomes,

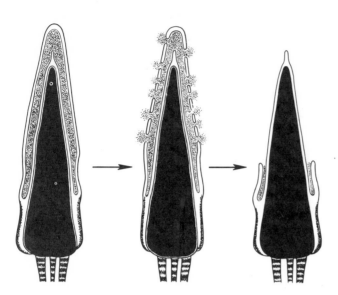

Figure 31.6 Schematic representation of the mammalian acrosome reaction. The outer acrosomal membrane fuses with the plasma membrane at multiple sites creating openings through which the enzyme-rich contents of the acrosome escape. This process leads ultimately to complete loss of the cell membrane over the anterior half of the head. The limiting membrane of the sperm head in this region is the inner acrosomal membrane. The equatorial segment of the acrosome persists. Its function is still poorly understood.

including acid phosphatase, β glucuronidase, n-acetylglucosaminidase (28, 3), and a trypsinlike protease, acrosin (110, 106, 109, 128). These findings have led to a concept of the acrosome as a highly specialized lysosome and to the suggestion that sperm penetration might be prevented by stabilization of the acrosomal membrane to prevent release of its hydrolytic enzymes or by development of specific inhibitors or antibodies that would inactivate its enzymes (108).

The release of enzymes during the acrosome reaction is believed to disperse the cells of the cumulus oophorus and facilitate access of the sperm head to the zona pellucida. A puzzling aspect of the problem, however, is the fact that virtually all of the acrosomal contents are released during this early stage of fertilization, leaving behind little or no acrosomal substance for dissolution of the thick zona pellucida, which would seem to be the principal barrier to sperm penetration. Since the equatorial segment is still present on spermatozoa in the perivitelline space and is apparently unchanged, it has been concluded that if acrosomal proteases are involved in penetration of the zona, they must reside in the inner acrosomal membrane. Some information exists on localization of enzymes within the acrosome. The observation that in traversing the zona, the sperm cuts only a narrow path, no larger than the greatest diameter of the head (29), seems consistent with the interpretation that the enzyme involved is bound to the inner membrane. Evidence favoring this interpretation has also been adduced from selective binding of fluorescein-labeled trypsin inhibitors to this membrane (110); from localization of antibody against acrosin on this membrane (73); and from biochemical detection of enzymatic activity on sperm experimentally denuded of the outer acrosomal membrane and acrosomal contents (20).

Nevertheless, some investigators studying sperm penetration with the electron microscope find it difficult to reconcile the idea of a purely enzymatic mechanism with the narrowness of the opening in the zona and the sharpness of the discontinuity in density along the edge of the path made by the sperm head, and they entertain the possibility that the firm wedge-shaped sperm nucleus advanced by vigorous motility may also play a significant mechanical role. The participation of the equatorial segment of the acrosome has not been ruled out, but it is unlikely since it appears to undergo no loss of substance or other morphological change in the process of sperm penetration. It has also been suggested that the equatorial segment may be involved later in sperm-egg fusion, but at present this is purely conjectural.

The interpretation of the acrosome as a lysosome seemed to raise serious doubts as to the feasibility of fertility control through inhibition or immunosuppression of its enzymes, for the reason that lysosomes are so widespread in the body and so essential to normal physiological processes that a general inhibition of their hydrolases might have far-reaching and intolerable effects outside of the reproductive system. Recent studies have demonstrated, however, that acrosomal hyaluronidase is a sperm-specific isoenzyme distinct from lysosomal hyaluronidase (127), and inhibition of hyaluronidase by antibody has been shown to be highly species-specific and tissue-specific and capable of inhibiting fertilization in vitro (71). These evidences of specificity keep alive the possibility of fertility control by enzyme inhibitors or isoimmunization.

Between the apical segment of the acrosome and the tip of the nucleus is a subacrosomal space (Figure 31.5), which in most mammalian species is quite small and generally devoid of contents after preparation for electron microscopy. In spermatozoa of rats and mice this space is more capacious and is occupied by a moderately dense, resistant structure that is often called the *perforatorium*. This is an unfortunate term in that it implies an undemonstrated mechanical function. The perforatorium of rat spermatozoa has been isolated and its protein composition determined. It is composed of a single polypeptide with a molecular weight of 13,000 (83).

The Postacrosomal Region and the Nuclear Envelope

Much interest has been centered in the region of the sperm head behind the posterior margin of the acrosome, for it is in this region that attachment and fusion of the sperm and egg membranes takes place (10, 111, 123, 124). In electron micrographs of thin sections the plasma membrane of this region has the usual trilaminar appearance, but it is underlain by a thin dense layer called the *postacrosomal dense lamina* or the *postacrosomal sheath* (36, 38). This corresponds to the structure formerly called the *postnuclear cap*. It courses parallel to the membrane at a distance of 150 to 200 Å, and regular periodic densities about 120 Å apart project from its outer aspect to the inner surface of the cell membrane (36, 38). Tangential sections indicate that these densities are cross-sectional profiles of circumferentially oriented parallel ridges on the postacrosomal sheath (89). A narrow clear space between the sheath and the nucleus is closed behind by the *posterior ring*, a narrow circumferential band of fusion of the plasmalemma to the underlying nuclear envelope (120, 88, 46).

The nuclear envelope of the mature sperm head is exceptional in several respects. Its entire area under the acrosomal cap and in the postacrosomal region is devoid of nuclear pores, and the two membranes of the envelope are separated by only 70–100 Å. Behind the posterior ring, however, the two membranes diverge to the usual 400–600 Å distance. Diverging from the surface of the condensed chromatin, the nuclear envelope forms a fold that extends for a variable distance back into the neck region (44). In contrast to the rest of the nuclear envelope, this redundant portion behind the posterior ring has a large number of typical nuclear pores in close hexagonal array. These are seen to best advantage after the freeze-cleaving technique. The area bounded by this fold of the nuclear envelope has been designated the *posterior nuclear space*. It is usually devoid of chromatin and appears empty in electron micrographs.

The recurrent limb of the neck fold again comes into contact with the condensed chromatin on the posterior surface of the nucleus. There again the pores are absent and the membranes are in close apposition. This portion of the nuclear envelope lines the implantation fossa, the site of attachment of the tail to the head (Figures 31.5, 31.7). Within the implantation fossa the narrow interspace (60–70 Å) between the two nuclear membranes is transversed by regular periodic densities about 60 Å wide and 60 Å apart (Figure 31.8). This periodic structure is seen only in favorably oriented

thin sections, and it may not extend over the entire area of head-to-tail attachment. Freeze-fracturing reveals that the portion of the nuclear envelope lining the implantation fossa is highly specialized within the plane of the membranes (46). A particle-free, relatively smooth region of membrane is found in the central portion of the fossa, but on either side of this featureless area is a very dense population of relatively large (15nm) intramembranous particles spaced about 20 nm apart (Figures 31.9, 31.10). These particles may be shared by both of the closely applied membranes, and they may correspond to the periodic densities observed traversing in the interspace between the membranes in thin sections. This region of the nuclear envelope is covered on its outer surface by a thick layer of very dense material, the basal plate, which lines the fossa and provides attachment for a large number of fine filaments that extend into it from the articular surface of the connecting piece (Figure 31.7).

31.3 The Sperm Tail

The principal structural components of the sperm tail were described soon after the introduction of the electron microscope some 20 years ago (Figures 31.2 –31.4), and the research of the past decade has been devoted to details of their ultrastructure and to their chemical dissection in an effort to discover the mechanism for generation of bending waves and their propagation along the tail. Since there is no fertility without sperm motility, the mechanism of sperm propulsion continues to be a subject of potential importance for population control.

The Connecting Piece

Immediately behind the sperm head is the connecting piece. This complex structure has a dense, convex articular region called the *capitulum,* which conforms to the concavity of the implantation fossa in the nucleus (Figures 31.7, 31.11, 31.12). Fine filaments traversing the narrow, electron-lucent space between the capitulum and the basal plate appear to be the structures mainly responsible for attachment of the head to the tail. These filaments are probably dissolved by reagents that separate the tails from heads (30). Extending backward from the capitulum are nine segmented columns one or two microns in length. At their caudal end these overlap the tapering anterior ends of the nine dense fibers of the flagellum, to which they are firmly united (Figure 31.7). The columns of the connecting piece therefore appear to be continuous with the outer dense fibers, but the two are of different origin (39), and a careful examination of the region at high magnification reveals an oblique line along which they have fused secondarily. In longitudinal sections the col-

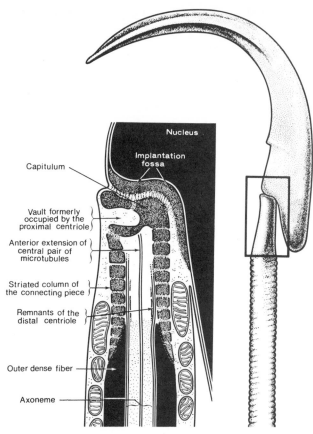

Figure 31.7 Drawing of a rat sperm head. At left is a diagram of the structures of the neck region (enclosed in the rectangle on the right-hand figure) as it would appear at higher magnification in an electron micrograph. The relationship of the connecting piece to the implantation fossa and to the outer fibers of the tail are shown, as well as the absena, in this species, of both centrioles. The main features of the diagram apply to all mammalian sperm, but in most species a proximal centriole is retained in a niche beneath the capitulum. From (120).

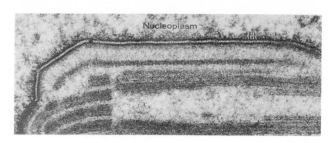

Figure 31.8 Electron micrograph of a thin section through the implantation fossa of a late Chinese hamster spermatid, showing the close apposition of the membranes of the nuclear envelope and the periodic densities that traverse the narrow cleft between them (see at arrows). From (37).

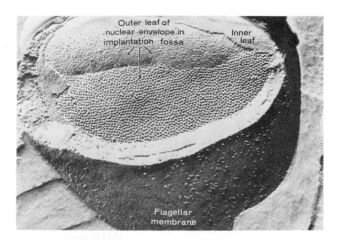

Figure 31.9 Freeze-cleaving preparation of rat sperm in which the fracture line has passed obliquely across the base of the flagellum. It illustrates a particle-poor area in the center of the implantation fossa, surrounded by an area of closely packed particles. The relation of these particles to the periodic densities seen between the leaves of the nuclear envelope in thin sections (see Figure 31.8) is not clear. From (45).

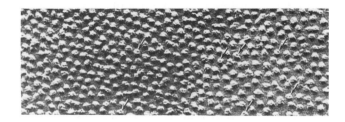

Figure 31.10 Higher magnification of the intramembranous particles in the nuclear envelope lining the implantation fossa. Some of the particles appear to have a central hole or pore (at arrows).

umns of the connecting piece seem to be composed of dense segments alternating with narrower light bands. The light bands are bisected by a very thin intermediate line. In favorable thin sections 11 fine transverse striations can be resolved within each dark segment. The chemical nature of the cross-banded columns of the connecting piece has not been established, but they are believed to be analogous to the cross-striated rootlets associated with the basal bodies of epithelial cilia.

A transverse or obliquely oriented proximal centriole usually occupies a niche or vault in the dense substance of the connecting piece (Figures 31.11, 31.12). During tail development there is also a distal centriole at the base of the axoneme, oriented approximately at a right angle to the proximal centriole. Concurrently with the development of the connecting piece the distal centriole disintegrates, but remnants of its nine triplets may be found in mature sperm adhering to the inner aspect of some of the nine segmented columns (39). Late in development the central pair of microtubules of the axoneme usually extend through the interior of the connecting piece as far anteriorly as the proximal centriole (128).

The neck region is usually quite slender and devoid of organelles except for the fold or scroll of redundant nuclear envelope and one or two longitudinally oriented mitochondria that project forward from the mitochondrial sheath of the midpiece. The neck of the human sperm is somewhat atypical in that it is very of-

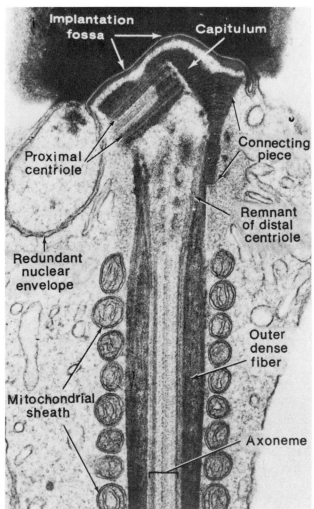

Figure 31.12 Neck region of a nearly mature boar spermatozoon from the testis showing the persistence of the proximal centriole in a niche within the connecting piece. The centriolar adjunct has disappeared, and only traces of the distal centriole remain. The axoneme of the sperm flagellum thus has no basal body comparable to those of cilia.

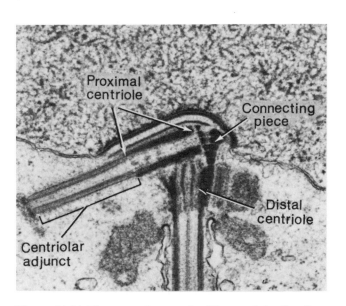

Figure 31.11 Electron micrograph of base of the flagellum and adjacent nucleus in a spermatid illustrating the presence of both proximal and distal centrioles. The proximal centriole at this stage has a prolongation called the centriolar adjunct. The distal centriole is beginning to disintegrate concurrently with formation of the connecting piece. From (37).

361   Structure of the Spermatozoon

ten surrounded by a rather large fusiform mass of residual cytoplasm that may extend forward around the base of the sperm head as far as the posterior ring.

Ultrastructural studies of the neck region of the spermatozoon have overturned two strongly held beliefs of classical cytologists. One of these was that all motile flagella must have a centriole or basal body to serve as a kinetic center and site of origin of the beat. It is now evident that a centriole is necessary as an organizing center or template during formation of the axoneme, but once the flagellum is formed it is not needed for the initiation or propagation of bending waves along the tail (122). This conclusion from morphological observations is borne out by the experimental demonstration that segments of sperm tails dissected away from the head and neck possess the ability to initiate and coordinate waves in the absence of a centriole (69).

The second time-honored belief was that the contribution of a centriole by the spermatozoon was necessary for formation of the first cleavage spindle and initiation of development. Although the proximal centriole does enter the egg with the sperm in most mammalian species, it has been found that neither centriole is present in the mature sperm in the rat (122). Thus it seems that the proximal centriole is not essential for fertilization and cleavage.

The Axoneme

The motor apparatus of the sperm tail is the *axoneme* or axial filament complex. It consists of two central microtubules surrounded by a row of nine evenly spaced doublet microtubules (Figure 31.13), and this 9 + 2 pattern is found in cilia and flagella throughout the plant and animal kingdoms. Rapid advances have been made recently in our understanding of its chemical nature and mode of assembly, and we may soon be able to interpret the mechanism of flagellar motion.

The doublets consist of two subunits: subfiber A, which is a complete microtubule, circular in cross section and about 26 nm in diameter; and subfiber B, which is C-shaped in section with its ends attached to the wall of subfiber A. The cylindrical wall of subfiber A is made up of 13 straight protofilaments 3.5 nm in diameter, each composed of 80 Å dimers of the protein tubulin. These dimers are associated end-to-end (56, 4), and those of adjacent protofilaments are believed to be in staggered array. Subfiber B is composed of similar dimeric units of tubulin in about 10 protofilaments (116, 117). In cross sections subfiber A is seen to provide attachment for two diverging arms that project toward the next doublet in the row (1). The arms consist mainly of dynein, a protein with ATPase activity (49, 50, 51). Also attached to each subfiber A are two slender nexin links that connect it to the adjacent doublets

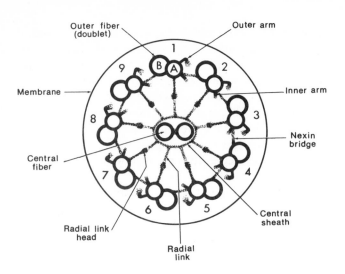

Figure 31.13 Schematic representation of the current interpretation of the organization of the axoneme of cilia and flagella. Based upon work of Linck, Stephens, Satir, Warner, and others.

(113) and a radial spoke that joins it to a helical sheath around the central pair of microtubules. The arms of the doublets are spaced at regular intervals of 240 Å along subfiber A (23, 66, 67), and the radial spokes, studied by negative staining of dissociated axonemes, are grouped into pairs or triplets (58, 117, 100). The members of the central pair of microtubules in the 9 + 2 are each composed of 13 protofilaments, like subfiber A of the doublets. The two central tubules are joined along their length by regularly spaced bridges about 135 Å apart (87, 88, 89), and they are enclosed in a sheath, said by some to be formed of a helically wound 60 Å filament (Figure 31.14).

The tubulin that is the principal structural protein of the flagellar microtubules is probably nearly identical to that of microtubules found in the spindle apparatus of dividing cells and in the interphase cytoplasm of cells generally. It occurs as a dimer with a molecular weight of about 110,000, made up of subunits of molecular weight 55,000 (96), each of which has one molecule of guanine nucleotide associated with it. The dimer of tubulin has the property of binding one molecule of the alkaloid colchicine (104). Advantage is taken of this affinity in the isolation of tubulin. Two fractions of tubulin can be distinguished electrophoretically—tubulin α and tubulin β. The dimers in the doublets probably have one subunit of each. Evidence is accumulating to suggest additional heterogeneity of tubulins in that the A and B subfibers of flagellar doublets and their subunits have different solubility properties (16, 66, 112). Heating doublets at 37°C results in selective solubilization of the B subfiber or tubule. After treatment with Sarkosyl the walls of the tubules

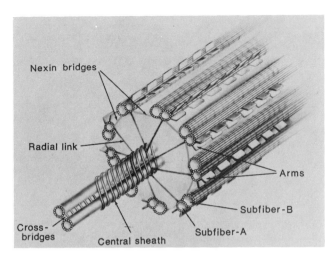

Figure 31.14 Highly schematic three-dimensional reconstruction of the axoneme and its associated structures. There is no basis for depicting the arms as rectangular; it simply indicates that they are periodic and not continuous along the doublets. The details of the attachments of the nexin bridges and radial links remain to be worked out.

are solubilized except for a more stable unit consisting of three protofilaments (119, 72). This was considered to be the segment comprising the wall between the tubules of the doublet, but this interpretation has now been challenged (68). Doublet tubule preparations contain at least nine minor protein components accounting for 25 to 35 percent of the total protein (68). Some of these may be involved in attachment of the B to the A subfiber or in the attachment of the arms, radial spokes, or nexin links. It is not clear whether these proteins reside in specific protofilaments or in the associated layer of material that is stained after fixation in solutions containing tannic acid.

The flagellar protein principally concerned with converting chemical energy into mechanical movement is dynein, a large molecule with a molecular weight of about 500,000, possessing ATPase activity. As in the case of tubulin, it is heterogeneous and can be separated electrophoretically into A_1, A_2, and B fractions (50). The A fractions, comprising two-thirds of the total, are located in the arms on the doublets; the location of the B fraction is still unclear.

In the reductionist approach to biology it is always gratifying, after one has "taken the alarm clock apart," to be able to begin putting it back together. Conditions have now been defined under which tubulin in solution can be repolymerized into microtubules in vitro (81). Also, after dynein has been extracted from flagella, subsequent electron micrographs show that the arms have been removed from the doublets, and when extracted axonemes are then exposed to so-

lutions of dynein under the appropriate conditions, the arms are restored to the doublets (48, 51).

The details of the mechanism by which the 9 + 2 complex of microtubules produce flagellar movement still elude us, but a satisfactory explanation is probably not far off. It is generally agreed that microtubules are incapable of shortening to produce bending. The most reasonable alternative is for localized sliding to take place between neighboring doublets. In favor of this is the morphological observation that the length of the doublets remains constant during bending (101). Compelling experimental evidence for sliding has now been adduced. When ATP is added to segments of demembranated flagella that have also been subjected to mild trypsin treatment, doublets move out opposite ends of the axoneme, thus providing direct evidence of sliding (114). Therefore it is now widely accepted that flagellar movement involves a sliding tubule mechanism analogous to the sliding filament mechanism of skeletal muscle. How the arms on one doublet interact with the neighboring doublet to generate the local shearing movements remains to be worked out, as well as the mechanism responsible for propagation of the bending wave along the tail.

That these details of axonemal structure are not solely of theoretical interest is apparent from the recent reports (90, 2) of certain infertile humans with adequate numbers of sperm that appear normal by light microscopy but have no motility. When examined by electron microscopy the axonemes were found to lack arms on the doublets, suggesting a genetic inability to synthesize the dynein necessary to convert the chemical energy of ATP to mechanical movement.

Outer Dense Fibers

An understanding of the motor mechanism for the simple flagella of invertebrate sperm does not seem far beyond our reach, but the problem is made more complex by additional fibrous components and circumferential sheaths of the mammalian sperm tail that seem to impose restraints to bending and to the sliding of the axonemal fibers. For a major part of the length of the mammalian sperm tail, the axoneme is surrounded by nine outer dense fibers, thus creating a 9 + 9 + 2 cross-sectional pattern (Figures 31.3, 31.15). Each dense fiber is continuous anteriorly with one of the segmented columns of the connecting piece and courses longitudinally just peripheral to each of nine doublets of the axoneme. Unlike the doublet microtubules, which all appear identical, the nine associated dense fibers differ from one another in size and cross-sectional shape. Fibers 1, 5, and 6 are usually distinctly larger than the others, and their cross-sectional configuration may be highly characteristic of a given species. There are also marked interspecies differences in the prominence of the outer fibers. In some species the outer fibers are very thick and extend the full length of the principal piece, while in others they are relatively thin and terminate in the anterior half of this segment. Near their termination each fiber appears to be fixed to the wall of the corresponding doublet. Herein lies one of the serious problems of explaining mammalian sperm tail motility by a sliding mechanism. The outer fibers are fixed to the nucleus anteriorly via the connecting piece and are attached to the doublets of the axoneme at their caudal end. This would seem to impose a serious restraint to sliding of axonemal components, unless they are either contractile or freely distensible.

The dense fibers have a thick medulla and a thin cortical layer, which is continuous over the abaxial surface but is usually absent on the side nearer the axoneme (Figures 31.15, 31.16). The cortex stains heavily with phosphotungstic acid (55). Surface replicas of outer dense fibers exhibit an oblique striation in the cortex, which appears to be composed of globular subunits (121, 82). In very thin longitudinal sections, a very fine 40–50 Å periodicity is sometimes detectable in the medulla (89).

The sperm of primitive aquatic animals have only a simple 9 + 2 flagellum and a single ring of mitochondria. The appearance of the outer fibers during phylogeny seems to have coincided with the development of internal fertilization. Associated with their develop-

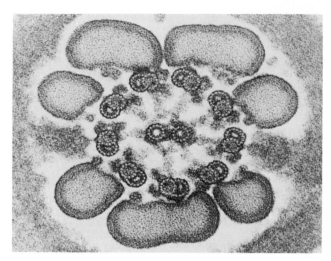

Figure 31.16 Axoneme and associated fibers in the principal piece of a spermatozoon after fixation in glutaraldehyde containing tannic acid. After this treatment the protofibrils in the walls of the central microtubule and the doublets are visible in negative image. The cortex and medulla of the outer fibers are also clearly differentiated. Electron micrograph courtesy of D. Phillips.

ment was a great increase in the number of mitochondria. These observations led to the speculation that the outer fibers were accessory motor elements evolved to overcome the greater resistance to locomotion in the female reproductive tract (36, 38). The concurrent development of a long mitochondrial sheath closely applied to the outer dense fibers has been interpreted as an adaptation to provide the necessary energy for contraction of the outer fibers. Consistent with the belief that these fibers were contractile was the observation that the asymmetry in their size and position seemed to correlate with observed directional differences in the speed and force of tail bending. Moreover, immunohistochemical studies were reported suggesting that the outer fibers possessed both ATPase activity (74) and antigenic similarities to actomyosin (75, 76). These observations further strengthened the belief that the outer fibers were contractile, but the validity of this conclusion is now seriously questioned as a result of recent chemical analyses of isolated outer fibers (97, 98, 7).

The outer fibers are resistant to solubilization by any of the methods commonly used for extraction of contractile proteins, but they can be put into solution by treatment with dithiothreitol and sodium dodecyl sulfate. Upon electrophoresis of outer fibers from rat sperm, four bands are detected, corresponding to polypeptides of molecular weights 40,000, 25,000, 12,000, and 11,000, with the 25,000 MW polypeptide accounting for 58 percent of the total (98). Similar studies on bull sperm from another laboratory yielded

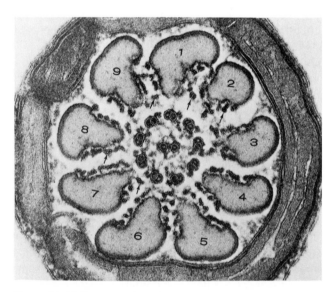

Figure 31.15 Cross section of the middle piece of a guinea pig spermatozoon after tannic acid fixation. The cortex of the outer dense fibers is heavily stained as well as numerous satellite fibrils (at arrows) around the adaxial surfaces of the dense fibers. These structures are found in many mammalian species, but their chemical nature and functional significance remain unknown. Micrograph courtesy of D. Friend.

somewhat different results, with three major bands corresponding to molecular weights of 55,000, 30,000, and 15,000, of which the 30,000 MW polypeptide was the most abundant (7). Amino acid analysis in both studies revealed a high content of cysteine. A surprising finding was the appreciable content of bound triglyceride (103 μg/mg protein). The reports are in disagreement concerning carbohydrates, with one recording (7) and the other denying (98) their presence in the fiber cortex. There is agreement on the absence of ATPase activity (95, 7, 98). The absence of phosphorus would also seem to indicate that energy-yielding nucleotides are not a part of these fibers.

The main thrust of these biochemical studies seems to suggest little chemical resemblance between the outer dense fibers and any known contractile proteins. Therefore it now seems somewhat unlikely that they are active motor elements. Being proteins that are stabilized by abundant disulfide cross-linking, they probably have significant passive elastic properties. Comparative cinematographic studies of sperm motility suggest that sperm tails of the species that have larger outer fibers are stiffer and have bending waves of lower amplitude than those with smaller outer fibers (92).

Mitochondrial Sheath

The mitochondrial sheath of the middle piece is believed to generate the energy for sperm locomotion. Its topographical relationships would suggest that the mitochondria might be especially important as an energy source for the outer fibers. But if these are not contractile, as the biochemical evidence now suggests, then the functional significance of the long mitochondrial sheath of mammalian sperm is far from clear; a very few mitochondria are needed for simple 9 + 2 flagella.

There is wide variation among mammals in the extent of the middle piece. It may be quite short, comprising as few as 15 gyres of mitochondria in man or as many as 300 in some rodents. If one accepts that the conditions encountered by spermatozoa in the female reproductive tract do not vary greatly from species to species and that the investments of the egg are very similar in most species, then there is no satisfactory explanation for the broad variation observed in the extent of the energy-generating apparatus.

In general the middle piece is invested by mitochondria arranged end-to-end to form a tight helix around the longitudinal fibrous elements of the tail. The end-on junctions of the mitochondria usually occur at random along the course of the helix, but in some species there is a remarkable regularity in their disposition. These examples of specific arrangement and precise order present fascinating problems of morphogenesis and pose challenging questions concerning the factors that control the assembly of the mitochondrial sheath. In some *Chiroptera* (*Myotis*) there are two mitochondria of identical size in each turn of the sheath, and their ends always meet on the plane passing through the central pair of microtubules in the axoneme (38). Therefore the end-to-end junctions of mitochondria in successive turns are aligned in register along the dorsal and ventral aspects of the midpiece for its entire length. In some rodents there are two mitochondria in each ring, but their end-to-end contacts in successive turns are offset by 90 degrees so that in surface replicas, the junctions in every other turn are aligned. A similar staggered arrangement is seen in successive rings of four mitochondria in the sperm of certain marsupials (*Didelphys* or *Caluromys*). This represents a rotation of 45 degrees from row to row. To maintain the precise alignment of junctions over the whole length of the midpiece in these species, the mitochondria must be nearly identical in size. Such uniformity in dimensions of this organelle in other cell types is rare, and there is no ready explanation as to how it is achieved in spermatid differentiation. Nor is it obvious what advantage for motility would be conferred by such a high degree of order and symmetry in the mitochondrial sheath.

The internal structure of mitochondria in the sperm midpiece usually does not differ significantly from that of mitochondria in other cell types, but there are exceptions. In marsupials there are remarkable concentric systems of membranes that fill the interior of the mitochondria (36, 91), and in at least one desert rodent a granular material of unknown nature accumulates in the space between the inner and outer membranes on the abaxial side of each mitochondrion in the midpiece (94).

The Fibrous Sheath

The fibrous sheath of the principal piece is a structural component peculiar to mammalian spermatozoa; it begins immediately posterior to the annulus, which marks the caudal limit of the midpiece. It consists of a series of circumferentially oriented ribs that pass halfway around the tail and terminate in two longitudinal columns, which run along opposite sites of the tail for its entire length (Figure 31.4). The closely spaced ribs of the sheath occasionally branch and anastomose with neighboring ribs. The columns consist of longitudinally oriented filamentous subunits that appear, in transverse section, as punctate densities. The ribs also exhibit a filamentous substructure, but its subunits are thinner than those of the longitudinal columns. In its initial portion the sheath is fixed to outer dense fibers 3 and 8. These fibers, which are approximately in the plane of the central pair of axonemal tubules, then terminate abruptly, leaving the other seven fibers to continue through the principal piece. Posterior to the termination of fibers 3 and 8, the adaxial side of the longitudinal columns tapers to a thin edge, which extends inward and appears to attach to a small ridge projecting from the wall of the doublets 3 and 8 (Figures 31.4, 31.16). As the sperm tail tapers along its length, the longitudinal columns become smaller and the ribs become thinner. Several microns from the tip of the tail, the fibrous sheath ends abruptly, marking the junction of the principal and end pieces. The longitudinal columns may continue a short distance into the end piece as ill-defined densities between axonemal doublets 3 and 8 and the flagellar membrane.

The attachment of doublets 3 and 8 of the axoneme to the longitudinal columns of the fibrous sheath would seem to prevent their participation in the sliding movements that are believed to be responsible for flagellar bending. The thick longitudinal columns of the sheath would also seem to impose considerable mechanical restraint upon bending in the plane of the central pair. But there should be little restraint to bending perpendicular to this plane, because it would only involve lateral bending of the columns and a widening or narrowing of the interspaces between successive ribs of the sheath. It remains paradoxical that these morphological considerations suggest specialization of the mammalian sperm tail for two-dimensional bending movements in the plane perpendicular to the central pair of microtubules, while cinematographic studies seem to demonstrate that the propagated waves are three-dimensional in the distal part of the tail.

The basic organization of the fibrous sheath is similar in all mammals, but there are variations in the size and shape of the columns and in the frequency of anastomosis of the ribs. In sperm of some rodents the ends of the ribs are bifid, so that a light interspace is visible between the longitudinal columns and the diverging heads of the ribs. In marsupials the ribs of the fibrous sheath are hollow near their ends, and therefore in parasagittal sections they often present open rectangular profiles.

The fibrous sheath has now been isolated in bulk from rat spermatozoa and characterized chemically. It consists predominantly of a single polypeptide with a molecular weight of 80,000 (84). One of the obstacles to an immunological approach to fertility control in the male has been the paucity of antigens specific for sperm. Clearly antibody to tubulin would have far-reaching undesirable effects upon cilia and flagella throughout the body. On the other hand, the proteins of the outer fibers and the fibrous sheath may prove to be unique to spermatozoa. If this is true, these antigenic proteins might be used as the basis for selective immunosuppression of spermatogenesis or sperm motility.

31.4 The Surface of the Spermatozoon

The plasma membrane of the spermatozoon is of primary importance for sperm-egg interaction and for the maintenance of sperm motility. It is to be expected therefore that application of specific agglutinins, freeze-fracture electron microscopy, and other modern methods of the membrane biologist will yield information about the internal organization and surface properties of the sperm membrane that may provide a basis for contraceptive development. There are few cell types in which regional specializations of the surface for particular functions are as sharply defined or as well known as they are for the spermatozoon. Its anterior region is concerned with secretion of acrosomal enzymes, the postacrosomal region is specialized for recognition and attachment to the egg, and the membrane of the tail is necessary for maintenance of motility. Spermatozoa are free-swimming, individual cells whose entire surface is accessible without applying dissociation procedures that might alter membrane properties. Their motility is a convenient visual indicator of viability. They thus provide the cell biologist with exceptionally favorable material for the correlation of particular patterns of membrane organization with specific functions.

Among the first explorations of the properties of the sperm surface were studies in which immobilized bull and rabbit spermatozoa placed in an electrophoretic field were observed to migrate toward the anode with their tails foremost, thus suggesting that the cells have a net negative charge on their surface, with the tail more strongly charged than the head (77). It was subsequently shown that the electrophoretic properties of rabbit spermatozoa change as they mature, becoming more negative as they pass through the epididymis (11).

In recent years there has been a recrudescence of interest in the surface charge on sperm and particularly in morphological methods for its visual demonstration. In electron micrographs of thin sections of spermatozoa, the plasmalemma has the usual trilaminar unit-membrane structure and there are no readily discernible regional differences in its appearance. By means of various cytochemical techniques, however, it has been possible to demonstrate a carbohydrate-rich cell coat or glycolemma (41, 42), and this seems to be developed to different degrees in the several regions of the cell surface.

A relatively crude approach to the determination of surface charge has involved the binding of electron-opaque particles of colloidal iron hydroxide to the sperm surface and the subsequent study of their localization in electron micrographs of thin sections (25, 125, 41). In this approach sperm tails were generally found to be more intensely labeled than heads—a finding consistent with the earlier electrophoretic studies. The distribution of iron particles was rather uniform within a particular segment, but abrupt changes in particle concentration were sometimes observed at junctions between segments. The patterns were consistent within species but not between species. In the rabbit, for example, the heads were relatively free of label, the midpiece was lightly labeled, and the remainder of the tail was heavily labeled. In the guinea pig, on the other hand, all of the surface was labeled, but the principal and end pieces were labeled most heavily. The acrosomal region was more heavily labeled than the postacrosomal segment (125). The abrupt changes observed from one region of the sperm to another were interpreted as indicating significant changes in biochemical properties of the membrane at these junctions. This conclusion may well be justified, but since the binding of colloidal iron is carried out on glutaraldehyde-fixed sperm at pH 1.6–2.0, the validity of the method as an index of charge density and distribution in the living spermatozoon can be seriously questioned.

A more physiological and biochemically meaningful approach has taken advantage of a group of agglutinins of plant origin (lectins) that are capable of binding specifically to certain saccharide residues on the membranes of mammalian cells. By coupling fluorescein isothiocyanate or ^{125}I to these lectins, fluorescence microscopy or autoradiography can demonstrate the distribution of specific saccharide-binding sites on the cell surface. If ferritin is coupled to the lectin, the electron density of the iron can be used to localize the binding sites with the greater resolution afforded by the electron microscope. For example, the lectin concanavalin A, at pH 7.4, consists of a tetramer of which each protomer binds to an α-D-mannose group. When it is added to a suspension of living, motile sperm, it results in their immediate agglutination, indicating that exposed α-D-mannose residues are present on the glycoproteins of the sperm membrane. These residues, as revealed by use of labeled lectins, are not uniformly distributed over the whole sperm but are concentrated over the acrosomal region of the head (30). D-galactose residues are also more abundant on the head. From the head-to-head sperm agglutination induced with Sendai (32) or influenza virus (79), it can be inferred that N-acetylneuraminic acid is prevalent on heads of rabbit and hamster sperm but is less abundant or absent on the tail.

The development of the method of freeze-fracturing for electron microscopy has now made it possible to examine the internal organization of cell membranes. Applied to spermatozoa, this method has provided the most dramatic demonstrations to date of regional differences in membrane structure (63, 64, 43, 46). In this procedure, cells very briefly fixed and exposed to glycerol as a cryoprotectant are instantaneously frozen in liquid freon or nitrogen and fractured in the frozen state. The fracture plane is not entirely random but preferentially passes through the lipid bilayer of cell membranes, thus splitting the membrane in half. By evaporating carbon onto the frozen surface, a coherent replica of the interior of the membrane is produced. This is examined in the electron microscope after metal has been deposited on its surface at an angle to increase the contrast and to produce a three-dimensional image of small variations in surface contour.

Two kinds of images are seen in these replicas of the inner surfaces of a membrane. On the outwardly directed inner half of a typical cell membrane, a large number of 60–90 Å particles are randomly distributed in a featureless background. These are believed to represent the protein constituents of the membrane and are called membrane-intercalated particles or intramembrane particles. The inwardly directed outer half-membrane has very few of these particles and appears relatively smooth, but in high-fidelity replicas one may observe shallow pits corresponding to the particles on the opposing face (19). Why the particles tend to remain attached to the inner half-membrane is not understood.

The particle-rich inner half-membrane is called the *A face* (or PF face). The particle-poor outer half is the *B face* (or EF face). There is compelling evidence that the particles can move about within the lipid bilayer, which is fluid at body temperature (47, 103). Thus the particles are free to associate in particular patterns and to dissociate again. As yet we know very little about how these alterations in distribution of particles affect the local physiological properties of the membrane. Only a few local specializations of epithelial cell surfaces that are concerned with cell adhesion or cell communication have been studied in any detail. For example, at the nexuses or gap junctions between epithelial cells and at electrical synapses in the nervous system, particles in the opposing membranes are closely aggregated, often in hexagonal array (54, 70). At occluding junctions (*zonulae occludentes*) there is a network of anastomosing strands or rods on the A face and a corresponding pattern of grooves on the B face (107). Relatively few other local specializations of membranes have been described. Freeze-cleaving studies of spermatozoa reveal a number of interesting internal specializations of their membrane that have thus far not been seen in other cell types.

In regions of contact between the successive acrosomes in rouleaux of guinea pig spermatozoa (Figures 31.17, 31.18), the opposing membranes are precisely parallel and separated by an interspace of about 10 nm. This space is traversed by very evenly spaced linear densities that have been likened to the septate junctions of invertebrate tissues (21). At high magnifications (Figure 31.19) the regularly repeating structures extending between the unit membranes are double-contoured and of distinctly lower density than the membranes. This lattice between the adhering membranes seems to be a special configuration of glycocalyx in which the glycoproteins are more highly ordered than they are on other parts of the cell surface.

When the cell membrane overlying the guinea pig acrosome is examined by freeze-fracturing, the A face exhibits areas of irregular outline with a quilted pattern separated by narrow strips of particle-studded membrane of more orthodox appearance (Figure 31.20). These highly ordered plaques or crystalline domains within the membrane do not appear to be formed by a close packing and an ordering of the ordinary membrane-intercalated particles, and no explanation of their molecular organization or significance can be offered at present (46). It seems likely, however, that the order observed in the structures traversing the interspace between the opposed membranes, in thin sections, is a reflection of the crystalline lattice seen within the membrane by freeze-cleaving. This cannot be interpreted as a specialization for adhesion peculiar to guinea pig sperm because very similar crystalline areas are observed in the cell membrane over the acrosome in rat spermatozoa, which do not associate in rouleaux (Figure 31.21). As other species are studied, this high degree of internal order may prove to be a common feature of the acrosomal region of the sperm membrane. If so, this will support the speculation that this unique structure of the membrane is related in

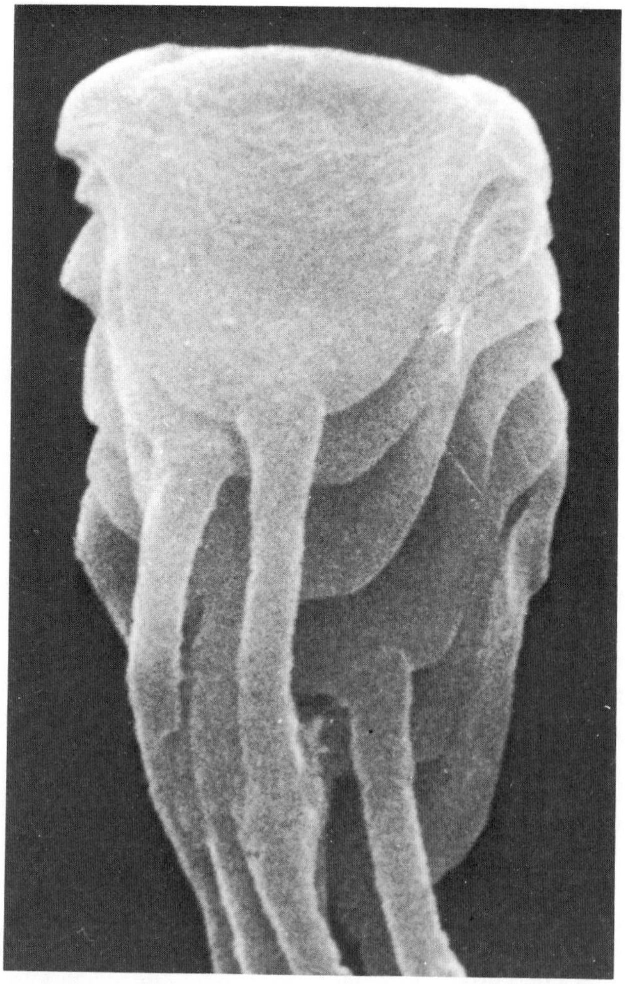

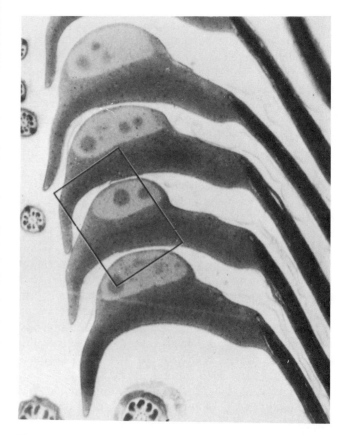

Figure 31.17 Scanning micrograph of guinea pig spermatozoa associated in a stack or rouleau as they commonly occur in the epididymis. This involves a conformity of shape of the acrosomes and a cohesion of the surface membranes.

Figure 31.18 A thin sagittal section through a rouleau of sperm heads shows the inhomogeneity in density of the acrosomal contents and the close contact of the convexity of one sperm head with the concavity in the next.

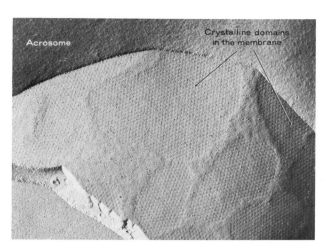

Figure 31.20 Freeze-cleaving preparation of the cell membrane overlying the concave surface of a guinea pig acrosome. Crystalline domains of varying size within the membrane are separated by areas of more orthodox appearance. From (45).

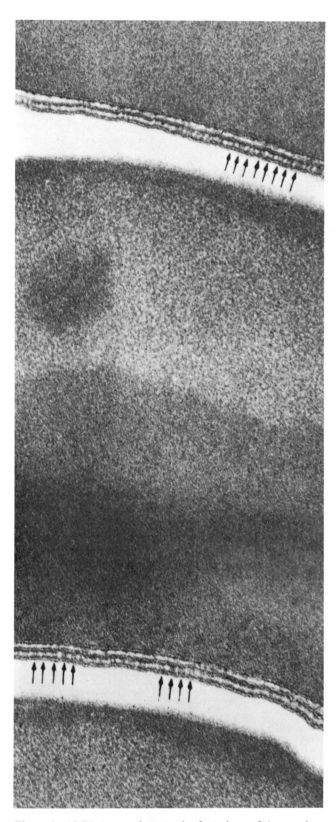

Figure 31.19 Electron micrograph of portions of three cohering guinea pig acrosomes. The apposed membranes are quite close and the narrow interspace between these is traversed by very regularly spaced densities. These are interpreted as a highly ordered area of the carbohydrate-rich cell coat or glycolemma. Micrograph by D. Friend.

some way to the participation of this region of the cell surface in the acrosome reaction.

Freeze-cleaving studies of the postacrosomal region of the spermatozoon have not been especially rewarding. There are no crystalline areas. There does, however, seem to be a greater number of intramembrane particles per unit area than in the membrane over the acrosome (Figure 31.22). If the generalization is true that the number of particles is correlated with the degree of metabolic activity of the membrane (19), then this finding is consistent with the importance usually attached to this region in sperm-egg interaction. In some species there are conspicuous intramembranous strands or rods that run obliquely forward from the posterior ring in the caudal part of the postacrosomal region (63, 43, 46). In other species there are in this same region well-ordered geometric arrays of very small particles (46). As yet, no clues have shed light on the significance of these unusual differentiations in relation to the specific role of this region in gamete fusion. The unique properties of the postacrosomal region essential for gamete attachment and fusion may not reside within the membrane proper but in the underlying dense lamina or more likely in the outer surface of the membrane, which is not seen in freeze-cleaving. The isozyme of lactic dehydrogenase that is specific for spermatozoa (LDH-X) is reported to be localized by electron microscopic immunocytochemistry in higher concentration on the postacrosomal membrane than elsewhere on the surface of mouse sperm (31). In view of the observation that female animals immunized against this isozyme exhibit defective fertilization (53), the localization of the enzyme in the postacrosomal region may be significant. An antigen

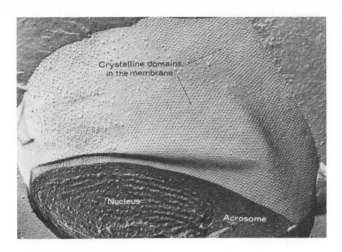

Figure 31.21 Freeze-cleaving preparation of a rat sperm head showing areas of highly ordered structure within the plasma membrane overlying the acrosome. Other areas of the same membrane have the usual random distribution of membrane-intercalated particles. Where the plane of fracture has broken across the nucleus a lamellar organization of the condensed chromatin is evident. From (45).

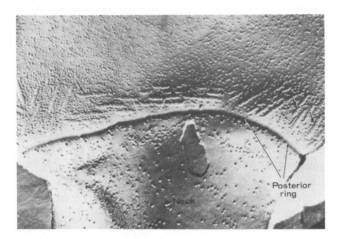

Figure 31.22 Freeze-cleaving preparation showing the intramembranous differentiations of the postacrosomal region in a rabbit spermatozoon. The great abundance of particles in the postacrosomal region can be compared with the relatively sparse population in the neck region. The posterior ring appears here as a distinct groove at the boundary between head and neck. Rods or linear aggregations of particles are characteristic of the postacrosomal membrane near the posterior ring in this species. Micrograph courtesy of J. E. Flechon.

peculiar to a primitive teratocarcinoma and other early embryonic cells has also been localized in the postacrosomal region of human spermatozoa (40).

Particular oligosaccharide residues of the surface membrane may prove to be important in gamete recognition and attachment, and specific enzymes may be involved in gamete fusion, but much more work is needed on this region of the spermatozoon to determine how these surface properties are related to the deeper membrane-intercalated particles and rods revealed by freeze-fracturing.

Of special interest is the circumferential groove in the plasmalemma—the posterior ring (120)—which marks the boundary between the head and the neck of the spermatozoon. Electron micrographs of thin sections show this to be a line of fusion of three membranes (Figure 31.23). In freeze-fracture preparations the groove shows a very fine transverse striation—another local differentiation of the cell membrane thus far found only on spermatozoa (46). Fusion of the membranes along this line is thought to effectively isolate the perinuclear compartment from the remainder of the cell. Experimental damage to the cell membrane is well known to cause immediate immobilization and death of the spermatozoon; yet in the acrosome reaction, the membrane over the entire anterior half of the sperm head is lost without any ill effect upon sperm motility. The explanation for this paradox seems to reside in the posterior ring. The naturally occurring, extensive disruption of the cell surface during the acrosome reaction probably could not be tolerated were it not for the fact that the perinuclear compartment is sealed off from the tail by membrane fusion along the posterior ring.

The membrane of the sperm midpiece in many species shows the usual randomly distributed population

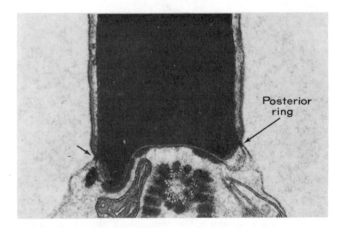

Figure 31.23 Thin section of the posterior part of a monkey sperm head showing the location and appearance of the posterior ring—a circumferential groove where the plasma membrane is fused to the underlying nuclear membranes.

of membrane-intercalated particles. In the guinea pig, however, the A face of the membrane displays extensive linear arrays of 60–80 Å particles generally oriented circumferentially (Figure 31.24) (46, 64). Corresponding rows of shallow pits are seen on the B face. These beaded strands are not uniformly distributed but are more abundant and more closely aggregated where the membrane overlies the gyres of the mitochondrial helix (Figures 31.25, 31.26). The membrane overlying the grooves or interstices between mitochondria contains only scattered 80 Å single particles or short rows. This is an interesting example of differentiation within the plane of a cell membrane that has a clear topographical relationship to an organelle in the subjacent cytoplasm. That the alignment of particles and their circumferential orientation depends upon proximity to the mitochondria is indicated by the fact that where the membrane diverges from the mitochondrial

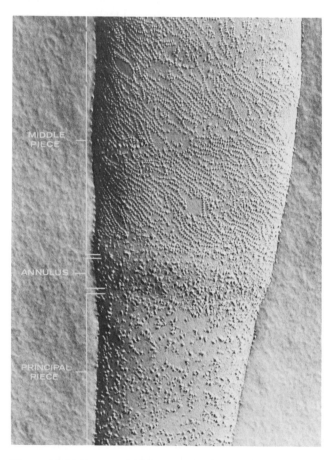

Figure 31.24 Freeze-cleaving preparation of the outwardly directed inner half of the plasma membrane from the junctional region between the middle and principal pieces of a guinea-pig spermatozoon. The beaded strands of small particles in the middle piece end abruptly at the annulus. The membrane of the principal piece contains a population of randomly distributed larger particles. Micrograph by D. Friend.

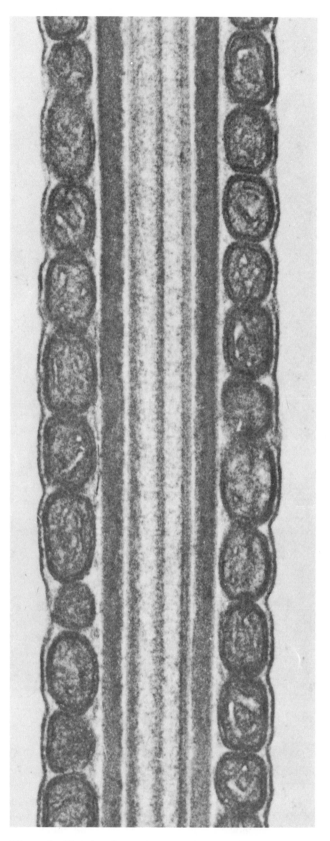

Figure 31.25 A longitudinal thin section of the middle piece of a mammalian spermatozoon. The circumferentially oriented mitochondria are cut transversely. Note how closely the cell membrane is apposed to the underlying mitochondria.

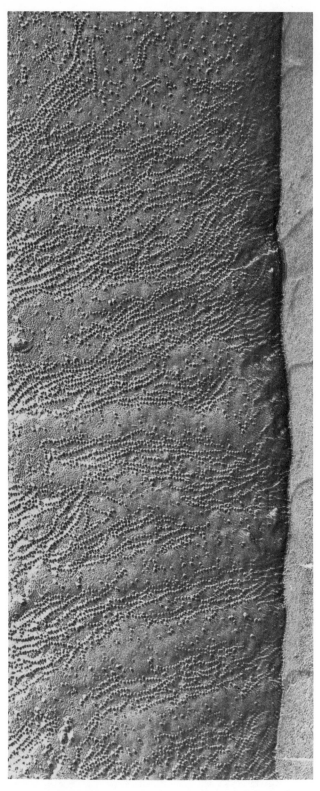

Figure 31.26 Freeze-cleaving preparation of the membrane of the middle piece from a guinea pig reveals linear arrays of intramembranous particles oriented circumferentially and concentrated over the mitochondria. The membrane over interstices in the mitochondrial sheath is relatively free of particles. These highly ordered arrays of particles are not found in the corresponding regions of sperm from other species.

helix to enclose the cytoplasmic droplet, the beaded strands within the membrane become disoriented and largely dispersed into single particles (46).

The linear arrays of intramembrane particles in the guinea pig midpiece terminate abruptly at the annulus, and the membrane of the principal piece has a random pattern of particles on its A face not unlike that of other cell membranes (Figure 31.24). A distinctive feature, however, is a double row of staggered 90 Å particles that runs longitudinally in the membrane over outer dense fiber 1 (Figure 31.27C). This zipperlike differentiation is always found in the same location and extends throughout the anterior half of the principal piece and possibly farther. In thin cross sections of guinea pig sperm tails, a slight thickening of the membrane can be detected in this position, and a local density is sometimes seen between the membrane and the underlying ribs of the fibrous sheath (Figure 31.27). In freeze-cleaving preparations of rat spermatozoa, a single row of more widely spaced 80–90 Å particles is seen in the same location (46). A localized thickening of the membrane over outer fiber 1 has now been observed in thin sections of sperm tails in other species, and it seems likely that a longitudinally oriented linear array of intramembrane particles will prove to be a common feature of the principal piece of mammalian spermatozoa studied by freeze-cleaving.

The significance of this structure is by no means clear. It bears some resemblance to the so-called necklaces of intramembranous particles that course circumferentially around the base of epithelial cilia (52) and around the base of the flagellum of certain invertebrate spermatozoa (17, 119). To date the only comparable example of a longitudinally oriented particle array in a flagellar membrane is found in the undulating membrane of trypanosomes, along the line of attachment of the flagellar membrane to the cell membrane (85). There are associated densities in the matrix of the flagellum and the cytoplasm. In this case the aligned intramembranous particles are clearly associated with a line of membrane-to-membrane attachment. This suggests that the row of particles over fiber 1 in the mammalian sperm tail may be a specialization for attachment of the membrane to the ribs of the underlying fibrous sheath. The unrestrained bending of the axoneme and its associated sheaths would seem to require some slack in the membrane and some degree of freedom of movement over the underlying structures of the tail. On the other hand, it could be argued that the tail probably functions more efficiently as a locomotor organ with its membrane fixed to the underlying structures than it would if the bending movements were taking place in a loose unattached sleeve. Why the attachment is situated over the ribs and fiber 1 instead of over one of the continuous columns of the fi-

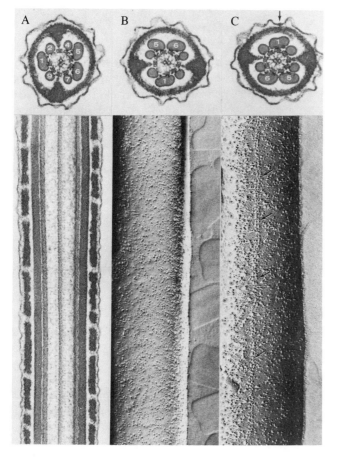

Figure 31.27 A. Longitudinal section through the principal piece of a sperm tail, approximately in the plane passing through fibers 2 and 7 or 9 and 4 of the cross section shown above. The section includes two doublets and one of the central pair of axonemal microtubules, two outer fibers, and groups of partially fused ribs of the fibrous sheath.

B. Freeze-cleaving preparation of the membrane on the side of the principal piece over the major compartment containing outer fibers 4 to 7. There is a high concentration of randomly distributed membrane-intercalated particles.

C. Freeze-cleaving preparation of the membrane on the side of the minor compartment containing fibers 9, 1, and 2. A double row of large particles runs longitudinally within the membrane overlying fiber 1. A slight thickening of the membrane at this site is evident (at the arrow) in the cross section shown above.

brous sheath, where it would be subject to the least tension in bending, defies explanation.

The finding of consistent regional differences in the patterns of internal organization of the sperm plasma membrane has interesting implications for the currently popular fluid mosaic model of membrane structure. There is evidence from nuclear magnetic resonance studies that lipid components of cell membranes may undergo rapid lateral movements (103). The glycoprotein surface antigens and binding sites for lectins have also been shown capable of movement to one pole of cells in the phenomenon called capping (115, 61). These observations have given rise to the concept that the plasma membranes of cells are dynamic fluid structures (105). Experiments on spermatozoa with ferritin-conjugated lectins have recently provided evidence for regional differences in the mobility of receptors, greater mobility being demonstrated in the postacrosomal than in the acrosomal or tail regions of the plasma membrane (80). On the other hand, the sharply demarcated and consistent regional differentiations demonstrated in sperm membranes by freeze-cleaving indicates that in this cell there must also be effective restraints to movement from one segment to another. In the case of the circumferentially oriented linear arrays of particles in the midpiece of guinea pig spermatozoa there is strongly suggestive evidence that proximity of the membrane to the mitochondria determines the degree of aggregation and orientation of the beaded strands of particles. The abrupt change of pattern from midpiece to principal piece suggests that the binding of the annulus to the membrane may prevent the free movement of membrane-intercalated particles from one region to the other. And finally, the maintenance of a longitudinal alignment of intramembranous particles in constant topographical relationship to a landmark in the interior of the tail represents yet another example of extraneous restraints to mobility of integral protein components of the membrane.

31.5 Important Gaps in Our Knowledge

The spermatozoon is certainly one of the most complex and highly specialized of all mammalian cells. Our knowledge of its structure is possibly also more detailed than that concerning any other cell type. Yet there remain important gaps in our understanding of its chemistry and physiology.

At the level of clinical evaluation of semen quality, we note the prevalence of large nuclear vacuoles in human sperm and numerous examples of incompletely condensed chromatin, but since sperm of this kind represent only a fraction of the millions normally present in an ejaculate, we do not know whether these structural or maturational defects affect the fertilizing capacity of the sperm. During sperm development, the chromatin of the nucleus undergoes a poorly understood process of condensation that results in a highly compacted, metabolically inert sperm head that is resistant to efforts at in vitro solubilization by any treatment but strong detergents and disulfide reducing agents. But one of the most remarkable phenomena in reproductive biology is the rapid decondensation of the sperm nucleus in the cytoplasm of the fertilized egg. Further work is needed to explain the biochemical mechanisms of chromatin condensation, its biological significance, and its rapid reversal to form the male pronucleus.

Much has been learned about the acrosomal enzymes. Their importance in ensuring access of the spermatozoa to the egg surface for fertilization is generally accepted. But we remain ignorant of the factors that normally trigger the acrosome reaction when sperm reach the vicinity of a recently ovulated egg. The enzymes released are credited with dispersing the cumulus cells. Nevertheless, it is puzzling that the entire content of the acrosomal cap is lost in this process before the sperm reaches the principal barrier in its path—the zona pellucida. It is not at all clear why so much enzyme is required to disperse the loosely organized cumulus cells, while the small amount of enzyme bound to the inner acrosomal membrane apparently suffices to lyse a path through the zona. The relative importance of zona lysis in mechanical penetration by a motile sperm needs further study.

It is assumed that the fertilizing spermatozoon induces release of cortical granules which in turn cause physicochemical changes in the zona pellucida that discourage the entry of additional sperm, but neither the nature of the cortical granules nor the mechanism by which they block polyspermy is adequately understood. A better understanding of the process might suggest ways of simulating this natural block in order to prevent fertilization.

There are recent indications that some of the acrosomal hydrolases are chemically distinct from the corresponding enzymes of lysosomes. This suggests the need for further characterization of the antigenic properties of these enzymes to determine the feasibility of specific immunosuppression of their activity without undesirable consequences outside of the reproductive tract.

Electron-microscopic study of fertilization has established that spermatozoa present the flat surface of their head to the egg and fusion occurs specifically in the postacrosomal region. The ultrastructure of this region is now fairly well documented, and there is evidence of greater mobility of surface receptors and of localization of at least one enzyme there. Still largely unknown is the chemical basis for the specificity of

this segment of the sperm suface and the molecular mechanisms involved in gamete attachment and fusion.

Detachment of sperm heads from sperm tails is observed as a genetic defect in some animals and can be induced in vitro by relatively brief exposure to endopeptidases. As a vulnerable site in the structural integrity of the spermatozoon, the nature of this linkage deserves additional study.

There has been rapid progress in the chemical dissection of the axoneme in the relatively simple sperm flagella of invertebrates. This fundamental research has been basic to the development of a sliding tubule hypothesis for the generation of flagellar waves. The isolation of tubulin—the principal molecular species in the axoneme—and dynein—the protein mainly involved in transduction of chemical energy to mechanical work in motility—have been landmark discoveries. There remain the more difficult tasks of characterization of the nexin links, radial spokes, and other minor components of the axoneme, and of fractionation of the doublets to identify the basis for the specific binding of dynein and spoke protein to particular protofilaments in the wall.

Any effort to develop a method of contraception based upon immunological or biochemical interference with sperm motility cannot be directed at the microtubular components of the axoneme, because their proteins are the same as those of cilia, mitotic spindles, and other microtubular components of somatic cells that have functions essential to life. It is important, therefore, to study the chemical nature and function of the fibrous components that are peculiar to spermatozoa, for these might yield a basis for developing destructive or suppressive methods having an acceptable degree of specificity.

The isolation and characterization of the outer fibers that are typical of mammalian sperm tails is a recent development. A little is now known about their composition, but it is still not possible to state with certainty whether they are or are not contractile. If they are not, then further work must be done to explain their universal occurrence in mammals, their effect upon the pattern of motility, and their relation to a long mitochondrial sheath, which appeared in phylogeny concurrently with the evolution of the outer dense fibers.

The past decade has seen a remarkable change in our concept of the cell membrane. The former emphasis on its structural uniformity and its passive role as a semipermeable cell boundary has given way to a dynamic view of membranes that recognizes their rapid turnover, their structural and chemical diversity, and their capacity for rapid change. There has been a growing appreciation of the fact that most important physiological processes take place at membranes, whether within cells or at their interface with their environment. This is probably no less true of spermatozoa than it is of cells organized into tissues and organs. There is already abundant evidence for a central role of membranes in capacitation, in the acrosome reaction, and in the recognition and attachment of the gametes.

To gain more insight into these phenomena, the reproductive biologist may have to put aside the time-honored methods of endocrinology and steroid biochemistry and adopt the methods of the membrane biologist, the immunologist, and the molecular pharmacologist. We need to know more about the significance of the unique patterns revealed by freeze-cleaving within the lipid bilayer in different regions of the sperm membrane. There is need for more work to ascertain how the membrane-intercalated particles are related to the oligosaccharides on the outer surface, which seem to be the basis for the regional specificity of the sperm membrane. More information is needed on the internal organization of the membrane in different stages of maturation and in the different environments encountered in the male and female reproductive tracts.

References

1. Afzelius, B. A. Electron microscopy of the sperm taii. J. Biophys. Biochem. Cytol. 5:269, 1959.

2. Afzelius, B. A., R. Eliasson, Ø. Johnson, and C. Lindholmer. Lack of dynein arms in immotile human spermatozoa. J. Cell Biol. 66:225, 1975.

3. Allison, A. C., and E. F. Hartree. Lysosomal enzymes in the acrosome and their possible role in fertilization. J. Reprod. Fertil. 21:501, 1970.

4. Amos, L., and A. Klug. Arrangement of subunits in flagellar microtubules. J. Cell Sci. 14:523, 1974.

5. Austin, C. R. Function of hyaluronidase in fertilization. Nature 162:63, 1948.

6. Austin, C. R., and M. W. H. Bishop. Role of the rodent acrosome and perforatorium in fertilization. Proc. R. Soc. Lond. [Biol.] 149:241, 1958.

7. Baccetti, B., V. Palline, and A. G. Burrini. Accessory fibers of the sperm tail. I. Structure and chemical composition of the bull "coarse fibers." J. Submicrosc. Cytol. 5:237, 1973.

8. Barlow, P., and C. G. Vosa. The Y chromosome in human spermatozoa. Nature 226:961, 1970.

9. Barros, C., J. M. Bedford, L. E. Franklin, and C. R. Austin. Membrane vesiculation as a feature of the mammalian acrosome reaction. J. Cell Biol. 34:C_1, 1967.

10. Barros, C., and L. Franklin. Behavior of the gamete membranes during sperm entry into the mammalian egg. J. Cell Biol. 37:C_{13}, 1968.

11. Bedford, J. M. Changes in the electrophoretic properties of rabbit spermatozoa during passage through the epididymis. Nature 200:1178, 1963.

12. Bedford, J. M. Ultrastructural changes in the sperm head during fertilization in the rabbit. Am. J. Anat. 123:329, 1968.

13. Bedford, J. M. An electron microscopic study of sperm penetration into the rabbit egg after natural mating. Am. J. Anat. 133:213, 1971.

14. Bedford, J. M., G. W. Cooper, and H. L. Calbin. Postmeiotic changes in the nucleus and membranes of mammalian spermatozoa. Proc. Int. Symp., *The genetics of the spermatozoon*, eds. R. A. Beatty and S. Glueckeon-Waelsch, p. 69. Edinburgh, 1971.

15. Bedford, J. M., H. Calvin, and G. W. Cooper. The maturation of spermatozoa in the human epididymis. J. Reprod. Fertil. Suppl. 18:199, 1970.

16. Behnke, D., and A. Forer. Evidence for four classes of microtubules in individual cells. J. Cell. Biol. 2:169, 1967.

17. Bergstrom, B. H., and C. Henley. Flagellar necklaces: Freeze-etch observations. J. Ultrastruct. Res. 42:551, 1973.

18. Blom, E. The evaluation of bull semen with special references to its employment for artificial insemination. Thesis Carl Fr. Mortensen, Copenhagen, 1950.

19. Branton, D. Fracture faces of frozen membranes. Proc. Natl. Acad. Sci. USA 55:1048, 1966.

20. Brown, C. R., and E. F. Hartree. Distribution of a trypsin-like proteinase in the ram spermatozoon. J. Reprod. Fertil. 36:195, 1974.

21. Burgos, M. H., J. Blaquier, M. S. Cameo, and L. Gutierrez. Morphological maturation of spermatozoa in the epididymis. In *Biology of reproduction*, (III Panamerican Congress of Anatomy), eds. J. T. Velardo and B. H. Kasprow, p. 367. Mexico City: Bay Gráfica y Ediciones, 1972.

22. Calvin, H. I., and J. M. Bedford. Formation of disulfide bonds in the nucleus and accessory structures of mammalian spermatozoa during maturation in the epididymis. J. Reprod. Fertil. (Suppl.) 13:65, 1971.

23. Chasey, D. Subunit arrangement in ciliary microtubules from *Tetrahymena pyriforms*. Exp. Cell Res. 74:140, 1972.

24. Clermont, Y., R. C. Clegg, and C. P. Leblond. Presence of carbohydrates in the acrosome of the guinea pig spermatozoon. Exp. Cell Res. 8:453, 1955.

25. Cooper, G. W., and J. M. Bedford. Acquisition of surface charge by the plasma membrane of mammalian spermatozoa during epididymal maturation. Anat. Rec. 169:300, 1971.

26. Darzynkiewicz, A., B. L. Gledhill, and N. R. Ringertz. Changes in deoxyribonucleoprotein during spermiogenesis in the bull. Exp. Cell Res. 58:435, 1969.

27. Dobell, C. Antony van Leeuwenhoek and his "little animals." New York: Dover, 1960.

28. Dott, H. M., and J. T. Dingle. Distribution of lysosomal enzymes in the spermatozoa and cytoplasmatic droplets of bull and ram. Exp. Cell Res. 52:523, 1968.

29. Dziuk, P. G., and Z. Dickenann. Sperm penetration through the zona pellucida of the sheep egg. J. Exp. Zool. 158:237, 1965.

30. Edelman, G. M., and C. F. Millette. Molecular probes of spermatozoon structure. Proc. Natl. Acad. Sci. USA 68: 2436, 1971.

31. Erickson, R. P., D. S. Friend, and D. Tennebaum. Localization of lactate dehydrogenase-X on the surfaces of mouse spermatozoa. Exp. Cell Res. (in press).

32. Ericsson, R. J., D. A. Buthala, and J. F. Norland. Fertilization of rabbit ova in vitro by sperm with absorbed Sendai virus. Science 173:54, 1971.

33. Evans, H. L. Properties of human X and Y sperm. In Proc. Int. Symp., *The genetics of the spermatozoon*, eds. R. A. Beatty and S. Glueckeon-Waelsch, p. 144. Edinburgh, 1971.

34. Fawcett, D. W. The structure of the mammalian spermatozoan. Int. Rev. Cytol. 7:195, 1958.

35. Fawcett, D. W. The anatomy of the mammalian spermatozoan with particular reference to the guinea pig. Z. Zellforsch. 67:279, 1965.

36. Fawcett, D. W. A comparative view of sperm ultrastructure. Biol. Reprod. (Suppl.) 2:90, 1970.

37. Fawcett, D. W., and R. Hollenberg. Changes in the acrosome of guinea pig spermatozoa during passage through the epididymis. Z. Zellforsch. 60:276, 1963.

38. Fawcett, D. W., and S. Ito. The fine structure of bat spermatozoa. Am. J. Anat. 116:567, 1965.

39. Fawcett, D. W., and D. M. Phillips. The fine structure and development of the neck region of the mammalian spermatozoon. Anat. Rec. 165:153, 1969.

40. Fellous, M., G. Gachelin, M. H. Buc-Caron, P. Dubois, and F. Jacob. Similar location of an early embryonic antigen on mouse and human spermatozoa. Dev. Biol. (in press).

41. Flechon, J. E. La membrane du spermatozoide de lapin. Repartition et nature des glycoproteines de la surface cellulaire. J. Microscopie 11:53, 1971.

42. Flechon, J. E. Étude ultrastructurale et cytochimique de constituants de la téte et de la surface du spermatozoide de lapin. Modifications au cours de la maturation et de la capacitation *in utero*. Thesis, University of Paris, 1973.

43. Flechon, J. E. Freeze-fracturing of rabbit spermatozoa. J. Microscopie 19:59, 1974.

44. Franklin, L. E. Formation of the redundant nuclear envelope in monkey spermatids. Anat. Rec. 161:149, 1968.

45. Franklin, L. E., C. Barros, and E. N. Fussell. The acrosome region and the acrosome reaction in sperm of the golden hamster. Biol. Reprod. 3:180, 1970.

46. Friend, D. S., and D. W. Fawcett. Membrane differentiations in freeze-fractured mammalian sperm. J. Cell Biol. 63:641, 1974.

47. Frye, C. D., and M. Edidin. The rapid intermixing of cell surface antigens after formation of mouse-human heterokaryons. J. Cell Sci. 7:319, 1970.

48. Gibbons, I. R. Chemical dissection of cilia. Arch. Biol. (Liege) 76:317, 1965.

49. Gibbons, I. R. Studies on the ATPase activity of 14S and 30S dynein from cilia of *Tetrahymena*. J. Biol. Chem. 241:5590, 1966.

50. Gibbons, I. R., and E. Fronk. Some properties of bound and soluble dynein from sea urchin flagella. J. Cell Biol. 54:365, 1972.

51. Gibbons, I. R., and A. J. Rowe. Dynein: A protein with ATPase activity from cilia. Science 149:424, 1965.

52. Gilula, N. B., and P. Satir. The ciliary necklace: A ciliary membrane specialization. J. Cell Biol. 53:494, 1972.

53. Goldberg, E. Infertility in female rabbits immunized with lactate dehydrogenase X. Science 181:458, 1973.

54. Goodenough, D. A., and J. P. Revel. A fine structural analysis of intercellular junctions in the mouse liver. J. Cell Biol. 45:272, 1970.

55. Gordon, M., and K. G. Benesch. Cytochemical differentiation of the guinea pig sperm flagellum with phosphotungstic acid. J. Ultrastruct. Res. 24:33, 1968.

56. Grimstone, A. V., and A. Klug. Observations on the substructure of flagella fibres. J. Cell Sci. 1:351, 1966.

57. Hartree, E. F., and P. N. Srivastava. Chemical composition of the acrosomes of ram spermatozoa. J. Reprod. Fertil. 9:47, 1965.

58. Hopkins, J. M. Subsidiary components of the flagella of *Chlamydomonas reinhardii*. J. Cell Sci. 7:823, 1970.

59. Inoue, S., and H. Sato. Arrangement of DNA in living sperm: A biophysical analysis. Science 136:1122, 1962.

60. Inoue, S., and H. Sato. Deoxyribonucleic acid arrangement in living sperm. In *Molecular architecture in cell physiology*, eds. T. Hayashi and A. Szent-Gyorgyi. Englewood Cliffs, N.J.: Prentice-Hall, 1966.

61. Karnovsky, M. J., E. R. Unanue, and M. Leventhal. Ligand-induced movement of lymphocyte membrane macromolecules. II. Mapping of surface moieties. J. Exp. Med. 136:907, 1972.

62. Koehler, J. K. Fine structure observations in frozen-etched bovine spermatozoa. J. Ultrastruct. Res. 16:359, 1966.

63. Koehler, J. K. A freeze-etching study of rabbit spermatozoa with particular reference to head structures. J. Ultrastruct. Res. 33:598, 1970.

64. Koehler, J. K. An unusual filamentous component associated with the guinea pig sperm middle piece. J. Microscopie 18:263, 1973.

65. Leblond, C. P., and Y. Clermont. Definition of the stages of the cycle of the seminiferous epithelium in the rat. Ann. NY Acad. Sci. 55:548, 1952.

66. Linck, R. W. Chemical and structural differences between cilia and flagella from the lamellibranch mollusc, Aequipecten irradians. J. Cell Sci. 12:951, 1973.

67. Linck, R. W., and L. A. Amos. The hands of helical lattices in flagella doublet microtubules. J. Cell Sci. 14:551, 1974.

68. Linck, R. W., and L. A. Amos. Flagellar doublet microtubules: Fractionation of minor components and α tubulin from specific regions of the A-tubule. J. Cell. Sci. 20:405, 1976.

69. Lindemann, C. B., and R. Rikmoenspoel. Sperm flagella: Autonomous oscillations of the contractile system. Science 175:337, 1972.

70. McNutt, N. S., and R. S. Weinstein. The ultrastructure of the nexus. A correlated thin-section and freeze cleave study. J. Cell Biol. 47:666, 1970.

71. Metz. C. B. Role of specific sperm antigens in fertilization. Fed. Proc. 32:2057, 1973.

72. Meza, I., B. Huang, and J. Bryan. Chemical heterogeneity of protofilaments forming the outer doublets from sea urchin flagella. Exp. Cell Res. 74:535, 1972.

73. Morton, D. B. Acrosomal enzymes: Immunochemical localization of acrosin and hyaluronidase in ram sperm. J. Reprod. Fertil. 375, 1975.

74. Nelson, L. Cytochemical sutdies with the electron microscope. I. Adenosine triphosphatase in rat spermatozoa. Biochem. Biophys. Acta 27:634, 1958.

75. Nelson, L. Actin localization in sperm. Biol. Bull. 123:468, 1962.

76. Nelson, L. Cytochemical aspects of sperm motility. In Spermatozoan motility, ed. D. W. Bishop, p. 171. Washington, D. C.: Am. Ass. Adv. Sci. 1962.

77. Nevo, A. C., I. Michaele, and H. Schindler. Electrophoretic properties of bull and of rabbit spermatozoa. Exp. Cell Res. 23:69, 1961.

78. Nieander, L., and A. Bane. The fine structure of boar spermatozoa. Z. Zellforsch. Mikrosk. Anat. 57:390, 1962.

79. Nicolson, G. L., and R. Yanagimachi. Terminal saccharides on sperm plasma membranes: Identification by specific agglutinins. Science 177:276, 1972.

80. Nicholson, G. L., and R. Yanagimachi. Mobility and restriction of mobility of plasma membrane lectin-binding components. Science 184:1295, 1974.

81. Olmsted. T. B., and G. G. Borisy. Microtubules. Ann. Rev. Biochem. 42:507, 1973.

82. Olson, G. Surface structure revealed by replicas of critical-point dried spermatozoa. J. Cell Biol. 59:254a, 1973.

83. Olson, G., D. W. Hamilton, and D. W. Fawcett. Isolation and characterization of the perforatorium of rat spermatozoa. J. Reprod. Fertil. 47:293, 1976.

84. Olson, G., D. W. Hamilton, and D. W. Fawcett. Isolation and characterization of the fibrous sheath of rat epididymal spermatozoa. Biol. Reprod. 14:517, 1976.

85. Paulin, J. J. Flagellar attachment in selected tryponosomes. In Proceedings of the 31st Meeting of the Electron Microscopical Society of America, ed. C. J. Arceneaus, p. 496. Baton Rouge, La.: Claitor's Publishing, 1973.

86. Pearson, P. L., and M. Bobrow. Fluorescent staining of the Y chromosome in meiotic stages of the human male. J. Reprod. Fertil. 22:177, 1970.

87. Pedersen, H. Observations on the axial filament complex of the human spermatozoon. J. Ultrastruct. Res. 33:457, 1970.

88. Pedersen, H. Further observations on the fine structure of the human spermatozoon. Z. Zellforsch. 123:305, 1972.

89. Pedersen, H. The human spermatozoon. Copenhagen: Costers Bogtrykkeri, 1974.

90. Pedersen, H. Ultrastructure of the sperm tail. In The physiology and genetics of reproduction, eds. E. M. Coutinho and F. Fuchs. New York: Plenum Press, 1974.

91. Phillips, D. M. Ultrastructure of spermatozoa of the wooly opossum Caluromys philander. J. Ultrastruct. Res. 33:397, 1970.

92. Phillips, D. M. Comparative analysis of mammalian sperm motility. J. Cell Biol. 53:561, 1972.

93. Phillips, D. M. Substructure of the mammalian acrosome. J. Ultrastruct. Res. 38:591, 1972.

94. Phillips, D. M. Spermiogenesis. New York: Academic Press, 1974.

95. Pihlaja, D. J., and L. E. Roth. Bovine sperm fractionation. II. Morphology and chemical analysis of tail segments. J. Ultrastruct. Res. 44:293, 1973.

96. Plattner, J. Bull spermatozoa: A re-investigation by freeze-etching using widely different cryofixation procedures. J. Submicrosc. Cytol. 3:19, 1971.

97. Price, J. M. Biochemical and morphological studies of outer dense fibers of rat spermatozoa. J. Cell Biol. 59:272a, 1973.

98. Price, J. M. Biochemical morphological characterization of outer dense fibers from rat spermatozoa. Thesis, Division of Medical Sciences, Harvard University, 1974.

99. Rowlands, I. W. Capacity of hyaluronidase to increase the fertilizing power of sperm. Nature 154:332, 1944.

100. Satir, P., and F. D. Warner. The structural basis of ciliary bend formation. J. Cell Biol. 59:304a (Abstract), 1973.

101. Satir, P. Studies on cilia. III. Further studies on the cilium tip and a "sliding filament" model of ciliary motility. J. Cell Biol. 39:77, 1968.

102. Sattler, C. A., and A. Staehelin. Ciliary membrane differentiations in Tetrahymena pyriformis. J. Cell Biol. 62:473, 1974.

103. Scandella, C. J., P. Devaus, and H. M. McConnell. Rapid lateral diffusion of phospholipids in rabbit sarcoplasmic reticulum. Proc. Natl. Acad. Sci. USA 69:2056, 1972.

104. Shelanski, M. L., and E. W. Taylor. Properties of the protein subunit of central-pair and outer-doublet microtubules of sea urchin flagella. J. Cell Biol. 38:304, 1968.

105. Singer, S. J., and G. L. Nicolson. The fluid mosaic model of the structure of cell membranes. Science 175:720, 1972.

106. Srivastava, P. N., C. E. Adams, and E. F. Hartree. Enzymic action of acrosomal preparations on the rabbit ovum in vitro. J. Reprod. Fertil. 10:61, 1965.

107. Staehelin, L. A., T. M. Mukharjee, and A. W. Williams. Freeze-etch appearance of tight junctions in the epithelium of small and large intestine of mice. Protoplasma 67:165, 1969.

108. Stambaugh, R., B. C. Brackett, and L. Mastroianni. Inhibition of in vitro fertilization of rabbit ova by trypsin inhibitors. Biol. Reprod. 1:223, 1969.

109. Stambaugh, R., and J. Buckley. Identification and subcellular localization of the enzymes effecting penetration of the zona pellucida by rabbit spermatozoa. J. Reprod. Fertil. 19:423, 1969.

110. Stambaugh, R., and J. Buckley. Histochemical subcellular localization of the acrosomal proteinase effecting dissolution of the zona pellucida using fluorescein-labelled inhibitors. Fertil. Steril. 23:348, 1970.

111. Stefanini, M., C. Oura, and L. Zambone. Ultrastructure of fertilization in the mouse. 2. Penetration of sperm into the ovum. J. Submicrosc. Cytol. 1:1, 1969.

112. Stephens, R. E. Thermal fractionation of outer fiber doublet microtubules into A- and B-fiber components. A- and B-tubulin. J. Molec. Biol. 47:353, 1970.

113. Stephens, R. E. Isolation of nexin, the linkage protein responsible for the maintenance of the 9-fold configuration of flagellar axonemes. Biol. Bull. 139:438, 1970.

114. Summers, K. E., and I. R. Gibbons. Adenosine triphosphate–induced sliding of tubules in Trypsin-heated flagella of sea-urchin sperm. Proc. Natl. Acad. Sci. USA 68:3092, 1971.

115. Taylor, R. B., W. P. N. Duffus, M. C. Raff, and S. de Petrio. Redistribution and pinocytosis of lymphocyte surface immunoglobulin molecules induced by auto-immunoglobulin antibody. Nature New Biol. 233:225, 1971.

116. Tilney, L. G., J. Bryan, D. J. Bush, K. Fujievara, M. S. Mooseker, B. Murphy, and D. H. Snyder. Microtubules: Evidence for 13 protofilaments. J. Cell Biol. 59:267, 1973.

117. Warner, F. D. New observations on flagella fine structure: The relationship between matrix structure and the microtubule component of the azoneme. J. Cell Biol. 47:159, 1970.

118. Wilkins, M. H. F., and J. T. Randall. Crystallinity in sperm heads: Molecular structure of nucleoprotein in vivo. Biochem. Biophys. Acta 10:192, 1953.

119. Witman, B. G., K. Carlson, J. Berliner, and J. L. Rosenbaum. Chlamydomonas flagella. J. Cell Biol. 54:507, 1972.

120. Woolley, D. M. A posterior ring in the spermatozoa of species of *Muridae*. J. Reprod. Fertil. 23:361, 1970.

121. Woolley, D. M. Striations in the peripheral fibers of rat and mouse spermatozoa. J. Cell Biol. 49:936, 1972.

122. Woolley, D. M., and D. W. Fawcett. The degeneration and disappearance of the centrioles during the development of the rat spermatozoon. Anat. Rec. 177:289, 1973.

123. Yanigamachi, R., and Y. D. Noda. Ultrastructural changes in the hamster sperm head during fertilization. J. Ultrastruct. Res. 31:465, 1970.

124. Yanigamachi, R., and Y. Noda. Electron microscope studies of sperm incorporation into the golden hamster egg. Am. J. Anat. 128:429, 1970.

125. Yanigamachi, R., Y. D. Noda, M. Fujimoto, and G. L. Nicolson. The distribution of negative surface charges on mammalian spermatozoa. Am. J. Anat. 135:497, 1972.

126. Zamboni, L., and M. Stefanini. The fine structure of the neck of mammalian spermatozoa. Anat. Rec. 169:155, 1971.

127. Zaneveld, L. J. D., K. L. Polakoski, and G. F. B. Schumadier. Properties of acrosomal hyaluronidase from bull spermatozoa. J. Biol. Chem. 248:564, 1973.

128. Zaneveld, L. J. D., P. N. Srivastava, and W. L. Williams. Relationship of a trypsin-like enzyme in rabbit spermatozoa to capacitation. J. Reprod. Fertil. 20:337, 1969.

32 The Metabolism of Mammalian Spermatozoa

R. A. P. Harrison

The biology of the male gamete occupies a central position in the field of reproduction. Although the spermatozoon is a terminal cell with an inactive nucleus and limited synthetic capabilities, its existence is nonetheless dynamic, not only because of its motility but also because of the continual process of change that characterizes its life span. In this latter sense the spermatozoon is little different from other cell types, but, paradoxically, the effects of these changes upon the sperm's functional capabilities are more profound by virtue of its lack of regenerative ability.

The field of sperm metabolism embraces all changes of a molecular nature that are associated with the sperm cell. In addition to the common aspects of intracellular metabolism, one must include changes affecting the spermatozoon as well as changes effected by it. The development of the field up to the early 1960s was reviewed by Mann (1964) in his classic monograph, which is still the standard reference work on the subject. A number of smaller reviews of more limited scope have been published since then, but few have covered the entire field.

Since the spermatozoon must not only fertilize the egg but must also first reach it by virtue of flagellar motility, I shall start by considering sperm metabolism under two headings: motility and fertilization. During its life span as a free cell, the spermatozoon also undergoes important changes: maturation, when it acquires the capacity for motility and fertilization; capacitation and the acrosome reaction, which prepare it for the actual process of egg penetration; and aging, when degenerative changes lead to loss of function and death of the cell.

32.1 Metabolism Associated with Motility

Metabolic Pathways

Motility is a necessity for fertilizing ability. Sperm flagellar motility is achieved by the transduction of chemical energy into mechanical energy, and the supply and application of this chemical energy form the largest part of the spermatozoon's metabolism, aside from the transduction process itself.

The immediate energy source in mammalian spermatozoa seems to reside in the pool of adenine nucleotides, ATP, ADP, and AMP; no traces of nonnucleotide high-energy storage compounds such as creatine phosphate have been found (Brooks 1971). ATP is formed by oxidative phosphorylation and by glycolysis and is utilized throughout the flagellum to produce mechanical energy. The ATP is "eked out" down the length of the flagellum by the adenylate kinase reaction—$2ATP \rightarrow 2ADP + 2P_i$; $2ADP \rightarrow ATP + AMP$; $ATP \rightarrow ADP + P_i$, and so on (Raff and Blum 1968; Young and Nelson 1969). The primary ATP supply is almost certainly formed only in the midpiece and must diffuse down the flagellum's length to supply all parts of it with energy (Nevo and Rikmenspoel 1970; Adam and Wei 1975).

To maintain this energy pool of ATP, the spermatozoon is able to metabolize a wide range of exogenous substrates: it can glycolyse glucose, mannose, and fructose; it can oxidize many simple substances such as lactate, pyruvate, volatile fatty acids, and citric acid cycle intermediates. In most sperm species the only proviso seems to be that these substances can readily enter the cell to reach their intracellular site of utilization (this proviso is not always borne in mind by investigators). The fact that the spermatozoon can utilize such a wide range of substrates implies that in none of its environments will it be seriously limited by lack of exogenous substrates. All parts of the male and female reproductive tracts in which the spermatozoon resides for any length of time are well vascularized and are thus supplied with a wide range of metabolites and oxygen (for the composition of tract fluids see reviews by Restall 1967; White 1973; Brackett and Mastroianni 1974). While the levels of many of these metabolites may be well below the optimum for some of the involved enzyme systems, all substrates will be metabolized eventually by the citric acid cycle (mostly via acetyl moieties); therefore this final metabolic pathway will almost certainly be saturated even when individual levels of exogenous substrates are low. One factor that might limit sperm energy metabolism is insufficiency of oxygen; this possibility has been suggested as a reason for the developed ability of mammalian spermatozoa to glycolyse anaerobically. But measurements of levels of oxygen required by spermatozoa for respiration and motility in vitro (Nevo 1965) and of oxygen tension in various parts of the male and female reproductive tracts imply that true anaerobic glycolysis in spermatozoa is not required and does not take place in vivo.

One sperm species, however, has a serious metabolic limitation: the human spermatozoon has a very poor oxidative capability and apparently relies entirely upon glycolysable sugars to maintain sufficient ATP levels for motility (Peterson and Freund 1970a). The reason for this low oxidative metabolism is as yet unclear, but recent evidence (Peterson and Freund 1974) suggests that there is within the human sperm mitochondria both a block at the level of NADH dehydrogenase and poor coupling of phosphorylation. Pyruvate is not metabolized alone, although pyruvate in the presence of succinate, fumarate, or malate yields high levels of citrate; succinate is readily oxidized but does not cause an increase in intracellular ATP levels. Thus pyruvate dehydrogenase and citrate synthetase are active, and the respiratory chain from succinate dehydrogenase to cytochrome oxidase is intact (although there is no coupling with phosphorylation). The only explanation for the low oxidative metabolism that seems to fit all the observations is that NADH cannot be reoxidized within the mitochondria via the respiratory chain; thus as soon as the $NADH/NAD^+$ ratio is sufficiently high, the citric acid cycle reactions involving intramitochondrial NAD^+ cease through lack of cofactor. Absolute dependence of motility on glycolysis appears uniquely a feature of human spermatozoa, for spermatozoa of the rhesus monkey (an assumedly related species) exhibit normal aerobic metabolism (Hoskins and Patterson 1968). Such a dependence offers a possible target for contraceptive development —reduction of glucose levels in the female tract, especially within the cervix where sperm motility seems essential (Thibault 1973). Accurate evaluation of available substrate levels in the human reproductive tracts will be of great interest.

Early work on energy metabolism in spermatozoa suggested that these cells contained an endogenous substrate, probably a form of lipid, which was used in the absence of exogenous substrates; later this endogenous material was reported to be a plasmalogen. More recently, however, analysis of sperm phospholipid during incubation of the cells in the absence of exogenous substrate has revealed little or no detectable changes in any of the phospholipid fractions under these conditions (Darin-Bennett et al. 1973a). The loss of phospholipid during the spermatozoon's maturation period in the epididymis had also been ascribed to its utilization as an energy source, but current ideas do not favor this theory (Poulos et al. 1973). In my view, a lot of evidence, both direct and indirect, suggests that spermatozoa can utilize long-chain fatty acids only very slowly compared with other substrates (Flipse 1959; Mills and Scott 1969; Storey and Keyhani 1974a; Casillas and Erickson 1975). Such inability to utilize the long-chain fatty acid products of any phos-

pholipid breakdown seriously weakens the concept of an endogenous phospholipid energy source.

Nevertheless, washed spermatozoa, especially those obtained from ejaculates, show quite high levels of endogenous respiration. What endogenous substrate is utilized? Recent work by Casillas and his colleagues offers an answer. Carnitine, which is well known to play an essential role in fatty acid metabolism, is found abundantly in the epididymis of several species (Casillas 1972) and is accumulated in large quantities (1–2 $\mu mol/10^9$ cells) by the spermatozoa as they pass through the organ (Casillas 1973). Measurements of the acetylation state of carnitine in spermatozoa under various conditions (Casillas and Erickson 1975) indicate that in the presence of substrates that yield acetyl moieties (fructose, lactate, acetate, etc.), a very large proportion of the considerable carnitine pool becomes acetylated. (Carnitine's normal function in the mitochondrion is as a carrier of acetyl and acyl groups.) The acetyl groups in this pool can be subsequently oxidized in the normal way via the citric acid cycle. Therefore spermatozoa, of several species at least, seem to have the ability to store large quantities of acetyl moieties "for future use," and this store is utilized in the absence of exogenous substrates.

The discovery of the carnitine pool and its function in spermatozoa appears to resolve the enigmatic role of the high levels of substrate such as fructose that are found in the seminal plasma of those species that deposit their spermatozoa in the vagina. These spermatozoa are not in contact with the seminal plasma for very long because the plasma does not pass through the cervix (Blandau 1973); therefore it cannot act as a long-term direct source of energy for the cells, as has often been believed. It now seems likely, however, that the spermatozoa can utilize the substrates, especially fructose, to accumulate a large acetyl store, as described above. This store may stand them in very good stead during their passage through the cervical mucus where substrate levels may be insufficient (Gibbons et al. 1974). Of course, the poor oxidative metabolism of human spermatozoa precludes the use of such a pool and highlights the possibly critical importance of cervical substrates in this particular species.

Sperm Enzymes
Studies on enzyme systems involved in energy production in spermatozoa have provided direct demonstrations of most of the enzymes involved in glycolysis, in the citric acid cycle, and in oxidative phosphorylation, as well as of other enzymes of intermediary metabolism. Some interesting features have emerged. Measurement of the total potential activities of individual key enzymes in glycolysis indicates that these activities are present in considerable excess compared with the

maximal overall glycolytic rates observed; thus the enzymes are by no means rate-limiting (Peterson and Freund 1970b; Harrison 1971). Certain well-known enzymes are conspicuous by their absence. For example, mammalian spermatozoa have been shown to lack an endogenous glycogen reserve (Mann 1964; Anderson and Personne 1970), and they also appear to lack the enzymic means to catabolize this energy source: neither phosphorylase (Castellano et al. 1968; Anderson and Personne 1970) nor phosphoglucomutase (R. A. P. Harrison, unpublished results) have been detected in them. Pentose phosphate pathway activity is extremely low in spermatozoa, as judged by the measurement of rates of metabolism of different specifically labeled glucose carbon atoms (Witters et al. 1966; O'Shea and Wales 1967; Murdoch and White 1968; Voglmayr et al. 1970), and the activity of one of the key enzymes of this pathway, glucose-6-phosphate dehydrogenase, is also almost undetectable in sperm extracts from domestic species (R. A. P. Harrison, unpublished results)—although some activity has been reported in human sperm extracts (Peterson and Freund 1970b).

The general absence of these enzyme systems from spermatozoa is hardly surprising from a biological point of view. As mentioned above, spermatozoa have little need of endogenous substrates; nor, as terminal cells with hardly any synthetic ability, do they require a source of nucleotide precursors or reducing power (NADPH) for synthetic reactions, as supplied by the pentose phosphate pathway. Yet these enzyme systems are highly active in other testicular cells; it is not known how the genes responsible for these enzymes are so effectively and specifically turned off in the germ cells.

A number of enzymes have been shown to exist in spermatozoa only or mainly in cell-specific forms. To date, the ST form of hexokinase (Harrison 1972), the X isoenzyme of lactate dehydrogenase (Markert 1971), hyaluronidase (Metz et al. 1972; Zaneveld et al. 1973), and acrosin (Polakoski and McRorie 1973) have all been shown to be sperm-specific. Phosphoglycerate kinase also appears to have a sperm-specific form (Vandeberg et al. 1973); and sorbitol dehydrogenase, if not cell-specific, is present in such large amounts in sperm cells that it has been used as a biochemical index of spermatogenesis (Bishop 1968). The precise functional significance of sperm-specific enzyme forms is at present unknown. Very little is known about their genetic relationships with the forms found in other tissues and about the mechanisms resulting in their expression. Some of the genes appear to be active only in the primary spermatocytes (see reviews by Blackshaw 1970; Markert 1971), but recent evidence suggests that others may be expressed later in spermatogenesis (Vandeberg et al. 1973).

Mechanisms of Environmental and Structural Maintenance

Maintenance of correct intracellular ion levels, so important to the functioning of any cell, is carried out by ion transport systems that are located in membrane structures and are usually energy-dependent. Such systems, well known in other cell types, have been shown to exist in the spermatozoon—for example, the ATP-dependent sodium-potassium pump (Quinn and White 1967a, 1968). What is particularly interesting with respect to these systems in spermatozoa is that the distribution of the ion pump sites over the membrane area of the (asymmetric) sperm cell is not uniform (O'Donnell and Ellory 1970; Gordon 1973). Such uneven distribution may well prove to be important with respect to physiological function.

The divalent cations, calcium and magnesium, are also important intracellular ions, especially in motile systems. While magnesium, together with potassium, is involved directly in flagellar movement (e.g., Lindemann and Gibbons 1975), calcium has recently been implicated both in the control of motility and in the initiation of the acrosome reaction (see below). Although relatively little attention has so far been devoted to the detailed biochemistry of this latter ion in spermatozoa, two recent discoveries deserve mention. First, Brooks and Siegel (1973) have found a specific calcium-binding phosphoprotein in bull spermatozoa, similar to one found in adrenal medulla and brain. Second, the mitochondria of rabbit spermatozoa have been shown to take up calcium only slowly, unlike the mitochondria of other tissues; moreover, the mitochondrial calcium-transport system in spermatozoa does not react in the same way to inhibitors or to phosphate ions as does the system in other tissues (Storey and Keyhani 1973, 1974b). The significance of these findings is as yet unknown.

The correct functioning of such transport systems, as well as many other important biochemical processes, depends upon the integrity of the cell membranes. This in turn depends largely upon the membranes' phospholipid components being intact. Natural auto-oxidation of fatty acid elements can occur in membranes via peroxide formation, and such oxidation affects the membranes adversely (e.g., Bidlack and Tappel 1973); the cell must be capable of replacing the damaged elements if it is to survive for any length of time. Recent work implies that such peroxide formation can occur in ram spermatozoa (Jones and Mann 1973), and it may therefore be of crucial importance to know whether and how the sperm cell can repair its sensitive membrane components if they become damaged. Its overall biosynthetic capabilities are severely limited. Protein and RNA synthesis may take place to a limited degree in the sperm mitochondria (Premkumar and Bhargava 1972), as has been found for these organelles in other tissues; however, even where true protein synthesis occurs in spermatozoa (see Busby et al. 1974), the amounts of synthesis involved are extremely small and their physiological import is unknown. Biosynthesis of phospholipids has been reported to take place in spermatozoa, but what has actually been demonstrated is that labeled carbon atoms in fatty acids and glucose can be incorporated into lipids and phospholipids. It appears that reactions can take place whereby fatty acids and glycerol moieties (from glucose) can be exchanged with their counterparts in phospholipid and lipid molecules (Minassian and Terner 1966; Scott et al. 1967; Neill and Masters 1972), but de novo synthesis has not been demonstrated and does not seem likely to occur.

Some information on lipid turnover in spermatozoa has been obtained by studying the incorporation of labeled fatty acids into different lipid classes (Mills and Scott 1969; Neill and Masters 1972, 1973, 1974). The results suggest that all the lipid classes are very stable insofar as little or no turnover occurs during epididymal transit, and that even in the presence of fatty acids, only phosphatidyl inositol and the diglycerides are labeled to any great extent; both of these lipid classes are minor components of the total sperm lipid, but apparently they can have a high turnover rate under certain conditions. It is not known whether these classes are preferentially utilized at any stage of the spermatozoon's life or whether they play some part in a possible membrane repair mechanism.

Control of Metabolism

Recent researches into the mechanisms controlling energy metabolism and motility in spermatozoa have produced some significant advances in our understanding of this field, although much remains to be elucidated. Careful and thorough work by the groups led by Hoskins and by Lardy has indicated that alterations in the intracellular cAMP levels almost certainly have a profound effect upon the motility of the sperm cell (Hoskins 1973; Garbers et al. 1973b). The cAMP level is the result of a dynamic balance between the activities of adenyl cyclase (which forms cAMP) and cyclic nucleotide phosphodiesterase (which breaks down cAMP). Alterations in the activity of either of these enzymes will alter the intracellular cAMP level. In vitro, caffeine and other inhibitors of the sperm phosphodiesterase have been used, together with exogenous cAMP, to effect changes in cAMP levels in spermatozoa: a rise in the level stimulates motility considerably and also stimulates both glycolysis and respiration.

Until this discovery, a singular lack of success had

been achieved in controlling sperm energy metabolism and motility. Gross treatments were successful in inducing changes in motility and metabolic rate—e.g., presence or absence of exogenous substrate, presence or absence of oxygen (using nonglycolysable substrates), environmental pH, metabolic inhibitors—but a Pasteur effect (in which glycolysis is reduced under aerobic conditions) could only be demonstrated in epididymal spermatozoa and even then not consistently. The reason for this lack of a Pasteur effect (and, as a corollary, the high glycolytic rates observed in spermatozoa under all conditions) appears to be the relatively low energy-charge ratio (ratio of [ATP] to [ADP] + [AMP]) in the motile spermatozoon (Hoskins et al. 1971). Under these conditions a controlling inhibition of phosphofructokinase is absent, and what little control of glycolytic rate there may be is imposed at the glyceraldehyde 3-phosphate dehydrogenase step, probably through the cytoplasmic $NADH/NAD^+$ ratio. The effect of cAMP on sperm metabolism and motility is therefore a most interesting discovery, particularly since investigations have demonstrated that the primary effect is mediated via motility. The effect on metabolism appears secondary, a consequence of lower energy-charge ratios resulting from increased ATP hydrolysis by the contractile processes.

In other tissues many of the physiological effects of cAMP are expressed through its activation of cAMP-dependent protein kinase. Considerable quantities of such a protein kinase have been demonstrated in spermatozoa, and the enzyme(s) has been isolated and characterized (Hoskins et al. 1972; Garbers et al. 1973c). The direct effect of cAMP on motility and the fact that the cAMP-dependent kinase may constitute as much as 10 percent of the sperm cytoplasmic protein has led naturally to the suggestion that this enzyme is involved in the control or even the mediation of ATP-induced motility. Although no direct evidence for this has yet been obtained, the case for the hypothesis has been strengthened recently by the discovery of equally large amounts of a phosphoprotein phosphatase in spermatozoa (Tang and Hoskins 1975). The phosphatase is apparently specific for proteins phosphorylated by the sperm cAMP-dependent kinase, and in a sperm extract, regulation of the activities of the kinase and phosphatase altered considerably the net incorporation of phosphate into protein.

Despite these seemingly clear-cut discoveries, it remains difficult to assess the degree to which cAMP is involved in changes in sperm activity observed in vivo. The original discoveries were made as a result of research into the cause of the almost instantaneous change from quiescence to activity shown by epididymal spermatozoa on ejaculation. In the hamster Morton and his colleagues (1974) have shown that spermatozoa removed from the epididymis are immotile until calcium ions are added, when the spermatozoa immediately become motile. Calcium ion activation is accompanied by a sudden increase in intracellular cAMP and a simultaneous decrease in the high levels of intracellular ATP. Thus one may suppose that because calcium is demonstrably absent from hamster epididymal fluid, the adenyl cyclase in the spermatozoa is inactive and hence cAMP levels are low; despite the high levels of ATP present, the spermatozoa are therefore immotile. On addition of calcium, the adenyl cyclase is activated, cAMP levels rise, and motility begins.

Unfortunately, such a requirement for calcium may be species-specific (Morita and Chang 1970). In many other species (including bull, boar, ram, and rabbit) the change from quiescence to activity appears to take place as soon as the spermatozoa are removed from the epididymis into direct contact with air, even when they remain in undiluted epididymal fluid. Such behavior suggests that quiescence is a result of lack of oxygen. On the other hand, as mentioned above, although oxygen tension in the epididymal lumen is low, conditions do not appear anaerobic. Moreover, quiescence through lack of oxygen would be mediated via insufficient levels of ATP, and it is difficult to comprehend how the required large quantities of ATP could be replenished as quickly as the activation is observed to take place. It can thus be seen that despite considerable advances, the general process of sperm activation during ejaculation is very far from being understood.

Another change in sperm activity that has been reported to take place in vivo is a considerable enhancement of motility and metabolism in the female tract as a result of capacitation. There is evidence that cAMP is involved in this change also. The time course of the activation resulting from capacitation is considerably slower than the almost instantaneous activation that occurs on ejaculation. The rapidity of the latter change has been a stumbling block with respect to the postulate of cAMP involvement, while the slow process of capacitation agrees better with such a hypothesis.

Nelson has investigated the possibility of the involvement of acetylcholine in the control of motility in spermatozoa, as a parallel to this compound's involvement in transmission of nerve impulses. Considerable acetylcholinesterase activity is present in many species of spermatozoa, and various neurochemical drugs have been shown to greatly affect sea urchin sperm motility, usually in a biphasic fashion causing stimulation at low concentrations and depression at high concentrations. Nelson has presented evidence for cholinoceptive sites in these spermatozoa (Nelson 1973). But there is no evidence to suggest any direct action of these compounds on sperm energy metabolism, and the relationship between acetylcholine metabolism and control of sperm motility is as yet undefined; its involvement in natural changes in sperm activity cannot even be guessed.

32.2 Metabolism Associated with Fertilization Processes

While sperm motility is a necessity for fertilizing ability (and indeed is enhanced in the vicinity of the egg, following capacitation), penetration through the egg investments and entry into the vitellus involves other considerable and specific enzymic action on the part of the spermatozoon. A great deal of research has been carried out lately into this aspect of sperm metabolism, and it has been comprehensively reviewed by McRorie and Williams (1974). Other important related reviews are those by Pikó (1969), Bedford (1970), Austin (1975), and Johnson (1975).

Location of Enzymes
Morphological observations have indicated that the acrosome, which surrounds the anterior of the sperm head, plays a vital role in the fertilization process. The enzymes implicated are hydrolases of various kinds (as far as is known at present), and they are believed to be located in the acrosomal region of the sperm head from whence they act to cut a passage for the spermatozoon through the various investments. A considerable array of hydrolytic enzymes has been detected in extracts from spermatozoa, including hyaluronidase, several proteinases, hexosaminidases, neuraminidase, mannosidase, β-galactosidase, phosphatases, and nonspecific esterases. Such extracts have often been termed *acrosomal extracts* because the acrosomes are disrupted during the procedure, and there has been a tendency to assume a role in the fertilization process for any hydrolase found in them. Unfortunately, other parts of the sperm cell are also extracted at the same time, as revealed by the concomitant presence of cytoplasmic and mitochondrial enzymes. The hydrolases cannot therefore be termed acrosomal in origin on this evidence, and in any case their presence would not be sufficient proof of participation in fertilization.

Some success has been achieved in locating hydrolases in or near the acrosome in spermatozoa. Acid phosphatase is apparently localized in the postacrosomal region and the subacrosomal space (Teichman and Bernstein 1971; Bryan and Unnithan 1973); at least two proteinases are localized in the acrosomal region (Gaddum and Blandau 1970; Yanagimachi and Teichman 1972; Garner et al. 1975) and so is hyaluronidase (Mancini et al. 1964; Fléchon and Dubois 1975). Esterases (Bryan and Unnithan 1973) and ATPases

(Gordon 1973) have also been found. Thus there is no doubt that the acrosomal region is rich in hydrolytic enzymes; moreover, it can be demonstrated that some of the sperm enzymes shown to play a part in fertilization are confined to that area in the cell.

As the spermatozoon passes through the egg investments (i.e., the cumulus and corona cells, the zona pellucida, and the vitelline membrane), changes occur in the sperm head membranes that apparently allow different groups of enzymes in sequence to come into contact with these egg investments. Initially, the surface membrane on the spermatozoon is the plasma membrane; then, during passage through the cumulus and corona cells, the outer acrosomal membrane and the plasma membrane fuse at sites all over the anterior region of the acrosome, and channels are formed to the acrosomal lumen. This is known as the *acrosome reaction*, and it results in the release of the contents of the acrosome into the immediate environs of the head. As the sperm cell approaches the surface of the zona pellucida, the membrane remnants vesiculate and slough off, leaving the inner acrosomal membrane as the new limiting membrane over the anterior part of the sperm head while the cell passes through the zona; during this time the equatorial segment and the postacrosomal region remain covered by the plasma membrane, which is confluent with the acrosomal membrane in the equatorial segment. Finally, at entry into the vitellus, fusion occurs between the vitelline membrane and the sperm plasma membrane in the equatorial and postacrosomal regions. All these morphological events must be borne in mind when interpreting the results of investigations into the possible roles played by the various sperm acrosomal enzymes.

Enzymes Implicated in Fertilization
In order to identify some of the roles, attempts have been made to interfere with sperm-egg interactions by using exogenous agents. At least four enzymes have so far been implicated. It has been known for a long time that hyaluronidase will disperse the cumulus cells surrounding freshly ovulated eggs in the same way as do capacitated spermatozoa. Considerable quantities of a cell-specific form of hyaluronidase have been detected in spermatozoa, apparently localized in the acrosomal region, and in rabbits, a species in which cumulus cells remain around the egg at the time of fertilization, treatment of the spermatozoa with species-specific univalent antisperm antibody will prevent cumulus dispersion, at the same time inhibiting the sperm hyaluronidase (Metz et al. 1972). On the other hand, in a number of animal species the cumulus and corona cells have largely or completely disappeared by the time the spermatozoa normally reach the egg (Restall 1967), yet much hyaluronidase is also found in

these species. This weakens the hypothesis of a specific cumulus-dispersing role for sperm hyaluronidase. Other recent findings suggest a multiple role for the enzyme, however. Metz and Anika (1970) observed that several sperm functions were blocked by univalent antisperm antibody; passage through the cervix and the uterotubal junction was prevented, as was fertilization itself, although the spermatozoa remained unagglutinated and motile. Also, Metz et al. (1972) found that only about half the hyaluronidase in the rabbit spermatozoa was inhibited by the antibody.

Since it is extremely unlikely that antibodies can penetrate the intact sperm plasma membrane, this finding suggested that the accessible hyaluronidase was on the outside surface of that membrane; more recently, O'Rand and Metz (1974), using an antihyaluronidase antibody, have detected the enzyme on the sperm surface. Moreover, the release of hyaluronidase from spermatozoa as a consequence of capacitation, which was previously thought to be a release of intraacrosomal enzyme following the acrosome reaction, has recently been shown to precede the acrosome reaction in hamster spermatozoa (see Talbot and Franklin 1974); this, too, implies that hyaluronidase is located on the outside of the sperm head. In this location the enzyme would be admirably placed to facilitate sperm passage through mucoprotein material such as cervical mucus and cumulus matrix material, and its inhibition might seriously hinder sperm passage: the observations of Metz and Anika (1970) would be entirely explained.

At the same time there is no doubt that hyaluronidase (perhaps a different form—see Morton 1973) is also located within the acrosome (Stambaugh and Buckley 1969, 1970). Brown (1975) and I have found that in media of low ionic strength, considerable quantities of hyaluronidase remain bound in sperm homogenates. These observations imply that much of the enzyme does not leak readily from spermatozoa, as has been widely believed, but remains bound to the inner acrosomal membrane, together with acrosin. Perhaps this hyaluronidase plays a role in zona penetration, either in conjunction or in sequence with acrosin.

A second enzyme that has been implicated in fertilization is the so-called corona-penetrating enzyme. Only Williams and his group have so far investigated this enzyme, and until recently only a single full research paper had been published concerning its properties (Zaneveld and Williams 1970). Now, however, further information has been published on the enzyme's properties and its presence in several sperm species (McRorie and Williams 1974). The unstable nature of the corona-penetrating enzyme, as well as its sensitivity to acrosin (Williams 1972), may perhaps explain why other independent reports of its presence have not been forthcoming. Since it is apparently specifically inhibited by decapacitation factor (see below) and by sialoproteins (Srivastava and Gould 1973), both of which substances can block fertilization, further investigation of this enzyme is certainly warranted. By inference, decapacitation factor acts while acrosomes are still intact, since it is supposed to be reversible in its function. Also, the acrosome reaction does not necessarily occur until after the spermatozoon has passed through the corona layer. One may therefore surmise that, like hyaluronidase, corona-penetrating enzyme is located on the surface of the sperm plasma membrane. Perhaps there is an array of such surface enzymes that cleave bonds in intercellular and secretory material to facilitate passage of the intact sperm cell in the female reproductive tract.

The best-known sperm enzyme with a role in egg penetration is the trypsinlike proteinase, acrosin. Acrosin has been isolated and purified from the spermatozoa of a number of mammalian species. It is a cell-specific enzyme, with catalytic properties akin to thrombin (Polakoski and McRorie 1973) and plasmin (Fritz et al. 1972b), and it seems to be located on the inner acrosomal membrane of all species so far investigated (Stambaugh and Buckley 1969, 1970; Brown and Hartree 1974). Treatment of spermatozoa with trypsin inhibitors blocks fertilization, apparently by preventing the spermatozoa from penetrating the zona pellucida; although the specific inhibition of acrosin in these spermatozoa has not actually been demonstrated, acrosin preparations dissolve the zona and are prevented from doing so when blocked by trypsin inhibitors. The actual nature of the enzyme's action in vivo is unknown; evidence suggests that the enzyme may attack certain specific trypsin-sensitive sites on the zona surface through which the spermatozoon then penetrates the investing layer (Hartmann and Gwatkin 1971; Hartmann and Hutchison 1974).

Neuraminidase activity has been detected in rabbit sperm extracts by one group of workers, although true neuraminidase activity is not found in crude extracts but appears during purification; however, neuraminidase treatment of rabbit eggs denuded of cumulus and corona cells completely inhibits their subsequent fertilization. Also, terminal residues similar to N-acetylneuraminic acid may be associated with the sperm-binding sites on the zona pellucida surface in hamster eggs (Oikawa et al. 1974); using a histochemical method, Soupart and Noyes (1964) could detect sialic acid in the zona pellucida and in the vitelline membrane of rabbit eggs. Thus there is some evidence for the involvement of sperm neuraminidase in egg penetration, perhaps in the initial recognition of the sperm-binding site on the zona.

Mode of Action of Enzymes

Naturally, enzymes other than these four are likely to play a role in sperm passage through the several egg investments; a wide range of possible participants has been detected in sperm extracts from a variety of species (for details see McRorie and Williams 1974). Enzymes may act in sequence or in concert on their respective substrates; some may function at one stage only while others function at several stages. Although some knowledge has been gained concerning the molecular biology of passage through the cumulus and corona mass and the zona pellucida, virtually nothing is known about passage through the vitelline membrane. Most of the complex process of egg penetration and fertilization remains a puzzle and requires much additional research.

With this in mind, some interesting points have recently emerged concerning the mode of action of the acrosomal enzymes. Originally the acrosomal enzymes were surmised to be released into the immediate vicinity of the sperm head following the occurrence of the acrosomal reaction and to act nearby. Observation of the path made by the spermatozoon through the zona pellucida, however, shows it to be a slit just wide enough to allow the sperm head to pass. This is what might be expected from the action of surface-bound enzymes (see Brown and Hartree 1974). There is no evidence of a general corrosive attack in the vicinity of the penetration slit, as might be expected from enzymes diffusing from the acrosome and as has been observed in marine invertebrates. Moreover, trypsin treatment (Hartmann and Gwatkin 1971) or neuraminidase treatment (Gould et al. 1971) of the zona pellucida blocked subsequent fertilization. Although similar treatment with solubilized acrosin does not seem to have been tested, similar results are likely to be obtained. If so, is it not likely that any acrosin and neuraminidase diffusing from the acrosome would act to block fertilization rather than to aid it? The circumstantial evidence suggests that the enzymes effecting sperm passage through the zona are necessarily tightly bound to the inner acrosomal membrane of the spermatozoon, which at that time is the surface membrane. Both the zona pellucida and the vitelline membrane appear to be involved in the species-specificity of fertilization (Hanada and Chang 1972; Yanagimachi 1972; Austin 1975). Perhaps the sperm enzymes involved in penetration are orientated correctly on membrane surfaces, first to effect binding of the spermatozoon to a specific site and then to cleave the various bonds as required to cut a passage through. Up to now, studies on these enzymes have almost exclusively used solubilized preparations. Consideration of the points discussed above implies that much more attention should be paid to their properties in the bound state.

Inhibitors in Seminal Plasma

A curious feature of the metabolism concerned with fertilization in mammals is the presence in seminal plasma of natural factors that will inhibit this process. Two have so far been described, the trypsin inhibitors and the so-called decapacitation factor. The proposal that this factor acts by inhibiting the corona-penetrating enzyme (Williams et al. 1970) is not widely accepted. The methods used to purify and characterize the factor were drastic, such that the end product was certainly not the same entity as the original native macromolecule. Moreover, as discussed above, the existence and action of the corona-penetrating enzyme, its reputed target, remain in question at present. The precise molecular action of the decapacitation factor has not yet been defined, but evidence to be discussed below suggests that it is unlikely to be a specific enzyme inhibitor.

On the other hand, protein trypsin inhibitors are well known to be present in considerable quantities in the seminal plasma of many species; these have been characterized and shown to be highly inhibitory toward purified acrosin (see the review by Fritz et al. 1973), and they can also block fertilization (presumably via inhibition of acrosin). The physiological role of the seminal plasma trypsin inhibitors is difficult to define. Measurements of kinetic constants of the acrosin-inhibitor complex (Fritz et al. 1972a; Zaneveld et al. 1973b) imply that under physiological conditions this complex formation is virtually irreversible. Yet the protein trypsin inhibitors do not affect sperm fertilizing ability unless the spermatozoa have been capacitated, whereas acrosin extracted from ejaculated spermatozoa is partially or completely inhibited. Thus it appears that trypsin inhibitors are present in semen and even in washed sperm suspensions (perhaps attached to the sperm surface), but they do not necessarily form complexes with the acrosin (see discussion by Zaneveld et al. 1973b). My own data suggest that acrosin is inhibited only in damaged spermatozoa, when external inhibitors can pass through the plasma membrane and outer acrosomal membrane, and that the physiological role of the seminal trypsin inhibitors is to block the fertilizing ability of damaged or defective spermatozoa in this way, thereby perhaps helping to obviate imperfections in the conceptus (Harrison 1975).

It is of interest in this respect that in humans and in rhesus monkeys, considerable amounts of certain serum trypsin inhibitors have been found in the secretions of the female reproductive tract as well as in the seminal plasma. Some of these inhibitors have been shown to inhibit acrosin strongly, and their levels in the female tract are hormonally regulated, falling to a minimum at the time of ovulation (Fritz et al. 1972c;

Stambaugh et al. 1974). Since in primates copulation occurs throughout the menstrual cycle, the presence of these inhibitors in the female tract may be a special natural device in this order for ensuring that aged (and thereby defective) spermatozoa, which have been deposited in the tract some time before ovulation, cannot fertilize eggs.

32.3 Long-Term or Irreversible Changes in Spermatozoa

In addition to the obvious manifestations of metabolism in spermatozoa described above, other more subtle metabolic processes occur in these cells. They result in changes in the spermatozoon itself and in its functional capabilities and are thus distinguishable from the control processes described earlier. Some changes occur naturally, usually over a relatively long time period (e.g., the process of sperm maturation that takes place in the epididymis), whereas others can be induced artificially and may take place very rapidly (e.g., changes resulting from cold shock).

Maturation

Spermatogenesis may be considered to terminate with the release of the spermatozoon into the seminiferous tubule. At this stage of its life, however, the spermatozoon is not yet capable of fertilizing an egg. A further process of development is required, known as *maturation*, which takes place as the spermatozoa pass from the rete testis through the length of the epididymis to its cauda (Orgebin-Crist 1969; White 1973). During this period the cells become biologically functional; as far as can be judged by insemination experiments with spermatozoa taken from different sections of the epididymis, the process is completed as the spermatozoa pass through the corpus region of the epididymis (Orgebin-Crist 1969; Overstreet and Bedford 1974). Of course, an enormous number of individual cellular functions are involved in the total fertilization process; up to the present, although many biochemical and morphological changes in the maturing sperm cell have been observed, it has been very difficult to correlate these changes either with each other or with the acquisition of fertilizing ability.

Perhaps the most obvious visible change during maturation is the attainment of motility. Spermatozoa removed from the rete testis are almost completely immotile, while spermatozoa from the cauda epididymidis are highly motile. At the same time, changes in metabolic pattern are observed (Setchell et al. 1969). Testicular spermatozoa show much lower rates of glycolysis and slightly lower rates of respiration than epididymal spermatozoa, and they also have greater synthetic ability, incorporating more carbon moieties from glucose into amino acids, into the glycerol moiety of certain phospholipids, and into inositol (which can then be used as a substrate). Testicular spermatozoa also show a pronounced Pasteur effect, the rate of glycolysis being considerably greater under anaerobic conditions than under aerobic conditions; this anaerobic rate can be as great as or greater than the maximum glycolytic rate observed in epididymal or ejaculated spermatozoa of the same species.

Although the suggestion does not appear to have been made elsewhere, it seems to me highly likely that the differences in metabolic pattern between immature and mature spermatozoa are largely a consequence of the immotility of the immature cells. Since all types of spermatozoa have little overall synthetic ability, total adenine nucleotide content per cell will be the same in all types. In the immotile immature cells, however, ATP will be utilized at a low rate because no contractile processes are occurring, and hence the intracellular energy-charge ratio will be relatively high under aerobic conditions. This will result in considerable inhibition of glycolysis, as well as in some inhibition of oxidative phosphorylation (low [ADP]). Under anaerobic conditions, when ATP cannot be synthesized so efficiently, the continuing low but constant demand for ATP (for ion pumps, for example) will have the effect of reducing the energy-charge ratio, thereby relieving the inhibition of glycolysis. Thus a Pasteur effect is observed in these immotile immature cells. In motile cells, on the other hand, the rate of overall ATP consumption is much higher, and the steady-state intracellular energy-charge ratio is therefore much lower. Little inhibition of glycolysis occurs under these conditions, and thus, under anaerobic conditions, when ATP is produced less efficiently, little effect on glycolytic rates is observed as a result of the further lowering of the energy-charge ratio. Support for this hypothesis is provided by the much lower ATP levels found in epididymal and ejaculated spermatozoa as compared with testicular spermatozoa (quoted by Hoskins 1973). Control of glycolysis in epididymal and ejaculated spermatozoa has been discussed in detail by Hoskins et al. (1971) and by Hoskins (1973).

The lower aerobic glycolytic rate observed in testicular spermatozoa may also account for the greater incorporation of glucose moieties into other molecules. The lower demands on glycolysis and the citric acid cycle as an indirect result of immotility would mean that the levels of some of the intermediates would be considerably higher; thus they could be diverted more efficiently from the main metabolic pathways.

Hence changes in metabolic pattern during maturation are probably due to the acquisition of motility. But what molecular processes result in motility? Re-

cently, in view of the postulated involvement of cAMP in sperm motility, Hoskins et al. (1974) investigated cAMP levels and cAMP-dependent protein kinase activity in immature and mature bull spermatozoa. They found a 40 percent increase in the intracellular cAMP levels during maturation but concluded that there was no difference in protein kinase activity. Moreover, the motility of immature spermatozoa could not be stimulated either by dibutyryl cAMP or by theophylline. The involvement of cAMP in the acquisition of motility is thus equivocal. Morphological changes in the flagellum are observed during sperm maturation: there is a migration and eventual loss of the cytoplasmic droplet, and structural alterations take place in the sperm mitochondria; the cell also loses phospholipid, lipid, protein, and water. None of these can at present be related to motility. On the other hand, Bedford and Calvin (1974a) have shown a considerable decrease in the number of sulphydryl groups in the tail during maturation; since they found concomitant dithiothreitol-sensitive structural stabilization, they concluded that intermolecular disulphide cross-links were formed in certain tail structures during maturation, and they suggested that the formation of the disulphide cross-links and the resultant structural stabilization were related to the acquisition of motility. Although no direct connection between the two events is known at present, these observations offer an exciting new basis for further investigations.

Changes also take place in the sperm head region during maturation. In many species (although not in humans) there are alterations in the size, shape, and internal structure of the acrosome. Subtle changes also occur in the state of the nucleoprotein of all eutherian mammals: the complex becomes more physically condensed and the binding characteristics of the histone to the nucleic acid alter (Gledhill 1971; Calvin and Bedford 1974). These changes are believed to be due to an increase in the intermolecular disulphide bonding in the sperm histone; a sperm-specific cysteine-arginine-rich histone replaces the normal somatic-cell-type histone in the germ cell nucleoprotein of eutherian mammals at the beginning of nuclear elongation in the spermatid (Loir and Hochereau-de Reviers 1972), and during the remaining period of spermatogenesis and subsequent sperm maturation all the cysteine sulphydryl groups in this histone are progressively transformed into intermolecular disulphide bonds (Marushige and Marushige 1975). It has been suggested that condensation of the nucleoprotein plays a significant part in the acquisition of fertilizing ability (Gledhill et al. 1966; Bedford et al. 1973).

Another possible change of obvious importance that might take place during maturation is the conversion of proacrosin to acrosin. Meizel and co-workers

(Huang-Yang and Meizel 1975; Mukerji and Meizel 1975) have discovered an inactive form of acrosin in rabbit testes that undergoes autoactivation at pH 8 to yield active acrosin. The reaction characteristics are typical of autocatalytic activation of a zymogen, and the inactive form has been duly called *proacrosin*. During autoactivation, the zymogen is first transformed to the active form without apparent change in molecular weight; subsequently the active form changes to a form equally active but half the size. Mukerji and Meizel (1975) suggest that proacrosin is either a dimer or a monomer attached to a membrane protein.

The existence of a zymogen form of acrosin seems established, but we do not know by what stage in the sperm's life sufficient active acrosin is formed to permit fertilization. Meizel et al. (1974) reported the presence of proacrosin in rabbit epididymal spermatozoa, and Polakoski (1974) found proacrosin in boar ejaculated spermatozoa. Schill and Fritz (1975) found that during incubation of human spermatozoa in vitro there was an increase in total extractable acrosin activity, which might have been due to autoactivation of a zymogen population. But no quantitative measurements appear to have been made of relative amounts of acrosin and proacrosin at different stages of maturation. This knowledge would obviously be of great interest.

A most important aspect of maturation is the extent to which the process is intrinsic to the spermatozoon, the extent to which it is influenced by exogenous factors in the epididymal tract, and how these factors are related to specific sections of the tract. This aspect is discussed in greater detail by others, but certain points are worth considering here. It is known that very little overall maturation occurs in vitro even in the presence of tract fluids (e.g., Setchell et al. 1969), so not much of the process is intrinsic (although few of the specific aspects of maturation mentioned above have been studied in this respect). If spermatozoa are confined to the initial (caput) segment of the epididymis by ligation, a motility capability and various morphological changes will develop in some species (cf. Gaddum and Glover 1965; Burgos and Tovar 1974), but fertilizing ability can never be developed in the caput segment (Bedford 1967; Orgebin-Crist 1969). Thus actual passage through the various epididymal regions is required.

During maturation, changes take place in the sperm-coating material and in the plasma membrane. Increased negative charge, increased ability to bind colloidal ferric oxide, and the appearance of concanavalin A receptors all indicate considerable changes in the sperm-coating material during passage through the epididymis (see Gordon et al. 1975). There is loss both of phospholipid, in particular phosphatidylcholine and phosphatidylethanolamine, and of lipid, mostly cholesterol—changes that perhaps result in more fluid and less stable membranes (Quinn and White 1967b; Poulos et al. 1973). Certainly during maturation spermatozoa become more susceptible to cold shock (see below). During capacitation—the process of incubation in the female reproductive tract required to prime the spermatozoon before it can take part in fertilization—further specific changes must take place in the sperm-coating material; also, during the fertilization process itself, the acrosome reaction must be able to occur. Thus it seems highly likely that the changes in the sperm coating and the plasma membrane that take place during maturation are such as will allow capacitation and the acrosome reaction to occur (see Johnson 1975). Coating material may be both added and removed; Killian and Amann (1973) found loss of some sperm-coating antigens and appearance of others during passage through the epididymis. Although the changes may be due to alteration of the molecules rather than to their replacement, it is likely to be through the action of specific segments of the epididymis rather than the result of storage. Perhaps it is in this aspect of maturation—the alteration of the sperm coating to allow subsequent capacitation—that the epididymis plays its most vital and specific role.

Capacitation and the Acrosome Reaction
Before they can penetrate the egg, spermatozoa require a period of incubation in the female reproductive tract, during which critical changes take place in the sperm cell. The process of change is termed *capacitation*. Such an important process has naturally received a great deal of attention, and the physiological aspects of capacitation have been extensively reviewed (Bedford 1970; Chang and Hunter 1975). Some of the biochemistry of the process has also been reviewed by Williams (1972), and an excellent discussion of some of its possible molecular events has been presented by Johnson (1975).

Initially, capacitation was considered to be a single complex process, beginning in the female tract after ejaculation and culminating in the initiation of egg penetration. When the acrosome reaction was first recognized, it was thought to be a part of capacitation, the final series of events in the process. It has become clear, however, that the acrosome reaction can be dissociated from capacitation (Bavister 1973; Mahi and Yanagimachi 1973; Bryan 1974), since it occurs as the result of a specific stimulus usually associated with the freshly ovulated egg. Leading workers in the field now consider capacitation to be the process that prepares the sperm cell so that the acrosome reaction will occur in response to the specific egg-associated stimulating factor (see, e.g., Bedford 1970; Yanagimachi and Usui

1974). This clear distinction between the acrosome reaction and capacitation is very important; before the distinction was made, much confusion and apparent contradiction existed in the literature.

The molecular events involved in the acrosome reaction are unknown: morphologically it can be observed that the plasma membrane and outer acrosomal membrane fuse at points all over the anterior acrosomal region, and holes through the two membranes appear at these points; eventually the entire region becomes detached from the sperm head and is lost. Johnson (1975) has discussed the possible changes in molecular organization that might take place and processes that might lead to the occurrence of such changes. There is no doubt that the acrosomal region is inherently unstable—acrosomal damage is a commonly used parameter in the assessment of treatments that might be detrimental to the cell. Such instability may either be a reflection of the properties of the coating material in that region—see Gordon et al. (1975) for discussion of local specificity of the sperm coating —or it may be an intrinsic property of the underlying membranes. As a prerequisite to membrane fusion, however, specific destabilization must apparently be brought about, probably by the removal or alteration of sperm-coating material.

Once destabilized, the membranes respond to a specific stimulus by undergoing the changes seen in the acrosome reaction. A stimulating factor has been studied: it seems to be a high-molecular-weight component, present in follicular fluid, though also found in blood (Yanagimachi 1969, 1970a; Bavister and Morton 1974). Evidence suggests that this factor is associated with the egg in some way, but it is probably a component of the follicular fluid, physically adsorbed to or trapped within the egg investments, rather than an intrinsic component of these investments. Of course, other factors may also be involved, for in some species the acrosome reaction can occur in the absence of follicular fluid or serum (Miyamoto and Chang 1973; Barros et al. 1973). Yanagimachi and Usui (1974) have shown that calcium ions will trigger the reaction in capacitated guinea pig spermatozoa, and others have found that the same ion enhances fertilization in the mouse and the rabbit, perhaps through a similar effect (see Davis et al. 1974).

Capacitation, therefore, is the process of destabilization of the sperm membranes that allows them to undergo the acrosome reaction when suitably stimulated. A great deal of evidence now suggests that the destabilization results from the removal or alteration of sperm-coating material. A number of workers have reported considerable changes in the sperm coating during capacitation, especially in the region of the head (Johnson and Hunter 1972; Oliphant and Brack-

ett 1973a; Gordon et al. 1975), and capacitation has been induced by treatments that apparently remove or modify coating material (Kirton and Hafs 1965; Gwatkin and Hutchison 1971; Johnson and Hunter 1972; Aonuma et al. 1973; Brackett and Oliphant 1975). Moreover, after removal of coating, further treatment with seminal plasma to replace it blocks the ability to undergo the acrosome reaction (Oliphant 1974).

The original report of the decapacitation factor in seminal plasma (Chang 1957) described its effect as reversible. Studies of the effect and the factor causing it have resulted in a vast and confused literature: some purification methods have resulted in highly degraded products whose physiological action is dubious; others have used a very crude seminal plasma pellet; most studies have failed to distinguish possible irreversible effects on spermatozoa undergoing the acrosome reaction from effects on the capacitation process per se. But Reyes et al. (1975) have now reported the partial purification and identification of a soluble glycoprotein from rabbit seminal plasma that reversibly blocks fertilization; they were able to show indirectly that the factor was a sperm-coating antigen.

It thus appears clear that capacitation is the specific removal and/or modification of sperm-coating glycoprotein substances that stabilize the sperm membranes, particularly in the acrosomal region; the decapacitation factor acts by recoating the sperm surface and restabilizing it. It can be inferred that the coating properties of the protein found by Reyes et al. (1975) would cause it to be found in large amounts on the particles so profuse in rabbit seminal plasma (Metz et al. 1968); in this species the coating protein would therefore be concentrated in a pellet obtained by high-speed centrifugation, whereas in species whose seminal plasma contains less particulate matter, such an effect would be less pronounced. The apparent contradictions between the work of Reyes et al. (1975), Davis (1974), and Williams et al. (1967) would thereby be explained. It may be that the antifertility effect of the sperm-coating material can be mimicked by other similar glycoprotein substances. Both fetuin and Cowper's gland mucin are reported to have an antifertility effect on capacitated rabbit spermatozoa (Srivastava and Gould 1973); although the authors claimed that these glycoproteins inhibited the corona-penetrating enzyme, it seems more likely that the antifertility action is mediated via a sperm-coating capability and a consequent restabilization of the capacitated sperm membranes.

In vivo, capacitation changes are almost certainly brought about enzymically. A number of different enzymes may be involved, either simultaneously or sequentially, and some sperm species may well have wider enzymic requirements than others—this would explain the considerable species variation in capacitation requirements (see Barros et al. 1973). Enzymes that have been shown to effect some degree of capacitation are β-amylase, β-glucuronidase, papain, trypsin, pronase, and neuraminidase (see Johnson 1975). Detailed study of enzymes in the female reproductive tract has not been carried out with respect to possible capacitatory action, although correlation between the capacitatory action of β-glucuronidase, its presence in the uterus, and uterine capacitatory function was discussed by Johnson and Hunter (1972). Some evidence suggests that a sequential action is required and that the relevant enzymes may be located in different regions of the female tract; capacitation is completed much more rapidly if spermatozoa are allowed to pass from the uterus to the oviducts, as in vivo, than if they are confined to either the uterus or the oviduct alone (see Bedford 1970; Chang and Hunter 1975). Future investigations of possible capacitating enzymes should take this observation into account.

In addition to conferring the ability to undergo the acrosome reaction, capacitation results in a considerable and peculiar enhancement of motility (Iwamatsu and Chang 1969; Yanagimachi 1970b; Barros et al. 1973) and an increase in energy metabolism (Hamner and Williams 1963; Mounib and Chang 1964; Iritani et al. 1969). Recently evidence has accrued to suggest that cAMP may be involved in these changes. Factors assumed to enhance the intracellular cAMP level can cause increases in oxygen consumption and motility when added to ejaculated spermatozoa; the effect of these factors is similar to the effect of incubation *in utero* (Hicks et al. 1972a,b; Garbers et al. 1973a; Schoenfeld et al. 1975). In addition, alterations in the properties of adenyl cyclase (which synthesizes cAMP) have been reported to occur after capacitation (Morton and Albagli 1973), and cAMP itself can speed up capacitation in vitro (Toyoda and Chang 1974; Rosado et al. 1974). Rogers and Morton (1973) have reported a decrease in ATP content in hamster spermatozoa during capacitation, which would agree with the postulated scheme for control of energy metabolism described above: cAMP enhances motility directly, which causes ATP to be utilized more rapidly; as a result, the energy-charge ratio decreases, and oxidative phosphorylation and glycolysis are thereby stimulated. A low-molecular-weight factor has been found in follicular fluid and serum that stimulates motility in capacitated hamster spermatozoa (Yanagimachi 1969; Morton and Bavister 1974; Bavister 1975); and Gaur and Talwar (1973) have described a low-molecular-weight factor from human seminal plasma that promotes fertilization. These factors may act by stimulating the sperm adenyl cyclase to produce increased intracellular levels of cAMP, thereby enhancing moti-

lity and metabolism as suggested above. It is of interest that calcium will cause the specific stimulation of motility in capacitated guinea pig spermatozoa (Yanagimachi and Usui 1974), for the same ion apparently stimulates adenyl cyclase in epididymal spermatozoa from this species (Morton et al. 1974).

The motility-stimulating factor is seemingly unable to act on the uncapacitated cell. An initial period of quiescence called the *preparatory phase* lasts for most of the process of capacitation (Mahi and Yanagimachi 1973); presumably it is during this time that the changes occur in the sperm coating. Only when the preparatory phase is completed does the peculiar intense motility pattern develop (*activation*). Perhaps removal of the coating unmasks binding sites for the motility-stimulating factor that were previously unavailable.

The complexity of capacitation and the ensuing acrosome reaction obviously makes biochemical study of the process very difficult. The sequence of events implies that careful consideration must be given to the timing of sampling, and the effects observed must be related to the physiological state of the cells. For example, studies on motility and metabolism must take into account a possible requirement for the preparatory phase before effects can be mediated. Moreover, it is well known that spermatozoa are more labile after capacitation (see Bedford 1970; Chang and Hunter 1975); great care must therefore be taken not to introduce artifactual effects of suboptimal media and handling techniques.

A physiological reason has not been ascertained for the special pattern of vigorous motility observed after capacitation. As suggested by Rogers and Morton (1973), however, enhanced motility may be necessary for or beneficial to penetration of the zona pellucida. Bedford and Calvin (1974b) have discussed the selecting effects of this resistant egg investment with respect to the development of a mechanically strong sperm head in eutherian mammals; an advantage may be similarly conferred by the special capacitated motility pattern. The metabolic results of the acrosome reaction with respect to the fertilization process have been discussed earlier. The hydrolases involved in fertilization are potentially damaging to structural elements in both the male and the female reproductive tracts. It would appear that the role of the acrosome is to sequester the hydrolases required for egg penetration within a membrane system that is unaffected by these enzymes, until the spermatozoon is in the immediate vicinity of the egg. Then, as a result of the ensuing acrosome reaction, the hydrolases are unmasked and rendered capable of acting upon the egg investments. The concept that the acrosome is a type of lysosome is now well established (Hartree 1975); it is therefore constructive to compare the behavior of the enzymes within the acrosome to those within somatic cell lysosomes and to liken the acrosome reaction to events such as the fusion of lysosomes with phagocytic vesicles. In this respect, the recent reports that calcium may be involved in triggering the acrosome reaction (Yanagimachi and Usui 1974; Davis et al. 1974) are of considerable interest, because this ion is believed to play an important role in membrane fusion events, especially those involving lysosomes (see Johnson 1975).

Senescence and Damage

Maturation is complete once the spermatozoon acquires fertilizing ability. But processes of change in the cell do not cease at this stage, for degenerative changes take place as a function of cell age. The general effect is known as *aging* and the resultant state as *senescence*. The characteristics of senescence in spermatozoa have been widely described and are set out in detail in a recent review (Mann and Lutwak-Mann 1975). On a gross scale, they consist of general degeneration and disintegration of membranes, particularly of the acrosome, accompanied by leakage of intracellular components. Yet previous to this extremity, a loss of fertilizing capacity occurs and changes are observed in glycolytic and respiratory rates and in the sperm nucleoprotein.

The molecular events involved in these observed changes and what causes their onset are not clear. As Mann and Lutwak-Mann (1975) have pointed out, the spermatozoon offers a particularly good model for studying aging processes because its nucleus is inactive and RNA is virtually absent; hence neither cell division nor protein synthesis occurs, and there is little regenerative ability to counteract degeneration. Detailed knowledge of the structural biochemistry of the spermatozoon is still scanty, however; changes that might take place in these structures can only be guessed with difficulty. Although mature spermatozoa are more prone than immature spermatozoa to become senescent, the processes that result in senescence are probably not a continuation of those that bring about maturation; more probably, maturation induces susceptibility to processes that cause senescence. Environment plays a considerable part in aging, as may be seen by comparing the fertile life span of rabbit spermatozoa in the cauda epididymidis (up to 49 days) with that in different regions of the female reproductive tract (no more than 32 hours) and with that in vitro (only a few moments, at high dilution). Thus the effect of artificial environment or treatment in causing senescence in spermatozoa is a most important field of study; moreover, the possibility of accidental damage to the cells may thereby be revealed so that future methodology can be modified.

There is no doubt that the cell-coating material plays an important part in the maintenance of viability. Coating material is readily eluted from spermatozoa by isotonic or slightly hypertonic saline solutions (Aonuma et al. 1973; Oliphant and Brackett 1973b; Brackett and Oliphant 1975), and treatments that would be expected to do this so that little coating material remains in the sperm environment are detrimental to these cells; such treatments include washing or dilution into a large volume, using solutions in which the osmolarity is maintained largely or wholly by ions. Protection is afforded by protein substances such as albumin, which may replace or prevent removal of the cell coating (Bredderman and Foote 1971b; Morton and Chang 1973; Lindholmer 1974). Similarly, capacitation, during which sperm coating material is removed, renders the cells very labile (see above), and there is evidence to suggest that capacitated spermatozoa can be stabilized in vitro by material that almost certainly contains sperm-coating substances (White et al. 1975). It is thought that coating substances act by stabilizing the plasma membrane. This latter structure is certainly a vulnerable part of the sperm cell, and its integrity is essential for motility and fertilizing ability.

Mechanisms involved in maintenance of the membrane structure are complex. In a series of fascinating studies, Bredderman and Foote (1969, 1971a, b) demonstrated that swelling and loss of motility, which reflect changes in the sperm plasma membrane, occurred in saline solutions in the absence of potassium ions or after a breakdown in the supply of intracellular ATP. Best maintenance of motility and protection against swelling were provided by inclusion of albumin, low levels of potassium, and an energy source in the saline medium. The functioning of the sodium-potassium pump therefore seems to be involved in the maintenance of the membrane structure. Later studies (Bredderman and Foote 1971c) showed that although calcium ions prevented swelling, they had a detrimental effect on motility; the investigators surmised that calcium competed for binding sites on the plasma membrane when the sodium-potassium pump was no longer functioning efficiently and thereby altered the properties of the membrane.

Obviously, spermatozoa can be damaged by treatments well known to be detrimental to cells: acid or alkaline conditions, detergents, reactive chemicals, osmotic shock, and deep-freezing, among others; the actions of these are generally well understood. Spermatozoa are also susceptible to sudden reductions of temperature below 15°C, however, even though freezing does not occur. This treatment, known as cold shock, results in a permanent loss of fertilizing ability and motility. Since low temperature storage of spermatozoa for artificial insemination involves exposure to this critical region of temperature (15°C–0°C), the phenomenon has been investigated extensively. Cold shock causes considerable measurable damage: morphological damage to the acrosome, increase in uptake of vital stains, loss of phospholipid-containing material, abolition of metabolic functions, leakage of intracellular enzymes, breakdown of intracellular metabolites, and alterations in intracellular ionic composition (for bibliography, see Darin-Bennett et al. 1973b; Mann and Lutwak-Mann 1975); some species of spermatozoa are more susceptible to cold shock than others.

The major result of cold shock is a breakdown of membrane structure and function; this catastrophe would bring about virtually all the measurable damage observed. Why a sudden reduction in temperature should cause such a breakdown is not clear. Many theories have been proposed, most of them focusing upon a particular event such as loss of specific phospholipids or uptake of calcium ions (both of which occur during cold shock) as the primary causative factor. It seems more likely that several factors are involved. Probably one of the primary events is a loss or loosening of sperm-coating material, which reduces the stability of the plasma membrane. At the same time the activity of the sodium-potassium pump is drastically reduced due to the fall in temperature, and this too renders the membrane labile. In combination, the two events would almost certainly result in immediate structural and functional degeneration of the membrane, followed by actual disruption. Most of the observable effects of cold shock, such as leakage of enzymes or loss of phospholipid material, are the result of the final disruption.

Cold shock may therefore affect spermatozoa by a mechanism identical to that of excessive dilution; the events and their result just occur much more rapidly. Supporting this hypothesis is the fact that spermatozoa can be protected to some degree against both treatments by low levels of potassium ions, maintaining ion pump function or at least structure (White 1953; O'Shea and Wales 1966), and by egg yolk (Cheng et al. 1949; see also Darin-Bennett et al. 1973b). Since the detailed effects of dilution upon the sperm plasma membrane have only recently been described, protection by phospholipids agaist dilution has not yet been tested; however, these compounds can protect effectively against cold shock. Butler and Roberts (1975) have shown that protection is specifically afforded by different phospholipids for different sperm species. These probably bind to the membrane itself and act to stabilize the structure under adverse conditions; Watson (1975) has shown that a high-molecular-weight, low-density lipoprotein component—which is the main cryoprotective agent in egg yolk (Pace and Gra-

ham 1974)—will compete for binding sites on the sperm plasma membrane.

To summarize, then, the structures in the spermatozoon most sensitive to suboptimal treatments appear to be the coating material and the plasma membrane. In the intact cell the coating plays an important part in maintaining the functional and structural integrity of the membrane and its components. Loss of the coating leads to instability of the membrane, and in the absence of the correct environment, degeneration and disruption quickly follow, with the resultant death of the cell. When handling spermatozoa in vitro, it is essential to maintain the integrity of the coating and membrane by correct ionic balance, avoidance of high ionic strengths, and inclusion of a coating factor in the sperm environment.

In vivo, damage to the spermatozoon is likely to occur along similar lines, but the agents are probably hydrolytic enzymes in the sperm environment. Glycosidases and proteinases could bring about changes in the sperm coating to render the cell intrinsically less stable (e.g., capacitation), after which phospholipases and proteinases might be capable of acting on the plasma membrane components, particularly if alterations in the membrane structure occurred. Masaki (1974) has found that phospholipase action on spermatozoa of several species is greatly enhanced after freezing and thawing. This suggests that sites sensitive to enzymic attack are protected in the intact cell; after damage, however, the sites are exposed. It is well known that epididymal spermatozoa are less susceptible to cold shock than are ejaculated spermatozoa, and a number of workers have reported the detrimental action of seminal plasma on these cells. Specific factors appear to be involved (Shannon 1965; Dott 1974), and these may come from particular accessory glands (Quinn et al. 1968; Morita and Chang 1970). From discussions above it is not unreasonable to assume that, because susceptibility to cold shock is induced, alterations in sperm-coating material are involved, brought about by specific enzyme action. Isolation and characterization of these seminal plasma factors could greatly improve our understanding of aging processes.

In addition to changes brought about by external factors, other intrinsic changes may take place within the sperm cell as a function of age. The active life of an enzyme can be terminated by loss of conformational structure resulting from molecular vibration. Statistically this situation could obviously occur even in an optimal environment, and the lack of synthetic ability in the spermatozoon would render it unable to replace inactivated enzyme molecules. If an essential enzyme were particularly sensitive to such inactivation, a finite functional life span would automatically be built into the sperm cells. Another possible cause of senescence not entirely unrelated to this concept is naturally occurring peroxide formation in lipids, which could have the effect of disturbing lipid conformation in membranes, thus leading to membrane degeneration. This was mentioned above in the section on energy metabolism and is discussed in detail with respect to aging by Mann and Lutwak-Mann (1975).

A factor damaging to spermatozoa that has been almost completely ignored by most workers is light. Norman et al. (1962) reported that light, in particular in the blue region, is toxic to spermatozoa, leading to a decline in motility and eventual cell death. The effect appeared to be mediated through peroxide formation since catalase, thiols, or lack of oxygen protected against it; because it was independent of temperature, the primary action was considered typical of photosensitized oxidation. Independently, Hamner and Williams (1961) described the stimulation of sperm respiration by even relatively short exposure of the cells to light, and later (1963) they showed that the stimulation of sperm respiration by incubation in utero could be largely masked by prior exposure to light.

Lack of interest in the effect of light on spermatozoa may stem from a possible implication by Mann (1964) that the observations reported by the two groups were due to two different and opposing processes, one detrimental and the other beneficial. Mann has always been at pains to point out, however, that stimulation of metabolism is not necessarily indicative of a beneficial effect (e.g., Mann 1964, p. 340). Thus the stimulation of sperm respiration by light may well be an uncoupling process. It is tempting to speculate that light can cause lipid peroxide formation in the membranes of the spermatozoon and thereby lead to structural and functional degeneration. While this may not be an important aging process in vivo, its relevance to the handling of spermatozoa both for experimental and for artificial insemination purposes cannot be doubted.

A great deal of research has been devoted to the effect of aging on sperm nucleoprotein. Although at one time such an effect was reported, more recent work has failed to show any changes in DNA content and has also failed to connect any observed changes in nucleoprotein characteristics with infertility. Changes that have been reported suggest merely a completion of the condensation process that takes place during maturation.

Some very recent observations on the state of acrosin in the spermatozoon offer a new and interesting line of investigation. In studies on the activation of proacrosin (the inactive zymogen of acrosin), Mukerji and Meizel (1975) observed an alteration in the molecular weight of acrosin that took place subsequent to activation and could be due to the loss of a membrane-binding component. Schill and Fritz (1975) reported an

activation and subsequent release of acrosin from human spermatozoa into the external media during prolonged incubation. Since in freshly prepared samples acrosin is very firmly bound to the head in all species so far studied (Stambaugh and Buckley 1970; Brown and Hartree 1974), one is tempted to interpret the observations of Schill and Fritz in the light of Mukerji and Meizel's findings—that is, a release of acrosin from the inner acrosomal membrane followed by leakage of this free enzyme from degenerating acrosomes into the external medium. The changes described by Schill and Fritz were temperature-dependent and therefore probably involved enzymic action, although they occurred more rapidly in saline media than in seminal plasma. If such a release from the acrosomal membrane takes place as a function of age in spermatozoa, it could explain early and specific loss of fertilizing ability observed during aging (e.g., Gulyas 1968) by the argument developed in the section on the mode of action of fertilization enzymes—free acrosin may actually prevent fertilization by reacting prematurely with the sperm-binding sites on the zona pellucida.

A discussion of sperm damage would not be complete without some mention of the effects of the antifertility agent α-chlorohydrin on spermatozoa. It appears that the primary antifertility action of the compound in vivo is on the spermatozoa themselves in the epididymis, where it rapidly produces depressed motility and metabolism (Brown and White 1973; Vickery et al. 1974; Brown-Woodman et al. 1975). A direct effect of α-chlorohydrin in vitro on the metabolism of spermatozoa has been demonstrated by Mohri et al. (1975). These workers found a dramatic and specific loss of glyceraldehyde 3-phosphate dehydrogenase activity in ram spermatozoa incubated in vitro with α-chlorohydrin, although the compound did not affect the isolated enzyme in assays in vitro. Mohri and his colleagues postulated that α-chlorohydrin was phosphorylated by the spermatozoon to 1-chloro-1-deoxyglycerol 3-phosphate and that this latter compound was the active agent, competitively inhibiting the sperm glyceraldehyde 3-phosphate dehydrogenase. Such an interpretation is not consistent with the known facts, however. First, such a process would be unlikely to reduce sperm motility under aerobic conditions as observed, for metabolic pathways other than glycolysis supply much of the energy under these conditions. Second, α-chlorohydrin has recently been shown to be rapidly dechlorinated in vivo, and it does not appear to interfere with glycerol metabolism (Edwards et al. 1975); a specific action of 1-chloro-1-deoxyglycerol 3-phosphate cannot be reconciled with these observations. Nevertheless the careful and important observations of Mohri and his colleagues may have provided the best clue to the action of α-chlorohydrin.

Jackson has investigated the considerable antifertility action of alkylating chemicals and has produced evidence to show that α-chlorohydrin is itself an alkylating agent and that it may act as such in vivo (Jones et al. 1969; Jackson et al. 1970). Such an action would be entirely consistent with the effects of α-chlorohydrin observed both in vivo and in vitro. Glyceraldehyde 3-phosphate dehydrogenase is an enzyme whose activity depends on a cysteine group in the active site (Mahler and Cordes 1971, pp. 509–511); it is very sensitive to thiol reagents (which include alkylating agents). The apparent specific sensitivity to α-chlorohydrin of the spermatozoa in the epididymis may be correlated with the large number of thiol groups found in the immature epididymal cells. These thiol groups disappear during maturation, an event that has been related to the acquisition of motility (Bedford and Calvin 1974a). Such thiol groups would naturally be targets for alkylating agents, and one can imagine that the prevention of specific thiol cross-linking during maturation, through blocking with alkylating agents, would interfere seriously with motility. Thus it seems quite likely that α-chlorohydrin acts in vivo and in vitro as an alkylating agent. Its primary targets in vivo are the alkyl-sensitive thiol groups in the immature sperm tail. Since in mature spermatozoa these thiol groups may have largely taken part in cross-linking, α-chlorohydrin acts on ejaculated spermatozoa in vitro by alkylating other sensitive thiol groups, of which glyceraldehyde 3-phosphate dehydrogenase contains a functionally important example.

32.4 Whither?

As one of the two principals in the reproductive process in higher organisms, the spermatozoon's importance can hardly be questioned. It also goes without saying that advances in our knowledge of sperm metabolism must immediately and fundamentally advance our knowledge of reproduction.

We now have a considerable grounding in the understanding of mammalian sperm metabolism, and it is timely in the present atmosphere of frugality to try to direct our further research efforts in the field toward the areas most likely to yield especially significant information for both basic knowledge and fertility control. In retrospect, I feel that the two most important individual contributions made in the field of sperm metabolism in the last decade have been, first, the discovery of the acrosomal proteinase acrosin and the demonstration of its essential role in egg penetration, and second, the recent demonstration that the primary control of motility is direct and not via the supply of energy. At the same time it would be both unfair and

invidious not to point out that very many other contributions, while possibly not as obviously important individually, have together advanced our understanding far more in overall terms.

The discovery of acrosin and its role in the penetration of the zona pellucida was the first clearly defined biochemical evidence for acrosomal lytic action during fertilization. Unfortunately, specific roles for other sperm enzymes in egg penetration have not been as clearly demonstrated. The obvious fundamental position of fertilization in sperm metabolism must therefore signpost one direction of further research. The enzymic processes directly involved in the spermatozoon's role in fertilization, particularly in egg penetration, must be defined as closely as possible. During such research it will be essential to correlate relevant enzyme activities with their location and state in or on the spermatozoon, and to compare this information as carefully as possible with known details of the penetration process. For example, if an enzyme thought to be involved in fertilization is found to be entirely in a free state within the acrosome, it would be extremely difficult to envisage its participation in fusion with the vitelline membrane.

Direct blocking of fertility by inhibition of an enzyme essential for egg penetration is certainly a plausible potential method of contraception. Nevertheless, at the present time it is difficult to see how this could be achieved on a practical basis. Low-molecular-weight materials introduced systemically would be likely to have toxic side effects by virtue of lack of target specificity. Direct treatment by deposition of agents intravaginally would be inconvenient from a practical standpoint as well as open to the same criticism of toxicity. High-molecular-weight inhibitors of acrosomal enzymes, such as protein trypsin inhibitors that inhibit acrosin, would almost certainly be ineffective, because it is unlikely that acrosomal enzymes are available to exogenous macromolecules until the acrosome reaction has occurred in the vicinity of the egg in the Fallopian tube. It is difficult to imagine how these macromolecular inhibitors could be induced in high concentration into this region of the female reproductive tract. As described in the section on fertilization metabolism, however, there is now some evidence that certain enzymes directly involved in fertilization processes may be located on the exterior of the sperm plasma membrane. Specific inhibition of these enzymes might be a more practical possibility, since they are likely to be readily accessible. Inhibition of one of them, using immunological methods, has already been shown to be associated with fertilization blocking. This sperm enzyme, hyaluronidase, appears to be a species-specific sperm antigen, and its specific inhibition by immunological means obviously offers a sensitive method of reducing fertility. In light of earlier remarks regarding the availability of fertilization enzymes to external macromolecules, it is of interest that hyaluronidase is the only acrosomal enzyme against which antibodies have proved to be effective inhibitors (Metz 1974, quoted by Austin 1975).

The demonstration that cAMP in spermatozoa stimulates motility directly and only affects metabolism secondarily via the resultant increased rate of ATP utilization has profound implications for future research on sperm metabolism. Obviously far more than enough ATP can be generated under aerobic conditions to supply the requirements for motility, and thus motility is not limited by energy supply in the presence of exogenous substrates. The wide metabolic capabilities of spermatozoa enable them to draw on a range of substrates (simultaneously, if need be), and it seems most likely that there is normally end-product inhibition of oxidative phosphorylation in these cells, both in vivo and in vitro, set by the intracellular ATP/ADP ratio acting at the final phosphorylation step, on citrate synthetase, and on isocitrate dehydrogenase (see Mahler and Cordes 1971, pp. 626–629). In other words, under in vivo conditions, levels of exogenous substrates would rarely, if ever, be so low as to limit energy supply. Therefore further work on substrate utilization in spermatozoa is likely to be relatively unproductive, offering few advances in reproductive knowledge and little possibility for fertility control—except perhaps in the human. The apparent inability of human spermatozoa to metabolize substrates via the citric acid cycle and oxidative phosphorylation suggests that these cells must rely exclusively on glycolysable sugars as energy sources. Since the cervix might be a critical region with respect to available substrates, investigation of methods to alter levels of glycolysable substrates in this region in humans may provide a fruitful possibility for contraceptive development.

The apparent direct effect of cAMP on sperm motility also offers an immediate starting point for further research into the control of sperm motility. The possible connection between cAMP and motility via cAMP-dependent protein kinase has already been suggested. Further research into the biochemistry of sperm motility, especially into the enzymology of energy transduction, should yield significant advances in reproductive knowledge. A particularly attractive possibility for the suppression of fertility is that unique control mechanisms for motility may exist in the spermatozoon, which can be acted upon specifically in vivo without the risk of nonspecific general toxicity due to systemic application. It is well known that permanently immotile spermatozoa are incapable of fertilizing ova.

Several other specific areas for future research have been delineated in the course of this review, and some of the speculative interpretations of known facts may suggest more ideas. But the most obvious gap in our understanding of sperm physiology lies in our lack of knowledge concerning the biology of the sperm investments—the sperm-coating material, the plasma membrane, the inner and outer acrosomal membranes, the postacrosomal cap, and the nuclear membrane. Membrane biology is currently assuming great importance, especially with respect to the spermatozoa. Many important sperm enzymes are membrane-bound. Great changes in the membranes of the head take place during the acrosomal reaction. The postacrosomal cap and equatorial region are implicated in sperm-egg fusion. Changes in the cell-coating material and the plasma membrane occur in vivo, during maturation, capacitation, and aging; and similar changes can be brought about as a result of cold shock or dilution in artificial media. It seems a strong possibility that low membrane permeability to certain substrates could account for the much lower overall rates of metabolism shown by some sperm species, notably the boar. And yet, despite their obvious fundamental importance in sperm function, research on the sperm investments has been directed mainly toward immediate solutions of practical problems (e.g., the freezing of semen for artificial insemination purposes) and has been largely empirical in approach. Thus detailed basic information should be gained concerning the biochemistry and physiology of the sperm investments. Apart from a great need to understand the roles played by them in reproduction, it seems highly likely that interference with the investments, perhaps by immunological means, will offer a specific and sensitive method of blocking fertility. Moreover, thorough understanding of the biology of the sperm membrane will certainly allow a more logical approach to improving fertility, particularly of stored semen.

References

Adam, D. E., and J. Wei. Mass transport of ATP within the motile sperm. J. Theor. Biol. 49:125, 1975.

Anderson, W. A., and P. Personne. Recent cytochemical studies on spermatozoa of some invertebrate and vertebrate species. In *Comparative spermatology*, ed. B. Baccetti, p. 431. London: Academic Press, 1970.

Aonuma, S., T. Mayuma, K. Suzuki, T. Noguchi, M. Iwai, and M. Okabe. Studies on sperm capacitation. I. The relationship between a guinea-pig sperm-coating antigen and a sperm capacitation phenomenon. J. Reprod. Fertil. 35:425, 1973.

Austin, C. R. Membrane fusion events in fertilization. J. Reprod. Fertil. 44:155, 1975.

Barros, C., M. Berrios, and E. Herrera. Capacitation in vitro of guinea-pig spermatozoa in a saline solution. J. Reprod. Fertil. 34:547, 1973.

Bavister, B. D. Capacitation of golden hamster spermatozoa during incubation in culture medium. J. Reprod. Fertil. 35:161, 1973.

Bavister, B. D. Properties of the sperm motility-stimulating component derived from human serum. J. Reprod. Fertil. 43:363, 1975.

Bavister, B. D., and D. B. Morton. Separation of human serum components capable of inducing the acrosome reaction in hamster spermatozoa. J. Reprod. Fertil. 40:495, 1974.

Bedford, J. M. Effects of duct ligation on the fertilizing ability of spermatozoa from different regions of the rabbit epididymis. J. Exp. Zool. 166:271, 1967.

Bedford, J. M. Sperm capacitation and fertilization in mammals. Biol. Reprod. Suppl. 2:128, 1970.

Bedford, J. M., M. J. Bent, and H. Calvin. Variations in the structural character and stability of the nuclear chromatin in morphologically normal human spermatozoa. J. Reprod. Fertil. 33:19, 1973.

Bedford, J. M., and H. I. Calvin. Changes in -S-S- linked structures of the sperm tail during epididymal maturation, with comparative observations in sub-mammalian species. J. Exp. Zool. 187:181, 1974a.

Bedford, J. M., and H. I. Calvin. The occurrence and possible functional significance of -S-S- crosslinks in sperm heads, with particular reference to eutherian mammals. J. Exp. Zool. 188:137, 1974b.

Bidlack, W. R., and A. L. Tappel. Damage to microsomal membrane by lipid peroxidation. Lipids 8:177, 1973.

Bishop, D. W. Sorbitol dehydrogenase in relation to spermatogenesis and fertility. J. Reprod. Fertil. 17:410, 1968.

Blackshaw, A. W. Histochemical localization of testicular enzymes. In The testis, Vol. 2, eds. A. D. Johnson, W. R. Gomes, and N. L. Vandemark, p. 73. New York: Academic Press, 1970.

Blandau, R. J. Sperm transport through the mammalian cervix: comparative aspects. In The biology of the cervix, eds. R. J. Blandau and K. S. Moghissi, p. 285. Chicago: The University of Chicago Press, 1973.

Brackett, B. G., and L. Mastroianni. Composition of oviducal fluid. In The oviduct and its functions, eds. A. D. Johnson and C. W. Foley, p. 133. New York: Academic Press, 1974.

Brackett, B. G., and G. Oliphant. Capacitation of rabbit spermatozoa in vitro. Biol. Reprod. 12:260, 1975.

Bredderman, P. J., and R. H. Foote. Volume of stressed bull spermatozoa and protoplasmic droplets, and the relationship of cell size to motility and fertility. J. Anim. Sci. 28:496, 1969.

Bredderman, P. J., and R. H. Foote. Alteration of cell volume in bull spermatozoa by factors known to affect active cation transport. Exp. Cell Res. 66:190, 1971a.

Bredderman, P. J., and R. H. Foote. Factors stabilizing bull sperm cell volume and prolonging motility at high dilution. Exp. Cell Res. 66:458, 1971b.

Bredderman, P. J., and R. H. Foote. The effect of calcium ions on cell volume and motility of bovine spermatozoa. Proc. Soc. Exp. Biol. Med. 137:1440, 1971c.

Brooks, D. E. Examination of bull semen and of the bull and rabbit testis for the presence of creatine phosphate and arginine phosphate. J. Reprod. Fertil. 26:275, 1971.

Brooks, J. C., and F. L. Siegel. Calcium-binding phosphoprotein: The principal acidic protein of mammalian sperm. Biochem. Biophys. Res. Commun. 55:710, 1973.

Brown, C. R. Distribution of hyaluronidase in the ram spermatozoon. J. Reprod. Fertil. 45:537, 1975.

Brown, C. R., and E. F. Hartree. Distribution of a trypsin-like proteinase in the ram spermatozoon. J. Reprod. Fertil. 36:195, 1974.

Brown, P. D. C., and I. G. White. Studies on the male antifertility drug 3-chloro-1,2-propanediol. J. Reprod. Fertil. 32:337, 1973.

Brown-Woodman, P. D. C., I. G. White, and S. Salamon. Effect of α-chlorohydrin on the fertility of rams and on the metabolism of spermatozoa in vitro. J. Reprod. Fertil. 43:381, 1975.

Bryan, J. H. D. Capacitation in the mouse: The response of murine acrosomes to the environment of the female reproductive tract. Biol. Reprod. 10:414, 1974.

Bryan, J. H. D., and R. R. Unnithan. Cytochemical localization of nonspecific esterase and acid phosphatase in the spermatozoa of the mouse (Mus musculus). Histochemie 33:169, 1973.

Burgos, M. H., and E. S. Tovar. Sperm motility in the rat epididymis. Fertil. Steril. 25:985, 1974.

Busby, W. F., P. Hele, and M. C. Chang. Apparent amino acid incorporation by ejaculated rabbit spermatozoa. Biochim. Biophys. Acta 335:246, 1974.

Butler, W. J., and T. K. Roberts. Effects of some phosphatidyl compounds on boar spermatozoa following cold shock or slow cooling. J. Reprod. Fertil. 43:183, 1975.

Calvin, H. I., and J. M. Bedford. Stimulation of actinomycin D-binding to eutherian sperm chromatin by reduction of disulphide bonds. J. Reprod. Fertil. 36:225, 1974.

Casillas, E. R. The distribution of carnitine in male reproductive tissues and its effect on palmitate oxidation by spermatozoal particles. Biochim. Biophys. Acta 280:545, 1972.

Casillas, E. R. Accumulation of carnitine by bovine spermatozoa during maturation in the epididymis. J. Biol. Chem. 248:8227, 1973.

Casillas, E. R., and B. J. Erickson. The role of carnitine in spermatozoan metabolism: Substrate-induced elevations in the acetylation state of carnitine and coenzyme A in bovine and monkey spermatozoa. Biol. Reprod. 12:275, 1975.

Castellano, M. A., N. I. Germino, M. Micucci, A. Godoy, and V. Grau. Ram spermatozoa studied with techniques for the cytochemical detection of phosphorylase and succinic dehydrogenase. J. Reprod. Fertil. 17:149, 1968.

Chang, M. C. A detrimental effect of seminal plasma on the fertilizing capacity of sperm. Nature 179:258, 1957.

Chang, M. C., and R. H. F. Hunter. Capacitation of mammalian sperm: Biological and experimental aspects. In Hand-

book of physiology, Section 7: *Endocrinology*, Vol. 5, eds. D. W. Hamilton and R. O. Greep, p. 339. Baltimore: Williams & Wilkins, 1975.

Cheng, P., L. E. Casida, and G. R. Barrett. Effects of dilution on motility of bull spermatozoa and the relation between motility in high dilution and fertility. J. Anim. Sci. 8:81, 1949.

Darin-Bennett, A., A. Poulos, and I. G. White. A re-examination of the role of phospholipids as energy substrates during incubation of ram spermatozoa. J. Reprod. Fertil. 34:543, 1973a.

Darin-Bennett, A., A. Poulos, and I. G. White. The effect of cold shock and freeze-thawing on release of phospholipids by ram, bull, and boar spermatozoa. Aust. J. Biol. Sci. 26: 1409, 1973b.

Davis, B. K. Decapacitation and recapacitation of rabbit spermatozoa treated with membrane vesicles from seminal plasma. J. Reprod. Fertil. 41:241, 1974.

Davis, B. K., D. M. Hunt, and M. C. Chang. Influence of calcium ions on fertilization in the rabbit. Proc. Soc. Exp. Biol. Med. 147:479, 1974.

Dott, H. M. The effects of bovine seminal plasma on the impedance change frequency and glycolysis of bovine epididymal spermatozoa. J. Reprod. Fertil. 38:147, 1974.

Edwards, E. M., A. R. Jones, and G. M. H. Waites. The entry of α-chlorohydrin into body fluids of male rats and its effect upon the incorporation of glycerol into lipids. J. Reprod. Fertil. 43:225, 1975.

Fléchon, J.-E., and M. P. Dubois. Localisation immunocytochimique de la hyaluronidase dans les spermatozoïdes de mammifères domestiques. C. R. Acad. Sci. [D] (Paris) 280: 877, 1975.

Flipse, R. J. Oxidation of fatty acids by bovine spermatozoa. J. Dairy Sci. 42:938, 1959.

Fritz, H., B. Förg-Brey, E. Fink, H. Schiessler, E. Jaumann, and M. Arnhold. Charakterisierung einer Trypsin-ännlichen Proteinase (Akrosin) aus Eberspermien durch ihre Hemmbarkeit mit verschiedenen Protein-Proteinase-Inhibitoren. I. Seminale Trypsin-Inhibitoren und Trypsin-Kallikrein-Inhibitor aus Rinderorganen. Hoppe-Seyler's Z. Physiol. Chem. 353:1007, 1972a.

Fritz, H., B. Förg-Brey, H. Schiessler, M. Arnhold, and E. Fink. Charakterisierung einer Trypsin-ännlichen Proteinase (Akrosin) aus Eberspermien durch ihre Hemmbarkeit mit verschiedenen Protein-Proteinase-Inhibitoren. II. Inhibitoren aus Blutegeln, Sojabohnen, Erdnüssen, Rindercolostrum und Seeanemonen. Hoppe-Seyler's Z. Physiol. Chem. 353:1010, 1972b.

Fritz, H., N. Heimburger, M. Meier, M. Arnhold, L. J. D. Zaneveld, and G. F. B. Schumacher. Humanakrosin: Zur Kinetik der Hemmung durch Human-Seruminhibitoren. Hoppe-Seyler's Z. Physiol. Chem. 353:1953, 1972c.

Fritz, H., H. Schiessler, and W. D. Schleuning. Proteinases and proteinase inhibitors in the fertilization process: New concepts of control? Adv. Biosci. 10:271, 1973.

Gaddum, P., and R. J. Blandau. Proteolytic reaction of mammalian spermatozoa on gelatin membranes. Science (NY) 170:749, 1970.

Gaddum, P., and T. D. Glover. Some reactions of rabbit spermatozoa to ligation of the epididymis. J. Reprod. Fertil. 9:119, 1965.

Garbers, D. L., N. L. First, S. K. Gorman, and H. A. Lardy. The effects of cyclic nucleotide phosphodiesterase inhibitors on ejaculated porcine spermatozoan metabolism. Biol. Reprod. 8:599, 1973a.

Garbers, D. L., N. L. First, and H. A. Lardy. The stimulation of bovine epididymal sperm metabolism by cyclic nucleotide phosphodiesterase inhibitors. Biol. Reprod. 8:589, 1973b.

Garbers, D. L., N. L. First, and H. A. Lardy. Properties of adenosine 3′,5′-monophosphate-dependent protein kinases isolated from bovine epididymal spermatozoa. J. Biol. Chem. 248:875, 1973c.

Garner, D. L., M. P. Easton, M. E. Munson, and M. A. Doane. Immunofluorescent localization of bovine acrosin. J. Exp. Zool. 191:127, 1975.

Gaur, R. D., and G. P. Talwar. Isolation of a factor from human seminal plasma that promotes fertilization. Nature 244: 450, 1973.

Gibbons, R., K. Collis, and R. Sellwood. Exogenous energy sources for spermatozoa in cervical mucus of the cow at oestrus. J. Reprod. Fertil. 40:187, 1974.

Gledhill, B. L. Changes in deoxyribonucleoprotein in relation to spermateliosis and the epididymal maturation of spermatozoa. J. Reprod. Fertil. Suppl. 13:77, 1971.

Gledhill, B. L., M. P. Gledhill, R. Rigler, and N. R. Ringertz. Atypical changes of deoxyribonucleoprotein during spermiogenesis associated with a case of infertility in the bull. J. Reprod. Fertil. 12:575, 1966.

Gordon, M. Localization of phosphatase activity on the membranes of the mammalian sperm head. J. Exp. Zool. 185:111, 1973.

Gordon, M., P. V. Dandekar, and W. Bartoszewicz. The surface coat of epididymal, ejaculated and capacitated sperm. J. Ultrastruct. Res. 50:199, 1975.

Gould, K. G., P. N. Srivastava, E. M. Cline, and W. L. Williams. Inhibition of in vitro fertilization of rabbit ova with naturally occurring antifertility agents. Contraception 3:261, 1971.

Gulyas, B. J. Effects of aging on fertilizing capacity and morphology of rabbit sperm. Fertil. Steril. 19:453, 1968.

Gwatkin, R. B. L., and C. F. Hutchison. Capacitation of hamster spermatozoa by β-glucuronidase. Nature 229:343, 1971.

Hamner, C. E., and W. L. Williams. The effect of light on the respiration of spermatozoa. Biochem. Biophys. Res. Commun. 5:316, 1961.

Hamner, C. E., and W. L. Williams. Effect of the female reproductive tract on sperm metabolism in the rabbit and fowl. J. Reprod. Fertil. 5:143, 1963.

Hanada, A., and M. C. Chang. Penetration of zona-free eggs by spermatozoa of different species. Biol. Reprod. 6:300, 1972.

Harrison, R. A. P. Glycolytic enzymes in mammalian spermatozoa. Activities and stabilities of hexokinase and phosphofructokinase in various fractions from sperm homogenates. Biochem. J. 124:741, 1971.

Harrison, R. A. P. Interconversion of hexokinase isoenzymes in mammalian spermatozoa. J. Reprod. Fertil. 31:510, 1972.

Harrison, R. A. P. Aspects of the enzymology of mammalian spermatozoa. In *The biology of the male gamete*, eds. J. G. Duckett and P. A. Racey, p. 301. London: The Linnean Society and Academic Press, 1975.

Hartmann, J. F., and R. B. L. Gwatkin. Alteration of sites on the mammalian sperm surface following capacitation. Nature 234:479, 1971.

Hartmann, J. F., and C. F. Hutchison. Nature of the prepenetration contact interactions between hamster gametes in vitro. J. Reproduc. Fertil. 36:49, 1974.

Hartree, E. F. The acrosome-lysosome relationship. J. Reprod. Fertil. 44:125, 1975.

Hicks, J. J., J. Martinez-Manautou, N. Pedron, and A. Rosado. Metabolic changes in human spermatozoa related to capacitation. Fertil. Steril. 23:172, 1972a.

Hicks, J. J., N. Pedron, and A. Rosado. Modifications of human spermatozoa glycolysis by cyclic adenosine monophosphate (cAMP), estrogens, and follicular fluid. Fertil. Steril. 23:886, 1972b.

Hoskins, D. D. Adenine nucleotide mediation of fructolysis and motility in bovine epididymal spermatozoa. J. Biol. Chem. 248:1135, 1973.

Hoskins, D. D., E. R. Casillas, and D. T. Stephens. Cyclic AMP–dependent protein kinases of bovine epididymal spermatozoa. Biochem. Biophys. Res. Commun. 48:1331, 1972.

Hoskins, D. D., and D. L. Patterson. Metabolism of rhesus monkey spermatozoa. J. Reprod. Fertil. 16:183, 1968.

Hoskins, D. D., D. T. Stephens, and E. R. Casillas. Enzymic control of fructolysis in primate spermatozoa. Biochim. Biophys. Acta 237:227, 1971.

Hoskins, D. D., D. T. Stephens, and M. L. Hall. Cyclic adenosine 3':5'-monophosphate and protein kinase levels in developing bull spermatozoa. J. Reprod. Fertil. 37:131, 1974.

Huang-Yang, Y. H. J., and S. Meizel. Purification of rabbit testis proacrosin and studies of its active form. Biol. Reprod. 12:232, 1975.

Iritani, A., W. R. Gomes, and N. L. Vandemark. The effect of whole, dialysed and heated female genital tract fluids on respiration of rabbit and ram spermatozoa. Biol. Reprod. 1:77, 1969.

Iwamatsu, T., and M. C. Chang. In vitro fertilization of mouse eggs in the presence of bovine follicular fluid. Nature 224:919, 1969.

Jackson, H., I. S. C. Campbell, and A. R. Jones. Is glycidol an active intermediate in the antifertility action of α-chlorhydrin in male rats? Nature 226:86, 1970.

Johnson, M. H. The macromolecular organization of membranes and its bearing on events leading up to fertilization. J. Reprod. Fertil. 44:167, 1975.

Johnson, W. L., and A. G. Hunter. Seminal antigens: Their alteration in the genital tract of female rabbits and during partial in vitro capacitation with beta amylase and beta glucuronidase. Biol. Reprod. 7:332, 1972.

Jones, A. R., P. Davies, K. Edwards, and H. Jackson. Antifertility effects and metabolism of α and epi-chlorhydrins in the rat. Nature 224:83, 1969.

Jones, R., and T. Mann. Lipid peroxidation in spermatozoa. Proc. R. Soc. [Biol.] 184:103, 1973.

Killian, G. J., and R. P. Amann. Immunoelectrophoretic characterization of fluid and sperm entering and leaving the bovine epididymis. Biol. Reprod. 9:489, 1973.

Kirton, K. T., and H. D. Hafs. Sperm capacitation by uterine fluid or beta-amylase in vitro. Science (NY) 150:618, 1965.

Lindemann, C. B., and I. R. Gibbons. Adenosine triphosphate–induced motility and sliding of filaments in mammalian sperm extracted with Triton X-100. J. Cell Biol. 65:147, 1975.

Lindholmer, C. The importance of seminal plasma for human sperm motility. Biol. Reprod. 10:533, 1974.

Loir, M., and M. T. Hochereau-de Reviers. Deoxyribonucleoprotein changes in ram and bull spermatids. J. Reprod. Fertil. 31:127, 1972.

Mahi, C. A., and R. Yanagimachi. The effects of temperature, osmolality and hydrogen ion concentration on the activation and acrosome reaction of golden hamster spermatozoa. J. Reprod. Fertil. 35:55, 1973.

Mahler, H. R., and E. H. Cordes. *Biological chemistry*, 2nd ed. New York: Harper & Row, 1971.

Mancini, R. E., A. Alonso, J. Barquet, B. Alvarez, and M. Nemirovsky. Histo-immunological localization of hyaluronidase in the bull testis. J. Reprod. Fertil. 8:325, 1964.

Mann, T. *The biochemistry of semen and of the male reproductive tract*. London: Methuen, 1964.

Mann, T., and C. Lutwak-Mann. Biochemical aspects of aging in spermatozoa in relation to motility and fertilizing ability. In *Aging gametes—their biology and pathology*, ed. R. J. Blandau, p. 122. Basel: S. Karger, 1975.

Markert, C. L. Isozymes and cellular differentiation. Adv. Biosci. 6:511, 1971.

Marushige, Y., and K. Marushige. Transformation of sperm histone during formation and maturation of rat spermatozoa. J. Biol. Chem. 250:39, 1975.

Masaki, J. Phospholipids and their hydrolysing enzymes in bull semen as a factor concerned with sperm motility. Jap. Agric. Res. Quart. 8:54, 1974.

McRorie, R. A., and W. L. Williams. Biochemistry of mammalian fertilization. Ann. Rev. Biochem. 43:777, 1974.

Meizel, S., S. K. Mukerji, and Y. H. J. Huang-Yang. Biochemical studies of rabbit testes and epididymal sperm proacrosin. J. Cell Biol. 63:222a, 1974.

Metz, C. B., and J. Anika. Failure of conception in rabbits inseminated with nonagglutinating, univalent antibody-treated semen. Biol. Reprod. 2:284, 1970.

Metz, C. B., G. W. Hinsch, and J. L. Anika. Ultrastructure and antigens of particles from rabbit semen. J. Reprod. Fertil. 17:195, 1968.

Metz, C. B., A. C. Seiguer, and A. E. Castro. Inhibition of the cumulus dispersing and hyaluronidase activities of sperm by heterologous and isologous antisperm antibodies. Proc. Soc. Exp. Biol. Med. 140:776, 1972.

Mills, S. C., and T. W. Scott. Metabolism of fatty acids by testicular and ejaculated ram spermatozoa. J. Reprod. Fertil. 18:367, 1969.

Minassian, E. S., and C. Terner. Biosynthesis of lipids by human and fish spermatozoa. Am. J. Physiol. 210:615, 1966.

Miyamoto, H., and M. C. Chang. The importance of serum albumin and metabolic intermediates for capacitation of spermatozoa and fertilization of mouse eggs in vitro. J. Reprod. Fertil. 32:193, 1973.

Mohri, H., D. A. I. Suter, P. D. C. Brown-Woodman, I. G. White, and D. D. Ridley. Identification of the biochemical lesion produced by α-chlorohydrin in spermatozoa. Nature 255:75, 1975.

Morita, Z., and M. C. Chang. The motility and aerobic metabolism of spermatozoa in laboratory animals with special reference to the effects of cold shock and the importance of calcium for the motility of hamster spermatozoa. Biol. Reprod. 3:169, 1970.

Morton, B., and L. Albagli. Modification of hamster sperm adenyl cyclase by capacitation in vitro. Biochem. Biophys. Res. Commun. 50:697, 1973.

Morton, B., and T. S. K. Chang. The effect of fluid from the cauda epididymidis, serum components and caffeine upon the survival of diluted epididymal hamster spermatozoa. J. Reprod. Fertil. 35:255, 1973.

Morton, B., J. Harrigan-Lum, L. Albagli, and T. Jooss. The activation of motility in quiescent hamster sperm from the epididymis by calcium and cyclic nucleotides. Biochem. Biophys. Res. Commun. 56:372, 1974.

Morton, D. B. Purification and properties of ovine testicular hyaluronidase. Biochem. Soc. Trans. 1:385, 1973.

Morton, D. B., and B. D. Bavister. Fractionation of hamster sperm-capacitating components from human serum by gel filtration. J. Reprod. Fertil. 40:491, 1974.

Mounib, M. S., and M. C. Chang. Effect of in utero incubation on the metabolism of rabbit spermatozoa. Nature 201:943, 1964.

Mukerji, S. K., and S. Meizel. The molecular transformation of rabbit testis proacrosin into acrosin. Arch. Biochem. Biophys. 168:720, 1975.

Murdoch, R. N., and I. G. White. Metabolic studies of testicular, epididymal, and ejaculated spermatozoa of the ram. Aust. J. Biol. Sci. 21:111, 1968.

Neill, A. R., and C. J. Masters. Metabolism of fatty acids by bovine spermatozoa. Biochem. J. 127:375, 1972.

Neill, A. R., and C. J. Masters. Metabolism of fatty acids by ovine spermatozoa. J. Reprod. Fertil. 34:279, 1973.

Neill, A. R., and C. J. Masters. The distribution of ^{14}C-label in the lipids of ram semen following the intratesticular injection of [1-^{14}C] palmitic acid. J. Reprod. Fertil. 38:311, 1974.

Nelson, L. Preliminary evidence for cholinoceptive sites in the excitability of spermatozoa. Nature 242:401, 1973.

Nevo, A. C. Dependence of sperm motility and respiration on oxygen concentration. J. Reprod. Fertil. 9:103, 1965.

Nevo, A. C., and R. Rikmenspoel. Diffusion of ATP in sperm flagella. J. Theor. Biol. 26:11, 1970.

Norman, C., E. Goldberg, and I. D. Porterfield. The effect of visible radiation on the functional life-span of mammalian and avian spermatozoa. Exp. Cell Res. 28:69, 1962.

O'Donnell, J. M., and J. C. Ellory. The binding of cardiac glycosides to bull spermatozoa. Experientia 26:20, 1970.

Oikawa, T., G. L. Nicolson, and R. Yanagimachi. Inhibition of hamster fertilization by phytoagglutinins. Exp. Cell Res. 83:239, 1974.

Oliphant, G. Role of the seminal plasma in sperm capacitation. Fed. Proc. 33:289, 1974.

Oliphant, G., and B. G. Brackett. Immunological assessment of surface changes of rabbit sperm undergoing capacitation. Biol. Reprod. 9:404, 1973a.

Oliphant, G., and B. G. Brackett. Capacitation of mouse spermatozoa in media with elevated ionic strength and reversible decapacitation with epididymal extracts. Fertil. Steril. 24:948, 1973b.

O'Rand, M. G., and Metz, C. B. Tests for rabbit sperm surface iron-binding protein and hyaluronidase using the "exchange agglutination" reaction. Biol. Reprod. 11:326, 1974.

Orgebin-Crist, M. C. Studies on the function of the epididymis. Biol. Reprod. Suppl. 1:155, 1969.

O'Shea, T., and R. G. Wales. Effect of casein, lecithin, glycerol, and storage at 5°C on diluted ram and bull semen. Aust. J. Biol. Sci. 19:871, 1966.

O'Shea, T., and R. G. Wales. The metabolism of ram, bull, dog, and rabbit spermatozoa after cooling to 5°C. Aust. J. Biol. Sci. 20:447, 1967.

Overstreet, J. W., and J. M. Bedford. Transport, capacitation and fertilizing ability of epididymal spermatozoa. J. Exp. Zool. 189:203, 1974.

Pace, M. M., and E. F. Graham. Components in egg yolk which protect bovine spermatozoa during freezing. J. Anim. Sci. 39:1144, 1974.

Peterson, R. N., and M. Freund. ATP synthesis and oxidative metabolism in human spermatozoa. Biol. Reprod. 3:47, 1970a.

Peterson, R. N., and M. Freund. Profile of glycolytic enzyme activities in human spermatozoa. Fertil. Steril. 21:151, 1970b.

Peterson, R. N., and M. Freund. Citrate formation from exogenous substrates by washed human spermatozoa. J. Reprod. Fertil. 38:73, 1974.

Pikó, L. Gamete structure and sperm entry in mammals. In Fertilization, Vol. 2, eds. C. B. Metz and A. Monroy, p. 325. New York: Academic Press, 1969.

Polakoski, K. L. Partial purification and characterization of proacrosin from boar sperm. Fed. Proc. 33:1308, 1974.

Polakoski, K. L., and R. A. McRorie. Boar acrosin. II. Classification, inhibition, and specificity studies of a proteinase from sperm acrosomes. J. Biol. Chem. 248:8183, 1973.

Poulos, A., J. K. Voglmayr, and I. G. White. Phospholipid changes in spermatozoa during passage through the genital tract of the bull. Biochim. Biophys. Acta 306:194, 1973.

Premkumar, E., and P. M. Bhargava. Transcription and translation in bovine spermatozoa. Nature New Biol. 240: 139, 1972.

Quinn, P. J., S. Salamon, and I. G. White. The effect of cold shock and deep-freezing on ram spermatozoa collected by electrical ejaculation and by an artificial vagina. Aust. J. Agric. Sci. 19:119, 1968.

Quinn, P. J., and I. G. White. Active cation transport in dog spermatozoa. Biochem. J. 104:328, 1967a.

Quinn, P. J., and I. G. White. Phospholipid and cholesterol content of epididymal and ejaculated ram spermatozoa and seminal plasma in relation to cold shock. Aust. J. Biol. Sci. 20:1205, 1967b.

Quinn, P. J., and I. G. White. The transport of cations by ram and bull spermatozoa. Aust. J. Biol. Sci. 21:781, 1968.

Raff, E. C., and J. J. Blum. A possible role for adenylate kinase in cilia: Concentration profiles in a geometrically constrained dual enzyme system. J. Theor. Biol. 18:53, 1968.

Restall, B. J. The biochemical and physiological relationships between the gametes and the female reproductive tract. Adv. Reprod. Physiol. 2:181, 1967.

Reyes, A., G. Oliphant, and B. G. Brackett. Partial purification and identification of a reversible decapacitation factor from rabbit seminal plasma. Fertil. Steril. 26:148, 1975.

Rogers, B. J., and B. Morton. ATP levels in hamster spermatozoa during capacitation in vitro. Biol. Reprod. 9:361, 1973.

Rosado, A., J. J. Hicks, A. Reyes, and I. Blanco. Capacitation in vitro of rabbit spermatozoa with cyclic adenosine monophosphate and human follicular fluid. Fertil. Steril. 25:821, 1974.

Schill, W. B., and H. Fritz. N^{α}-benzoyl-L-arginine ethyl ester splitting activity (acrosin) in human spermatozoa and seminal plasma during aging in vitro. Hoppe-Seyler's Z. Physiol. Chem. 356:83, 1975.

Schoenfeld, C., R. D. Amelar, and L. Dubin. Stimulation of ejaculated human spermatozoa by caffeine. Fertil. Steril. 26: 158, 1975.

Scott, T. W., J. K. Voglmayr, and B. P. Setchell. Lipid composition and metabolism in testicular and ejaculated ram spermatozoa. Biochem. J. 102:456, 1967.

Setchell, B. P., T. W. Scott, J. K. Voglmayr, and G. M. H. Waites. Characteristics of testicular spermatozoa and the fluid which transports them into the epididymis. Biol. Reprod. Suppl. 1:40, 1969.

Shannon, P. Presence of a heat-labile toxic protein in bovine seminal plasma. J. Dairy Sci. 48:1362, 1965.

Soupart, P., and R. W. Noyes. Sialic acid as a component of the zona pellucida of the mammalian ovum. J. Reprod. Fertil. 8:251, 1964.

Srivastava, P. N., and K. G. Gould. Inhibition of the fertilizing capacity of rabbit spermatozoa by sialoproteins. Contraception 7:65, 1973.

Stambaugh, R., and J. Buckley. Identification and subcellular localization of the enzymes effecting penetration of the zona pellucida by rabbit spermatozoa. J. Reprod. Fertil. 19:423, 1969.

Stambaugh, R., and J. Buckley. Comparative studies of the acrosomal enzymes of rabbit, rhesus monkey, and human spermatozoa. Biol. Reprod. 3:275, 1970.

Stambaugh, R., H. M. Seitz, and L. Mastroianni. Acrosomal proteinase inhibitors in rhesus monkey (Macaca mulatta) oviduct fluid. Fertil. Steril. 25:352, 1974.

Storey, B. T., and E. Keyhani. Interaction of calcium ion with the mitochondria of rabbit spermatozoa. FEBS Letters, 37:33, 1973.

Storey, B. T., and E. Keyhani. Energy metabolism of spermatozoa. II. Comparison of pyruvate and fatty acid oxidation by mitochondria of rabbit epididymal spermatozoa. Fertil. Steril. 25:857, 1974a.

Storey, B. T., and E. Keyhani. Energy metabolism of spermatozoa. III. Energy-linked uptake of calcium ion by the mitochondria of rabbit epididymal spermatozoa. Fertil. Steril. 25:976, 1974b.

Talbot, P., and L. E. Franklin. The release of hyaluronidase from guinea-pig spermatozoa during the course of the normal acrosome reaction in vitro. J. Reprod. Fertil. 39:429, 1974.

Tang, F. Y., and D. D. Hoskins. Phosphoprotein phosphatase of bovine epididymal spermatozoa. Biochem. Biophys. Res. Commun. 62:328, 1975.

Teichman, R. J., and M. H. Bernstein. Fine structure localizations of acid phosphatase in rabbit and bull sperm heads. J. Reprod. Fertil. 27:243, 1971.

Thibault, C. Sperm transport and storage in vertebrates. J. Reprod. Fertil. Suppl. 18:39, 1973.

Toyoda, Y., and M. C. Chang. Capacitation of epididymal spermatozoa in a medium with high K/Na ratio and cyclic AMP for the fertilization of rat eggs in vitro. J. Reprod. Fertil. 36:125, 1974.

Vandeberg, J. L., D. W. Cooper, and P. J. Close. Mammalian testis phosphoglycerate kinase. Nature New Biol. 243: 48, 1973.

Vickery, B. H., G. I. Erickson, and J. P. Bennett. Mechanism of antifertility action of low doses of α-chlorohydrin in the male rat. J. Reprod. Fertil. 38:1, 1974.

Voglmayr, J. K., L. H. Larsen, and I. G. White. Metabolism of spermatozoa and composition of fluid collected from the rete testis of living bulls. J. Reprod. Fertil. 21:449, 1970.

Watson, P. F. The interaction of egg yolk and ram spermatozoa studied with a fluorescent probe. J. Reprod. Fertil. 42: 105, 1975.

White, I. G. The effect of potassium on the washing and dilution of mammalian spermatozoa. Aust. J. Exp. Biol. 31:193, 1953.

White, I. G. Biochemical aspects of spermatozoa and their environment in the male reproductive tract. J. Reprod. Fertil. Suppl. 18:225, 1973.

White, I. G., J. C. Rodger, R. N. Murdoch, W. L. Williams, and T. O. Abney. Effect of decapacitation factor on the oxygen uptake of rabbit spermatozoa recovered from the uterus. Experientia 31:80, 1975.

Williams, W. L. Biochemistry of capacitation of spermatozoa. In *Biology of mammalian fertilization and implantation*, eds. K. S. Moghissi and E. S. E. Hafez, p. 19. Springfield, Ill.: Charles C Thomas, 1972.

Williams, W. L., T. O. Abney, H. N. Chernoff, W. R. Dukelow, and M. C. Pinsker. Biochemistry and physiology of decapacitation factor. J. Reprod. Fertil. Suppl. 2:11, 1967.

Williams, W. L., R. T. Robertson, and W. R. Dukelow. Decapacitation factor and capacitation. Adv. Biosci. 4:61, 1970.

Witters, W. L., C. W. Foley, and R. E. Erb. Metabolic characteristics of washed boar spermatozoa. J. Anim. Sci. 25:348, 1966.

Yanagimachi, R. In vitro acrosome reaction and capacitation of golden hamster spermatozoa by bovine follicular fluid and its fractions. J. Exp. Zool. 170:269, 1969.

Yanagimachi, R. In vitro capacitation of golden hamster spermatozoa by homologous and heterologous blood sera. Biol. Reprod. 3:147, 1970a.

Yanagimachi, R. The movement of golden hamster spermatozoa before and after capacitation. J. Reprod. Fertil. 23:193, 1970b.

Yanagimachi, R. Penetration of guinea pig spermatozoa into hamster eggs in vitro. J. Reprod. Fertil. 28:477, 1972.

Yanagimachi, R., and R. J. Teichman. Cytochemical demonstration of acrosomal proteinase in mammalian and avian spermatozoa by a silver proteinate method. Biol. Reprod. 6:87, 1972.

Yanagimachi, R., and N. Usui. Calcium dependence of the acrosome reaction and activation of guinea pig spermatozoa. Exp. Cell Res. 89:161, 1974.

Young, L. G., and L. Nelson. Divalent cation activation of flagellar ATP-phosphohydrolase from bull sperm. J. Cell Physiol. 74:315, 1969.

Zaneveld, L. J. D., K. L. Polakoski, and G. F. B. Schumacher. Properties of acrosomal hyaluronidase from bull spermatozoa. Evidence for its similarity to testicular hyaluronidase. J. Biol. Chem. 248:564, 1973a.

Zaneveld, L. J. D., G. F. B. Schumacher, H. Fritz, E. Fink, and E. Jaumann. Interaction of human sperm acrosomal proteinase with human seminal plasma proteinase inhibitors. J. Reprod. Fertil. 32:525, 1973b.

Zaneveld, L. J. D., and W. L. Williams. A sperm enzyme that disperses the corona radiata and its inhibition by decapacitation factor. Biol. Reprod. 2:363, 1970.

33 The Mammalian Accessory Sex Glands: A Morphological and Functional Analysis

L. F. Cavazos

The structure and physiology of the accessory sex glands of the male has been known for some time, but the details and the exact mechanism by which they interact in the reproductive process is still not clear. Numerous investigators have determined that the secretions of the seminal vesicle, the prostate gland (and coagulating gland in rodents), and the bulbourethral glands contribute the bulk of major component of semen. The other portion of semen, spermatozoa, when mixed with the secretions of the accessory sex glands, become motile. A vast literature has also accumulated demonstrating that these glands are directly or indirectly dependent upon the titer of circulating androgen; therefore the accessory sex glands are delicate indicators of the presence of the male sex hormone. Fall of testosterone levels in the mammal are reflected almost immediately in the epithelia of the accessory sex glands by a marked decrease in epithelial cell height, termination of secretory activity, and reduction of nuclear volume and nuclear pyknosis.

As early as the eighteenth century, the dependence of the accessory sex glands on the gonads was suspected. John Hunter (1786), the English anatomist, described the seminal vesicles of the rat and noted a direct relationship between the testis and the accessory sex glands. The classical investigation that truly established the endocrine role of the testis in maintenance of accessory sex gland function was carried out by Moore and co-workers (1930a,b). They demonstrated the atrophy and dysfunction of the seminal vesicles and the prostate gland of the rat after castration and the enlargement and secretion of these glands following injection of a steroid extract prepared from bull testes.

In more recent times, a considerable volume of literature has been generated on the structure and function of the accessory sex glands. The studies elucidating the action of androgens on the seminal vesicles, prostate gland, and the bulbourethral glands have involved chiefly biochemical, histochemical, and fine structural techniques (Mann 1954, 1956, 1964; Cavazos and Melampy 1954). A number of reviews have recently appeared on the sex accessory glands (Mann and Lutwak-Mann 1951; Price and Williams-Ashman 1961; Cavazos 1975). Brandes (1966) and Brandes and Groth (1963) have reported the fine structure and histochemistry of the prostate gland of the rat, mouse,

dog, and man. The metabolism of normal and neoplastic prostate gland and some of the effects on morphological changes occurring after castration, estrogen treatment, and aging have been described and reviewed by others (Ofner 1968; Leav and Cavazos 1975; Ofner et al. 1974).

All of the accessory sex glands depend in a precise and delicate fashion on the level of testosterone or its metabolites. This is particularly important because in the past few years, evidence has accumulated which strongly suggests that male sex hormone effects on accessory reproductive organs are mediated partly or entirely by intracellular metabolites of the circulating androgens (Williams-Ashman and Reddi 1971; Ofner 1971). Baulieu (1973) has recently reviewed the mode of action of steroid hormones.

33.1 Seminal Vesicles

The seminal vesicles are paired glands positioned dorsal to the trigonal area of the urinary bladder. Each seminal vesicle is close and almost parallel to the ampulla of the ductus deferens of the same size. The seminal vesicles of rodents and swine are large with respect to the other glands, while in humans they are relatively small. As would be expected, functional differences also occur between species. The manner in which they secrete into the duct system is also variable. In the adult rat, this gland empties its secretion into the ejaculatory duct (Walker 1910). In other animals in which an ejaculatory duct is absent, the seminal vesicles pour their secretion directly into the pelvic urethra (Price and Williams-Ashman 1961).

Embryologically, the seminal vesicles of rodents are derived from an evagination of a saccule from the distal end of each mesonepheric or Wolffian duct (Burnes 1961; Price 1936; Wiesner 1934). In the case of the human, the anlage of the seminal vesicle develops at the end of the first trimester, when it is seen as a small appendage and evagination of the ductus deferens. During the whole process, the rudiments of the developing seminal vesicle have a lumen.

Cytological Structure
The epithelium of rodents and primates is variable, ranging from a simple columnar shape with basal cells to a pseudostratified columnar shape (Lyman and

Dempsey 1951; Melampy and Cavazos 1953; Feagans et al. 1961; Cavazos et al. 1961). In terms of light microscopy and histochemistry, the seminal vesicles are characterized by the presence of an intense basophilia in the perinuclear and apical cytoplasm. This reaction is abolished by ribonuclease hydrolysis prior to staining with toluidine blue (Deane and Porter 1960; Melampy and Cavazos 1953). At the fine structural level, these sites of basophilia are occupied by abundant cisternae of granular endoplasmic reticulum (Fugita 1959; Deane and Porter 1960; Szirmai and van der Linde 1962; Cavazos et al. 1964; Deane and Wurzelmann 1965; Toner and Baillie 1966).

Following the periodic acid-Schiff reaction there is a moderate reaction in the cytoplasm of the epithelium of the hamster seminal vesicle (Feagans et al. 1961) but only a slight coloration in that of the rat (Leblond 1950; Melampy and Cavazos 1953). Other histochemical characteristics of the epithelial cytoplasm are a diffuse sudanophilia (Cavazos et al. 1954), abundant plasmalogen (Belt 1950), and apical granules of acid phosphatase (Deane and Dempsey 1945).

As is typical of most cells secreting high volumes of proteins, the epithelium of the seminal vesicle has a large and elaborate Golgi apparatus. The Golgi complex consists of flattened membranous sacs, vesicles, and large vacuoles. Secretory material is often seen packaged into the vacuoles. Additionally, these secretory granules are distributed in the cytoplasm up to the free apical margin of the cell. Mitochondria are dispersed throughout the cytoplasm. In addition to a copious granular endoplasmic reticulum, there are many free ribosomes in the cytoplasm, occurring in rosettes or singly.

Of especial interest is the presence of numerous lysosomes in the supranuclear area in the epithelium of the hamster seminal vesicle. These are large electron-dense structures of variable size. When viewed by light microscopy, the larger structures are probably a lipofuscin pigment. At the level of the electron microscope, these lysosomes are the sites of focal cytoplasmic degradation and have a considerable reaction to acid phosphatase (Cavazos 1963; Belt and Cavazos 1967; Kovacs 1968).

Morphological Indicators of Endocrine Imbalance
The seminal vesicle epithelium responds rapidly to decreases in circulating testosterone. The sensitivity of the rat seminal vesicle epithelium to castration was reported in a cytometric study (Cavazos and Melampy 1954). Within six hours after castration there was a statistically significant reduction in cell height. Nuclear diameter in castrates treated with testosterone propionate increased within 12 hours, and the epithelial

cell height followed with an increase within 24 hours. Effects of castration on the fine structure of the seminal vesicles have been reported by a number of investigators (Allison 1964; Deane 1963; Deane and Porter 1960; Szirmai and van der Linde 1962). For a comprehensive literature review on this topic see Cavazos (1975). In all rodents studied, the indicators of cytological secretory activity were eliminated or markedly depressed after castration. There was loss of the granular endoplasmic reticulum, reduction in size and structural organization of the Golgi complex, loss of secretory vesicles, accumulation of lysosomes, and reduction in nucleolar size. The nucleus was small, and there was an increase in heterochromatin. There was often depletion of the number of mitochondria. Following treatment of the castrates with testosterone, the typical cellular fine structure seen in the intact rat seminal vesicle was quickly restored.

Exogenous hormones such as diethylstilbestrol, estrone alpha estradiol, and ethinyl estradiol are known to have a marked degenerative effect on the epithelium of the seminal vesicles of the hamster (Feagans et al. 1961), including loss of secretion, reduction in basophilia, diminution of the Golgi apparatus, and a marked increase in lipofuscin granules. Results obtained on the effects of diethylstilbestrol on the seminal vesicle were confirmed at the fine structural level (Cavazos 1963; Belt and Cavazos 1967). There was a marked depletion of the granular endoplasmic reticulum, loss of secretory vesicles, and virtual elimination of the Golgi complex. Lysosomes were numerous. Cytoplasmic structures such as endoplasmic reticulum, mitochondria, and secretory granules could be observed to be enclosed by the limiting membrane of the autophagic vacuoles. As previously mentioned, these lysosomes were comparable to lipofuscin pigment seen by light microscopy. A review of the formation of cytoplasmic lipofuscin pigments induced by aging and their formation from lysosomes (Toth 1968) suggests that all organelles of the cell can serve as potential sites of origin of lipofuscin pigments.

Special Biochemical Characteristics
A property of the seminal vesicle in man is its high content of fructose (approximately 315 mg/100 ml). This sugar accounts for almost all of the reducing capacity of human seminal plasma. Fructose metabolism of the seminal vesicles has been used as an indicator of androgenic activity (Ortiz et al. 1956). Inositol and sorbitol are also found in the seminal vesicles and respond to changes in levels of circulating testosterone. It appears that fructose, inositol, and sorbitol are fashioned in the cisternae of the endoplasmic reticulum. In a study on the postnatal differentiation of the seminal

vesicle epithelium of the mouse, Deane and Wurzelmann (1965) found that distension of the ergastoplasm was inversely related to the osmolarity of the fixative employed. They suggested that the ergastoplasmic cisternae housed considerable amounts of small, osmotically active substances. Deane and Wurzelmann (1965) have reported that the mature Golgi complex vacuoles have a large perigranular space that might contain hexoses, polyols, and organic ions. A considerable quantity of citric acid and fructose have been found in seminal vesicles of the boar (Mann 1974). These substances are also responsive to male sex hormone titers (Mann 1964). Price and Williams-Ashman (1961) have reported that ascorbic acid is added to semen by the seminal vesicles of rat and quinea pig. The localization of ascorbic acid in the guinea pig seminal vesicles has been observed histochemically (Kocen and Cavazos 1958).

The levels of acid and alkaline phosphatase in seminal vesicles have been determined by chemical procedures (Stafford et al. 1949; Porter and Melampy 1952). Injections of testosterone into castrate rats resulted in an increase over the castrate levels of these enzymes of 1,061 percent in alkaline phosphatase and 520 percent in acid phosphatase (Porter and Melampy 1952).

In recent years, a group of unsaturated C20 fatty acids characterized by the presence of the cyclopentanone rings and capable of stimulating smooth-muscle contraction have been isolated from human seminal plasma. These substances, known as prostaglandins, were thought to originate in the prostate gland but are now known to be secreted by the seminal vesicle. The seminal vesicle prostaglandins probably account for most of the smooth-muscle-stimulating activity of human seminal plasma (Mann 1974). It has been suggested that one function of seminal plasma prostaglandins is to bring about contractions of the oviduct muscularis and thereby facilitate sperm transport.

For additional information on the biochemistry of semen and the specific secretions of the seminal vesicle, see the reviews by Mann and Lutwak-Mann (1951) and Mann (1964, 1974).

33.2 Prostate Gland

The prostate gland develops from the urogenital sinus, and the embryology and origin of each of its individual lobes has been studied in the rat by Price (1936, 1963). In the mature rodent the gland is formed by a complex arrangement of lobes which pour their secretion into the prostatic urethra through a number of ducts opening near the prostatic utricle on the colliculus seminalis. According to Price (1936), the prostate gland of the sexually mature rat is formed by discrete, paired, ven-

tral lobes at the neck of the urinary bladder and a cranial or anterior lobe (coagulating gland) adjacent to and in the curvature of the seminal vesicle.

The heterogeneous nature of the developing human prostate gland was noted by Lowsley (1912). The gland develops at the third fetal month, and solid epithelial outgrowths form from five distinct parts of the prostatic urethra. From these five points of origin arise five groups of tubules. As they develop, they become encased in stroma, and depending upon their anatomic relationship to the urethra, urinary bladder, or ejaculatory duct, they form the five lobes of the adult human prostate gland: middle, right, and left lateral, posterior, and anterior lobes. As these lobes undergo development, the boundaries between them become somewhat indistinct and they merge, forming what appears to be a homogeneous gland. It is of interest, however, that the vast majority of prostatic cancers arise in the posterior lobe.

McNeal (1969) considers the adult prostate a heterogeneous organ formed by three separate and distinct glandular structures within a single capsule. Two of these glands are designated *true prostate* and are termed *central* and *peripheral* zones. The third glandular entity is the periurethral gland. McNeal (1969) finds carcinoma of the prostate in the peripheral zone, while benign prostatic hyperplasia appears to originate in the periurethral glands.

The structure and physiological activity of the accessory reproductive glands of mammals have been reviewed, and considerable information has been obtained on the cytology and histochemistry of the prostate gland (Price and Williams-Ashman 1961). The prostate gland is a compound tubuloalveolar gland with 18 to 20 ducts that open separately onto the colliculus seminalis. The simple columnar epithelium rests upon a thin basement membrane, and numerous basal cells are present. As in all accessory sex gland epithelia that are highly dependent upon the level of circulating androgen, castration results in epithelial atrophy or regression (Moore et al. 1930b).

Cytological Characteristics

Although a recent review of the fine structure of the prostate gland detailed the cytological differences between the prostates of various species and the microscopic structure of the prostatic lobes in the same species, a general cytological pattern exists for all lobes. Secretion is elaborated from 30 to 50 compound tubuloalveolar glands. These large alveolar cavities are lined with an epithelium that varies from low to cuboidal or even squamous in shape, but in most places it is pseudostratified columnar in form. In the rat and mouse prostate gland, especially in the ventral lobe, a granular endoplasmic reticulum is well developed not only in the perinuclear area but also throughout the cell (Brandes 1966; Brandes and Groth 1961, 1963; Harkin 1957, 1963; Dahl et al. 1973). The typical feature of the epithelium of the lateral lobe is an extremely well developed brush border. The dorsal lobe and the coagulating gland epithelium are characterized by the configuration of the granular endoplasmic reticulum, which is composed of widely dilated cisternae. The rest of the organelles are typical of protein-synthesizing cells in that the cytoplasm contains a large and prominent Golgi complex and numerous secretory granules.

In a recent study on the prostate gland of the dog most sections seen were hyperplastic and characterized by tortuous infolds of acinar lining that projected into the dilated or cystic acini. The cytoplasm of the epithelium was filled with cisternae of granular endoplasmic reticulum, and numerous free ribosomes were seen dispersed in the cytosome. The cytoplasm contained many large membrane-limited secretory droplets (Leav et al. 1971, 1974). The fine structure of the human prostate gland is quite similar, with the exception that the secretion appears to be almost totally extracted from the secretory droplet instead of appearing homogeneous as it does in rodents and the dog (Fischer and Jeffrey 1965; Takayasu and Yamaguchi 1962).

Other structural features of the prostatic epithelium include numerous lysosomes identified by light- and electron-microscopic histochemical techniques (Brandes 1966; Brandes and Groth 1963; Helminen and Ericsson 1970). This is to be expected, because in man a striking feature of the prostatic secretion is the extraordinarily high concentration of acid phosphatase (Mann 1974).

Endocrine Defects and Morphological Changes
The effects of gonadectomy on the prostate gland epithelium have been recorded by many investigators. It has become standard practice to use antiandrogenic measures in patients with adenocarcinoma of the prostate gland, since the lobes of the human prostate differ in responsiveness to sex hormones and adenocarcinoma originates in the androgen-sensitive zones (Huggins and Webster 1948). After gonadectomy of the rat, the epithelium of the prostate atrophies. At the fine structural level there is a gradual collapse of the granular endoplasmic reticulum and loss of the amorphous content of the cisternae. This is followed by fragmentation of the endoplasmic reticulum, loss of ribosomes, and acceleration of lysosome production (Brandes 1966; Harkin 1963). Lipofuscin pigment accumulates as the cell undergoes total regression.

The effects of gonadectomy on the dog prostate have been reported (Leav et al. 1971). The dog is of special interest because the canine prostate shares with the human prostate gland an age-dependent tendency to develop benign prostatic hyperplasia (Ofner 1968) and adenocarcinoma (Leav et al. 1974). Castration resulted in striking alterations in the fine structure of the prostatic epithelial cells. There was almost complete loss of the granular endoplasmic reticulum, accumulation of free ribosomes, an apparent decrease in mitochondria, and many lysosomes in the cytoplasm.

Dogs treated with estradiol-17β cyclopentane-propionate had a squamous metaplasia of the prostate gland and aspermatogenesis (Leav et al. 1971). The cytoplasm of the prostatic epithelial cells of estrogen-treated dogs had an almost complete loss of granular endoplasmic reticulum, and in some cases, large dilated vesicles rimmed with ribosomes remained. The considerable amount of heterochromatin present was massed near the nuclear membrane, and often the perinuclear cisternae appeared dilated. There were also fewer mitochondria, and the Golgi complex was quite small.

Secretory Function of the Prostate
The secretion of the human prostate is a thin, clear fluid with a slightly acid pH (6.5). It has a content of citric acid and acid phosphatase (Mann 1974). Both constituents are directly dependent on the level of circulating androgen. These substances increase at puberty, and thus acid phosphatase and citric acid levels and metabolism can be considered as secondary sex characteristics. It is known that acid phosphatase is assembled on the granular endoplasm reticulum and transferred to the Golgi complex for segregation, where two varieties of the enzyme are prepared. One, the major component, remains in the cytoplasm as a precursor of lysosomal activity. The other component is secreted directly into the prostatic lumen.

The highest concentrations of zinc in the human body occur in the epithelium of the lateral lobe of the prostate (Gunn and Gould 1956). The function of this high zinc concentration in human seminal plasma is not known. Additionally, the prostatic secretion contains several protolytic enzymes, β glucuronidase and diastase. The oldest known organic constituent of human seminal plasma, spermine, is produced in the prostate (Mann 1974).

It must be emphasized that all of the above-mentioned secretory products and others of the prostate are dependent upon the levels of circulating androgen; therefore, a decrease of these substances in the seminal plasma indicates a fall in androgen level or blockage of hormone action at the cellular level. Such a decrease might be a test of the effectiveness of certain chemical compounds in altering the function of the prostate gland.

33.3 Coagulating Gland

The coagulating gland is considered a part of the rodent prostatic complex. There is also a homologous relationship between the middle lobe of the human prostate and the coagulating gland (Price 1963). Like the other accessory sex glands, the coagulating gland responds sensitively to decreased androgen; the epithelium undergoes a rapid involution and atrophy. After injection of 50 μg testosterone propionate daily for 20 days into castrate rats, the epithelium demonstrates a histochemical appearance comparable to that seen in intact sexually mature rats (Cavazos and Melampy 1956).

The coagulating gland epithelium is characterized at the fine structural level by many short microvilli on the luminal surface (Brandes et al. 1959). The granular endoplasmic reticulum is extensively developed and dilated, and the cisternae form large cavities. Gonadectomy is followed by a partial collapse of the dilated endoplasmic reticulum, decreased numbers of vacuoles in the Golgi complex region, and accentuation of the nuclear indentations. Although little information is available on the secretory functions and mechanisms of this gland, it is known to produce fructose (Mann 1974). Its organ-specificity and androgen-responsiveness are so characteristic that it can be reproduced in transplanted tissues. Lutwak-Mann et al. (1949) transplanted minute fragments of coagulating gland subcutaneously into a female rat. These fragments of tissue grew in response to injection of testosterone, and they produced fructose in high concentrations. The coagulating gland epithelium produces an enzyme known as *vesiculase,* which acts upon a coagulable protein secreted by the seminal vesicle. This action forms the copulatory or vaginal plug.

33.4 Bulbourethral Glands

The paired bulbourethral glands (Cowper's glands) are derived from the phallic portion of the embryonic urogenital sinus (Price and Williams-Ashman 1961). The adult gland is a compound tubuloalveolar gland that empties its mucous secretion directly into the membranous or penile urethra. The cells of the bulbourethral gland are pyramidal to columnar, and the nucleus is usually flattened and basally located. Numerous secretory droplets, which fill the cytoplasm, are positive for Hale's colloidal iron reaction indicating acid mucopolysaccharides (Feagans et al. 1961). Like other accessory sex glands, the bulbourethral gland can be used as an indicator of the level of circulating androgen (Heller 1930, 1932). A study on the effects of estrogens on male hamsters (Feagans et al. 1961) found that the bulbourethral gland was the most sensitive indicator of decreasing androgen activity of all of the accessory sex organs.

In the fine structure of the epithelial cells of the bulbourethral gland of the hamster, the apical plasmalemma had numerous microvilli. Only a few profiles of the granular endoplasmic reticulum were present. Most of the cytological features were obliterated by the massive accumulation of secretion droplets (Feagans et al. 1963). In the same study the bulbourethral gland epithelium of 10-day-old hamsters contained an organized Golgi complex, and even at this early time there was evidence of secretory formation. Thus it appears that the bulbourethral gland in the hamster is even more sensitive to levels of circulating androgen than is the seminal vesicle.

Gonadectomy of the hamster resulted in sloughing of many of the epithelial cells of the bulbourethral gland. Most of the remaining cells were vacuolated, possibly from coalescence of mucous secretory droplets. Remains of many cells also indicated fragmentation of much of the epithelium. Dense bodies or lysosomes were not observed in the epithelium. Histochemical studies of hamster bulbourethral glands reported no increase in residual bodies or lipofuscin pigment after castration. It has been emphasized that the accessory sex glands that secrete protein undergo lysosome formation as a consequence of endocrine imbalance. In the bulbourethral gland the secretion is mucous, and the atrophy of the cell, because of decrease in androgen levels, must be mediated through an unknown mechanism.

Secretory Products

The mucopolysaccharide in the bulbourethral gland secretion is composed of galactose, galactosamine, galactouronic acid, sialic acid, and methylpentose. Hart and Greenstein (1964) suggested that the galactose is a nutrient source for spermatozoa. Hartree (1962) reported that the sialic acid levels in the semen of the boar could be used as an accurate indicator of the secretory activity of the bulbourethral gland.

Little is known of the mechanism that results in the secretory process of the epithelium of the bulbourethral gland. The accumulation of mucus in the epithelium of this gland is probably similar to the apocrine type of secretory mechanism seen in the goblet cell.

33.5 Discussion

Androgen Dependency

The action of androgen in the maintenance of the accessory sex organs has been emphasized. It is well established that testosterone production is required for the differentiation and function of the accessory sex gland at the time of puberty. It follows that after this differentiation, any decrease in levels of circulating androgen results in cellular dysfunction, which is reflected both morphologically and chemically. The loss of secretion in castrated animals is tied directly to the functional failure of the endoplasmic reticulum. This, in turn, is related to blockage of mRNA and other biochemical events until the secretory mechanism is destroyed and the cell is essentially incapable of carrying out its function. All of these changes can be reversed quite rapidly by the administration of testosterone.

Light and electron microscopy can determine that the cell is undergoing atrophy and that the secretory mechanism is affected. Decreases measured by biochemical methods in levels of citric acid, fructose, acid phosphatase, and many other chemical constituents of semen quickly reveal the endocrine milieu that affects the accessory sex glands.

It is known that the general indirect hormonal control of the accessory sex glands is via the testis-hypothalamic-pituitary axis, but only limited information is available on the localization of androgens in the sex accessory glands. Considerable research is being carried out on the mode of action of testosterone at the cellular level. A body of evidence suggests that male hormone effects on the epithelium of the accessory sex organs are mediated partly or perhaps entirely by intracellular metabolites of circulating androgens (Short 1967; Armstrong 1970; Ofner 1968, 1971; Wilson and Gloyna 1970). Testosterone in the rat is reduced to dihydrotestosterone by prostatic nuclei, and the cytosol contains soluble proteins with specific binding activity for 5α-dihydrotestosterone (17β-hydroxy-5α-androstan-3-one) (Bruchovsky and Wilson 1968a,b; Anderson and Liao 1968). In a variety of androgen-dependent tissues of several species, testosterone is converted first to 5α-reduced 17β-hydroxysteroid metabolites. These metabolites appear to be the major factors responsible for growth, secretion, and maintenance of the accessory sex organs (Gloyna and Wilson 1969; Robel et al. 1971; Ofner et al. 1974).

One of the recent techniques developed for study of hormone action has been the use of organ cultures (Lasnitzki et al. 1974). In organ cultures of rat ventral prostates, 5α-dihydrotestosterone and 5α-androstane-3β, 17β-diols were much more effective than testosterone in stimulating cell growth and secretion. When studied with electron microscopy, the organ cultures were comparable in every way to those in the intact animal (Robel et al. 1971). Therefore it appears that circulating testosterone, elaborated by the Leydig cells of the testis, enters the epithelium of the sex accessories and in the cytoplasm follows a largely reductive metabolic pathway, which results in the formation of biologically active products. The hormonal compound 5α-dihydrotestosterone is bound to a specific intracytoplasmic protein receptor, and the resultant protein-hormone complex is translocated to the nucleus of the cell, where it is bound to acidic proteins in the nuclear chromatin. It is now thought to result in new RNA synthesis, although this is not clearly demonstrated. Thus 5α-reductase and 3α- and 3β-oxidoreductases, the enzymes that convert testosterone to 5α-dihydrotestosterone and then to 5α-androstone-3β,17β-diol and 5α-androstone-3α-17β-diol, appear to have an essential and major function in regulation of hormone responsiveness in the accessory sex organs.

Investigations are needed on the possibility of controlling accessory sex organ function by blocking some of the enzymes that are responsible for the metabolic transformation of testosterone. Although cyproterone acetate is thought to compete with testosterone for the cytoplasmic receptor, little is known about the possibility of blocking enzymes with an antimetabolite. This could result in shifts from the reductive to the oxidative pathways. If dihydrotestosterone is not formed, the 3α- and 3β-diols will not be produced. It is thought that the diols have their site of activity in the cytoplasm and are responsible for the formation of secretion in the epithelium of the accessory sex organs. There is a need for more comprehensive studies of the enzymes in accessory sex organs that are responsible for the biosynthesis of the male hormone; its transformation into intracellular metabolites is basic to the understanding of the mechanism of androgen action.

Efforts should also be directed to producing compounds that compete against the cytoplasmic receptor of testosterone and will lock subsequent metabolism of androgen. Additional information must be obtained upon the direct role of the accessory sex glands in this fertilization process. Spermatozoa taken from the epididymis and used for artificial insemination are capable of fertilizing ova. The seminal vesicles are absent in the canine, and the coagulating gland appears only in rodents. Even if the functions of the accessory sex glands became blocked, information should be gathered on the effects of this fertility blockage.

Action of Estrogens
Estrogens are directly and indirectly antagonistic to testosterone effects on the accessory sex organs. The indirect effects of estrogens are probably by the inhibition of pituitary gonadotropins, which in turn results in suppression of testosterone. This steroid is produced by the smooth endoplasmic reticulum of the Leydig cells of the testis. As a consequence of the estrogen blockage of testosterone production, the level of circulating androgen decreases. In a study on the effects of estradiol on dogs (Leav et al. 1971), the results obtained on prostatic C19-steroid metabolism provided support for the reported estrogen-induced inhibition of

the 17β-hydroxysteroid pathway and concurrent stimulation of the 17-ketosteroid pathway of in vivo testosterone metabolism reported by others in men.

Estrogen therapy in intact dogs and men results in squamous metaplasmia of the prostatic epithelium. This transformation of the epithelium into a squamous form is thought to be due to proliferation of the basal cells into squamous epithelium.

Thus it is known that estrogens suppress spermatogenesis and bring about atrophy of the seminal vesicles and bulbourethral glands. If the dose of estrogen is high enough, it will produce an epithelial atrophy comparable to that seen following castration. Additional research should be carried out on the differential effects of estrogens on the accessory sex glands.

The Cell Surface
One of the characteristics of all the epithelia of the accessory sex glands is the presence of a fine glycocalyx (Bennett 1963) on the apical plasma membrane of the epithelium. When examined with the light microscope, this epithelium has a positive periodic acid-Schiff reaction at the cell apex (Feagans et al. 1961; Jeffrey et al. 1967). At the fine structural level, this glycocalyx is seen as a short, fine, filamentous substance attached to the microvilli of the apical plasma membrane of the sex accessories. This mucopolysaccharide substance at the cell apex does not attain the length, nor has it the complexity, of that found on the brush border of the cat intestine (Ito 1965). In the intestine this surface layer acts as a barrier to large particles while allowing emulsified lipid, colloidal particles, and substances in solution to pass freely through its meshes and into the clefts between the microvilli.

The glycocalyx is quite resistant to many proteolytic and potent mucolytic agents. The significance of the localization of this carbohydrate coat on the epithelium of the accessory sex glands and its function in reproductive physiology is certainly not understood and should be investigated further for its possible role in fertility or sterility. One possibility is the induction of infertility by obliterating the mucopolysaccharide layer with a chemical agent. It must be emphasized, however, that there is only limited information on the role of the apical plasma membrane in reproductive physiology. Few have looked at the problem, possibly because of the many technical difficulties in working with these membranes. Perhaps an evaluation and understanding of these membranes could be obtained with stereoelectron microscopy or highly sophisticated biochemical procedures that could isolate these apical membranes and their glycocalyx.

Methodological Resources
The accessory sex glands are ideal systems in which to study the biological effects of hormones on a cell complex. The classical techniques of castration and hormone replacement have been used a long time, and a considerable amount of information has been obtained. Yet a number of techniques have recently been developed that will extend our knowledge of the interaction of androgens on the accessory sex glands:

1. Explant techniques or organ cultures are being used to study the mechanism of androgen uptake and concentration by the prostate and seminal vesicles and to examine benign prostatic hyperplasia. These techniques would also be excellent for study of the direct effects of antifertility agents on the accessory sex glands, since the multitude of biological factors that mask or cloud the results would be eliminated.

2. Radioactive steroids are being used for radioautographic studies to locate hormones in frozen sections. The localization of sites of activity has been precise, and the results and procedures could be extended to identify sites of concentration of radioactive antifertility agents at the cytological level.

3. Implant techniques have been developed that allow sex accessory tissues to be implanted in host animals.

4. There is a need to more fully develop tissue-fractionation techniques in order to determine the biological activity of a variety of cells and tissues that relate to the secretory epithelium and are probably under the influence of androgen. For lack of more precise techniques, little is known of the role of the connective tissues, basal cells, and smooth-muscle coats of the accessory sex glands.

References

Allison, V. F. Ultrastructural changes in the seminal vesicle epithelium of the rat following castration and androgen administration. Anat. Rec. 148:254 (Abstract), 1964.

Anderson, K. M., and S. H. Liao. Selective retention of dihydrotestosterone by prostate nuclei. Nature 219:277, 1968.

Armstrong, D. T. Reproduction. Ann. Rev. Physiol. 32:439, 1970.

Baulieu, E.-E. Survey of the mode of action of steroid hormones. *Endocrinology*, Proc. Fourth Int. Cong. Endocrinol., ed. R. Scow, Int. Cong. Series No. 273, p. 30. New York: American Elsevier, 1973.

Belt, W. D. Distribution of carbonyl lipids in the adult white rat. M.Sc. Thesis, Ohio State University, 1950.

Belt, W. D., and L. F. Cavazos. Fine structural alterations of the epithelium of the hamster seminal vesicle following treatment with diethylstilbestrol. Anat. Rec. 157:212 (Abstract), 1967.

Bennett, H. S. Morphological aspects of extracellular polysaccharides. J. Histochem. Cytochem. 11:14, 1963.

Brandes, D. The fine structure and histochemistry of prostatic glands in relation to sex hormones. Int. Rev. Cytol. 20:2, 1966.

Brandes, D., and D. Groth. The fine structure of the rat prostatic complex. Exp. Cell Res. 23:159, 1961.

Brandes, D., and D. Groth. Functional ultrastructure of rat prostatic epithelium. Natl. Cancer Inst. Monogr. 12:47, 1963.

Brandes, D., W. D. Belt, and G. Bourne. Preliminary remarks concerning the fine structure of the epithelium of the coagulating gland. Exp. Cell Res. 16:683, 1959.

Bruchovsky, N., and J. D. Wilson. The conversion of testosterone and 5α-androstan-17β-ol-3-one by rat prostate in vivo and in vitro. J. Biol. Chem. 243:2012, 1968a.

Bruchovsky, N., and J. D. Wilson. The conversion of testosterone to 5α-androstan-17β-ol-3-one by rat prostate. J. Biol. Chem. 243:5953, 1968b.

Burnes, R. K. Role of hormones in the differentiation of sex. In *Sex and internal secretions*, ed. W. C. Young, p. 76. Baltimore: Williams & Wilkins, 1961.

Cavazos, L. F. Effects of stilbestrol on the fine structure of the hamster seminal vesicle. Anat. Rec. 145:215 (Abstract), 1963.

Cavazos, L. F. Fine structure and functional correlates of male accessory sex glands of rodents. In *Handbook of physiology*, Section 7: *Endocrinology*, Vol. 5: *Male reproductive system*, eds. R. O. Greep and D. W. Hamilton. Baltimore: Williams & Wilkins, 1975.

Cavazos, L. F., and R. M. Melampy. Cytological effects of testosterone proprionate on epithelium of rat seminal vesicles. Endocrinology 54:640, 1954.

Cavazos, L. F., and R. M. Melampy. Effects of differential testosterone proprionate levels on rat accessory gland activity. Iowa State Coll. J. Sci. 31:19, 1956.

Cavazos, L. F., W. D. Belt, M. N. Sheridan, and W. M. Feagans. The fine structure of the hamster seminal vesicle with special reference to pigment formation. Z. Zellforsch. 63: 179, 1964.

Cavazos, L. F., J. E. Jeffrey, and W. M. Feagans. Effects of DL-ethionine on the cytochemistry of the male reproductive tract. Acta Anat. 45:252, 1961.

Cavazos, L. F., J. C. Porter, and R. M. Melampy. Composition of rat seminal vesicles and effects of testosterone propionate on lipid distribution. Proc. Soc. Exp. Biol. Med. 85:511, 1954.

Dahl, E., A. Kjaerheim, and K. J. Iveter. The ultrastructure of the accessory sex organs of the male rat. I. Normal structure. Z. Zellforsch. 137:345, 1973.

Deane, H. W. Electron microscopic observations on the mouse seminal vesicle. Natl. Cancer Inst. Monogr. 12:63, 1963.

Deane, H., and E. Dempsey. The localization of phosphatases in the Golgi region of intestinal and other epithelial cells. Anat. Rec. 93:401, 1945.

Deane, H. W., and K. R. Porter. Response of the epithelium of mouse vesicular glands to altered levels of circulating androgen. Proc. First Int. Cong. Endocrinol., p. 971. Copenhagen, 1960.

Deane, H. W., and S. Wurzelmann. Electron microscopic observations on the postnatal differentiation of the seminal vesicle epithelium of the laboratory mouse. Am. J. Anat. 117:91, 1965.

Feagans, W. M., W. D. Belt, and M. Sheridan. Fine structure of the acinar cell in the hamster bulbourethral gland. Acta Anat. 52:273, 1963.

Feagans, W. M., L. F. Cavazos, and A. T. Ewald. A morphological and histochemical study of estrogen-induced lesions in the hamster male reproductive tract. Am. J. Anat. 108:31, 1961.

Fischer, E., and W. Jeffrey. Ultrastructure of human normal and neoplastic prostate. Am. J. Clin. Pathol. 44:119, 1965.

Fugita, M. The fine structure of the epithelial cell of the mouse seminal vesicle studied with the electron microscope. J. Kurume Igakkai Zasshi 22:536, 1959.

Gloyna, R. E., and J. D. Wilson. A comparative study of the conversion of testosterone to 17β-hydroxy-5α-androstan-3-one (dihydrotestosterone) by prostate and epididymis. J. Clin. Endocrinol. Metab., 29:970, 1969.

Gunn, S., and T. Gould. Differences between dorsal and lateral components of the dorsolateral prostate of rat in Zn65 uptake. Proc. Soc. Exp. Biol. Med. 92:17, 1956.

Harkin, J. C. An electron microscope study of the castration changes in rat prostate. Endocrinology 60:185, 1957.

Harkin, J. C. Prostatic ultrastructure. Natl. Cancer Inst. Monogr. 12:85, 1963.

Hart, R., and J. S. Greenstein. An analysis of Cowper's gland secretion in the adult male albino rat. Am. Zool. 4:260 (Abstract), 1964.

Hartree, E. F. Sialic acid in the bulbo-urethral glands of the boar. Nature 196:483, 1962.

Heller, R. E. Cowper's gland as a testis hormone indicator. Proc. Soc. Exp. Biol. Med. 27:752, 1930.

Heller, R. E. Cowper's gland and its reaction to castration and to different sex hormone conditions. Am. J. Anat. 50:73, 1932.

Helminen, H. J., and J. L. E. Ericsson. On the mechanism of lysosomal secretion. Electron microscopic and histochemical studies on the epithelial cells of the rat's ventral prostate lobe. J. Ultrastruct. Res. 33:528, 1970.

Huggins, C., and W. O. Webster. Duality of human prostate in response to estrogen. J. Urol. 59:258, 1948.

Hunter, J. Observations on certain parts of the animal oeconomy. London: Leicester Square, 1786.

Ito, S. The enteric surface coat on cat intestinal microvilli. J. Cell Biol. 27:475, 1965.

Jeffrey, J., L. F. Cavazos, W. M. Feagans, and F. Schmidt. The interaction of estrogen, testosterone and chorionic gonadotropin (HGG) on the reproductive system of the male hamster. Acta Anat. 66:387, 1967.

Kocen, B. P., and L. F. Cavazos. Cytochemistry of male reproductive tract in scurvy and inanition. Proc. Soc. Exp. Biol. Med. 98:485, 1958.

Kovacs, J. Focal cytoplasmic degradation and lysosome formation in the epithelial cells in the seminal vesicles of the mouse. Acta Biol. Acad. Sci. Hung. 19:23, 1968.

Lasnitzki, I., H. R. Franklin, and J. D. Wilson. The mechanism of androgen uptake and concentration by rat ventral prostate in organ culture. J. Endocrinol. 60:81, 1974.

Leav, I., and L. F. Cavazos. Some morphologic features of normal and pathologic canine prostate. In *Normal and abnormal growth of the prostate*, ed. M. Goland, pp. 69–101. Springfield, Ill.: Charles C Thomas, 1975.

Leav, I., L. F. Cavazos, and P. Ofner. Fine structure and C_{19}-steroid metabolism of spontaneous adinocarcinoma of the canine prostate. J. Natl. Cancer Inst. 52:789, 1974.

Leav, I., R. Morfin, P. Ofner, L. F. Cavazos, and E. B. Leeds. Estrogen and castration-induced effects on canine prostatic fine structure and C_{19}-steroid metabolism. Endocrinology 89:465, 1971.

Leblond, C. P. Distribution of periodic acid-reactive carbohydrates in the adult rat. Am. J. Anat. 86:1, 1950.

Lowsley, O. S. Development of the human prostate gland with reference to the development of other structures at the néck of the urinary bladder. Am. J. Anat. 13:299, 1912.

Lutwak-Mann, C., T. Mann, and D. Price. Metabolic activity in tissue transplants. Hormone induced formation of fructose and citric acid in transplants from accessory glands of reproduction. Proc. R. Soc. [Biol] 136:461, 1949.

Lyman, C., and E. Dempsey. The effect of testosterone on the seminal vesicles of castrated, hibernating hamsters. Endocrinology 49:647, 1951.

McNeal, J. E. Origin and development of carcinoma in the prostate. Cancer 23:24, 1969.

Mann, T. *The biochemistry of semen*, London: Methuen, 1954.

Mann, T. Male sex hormone and its role in reproduction. Recent Prog. Horm. Res. 12:353, 1956.

Mann, T. *The biochemistry of semen and of the male reproductive tract*. London: Methuen, 1964.

Mann, T. Secretory function of the prostate, seminal vesicle and other male accessory organs of reproduction. J. Reprod. Fertil. 37:179, 1974.

Mann, T., and C. Lutwak-Mann. Secretory function of male accessory organs of reproduction in mammals. Physiol. Rev. 31:27, 1951.

Melampy, R. M., and L. F. Cavazos. Effects of testosterone propionate on histochemical reactions of rat seminal vesicles. Endocrinology 52:173, 1953.

Moore, C. R., W. Hughes, and T. F. Gallagher. Rat seminal-vesicle cytology as a testis-hormone indicator and the prevention of castration changes by testis-extract injection. Am. J. Anat. 45:109, 1930a.

Moore, C. R., D. Price, and T. F. Gallagher. Rat-prostate cytology as a testis-hormone indicator and the prevention of castration changes by testis-extract injection. Am. J. Anat. 45:71, 1930b.

Ofner, P. Effects and metabolism in normal and neoplastic prostate tissue. Vitam. Horm. 26:237, 1968.

Ofner, P. Recent developments in the study of hormone effects and metabolism in prostate tissue. Symp. Dtsch. Ges. Endokrinol. 17:147, 1971.

Ofner, P., I. Leav, and L. F. Cavazos. C_{19}-steroid metabolism in male accessory sex gland. Correlation of changes in fine structure and radiometabolite patterns in the prostate of the androgen-deprived dog. In *Male accessory sex organs: Structure and function in mammals*, ed. D. Brandes. N.Y.: Academic Press, 1974.

Ortiz, E., D. Price, H. G. Williams-Ashman, and J. Banks. Influence of androgen on the male accessory reproductive glands of the guinea pig. Endocrinology 59:479, 1956.

Porter, J. C., and R. M. Melampy. Effects of testosterone propionate on the seminal vesicles of the rat. Endocrinology 51:412, 1952.

Price, D. Normal development of the prostate and seminal vesicles of the rat with a study of experimental postnatal modifications. Am. J. Anat. 60:79, 1936.

Price, D. Comparative aspects of development and structure in the prostate. Natl. Cancer Inst. Monogr. 12:1, 1963.

Price, D., and H. G. Williams-Ashman. The accessory reproductive glands in mammals. In *Sex and internal secretions*, 3rd ed., ed. W. C. Young, p. 366. Baltimore: Williams & Wilkins, 1961.

Robel, P., I. Lasnitzki, and E.-E. Baulieu. Hormone metabolism and action: Testosterone and metabolites in prostate organ culture. Biochimie 53: 81, 1971.

Short, R. V. Reproduction. Ann. Rev. Physiol. 29:373, 1967.

Stafford, R. O., I. Rubinstein, and R. K. Meyer. Effect of testosterone propionate on phosphatases in the seminal vesicle and prostate of the rat. Proc. Soc. Exp. Biol. Med. 71:353, 1949.

Szirmai, J., and P. C. van der Linde. The fine structure of the seminal vesicles in normal and castrated rats. Electron Microsc. 2:TT-9, 1962.

Takayasu, H., and Y. Yamaguchi. An electron microscopic study of prostate cancer cell. J. Urol. 87:935, 1962.

Toner, P., and A. Baillie. Biochemical, histochemical and ultrastructural changes in the mouse seminal vesicle after castration. J. Anat. 100:173, 1966.

Toth, S. E. The origin of lipofuscin age pigments. Exp. Gerontol. 3:19, 1968.

Walker, G. A special function discovered in a glandular structure hitherto supposed to form a part of the prostate gland in rats and guinea pigs. Bull. Johns Hopkins Hosp. 21:182, 1910.

Wiesner, B. The post-natal development of the genital organs in the albino rat. J. Obstet. Gynaecol. Br. Empire 41:867, 1934.

Williams-Ashman, H. G., and A. H. Reddi. Actions of vertebrate sex hormones. Ann. Rev. Physiol. 33:31, 1971.

Wilson, J. D., and R. E. Gloyna. The intranuclear metabolism of testosterone in the accessory organs of reproduction. Recent Prog. Horm. Res. 26:309, 1970.

The Epididymis   David W. Hamilton

The epididymis is an organ whose sole function seems to be the post-testicular maturation of sperm. Controversies as to whether sperm maturation is inherent in the sperm or is brought about by action of the epididymis have largely been resolved today with the recognition that the maturation process is a cooperative phenomenon that requires interaction among sperm, luminal fluid, the epididymal epithelium, and the blood and lymph vascular compartments.

34.1 Sperm Maturation

Spermatozoa are formed in the seminiferous tubules and are transported from the testis, via the rete testis, into the excurrent duct system. This system is comprised of several ductuli efferentes that empty into a single, high-coiled ductus epididymidis, which ends as the straight ductus deferens. Sperm remain in the duct system for varying periods of time before being ejaculated, and during this time they change from functionally immature cells that are unable to fertilize an egg to cells with full fertilizing capacity. Experimental evidence for the phenomenon is available for all species that have been studied to date (i.e., guinea pig: Young 1931; rabbit: Nishikawa and Waide 1952, Fulka and Koefoed-Johnson 1966, Bedford 1966, Orgebin-Crist 1967, 1969, Glover 1969; rat: Blandau and Rumery 1964; hamster: Horan and Bedford 1972; human: Bedford et al. 1973b). The rabbit has been the most extensively studied species; Table 34.1 summarizes some of the data of Orgebin-Crist (1969). As is clear, the ability of sperm to fertilize ova increases along the length of the duct. In the rabbit the lower corpus seems to be the point at which maturation is finally achieved, since sperm in the proximal cauda are fully mature.

Morphological Features

The most obvious morphological change observable as sperm progress through the epididymis is the caudal migration of the cytoplasmic droplet. This was first reported by Redenz (1924), but it has subsequently been mentioned by numerous authors, and the mode of its formation has been studied by electron microscopy (Bloom and Nicander 1961; Fawcett and Phillips 1969). Sperm in which the cytoplasmic droplet does not migrate are generally not expected to be able to fertilize an ovum (Dott and Dingle 1968), but no experimental evidence exists for this. The cytoplasmic droplet contains hydrolytic enzymes (Dott and Dingle 1968) and may be a lysosome, but the functional implications of this and the causative factors in its migration are completely obscure.

Other than cytoplasmic droplet migration, acrosome changes are the only well-documented morphological changes that take place in sperm in the epididymis. Fawcett and Phillips (1969) illustrated striking changes in acrosome shape in different portions of the epididymis in two hystricomorph rodents, the guinea pig and the chinchilla; these changes involved remodeling of the acrosome from an initially flattened structure to

Table 34.1 Fertilizing ability of sperm from various epididymal segments in the rabbit (after Orgebin-Crist 1969)

	Caput	Upper Corpus (Proximal Corpus)	Lower Corpus (Distal Corpus)	Proximal Cauda	Distal Cauda
% fertilization by sperm from this segment	—	1	63.3	92.7	92.4
% fertilization after 12 days of ligation of the corpus	0	—	—	—	60.4
% of fetuses developed from implants after fertilization by sperm from lower corpus and distal cauda (Day 28)	—	—	69.0	—	78.0
% of fetuses developed from implants after fertilization by sperm retained in the upper corpus by 24-hr ligation (Day 28)	—	55.5	—	—	91.1

one of considerable complexity. Bedford (1965) noted somewhat simpler changes in the rabbit in the disposition of the plasma membrane over the sperm head as it progressed through the epididymis, and he related this to osmotic phenomena probably produced by electrolyte changes along the length of the duct. As with the cytoplasmic droplet, however, the acrosome changes cannot be related either to processes inherent in the sperm or to the influence of the epididymis.

One morphological change that may be related to both biochemical and physiological changes in many species is the disposition of the plasmalemma in sperm from caudal regions of the duct. Bedford (1965) showed that in sperm from the cauda epididymidis in rabbits, the plasmalemma over the acrosome gives the appearance of having swelled when compared with the plasmalemma in sperm from more proximal parts of the duct. He suggested that this might indicate osmotic swelling produced by changes in the membrane as it proceeds down the duct. The earliest and most direct evidence suggesting that the plasmalemma of the sperm changes along the duct was that sperm in distal portions were more susceptible to histological stains than were those in the caput (Glover 1960, 1962; Ortavant 1953), which implied that some of the permeability properties of the sperm were different in the two regions. The properties of phospholipids are generally felt to be important in determining passive permeability, whereas active transport involves enzyme mediated transfer from the extracellular to the intracellular compartment. There is ample evidence from a number of species showing that sperm phospholipids change from the caput to the cauda, which offers support to the idea of related permeability changes similar to those seen in other cell types (van Deenen et al. 1963). It can also be shown (Quinn and White 1967; Mann 1964) that sperm from the caput are more resistant to cold shock than caudal sperm, but the response to cold shock in caudal sperm can be masked by added phospholipids.

These results suggest that the plasmalemma of sperm is very important in their maturation. Bedford and his colleagues have recently been interested in changes in the sperm membrane as the sperm traverse the duct. With electron microscopy, Bedford and Nicander (1971) described specific differences between capital and caudal sperm in the acrosomal membrane of the rabbit and the monkey. The membrane thicknesses differed in the outer and inner leaflets. Cooper and Bedford (1971) showed that the sperm plasmalemma accumulates a net negative surface charge as the sperm proceed along the epididymis. This can be correlated with other observations involving changes in the surface of the sperm.

Barker and Amann (1969) and Johnson and Hunter (1970) have presented evidence that a portion of sperm-associated antigens originate in the epididymis, and Johnson and Hunter (1970) and Crabo and Hunter (1975) suggest that some of these antigens coat the sperm during its passage through the epididymis in the rabbit. These observations may help explain the differences in electrophoretic response that Bedford (1963) notes between capital and caudal rabbit sperm and also the progressive agglutination that occurs between sperm in some species. Bedford's 1963 experiments showed that capital sperm were primarily oriented with the head toward the anode in his electrophoretic system and that as one proceeded along the duct, the polarity reversed so that caudal sperm were primarily tail-oriented toward the anode. Bedford interpreted this to indicate a net increase in negative charge over the surface of the tail. This agrees with the data of Nevo et al. (1961) showing a higher net surface charge on isolated bull sperm tails than on sperm heads. The negative surface charge might possibly be attributable to a glycoprotein coat acquired in the epididymis which acts as a sperm-specific antigen, possibly like those revealed by the immunological studies of Johnson and Hunter (1970). Moreover, Bey (1965) has shown that neuraminidase releases measurable amounts of sialic acid from bull sperm; this release is parallel over time to a decrease in the sperm's electrophoretic mobility.

Physiology and Biochemistry
The voluminous literature on the physiology of maturing sperm has been reviewed by Bishop (1961), Bishop and Walton (1960), and Orgebin-Crist (1969). Epididymal sperm in situ are not motile (Simeone 1933; Gunn 1936; Walton 1956; Lardy et al. 1945; Hartman 1939), but as they move along the epididymis they develop the capacity for normal progressive motility. Thus Blandau and Rumery (1964), Gaddum (1969), and Voglmayr et al. (1967) have shown that sperm removed from the caput exhibit disoriented circular swimming motions, whereas caudal sperm have the progressive movement characteristic of ejaculated spermatozoa. The suggestion has been made that migration of the cytoplasmic droplet affects motility, but Bedford (1967) has shown that this is not true. Voglmayr et al. (1967) reported that freshly collected rete testicular spermatozoa were immotile, and they explored the possibility that this condition was due to a lack of ATP. They found that the ATP content of testicular sperm was similar to that in ejaculated cells. Similarly, Morton et al. (1973) showed that the immotility in quiescent hamster epididymal spermatozoa was not due to a lack of ATP. In addition, the immotility of ram testicular spermatozoa is apparently unrelated to differences between the activity of ATP in these cells and that in ejaculated cells (Voglmayr et al. 1969).

Recent reports from several laboratories have noted the multiple effects of cAMP-phosphodiesterase modulators and dibutyryl cAMP on spermatozoan metabolism motility and cyclic nucleotide content (reviewed by Hoskins and Casillas 1973). These studies have demonstrated the involvement of cAMP in the motile process of mammalian spermatozoa and have also provided a framework for a detailed study of the interrelationship between the cellular components involved in motility and those involved in the production of energy. Briefly, with regard to epididymal spermatozoa, it has been shown that phosphodiesterase inhibitors or dibutyryl cAMP stimulate motility in quiescent bovine caput (D. D. Hoskins, unpublished) and caudal sperm (Garbers et al. 1971, 1972; Hoskins et al. 1971, 1974; Hoskins 1973) and in hamster sperm (Morton et al. 1973). How phosphodiesterase inhibitors stimulate motility is largely unknown, but it is clear that intracellular cAMP levels increase within minutes after their addition to spermatozoa (Garbers et al. 1973a). The fact that the cAMP-dependent protein kinase is present in exceptionally large amounts in bovine epididymal (Hoskins et al. 1972, 1974; Garbers et al. 1973b) and monkey ejaculated spermatozoa (Hoskins et al. 1972) suggests that this enzyme is also involved in the motile process. Although phosphodiesterase inhibitors stimulate sperm respiration (Garbers et al. 1971; Hicks et al. 1972) and fructolysis (Hoskins 1973), these effects occur after the increase in cAMP levels and are therefore probably indirect and related to motility-induced changes in the composition of the intracellular adenylate pool (see Hoskins and Casillas 1973 for details). The involvement of cAMP in spermatozoon motility may be pertinent to the development of motility within the epididymis, especially since cAMP levels in bovine sperm increase nearly two-fold during epididymal transit (Hoskins et al. 1974). In other cells cAMP levels usually rise in response to a specific hormonal activation of the enzyme adenyl cyclase. Although the enzyme is present in mammalian spermatozoa (Casillas and Hoskins 1970, 1971), and in monkey sperm it is significantly stimulated by triiodothyronine (Casillas and Hoskins 1970), treatment of spermatozoa with various hormones has usually been ineffective in increasing intracellular cAMP levels. Whether activators of spermatozoon adenyl cyclase exist in epididymal or female genital tract fluids is unknown and is a problem that should be pursued.

The permeability properties that have been studied morphologically are mirrored by changes in ion permeability as sperm travel through the epididymis. Crabo (1965) measured ion concentration in sperm and epididymal plasma in bulls and found that as sperm progressed along the epididymis, there was a slow, passive extrusion of K^+.

Until recently, chemical changes during spermatozoon maturation were noted only in the lipid fractions (Dawson and Scott 1964; Grogan et al. 1966; Picket and Komarek 1967; Picket et al. 1967; Quinn and White 1967). It has now been shown, however, that proteins also change (Lavon et al. 1971). There is not only nonnuclear loss of protein but also qualitative changes in the proteins due to shifts in the proportions of amino acids that are present. Lavon et al. (1971) conclude that most of the changes they report result from changes in sperm lipoprotein. This correlates with losses of the phospholipids and cholesterol that have been reported (see above references in addition to Scott et al. 1963a,b,c; Scott and Dawson 1968) and implicates the plasma membrane as one site of the biochemical changes. An alternative explanation could be that the changes are in the enzymes necessary for motility.

New observations by Bedford and his colleagues (Bedford et al. 1972, 1973a; Bedford and Calvin 1974) have focused attention on the increase in disulfide bonds that occurs in both the nucleus and the tail of a sperm as it traverses the epididymis. Nuclear disulfide bond formation is presumably associated with continuing condensation of the nucleus in the epididymis, and this has been shown to be true in the human as well as in animal species. Increased numbers of disulfide bonds in the sperm tail are apparently related to the outer dense fibers, but the functional implications of this are obscure.

In addition to changes in the biochemical constituents of sperm as they proceed along the epididymis, numerous reports identify metabolic changes between testicular and epididymal sperm (Henle and Zittle 1942; Lardy et al. 1949; Voglmayr et al. 1966, 1967; Setchell et al. 1969; many others). Specifically Frenkel et al. (1973) and Hoskins (unpublished) have shown increased glycolytic and fructolytic rates in caudal epididymal sperm in comparison with sperm from the caput.

Sperm maturation thus has many facets and some of these are relatively completely worked out. For the most part, however, we know little about the process and, indeed, little about the interrelationships among the data that already exist. Table 34.2 summarizes the various aspects of sperm maturation that have been discussed here and draws comparisons between morphological, biochemical, and physiological observations in an attempt to provide correlations between the three approaches to study of the phenomenon.

34.2 Physiology of the Epididymis

The epididymal epithelium has all of the attributes of being very metabolically active. Two specific func-

Table 34.2 Maturational changes in sperm during epididymal transit (modified from Hamilton 1975)

Biochemical	Morphological	Physiological
Phospholipids ↓	Membranes	Cold shock susceptibility ↑
Proteins (non nuclear) ↓		Permeability ↑
Cholesterol ↓		Negative charge ↑
Water and some electrolytes ↑	?	Specific gravity ↑
-S-S- bonds* ↑	Nucleus	?
-S-S- bonds* ↑	Outer dense fibers	Motility pattern changes
cAMP ↑	?	
Carnitine ↑	–	Energy substrate utilization potential ↑
Rates of glycolysis and fructolysis in vitro ↑		
?	Acrosome	?
?	Cytoplasmic droplet migration	?

↓ = decrease.   ↑ = increase.   ? = unknown.   – = no effect.
*disulfide bonds.

tions that have been described are absorption and secretion.

Absorption
In the ductuli efferentes and portions of the epididymis the epithelium has the functions of transferring fluid from the lumen into the interstitium and of absorbing and digesting particular (or macromolecular) material.

The anatomy of absorption of particulate material from the lumen of the duct has been studied for many years (Clubb 1969; Mollendorff 1920; Shaver 1954; Wagenseil 1928; Young 1933; Mason and Shaver 1952), and recently it has been shown with the electron microscope that material is absorbed by the epithelium of the ductuli efferentes (Burgos 1964; Sedar 1966), by the head (Nicander 1965) and tail (Friend 1969; Nicander et al. 1965) of the epididymis, and by the vas deferens (Friend and Farquhar 1967) from a variety of species. The structural details of this activity do not differ significantly from similar processes in other cell types.

The tracer materials that have been used in these studies (colloidal mercuric sulfide, India ink, iron dextran, horseradish peroxidase) are not normally found in the epididymis and thus constitute an unnatural and unphysiological situation. It is not unreasonable to speculate, however, that similar processes also function under normal circumstances in absorbing material from the lumen, although the actual process of absorption that has been described as a result of tracer studies has not been observed in normal animals. Occasionally, vacuoles and multivesicular bodies contain a flocculent, electron-dense precipitate that may represent absorbed material undergoing dehydration, but even in these instances micropinocytosis of similar material is not seen at the apices of the cells. Under some experimental conditions, epithelial cells in various parts of the epididymis are capable of absorbing portions of spermatozoa. Hoffer et al. (1975) have found that when spermatoceles form after a lesion-producing dose of the drug U5897 or after mechanical obstruction of the epididymis, principal cells of the ductuli absorb degenerating spermatozoa and sequester them in large multivesicular bodies. This is an unnatural situation, however, and in the normal state one rarely finds evidence of epithelial spermiophagy (Nicander 1965).

The processes described above are directed toward cellular digestion of the absorbed material. Fluid transport, on the other hand, is apparently directed toward moving the fluid out of the luminal and epithelial compartments and into the interstitial vessels. The volume of fluid produced by the ram's testis each day (Setchel et al. 1969; Voglmayr et al. 1966, 1967) is approximately 100 times that which leaves the epididymis in a sexually active animal (Waites and Setchell 1969), which clearly means that epididymal fluid resorption takes place. Crabo (1965) estimates that more than 90 percent of the fluid that leaves the testis in the bull or boar is resorbed in the ductuli efferentes and first part of the epididymis, but no one has studied the morphological correlates of fluid transport in this organ. The processes involved here are probably similar to those described by Kaye et al. (1966) for gallbladder epithelium, which actively moves fluid from the lumen to the interstitial capillaries. Kaye et al. show that during active water transport there is great distension of the intercellular spaces and apparent shrinkage of the basal parts of the cells. The apical portions remain essentially normal, and intercellular distension does not affect the apical junctional complexes.

The initial stages of fluid movement probably involve micropinocytosis at the luminal plasmalemma. Whether osmotic gradients also play a part here is not known. If the standing osmotic gradient theory of Diamond and Tormey (1966) is correct, a solute pump exists along the lateral plasmalemma, though not seen morphologically, which serves to produce an osmotic gradient that forces water out of the cell. Probably particulate absorption and fluid transport function in a complementary manner. Thus by "drinking" the epididymal plasma, the cell would take up not only water and ions but macromolecules of various types. While the ions and water may be moved out of the cell, the macromolecules might be sequestered and digested. It is not known why water transport occurs only in certain places along the duct, while particulate absorption apparently happens all along.

Secretion

Considerable evidence shows that the epididymis can synthesize certain compounds, and some evidence suggests that some of them are secreted into the epididymal lumen.

Glycerylphosphorylcholine (GPC) Dawson et al. (1957) first noted that the epididymis contains a large amount of GPC, and their observations have been confirmed and extended by numerous investigators. Subsequently Dawson and Rowlans (1959) and others (Scott and Dawson 1968; Scott et al. 1963b; Wallace et al. 1966) showed that ^{32}P-orthophosphate is incorporated into epididymal GPC both in vivo and in vitro, and Scott et al.(1963c) provided convincing proof that the epididymis, not the testis, is the major source of this compound in semen.

The physiological role of GPC in epididymal semen is still unknown, but it may have a stabilizing effect on sperm, and it may play a role in maintaining osmotic pressure balance in the lumen as NaCl is absorbed (Scott et al. 1963c). Sperm are not able to metabolize exogenous GPC, and this, coupled with the fact that no GPC diesterase exists in the epididymis (although alkaline phosphatases and aliesterase have been demonstrated by Allen and Slater 1957), probably accounts for its accumulation along the duct. Wallace et al. (1966) estimate that 20 per cent of the GPC can be accounted for as phospholipid metabolite of the sperm.

Carbohydrates In their study of GPC, Scott et al. (1963c) made the incidental observation that approximately half of the orcinolreactive carbohydrate in ram epididymal fluid is precipitable with trichloracetic acid, thus suggesting that it is protein-bound. Carbohydrate moiety may be produced by the epididymis since the epididymis contains a number of enzymes for carbohydrate metabolism and synthesis, and many of these have been localized in the epithelium histochemically. Possibly the protein moiety is also synthesized here (Gustafsson 1966).

The most direct evidence for epithelial involvement in the synthesis of complex carbohydrates is derived from two sources. In 1966 Neutra and Leblond noted that 10 minutes after administration of ^{3}H-galactose to male rats, tritium can be localized radioautographically over the Golgi region in epididymal epithelial cells.

After 30 minutes silver grains are found over the luminal surfaces of the cells. They did not pursue the activity but suggested that it would eventually enter the lumen. They purposely chose galactose as their tracer since it is mostly converted to complex carbohydrates, in contradistinction to glucose, which may be metabolized in many ways. Direct biochemical evidence of the importance of galactose in the epididymis came in 1969 when Fleischer et al. isolated the Golgi apparatus from bull epididymides and showed that it has an extremely active galactosyltransferase. Fleischer et al. suggest that the enzyme is directed toward glycoprotein production, similar to other tissues that are rich in glycosyltransferases. Further evidence bearing on this is the report by Rambourg et al. (1969) that a dense deposit is localized in Golgi saccules of rat principal cells after thin sections are subjected to the chromic acid–phosphotungstic acid stain for complex carbohydrates. In addition, a thiamine pyrophosphatase (which may be a general nucleoside diphosphatase according to Fleischer et al. 1969) is found in epididymal Golgi in rat, mouse, and bull (Friend and Farquhar 1967; Allen and Slater 1957; Fleischer et al. 1969).

The direct involvement of the Golgi apparatus is the only piece of evidence relating glycoprotein production to cell morphology in the epididymis. One suspects that the protein moiety is formed in the rough endoplasmic reticulum, but there is no morphological evidence to show how the compounds are secreted here. It is possible, considering the action in other tissues, that the Golgi apparatus is involved in some way.

The identification of the non-acid-soluble carbohydrate has not been attempted, but it cannot be glycolyzable sugars (Scott et al. 1963c) such as glucose or fructose, since these are not present in epididymal semen (Scott et al.1963c; Mann and Glover 1954). It is possible that this fraction is bound to lipid or polysaccharide.

As mentioned above, fructose, glucose, and citric acid have been reported to be virtually nonexistent in epididymal plasma (Mann 1964). The absence of reducing sugars (White and Wales 1961) and a low concentration of short-chain fatty acids (Scott et al. 1962) were also reported in epididymal plasma, giving rise to the question of the substrate for metabolism of epididymal spermatozoa. Wu et al. (1959) reported that epididymal spermatozoa utilize glucose via the Embden-Meyerhof pathway in vitro. Scott et al. (1962) found that ram and bull spermatozoa oxidize acetate in preference to glucose in vitro and stated that this preferential oxidation of acetate indicated a greater ability to activate acetate in the presence of pyruvate. Annison et al. (1963) and Setchell and Waites (1964) examined in vivo uptake of glucose and oxygen in the ram, but their studies necessarily involved only whole-organ observations and could give no estimates of differences in metabolism of sperm cells versus actual epididymal tissue. Allen and Slater (1961) located lactic dehydrogenase in the apical portion of the epididymal epithelial cells of the rat. Blackshaw and Samisoni (1965) confirmed this in the bull, and Elliot (1965a) pursued the idea and subsequently proposed that either spermatozoa or the epididymal fluid may have some controlling mechanism for the secretion of lactate by the epithelium. Scott et al. (1963c) had already noted the findings of Cross and Silver (1962) regarding the possibility of aerobic conditions in the epididymal duct and had indicated that their finding of high lactate concentrations in epididymal plasma might suggest lactate as the main energy substrate for epididymal spermatozoa. This possibility was reiterated by Wales et al. (1966).

The in vitro studies of Elliot (1965a,b) showed the primarily glycolytic activity of epididymal tissue. Johnson and Turner (1971), using epididymal tissue of the mouse, rat, and rabbit, investigated the existence of pentose-shunt (hexose monophosphate shunt) activity in the epididymis. They found it to exist in all three species. Kraft and Johnson (1972), using the same three species, found evidence of pentose-shunt activity but reported that glucose metabolism in epididymal tissue was mainly via the Embden-Meyerhof and Krebs-cycle pathways. Turner and Johnson (1972; 1973a,b) reported the carbohydrate metabolism along the length of the bovine epididymis. These workers again found evidence of pentose-cycle activity but with the Embden-Meyerhof and Krebs pathways much more prevalent. In their work the proximal caput and midcorpus were indicated as areas of potential physiological importance because of the high rates of carbohydrate metabolism found in these areas.

The respiratory activity of rabbit caput epididymal tissue has been reported to be low in comparison to other mammalian tissues (Wallace et al. 1966). Kraft and Johnson (1972) likewise found higher rates of glycolysis than of respiration in epididymal tissues from rats, mice, and rabbits. Patterns of $^{14}CO_2$ evolution from specifically labeled glucose also indicates that glucose was metabolized via the pentose cycle. Other studies have indicated significant epididymal pentose-cycle activity (Lunaas et al. 1968; Johnson and Turner 1971; Turner and Johnson 1973a; Sholl and Leathem 1973).

Metabolic activity has also been studied following isolation of the epididymis from the testis. Elliot (1965b) reported that efferentiectomy reduced the rate of glycolysis and respiration of mouse epididymal homogenates; however, the loss of spermatozoa could account for the decreased respiration and for the lowered glycolytic rate. Turner and Johnson (1973a, b)

found a significantly higher utilization of glucose and Krebs-cycle intermediates by the intact than by the isolated bull epididymis.

Proteins Study of epididymal proteins per se has not been extensive, although recently considerable interest has developed in this subject. In studies on boar epididymal proteins, Sedláková et al. (1968) identified serum albumin in the epididymal fluid and assumed that blood serum is the source of proteins in epididymal plasma. Likewise, in the ram, Alumot et al. (1971), using immunoelectrophoresis, found that most proteins of epididymal fluid and seminal plasma have antigens in common with blood serum.

Huang and Johnson (1975) have demonstrated the presence of several proteins unique to epididymal fluid in different species, suggesting that the tissue of the epididymis can secrete specific proteins into the lumen of the epididymal duct. Similar evidence has been presented by Crabo and Hunter (1975). Secretion of proteins by the epididymis is further supported by evidence showing changes in the relative concentrations of the unique proteins from caput to cauda epididymidis. When the epididymal tube becomes free of sperm, the relative protein concentration changes, suggesting that the presence of sperm in the lumen of the epididymal duct can affect the production or accumulation of these unique proteins.

Besides the epididymal plasma unique proteins, the relative concentrations of other proteins in epididymal fluid also change from zone to zone. This suggests that tissues of the epididymal duct of different areas may have the selective ability, not only qualitatively but also quantitatively, to take up certain proteins from blood serum and discharge them into the lumen of the epididymal duct. Conversely, the evidence may indicate selective absorption of proteins along the length of the duct. In either case, these observations point to a fundamental difference between epididymis and testis. The blood-testis barrier acts as an effective block for movement of proteins into the lumen of the seminiferous tubule. In the epididymis, however, no effective barrier to movement of large-molecular-weight compounds seems to exist.

Carnitine Marquis and Fritz (1965a,b,c) were the first to report the exceedingly high concentration of carnitine and carnitine acetyltransferase in the epididymis. Their work showed that carnitine in the rat epididymis is predominantly found in the epididymal fluid, whereas sperm contain the highest activity of the transferase found in the body. Their observations remained relatively unnoticed for many years by reproductive biologists, although the high concentration of carnitine in the rat epididymis was confirmed by Pearson and Tubbs (1967). Recently, however, considerable interest has developed in epididymal carnitine

(Brooks et al. 1973, 1974; Casillas 1972, 1973), and new observations have contributed significantly to our understanding of epididymal physiology. One theoretical basis for interest in carnitine is the fact that carnitine and GPC are present in the rat epididymal fluid in almost equimolar concentrations (63mM carnitine, 41mM GPC), and it could be postulated that the fatty acids derived from lecithin (during its metabolism to GPC) could act as an energy substrate for sperm in the epididymis. The breakdown of lecithin could take place either in the sperm or in the epididymal epithelial cells. Aside from data briefly mentioned below, no published evidence supports this hypothesis.

The experiments of Marquis and Fritz (1965b) showed that carnitine concentration in the rat epididymis increases with age, and they speculated that this might mean that the epididymis synthesizes carnitine. Brooks et al. (1973) and Bøhmer (1974) were unable to find synthetic activity in the epididymis; however, Brooks et al. (1973) showed that blood-borne radioactive L-carnitine accumulates preferentially in the epididymis.

It has been known for years that some drugs, as well as some nonpharmacological compounds, accumulate in semen (e.g., Mann, 1964, 1968), but little attention has been given to how or where the accumulation takes place. Crabo and Appelgren (1972) showed autographically that 3-chloro-1,2-propanediol accumulates in the lumen of the rat cauda epididymidis after intravenous injection, as well as in other organs. In their experiment, rats were sacrificed at varying intervals after administration of the drug. They illustrated only two intervals, 24 hours and four days, but their illustrations are interesting in light of the work on L-carnitine accumulation by the rat epididymis. The α-chlorohydrin is seen at 24 hours to be present in the lower middle segment of the epididymis (Glover and Nicander 1971) as well as in the cauda epididymidis. At four days, the compound is found only in the cauda.

The correspondence between the results of work in carnitine and that on α-chlorohydrin by Crabo and Appelgren (1972) is impressive, and two further comparisons suggest that these observations may be of fundamental importance in epididymal physiology. Glover and Nicander (1971), after careful study of the comparative anatomy and evolution of the male excurrent ducts, have proposed a new terminology based primarily on the distribution of function along the length of the duct. They recognize clearly that the cauda epididymidis is an area of sperm storage (their terminal segment) and that sperm maturation occurs throughout the most proximal parts of the duct.

They recognize an initial segment (Benoit 1926), because it is histologically and ultrastructurally unique (Hoffer et al. 1973), but they place the remainder of the duct, as suggested also by the observations of Hamilton (1972), into a single middle segment. The junction between the middle segment and terminal segment is the point at which sperm are first recognized to be mature (i.e., the old lower corpus designation). Thus carnitine is taken up in the middle segment of the rat epididymis and moves distally to the terminal segment. Casillas (1973) has studied uptake of carnitine by bovine sperm removed from specific segments of the bull epididymis, and he has found that the sperm accumulate carnitine along the middle segment of the bull epididymis, as defined by Glover and Nicander (1971). Earlier work (Casillas 1972) showed that in vitro palmitic acid oxidation by isolated mitochondria from bull epididymal sperm is stimulated up to 40-fold by the addition of carnitine to the incubation medium. Since fatty acid oxidation is thought to play a major role in energy metabolism of epididymal spermatozoa (Hartree and Mann 1959), carnitine accumulation by sperm along the length of the epididymis is probably important to their metabolism during their prolonged stay in the epididymis and is probably associated with their maturation process.

Steroids Testosterone is present in rete testis fluid (Waites and Setchell 1969), and testosterone and dehydroepiandrosterone (DHEA) have been found in epididymal (White and Hudson 1968) as well as in ejaculated semen (Mullen et al. 1968; Steeno et al. 1966; Dirscherl and Breuer 1963; Dirscherl and Knuchel 1950; Oertel and Treiber 1967). It has been thought that the testis is the sole source of these seminal androgens, as well as the seminal estrogens when present, but recent evidence indicates that the epididymis can synthesize steroids in vitro in addition to metabolizing testosterone in normal response to testicular androgen stimulation (Gloyna and Wilson 1969).

The first indication that the epididymis might have the ability to synthesize steroids was the biochemical demonstration of hydroxysteroid dehydrogenases in hamster epididymis by McGadey et al. (1966). This was subsequently borne out biochemically by a number of investigators working independently. Hamilton et al. (1968, 1969) showed that mouse epididymis can synthesize cholesterol from [1-^{14}C] acetate, and Frankel and Eik-Nes (1970a) found that rabbit epididymis synthesizes DHEA from pregnenolone. In a large study of epididymal steroid metabolism, Inano et al. (1969) reported that small quantities of testosterone are formed by substrates of pregnenolone, progesterone, 17α hydroxyprogesterone, and androstenedione in cell-free homogenates of rat epididymis; Hamilton and Fawcett (1970) subsequently showed [1-^{14}C] acetate incorporation into testosterone and cholesterol in slices of rat epididymis and vas deferens. Other species, such as rabbit, ram, and hamster (Fawcett and

Hamilton 1970; Hamilton 1971, 1972) can also synthesize androgens from acetate, although Frankel and Eik-Nes (1970b), using different conditions than Hamilton (1971), were unable to show incorporation of cholesterol or acetate into DHEA or testosterone in rabbit epididymis. This difference in results is disturbing, but nevertheless there is no question that the epididymis can produce steroids in vitro. Until recently it was not known whether epididymal steroids were produced in vivo. Pierrepoint et al. (1974), however, showed that epididymal luminal steroids play an important role in the maintenance of prostate and seminal vesicles in gonadectomized animals.

34.3 Control of Epididymal Function

Androgen Control of the Epididymis
The epididymis is clearly dependent upon testicular hormones in early fetal life, since the presence of androgens determines whether the wolffian or the müllerian ducts predominate and thus whether the animal becomes a male or a female (Price and Ortiz 1965; Wilson 1973). Flickinger (1969) has shown that prior to the onset of hormone production by the fetal testis, wolffian duct cells are relatively undifferentiated. After 15 days of gestation, when testosterone is being produced, epithelial cells show obvious changes involving microvillar growth, increase in smooth endoplasmic reticulum and coated vesicle, and so forth, that presage the adult form. The Golgi apparatus (Flickinger 1969) and stereocilia (Leeson and Leeson 1964), however, do not reach their full development until after birth.

Hormone dependence continues into adult life, as has been amply documented (Maneely 1959; Risley 1963). Cavazos (1958), Allen and Slater (1957), and others have shown that maintenance of the normal histochemistry of the epithelium is dependent upon testosterone. Wislocki (1949) noted seasonal variations in alkaline phosphatase activity in epididymides of the Virginia deer that can be correlated with sexual activity and thus with circulating testosterone levels (Lincoln et al. 1970). Aside from effects on enzymic mechanisms in the epididymis, testosterone is also essential in the maintenance of the morphology of the cells. In the mouse, Hamilton et al. (1969) showed that castration results in loss of microvilli, loss of mitochondria, reduction in the area of the Golgi, and almost total loss of smooth endoplasmic reticulum. Nuclear changes were not noted. Pharmacological doses of testosterone propionate (2 mg/kg) restores the cells almost to normal. It is interesting that the minimal dose of androgen required to maintain the epididymis at control values after castration is up to four times

greater than that required to maintain other male accessory sex organs (Prasad et al. 1973).

The studies on morphological effects of castration are complemented in part by physiological observations. Thus after castration almost all assayable compounds decrease in concentration, and testosterone replacement results in an increase over concentrations found in castrates. Often, however, in the castrated testosterone-treated animals the concentration does not reach normal levels. Thus carnitine restoration was only 65 percent of normal in the head and 49 percent of normal in the tail of the rat epididymis in the experiments of Marquis and Fritz (1965c). These observations are not inconsistent with a hypothesis of hormonal control of the epididymis, but they do suggest that factors other than circulating androgen play a significant role in creating a normal environment in the epididymis.

The effects of circulating androgens on the epididymal epithelium are mirrored to a great degree by their functional effects on epididymal spermatozoa. Benoit (1926) and Moore (1928) showed that epididymal spermatozoa stay motile longer if one or both testes are present. Orgebin-Crist et al. (1973) and Lubicz-Nawrocki and Chang (1973) indicate that steroids can maintain both fertilizing capacity and motility of epididymal sperm from castrated animals for up to 12 days. In nonmaintained castrate animals, normal sperm function is lost by three days. Lubicz-Nawrocki and Chang (1973) have found that exogenous 5α-androstane-$3\alpha,17\beta$-diol is much more effective in maintenance of caudal sperm viability than either testosterone or dihydrotestosterone.

Innumerable examples show epididymal dependence upon androgens, but many of them are too peripheral to the main thrust of this review to warrant citation here. The most important question to be asked is: How do androgens interact with the epididymis to produce their effect?

Androgen Metabolism by the Epididymis
This field has a very brief history. Much of the work published since the first papers appeared in 1968–1969 has been influenced by developments in the general understanding of androgen metabolism and action in male accessory reproductive glands. Even at present little precise information exists regarding the relation of epididymal steroid metabolism to specific functions of the organ under physiological conditions. In particular, little is known about how and which of the intracellular metabolites of the circulating androgens formed in specific segments of the epididymis reach the close proximity of the spermatozoa, in what manner the metabolite(s) is then assimilated, and which are

the active free or receptor-bound species in the spermatozoa that may be held responsible for initiation of the maturation process.

Evidence for the view that the circulating systemically active C19-steroids exert their androgenicity in accessory reproductive organs through intracellular metabolites has been reviewed by Williams-Ashman and Reddi (1971), Ofner (1971), and Ofner et al. (1975). A consensus of opinion favors the existence of a common mechanism of activation of circulating testosterone in accessory sex glands by the action of an NADPH-linked 4-ene-3-oxosteroid 5α-reductase and of translocation of the resulting 5α-dihydrotestosterone, as a complex with a specific cytoplasmic receptor protein, to a specific nuclear site.

In a study comparing the distribution of radioactivity in various rat accessory sex organs of the 24-hour castrate after intramuscular administration of ^{3}H-testosterone one hour before sacrifice, Tveter and Aakvaag (1969) found 22 percent of the label in the "conjugated fraction" of the epididymis, whereas none was found in this fraction in the ventral and lateral prostate. The fraction designated *conjugated* consisted of the metabolites that could not be extracted into ether from aqueous organ extracts and might therefore also have contained highly polar free steroids.

Continuing this line of investigation, Djøseland et al. (1973) administered ^{3}H-testosterone by intramuscular injection into intact rats 30 minutes before decapitation. Guided by the aforementioned finding of epididymal radiosteroid conjugates, they separated the raw extracts into free and water-soluble fractions and found 10 percent of the epididymal radioactivity in the water-soluble fraction. The identification (and pattern) of radiometabolites derived by chromatographic resolution of the free fraction demonstrated the presence of 4-ene-3-oxosteroid 5α-reductase and 3α-, 3β-, and 17β-hydroxysteroid oxidoreductases in the rat epididymis; documentation of the absence of blood-borne 5β-androstane derivatives or of other hepatic radiosteroid markers was not provided. The distinctive features of the pattern of in vivo ^{3}H-testosterone metabolism in the rat epididymis, then, are the predominance of the 5α-reductive 17β-hydroxysteroid pathway over the 17-oxosteroid pathway, of 5α-dihydrotestosterone (47 percent of the free fraction) over the other metabolites, and extensive transformation of this metabolite to the 5α-androstane-diol epimers. There was a fivefold preponderance of 5α-androstane-3α,17β-diol over 5α-androstane-3β,17β-diol, which brings us back to the observation noted above that the 3α epimer is more effective in maintaining caudal sperm viability than either testosterone or dihydrotestosterone.

Simultaneously with publication of the work of Djøseland et al. (1973), Ofner et al. reported data of an analogous study of comparative radiotestosterone metabolism in the canine prostate and epididymis in vivo. This study revealed extensive epididymal transformation of the substrate to the 5α-androstanediol epimers. The radiometabolite patterns in the canine provide evidence of (1) striking predominance of 5α-reduced 17β-hydroxysteroid over 17-oxosteroid metabolites in both prostate and epididymis; (2) significantly greater transformation of the substrate to the 5α-androstane-3α(and 3β),17β-diol epimers in epididymis than in prostate; and (3) preponderance of 3β-hydroxy over 3α-hydroxysteroid radiometabolites on infusion of 50 μg of substrate, but epididymal formation of approximately equal quantities of the epimeric diols at 0.5 μg of administered testosterone. The radiometabolite patterns suggest that protein binding of testosterone in the epididymis plays a smaller part in the control of its 5α-reduction than in the prostate.

Interest in the epididymal role of 5α-androstane-3α,17β-diol is heightened by the work of Sowell and Eik-Nes (1972), who used an isolated preparation of canine epididymis to study the uptake and metabolism of ^{3}H-testosterone infused at a constant rate via the epididymal artery in dog's oxygenated arterial blood. Labeled testosterone, androstenedione, and 5α-dihydrotestosterone, but no 5α-androstane-3α,17β-diol, were isolated from the effluent epididymal venous blood; 5α-androstane-3α,17β-diol was the predominant radiometabolite in the epididymal tissue, considerably exceeding the content of [3]H-5α-dihydrotestosterone and ^{3}H-androsterone. Thus, under the conditions of the infusion, 5α-dihydrotestosterone and androstenedione were secreted, and 5α-androstane-3α,17β-diol was retained.

Steroid-Spermatozoa Interactions

Sperm are bathed in steroids from the time they first leave the seminiferous tubules (Harris 1973) until ejaculation (Steeno et al. 1966; Mullen et al. 1968; White and Hudson 1968; others). To date, very little is known of the kinetics of interaction between steroids and sperm, even though a reasonable amount of work has been done in this area. The steroids that have been identified either in ejaculates or in samples of epididymal semen are testosterone, DHEA and its sulfate (DHEA-S), estrone, estradiol-17β, and estriol. The androgens are present in concentrations about 200 times higher than estrogens. Estrogen content of semen is particularly surprising, although Ericsson and Baker (1966) and Banerjee (1968) have shown that exogenously administered estrogens can be carried to the female at copulation and inhibit pregnancy.

Of particular interest here is the observation by

Diczfaluzy (1954) that human-ejaculated semen contains 60 ng/ml estrone, 10 ng/ml estradiol, and 30 ng/ml estriol. Diczfaluzy did not attempt to separate sperm from seminal plasma, but Schaffenburg and McCullagh (1954) paid particular attention to the distribution of estrogenic substances and showed by bioassay that all of the activity is associated with the sperm fraction and no estrogenic activity can be found in plasma.

The in vitro steroid-binding experiments of Ericsson et al. (1967) seem to have been the first publications on this subject. Ericsson et al. (1967) further found that after injection of ^{3}H-estradiol-17β the epididymis contained a significantly greater amount of radioactivity than the testis, and about 11 percent of the total was bound to epididymal spermatozoa. From this, they conclude that exogenous estrogens gain access to semen by way of the accessory sex glands.

Blaquier (1971) reported experiments in which radiolabeled testosterone or 5α-dihydrotestosterone was injected into live rats and the uptake and metabolism were studied in various fractions of the epididymis. His results showed conclusively that sperm do bind exogenous steroids, but in addition, he reported the interesting fact that 10 percent of the sperm-associated tritium were present as 5α-androstane-3α,17β-diol after injection of ^{3}H-testosterone, 50 percent was present as 5α-dihydrotestosterone, and 21 percent was unchanged testosterone. He concluded that sperm do not concentrate steroids, but his experiments did not take into consideration endogenous pools of steroids within sperm that probably compete with the exogenous compounds. Nonetheless, his results point once again to the androstanediol epimers as compounds that may well have important effects in the epididymis, possibly directly upon sperm.

The nature of steroid influence on sperm is not at all clear. Seamark and White (1964), Scott et al. (1963a), Hathaway and West (1964), Hathaway (1967), Hathaway and Chamberlain (1970), Murdoch et al. (1970), and Wester and Salisbury (1972) have all studied the effects of various steroids on sperm respiration. Without exception, the concentrations of steroid necessary to elicit a response are two to five times greater than physiological concentrations. Some investigators have suggested that in vivo mechanisms may exist for increasing local concentrations of steroids near epididymal sperm. The sperm steroid-binding property may well be a mechanism for concentration of steroids in sperm. Hamilton (unpublished) has shown for rat sperm that the binding is not saturable up to 10^{-5} molar substrate concentration and that as the number of sperm increases, the total amount of bound steroid increases. Presumably, then, if in vivo steroid concentrations are kept constant in the epididymal plasma, sperm uptake will be continuous. Since the system is

not saturable, equilibrium will never be reached, and high concentrations of steroid could theoretically be attained by sperm. If one assumes, however, that the figures quoted above for steroid concentrations reflect the total steroid present, then even assuming that all of it is bound to sperm, one still comes out with figures two or more orders of magnitude less than the minimum amount of steroid that elicits a metabolic response in vitro.

Steroid-Binding Proteins
Two steroid-binding proteins have been characterized in the rat epididymis (Hansson et al. 1975). The properties of one of these are very similar to those of the rat ventral prostate receptor in that it is specific for 5α-dihydrotestosterone, it is elucted in the void volume from a column of Sephadex G-200, and it does not survive charcoal treatment. This protein is presumably involved in the translocation of the steroid to the nuclear binding sites mentioned above.

The other protein, androgen-binding protein (ABP), has high affinity for both 5α-dihydrotestosterone and testosterone. It is retarded on a column of Sephadex G-200 (eluting between IgG and albumin), and it is not affected by charcoal treatment or heating (50°C for 30 minutes). There is strong evidence that ABP is synthesized in the testis on stimulation by FSH, and it is carried to the epididymis via the rete testis and ductuli efferentes. A preponderance of published evidence suggests that ABP is either lost or deactivated as it moves along the epididymis (Hansson et al. 1974, 1975; Danzo et al. 1973), since binding to cytosol from whole epididymal homogenates decreases along the epididymis. If one assumes one binding site per ABP molecule, then all of the testosterone entering the epididymis via rete testis fluid would be bound to ABP and presumably would be metabolically inactive. Hansson and his colleagues (1974, 1975) have postulated that the ABP-steroid complex interacts with cells lining the first portions of the epididymis, and this interaction may shunt luminal testosterone into the metabolic pools of the cells. This is an attractive hypothesis and could account for the discrepancy noted earlier between epididymis and other accessory sex organs with respect to the minimum amounts of steroid needed to maintain the epididymis in castrate animals at control levels, since luminal testosterone would presumably be absent. Some question can be raised about this explanation, however, since Blaquier (1971) has shown that intravenously administered ^{3}H-testosterone crosses the epididymal epithelium to the duct lumen and binds to sperm. It is not clear why a similar movement of blood-borne testosterone would not occur in castrate animals.

Blaquier and Calandra (1973) have revealed certain

peculiarities of epididymal androgen metabolism in the rat that require further investigation. Apparently the epididymal cytoplasmic 4-ene-3 oxosteroid 5α-reductase is much more resistant to heparin inhibition than the prostatic enzyme. Evidence for ^{3}H-steroid translocation to the nucleus can only be obtained with minced epididymal preparations (from hemicastrate rats); if the homogenates or cytosol are charged with ^{3}H-testosterone, no transfer occurs. Cellular integrity appears to be required under the given experimental conditions. This behavior applies only to epididymal nuclei; ^{3}H-steroid-charged epididymal cytosol transfers protein-bound steroid radioactivity to rat ventral-prostate nuclei under identical conditions. [3]H-5α-dihydrotestosterone is not translocated per se but has to be generated from ^{3}H-testosterone in the minced preparation. Curiously, incubations of 5α-androstane-3α, 17β-diol with minced epididymal cytosol effected translocation to yield a protein-bound 3.5S nuclear species. This transfer is apparently not mediated by prior conversion to 5α-dihydrotestosterone.

Acknowledgment

In the course of writing this review the author asked a number of consultants to write short summaries of their fields. Portions of some of these summaries have been incorporated into this chapter, although the final wording is the responsibility of the author. The author wishes to acknowledge the following consultants: A. D. Johnson, M. R. N. Prasad, E. R. Casillas, T. D. Glover, I. G. White, P. Ofner, H. Jackson, and A. F. Holstein.

References

Allen, J. M., and J. J. Slater. A chemical and histochemical study of alkaline phosphatase and aliesterase in the epididymis of normal and castrate mice. Anat. Rec. 129:255, 1957.

Allen, J. M., and J. J. Slater. A cytochemical study of Golgi associated thiamine pyrophosphatase in the epididymis of the mouse. J. Histochem. Cytochem. 9:418, 1961.

Alumot, E., Y. Lensky, and H. Schindler. Separation of proteins in the epididymal fluid of the ram. J. Reprod. Fertil. 25:349, 1971.

Annison, E. F., T. W. Scott, and G. M. H. Waites. The role of glucose and acetate in the oxidative metabolism of the testis and epididymis of the ram. Biochem. J. 88:482, 1963.

Banerjee, B. N. The effect of oestrogen on the fertility of the rat when transferred through the semen during mating. J. Reprod. Fertil. 17:157, 1968.

Barker, L. D. S., and R. P. Amann. Sperm antigens and their localization within the bovine epididymal epithelium. J. Reprod. Fertil. 18:155, 1969.

Bedford, J. M. Morphological changes in rabbit spermatozoa during passage through the epididymis. J. Reprod. Fertil. 5:169, 1963.

Bedford, J. M. Changes in the fine structure of the rabbit sperm head during passage through the epididymis. J. Anat. 99:891, 1965.

Bedford, J. M. Development of the fertilizing ability of spermatozoa in the epididymis of the rabbit. J. Exp. Zool. 163:319, 1966.

Bedford, J. M. Effects of duct ligation on the fertilizing ability of spermatozoa from different regions of the rabbit epididymis. J. Exp. Zool. 166:271, 1967.

Bedford, J. M., M. J. Bent, and H. C. Calvin. Variations in the structural character and stability of the nuclear chromatin in morphologically normal human spermatozoa. J. Reprod. Fertil. 33:19, 1973a.

Bedford, J. M., and H. C. Calvin. Changes in -S-S- linked structures of the sperm tail during epididymal maturation, with comparative observations in sub-mammalian species. J. Exp. Zool. 187:181, 1974.

Bedford, J. M., H. C. Calvin, and G. W. Cooper. The maturation of spermatozoa in the human epididymis. J. Reprod. Fertil. Suppl. 18:199, 1973b.

Bedford, J. M., G. W. Cooper, and H. I. Calvin. Post-meiotic changes in the nucleus and membranes of mammalian spermatozoa. In Genetics of the spermatozoon, eds. R. A. Beatty and S. Gluecksohn-Waelsch, p. 69. Copenhagen: Bogtrykkiert Printer, 1972.

Bedford, J. M., and L. Nicander. Ultrastructural changes in the acrosome and sperm membranes during maturation of spermatozoa in the testis and epididymis of the rabbit and monkey. J. Anat. 108:527, 1971.

Benoit, M. J. Recherches anatomiques, cytologiques et histophysiologiques sur les voies excretrices du testicle, chez les mammifères. Arch. Anat. Histol. Embryol. (Strasbourg) 5:173, 1926.

Bey, E. The electrophoretic mobility of sperm cells. In Cell electrophoresis, ed. E. J. Ambrose, p. 142. London: Churchill, 1965.

Bishop, D. W. Biology of spermatozoa. In Sex and internal secretions, Vol. 2, ed. W. C. Young, p. 707. Baltimore: Williams & Wilkins, 1961.

Bishop, M. W. H., and A. Walton. Spermatogenesis and the structure of mammalian spermatozoa. In Marshall's physiology of reproduction, 3rd ed., Vol. 1, ed. A. S. Parkes, p. 1. London: Longmans, Green, 1960.

Blackshaw, A. E., and J. I. Samisoni. Histochemical localization of some dehydrogenase enzymes in the bull testis and epididymis. J. Dairy Sci. 50:747, 1965.

Blandau, R. J., and R. E. Rumery. The relationship of swimming movements of epididymal spermatozoa to their fertilizing capacity. Fertil. Steril. 15:571, 1964.

Blaquier, J. Selective uptake and metabolism of androgens by rat epididymis. The presence of a cytoplasmic receptor. Biochem. Biophys. Res. Commun. 45:1076, 1971.

Blaquier, J. A., and R. S. Calandra. Intranuclear receptor for androgens in rat epididymis. Endocrinology 93:51, 1973.

Bloom, G., and L. Nicander. On the ultrastructure and development of the protoplasmic droplet of spermatozoa. Z. Zellforsch. 55:833, 1961.

Bøhmer, T. Conversion of butyrobetaine to carnitine in the rat in vivo. Biochim. Biophys. Acta 343:551, 1974.

Brooks, D. E., D. W. Hamilton, and A. H. Mallek. The uptake of L-[methyl-^{3}H] carnitine by the rat epididymis. Biochem. Biophys. Res. Commun. 52:1354, 1973.

Brooks, D. E., D. W. Hamilton, and A. H. Mallek. Carnitine and glycerylphosphorylcholine in the reproductive tract of the male rat. J. Reprod. Fertil. 36:141, 1974.

Burgos, M. H. Uptake of colloidal particles by cells of the caput epididymidis. Anat. Rec. 148:517, 1964.

Casillas, E. R. The distribution of carnitine in male reproductive tissues and its effect on palmitate oxidation by spermatozoal particles. Biochim. Biophys. Acta 280:545, 1972.

Casillas, E. R. Accumulation of carnitine by bovine spermatozoa during maturation in the epididymis. J. Biol. Chem. 248:8227, 1973.

Casillas, E. R., and D. D. Hoskins. Activation of monkey spermatozoal adenyl cyclase by thyroxine and triiodothyronine. Biochem. Biophys. Res. Commun. 40:255, 1970.

Casillas, E. R., and D. D. Hoskins. Adenyl cyclase activity and cyclic 3', 5'-AMP content of ejaculated monkey spermatozoa. Arch. Biochem. Biophys. 147:148, 1971.

Cavazos, L. F. Effects of testosterone propionate on histochemical reactions of epithelium of rat ductus epididymis. Anat. Rec. 132:209, 1958.

Clubb, R. W. A study of epididymal transport of India ink and related epithelial reactions. Thesis, University of Rochester. Cited from Orgebin-Crist (1969).

Cooper, G. W., and J. M. Bedford. Acquisition of surface change by the plasma membrane of mammalian spermatozoa during epididymal maturation. Anat. Rec. 169:300, 1971.

Crabo, B. Studies on the composition of epididymal content in bulls and boars. Acta Vet. Scand. 6 (Suppl. 5):1, 1965.

Crabo, B., and L. E. Appelgren. Distribution of ^{14}Cα-chlorohydrin in mice and rats. J. Reprod. Fertil. 30:161, 1972.

Crabo, B., and A. Hunter. Sperm maturation and epididymal function. In Control of male fertility, eds J. Sciarra, C. Markland, and J. Speidel, p. 2. New York: Harper & Row, 1975.

Cross, B. A., and I. A. Silver. Neurovascular control of oxygen tension in the testis and epididymis. J. Reprod. Fertil. 3:377, 1962.

Danzo, B. J., M. C. Orgebin-Crist, and D. O. Toft. Characterization of acytoplasmic receptor for 5α-dihydrotestosterone in the caput epididymis of intact rabbits. Endocrinology 92:310, 1973.

Dawson, R. M. C., T. Mann, and I. G. White. Glycerylphosphorylcholine and phosphorylcholine in semen, and their relation to choline. Biochem. J. 65:627, 1957.

Dawson, R. M. C., and I. W. Rowlands. Glycerylphosphorylcholine in the male reproductive organs of rats and guinea pigs. Quart. J. Exp. Physiol. 44:26, 1959.

Dawson, R. M. C., and T. W. Scott. Phospholipid composition of epididymal spermatozoa prepared by density gradient centrifugation. Nature 202:292, 1964.

Diamond, J., and J. Tormey. Studies on the structural basis of water transport across epithelial membranes. Fed. Proc. 25:1458, 1966.

Diczfaluzy, E. Characterization of the oestrogens in human semen. Acta Endocrinol. 15:317, 1954.

Dirscherl, W., and H. Breuer. Isolierung von Dehydroepiandrosteron aus menschlichem Sperma. Acta Endocrinol. 44: 403, 1963.

Dirscherl, W., and W. Knüchel. Wirkungvon testosteronproprionate und oestron auf atmung und glykolyse von leber und zwerchfell junger mäuse beiderlei geschlechts. Biochem. Z. 320:228, 1950.

Djøseland, O., V. Hansson, and H. Haugen. Androgen metabolism by rat epididymis. L. Metabolic conversion of ^{3}H-testosterone in vivo. Steroids 21:773, 1973.

Dott, H. M., and J. T. Dingle. Distribution of lysosomal enzymes in the spermatozoa and cytoplasmic droplets of bull and ram. Exp. Cell Res. 52:523, 1968.

Elliot, P. R. The metabolism of homogenates of the mouse epididymis. J. Cell Physiol. 66:281, 1965a.

Elliott, P. R. The effect of efferentiectomy and orchidectomy on the metabolism of the epididymis of the mouse. J. Cell Physiol. 66:294, 1965b.

Ericsson, R. J., and V. Baker. Transport of oestrogens in semen to the female rat during mating and its effect on fertility. J. Reprod. Fertil. 12:381, 1966.

Ericsson, R. J., J. Cornette, and D. Buthala. Binding of sex steroids to rabbit sperm. Acta Endocrinol. 56:424, 1967.

Fawcett, D. W., and D. W. Hamilton. Electron and microscopical and biochemical evidence for steroid biosynthesis by the mammalian epididymis and vas deferens. In Morphological aspects of andrology, eds. A. F. Holstein and E. Horstmann, p. 119. Berlin: Grosse Verlag, 1970.

Fawcett, D. W., and D. M. Phillips. Observations on the release of spermatozoa and on changes in the head during passage through the epididymis. J. Reprod. Fertil. Suppl. 6:405, 1969.

Fleischer, B., S. Fleischer, and H. Ozawa. Isolation and characterization of Golgi membranes from bovine liver. J. Cell Biol. 43:59, 1969.

Flickinger, C. J. Fine structure of the wolffian duct and cytodifferentiation of the epididymis in fetal rats. Z. Zellforsch. 96:344, 1969.

Frankel, A. I., and K. B. Eik-Nes. Testosterone and dehydroepiandrosterone in the epididymis of the rabbit. J. Reprod. Fertil. 23:441, 1970a.

Frankel, A. I., and K. B. Eik-Nes. Metabolism of steroids in the rabbit epididymis. Endocrinology 87:646, 1970b.

Frenkel, G., R. N. Peterson, and M. Freund. Changes in the metabolism of guinea pig sperm from different segments of the epididymis. Proc. Soc. Exp. Biol. Med. 143:1231, 1973.

Friend, D. S. Cytochemical staining of multivesicular body and Golgi vesicles. J. Cell Biol. 41:269, 1969.

Friend, D. S., and M. G. Farquhar. Functions of coated vesicles during protein absorption in the rat vas deferens. J. Cell Biol. 35:357, 1967.

Fulka, J., and H. H. Koefoed-Johnson. The influence of epididymal passage in rabbits on different spermatozoan characteristics including fertilizing capacity. Ann. Rep. R. Vet. Agric. Coll. Steril. Inst., Copenhagen, p. 213, 1966.

Gaddum, P. Sperm maturation in the male reproductive tract: Development of motility. Anat. Rec. 161:471, 1969.

Garbers, D. L., N. L. First, and H. A. Lardy. The stimulation of bovine epididymal sperm metabolism by cyclic nucleotide phosphodiesterase inhibitors. Biol. Reprod. 7:132 (Abstract), 1972.

Garbers, D. L., N. L. First, and H. A. Lardy. The stimulation of bovine epididymal sperm metabolism by cyclic nucleotide phosphodiesterase inhibitors. Biol. Reprod. 8:589, 1973a.

Garbers, D. L., N. L. First, and H. A. Lardy. Properties of adenosine 3', 5'-monophosphate-dependent protein kinases isolated from bovine epididymal spermatozoa. J. Biol. Chem. 248:875, 1973b.

Garbers, D. L., W. D. Lust, N. L. First, and H. A. Lardy. Effects of phosphodiesterase inhibitors and cyclic nucleotides on sperm respiration and motility. Biochem. J. 10:1825, 1971.

Glover, T. D. Spermatozoa from the isolated cauda epididymis of rabbits and some effects of artificial cryptorchidism. J. Reprod. Fertil. 1:121, 1960.

Glover, T. D. The reaction of rabbit spermatozoa to nigrosin eosin following ligation of the epididymis. Int. J. Fertil. 7:1, 1962.

Glover, T. D. Some aspects of function in the epididymis. Experimental occlusion of the epididymis in the rabbit. Int. J. Fertil. 14:216, 1969.

Glover, T. D., and L. Nicander. Some aspects of structure and function in the mammalian epididymis. J. Reprod. Fertil. Suppl. 13:39, 1971.

Gloyna, R. E., and J. D. Wilson. A comparative study of the conversion of testosterone to 17α-hydroxy-5α-androstane-3one (dihydrotestosterone) by prostate and epididymis. J. Clin. Endocrinol. Metab. 29:970, 1969.

Grogan, D. E., D. T. Mayer, and J. D. Sikes. Quantitative differences in phospholipids of ejaculated spermatozoa and spermatozoa from three levels of the epididymis of the boar. J. Reprod. Fertil. 12:431, 1966.

Gunn, R. M. C. Fertility in sheep. Artificial production of seminal ejaculation and the characters of the spermatozoa contained therein. Bull. Counc. Sci. Ind. Res. Aust. 94:1, 1936.

Gustafsson, B. Luminal contents of the bovine epididymis under conditions of reduced spermatogenesis, luminal blockage certain sperm abnormalities. Acta Vet. Scand. Suppl. 17:1, 1966.

Hamilton, D. W. Steroid function in the mammalian epididymis. J. Reprod. Fertil. Suppl. 13:89, 1971.

Hamilton, D. W. The mammalian epididymis. In Reproductive biology, eds. H. Balin and S. Glasser, p. 268. Amsterdam: Excerpta Medica, 1972.

Hamilton, D. W. Structure and function of the epithelium lining the ductuli efferentes, ductus epididymis and ductus deferens in the rat. In Handbook of physiology, Section 7: Endocrinology, Vol. 5, eds. D. W. Hamilton and R. O. Greep, p. 259. Baltimore: Williams & Wilkins, 1975.

Hamilton, D. W., and D. W. Fawcett. In vitro synthesis of cholesterol and testosterone from acetate by rat epididymis and vas deferens. Proc. Soc. Exp. Biol. Med. 133:693, 1970.

Hamilton, D. W., A. L. Jones, and D. W. Fawcett. Sterol biosynthesis from (1-¹⁴C) acetate in the epididymis and vas deferens of the mouse. J. Reprod. Fertil. 18:156, 1968.

Hamilton, D. W., A. L. Jones, and D. W. Fawcett. Cholesterol biosynthesis in the mouse epididymis and ductus deferens: A biochemical and morphological study. Biol. Reprod. 1:167, 1969.

Hansson, V., E. M. Ritzen, F. S. French, and S. Nayfeh. Androgen transport receptor mechanisms in testis and epididymis. In Handbook of physiology, Section 7: Endocrinology, Vol. 5, eds. D. W. Hamilton and R. O. Greep, p. 173. Baltimore: Williams & Wilkins, 1975.

Hansson, V., O. Trygstad, F. S. French, W. S. McLean, A. A. Smith, D. J. Tindall, S. C. Weddington, P. Petrusz, S. N. Nayfeh, and E. M. Ritzen. Androgen transport and receptor mechanisms in testis and epididymis. Nature 250:387, 1974.

Harris, M. Concentration of testosterone in testis fluid of the rat. Proc. Soc. Study Fertil. (USA) Sixth Annual Meeting, 61 (Abstract), 1973.

Hartman, C. G. Ovulation, fertilization and the transport and viability of eggs and spermatozoa. In Sex and internal secretions, 2nd ed., eds. E. Allan, C. H. Danforth, and E. A. Doisy, p. 719. Baltimore: Williams & Wilkins, 1939.

Hartree, E. F., and T. Mann. Plasmalogen in ram semen, and its role in sperm metabolism. Biochem. J. 71:423, 1959.

Hathaway, R. R. Estradiol metabolism and its inhibition in bull semen. J. Dairy Sci. 50:1831, 1967.

Hathaway, R., and E. Chamberlain. Bull seminal plasma and the regulation of 17β-estradiol dehydrogenase activity in spermatozoa. Biol. Reprod. 2:164, 1970.

Hathaway, R. R., and C. D. West. Conversion of 17α-estradiol to estrone by spermatozoa. Endocrinology 75:616, 1964.

Heap, R. B., A. M. Symons, and J. C. Watkins. An interaction between oestradiol and progesterone in aqueous solutions and a model membrane system. Biochim. Biophys. Acta 233:307, 1971.

Henle, G., and C. A. Zittle. Studies of metabolism of bovine epididymal spermatozoa. Am. J. Physiol. 136:70, 1942.

Hicks, J. J., N. Pedron, and A. Rosado. Modifications of human spermatozoa glycolysis by cyclic adenosine monophosphate (cAMP), estrogens, and follicular fluid. Fertil. Steril. 23:886, 1972.

Hoffer, A. P., D. W. Hamilton, and D. W. Fawcett. The ultrastructure of the principal cells and intraepithelial leucocytes in the initial segment of the rat epididymis. Anat. Rec. 175:169, 1973.

Hoffer, A. P., D. W. Hamilton, and D. W. Fawcett. Phagocytosis of sperm by the epithelial cells of the rat ductuli efferentes under experimental conditions. J. Reprod. Fertil. 44:1, 1975.

Horan, A. H., and J. M. Bedford. Development of the fertilizing ability of spermatozoa in the epididymis of the Syrian hamster. J. Reprod. Fertil. 30:417, 1972.

Hoskins, D. D. Adenine nucleotide mediation of fructolysis and motility in bovine epididymal spermatozoa. J. Biol. Chem. 248:1135, 1973.

Hoskins, D. D., and E. R. Casillas. Hormones, second messengers, and the mammalian spermatozoon. In *Advances in sex hormone research*, Vol. 1, eds. R. L. Singhal and J. A. Thomas. Baltimore: University Park Press, 1973.

Hoskins, D. D., E. R. Casillas, and D. T. Stephens. Cyclic AMP-dependent protein kinases of bovine epididymal spermatozoa. Biochem. Biophys. Res. Commun. 48:1331, 1972.

Hoskins, D. D., D. T. Stephens, and E. R. Casillas. Enzymic control of fructolysis in primate spermatozoa. Biochim. Biophys. Acta 237:227, 1971.

Hoskins, D. D., D. T. Stephens, and M. L. Hall. Cyclic adenosine 3′,5′-monophosphate and protein kinase levels in developing bovine spermatozoa. J. Reprod. Fertil. 37:131, 1974.

Huang, H. F. S., and A. D. Johnson. Amino acid composition of epididymal plasma of mouse, rat, rabbit and sheep. Comp. Biochem. Physiol. 50:359, 1975.

Inano, H., A. Machino, and B.-I. Tamaoki. In vitro metabolism of steroid hormones by cell-free homogenate of epididymides of adult rats. Endocrinology 84:997, 1969.

Johnson, A. D., and P. C. Turner. Epididymal carbohydrate metabolism. I. Glucose-1-^{14}C and glucose-6-^{14}C metabolism by mouse, rat, and rabbit tissues. Comp. Biochem. Physiol. 39A:599, 1971.

Johnson, W. C., and A. G. Hunter. Immunofluorescent changes associated with maturation of rabbit sperm. Proc. Soc. Study Reprod. (USA) 3:8 (Abstract), 1970.

Kaye, G. I., H. O. Wheeler, R. T. Whitlock, and N. Lane. Fluid transport in the rabbit gall bladder. A combined physiological and electron microscopic study. J. Cell Biol. 30:237, 1966.

Kraft, L. A., and A. D. Johnson. Epididymal carbohydrate metabolism. II. Substrates and pathway utilization of caput and cauda epididymal tissue from the rabbit, rat and mouse. Comp. Biochem. Physiol. 42B:451, 1972.

Lardy, H. A., D. Ghosh, and G. W. E. Plaut. A metabolic regulator in mammalian spermatozoa. Science 109:365, 1949.

Lardy, H. A., R. G. Hansen, and P. H. Phillips. Metabolism of bovine epididymal spermatozoa. Arch. Biochem. 6:41, 1945.

Lavon, R., R. Volgani, and D. Danon. The proteins of bovine spermatozoa from the caput and cauda epididymis. J. Reprod. Fertil. 24:219, 1971.

Leeson, T., and C. Leeson. An electron microscope study of the postnatal development of the ductus epididymis in the rat. Anat. Anz. 114:168, 1964.

Lincoln, G. A., R. W. Youngson, and R. V. Short. The social and sexual behavior of the red deer stag. J. Reprod. Fertil. Suppl. 11:71, 1970.

Lubicz-Nawrocki, C. M., and M. C. Chang. The comparative efficacy of testosterone, progesterone and dehydroepiandrosterone for the maintenance of fertilizing capacity in castrated hamsters. Biol. Reprod. 9:295, 1973.

Lunaas, T., R. L. Baldwin, and P. T. Cupps. Levels of certain soluble dehydrogenases in the rat testis and epididymis. J. Reprod. Fertil. 17:177, 1968.

McGadey, J., A. H. Baillie, and M. M. Ferguson. Histochemical utilization of hydroxysteroids by the hamster epididymis. Histochemie 7:211, 1966.

Maneely, R. B. Epididymal structure and function: A historical and critical review. Acta Zool. (Stockholm) 40:1, 1959.

Mann, T. *The biochemistry of semen and of the male reproductive tract*. London: Methuen, 1964.

Mann, T. Effects of pharmacological agents on male sexual functions. J. Reprod. Fertil. Suppl. 4:101, 1968.

Mann, T., and T. Glover. Contribution of the seminal vesicles towards the composition of whole semen. Endocrinology 10:iv (Abstract), 1954.

Marquis, N. R., and I. B. Fritz. Distribution of carnitine, acetylcarnitine and carnitine acetyltransferase in rat tissue. In *Recent research on carnitine*, ed. G. Wolf, p. 27. Cambridge, Mass.: MIT Press, 1965a.

Marquis, N. R., and I. B. Fritz. The distribution of carnitine, acetylcarnitine and carnitine acetyltransferase in rat tissues. J. Biol. Chem. 240:2193, 1965b.

Marquis, N. R., and I. Fritz. Effects of testosterone on the distribution of carnitine, acetylcarnitine, and carnitine acetyltransferase in tissues of the reproductive system of the male rat. J. Biol. Chem. 240:2197, 1965c.

Mason, K. E., and S. L. Shaver. Some functions of the caput epididymis. Ann. N.Y. Acad. Sci. 55:585, 1952.

Mollendorff, W. von. Vitale Farbungen an tierischen Zellen. Arundlagen Ergebnisse und zeile biologischer Farbstoff versuche. Ergeb. Physiol. 18:141, 1920.

Moore, C. R. On the properties of the gonads as controllers of somatic and physical characteristics. X spermatozoon activity and the testis hormone. J. Exp. Zool. 50:455, 1928.

Morton, B., J. Harrigan, and T. Jooss. The activation of motility in quiescent hamster sperm from the epididymis. Biol. Reprod. 9:71 (Abstract), 1973.

Mullen, J. O., K. H. Moon, and M. E. Yannone. Estimation of androgens in human seminal plasma by gas-liquid chromatography. Invest. Urol. 6:143, 1968.

Murdoch, R. N., I. G. White, and R. F. Seamark. Oxidative and glycolytic activity of ejaculated ram sperm in the presence of steroid hormones. Acta Endocrinol. 64:557, 1970.

Neutra, M., and C. P. Leblond. Radioautographic comparison of the uptake of galactose-^{3}H and glucose-^{3}H in the Golgi region of various cells secreting proteins or mucopolysaccharides. J. Cell Biol. 30:137, 1966.

Nevo, A. C., I. Michaeli, and H. Schindler. Electrophoretic properties of bull and rabbit spermatozoa. Exp. Cell Res. 23:69, 1961.

Nicander, L. An electron microscopal study of absorbing cells in the posterior caput epididymis of rabbits. Z. Zellforsch 66:829, 1965.

Nicander, L., S. Paulsson, and U. Selander. An electron microscopal study of iron absorption in the epididymal tail of rabbits. Rep. Fourth Scand. Cong. Cell Res., 51, 1965.

Nishikawa, Y., and Y. Waide. Studies on the maturation of spermatozoa. I. Mechanism and speed of transition of spermatozoa in the epididymis and their function changes. Bull. Nat. Inst. Agr. Sci. (Series G.) 3:69, 1952.

Oertel, G. W., and L. Treiber. Excretion of C19-steroids in human seminal fluid. Experientia 24:71, 1967.

Ofner, P. Recent developments in the study of hormone effects and metabolism in prostate tissue. Symp. Dtsch. Ges. Endokrinol. 17:147, 1971.

Ofner, P., I. Leav, and L. F. Cavazos. C_{19} steroid metabolism in sex accessory organs. Correlation of changes in metabolite patterns and fine structural alterations in the prostate of the androgen deprived dog. In *Male accessory sex organs, structure and function in mammals*, ed. D. Brandes, p. 267. New York: Academic Press, 1974.

Ofner, P., R. L. Vena, R. F. Morfin, M. A. Aliapoulios, and I. Leav. In vivo metabolism of C_{19}-steroids in prostatic tissue. In *Normal and abnormal growth of the prostate*, ed. M. Goland. Springfield, Ill.: Charles C Thomas, 1975.

Orgebin-Crist, M.-C. Maturation of spermatozoa in the rabbit epididymis: Fertilizing ability and embryonic mortality in does inseminated with epididymal spermatozoa. Ann. Biol. Anim. Biochim. Biophys. 7:373, 1967.

Orgebin-Crist, M.-C. Studies on the function of the epididymis. Biol. Reprod. Suppl. 1:155, 1969.

Orgebin-Crist, M.-C., J. Davies, and P. Tichenor. Maturation of spermatozoa in the rabbit epididymis: Effect of hypophysectomy and castration. In *The regulation of mammalian reproduction*, p. 189. Springfield, Ill.: Charles C Thomas, 1973.

Ortavant, R. Existence d'une phase critique dans la maturation epididymaire des spermatozoides de belier et de taureau. C. R. Soc. Bio. (Paris) 147:1552, 1953.

Pearson, D. J., and P. K. Tubbs. Carnitine and derivatives in rat tissues. Biochem. J. 105:953, 1967.

Picket, B. W., and R. J. Komarek. Lipid and dry weight of bovine seminal plasma and spermatozoa from first and second ejaculates. J. Dairy Sci. 50:742, 1967.

Picket, B. W., R. J. Komarek, M. R. Gebauer, R. W. Benson, and E. W. Gibson. Lipid and dry weight of ejaculated, epididymal and post-castrate semen from boars. J. Anim. Sci. 26:792, 1967.

Pierrepoint, C. G., P. Davies, and D. W. Wilson. The role of the epididymis and ductus deferens in the direct and unilateral control of the prostate and seminal vesicles of the rat. J. Reprod. Fertil. 41:413, 1974.

Prasad, M. R. N., M. Rajalakshmi, G. Gupta, and T. Karkun. Control of epididymal function. J. Reprod. Fertil. Suppl. 18:215, 1973.

Price, D., and E. Ortiz. The role of fetal androgen in sex differentiation in mammals. In *Organogenesis*, eds. R. L. de-

Haan and H. Ursprung, p. 629. New York: Holt, Rinehart & Winston, 1965.

Quinn, P. J., and I. G. White. Phospholipid and cholesterol content of epididymal and ejaculated ram spermatozoa and seminal plasma in relation to cold shock. Aust. J. Biol. Sci. 20:1205, 1967.

Rambourg, A., W. Hernandez, and C. P. Leblond. Detection of complex carbohydrates in the golgi apparatus of rat cells. J. Cell Biol. 40:395, 1969.

Redenz, E. Versuch einer biologischen Morphologie des Nebenhodens. Arch. Mikrosk. Anat. Entwicklungsmech. 103: 593, 1924.

Risley, P. L. Physiology of the male accessory organs. In *Mechanisms concerned with conception*, ed. C. C. Hartmann, p. 73. New York: Pergamon Press, 1963.

Schaffenburg, C. A., and E. P. McCullagh. Studies in sperm hormones: demonstration of estrogenic activity. Endocrinology 54:296, 1954.

Scott, T. W., B. Baggett, and I. G. White. Metabolism of testosterone by semen and the effect of testosterone on oxidative metabolism of spermatozoa. Aust. J. Exp. Biol. 41:363, 1963a.

Scott, T. W., B. Baggett, and I. W. Rowlands. Phospholipid interrelationships in rat epididymal tissue and spermatozoa. Biochem. J. 87:507, 1963b.

Scott, T. W., and R. M. C. Dawson. Metabolism of phospholipids by spermatozoa and seminal plasma. Biochem. J. 108: 457, 1968.

Scott, T. W., R. G. Wales, J. C. Wallace, and I. G. White. Composition of ram epididymal and testicular fluid and the biosynthesis of glycerylphosphorylcholine by the rabbit epididymis. J. Reprod. Fertil. 6:49, 1963c.

Scott, T. W., I. G. White, and E. F. Annison. Glycose and acetate metabolism by ram, bull, dog and fowl spermatozoa. Biochem. J. 83:398, 1962.

Seamark, R. F., and I. White. The metabolism of steroid hormones in semen. J. Endocrinol. 30:307, 1964.

Sedar, W. W. Transport of exogenous peroxidase across the epithelium of the ductuli efferentes. J. Cell Biol. 31:201A, 1966.

Sedláková, E., J. Dostál, and J. Matoušek. Serum albumin in pig epididymis. Comp. Biochem. Physiol. 26:143, 1968.

Setchell, B. P., T. W. Scott, J. K. Voglmayr, and G. M. H. Waites. Characteristics of testicular spermatozoa and the fluid which transports them into the epididymis. Biol. Reprod. Suppl. 1:40, 1969.

Setchell, B. P., and G. M. H. Waites. Blood flow and the uptake of glucose and oxygen in the testis and epididymis of the ram. J. Physiol. 171:411, 1964.

Shaver, S. L. Role of stereocilia in removing India ink particles from lumen of rat epididymis. Anat. Rec. 119:177, 1954.

Sholl, S. A., and J. H. Leathem. Effects of postnatal maturation and castration on rat epididymal carbohydrate metabolism. Proc. Soc. Exp. Biol. Med. 142:635, 1973.

Simeone, F. A. A neuromuscular mechanism in the ductus epididymidis and its impairment by sympathetic denervation. Am. J. Physiol. 103:582, 1933.

Sowell, J. G., and K. B. Eik-Nes. Formation in vivo of 5-dihydrotestosterone by the canine epididymis. Proc. Soc. Exp. Biol. Med. 141:827, 1972.

Steeno, O., C. Schirren, W. Heyns, and P. deMoor. Dehydroepiandrosterone in human seminal plasma. J. Clin. Endocrinol. 26:353, 1966.

Turner, T. T., and A. D. Johnson. Glucose metabolism of bovine epididymal tissue. J. Anim. Sci. 35:256 (Abstract), 1972.

Turner, T. T., and A. D. Johnson. The metabolic activity of the bovine epididymis. I. Utilization of glucose and fructose. J. Reprod. Fertil. 34:201, 1973a.

Turner, T. T., and A. D. Johnson. The metabolic activity of the bovine epididymis. II. Utilization of acetate, succinate, pyruvate, lactate and glucose. J. Reprod. Fertil. 35:445, 1973b.

Tveter, K. J., and A. Aakvaag. Uptake and metabolism in vivo of testosterone-1, 2-^{3}H by accessory sex organs of male rats: Influence of some hormonal compounds. Endocrinology 85:683, 1969.

van Deenen, L. L. M., J. de Gier, U. Houtsmuller, A. Montfoort, and E. Mulder. Dietary effects on the lipid composition of biomembranes. In *Biochemical problems of lipids*, ed. A. Frazier, p. 404. Amsterdam: Elsevier, 1963.

Voglmayr, J. K., T. W. Scott, B. P. Setchell, and G. M. H. Waites. Metabolism of testicular spermatozoa and characteristics of testicular fluid collected from conscious rams. J. Reprod. Fertil. 14:87, 1967.

Voglmayr, J. K., G. M. H. Waites, and B. P. Setchell. Studies on spermatozoa and fluid collected directly from the testis of the conscious ram. Nature 210:861, 1966.

Voglmayr, J. K., I. G. White, and P. J. Quinn. A comparison of adenosinetriphosphatase activity in testicular and ejaculated spermatozoa of the ram. Biol. Reprod. 1:121, 1969.

Wagenseil, F. Experimentaluntersuchungen am Nebenhoden der Maus. Z. Zellforsch 7:141, 1928.

Waites, G. M. H., and B. P. Setchell. Physiology of the testis, epididymis and scrotum. In *Advances in reproductive biology*, Vol. 4, ed. A. McLaren, p. 1. London: Logos Press, 1969.

Wales, R. G., J. C. Wallace, and I. G. White. Composition of bull epididymal and testicular fluid. J. Reprod. Fertil. 12: 139, 1966.

Wallace, J. C., R. G. Wales, and I. G. White. The respiration of the rabbit epididymis and its synthesis of glycerylphosphorylcholine. Aust. J. Biol. Sci. 19:849, 1966.

Walton, A. The initiation of motility in mammalian spermatozoa. Stud. Fertil. 8:53, 1956.

Wester, R. C., and G. W. Salisbury. Effect of testosterone, estradiol-17β and progesterone on the oxygen uptake by bovine semen, washed spermatozoa and epididymal-like spermatozoa. Biol. Reprod. 7:25, 1972.

White, I. G., and B. Hudson. The testosterone and dehydroepiandrosterone concentration in fluids of the mammalian male reproductive tract. J. Endocrinol. 41:291, 1968.

White, I. G., and R. G. Wales. Comparison of epididymal and ejaculated semen of ram. J. Reprod. Fertil. 2:225, 1961.

Williams-Ashman, H. G., and A. H. Reddi. Actions of vertebrate sex hormones. Ann. Rev. Physiol. 33:31, 1971.

Wilson, J. D. Testosterone uptake by the urogenital tract of the rabbit embryo. Endocrinology 92:1192, 1973.

Wislocki, G. B. Seasonal changes in the testes, epididymides and seminal vesicles of deer investigated by histochemical methods. Endocrinology 44:167, 1949.

Wu, S. H., F. F. McKenzie, S. C. Fang, and J. S. Butts. Pathways of glucose utilization in epididymal and testicular sperm cells. J. Dairy Sci. 42:110, 1959.

Young, W. C. A study on the function of the epididymis. III. Functional changes undergone by spermatozoa during the passage through the epididymis and vas deferens in the guinea-pig. J. Exp. Biol. 8:151, 1931.

Young, W. C. Die Resorption in den Ductuli efferentes der Maus und ihre Bedeutung fur das Problem der Unterbindung im Hoden-Nebenhodensystem. Z. Zellforsch. 17:729, 1933.

35 Semen: Metabolism, Antigenicity, Storage, and Artificial Insemination

Thaddeus Mann

35.1 Present Trends in Research on Semen

Considerable progress has been made within the last decade in research concerned with the composition and function of semen. Among the various problems that have been successfully tackled, the following can serve as particularly good examples of the ways along which the entire area is developing: (1) the mechanisms underlying the interaction between the two main components of ejaculated semen, the spermatozoa and the seminal plasma, (2) the correlation between the two main functions of the live spermatozoon, motility and fertilizing ability, and especially the link-up with the fine structure of the various sperm organelles, (3) the long-term storage of deep-frozen semen for artificial insemination, and (4) the application of semen analysis to the clinical evaluation of male fertility.

Much that has been achieved, particularly in regard to the first two problems, has been made possible by the growing awareness among investigators that meaningful solutions in the biology of reproduction can be obtained only by a close integration of morphological, biochemical, biophysical, and other expert scientific endeavor. The rewards from combined structural and functional studies have been particularly evident in research aimed at defining the mode of action of the various sperm organelles, such as the plasma membrane, acrosome, nucleus, mitochondrial sheath, cytoplasmic droplet, and the axoneme of the flagellum. The fruitfulness of such joint studies is best illustrated by the new information on the role played by the sperm acrosome and its lysosomal enzymes in the process of sperm penetration into the ovum and subsequent fertilization. Further gratifying examples of this kind are found in the results of studies on the relation of sperm mitochondria to energy utilization by spermatozoa and on the role of axonemal tubular elements in the propagation of flagellar movements.

The shift toward collaborative studies, aimed at correlating the structural and functional characteristics of the spermatozoon, has also been extended to investigations of the male reproductive tract as a whole and is clearly reflected in the tendency to correlate, at the cytochemical level, the characteristics of various organelles in the cells of the testis, epididymis, prostate, and seminal vesicle with specific functions of these organs, such as androgen production by the Leydig cells, sperm maturation in the epididymal tubules, and the secretory activity of the epithelial cells lining the male accessory organs, which is ultimately responsible for the formation of seminal plasma.

The widespread use of deep-frozen semen for artificial insemination and the application of semen analysis for the purpose of evaluating fertility in individual males owe their spectacular progress largely to the adoption by investigators of a comparative approach. This approach increasingly involves conclusions drawn from comparative studies in which the experimental objects are no longer restricted merely to humans and small laboratory animals, but include an impressive and steadily growing range of other, mostly large, animal species.

Studies on the semen of farm animals such as the bull, ram, boar, and stallion have been largely responsible for the rapid advances in the techniques of long-term storage of deep-frozen semen. They were equally instrumental in successful development of various analytical parameters, both morphological and chemical, which are now widely employed in the assessment of the quality of semen and of male fertility in general.

Another interesting trend in modern research on semen and male reproductive functions has been the shift of emphasis from purely physiological to pathological studies, reflected in recent attempts to link certain forms of male infertility to definite ultrastructural and cytochemical abnormalities in ejaculated spermatozoa. *Knobbed acrosome*, *pseudodroplet*, *corkscrew mitochondrial sheath*, and *nuclear pouch* are a few examples of the types of sperm abnormalities that have been studied in recent years. Increased knowledge of such abnormalities will doubtlessly enable further important advances to be made in the area of semen pathology.

From this brief outline of present trends in semen research it may be concluded that further gains in knowledge will certainly depend upon (1) support for collaborative efforts of structural, chemical, and physical biologists, directed toward the elucidation, at cellular and subcellular level, of the relationships between the various sperm organelles and the motility, viability, energetics, and fertilizing potential of spermatozoa, (2) recognition for the fundamental value of imaginatively conceived comparative studies on semen and the male reproductive functions, particularly by research teams concerned with fertility problems in humans and large farm animals, and (3) encouragement of investigations in the pathology of semen and male reproduction, with the goal of evolving abnormal "spermiograms" that would help the diagnosis of defective testicular and epididymal function and developing more precise biochemical methods of seminal plasma analysis as a basic criterion of the functional status of the prostate, seminal vesicle, and other male accessory organs of reproduction.

35.2 Metabolism of Semen

Nature has endowed the spermatozoa with the means of efficient utilization of extraneous sources of energy, such as are available to the sperm cells in their natural environment. During sperm passage in the male reproductive tract, the environment is provided by the male accessory secretions, which contain a few substances that can be utilized by spermatozoa. Not all accessory secretions, however, are of potential use in this respect. Chemically, the environment provided by the testicular plasma for testicular spermatozoa in the rete testis and efferent ducts, or by the epididymal plasma for epididymal spermatozoa, substantially differs from the medium in which the spermatozoa are actually ejaculated, that is, the seminal plasma in whole semen. We also know that during passage within the same organ, the character of the extracellular medium can undergo remarkable fluctuations. This phenomenon has been studied with particular care in the epididymis by Crabo and Gustafsson in Sweden, White and his colleagues in Australia, Glover and Jones in England, and others. In the epididymis, there are marked differences in the composition of fluids produced by the caput, corpus, and cauda epididymidis with regard to secretory products such as lipids, glycerylphosphorylcholine, glycerylphosphorylinositol, hypotaurine, carnitine, certain enzymes (notably glycosidases), and several ions, particularly potassium and sodium.

In the unit in Cambridge University the main effort has been directed toward elucidating the mechanisms that control the metabolism of whole (i.e., ejaculated) semen. The two fundamental processes that have been studied in mammalian semen are respiration and fructolysis. The respiratory activity of ejaculated spermatozoa can proceed up to a point in the absence of seminal plasma, but fructolysis is possible only if fructose is made available to the spermatozoa by the seminal plasma. In humans this sugar is contributed mainly by the seminal vesicles. The importance of exogenous fructose is evident especially under anaerobic conditions, when because of the absence of oxygen, the spermatozoa can no longer use their endogenous substrates but must depend instead upon anaerobic fruc-

tolysis, that is, the conversion of extracellular fructose to lactic acid.

Various aspects of the metabolic processes in mammalian semen are now much better understood than they were a decade ago, particularly in regard to details of both glycolytic and oxidative enzymic pathways. Answers are now available to questions concerning the metabolism of substances other than fructose, such as glucose, sorbitol, lactate, pyruvate, acetate, acetoacetate, and many other metabolites. Much new information has been obtained in relation to effects of enzyme inhibitors, spermicidal agents, and cold shock (sperm immobilization resulting from quick cooling of semen to temperatures slightly above 0°C) on the metabolism of semen. A great deal has also been learned, particularly in the last few years, about the regulatory influence that sperm coenzymes—such as adenosine triphosphate (ATP), nicotinamide-adenine dinucleotide (NAD), and cyclic adenosine-3'5'-monophosphate (cAMP)—exert on the energy-yielding and energy-utilizing processes in semen. The ways in which these coenzymes link catalytic processes in semen to motility and survival of spermatozoa are gradually becoming clearer, not only as a result of the unit's efforts, but thanks to extensive studies in several other laboratories, in particular those of Lardy at the University of Wisconsin and Hoskins at the Oregon Primate Research Center.

In addition to carbohydrates, other extracellular metabolites have been identified in recent years in catalytic processes in the spermatozoa. A good example is provided by the metabolic behavior of carnitine (β-oxo-α-butyrobetaine), a substance discovered in 1965 by Marquis and Fritz in the epididymal plasma and shown to be acetylated by spermatozoa to acetylcarnitine. Carnitine and acetylcarnitine probably play an essential role in the metabolism of semen, perhaps in the oxidation of fatty acids.

Fatty acids constitute a particularly interesting group of seminal constituents, especially in human semen. Among the fatty acids present in human seminal plasma the prostaglandins have attracted special attention on account of their manifold physiological and pharmacological properties. At least 13 prostaglandins have so far been identified in human semen by Bergström, Samuelsson, and their collaborators, but the physiological role in reproduction of only a few of these has so far been studied to any extent.

In general, as a result of the various metabolic studies carried out with semen, we know that any damage to mammalian spermatozoa that leads to declining mobility and shortened survival is bound to be reflected in a decline of their metabolic activity, particularly fructolysis. Such a decline is accompanied by an increased permeability of the sperm membranes, leading to a leakage of vital intracellular sperm constituents into the surrounding medium. This leakage phenomenon, which as yet is incompletely understood, represents one of the most characteristic changes associated with the processes of so-called aging of spermatozoa. It affects a wide range of sperm constituents, varying from ions (particularly potassium) and low-molecular-weight organic substances (such as the vitally important coenzyme cAMP) to high-molecular-weight sperm components, such as lipoproteins, certain intracellular enzymes, and cytochrome c. What role, if any, is allotted to the seminal plasma in the leakage phenomenon is a question in need of much further study. Two interesting but as yet largely unexplored observations may be relevant to this question. One is that the presence of seminal plasma in stored semen may in certain situations accelerate the decay processes in spermatozoa. The other, diametrically opposed and equally disputed, is that in certain infertile individuals the spermatozoa can be rendered fertile by suspending them in "good" seminal plasma, obtained from fertile males. One must assume, of course, that the samples of "good" seminal plasma with which successes have been claimed in artificial insemination have been conscientiously checked for complete absence of spermatozoa prior to mixing with low-quality semen!

One more observation may also be relevant to the problem of metabolic interactions between plasma and spermatozoa. As is well known from studies by Leone in Naples and by others, mammalian seminal plasma is remarkably rich in nucleolytic enzymes. Could it be that some of the hydrolytic enzymes present in the seminal plasma (e.g. nucleases and nucleotidases and possibly also phosphodiesterases and proteases) play some physiological role in the "disposal" of aging spermatozoa that are already in the process of losing their vital intracellular constituents as part of the leakage phenomenon?

Solutions are also needed to two further questions concerning semen metabolism, namely, (1) the ways in which drugs and other toxic substances affect the various intermediary reactions of fructolysis and respiration in vitro and (2) the possibility of influencing the metabolic activity as well as the motility and fertilizing ability of spermatozoa by substances capable of passing into semen after administration in vivo.

In regard to drugs that affect spermatozoa in vitro, a clear distinction must be drawn between spermiostatic agents such as metabolic inhibitors, which arrest sperm motility and metabolism in a reversible fashion, and spermicidal agents such as the various sulfhydryl-binding and surface-active drugs, which inactivate the spermatozoa irreversibly. It is also necessary to distinguish between substances such as certain radiomimetic agents, which render the spermatozoa infertile

without necessarily depriving them of either motility or metabolic activity, and other substances that affect not only fertility but also motility and metabolism.

In terms of the possibility of influencing spermatozoa by means of substances administered orally or parenterally, it must not be forgotten that the tissues that compose the reproductive tracts of male and female do not constitute an absolute barrier to extraneously administered agents. A wide variety of substances such as alcohol, salicylates, sulfonamides, thalidomide, tetracyclines, etc., penetrate into male accessory secretions and semen after ingestion or injection. Certain steroid hormones can also apparently enter into semen, as can ergothioneine, a substance normally occurring in semen, which passes readily into semen after oral administration. Some of the drugs examined, for instance thalidomide and tetracycline, are actually capable of binding to spermatozoa. But none of the chemical agents that enter only into the seminal plasma could exert the effect indicated by the observation that in humans aspirin administration leads to a reduction in the level of prostaglandins in semen.

More research on the passage of drugs into semen would be of great scientific as well as clinical interest, particularly in relation to the problem of controlling male fertility.

What other major gaps are there in our knowledge of semen metabolism, and how could they be filled?

Earlier in this chapter several suggestions have been made stressing the need for further investigations on questions relating to the metabolism of aging spermatozoa, the probable role of certain enzymes in the seminal plasma, and the possibility of influencing spermatozoa in vivo by means of orally or parenterally administered drugs. Special emphasis was placed on the fact that the physiological environment that nature provides for the spermatozoa is subject to considerable fluctuations; the testicular plasma, for example, exhibits a composition differing from that of the plasma secreted in the various segments of the epididymidis and also from that of the other secretory fluids produced in the male or female genital organs. The spermatozoa themselves, as is well known, also undergo profound changes during their passage from the testes to the site of fertilization.

In recent years several new cannulation techniques have been worked out permitting the collection of spermatozoa separately from the seminiferous tubules, rete testis, and the various segments of the epididymis. Especially promising is the technique for the collection of testicular semen developed by Voglmayr and his colleagues in Australia, which can be applied to large animals such as the ram or bull over periods of several weeks without interfering with other functions of these animals. These methods deserve to be perfected because they are likely to contribute to a better understanding of the physiological mechanisms that enable the spermatozoa to acquire their motility, metabolic peculiarities, and fertilizing ability during the passage in the reproductive tract. Testicular spermatozoa, collected directly from the rete testis of a ram or bull, though perfectly shaped, are neither motile nor fertile. But in the epididymis, as a result of the "ripening" process, they acquire both these properties. Much effort is now being devoted to developing new, often ineffective or unacceptable, antispermatogenic agents. It might be much more productive to concentrate instead on methods of preventing the testicular spermatozoa from becoming fertile in the first place.

35.3 Antigenicity of Spermatozoa and Seminal Plasma

Great hopes were pinned at one time on the possibility of utilizing semen antigens for the purpose of immunizing the human male or female against spermatozoa and thereby providing an effective method of immunological contraception. This approach to the problem of fertility control has not been particularly successful, and the various measures suggested did not turn out to be nearly as effective as, for example, steroidal contraception, tubal ligation, or vasectomy. Insufficient notice was taken by the early investigators of the fact that many so-called sperm antigens are not specific to spermatozoa but occur in other parts of the body, and that some of them are actually "deposited" on the sperm cells by the male accessory secretions. The antigenicity of semen, like semen metabolism, is greatly influenced by sperm–seminal plasma interactions.

Two good examples of sperm-coating antigens in human semen are (1) the ABO blood group antigens, present in the prostatic secretion of so-called secretor males (individuals who also secrete these antigens in the saliva) and (2) Weil's sperm-coating antigen of the seminal vesicle secretion. The latter is a particularly powerful antigen, and we know more about it than about the others. Attempts to elucidate its chemical nature were unsuccessful at first but later were greatly helped by the discovery of an antigen with closely similar properties in human milk and the subsequent demonstration that milk lactoferrin also has sperm-coating antigenic properties. Like the lactoferrin of human milk, the vesicular antigen has a molecular weight of about 70,000 and the capacity to bind two atoms of iron to each molecule. Its concentration is about the same in human semen and milk, around 0.5–1.0 mg/ml. But the electrophoretic mobility of the seminal iron-binding protein is somewhat different from that of milk lactoferrin, and on this and certain other accounts Roberts and Boettcher prefer to call it *scaferrin*. Experiments performed with the fluorescent antibody technique have shown that the lactoferrinlike antigen is characteristic of ejaculated spermatozoa but is absent from testicular spermatozoa: the staining reaction in the acrosomal region of the sperm head, resulting from the use of either milk antiserum or seminal plasma antiserum, is strongly positive in ejaculated spermatozoa but negative in testicular spermatozoa.

When considering the events associated with coating and decoating of spermatozoa by antigens, one must note a certain analogy between these reactions and the events that form part of the capacitation and decapacitation processes. Capacitation is probably a decoating phenomenon, dependent on the removal in the female reproductive tract of a decapacitation factor with which the spermatozoa have been coated during their passage through the male reproductive tract.

It would be wrong, however, to say that all antigens in semen are shared by spermatozoa and seminal plasma. On the contrary, there is good evidence, derived from studies by Behrman, Menge, Mancini, Shulman, Quinlivan, Metz, and others, for distinct differences in the antigenic properties of spermatozoa and seminal plasma, as well as between testicular antigens and those produced in the epididymis, prostate, seminal vesicle, and other male accessory organs of reproduction. But only a few of these antigens have so far been properly purified and identified. The so-called LDH-X isozyme of lactate dehydrogenase, crystallized by Goldberg, provides a good example of an antigenic protein that is unique to spermatozoa and absent from seminal plasma. Sperm hyaluronidase, certain acrosomal proteases, and sorbitol dehydrogenase provide similar examples. It has been reported that immunization of laboratory animals with some of these enzymes lowers the pregnancy rate, but the phenomenon does not occur on a scale that would justify the use of such antigens and the respective antibodies as antifertility agents.

The antigens of seminal plasma may be distributed into three broad categories: (1) blood serum proteins, such as the various albumins, globulins, immunoglobulins, and immunoglobulin fragments; (2) antigens common to semen and other organs in the body; and (3) seminal plasma-specific antigens, such as the 3.72S protein of vesicular origin and the three antigenic compounds specific to the human prostate.

At present it seems more realistic to use the seminal antigens as diagnostic aids in certain forms of infertility due to immunological pathogenesis than to use them as contraceptive agents. This assessment has attracted the attention of many investigators since Wilson and Rümke independently reported in 1954 the presence of sperm agglutinins in the blood sera of some sterile patients. The present interest is due largely to the rapidly accumulating evidence that autoimmunity to spermatozoa, expressed as a high titer of sperm agglutinins in blood serum, can develop as a sequel to vasectomy, presumably caused by extravasation of spermatozoa and the formation of spermatic granulomas. The significance of sperm autoimmunity in infertile patients who have not undergone vasectomy is more difficult to explain and is yet another of the many unsolved questions in the area of semen antigenicity.

The major problem that should be given priority is that of separating and identifying both chemically and immunologically further antigens of spermatozoa and obtaining the respective antibodies. Perhaps when progress has been made in this direction, it will be easier to understand the relationship of the various antigens and antibodies to sperm motility, cervical mucus penetration, and other steps in reproduction and fertility, including the intriguing possibility to which Metz, Brackett, and others have drawn attention, that the antigenicity of ejaculated spermatozoa changes during sperm ascent in the female reproductive tract and capacitation.

Another possibility that merits attention is the use of sperm antigens for the purpose of separating X and Y spermatozoa. A modest success in shifting the sex ratio of mice offspring in favor of the female sex has recently been reported by Bennett and Boyse, with spermatozoa preincubated in antisera against the Y antigen.

35.4 Artificial Insemination

The practice of artificial insemination as a means of breeding farm animals has long provided the main incentive to laboratory workers for developing improved media, pabula, dilutors, and extenders, in which to store semen prior to transportation and insemination. An early step forward in this area was the introduction in 1939 of the egg-yolk phosphate-diluent, which soon became accepted as a popular medium for storing bovine semen for periods of several days at temperatures slightly above $0°C$. Another major advance occurred 10 years later with the introduction of glycerol as an agent capable of protecting spermatozoa from damage during freezing in solid CO_2 ($-79°C$) and thawing. Within a year of that discovery a bank of glycerol-frozen bull semen was set up in England, providing samples for artificial insemination. At present, that same batch of glycerol-frozen semen is still being used successfully for the production of live and perfectly normal calves. During the intervening years the technique of semen storage has greatly improved. Other protective additives such as dimethylsulfoxide have come

into use, and solid CO_2 has been replaced by liquid nitrogen ($-196°C$).

Attempts to freeze semen from animals other than bulls have not met with the same immediate success, and the pregnancy rate obtainable with frozen semen of rams, boars, stallions, or for that matter, men, is by no means as high as with bovine semen. But even among bulls certain individuals are characterized by a poor "keeping quality" of their frozen semen, and at the present time these individual variations are not well understood. Whether human or animal, the thawed spermatozoa seem often to recover their motility much more readily than their fertilizing ability. This dissociation of motility and fertilizing properties in a way resembles the behavior of spermatozoa following exposure to short-wave irradiation. This can also result in a loss of fertilizing capacity but not necessarily of motility.

How the two fundamental sperm functions—motility and fertilizing ability—are linked with each other is a question to which as yet there is no adequate answer. An answer will have to be found before an explanation can be offered for why under any given storage condition, in vitro or in vivo, the spermatozoa should be capable of preserving their motility much more efficiently than their fertilizing ability.

It is of course possible, as has been suggested by several investigators, that the chromatin of the sperm nucleus is much more sensitive to freezing and thawing than is the sperm tail. But the sperm tail is not entirely insensitive to freezing and thawing, and its movements can also be affected, except that the decrease in motility is slower than the loss in fertilizing function. In other words, in a given sample of frozen semen, the spermatozoa that exhibit good motility when examined microscopically immediately after thawing may be losing their capacity for survival too soon and therefore no longer possess full motility at the time they reach the site of fertilization in the oviducts. Polge, Salamon, and Wilmut at the Cambridge unit have shown that if boar semen is diluted with a yolk-glucose-glycerol medium and stored in liquid nitrogen for a month or two, the thawed spermatozoa are motile but incapable of inducing a pregnancy after the usual intrauterine artificial insemination. Yet the same spermatozoa manage to fertilize pig eggs successfully, provided the thawed semen is surgically introduced directly into the oviducts, near the site of fertilization.

Marked differences in storage quality of frozen semen between individual men can also be illuminated by observations on farm animals. In recent experiments by Stewart, Beatty, Hancock, and their colleagues in Great Britain, using the method called heterospermic insemination, fresh semen from four bulls was mixed and used for inseminating cattle; the number of calves sired per bull was in a ratio close to 1:1:1:1. However, when the mixed semen was first subjected to deep-freezing at −196°C prior to insemination, then one bull sired about 50 per cent of all the progeny. Obviously the ability of semen from this particular bull to withstand deep-freeze storage must have been far superior to that of sperm from the three other animals. It would be of great interest to find out how and why the semen of the superior bull differs from that of the three other animals in other respects, including metabolism of the spermatozoa.

The question why some but not other specimens of initially fertile semen fail to fertilize after freezing and thawing is particularly relevant to problems in humans. For this reason the development of reliable criteria (ultrastructural, metabolic, etc.) that could be used for predicting the fertilizing potential of frozen human semen is of utmost importance if human sperm banks are to fulfill their expected role in artificial insemination. As is amply evident from recent extensive reviews on this subject by Behrman, Sherman, Tyler, and others, the techniques of storing frozen human semen have improved considerably over the last decade, particularly since liquid nitrogen (−196°C) has replaced other refrigerants, but the freezing and thawing techniques, as well as the criteria for assessing the fertilizing potential of thawed spermatozoa, need further elaboration, particularly in regard to the feasibility of (1) concentrating the sperm specimens by centrifugation prior to freezing, (2) replacing glycerol by other cryoprotective agents, and (3) defining more strictly the optimal rates for freezing and thawing. One other aspect of the problem of storing frozen human semen that should not be overlooked in future research relates to the possibility that some genetic damage, and consequently fetal abnormalities or death, may occasionally arise as a result of either freezing, storage, or thawing. Most authorities on this subject seem to agree that the risk is either very small or nonexistent; however, the series of pregnancies on which these optimistic claims have been based is not sufficiently large to convincingly allay all the fears.

Ultimately the fate of the human sperm banks will depend upon their acceptance by the public. In view of the present popularity of vasectomy and the concern being expressed about the chances of reversing the consequences of this operation, a real need for human sperm banks may arise. There are, however, major psychological as well as legal complicating factors inherent in the use of human sperm banks. One of the many unanswered questions is: What would be society's attitude to the social position, legal status, and inheritance rights of a child born following artificial insemination with a sample of semen that had been collected a decade or two earlier?

Key References

Metabolism

Garbers, D. L., N. L. First, and H. A. Lardy. The stimulation of bovine epididymal sperm metabolism by cyclic nucleotide phosphodiesterase inhibitors. Biol. Reprod. 8:589, 1973.

Horton, E. W., R. L. Jones, and C. G. Marr. Effect of aspirin on prostaglandin and fructose levels in human semen. J. Reprod. Fertil. 33:385, 1973.

Hoskins, D. D., and E. R. Casillas. Hormones, second messengers, and the mammalian spermatozoon. Adv. Sex Horm. Res. 1, 1974.

Mann, T. The biochemistry of semen and of the male reproductive tract. London: Methuen, 1964.

Mann, T. Sperm metabolism. In Fertilization, Vol. 1, eds. C. B. Metz and A. Monroy, p. 99. New York: Academic Press, 1967.

Mann, T. Energy requirements of spermatozoa and the cervical environment. In The biology of the cervix, eds. R. J. Blandau and K. Moghissi, p. 329. Chicago: Univ. of Chicago Press, 1967.

Marquis, N. R, and I. B. Fritz. Effects of testosterone on the distribution of carnitine and carnitine acetyltransferase in tissues of the reproductive system of the male rat. J. Biol. Chem. 240:2197, 1965.

Setchell, B. P., T. W. Scott, J. K. Voglmayr, and G. M. Waites. Characteristics of testicular spermatozoa and the fluid which transports them into the epididymis. Biol. Reprod. Suppl. 1:40, 1969.

Voglmayr, J. K., T. W. Scott, B. P. Setchell, and G. M. H. Waites. Metabolism of testicular spermatozoa and characteristics of testicular fluid collected from conscious rams. J. Reprod. Fertil. 14:87, 1967.

White, I. G. Biochemical aspects of spermatozoa and their environment in the male reproductive tract. J. Reprod. Fertil. Suppl. 18:225, 1973.

Antigenicity

Bennett, D., and E. A. Boyse. Sex ratio in progeny with H-Y antiserum. Nature 246:308, 1973.

Boettcher, B. Antigens of the male tract. J. Reprod. Fertil. Suppl. 18:77, 1973.

Erickson, R. P. An antiglobulin test for the detection of surface antigens of mouse spermatozoa. J. Reprod. Fertil. 28: 109, 1972.

Goldberg, E. Infertility in female rabbits immunized with lactate dehydrogenase X. Science 181:458, 1973.

Hekman, A., and P. Rümke. The antigens of human seminal plasma with special reference to lactoferrin as a spermatozoa-coating antigen. In Protides of the biological fluids, ed. H. Peeters, p. 549. Oxford: Pergamon Press, 1968.

Johnson, W. L., and A. G. Hunter. Seminal antigens: Their alteration in the genital tract of female rabbits and during partial in vitro capacitation with amylase and glucuronidase. Biol. Reprod. 1:332, 1972.

Li, T. S., and S. J. Behrman. The sperm- and seminal plasma-specific antigens of human semen. Fertil. Steril. 21:565, 1970.

Mancini, R. E., O. Gutierrez, and F. E. Collazo. Immunohistochemical localization of antigens in human spermatozoa. Fertil. Steril. 22:475, 1971.

Masson, P. L., J. F. Heremans, and Ch. Dive. An iron-binding protein common to many external secretions. Clin. Chim. Acta, 14:735, 1966.

Menge, A. C. Immune reactions and infertility. J. Reprod. Fertil. Suppl. 10:171, 1970.

Metz, C. B. Role of specific sperm antigens in fertilization. Fed. Proc. 32:2057, 1973.

Metz, C. B. Gamete surface components and their role in fertilization. In *Fertilization*, Vol. I, eds. C. B. Metz and A. Monroy, p. 163. New York: Academic Press, 1967.

Oliphant, G., and B. G. Brackett. Immunological assessment of surface changes in rabbit sperm undergoing capacitation. Biol. Reprod. 9:404, 1973.

Roberts, I. K., and B. Boettcher. Identification of human sperm-coating antigen. J. Reprod. Fertil. 18:347, 1969.

Shulman, S. Antigenic analysis of the male tract. In *Immunology and reproduction*, ed. R. G. Edwards, p. 109. London: Int. Planned Parenthood Fed., 1969.

Shulman, S., A. Hekman, and C. Pann. Antibodies to spermatozoa. II. Spermagglutination techniques for guinea pig and human cells. J. Reprod. Fertil. 27:31, 1971.

Weil, A. J. Antigens of the seminal plasma. J. Reprod. Fertil. Suppl. 2:25, 1967.

Storage and Artificial Insemination

Behrman, S. J., and D. R. Ackerman. Freeze preservation of human sperm. Am. J. Obstet. Gynecol. 103:654, 1969.

Ingelman-Sundberg, A., and N.-O. Lunell, eds. *Current problems in fertility*. (Articles by S. J. Behrman, J. Friberg, and O. Nilsson.) New York: Plenum Press, 1971.

Pedersen, H., and P. E. Lebeck. Ultrastructural changes in the human spermatozoon after freezing for artificial insemination. Fertil. Steril. 22:125, 1971.

Polge, C., S. Salamon, and I. Wilmut. Fertilizing capacity of frozen boar semen following surgical insemination. Vet. Rec. 87:424, 1970.

Report of panel on human artificial insemination (Appendix V to the Annual Report of the Med. Council). Br. Med. J. Suppl., April 7, 1973.

Richardson, D. W., and R. M. Sadleir. The toxicity of various non-electrolytes to human spermatozoa and their protective effects during freezing. J. Reprod. Fertil. 14:439, 1967.

Rowson, L. E. A. The role of reproductive research in animal production. J. Reprod. Fertil. 26:113, 1971.

Sherman, J. K. Synopsis of the use of frozen human semen since 1964: State of the art of human semen banking. Fertil. Steril. 24:397, 1973.

Stewart, D. L., R. L. Spooner, G. H. Bennett, R. A. Beatty, and J. L. Hancock. A second experiment with heterospermic insemination in cattle. J. Reprod. Fertil. 36:107, 1974.

Tyler, E. The clinical use of frozen semen banks. Fertil. Steril. 24:413, 1973.

36 Capacitation of Spermatozoa and Fertilization in Mammals

M. C. Chang, C. R. Austin,
J. M. Bedford, B. G. Brackett,
R. H. F. Hunter, and R. Yanagimachi

36.1 Introduction and Summary (M. C. Chang)

The connection between reproduction and sex has always evoked a degree of emotional inhibition in both Western and Eastern countries. In early times, except for a few embryologists, the study of reproduction was in the hands of animal breeders and gynecologists interested in improvement of fertility or the cure of sterility. The publication of *Physiology of reproduction* by F. H. A. Marshall in 1910 and the serious challenge to American law in 1913 by Margaret Sanger placed reproductive biology in a respected position both for scientific inquiry in academic institutions and for contraceptive development for the emancipation of women and for family planning. Since the post–World War II growth of awareness of the population explosion, the importance of population control has been stressed everywhere for the very survival of the human race. Thus various government agencies in different countries and many philanthropic foundations such as the Ford Foundation have supported scientific research on reproduction in the hope of developing effective and efficient measures for the control of human fertility.

The capacitation of spermatozoa, recognized only in 1951 but commonly mentioned in present literature, refers to the preparation in the female of spermatozoa for fertilization. Fertilization, the union of a spermatozoon and the egg, is the beginning of the development of an individual. It is also a primary determining factor of sterility and fertility.

This report was prepared by several scientists who hold academic positions but are actively working on capacitation and fertilization. Our academic research during the past 10 years has been directly or indirectly aided by the Ford Foundation, to which we are grateful for support that, at least in part, has enabled us to satisfy our scientific curiosity. The rapid progress in these studies during the past decade makes it difficult for one person to write a report without bias or without neglecting certain aspects. Thus a different topic is described here by each participant. The scientists who have contributed to our present knowledge and the sources of their reports are not all listed because of the nature of this report.

By reading and discussing each other's contributions, we came to various conclusions:

In spite of the important progress made in recent years, the acquisition of basic knowledge in reproductive biology is still of fundamental importance if we are to develop suitable measures for the regulation of fertility, either to improve animal fertility for food production or to decrease human fertility.

Sperm capacitation is a general characteristic of many mammalian species, including humans. This preparation for the final penetration of the egg membranes is achieved synergistically and efficiently in the female tract in the sequential routes, although it can also be achieved outside the female tract in many species, including humans, under various experimental conditions. Capacitation involves physiological changes in sperm at a molecular level, probably as a result of removing components attached to the surface and release or activation of some enzymes in the acrosome on the sperm head. These changes facilitate or ultimately allow a morphological change of the acrosome that is a prerequisite for penetration of the coat of the egg. During capacitation, the metabolic activity and motility of sperm increase for the final penetration of the egg, but this increased activity limits the survival time of sperm.

The process of fertilization has been difficult to analyze scientifically in mammals because it occurs inside the body; however, fertilization of eggs from many laboratory animals and humans can now be routinely performed in a watchglass. From electron-microscopic study of capacitiation and fertilization inside and outside the body, we now know many of the fine structural details of the morphological events from the time that sperm approaches the egg until the time of the first cleavage. The biochemical and physiological changes during fertilization, such as the species-specificity of the egg coat, the release of cortical granules from the egg proper which change the property of the zona pellucida to prevent the further entry of sperm, the enlargement of the sperm head in eggs at an appropriate stage of maturity, and the replication of DNA in the male and female pronuclei, have all been identified and studied to some degree.

There are many potential leads for contraceptive development. For instance, by hormonal or chemical manipulation of regions of the female tract, such as the cervix or Fallopian tube, or of the secretion of the female tract, it is possible to interfere with sperm transport, capacitation, and survival. The enzyme activity of the sperm head can be suppressed to prevent sperm entry into the egg. The effect of decapacitation factor present in the male tract can be mimicked in the female tract by immunological or other means. Since the zona pellucida is so sensitive to the contents of the cortical granules and since many plant extracts, such as agglutinins, can be used to harden the zona pellucida, immunological and other means can be utilized to prevent sperm penetration. These illustrate only a few possible areas for the development of contraceptives in the future. If more fundamental knowledge on capacitation and fertilization can be gained during the next few years, it is possible that a variety of effective and efficient contraceptives will be produced by pharmaceutical houses throughout the world. Moreover, by perfecting our ability to achieve fertilization outside the body we will be able to fertilize eggs of genetically desirable domestic animals in a dish, store them in a frozen condition, and transfer them to recipient animals, thereby improving our food production system.

36.2 Capacitation of Spermatozoa (J. M. Bedford)

That mammalian sperm finally become competent to penetrate the egg only when in the female tract was first recognized by Austin (1951) and by Chang (1951), independently. Subsequently it has been proved that all eutheria examined display the need for capacitation of their sperm in the female before fertilization can occur, and it now seems reasonable to think that this phenomenon is a general characteristic of the conception process in eutherian mammals, including humans. At the time of this writing many facets of capacitation are not understood and are difficult to ascertain. The difficulty of investigation in this area is explained at least partly by the relatively small numbers of capacitated spermatozoa in either the uterus or Fallopian tube and the presence of dead sperm, leucocytes, other cells, and tissue debris mixed with them in flushings of the female tract after mating. This task has been further complicated by species variation and the suspicion that different sperm in a given population may become capacitated at different rates in the same environment.

Morphological and Physiological Aspects of Capacitation

There is now a reasonable consensus that capacitation as such does not involve a change in the sperm cell that is visible in the electron microscope and that capacitation should be distinguished from the ensuing acrosome reaction, for which capacitation is a prerequisite. Although capacitation per se does not involve morphological change in the sperm, it does facilitate the occurrence of the acrosome reaction under appropriate environmental conditions. Since the acrosome reaction is characterized by a fusion and breakdown of the cell membrane and outer acrosomal membrane, the sperm head membranes may be modified at the molecular level during capacitation. Experimental evidence suggests that the acrosome reaction then propagates change in the nature of the still intact surface of the postacrosomal region of the sperm head and that such changes determine the success of the sperm in fusing with the vitelline surface after passing through the zona pellucida.

Other evidence suggesting that the sperm surface is modified in the female includes the absence of agglutination behavior in the presence of antisperm antibody, the killing of rabbit uterine sperm by an agglutinating seminal plasma that was innocuous to ejaculated sperm, changes in the electrophoretic behavior of sperm after residence in the uterus, and changes in the phagocytic response of leucocytes to intact but capacitated (uterine) spermatozoa. It has seemed likely to many investigators that surface changes in sperm in the female tract simply reflect the removal of components of seminal plasma or of epididymal secretions adsorbed by the sperm after leaving the testis.

While various fragments of evidence point to this conclusion, such a simple concept does not satisfy the findings of various experimental studies which suggest that capacitation involves more than a single change in the sperm cell. Clearly there is a pressing need for more information about the chemistry of the sperm surface and the changes that occur there as a concomitant of capacitation. A further question concerns the nature of the trigger that evokes the acrosome reaction in the capacitated or "prepared" spermatozoon. Although there is ample evidence that this is a diffusible element of the egg coat, termed *fertilizin*, in some invertebrates, there is as yet no evidence as to whether the egg and/or the granulosa cell mass is the source of the stimulus for the acrosome reaction in eutherian mammals.

Not only is the likelihood strong that functionally important changes occur over some regions of the sperm surface during capacitation, but there is also evidence of the involvement of other systems of the sperm, in particular those concerned with motility. The initial report of changes in the pattern of energy metabolism (O_2 uptake, glucose utilization) of rabbit spermatozoa after their incubation in the uterus has been confirmed in other species such as the sheep and pig, and there are reports of increased adenyl cyclase and, inferentially, cAMP synthesis during capacitation of hamster spermatozoa in vitro. In the hamster and guinea pig the spermatozoa have been observed to adopt what might be described as a more energetic or urgent pattern of motility, perhaps as a reflection of such metabolic changes. Thus it appears that in some species at least the spermatozoon develops its maximum thrust following capacitation, that is, immediately before it might expect to begin to penetrate the zona pellucida. This and the uniquely tough nature of the eutherian sperm head suggest that the forward thrust of the sperm rather than a digestive lysin may be the major factor that assists its passage through the zona pellucida, though it is perhaps inappropriate to assign relative degrees of importance to the different aspects of such a coordinated function.

Investigations by Williams and co-workers at the University of Georgia have produced evidence for the idea that at least some acrosomal enzymes exist in an inhibited state in ejaculated spermatozoa and that the naturally occurring inhibitors are removed during sperm transport through the female tract. As yet no direct evidence links such claims to the process of functional capacitation, and many questions remain about the means whereby inhibitors are removed and pass through the intact membranes enveloping the acrosomal content. Nonetheless this is an area that should be pursued in an effort to establish the role of these inhibitors in the whole scheme of fertilization, including the reason for their existence in the rete testis fluids and in the ejaculate.

Transport and Survival of Sperm in the Female Tract
Sperm transport into the cervix is rapid—from 90 to 180 seconds after coitus in both humans and rabbits. Thereafter, in the rapid phase, sperm may be transported to the site of fertilization in a matter of minutes after coitus in the domestic ruminants, and studies in women indicate that a few motile sperm can appear there within five minutes of vaginal instillation, the rapid phase of transport presumably being effected mainly by the tract rather than by the motility of the sperm.

The subsequent and slower phase of sperm transport in which sperm pass to the tubal ampulla over a period of several hours demands the presence of a cervical sperm reservoir, which itself depends on the innate motility of the sperm. It also seems that sperm transport through the Fallopian tube is not simply a question of constant contractions of this region supported by the innate motility of the sperm. Some evidence also exists of correlation between the tubal passage of sperm to the ampulla and the timing of ovulation or the presence of the products of ovulation in the tubal ampulla. Transport is minimized in progesterone-dominated females, probably as a result of change in the receptivity of the cervical mucus and of the contractile activity of the walls of the tract.

Although stress is sometimes placed on the rapidity of sperm transport after coitus in some species, it is not certain that this can have much import in normal fertility situations. First, the spermatozoa of all mammals examined probably have a capacitation requirement of at least one hour or longer before they begin to penetrate an egg. Second, in most feral animals and in efficient farming operations the period of receptivity to the male is normally detected early in estrus, and insemination is most likely to take place some hours before ovulation.

The question of the longevity of sperm in the female has an obvious bearing on the efficacy of the rhythm method of contraception, and any significant reduction in the length of sperm viability would clearly go far to reduce the conception rate within a population.

Although the synchrony between sexual receptivity and the ovulatory phase has been virtually lost in women, in most spontaneous ovulators there is a correlation between the length of estrus plus the fertile life of the egg on the one hand and the viable life of sperm in the female on the other, and in induced ovulators the fertile life of sperm is approximately twice as long as the period that elapses between coitus and deterioration of the unfertilized egg.

Among mammals in general, a considerable species variation has been found in the viable life of sperm in the female. For example, most rodent sperm remain motile for a relatively short period of 12 to 15 hours, whereas those of the dog can remain motile for up to 11 days after insemination. The life of the sperm lies between these extremes in most other mammals (rabbit, about 30 hours; ferret, about 126 hours; sheep, 30 to 40 hours). At present there is no information about the viability or fertile life of sperm in female subhuman primates or humans. Motile human spermatozoa have been observed in material collected from the cervix up to six days after intercourse, but the bulk of (indirect) evidence indicates that their fertile life is considerably less than six days—perhaps 36 to 48 hours. In some animals, as suggested above for humans, the motility of sperm may persist for some time after fertilizing ability has declined, and in some species the evidence indicates that fertilizing ability has a limited span once capacitation has occurred. We have no idea at present as to the nature of the initial lesion in the sperm whereby fertilizing ability clearly is lost before motility. At present very little is known about the biochemical dependence of sperm metabolism upon elements in the female tract. Nor are there currently any leads that seem to offer a means of deliberately curtailing the survival of sperm once they have entered the female. Spermatozoa may be removed or disposed of more quickly in the female tract immunized against sperm antigens, but there is no clear evidence to prove this point.

Analysis of the Factors Required for Capacitation

The relative importance of different regions of the female tract for capacitation appears to be at least partially linked to the site of deposition of semen at coitus. In the species whose whole semen passes in bulk to the uterine lumen, complete capacitation is rarely achieved in the uterus alone. Synergism between uterus and tube appears as a definite phenomenon in the rabbit, and sperm are then transported through the uterus to the oviduct. In the rabbit, in contrast to rodents, spermatozoa can readily be capacitated completely in the uterus alone, as judged by their ability to penetrate eggs there, or in vitro, where the eggs have been denuded of granulosa cells. Nonetheless, complete capacitation in the rabbit uterus or oviduct requires much longer than the four hours needed when sperm pass through both uterus and tube. This suggests that in such species there is a synergism between uterus and oviduct in the accomplishment of capacitation.

Thus in some species both uterus and tube show the ability to capacitate sperm, though a combination of the two seems to provide the optimal conditions for its accomplishment. In many species the uterus is probably less important than the tube for capacitation, particularly in species whose whole semen is deposited into the uterus at coitus.

Initial observations by Chang in 1958 showed that the capacitation environment in the female may vary drastically according to the endocrine state of the female; this gave rise to hopes of an easy route for control of capacitation. But although it was clear that the capacitation potential of the rabbit uterus essentially disappeared in the progestin-dominated state, the Fallopian tube retained its capacitation ability in progestin-dominated females. Subsequent extensions of Chang's studies by Bedford, Soupart, and Hamner have demonstrated that the capacitation potential of the uterus is markedly reduced though not extinguished in the estrogen-deficient rabbit and that the rabbit Fallopian tube essentially retains its capacitation potential regardless of the steroid status of the female.

Further investigation seems worthwhile in this area, first because the above conclusions are derived from only one species, the rabbit, and second because rabbits and primates distinctly differ in the response of the oviduct to steroids or to their deficiency. The cilia in the rabbit oviduct seem largely independent of the steroid status of the female. It may well prove, therefore, that the refractoriness of the rabbit oviduct is unique in this respect and that the capacitation potential of the primate oviduct, like the cilia, can be modified by endocrine manipulation.

Little has been learned from in vivo experiments about the specific nature of factors required for capacitation. Rabbit sperm seem to have a rather close dependence upon the specific female environment for complete capacitation, but some degree of capacitation has been achieved, in a temporal sense, in a foreign uterus and in extrareproductive sites. Since the spermatozoa can be capacited in vitro in several rodents, cats, and humans, extrareproductive methods will probably provide one means by which to study the precise requirement for capacitation.

Since capacitation itself may be a composite change (surface, motility/metabolic), at least two factors may be important, and Yanagimachi (1969b) has shown the existence of two relevant and separate capacitating components in bovine follicular fluid. Undoubtedly species differ in this respect. For instance, among the rodents, homologous rather than heterologous serum or follicular fluid provides the better capacitation medium, though use of the latter does not necessarily prevent but merely lowers the efficiency of capacitation, as judged ultimately by fertilization rate. Gwatkin et al. (1972) claim a special role in capacitation for the cumulus oophorus and state that the capacitating activity of the hamster oviduct contents depends entirely on this component, with both cells and matrix seeming to be critical. In view of positive evidence of fertilization of granulosa-denuded eggs by sperm capacitated in vitro in serum-containing and other media, which does not receive any detailed consideration in the position of Gwatkin and his colleagues, it is difficult to accept without reservation their contention that cumulus cells have a special role in the capacitation of sperm. Bavister (1973), in distinguishing between conditions in which hamster sperm can be capacitated and can undergo the acrosome reaction, has provided some evidence that capacitation can be achieved in Tyrode's solution supplemented only by bovine serum albumin.

Decapacitation and Recapacitation

The initial observation by Chang in 1957 that the fertilizing ability of capacitated rabbit spermatozoa can be reversibly inhibited by exposure to seminal plasma, and the subsequent demonstration that the decapacitation factor (DF) can be removed by centrifugation at 105,000 G, has stimulated attempts to isolate and characterize the active moiety. But after about 20 years not only is there no consensus as to the nature of the active inhibitory fraction, there is also no clear idea of how its inhibitory effect is mediated.

The active factor in seminal plasma is obviously stable to storage and to various physical treatments and is relatively nonspecific, though it does not act to inhibit the acrosome reaction of sea urchin sperm. The work of Williams's group claims active DF as a small lysine-containing peptide. The work of Davis, on the other hand, suggests that the DF activity resides in one glycoprotein fraction of seminal plasma and that a relatively large molecule is involved.

It should be remembered that *decapacitation* is a functional term and that there may be more than one substance in seminal plasma that can act to reversibly inhibit the fertilizing ability of capacitated sperm. In recent years, Williams and others have claimed that a major acrosomal protease—which they term *acrosin*—is inhibited by DF added to the sperm during ejaculation and is subsequently removed during incubation in the female tract. Although they feel that such a lifting of the enzyme inhibition constitutes (a phase of) capacitation, their interpretation is questionable. According to their own work, the enzyme in rabbit epididymal sperm is not inhibited, yet such sperm require the same time and conditions as do ejaculated sperm for successful capacitation. More likely is the possibility that DF acts at the sperm surface, and by binding there it masks sites of importance in the induction of the acrosome reaction. I have shown that prior mixing of rabbit uterine sperm with small amounts of seminal plasma inhibits the ability of follicular fluid to produce acrosomal disruption in these sperm. Aonuma et al. (1973) reported the elution from epididymal guinea pig spermatozoa of a sperm-coating antigen that possesses decapacitation properties. This and earlier work by Weinman and Williams suggests that an active inhibitory factor is present in the epididymis and that sperm are in a sense decapacitated before they come into contact with seminal plasma at ejaculation.

Effects of Chemical Agents and Hormones
Since we do not understand the nature of capacitation, rational study has not been applied to the action of many agents that might affect capacitation. Claims for capacitation in vitro by enzymes such as β-amylase have not been confirmed, and no other enzymes have been shown to be instrumental in the accomplishment of functional capacitation. The demonstration of the decapacitation action of seminal plasma indicates that the inhibition of the capacitated state by nontoxic agents is feasible, but not enough effort has been made to test known carbohydrates of lipoproteins and glycoproteins for such activity. We still do not understand the identity of the factors that have been shown to be active in in vitro capacitation systems.

In Chang's laboratory in 1966 I discovered that the seminal plasma of a fertile male rabbit had strong agglutinating properties and that this particular fluid would kill rabbit spermatozoa, but only after they had been in the female tract for several hours. This shows that not only the functional state but also the susceptibilities of sperm may change after capacitation. Thus possible inhibitory agents, particularly those aimed at inhibition of motility, should perhaps be tested routinely on capacitated as well as on ejaculated spermatozoa.

Prospects for Control of Capacitation
The prospects for control of capacitation are ultimately promising. The most likely immediate possibility is that capacitation control can be achieved or is being achieved by low-level progestins, either completely or partially. Although the capacitation potential of the rabbit oviduct resists such manipulation, nothing is known of the response of the oviduct of the subhuman primate or human. As noted earlier, the cilia of the primate oviduct show a dependence on estrogen that is largely absent in the rabbit, and it may well be, therefore, that the capacitation activity of the primate oviduct shows a greater dependence on the steroid status of the female than does that of the rabbit oviduct. Present evidence suggests that changes occur in the sperm surface, in the motility mechanisms, and possibly in the state of the acrosomal enzymes as functional concomitants of capacitation.

A tempting view held by several investigators is that capacitation simply involves an ordered removal of the seminal coating laid down in the epididymis or at ejaculation, but this is almost certainly a simplification and does not explain the possibility of partial capacitation or the synergistic activity of uterus and tube. The reversible inhibition of capacitation by elements in epididymal fluids and in the seminal plasma shows that a block of the capacitated state can be achieved by nontoxic substances, but the true nature of this molecule or its active site must be established before there can be any prospect or consideration of delivering it to the site of fertilization.

Before a rational approach to capacitation control becomes possible, further characterization must be achieved of the chemical nature of the cell surface and of the changes occurring in this surface in the epididymis and in the female tract. This must involve intensive experimental work in a few species of laboratory animals to firmly establish the functionally relevant changes in capacitation per se as a basis for comparison with primates and humans, where, initially, this work will be less easily performed. This type of work was not previously possible because the technical probes were not available and the general concepts of biological membrane structure and function were not as clear as they are now becoming. It seems imperative to attract into the field biochemists who are skilled in the handling, isolation, and study of membrane components. Since it appears likely that capacitation involves change in the motility patterns of spermatozoa, the control points in the metabolic pathway(s) should be thoroughly characterized. There is no good evidence of any change in the stage of the sperm nucleus during capacitation: it appears to be completely suppressed, being turned on only in the hours following its decondensation inside the egg.

There has been much loose, uncritical work in this whole field, and the biochemists involved have often seemed ignorant of its biology. Perhaps the most pressing need is for a clear definition of the functional changes occurring in the sperm that confer on it the ability to undergo the acrosome reaction and penetrate the egg. Simultaneously, it should be recognized that we are studying a phenomenon whose biological significance we still do not understand.

36.3 Sperm Capacitation (C. R. Austin)

Progress in the Past Decade
In 1964 an important milestone was achieved, namely the report by Yanagimachi and Chang on the fertilization of the hamster egg in vitro. Not only was this the first time that rodent eggs had been fertilized in vitro, but some success was achieved with spermatozoa deriving directly from the epididymis. Up to this time work had been restricted to the rabbit, and the spermatozoa used had always undergone prior capacitation in the female tract. Capacitation was also occurring in the experiments of Yanagimachi and Chang, as shown by the fact that there was a delay of several hours between placing the gametes together and observing the first penetrated eggs. So it was clear that the factors normally responsible for the capacitation of spermatozoa could be isolated from the female tract and maintained in an experimentally controllable environment. All that was recovered from the oviducts were eggs in cumulus and traces of incidentally included oviduct secretions, so the search for the substances or conditions responsible for capacitation was significantly narrowed by this work.

The next step was the observation by Barros and Austin in 1967 that fertilization in vitro could be obtained with follicular oocytes and epididymal spermatozoa, the oocytes being recovered shortly before ovulation. This meant that the factors responsible for sperm capacitation were not restricted to the female tract but also accompanied the eggs and cumulus cells; indeed the association with the eggs and cumulus must have been intimate, for it survived several transfers of the cells to fresh media. As in Yanagimachi and Chang's experience, an interval of a little more than three hours occurred between mixing the gametes and the appearance of penetrated eggs. If spermatozoa were incubated for four to five hours with follicular oocytes in cumulus and then transferred to fresh oocytes they would promptly proceed to penetrate; preincubation of spermatozoa in various media lacking oocytes did not produce such a result. Barros and Austin also found that in preparations promoting fertilization the visible occurrence of the acrosome reaction in freely swimming spermatozoa coincided with the start of sperm penetration into the eggs, and acrosome reactions were not seen when the spermatozoa were incubated in the absence of eggs. The inference drawn was that capacitation and the acrosome reaction were two separate phenomena, the first being the necessary preliminary to the second.

Human spermatozoa have also been induced to undergo capacitation in vitro in media containing follicular fluid, and fertilization of follicular oocytes has ensued also in vitro, as reported by Bavister et al. (1969).

Yanagimachi (1969a,b) investigated the hamster follicular contents and found that follicular fluid by itself was highly effective in inducing capacitation and the acrosome reaction. Fractionation of the components of follicular fluid revealed a heat-stable low-molecular-weight compound, which favored prolonged motility of spermatozoa, and a heat-labile high-molecular-weight compound, which eventually evoked the acrosome reaction in spermatozoa that had maintained motility for four to five hours. Factors with the same properties were also found in blood serum by Yanagimachi in 1970. Results obtained by Bavister showed that the function of Yanagimachi's low-molecular-weight compound in sustaining motility was probably nonspecific, in the sense that the effect could be achieved in a carefully balanced, fully defined medium. The point was further made that the changes occurring during the long motile phase corresponded to capacitation, which could be regarded as an endogenous change in the spermatozoon that ensued under appropriate environmental conditions, while the acrosome reaction still required the stimulus of some substance of an apparently specific nature and normally present in both follicular fluid and blood serum (Austin et al. 1973).

Prospects for Contraceptive Development
The best-established fact is that spermatozoa need to be sustained at a high level of motility for several hours for capacitation to be achieved. Interference here would seem to offer some possibilities in future contraceptive development. To achieve such a result the essential requirement would be a means of altering the properties of female tract secretions. Appropriate means could involve administration of hormones or

other physiological or pharmacological agents, conveyed by systemic injection, medicated IUD, etc. Existing contraceptive methods involving steroid hormones and IUDs may owe their effect, at least in part, to interference with capacitation in this way. Other longer-term possibilities for contraceptive development can also be envisaged whereby agents are used to interfere with the properties of the sperm membranes in such a way as to preclude the acrosome reaction. Appropriate agents might include specific antibodies against spermatozoa, plant lectins, and perhaps even simple chemicals such as magnesium or copper ions; a vehicle for these agents could be a modification of the medicated IUD.

36.4 Capacitation and Fertilization in Vitro (B. G. Brackett)

Methods and Procedures for In Vitro Capacitation and Fertilization
Rabbit experiments The rabbit was commonly used for the study of capacitation and fertilization before the achievement of in vitro fertilization of hamster eggs by Yanagimachi and Chang in 1964. The assay used in early efforts to accomplish in vitro capacitation of rabbit sperm involved tubal insemination of treated sperm. It is now widely held that only partial capacitation was achieved in the earliest examples of in vitro capacitation. In 1965 Kirton and Hafs tubally inseminated rabbit sperm cultured in the uterine fluid or treated with β-amylase and claimed the capacitation of sperm in vitro, while in 1969 Ericsson also reported the partial capacitation of rabbit sperm in vitro by the treatment with mule eosinophils. These claims, however, were neither confirmed nor repeated.

In 1971 Ericsson et al. reported fertilization of rabbit eggs in vitro following treatment of epididymal sperm with Sendai virus. Sendai virus was mixed with sperm and kept at room temperature for 15 minutes before incubation with eggs. Controls included eggs with virus plus eggs and sperm without virus. In 10 experiments, 49 percent of 185 eggs cultured with virus-treated sperm cleaved into two to eight cells, while none of 85 eggs cultured with untreated sperm cleaved. Ericsson et al. speculated that the Sendai virus might have acted to induce a combination capacitation and acrosome reaction by the viral enzymatic splitting off of a negatively charged molecule, thereby drastically changing the sperm surface.

In 1972 Brackett et al. reported preliminary efforts to capacitate rabbit sperm in vitro using various enzymes and biological fluids prior to incubating the sperm with ovulated eggs in vitro. The best results were obtained when uterine fluid was used after 24 hours of refrigeration. Careful examination of the data

from these experiments led to the suggestion that increasing volumes of uterine fluid per million sperm resulted in improved proportions of egg cleavage.

In 1971 Ogawa et al. reported that some of the rabbit eggs following in vitro fertilization by epididymal sperm could develop into blastocysts in culture and that sperm were capacitated in a very complicated but chemically defined medium. Ogawa and his colleagues suggested that the concept of capacitation should be radically changed because incubation in a synthetic medium causes rabbit epididymal sperm to develop an increased capacity for fertilization. They suggested that hormonal pretreatment of the male rabbit has a favorable effect on the sperm. Their positive results, however, might have been due to the increased osmolarity of the medium (see below).

Recent emphasis in several laboratories has been directed toward defining the mechanism of the capacitation process in the rabbit. In view of these efforts, it is now clear that seminal plasma components coating the surface of the sperm cells are removed or altered during the process of capacitation. In 1973 Oliphant and Brackett developed a radioimmunoassay to follow the progress of the capacitation process in the rabbit. This assay involves the recognition of sperm coating antigens by ^{14}C-labeled antibodies. An inverse relationship between the binding of antibodies and the fertilizing capacity of sperm has been demonstrated. Following capacitation, it is possible to restore the sperm-coating antigens by treatment of capacitated sperm with seminal plasma or decapacitation factor. These findings led to a search for a means of removing the coating of seminal plasma components on the sperm surface that would effect capacitation in vitro. Since mouse epididymal spermatozoa have been shown to undergo capacitation in a simple medium (Toyoda et al. 1971), mouse in vitro experiments based on the assumption that capacitation involves removal of sperm-coating antigens were carried out by Oliphant and Brackett in 1973. Sperm were treated with Toyoda's medium supplemented with increasing amounts of NaCl in an effort to remove the sperm-coating antigens. This study demonstrated that increased ionic strength increased the rate of sperm capacitation. Additional protein could be washed from the epididymal sperm by further washing with a medium of high ionic strength. Moreover, additional washings eluted from epididymal sperm preparations had decapacitation activity. The sperm could be recapacitated by an additional incubation in the high-ionic-strength medium. These findings in the mouse, coupled with the previous findings in the rabbit, suggest a similar mechanism for sperm capacitation among mammalian species.

Recent work on the rabbit in our laboratory has revealed that ejaculated spermatozoa can be capacitated in vitro in media of elevated ionic strength. In brief, the procedure involves washing the sperm cells once in a pyruvate-supplemented medium used for in vitro fertilization, then incubation for 15 minutes at 38°C in the medium with increased NaCl (380 mosm/L.), followed by recentrifugation for an additional five minutes and resuspension in the defined medium. Approximately a million sperm cells are added to 4.0 ml of fertilization medium containing recently ovulated eggs recovered from the ovarian surface of superovulated rabbits. Evidence of fertilization includes sperm inside the perivitelline space, the presence of pronuclei, cleaved eggs, and normal development of two males following transfer of cleaved eggs from one of these experiments. Sperm of some bucks were found to be more easily capacitated in vitro, and day-to-day variability was also suggested in the tenacity with which ejaculated sperm from an individual buck bind seminal plasma components (Brackett and Oliphant 1975).

Subhuman primate experiments In 1973 Gould et al. reported the induction of ovulation and fertilization in vitro in the squirrel monkey (*Saimiri sciureus*). Sperm were collected by electroejaculation and suspended in TC-199 supplemented with fetal calf serum. The pH was adjusted to 7.2 with $NaHCO_3$, and an undetermined amount of follicular fluid was added with the eggs. Eggs were recovered from preovulatory follicles of PMS-treated females and suspended under mineral oil, and sperm were added. Four to six hours later, a second PMS-treated female was anesthetized, eggs were recovered and suspended in the culture medium, and sperm from the previously inseminated flask were added. Eleven of 17 mature eggs inseminated in the second flask showed some evidence of fertilization, and six eggs cleaved to two cells between 36 and 42 hours after insemination. These results suggest that the requirements for fertilization in vitro in this species are similar to those for the hamster and that capacitation occurred in vitro in the presence of biological fluids. Attempts in our laboratory to fertilize the eggs of rhesus monkeys in vitro have not been successful.

Human experiments Efforts to fertilize human eggs in vitro were reported in 1944 by Rock and Menkin, who observed cleavage of four eggs after insemination of follicular eggs cultured previously. Sporadic claims of fertilization of human eggs in vitro have been reported, but because parthenogenetic cleavage may occur in vitro, such claims have not been confirmed. Edwards et al. (1969) used a medium based on Tyrode's solution supplemented with bicarbonate and bovine serum albumin. The pH of the medium was 7.6 after equilibration with 5 percent CO_2 in air. Oocytes were recovered from ovarian follicles and cultured in droplets of medium under paraffin oil. After 38 hours, 34 of 56 oocytes had matured, as evidenced by the presence of the first

polar body. Ejaculated sperm were washed once in a medium and resuspended for insemination. Human follicular fluid was added to some samples of sperm before they were added to the oocytes. Spermatozoa were seen in the perivitelline space of five eggs, and in four of them the sperm were motile. Penetration of spermatozoa into the perivitelline space was first seen in eggs examined around seven hours after insemination, and pronuclei were observed at 11.5 hours with the possibility of polyspermy. The impression of Edwards et al. was that the preincubation of sperm with follicular fluid prior to insemination led to attachment of more sperm to the zona pellucida and to a higher incidence of penetrated and pronucleate eggs.

Subsequently Edwards et al. (1970) treated patients with human menopausal gonadotropin and hCG to induce follicular growth and egg maturation. Oocytes were recovered by aspiration of follicles 30 to 32 hours after the injection of hCG during laparoscopy, and the oocytes were suspended in droplets of follicular fluid or one of several media being tested for ability to support fertilization. Oocytes were incubated one to four hours at 37°C, then washed twice, and finally placed in sperm suspensions. Ejaculated spermatozoa were washed twice by gentle centrifugation before use, and 0.05 ml fertilization droplets were employed. The previously used medium was modified in this study by reducing the NaCl and increasing the KCl. A total of 38 eggs cleaved in culture. The blastomeres of many eggs that had cleaved normally possessed a single nucleus, as judged by phase-contrast microscopy. Edwards et al. commented on the likely role of follicular fluid in preparing sperm for capacitation and egg penetration. In addition, it was posulated that progesterone from human follicular fluid and/or synthesized by granulosa cells might play a role in the acrosome reaction.

In 1971 Seitz et al. reported the cleavage of eight human eggs following in vitro insemination with sperm incubated four to five hours in the uterus of the midcycle rhesus monkey. In these experiments, sperm were washed in calcium-free Kreb's Ringer phosphate solution twice before resuspension in Ham's F-10 medium. After incubation in the monkey uterus for various times and rewashing by centrifugation, the sperm sample was finally resuspended in Ham's F-10 supplemented with estrone and 20 percent human serum. Ovarian oocytes were cultured 24 hours prior to in vitro insemination. Since cleavage was not observed after insemination with twice-washed ejaculated sperm, incubation in the monkey uterus might have played a role for the capacitation of human sperm.

In 1971 Shettles claimed that human eggs developed to the blastocyst stage following insemination with a drop of semen together with follicular fluid, cervical mucus, and very small pieces of tubal fimbriae in a covered Petri dish. This work has not been validated, however.

In 1974 Soupart and Strong provided electron-microscopic evidence of sperm in the vitellus of human eggs. Immature oocytes were cultured for 48 hours in Ham's F-10 medium, to which sodium pyruvate and 17β-estradiol were added for the first four hours. Culture was continued for another four hours in the same medium but containing 17α-hydroxyprogesterone instead of estrogen. Insemination was carried out in Bavister's medium supplemented with heparin, penicillin, streptomycin, FSH, LH, and hCG. After equilibration with 5 percent CO_2 in air, the fertilization medium had a pH of 7.60 and a tonicity of 327 mosm/L. Sperm samples were obtained from the uppermost layer of a cylinder, diluted, and centrifuged for insemination. Final fertilization cultures consisted of a $50\,\mu l$ droplet of sperm suspension, and one oocyte was transferred to each $50\,\mu l$ of sperm suspension. This is basically the same procedure used by Edwards and by Wood in 1974, but like Hayashi and Seitz, Soupart and Strong added hormones to the medium.

In Vitro versus In Vivo
The evidence of sperm penetration through the zona pellucida either in vivo or in vitro following experimental treatment of ejaculated or epididymal sperm cannot be interpreted to mean that the physiological requirements for the process of sperm capacitation in vitro are the same as they are in vivo. A certain treatment may result in partial capacitation in vitro, with completion of the capacitation process in vivo, as probably occurred in many early experiments in the rabbit. The possibility of altering the egg to make it more easily penetrable must also be considered during in vitro fertilization. In this regard, it is also important to know that the physiological stage of the egg exposed to treated sperm is comparable to that of a normally ovulated egg. It is possible from in vitro treatments of spermatozoa, coupled with in vitro insemination of recently ovulated eggs, to gain insight into the mechanism of sperm capacitation. Removal of seminal plasma components coating the surface of the sperm cell might be effected in several ways, such as by treatment of sperm cells with high-ionic-strength medium or by treatment with enzymes.

The motility and metabolism of sperm change after capacitation. Both cAMP and phosphodiesterase inhibitors have been shown recently to increase sperm metabolism, and such factors may prove to facilitate capacitation in vitro. Certain factors found in the female reproductive tract are already known to greatly influence sperm metabolism. Among these are pyruvate and bicarbonate. Since in vitro experimentation is controllable to some extent, this approach can be considered as a reasonable guide for subsequent efforts to understand the basic physiological processes.

The definition of conditions that are favorable for gamete union in vitro is important for improving our understanding of the fertilization process, but the effects of conditions in vitro may not be comparable to the effects of similar conditions imposed on the physiological process in vivo. In the rabbit the sequence of events after sperm penetration was found to be comparable to the in vivo fertilization process when capacitated spermatozoa were used for in vitro fertilization. Since live offspring are produced from in vitro fertilized eggs of the mouse, rat, and rabbit, at least some of the eggs fertilized in vitro are completely normal and have the normal potential for subsequent development. Under certain experimental conditions, in vitro fertilization might result in embryonic development with slight phenotypic abnormality, as reported by Fraser and Dandekar (1973) for rabbits and by Toyoda and Chang (1974a) for rats. An important goal of scientists interested in fertilization in vitro is to adequately duplicate the in vivo environment and to ensure that fertilization and development are normal.

Suggestions for the Future
In vitro fertilization represents a useful research tool and a potentially practicable procedure. Studies of fertilization in vitro may well allow us to analyze more easily the factors involved in gamete union. It should be possible, eventually, to acquire sufficient knowledge of this process to develop means by which gamete union might be enhanced or inhibited. Such means can obviously be applied to infertility treatments or to contraception. Direct application of procedures for in vitro fertilization might receive widespread human medical usage in both genetics and fertility. Much more extensive animal experimentation will be required before this approach can be used in women to bypass blocked Fallopian tubes by fertilization and extracorporeal culture prior to transfer.

To this day no one has been able to achieve consistent extracorporeal fertilization with gametes of a large domestic species. Nevertheless, the application of in vitro fertilization can be expected to yield substantial improvements in animal breeding. Fertilization in vitro in cattle and other food-producing animals would provide a useful procedure for rapid dissemination of important blood lines. Moreover, the recent demonstration of normal young obtained following the transfer of frozen early embryos further stresses the importance of in vitro fertilization of cow eggs for the improvement of food production.

In vitro fertilization can be used for assessing the fertilizing capacity of individual ejaculates and for evaluating the fertilizability of eggs. More information is needed on the penetrability of eggs in various stages of maturation and also on the fertilizing ability of sperm. The present methods and procedures for in vitro fertilization are still too complicated; more standardized methods are needed for such purposes.

Accumulation of more basic knowledge is essential to any intelligent and serious attempts to inhibit sperm-egg interaction for contraception. Knowledge of sperm capacitation and the early stages of the fertilization process (the acrosome reaction, penetration through the zona pellucida, and pronuclear formation) would provide the best basis on which to develop ideal means for human contraception.

36.5 Sperm Capacitation in Some Domestic Animals (R. H. F. Hunter)

Following the discovery of the phenomenon of capacitation in laboratory mammals by Austin and by Chang in 1951, a number of studies attempted to extend this work to the domestic species, particularly the sheep, pig, and cow. Quite apart from the intrinsic value of the studies, one of the principal objectives was to obtain suitable preparations of sperm for use in experiments on in vitro fertilization. Prominent among the workers in this field were Thibault, Dauzier, Ortavant, and their colleagues at Jouy-en-Josas, France, and a series of publications summarized their experiments on capacitation and in vitro fertilization from 1956 to 1967 (e.g., Dauzier and Thibault 1956; Thibault 1959, 1967; Thibault and Dauzier 1961).

Circumstantial evidence of the need for capacitation by ram sperm is found in the 1961 study of Thibault and Dauzier, in which 3 of 51 sheep eggs were apparently fertilized in vitro when sperm were recovered from the uterus of estrous ewes. No success was obtained with freshly ejaculated sperm. The more direct approach of studying the time of fertilization after insemination has shown that ejaculated ram sperm deposited directly into the Fallopian tubes shortly after ovulation are capable of penetrating the zona pellucida within 90 minutes, as reported by Mattner in 1963. The minimum period that may elapse after natural mating until sperm penetration of sheep eggs is still unknown, however.

Systematic studies on the earlier stages of fertilization in the pig did not appear until the reports by Pitkjanen in 1955, Thibault in 1959, and Hancock in 1961. Although critical aspects of the timing of sperm penetration were not presented in Pitkjanen's work, the first evidence of fertilization recorded by Thibault was 5.75 hours after mating. In view of this interval, and because Du Mesnil du Buisson and Dauzier in 1955 had found boar spermatozoa in the upper half of the

Fallopian tubes within two hours of mating, Thibault suggested that the 5.75-hour delay might include a period of capacitation. On the other hand, Hancock saw no reason to invoke a period of capacitation for boar spermatozoa, interpreting his own observation of a 6-hour delay between mating and recovery of pronuclear eggs as the time needed for sperm to reach and penetrate the eggs. It is now clear, however, that boar spermatozoa do require capacitation and that the shortest interval for this process in vivo is 2 to 3 hours, as has been reported by Hunter and Dziuk in 1968.

Although sperm will complete capacitation after deposition directly into the Fallopian tubes of gilts or sows, recent studies have shown that the rate of capacitation is accelerated by some 2 hours if sperm are exposed sequentially to the uterine and tubal environments, as would occur after natural mating. This synergistic effect of different portions of the female reproductive tract upon the sperm cells had also been noted in the rabbit.

Several claims for in vitro fertilization of pig eggs were made by Harms and Smidt in 1970, suggesting the completion of capacitation in vitro, but this work has yet to be endorsed. In extensive studies on in vitro fertilization of pig eggs at Jouy-en-Josas a number of spontaneously activated pronuclear eggs were found, but sperm penetration of the zona pellucida was never seen.

The results with bull spermatozoa are much less precise because no chronological studies of fertilization are available, doubtless because of the difficulty in predicting the moment of ovulation. Nonetheless, since ovulation is known to occur a number of hours after the end of estrus, it may be inferred that a period of capacitation is also a requirement for bull sperm. Once again, an in vitro fertilization system would be valuable in assessing different suspensions of sperm, but no satisfactory progress has been made in attempts to fertilize cow eggs in culture. In experiments on the precocious induction of fertility, fertilized calf eggs were obtained after gonadotropic hormone treatment coupled with the intraperitoneal deposition of semen samples. This clearly suggests no absolute requirements for bull sperm to be exposed to the cervix and uterus as a preliminary to capacitation.

Further studies on capacitation and in vitro fertilization in these three domestic species will undoubtedly use samples of spermatozoa taken from the epididymis or vas deferens. Until recently, difficulty in procuring such sperm samples has retarded progress, but the technique of placing a fistula in the male tract is now well developed. Irrespective of the success obtained in such in vitro studies, it is unlikely that the process of capacitation will be accomplished more rapidly than following mating, when an integrated sequential action of the different regions of the female tract prepares the spermatozoa that will penetrate the eggs.

36.6 Recent Advances in the Study of Capacitation and Fertilization In Vitro (M. C. Chang)

Three years after the recognition of the phenomenon of sperm capacitation in 1951, Thibault and his associates reported cytological evidence for in vitro fertilization of rabbit eggs by capacitated sperm recovered from the uterus. The controversy surrounding the question of fertilization of mammalian eggs in vitro was perhaps resolved in 1959 when I obtained young developed from rabbit eggs fertilized in vitro and then transferred to recipient mothers. Yanagimachi and I were subsequently able to fertilize hamster eggs first with sperm recovered from the uterus, then in 1964 with epididymal sperm.

Further studies of in vitro fertilization in the hamster by Bavister (1969), in the mouse by Toyoda et al. (1971), and in the hamster, mouse, and rat in my laboratory from 1969, have shown that tissue fluids, such as follicular or tubal fluids or serum, are not necessary for in vitro fertilization if crystalline bovine serum albumin, sodium lactate, and sodium pyruvate are included in the culture medium. Thus the search for the substances or conditions responsible for the capacitation and fertilization of various mammalian eggs can now be analyzed in a chemically more defined situation.

The successful fertilization of mouse eggs by sperm recovered from the uterus was first reported by Whittingham in 1968, and later Iwamatsu and I were able to fertilize mouse eggs with epididymal sperm capacitated in vitro. Iwamatsu, Miyamoto, and I have determined various conditions affecting the fertilization in vitro of hamster and mouse eggs, such as osmolarity, pH value, the importance of serum albumin, and metabolic intermediates for capacitation and fertilization. We determined the importance of various conditions for fertilization, such as volume of the medium and the strain of animals providing the gametes. We also studied the fertilizability of eggs during maturation and at various times after ovulation and the fertilizability of eggs with or without follicular cells. In 1973 Toyoda, Miyamoto, and I were able to fertilize rat eggs first with uterine-capacitated and later on with treated epididymal sperm. The fertilization of rat eggs in vitro is more difficult, but fertilization appears to be normal because offspring were obtained after the transfer of such eggs into recipient mothers. Moreover, we have found that with a high ratio of K to Na and with cAMP in the medium, capacitation of rat sperm can be hastened (Toyoda and Chang 1974a,b).

Since mice and rats are very commonly used in laboratories throughout the world, we felt that this achievement was a breakthrough as a routine procedure for anyone interested in studying the mechanisms of fertilization or in evaluating the fertilizing capacity of sperm and the fertilizability of eggs. In 1974 Niwa and I were able to determine the optimal concentration of sperm and the total number of available sperm for in vitro fertilization of rat eggs.

Fertilization in vitro may differ considerably from fertilization in vivo. The most obvious difference is that in the hamster, mouse, and rat, where polyspermy is very rare when fertilization occurs in vivo but is abundant under present in vitro conditions. The number of sperm in the ampulla of each oviduct is about 45 in the rat at the time of fertilization—about 10 sperm for each egg. We have found, however, that it requires at least about 3 to 6,000 sperm for each egg under our experimental conditions. Thus the critical role played by the female tract in the selection, transportation, and capacitation of sperm can be appreciated.

Although the process of sperm capacitation is most efficient in the female tract of estrous animals, it can be achieved in vitro in many species, including humans, under experimental conditions. The capacitation of rabbit sperm in vitro appears to have been achieved by Brackett et al. (1972). For the past 20 years, fertilization of mammalian eggs in vitro has been considered a difficult task; its procedures are complicated and the results are irregular. Because of the labor of many scientists, however, in vitro fertilization of mammalian eggs can now be performed in a routine manner. The inhibition of fertilization by various means, as reported by Shivers et al. (1972), Metz (1973), and Oikawa et al. (1973), points to the possibility of control of fertilization per se. The pursuit of these studies will undoubtedly provide leads to contraceptive development. Twenty years ago our knowledge of fertilization was based mainly on the study of sea urchin eggs; now we are looking forward to a better understanding of the basic mechanisms of mammalian fertilization by an extensive use of the in vitro fertilization system.

36.7 Fertilization and Inhibition of Fertilization in Mammals (R. Yanagimachi)

Morphology and Physiology of Fertilization
Fertilization involves (1) penetration of the egg by a spermatozoon, (2) formation of the male pronucleus from a sperm nucleus and the female pronucleus from the egg nucleus, (3) growth and development of the pronuclei, (4) replacement of the pronuclei by chromosome groups, and (5) union of the two chromosome

groups. Morphological observations have shown a remarkable similarity in the basic patterns of fertilization in laboratory animals (Piko 1969; Austin 1961; Zamboni 1971) and humans, suggesting that the physiological mechanisms involved are common to most mammalian species. Although many details remain to be clarified, the outline of fertilization processes can now be summarized as follows.

When a capacitated spermatozoon approaches the egg or contacts the cumulus oophorus surrounding the egg, small perforations are produced in the acrosome wall for release of enzyme (including hyaluronidase), which enables the spermatozoon to depolymerize the matrix (hyaluronic acid complex) of the cumulus oophorus (Barros et al. 1967; Piko 1969). This structural change—the acrosome reaction—is believed to be triggered by some substance(s) or condition(s) in the oviducal fluid (secretory products of oviduct epithelium *plus* follicular fluid) and/or cumulus oophorus (Barros and Austin 1967; Piko 1969). By the time the spermatozoon reaches the zona pellucida or begins to pass through it, the spermatozoon loses its acrosomal elements except for the posterior (equatorial) segment and the inner acrosomal membrane (Yanagimachi and Noda 1970).

Lytic agents or enzymes bound to either the posterior segment of the acrosome or the inner acrosomal membrane are believed to assist the sperm passage through the zona pellucida (Piko 1969; Bedford 1970b). Once the spermatozoon passes through the zona pellucida, it quickly travels through the perivitelline space and becomes firmly attached to the vitelline surface. A process of fusion follows, involving the union of the plasma membranes of the spermatozoon and egg in such a way that the two cells come to be enclosed within the same envelope (Piko 1969; Yanagimachi and Noda 1970a; Zamboni 1971).

A series of dramatic morphological and physiological changes—activation of the egg—is provoked as the result of sperm-egg fusion. One of the first visible indications of activation is the extrusion of minute granules (cortical granules) from the egg cortex into the perivitelline space. The precise function of the cortical granules remains to be determined; it has been suggested that the material they release covers the surface of the egg plasma membrane and/or modifies the chemical characteristics of the zona pellucida, thus rendering the egg impenetrable to excess spermatozoa (Cooper and Bedford 1971; Piko 1969). Another visible indication of egg activation is the resumption of meiotic division of the egg nucleus, which ends with the formation of the second polar body. The chromosomes remaining within the egg develop into the female pronucleus. Meanwhile, the highly condensed sperm nucleus now within the egg quickly decondenses and

develops into a male pronucleus. Replication of DNA begins in both male and female pronuclei several hours after sperm entry into the egg. When the pronuclei are fully developed, they come into intimate contact in the center of the egg, the nuclear envelopes gradually disappear, and finally the chromosomes of both arrange themselves at the center of the first cleavage spindle (Longo 1973; Zamboni 1971).

Nature and roles of some structural components of the spermatozoon and egg in fertilization One of the structural components of the spermatozoon that is believed to play a central role in fertilization is the plasma membrane. Besides serving as a permeability barrier, it most likely contains the specific receptor sites that interact with complementary egg substances (Metz 1967; Piko 1969). The strong adsorption of antigenic macromolecules from the secretions of the epididymis and the accessory glands onto the sperm plasma membrane has been well established, and the belief prevails that the removal or alteration of such surface-adsorbed substances constitutes at least a part of the capacitation (Oliphant and Brackett 1973a; Piko 1969; Weinman and Williams 1964). Active studies are under way to elucidate the molecular configurations of the sperm plasma membrane, utilizing various newly developed techniques such as labeling with plant lectins (Nicolson and Yanagimachi 1972), labeling with hydrophobic fluorescent probes (Mercado and Rosado 1973), and freeze-etching or freeze-fracture (Koehler 1972).

The acrosome, one of the most characteristic sperm organelles, occurs almost universally in flagellated animal spermatozoa (Dan 1967). There is good reason to believe that its function is essentially the same in all these species: the enzymes and various other components it contains enable the spermatozoon to penetrate the outer egg envelopes and to contact the egg plasma membrane. The acrosomes of mammalian spermatozoa contain a variety of enzymes (Stambaugh 1972; Zaneveld et al. 1973), but the principal enzyme responsible for digesting the cumulus oophorus matrix is believed to be hyaluronidase, which is localized in the anterior segment of the acrosome. The zona lytic agents, if present in the spermatozoon, must be either on the inner acrosomal membrane or in the posterior (equatorial) segment of the acrosome (Bedford 1970b). A possible candidate for such lytic agents is a trypsin-like enzyme or acrosin (Stambaugh 1972).

The process by which these acrosomal enzymes (hyaluronidase, the trypsinlike enzyme, and others) are released or exposed to the outside of sperm cells to effect their lytic actions on the egg envelopes is the acrosome reaction, which involves multiple unions between the outer acrosomal membrane and the overlying sperm plasma membrane and the eventual detachment of these membranes from the sperm surface (Barros et al. 1967). The mechanisms that trigger the acrosome reaction are not fully understood. In some species (e.g., the rabbit) the reaction seems to be triggered by some specific substance (fertilizinlike?) from the cumulus oophorus or egg (Bedford 1970b). In other species (e.g., the hamster and guinea pig) the reaction can occur in the total absence of the cumulus oophorus or egg (Barros and Austin 1967), indicating that the factor(s) triggering the acrosome reaction is not restricted to these components. It is inferred that calcium ions and membrane-bound phosphatases are intimately involved in the initiation of the acrosome reaction.

The function of other structural components of the spermatozoa (excepting the nucleus) are not fully understood. For example, the postacrosomal dense lamina or postnuclear sheath, which shows a superficial similarity to septate desmosome, may be a purely structural device for maintaining firm cohesion between the plasma membrane and the nuclear envelope in this region, but it could also have roles in activating the egg or in the rapid breakdown of the surrounding membranes during sperm entry into the egg cytoplasm (Piko 1969). The sperm centriole axial filament and mitochondria, which in most mammals are all incorporated into the egg cytoplasm at fertilization (Austin 1961), are reported to undergo steady degeneration. Any direct contribution by them to embryonic development is unlikely; however, the possible participation of their components (e.g., mitochondrial DNA) in development has not been ruled out.

The cumulus oophorus (comprising granulosa cells, corona cells, and their matrix) is a barrier that the fertilizing spermatozoon must traverse before it reaches the surface of the egg. Austin (1961) suggested that the cumulus improves the chance of fertilization by providing a larger target for spermatozoa to encounter and by orienting the spermatozoa toward the egg, through the radial arrangement of the follicle cells. The presence of intact cumulus oophorus around the egg appears not to be essential for successful fertilization, but artificial removal of the cumulus oophorus from the egg often results in reduction of fertilizability of the egg (Miyamoto and Chang 1972). A claim that the cumulus oophorus is the principal component for sperm capacitation (Gwatkin et al. 1972) is difficult to accept. In vivo, it is possible that sperm capacitation is completed through the actions of the uterine and/or oviducal secretions before the spermatozoon penetrates the cumulus oophorus. The role of the cumulus could be either to trigger the acrosome reaction or to enhance the reaction of the capacitated spermatozoon.

The zona pellucida is another extracellular barrier through which the spermatozoon must pass before it reaches the egg cytoplasm. Considerable attention has been directed toward this structure, since it serves not only as mechanical protection for the fragile preimplantation embryos but also as an important site for the species- and tissue-specificity of fertilization, as well as a site of the mechanisms for preventing polyspermic fertilization (Austin 1961). The zona pellucida is a porous structure that is readily permeable to macromolecules such as albumin, peroxidase, ferritin, and even virus. Chemically it is glycoprotein or glycopeptide in nature. The presence of a considerable amount of lipid has also been reported. The zona pellucida is by no means static in its biological and biochemical characteristics. In many species the zona becomes less penetrable to spermatozoa soon after the first (fertilizing) spermatozoon has entered the egg cytoplasm—the zona reaction (Austin 1961). This is most probably due to changes in the molecular configuration of the zona pellucida caused by cortical granule material released from the egg cortex upon activation of the egg by the fertilizing spermatozoon. Gwatkin et al. (1973) have suggested that the cortical granules contain a trypsinlike proteinase that alters trypsin-sensitive sperm receptor sites on the zona surface. An increased resistance of the zona pellucida to zona-dissolving agents (e.g., proteolytic enzymes, acids, and disulfide-reducing agents) following fertilization has long been recognized, but little is known about the chemical basis of such changes.

Sperm-egg fusion and subsequent events in fertilization Morphological studies of fertilization processes utilizing light microscopy (Austin 1961) have provided the necessary background for more detailed studies employing the greater resolution achieved by electron microscopy (Longo 1973; Piko 1969; Zamboni 1971). Electron-microscopic studies have clearly shown that the initial fusion of the spermatozoon and the egg occurs between the egg plasma membrane and the plasma membrane of the sperm head. This situation in mammals is in marked contrast to that in most invertebrate species; in the latter the union between the spermatozoon and egg is initiated between the egg plasma membrane and the inner acrosomal membrane of the spermatozoon. There is experimental evidence to suggest that the characteristics of the sperm plasma membrane are modified during capacitation and/or the acrosome reaction in such a way that it becomes capable of uniting (fusing) with the egg plasma membrane (Yanagimachi and Noda 1970b). The fusion of sperm and egg plasma membranes transforms the egg from a semiquiescent state to a dynamic state characterized by a series of changes, referred to generally as activation of the egg. The physiology and biochemistry of egg activation have been studied almost exclusively in nonmammalian vertebrates and invertebrates. It is surprising that we know practically nothing of the physiology and biochemistry of the activation of mammalian eggs in view of the fact that a great amount of information on the physiology and biochemistry of preimplantation mammalian embryos has been accumulated during the past decade. The gap in this particular area is due not to a lack of interest in the problem but rather to a lack of attention by investigators.

In some species (e.g., the rabbit) the egg plasma membrane becomes incapable of uniting (fusing) with spermatozoa shortly after activation of the egg by the fertilizing spermatozoon. Apparently egg activation causes rapid physical or biochemical changes in or on the egg plasma membrane in such a way that the sperm-recognition or sperm-binding sites become inaccessible to spermatozoa. The precise chemical basis of such membrane changes is not known, but the possible involvement of N-acetyl-O-diacetylneuraminic acid residues has been suggested (Cooper and Bedford 1971). Concanavalin A binding sites (α-D-mannopyranosyl-like terminal saccharide residues) on the egg plasma membrane dramatically increase in density following fertilization of the egg.

So far little attention has been directed to the mechanism by which the sperm nucleus rapidly decondenses within the egg cytoplasm and develops into a male pronucleus. A study has suggested that in the hamster the factor(s) or substance(s) causing this decondensation (swelling) does not exist in the cytoplasm all the time. Instead it begins to appear about the time of breakdown of the germinal vesicle of ovarian oocytes, disappearing within a relatively short time after the oocyte (egg) has been penetrated by the fertilizing spermatozoon, and it reappears shortly before the first cleavage (Usui and Yanagimachi, 1976). The chemical nature of the sperm nucleus decondensation factor(s) is not known; it may be a disulfide-reducing agent or SH-rich protein (peptide) within the egg cytoplasm.

The final stage of fertilization (the development, migration, and union of male and female pronuclei, the disappearance of the nuclear envelopes, and the arrangement of the chromosomes at the center of the cleavage spindle) has been carefully studied by electron microscopy (Longo 1973; Szollosi 1965; Zamboni 1971), but the physiological and biochemical bases of these important stages of fertilization are totally unknown.

Studies of Inhibition of Fertilization

Since fertilization is a complex series of sequential events, one would expect inhibition of fertilization if any of the events or reactions involved is blocked.

Acrosomal enzymes are almost certainly involved in sperm penetration through the egg investments (cumulus oophorus and zona pellucida). The idea of blocking fertilization by inhibiting the acrosomal enzymes is not new. Pioneer workers reported a decrease in fertility following intravaginal insemination of rabbit females with spermatozoa admixed with hyaluronidase inhibitors. There is a report that ammonium aurine tricarboxylate, a hyaluronidase inhibitor, has an antifertility effect on the male rat when administrated orally. These reports, however, leave us in doubt whether the decreased fertility is actually due to inhibition of acrosomal hyaluronidase at the site of fertilization. Recent studies have shown that sperm hyaluronidase is immunologically highly species and tissue (sperm) specific, and attempts are in progress to inhibit fertilization by means of an antibody against a purified sperm hyaluronidase (Metz 1973).

Another acrosomal enzyme that has been intensively studied in the past several years is a trypsinlike proteinase often referred to as *acrosin* (Stambaugh 1972). This enzyme is capable of dissolving the zona pellucida and is believed by many workers to be responsible for zone penetration by the spermatozoon. Various trypsin inhibitors (e.g., soy bean trypsin inhibitor, trypsin inhibitor from seminal plasma, and synthetic trypsin inhibitors such as TLCK) prevent zona penetration by rabbit spermatozoa in vitro. TLCK effectively blocks fertilization when deposited in the vagina prior to the mating of animals (Zaneveld et al. 1970). The technique for purification of the trypsinlike enzyme has been advanced (Zaneveld et al. 1973), and the tissue (sperm) specificity of the enzyme has been documented, but the necessary tests for isoantigenicity and antibody inhibition of biological activity (sperm penetration of zona) have yet to be performed.

Inhibition of fertilization by isoimmunization of females with spermatozoa, semen, and even testicular tissue (extract) has long been reported. Treatment of spermatozoa with antisera produced against these antigenic materials also results in fertilization failure. It has not been clarified, however, whether such effects result from the direct action of the antibody on the fertilization process itself, from the general toxic effects of the antibody on spermatozoa, or from interference with other biological mechanisms such as sperm transport within the female genital tract. Lactic dehydrogenase-X is an interesting example of an apparently sperm-specific isoenzyme that is inhibited by antibodies of heterologous origin. Such antibodies are reported to produce pregnancy suppression following passive postcoital immunization of female rabbits (Goldberg and Lerum 1972). Here again, it is not certain at the present time whether the pregnancy-suppressing action of the antibodies results from their direct action on the fertilization process or their interference with other biological processes.

The zona pellucida of the eggs is a potential target for controlling or inhibiting fertilization. In many mammals the zona pellucida becomes impenetrable to spermatozoa soon after entry of the first (fertilizing) spermatozoon into the egg. The molecular basis of this change in the zona pellucida—the zona reaction—is yet to be determined. A recent study has suggested that cortical granule material contains a trypsinlike enzyme that alters the sperm-binding sites of the hamster zona pellucida (Gwatkin et al. 1973). Mild treatment of unfertilized hamster eggs with trypsin or chymotrypsin does render the zona pellucida completely impenetrable by spermatozoa. Treatment of the rabbit egg with neuraminidase also induces a change similar to a zona reaction. Probably any agents or conditions that alter the molecular configuration of the zona pellucida would cause alterations in its biochemical and biological characteristics. In fact, nonenzymatic agents such as plant lectins, which specifically bind to terminal saccharide residues of the zona material, are very effective agents in inducing changes similar to the zona reaction (Oikawa et al. 1973, 1974). Recent immunological studies have shown that the antibody raised against the ovary (zona pellucida) produces a strong precipitation of the zona surface that effectively prevents spermatozoa from entering (Shivers et al. 1972). The possibility of using such antibodies as antifertility vaccines is being investigated.

Prospects for Fertility Control
Every structural element of the spermatozoon and egg most probably plays a crucial role in the fertilization process at one time or another. A considerable amount of information has already been accumulated on the morphology of the structural elements of the spermatozoon and egg, but our knowledge concerning the chemical and molecular organization of these elements is still very limited. For example, the sperm plasma membrane, which plays crucial roles in sperm metabolism, capacitation, acrosome reaction, and sperm-egg fusion, has been described merely as a typical trilaminar structure. Practically nothing is known about its molecular configuration. Most probably the molecular configuration of the membrane changes drastically in response to the environment to which the spermatozoon is exposed. The egg plasma membrane, which plays important roles in egg metabolism and sperm-egg fusion, must also undergo significant physiological and biochemical changes during and after fertilization. If we learn more about the properties (physiological, biochemical, and immunological) of the sperm and egg membranes, a new means of fertility control through interference with sperm and egg physiology may emerge.

The sperm acrosome is a possible target for the development of agents or techniques for fertilization control. Any conditions or agents that specifically inhibit the acrosome reaction should effectively block fertilization. Environmental conditions (physical as well as biochemical) necessary for the acrosome reaction should be fully investigated. It has already been demonstrated that fertilization may be inhibited by acrosomal enzyme inhibitors; therefore, further intensive studies of the acrosomal enzymes and the search for highly potent enzyme inhibitors specific to the acrosomal enzymes could lead us to the development of highly effective contraceptive agents or techniques. An immunological approach to blocking fertilization by utilizing antibodies against highly purified acrosomal enzymes has shown considerable promise, and studies along this line should be encouraged.

The zona pellucida of the egg is another obvious target for attack in programs aimed at the development of contraceptive agents. An immunological approach to prevent zona penetration by spermatozoa utilizing antibodies against zona material has already shown promise, but we need more complete information on the physical and biochemical properties of the zona pellucida as well as the molecular basis for the native zona reaction in order to develop the most effective agents capable of preventing the spermatozoon from penetrating the egg.

As stated previously, fertilization is a complex series of sequential events. Agents or conditions that interfere with any of the events or interactions between the spermatozoon and egg should block fertilization and consequently cause infertility. Thus every step or event in the fertilization processes could be a potential target for the development of contraceptive agents or techniques. Studies that have already given rise to promising leads should continue, but other studies that may not have an immediate impact on fertility control should not be ignored or underestimated. New approaches to fertility control are dependent on the sound extension and balance of fundamental knowledge.

References

Aonuma, S., T. Mayumi, K. Suzuki, T. Noguchi, M. Iwai, and M. Okabe. Studies on sperm capacitation. I. The relationship between a guinea pig sperm-coating antigen and a sperm capacitation phenomenon. J. Reprod. Fertil. 35:425, 1973.

Austin, C. R. Observations on the penetration of the sperm into the mammalian egg. Aust. J. Sci. Res. B 4:581, 1951.

Austin, C. R. *The mammalian egg*. Springfield, Ill.: Charles C Thomas, 1961.

Austin, C. R., B. D. Bavister, and R. G. Edwards. Components of capacitation. In *The regulation of mammalian reproduction*, ed. S. J. Segal et al., p. 247. Springfield, Ill.: Charles C Thomas, 1973.

Barros, C., and C. R. Austin. In vitro fertilization and the sperm acrosome reaction in the hamster. J. Exp. Zool. 166:317, 1967.

Barros, C., J. M. Bedford, L. E. Franklin, and C. R. Austin. Membrane vesiculation as a feature of the mammalian acrosome reaction. J. Cell Biol. 34:C1, 1967.

Bavister, B. D. Environmental factors important for in vitro fertilization in the hamster. J. Reprod. Fertil. 18:544, 1969.

Bavister, B. D. Capacitation of Golden hamster spermatozoa during incubation in culture medium. J. Reprod. Fertil. 35:161, 1973.

Bavister, B. D., R. G. Edwards, and P. C. Steptoe. Identification of the midpiece and tail of the spermatozoon during fertilization of human eggs in vitro. J. Reprod. Fertil. 20:159, 1969.

Bedford, J. M. Limitations of the uterus in the development of the fertilizing ability (capacitation) of spermatozoa. J. Reprod. Fertil. Suppl. 8:19, 1969.

Bedford, J. M. Observations on some properties of a potent sperm-head agglutinin in the semen of a fertile rabbit. J. Reprod. Fertil. 22:193, 1970a.

Bedford, J. M. Sperm capacitation and fertilization in mammals. Biol. Reprod. Suppl. 2:128, 1970b.

Bedford, J. M. The rate of sperm passage into the cervix after coitus in the rabbit. J. Reprod. Fertil. 25:211, 1971.

Brackett, B. G., J. A. Mills, G. Oliphant, H. M. Seitz, Jr., G. G. Jeitles, Jr., and L. Mastroianni, Jr. Preliminary efforts to capacitate rabbit sperm in vitro. Int. J. Fertil. 17:86, 1972.

Brackett, B. G., and G. Oliphant. Capacitation of rabbit spermatozoa in vitro. Biol. Reprod. 12:260, 1975.

Chang, M. C. Fertilizing capacity of sperm deposited in the Fallopian tube. Nature 168:697, 1951.

Chang, M. C. A detrimental effect of seminal plasma on the fertilizing capacity of sperm. Nature 179:258, 1957.

Chang, M. C. Capacitation of rabbit spermatozoa in the uterus with special reference to the reproductive phases of the female. Endocrinology 63:619, 1958.

Chang, M. C. Fertilization of rabbit ova in vitro. Nature 184:466, 1959.

Chang, M. C. Fertilizing life of ferret sperm in the female tract. J. Exp. Zool. 158:87, 1965.

Cooper, G. W., and J. M. Bedford. Charge density change in the vitelline surface following fertilization of the rabbit egg. J. Reprod. Fertil. 25:431, 1971.

Dan, J. C. Acrosome reaction and lysins. In *Fertilization*, Vol. 1, eds. C. B. Metz and A. Monroy, p. 237. New York: Academic Press, 1967.

Dauzier, L., and C. Thibault. Quelques considérations sur la physiologie de la reproduction en rapport avec l'insémination artificielle. Proc. Third Int. Cong. Anim. Reprod., Cambridge 1:89, 1956.

Davis, B. K. Macromolecular inhibitor of fertilization in rabbit seminal plasma. Proc. Natl. Acad. Sci. USA 68:951, 1971.

Du Mesnil du Buisson,.F., and L. Dauzier. La remontée des spermatozoides du verrat dans le tractus génital de la Truie en oestrus. C. R. Soc. Biol. (Paris) 149:76, 1955.

Edwards, R. G., B. D. Bavister, and P. C. Steptoe. Early stages of fertilization in vitro of human oocytes matured in vitro. Nature 221:632, 1969.

Edwards, R. G., P. C. Steptoe, and J. M. Purdy. Fertilization and cleavage in vitro of pre-ovulatory human oocytes. Nature 227:1307, 1970.

Ericsson, R. J. Capacitation in vitro of rabbit sperm with mule eosinophils. Nature 221:568, 1969.

Ericsson, R. J., D. A. Buthala, and J. F. Norland. Fertilization of rabbit ova in vitro by sperm with adsorbed Sendai virus. Science 173:54, 1971.

Fraser, L. R., and P. V. Dandekar. The effects of aging on in vitro fertilization of rabbit eggs and subsequent embryonic development. J. Exp. Zool. 184:303, 1973.

Goldberg, E., and J. Lerum. Pregnancy suppression by an antiserum to sperm specific lactate dehydrogenase. Science 176;686, 1972.

Gould, K. G., E. M. Cline, and W. L. Williams. Observations on the induction of ovulation and fertilization in vitro in the squirrel monkey (*Saimiri sciureus*). Fertil. Steril. 24:260, 1973.

Gwatkin, R. B. L., O. F. Anderson, and C. F. Hutchinson. Capacitation of hamster spermatozoa in vitro: The role of cumulus components. J. Reprod. Fertil. 30:389, 1972.

Gwatkin, R. B. L., D. T. Williams, J. F. Hartmann, and M. Kniazuk. The zona reaction of hamster and mouse eggs: Production in vitro by a trypsin-like protease from cortical granules. J. Reprod. Fertil. 32:259, 1973.

Hamner, C. E., J. P. Jones, and N. J. Sojka. Influence of the hormonal state of the female on the fertilizing capacity of rabbit spermatozoa. Fertil. Steril. 19:137, 1968.

Hancock, J. L. Fertilization in the pig. J. Reprod. Fertil. 2:307, 1961.

Hunter, R. H. F., and P. J. Dziuk. Sperm penetration of pig eggs in relation to the timing of ovulation and insemination. J. Reprod. Fertil. 15:199, 1968.

Iwamatsu, T., and M. C. Chang. In vitro fertilization of mouse eggs in the presence of bovine follicular fluid. Nature 224:919, 1969.

Kirton, K. T., and H. D. Hafs. Sperm capacitation by uterine fluid or beta-amylase in vitro. Science 150:618, 1965.

Koehler, J. K. Human sperm head ultrastructure: A freeze-etching study. J. Ultrastruct. Res. 39:520, 1972.

Longo, F. L. Fertilization: A comparative ultrastructural review. Biol. Reprod. 9:149, 1973.

Mattner, P. E. Capacitation of rat spermatozoa and penetration of the ovine egg. Nature 199:772, 1963.

Mercado, E., and A. Rosado. Structural properties of the membrane of intact human spermatozoa: A study with fluorescent probes. Biochim. Biophys. Acta 298:639, 1973.

Metz, C. B. Gamete surface components and their role in fertilization. In *Fertilization*, Vol. 1, eds. C. B. Metz and A. Monroy, p. 163. New York: Academic Press, 1967.

Metz, C. B. Role of specific sperm antigens in fertilization. Fed. Proc. 32:2057, 1973.

Miyamoto, H., and M. C. Chang. Development of mouse eggs fertilized in vitro by epididymal spermatozoa. J. Reprod. Fert. 30:135, 1972.

Miyamoto, H., and M. C. Chang. The importance of serum albumin and metabolic intermediates for capacitation of spermatozoa and fertilization of mouse eggs in vitro. J. Reprod. Fertil. 32:193, 1973a.

Miyamoto, H., and M. C. Chang. In vitro fertilization of rat eggs. Nature 241:50, 1973b.

Nicolson, G. L., and R. Yanagimachi. Terminal saccharides on sperm plasma membranes: Identification by specific agglutinins. Science 177:276, 1972.

Niwa, K., and M. C. Chang. Optimal sperm concentration and minimal number of spermatozoa for fertilization in vitro of rat eggs. J. Reprod. Fertil. 40:471, 1974.

Ogawa, S., K. Sathoh, and H. Hashimoto. In vitro culture of rabbit ova from the single cell to the blastocyst stage. Nature 233:422, 1971.

Oikawa, T., G. L. Nicolson, and R. Yanagimachi. Inhibition of hamster fertilization by phytoagglutinins. Exp. Cell Res. 83:239, 1974.

Oikawa, T., R. Yanagimachi, and G. L. Nicolson. Wheat germ agglutinin blocks mammalian fertilization. Nature 241:256, 1973.

Oliphant, G., and B. G. Brackett. Immunological assessment of surface changes of rabbit sperm undergoing capacitation. Biol. Reprod. 9:404, 1973a.

Oliphant, G., and B. G. Brackett. Capacitation of mouse spermatozoa in media with elevated tonic strength and reversible decapacitation with epididymal extracts. Fertil. Steril. 24:948, 1973b.

Piko, L. Gamete structure and sperm entry in mammals. In *Fertilization*, Vol. 2, eds. C. B. Metz and A. Monroy, p. 325. New York: Academic Press, 1969.

Pitkjanen, I. G. Ovulation, fertilization and the first stages of embryonic development in pigs (in Russian). Izv. Akad. Nauk. SSSR [Biol.] 3:120, 1955.

Rock, J., and M. F. Menkin. In vitro fertilization and cleavage of human ovarian eggs. Science 100:105, 1944.

Seitz, H. M., G. Rocha, B. G. Brackett, and L. Mastroianni, Jr. Cleavage of human ova in vitro. Fertil. Steril. 22:255, 1971.

Shettles, L. B. Human blastocyst grown in vitro in ovulation cervical mucus. Nature 229:343, 1971.

Shivers, C. A., A. B. Dudkiewicz, L. E. Franklin, and E. N. Fussell. Inhibition of sperm-egg interaction by specific antibody. Science 178:1211, 1972.

Soupart, P. Studies on the hormonal control of rabbit sperm capacitation. J. Reprod. Fertil. Suppl. 2:49, 1967.

Soupart, P., and P. A. Strong. Ultrastructural observations on human oocytes fertilized in vitro. Fertil. Steril. 25:11, 1974.

Stambaugh, R. Acrosomal enzymes and fertilization. In *Biology of mammalian fertilization and implantation*, eds. K. S. Moghissi and E. S. E. Hafez, p. 185. Springfield, Ill.: Charles C Thomas, 1972.

Szollosi, D. Extrusion of nucleoli from pronuclei of the rat. J. Cell Biol. 25:545, 1965.

Thibault, C. Colloque sur la reproduction et l'insémination artificielle du porc. Ann. Zootech. D (Suppl.):188, 1959.

Thibault, C. A comparative analysis of fertilization and its anomalies in the ewe, cow and rabbit. Ann. Biol. Anim. Biochem. Biophys. 7:5, 1967.

Thibault, C., and L. Dauzier. Analyses des conditions de la fécondation in vitro de l'oeuf de la lapine. Ann. Biol. Anim. Biochem. Biophys. 1:277, 1961.

Toyoda, Y., and M. C. Chang. Fertilization of rat eggs in vitro by epididymal spermatozoa and the development of eggs following transfer. J. Reprod. Fertil. 36:9, 1974a.

Toyoda, Y., and M. C. Chang. Capacitation of epididymal spermatozoa in a medium with high K/Na ratio and cyclic AMP for the fertilization of rat eggs in vitro. J. Reprod. Fertil. 36:125, 1974b.

Toyoda, Y., M. Yokoyama, and T. Hosi. Studies on the fertilization of mouse eggs in vitro. I. In vitro fertilization of eggs by fresh epididymal sperm. Jap. J. Anim. Reprod. 16:147, 1971.

Usui, N., and R. Yanagimachi. Behavior of hamster sperm nuclei incorporated into eggs at various stages of maturation, fertilization, and early development. J. Ultrastruct. Res. 57:276, 1976.

Weinman, D. E., and W. L. Williams. Mechanism of capacitation of rabbit spermatozoa. Nature 203:423, 1964.

Whittingham, D. G. Fertilization of mouse eggs in vitro. Nature 220:592, 1968.

Williams, W. L. Biochemistry of capacitation of spermatozoa. In *Biology of mammalian fertilization and implantation*, eds. K. S. Moghissi and E. S. E. Hafez, p. 19. Springfield, Ill.: Charles C Thomas, 1972.

Wood, C. Treatment of tubal infertility by artificial fertilization. In *Year book of obstetrics and gynecology*, ed. J. P. Greenhill. Chicago: Year Book Medical Publishers, 1974–1975.

Yanagimachi, R. In vitro capacitation of hamster spermatozoa by follicular fluid. J. Reprod. Fertil. 18:275, 1969a.

Yanagimachi, R. In vitro acrosome reaction and capacitation of Golden hamster spermatozoa by bovine follicular fluid and its fractions. J. Exp. Zool. 170:269, 1969b.

Yanigimachi, R. In vitro capacitation of Golden hamster spermatozoa by homologous and heterologous blood sera. Biol. Reprod. 3:147, 1970.

Yanigimachi, R., and M. C. Chang. Sperm ascent through the oviduct of the hamster and rabbit in relation to the time of ovulation. J. Reprod. Fertil. 6:413, 1963.

Yanagimachi, R., and M. C. Chang. In vitro fertilization of Golden hamster ova. J. Exp. Zool. 156:361, 1964.

Yanagimachi, R., and Y. D. Noda. Ultrastructural changes in the hamster sperm head during fertilization. J. Ultrastruct. Res. 31:465, 1970a.

Yanagimachi, R., and Y. D. Noda. Physiological changes in the postnuclear cap region of mammalian spermatozoa: A necessary preliminary to the membrane fusion between sperm and egg cells. J. Ultrastruct. Res. 31:486, 1970b.

Zamboni, K. *Fine morphology of mammalian fertilization*. New York: Harper & Row, 1971.

Zaneveld, L. J. D., K. L. Polakoski, G. F. B. Schumacher. Properties of acrosomal hyaluronidase from bull spermatozoa. J. Biol. Chem. 248:564, 1973.

Zaneveld, L. J. D., R. T. Robertson, and W. L. Williams. Synthetic enzyme inhibitors as antifertility agents. FEBS Letters 11:345, 1970.

37 Sperm Motility   I. R. Gibbons

37.1 Introduction

Sperm motility is generally a result of undulatory bending waves that are propagated backward along the length of the flagellum so that a forward propulsive thrust is developed more or less along the axis of the sperm. The internal structure of the flagellum usually contains an axoneme with the familiar 9 + 2 pattern of filaments running along the length. In the primitive spermatozoa typically found in animals having external fertilization, the flagellum consists simply of this longitudinal axoneme surrounded by the cell membrane. In the more highly specialized spermatozoa characteristic of animals with internal fertilization, the flagellum has a more complex structure in which the 9 + 2 axoneme of the simple flagellum is supplemented by additional components within the cell membrane. Mammalian sperm flagella are the best-known example of the complex type: the axoneme is here supplemented by nine auxiliary fibers much larger than microtubules as well as by a fibrous sheath. Other types of complex flagella are common in spermatozoa of amphibians and insects.

Since mammalian sperm flagella appear to be specialized elaborations of the 9 + 2 axoneme, most workers studying the fundamental mechanisms of sperm motility have chosen to use primitive sperm containing the unelaborated axoneme. Sea urchin sperm have been particularly favored because they are available in large quantities and their movements are relatively constant and homogeneous. It is usually assumed that once the basic mechanism of flagellar movement has been elucidated with this simple material, it will be possible to extend the work to mammalian flagella without exceptional difficulty. Until quite recently, direct studies on mammalian sperm flagella have been confined to descriptions of their structure and pattern of movement; the experimental work essential for a full understanding has only just begun.

37.2 Primitive Sperm

In reviewing developments over the past decade, it is convenient first to consider work on the fine structure and protein composition of flagella and then to show how the knowledge from these techniques has been used to further direct studies of the mechanism of flagellar motility.

Structure

Detailed knowledge of flagellar fine structure began in 1959 with the discovery by Afzelius of accessory structures associated with the axonemal microtubules. Among the more important of these structures are the double row of projections (arms) ranged along one side of each doublet tubule, the radial connections (spokes) that join each doublet tubule to the sheath surrounding the two central tubules, and the circumferential connections (nexin links) that join adjacent doublet tubules. The packing arrangements of subunits in the walls of the flagellar tubules have been studied by optical diffractometry of electron micrographs by Amos and Klug, with results in 1974 indicating the presence of different packing arrangements in the A and B components of the doublet tubules. X-ray diffraction of isolated tubules has been attempted, but the patterns obtained have so far lacked sufficient detail to be fully interpretable.

Protein Composition

Early studies of flagellar proteins were handicapped by their apparent insolubility, and little was accomplished until 1963, when Gibbons demonstrated that this apparent insolubility resulted from enclosure of the structure by the flagellar membrane. After this membrane had been removed, the flagellar axoneme could be solubilized under mild conditions and studied by the usual techniques of protein chemistry. Two of the major axonemal proteins, tubulin and dynein, have been isolated and studied in detail, and preliminary work has been done on other protein components.

Tubulin is the principal structural protein of the flagellar tubules. The native protein is a dimer of molecular weight about 110,000, containing two similar subunits of molecular weight 55,000. Each subunit has one molecule of guanine nucleotide (GTP or GDP) associated with it. The native dimer has the characteristic property of binding tightly one molecule of the alkaloid, colchicine. The use of this affinity for colchicine as an identifying marker has permitted the isolation of tubulin from tissue culture cells, brain tissue, and other sources containing numerous cytoplasmic microtubules. Preparations of tubulin from all sources show microheterogeneity, with two major subfractions, tubulin α and tubulin β. It is probable, although not yet proved, that the native molecule is a heterodimer containing one tubulin α subunit and one tubulin β subunit. A more complex microheterogeneity may be present in preparations of tubulin from flagellar tubules, for the A and B components of the doublet tubules have different solubility properties and different packing arrangements of subunits. Preparations of soluble tubulin can be repolymerized into tubules in the presence of GTP and Mg^{++} at room temperature. The polymerization reaction is inhibited by traces of Ca^{2+} and so is usually performed in the presence of the chelating agent EGTA.

Dynein is the ATPase protein of the flagellar axoneme, and it is thought to play a major role in converting the chemical energy provided by dephosphorylation of ATP into the mechanical energy needed for flagellar movement. The dynein molecule is globular with a molecular weight of about 500,000. It contains one extremely long peptide subunit weighing 400,000 to 500,000 daltons and possibly other relatively small subunits. The size of the major dynein subunit makes it one of the longest peptide chains so far discovered. Dynein ATPase has a relatively high degree of specificity for ATP as substrate, and optimal activity is obtained with Mg^{2+} as the activating divalent cation. The variation of dynein ATPase activity with pH is sensitive to the structural position of dynein in the axoneme and changes considerably when the dynein is extracted into solution; the other enzymatic properties are little affected by solubilization. Preparations of dynein show microheterogeneity upon electrophoresis, and the different subfractions appear to be localized at different locations in the axonemal structure. Approximately two-thirds of the dynein A$_1$ and A$_2$ fractions is located in the outer and inner arms of the doublet tubules, while the remaining one-third (B fraction) may be associated with the radial spokes.

Flagellar Movement
The movements of sperm flagella can be recorded by flash photomicrography or, when necessary, by high-speed cinematography. The bending waves of sea urchin sperm flagella are easy to study because they are uniform, planar, and nearly symmetrical. Most observations have been made of sperm swimming close to the surface of a microscope slide, which prevents them from rotating and confines the flagellar bending to the plane of optical focus. Flagellar bending waves were thought to be sinusoidal, but the detailed work of Brokaw has shown that the waves can be more accurately represented as a series of circular arcs and straight lines. The departure from sinuosoidal form is most striking when the sperm are swimming against an abnormally high resistance, as in a medium of high viscosity or when the sperm head becomes stuck to the microscope slide.

The energy for sperm motility is normally provided by ATP, which diffuses down the flagellum from the mitochondria located near the base of the sperm head. In order to study the effects of varying chemical conditions on the properties of the motile apparatus, it is necessary to obtain preparations in which the selective permeability of the flagellar membrane has been destroyed. It has been known for some time that sperm in which the membrane has been rendered permeable by extraction with glycerol would regain motility if transferred to a suitable medium containing exogenous ATP; however, the usefulness of such glycerinated sperm was limited by their nonuniformity, with only 20 to 50 percent of the sperm becoming motile. A greatly improved procedure involving treatment of the flagellar membrane with the nonionic detergent Triton X-100 was developed in Gibbons's laboratory in 1967. When reactivated with ATP, the sperm demembranated with Triton become 95 to 100 percent motile and travel through the medium in a manner similar to that of live sperm. The availability of these motile demembranated sperm has made possible a number of experimental manipulations of the motile apparatus.

The rate of ATP hydrolysis by demembranated sperm under different conditions correlates with their degree of motility. Under optimal conditions 70 to 80 percent of the total ATP hydrolysis is coupled to motility. The nucleotide specificity and divalent cation requirements for reactivating bending waves resemble those for hydrolysis of ATP by the flagellar ATPase protein dynein. In suitable cases it is possible to reactivate bending waves in isolated axonemes detached from the sperm heads, thus demonstrating that the flagellar axoneme contains the complete apparatus necessary for normal motility.

The nature of the mechanical force induced in the flagellar axoneme by ATP has been studied by briefly digesting the isolated axonemes with trypsin. Subsequent addition of ATP to the trypsin-treated axonemes caused them to disintegrate into separate doublet tubules. Direct observation of this disintegration by light microscopy under dark-filled illumination has shown that it occurs principally as a result of active sliding movements that lead to the gradual extrusion of doublet tubules from the axoneme. The length after disintegration is often as much as six to eight times that of the original axoneme, indicating that sliding occurs between most or all pairs of adjacent doublet tubules. The rate at which trypsin sensitizes the axonemes to

ATP parallels the rate at which it disrupts the nexin links between adjacent doublets and the radial spokes running from the doublets to the central sheath. The dynein arms are relatively resistant to digestion and remain largely intact. These results demonstrate that the effect of ATP is to induce active sliding movements between the doublet tubules and suggest that these movements may be generated through the interaction of ATP with the dynein arms.

More direct evidence for the involvement of the dynein arms has been provided by briefly extracting demembranated sperm with 0.5 M KCl, which removes the outer arms from the doublet tubules while leaving the inner arms and other axonemal structures intact. The KCl-extracted sperm have a flagellar beat frequency only half that of control demembranated sperm, while the form of their flagellar bending waves remains unchanged. When the duration of KCl extraction is varied, the rate at which the beat frequency decreases parallels the rate of disappearance of the dynein arms. These results indicate that the beat frequency, which is equivalent under these conditions to the rate of sliding between tubules, varies in direct proportion to the number of dynein arms present.

The Mechanism of Motility
Mechanisms that have been proposed to account for flagellar movement have been of two general types: local contraction hypotheses in which bending results from a localized shortening of the tubules on one side of the flagellum and sliding filament hypotheses in which bending occurs as a result of active shearing forces between the tubules leading to localized sliding movements and the generation of a bending moment. The demonstration by Satir in 1968 that the length of ciliary tubules remains constant during bending and the observation by Summers and Gibbons in 1971 that ATP induces active sliding between the tubules in trypsin-treated flagellar axonemes have provided direct and substantial evidence favoring a mechanism of the sliding filament type, and this mechanism is now generally accepted.

It is a general characteristic of sliding filament mechanisms, in which the tubules are assumed to be inextensible and to run straight along the axoneme without twisting, that the angle of each bend in a wave will be determined by the total amount of sliding that has occurred between the tubules and on the inside and outside of the bend. For waves of a given form, the beat frequency will be proportional to the speed of sliding between tubules. The other wave parameters will be determined by the interaction of the active shearing force with the passive elastic and viscous resistances that oppose it. The theoretical mechanisms by which a balance of active and passive forces might give rise to propagated waves with the observed properties have been considered in detail by Brokaw, Lubliner and Blum, and Rikmenspoel.

When the arms on the doublet tubules were first described by Afzelius, he suggested that they might function to induce sliding movements between the tubules. This suggestion has been amply confirmed by more recent work. From the laboratory of Gibbons have come successive reports that the arms are composed of the ATPase protein, dynein, that the properties of dynein ATPase closely resemble the conditions for generating motility in demembranated flagella and for inducing active disintegration in trypsin-treated axonemes, and that the arms can be observed making cross-bridges between tubules. These reports have provided evidence that the sliding movements between tubules are generated through the interaction of the dynein arms with ATP. Particularly conclusive evidence has been provided by the recent finding that partial removal of the dynein arms causes a proportional decrease in beat frequency, indicating that the speed of sliding between tubules is proportional to the number of dynein arms present.

The details of the mechanisms by which the arms generate sliding movements remain to be determined. One possibility is that the binding and hydrolysis of ATP cause a cyclic change in the angle of the arms, which, coordinated with the repeated making and breaking of their attachment to successive binding sites along the length of the adjacent doublet tubule, results in the arms "walking" one doublet tubule along the other. Such a mechanism would be analogous to that which is thought to occur in muscle, where cyclic movements of the bridges on the myosin filaments cause sliding relative to the actin filaments.

Although the general basis of the mechanism generating the sliding movements between tubules seems to be reasonably clear, there is as yet little evidence concerning the mechanisms responsible for regulating these movements to produce propagated bending waves with the observed properties. The investigation of these regulatory mechanisms represents an area of intensive research activity at the present time.

37.3 Mammalian Sperm

Our store of knowledge concerning the mechanism of motility in mammalian sperm is far smaller than that concerning the mechanism of motility in primitive sperm. This imbalance arises from the greater structural complexity of mammalian sperm, from the considerable diversity in the pattern of movement of the sperm within a preparation, and from the difficulty in obtaining adequate quantities of fresh sperm in good condition. These difficulties have particularly tended to discourage quantitative studies of motility and studies on sperm protein composition. The work that has been accomplished tends to indicate that the basic mechanism of motility in mammalian sperm is not greatly different from that in primitive sperm.

Structure

The structure of mammalian sperm flagella has been studied particularly thoroughly in the laboratory of Fawcett. The flagella typically contains a normal 9 + 2 axoneme supplemented with nine large auxiliary fibers enclosed by a mitochondrial sheath in the proximal portion and a fibrous protein sheath in the distal portion. The whole structure is contained within the cell membrane.

Protein Composition

The composition of mammalian sperm flagella has been relatively little studied. The isolated flagella possess ATPase activity, and most of this activity can be solubilized by extraction with 0.5 M KCl; however, the solubilized ATPase protein has not yet been isolated or studied in sufficient detail to determine the extent of its resemblance to the axonemal ATPase, dynein, from simple sperm.

The only structural component isolated in pure form from mammalian sperm flagella has been the auxiliary fibers. The recent work of Price and of Bacetti and Pallini has shown that these fibers have a keratinlike structure and are composed of a major protein subunit of molecular weight about 30,000 with a high proportion of cysteine residues. The intact fiber contains a large number of intermolecular disulfide bridges. No ATPase activity has been found associated with the isolated fibers.

New techniques have recently been developed in Edelman's laboratory for separating mammalian sperm into their principal structural components (Millette et al. 1973), and it is possible that these techniques will encourage further work on chemical composition.

Movement

Gray was the first to analyze carefully the pattern of flagellar beating in mammalian sperm. He showed that the waves are largely planar in form, although a three-dimensional component appears toward the distal tip of the flagellum. The waveform is not sinuosoidal, but it can be approximated by a sine wave whose amplitude and wavelength change as the wave propagates along the flagellum.

The recent detailed studies of Rikmenspoel and coworkers have shown that the diversity of flagellar movement within a sperm preparation makes it necessary to use statistical procedures to obtain an adequate quantitative analysis of the movement. Such procedures have made it possible to show that increases in the viscosity of the medium have little effect upon the flagellar waveform, while the beat frequency decreases in approximate proportion to the square root of the viscosity.

A comparative analysis of sperm motility in several mammalian species has been made by Phillips. Three distinct forms of motile pattern were found in mouse sperm. The first type involved an asymmetrical beat that seemed to propel the sperm in circles. The second involved rotation of the sperm and appeared to allow them to maintain straight paths. In the third type of pattern, the sperm appeared to move by crawling on surfaces in a snakelike manner. This crawling pattern was observed only in sperm gathered from the female genital tract, and it is possible that it constitutes the predominant physiological pattern of movement, while the other motile patterns seen in vitro are the result of undirected flailing of sperm lacking a physiological substrate. It has not yet been possible, however, to determine how sperm actually do move in the female genital tract.

A striking variable in the sperm movement of different mammalian species is the degree of stiffness of the flagellum. In some species (e.g., mouse, human, and rabbit) the flagella appear relatively flexible and form arcs with a small radius of curvature as they beat. In other species (e.g., hamster and rat) the flagella appear very stiff when beating and always have a large radius of curvature. There is a close correlation between the apparent stiffness and the size of the auxiliary fibers. This correlation suggests that the auxiliary fibers are stiff elements that influence the form of beat by determining the elastic properties of the flagellum. The different-shaped beats in different species may be suited to specific conditions in the female reproductive tract.

Mammalian sperm obtained from the male storage organ, the epididymis, are not usually fully motile. In hamster sperm, for example, there is a marked activation of motility upon capacitation, while in mouse sperm the motility pattern of sperm obtained from the oviduct differs from that of epididymal or of freshly ejaculated sperm. Garbers et al. (1971) have demonstrated the importance of a cAMP-dependent protein phosphokinase in this activation process, but it is not yet clear whether this kinase acts directly on the motile apparatus or indirectly by influencing the sperm metabolism.

Mechanism of Movement

Present evidence suggests that the movement of mammalian sperm flagella is generated by a sliding filament mechanism similar to that found in simple axonemes. The role of the supplementary structures characteristic of mammalian sperm flagella has not yet been established.

Although it had earlier been reported that reactivated mammalian sperm were not capable of coordinated movement, more recent reports from several laboratories have indicated that propagated bending waves with progressive forward movement can be obtained with reactivated sperm of bulls, humans, and hamsters. The conditions for obtaining progressive motility appear to be more critical than that in primitive sperm, but if the proper balance of Mg^{++} and ATP is maintained, then Triton-extracted bull sperm can be reactivated to give beat frequencies and forward velocities similar to those of the live sperm. Studies by Lindemann and by Summers have shown that sliding movements of both the large auxiliary fibers and the doublet axonemal tubules are observed upon exposure to ATP after prior digestion with trypsin. It is not yet clear, however, whether all of the active force is generated by the dynein arms on the doublet tubules or whether the auxiliary fibers also play an active role in force generation.

The correlation between the flagellar stiffness and the size of the auxiliary fibers indicates that these fibers play a major role in determining the elastic properties of the flagellum, regardless of whether or not they also play an active role in force generation.

37.4 Major Gaps in Our Knowledge

There are five major gaps in our knowledge of the fundamental mechanisms of sperm motility:

1. The detailed manner by which dynein ATPase transforms the chemical energy released by hydrolysis of ATP into the mechanical energy of sliding tubules.

2. The coordination mechanisms responsible for regulating the sliding between tubules to produce propagated bending waves.

3. The nature of major protein components of mammalian sperm flagella. These proteins need to be isolated and characterized in order to determine the extent of their similarity to the proteins of simple flagella.

4. The function of the supplementary extra-axonemal structures in mammalian sperm flagella. More detailed knowledge of the chemistry of these structures will be a prerequisite to adequate understanding of their function.

5. The mechanisms responsible for changing the form of the flagellar beat as a response to differing physiological conditions. Such changes in beating pattern occur in the presence of chemotactic agents with some invertebrate sperm and upon capacitation with mammalian sperm.

References

Afzelius, B. A. Electron microscopy of the sperm tail. Results obtained with a new fixative. J. Biophys. Biochem. Cytol. 5:269, 1959.

Amos, B., and A. Klug. Arrangement of subunits in flagellar microtubules. J. Cell Sci. 14:523, 1974.

Bacetti, B., V. Pallini, and A. G. Burrini. The accessory fibers of the sperm tail. 1. Structure and chemical composition of the bull "coarse fibers." J. Submicrosc. Cytol. 5:237, 1973.

Blum, J. J., and J. Lubliner. Biophysics of flagellar motility. Ann. Rev. Biophys. Bioeng. 2:181, 1973.

Brokaw, C. J. Non-sinusoidal bending waves of sperm flagella. J. Exp. Biol. 43:155, 1965.

Brokaw, C. J. Effects of increased viscosity on the movements of some invertebrate spermatozoa. J. Exp. Biol. 45:113, 1966.

Brokaw, C. J. Bend propagation by a sliding filament model for flagella. J. Exp. Biol. 55:289, 1971.

Brokaw, C. J. Flagellar movement: A sliding filament model. Science 178:455, 1972.

Burnasheva, W. A. Properties of spermosin a contractile protein in sperm cells. Biokhimiya 23:558, 1958.

Fawcett, D. W. A comparative view of sperm ultrastructure. Biol. Reprod. (Suppl.) 2:90, 1970.

Garbers, D. L., W. D. Lust, N. L. First, and H. A. Lardy. Effects of phosphodiesterase inhibitor and cyclic nucleotides on sperm respiration and motility. Biochemistry 10:1825, 1971.

Gibbons, B. H., and I. R. Gibbons. Flagellar movement and adenosine triphosphatase activity in sea urchin sperm extracted with Triton X-100. J. Cell Biol. 54:75, 1972.

Gibbons, B. H., and I. R. Gibbons. The effect of partial extraction of dynein arms on the movement of reactivated sea urchin sperm. J. Cell Sci. 13:337, 1973.

Gibbons, I. R. Studies on the protein components of cilia from Tetrahymena pyriformis. Proc. Natl. Acad. Sci. USA 50:1002, 1963.

Gibbons, I. R. The molecular basis of flagellar motility. In Molecules and cell movement, eds. S. Inoue and R. E. Stephens, p. 207. New York: Raven Press, 1975.

Gibbons, I. R., and A. V. Grimstone. On flagellar structure in certain flagellates. J. Biophys. Biochem. Cytol. 7:697, 1960.

Gibbons, I. R., and A. J. Rowe. Dynein: A protein with ATPase activity from cilia. Science 149:424, 1965.

Gray, J. Introduction: Flagellar propulsion. In Spermatozoan motility, ed. D. W. Bishop, p. 1. Washington, D.C.: AAAS, 1962.

Lindemann, C. B., and I. R. Gibbons. Adenosine triphosphate–induced motility and sliding of filaments in mammalian sperm extracted with Triton X-100. J. Cell Biol. 65:147, 1975.

Lubliner, J., and J. J. Blum. Model of flagellar waves. J. Theor. Biol. 34:515, 1972.

Millette, C. F., P. G. Spear, W. E. Gall, and G. M. Edelman. Chemical dissection of mammalian spermatozoa. J. Cell Biol. 58:662, 1973.

Olmsted, J. B., and G. G. Borisy. Microtubules. Ann. Rev. Biochem. 42:507, 1973.

Phillips, D. Comparative analyses of mammalian sperm motility. J. Cell Biol. 53:561, 1972.

Price, J. M. Biochemical and morphological studies of the outer dense fibers of rat spermatozoa. J. Cell Biol. 59:272a, 1973.

Renaud, F. L., A. J. Rowe, and I. R. Gibbons. Some properties of the protein forming the outer fibres of cilia. J. Cell Biol. 36:79, 1968.

Rikmenspoel, R. Contractile mechanisms in flagella. Biophys. J. 11:446, 1971.

Rikmenspoel, R., A. C. Jacklett, S. E. Orris, and C. B. Lindemann. Control of bull sperm motility. Effects of viscosity, KCN and thiourea. J. Mechanochem. Cell Motil. 2:7, 1973.

Satir, P. Studies on cilia. III. Further studies on the cilium tip and a "sliding filament" model of ciliary motility. J. Cell Biol. 39:77, 1968.

Shelanski, M. L., and E. W. Taylor. Properties of the protein subunit of central-pair and outer doublet microtubules of sea urchin flagella. J. Cell Biol. 38:304, 1968.

Sleigh, M. L., ed. Cilia and flagella. New York: Academic Press, 1974.

Summers, K. E. ATP-induced sliding of microtubules in bull sperm flagella. J. Cell Biol. 60:321, 1974.

Summers, K. E., and I. R. Gibbons. Adenosine triphosphate–induced sliding of tubules in trypsin-treated flagella of sea-urchin sperm. Proc. Natl. Acad. Sci. USA 68:3092, 1971.

Summers, K. E., and I. R. Gibbons. Effects of trypsin digestion on flagellar structures and their relationship to motility. J. Cell Biol. 58:618, 1973.

Warner, F. D., and P. Satir. The structural basis of ciliary bend formation: Radial spoke positional changes accompanying microtubule sliding. J. Cell Biol. 63:35, 1974.

Weisenberg, R. C. Microtubule formation in vitro in solutions containing low calcium concentrations. Science 177:1104, 1972.

38 Regulation of Male Fertility   C. Alvin Paulsen

38.1 Male Contraceptive Development

In the past several years there has been renewed interest in developing methods for male contraception. The impetus for this activity has come from the consumer rather than from the scientific community, resulting partly from a sincere concern with possible adverse reactions associated with use of the "pill" by women, partly from a definite social trend toward a sharing of responsibility for family planning between partners, and partly from a desire expressed by many men to assume control over their own fertility.

To meet this need, funding agencies within the United States (Contraceptive Development Branch of the National Institute of Child Health and Human Development, Ford Foundation, Rockefeller Foundation) have expanded their activities to support basic research and to implement clinical trials based on available information. On a broader scale, the World Health Organization, through its expanded program, has earmarked a portion of its resources for a task force on methods for regulating male fertility.

In contrast to the situation with respect to females, where successful oral contraceptive agents are available, investigators are still searching for a satisfactory oral male contraceptive agent. Furthermore, the search for such contraceptive agents has been somewhat oblique compared to the direct approach in seeking such an agent for the female. The reasons for this are complex but in part relate to the psychology of the male. This attitude has been reflected in the decision-making of funding agencies, basic scientists, and clinical investigators. Therefore, consciously or unconsciously, much of the past work in the male, until just recently, has been directed primarily to understanding the fundamental control mechanisms involved in pituitary-hypothalmic-testicular interaction, with little attention to possible means of interfering with these mechanisms.

A widely quoted statistic has it that during one year in the early 1970s, 750,000 men submitted to bilateral vasectomy. Contrary to sporadic reports, this procedure should be considered *permanent*. It is clear, then, that alternate methods should be made available to the male that are safe, effective, and reversible. At present the condom fulfills these criteria in part, but to many men it is not acceptable for a variety of reasons.

The search for new methods has followed several pathways: use of steroids to interfere with gonadotropin secretion, agents to interfere with sperm maturation, and agents that might directly disrupt spermatogenesis.

Five major categories of compounds or agents have been evaluated in the male as positive contraceptives. These include plant extracts, antineoplastic agents, steroidal compounds, amebicides, and agents that interfere with sperm maturation.

Plant Extracts
Lithospermum ruderale has been the most extensively studied plant extract. Based on a report published in 1941 by Train, Henricks, and Archer that described the medicinal uses of plants by Indian tribes of Nevada (1), Cranston published in 1945 the first study on the effects of extracts from *Lithospermum ruderale* on the reproductive system of the rat (2). Both male and female rats received the extract and were examined in mating experiments. Extracts were also studied independently in female mice and rats and male rats. Finally, in vitro studies were carried out to further identify the antigonadotropic properties of *Lithospermum ruderale* extracts. It was concluded that this agent was antiestrous and probably worked by means of inactivating gonadotropins, since this property was demonstrated in vitro. Inhibition of ovarian and testicular function occurred following administration of such extracts orally to animals. Considerable work was carried out over the next 10 years, but interest in these extracts gradually declined, presumably due to unacceptable toxicity.

Antineoplastic Agents
Aside from their obvious role in the chemotherapy of malignant tumors, antineoplastic agents have been studied in animals for possible contraceptive properties. Although certain animal studies suggest that effective and nontoxic doses could be developed for humans, human trial studies have not been carried out. This is mainly due to a deep concern for the potential toxicity of this class of agents.

Steroidal Compounds
19-norsteroids   In the mid-1950s when interest in the 19-nor synthetic progestational agents as possible fe-

male contraceptives was rampant, these preparations were also examined for their effects in the male. Maddock, Leach, and Paulsen at Wayne State University and Heller's group at the University of Oregon Medical School carried out independent studies.

Studies in Detroit in 1955 led to the rather interesting conclusion that certain subcategories of the 19-nor compounds were inherently estrogenic. This property was easily identified in the male. Paulsen et al. (3) showed that the 19-nor compounds that possessed a 17α-ethynyl group were inherently estrogenic. In contrast, compounds such as norethandrolone (17α-ethyl-19-nortestosterone) or 17α-vinyl-19-nortestosterone were not estrogenic. Thus norethynodrel and norethindrone, being estrogenic, were unacceptable as male oral contraceptives despite the fact that they were effective in producing azoospermia.

Studies demonstrated that by the end of 4 weeks norethandrolone was capable of inducing a perceptible decrease in sperm output, and by the end of 8 to 12 weeks almost all of the men studied attained azoospermia. This compound was mildly androgenic, but this was not sufficient to maintain libido and sexual potential in the men who received it. Like all the compounds in this series, norethandrolone is a potent gonadotropin inhibitor, and it was eventually used in the treatment of men with idiopathic oligospermia and infertility. Norethandrolone was administered daily, and testosterone enanthate was administered intramuscularly every three weeks or so.

The C21-substituted progestins such as medroxyprogesterone acetate have not received appropriate attention. This is unfortunate, since the depo preparation has been used successfully in producing cessation of testosterone production in males with idiopathic precocious puberty.

Analogs of ethynyl testosterone—danazol (17α-pregn-4-en-20-yno-(2,3-d) isoxazol-17-ol) The effects of this interesting analog of ethynyl testosterone have been extensively studied since 1965 in normal adult males. When used orally, the preparation is effective in decreasing endogenous testosterone levels to those observed in normal adult females, without an attendant decrease in serum LH titers. Sherins et al. (4) concluded that this compound was an "incomplete" androgen and when administered at certain dosages had the ability to directly depress testicular function. As the dose of danazol was increased, hLH levels were suppressed. Very little change was seen in sperm production with danazol alone. This came as a surprise because of the marked depression of serum testosterone levels. The importance of normal endogenous androgen levels in supporting spermatogenesis is well recognized. In some of the men, though, there was a distinct downward trend in sperm concentration. In

light of this, Sherins and Paulsen ran preliminary studies to determine whether or not a small amount of exogenously administered testosterone in conjunction with the danazol would reverse the downward trend in sperm concentration. Just the reverse happened, however. They observed a strong synergistic action between danazol and testosterone; thus severe oligospermia was achieved when danazol, 600 mg per day, was administered orally in conjunction with testosterone propionate, 10 mg i.m. three times weekly. These data served as the basis to propose that a synergistic action exists between small doses of androgen and a progestational or an impeded androgenic compound. Each of these preparations, if administered by itself in such dosages, would not exert a depressive effect on spermatogenesis. Skoglund and Paulsen (5) published a preliminary report which established that oral danazol in conjunction with testosterone propionate or testosterone enanthate was effective in producing severe oligospermia or azoospermia. Currently, extensive studies are evaluating the effect on spermatogenesis of orally administered danazol plus methyltestosterone or intramuscularly administered testosterone enanthate.

When danazol—a weak androgen—is combined with a potent, long-acting androgen such as testosterone enanthate, a sharp reduction in sperm production occurs. Because these two compounds act synergistically in terms of gonadotropin suppression, it was possible to reduce testosterone administration to once a month while danazol was administered once a day. In one study involving about 200 volunteers, one dose combination showed 85 percent effectiveness in producing a state of temporary infertility. The time required for oligospermia to develop varied from 4 to 16 weeks. It is important to emphasize that this inhibitory process is 100 percent reversible within six months.

Cyproterone acetate Cyproterone acetate, an antiandrogen and antigonadotropin, is also being studied in the human. Animal studies have suggested that this preparation may prevent sperm maturation without altering sperm production.

Preliminary studies conducted in West Berlin and New Delhi have shown that this compound interferes with sperm production and maturation in a rather unusual manner. When administered in daily doses of 10 to 20 mg, modest oligospermia of 20 to 40 million/ml develops. Despite very little change in motility assessed by "wet-drop" methods, the sperm present in the ejaculate have lost their ability to penetrate cervical mucus. Cyproterone acetate possesses both antiandrogen and progestational properties, but in these two studies no significant or persistent decrease in libido or sexual potentia was observed. Clinical trials sponsored by the World Health Organization are being extended to Denmark, South Korea, Hong Kong, and Thailand.

Amebicides
Compounds characterized by the bis (dichloroacetyl) diamines synthesized by Surrey and Mayer (6, 7) were originally scheduled for the market as amebicides. During chronic toxicity studies, Coulston (8) demonstrated that certain of these compounds suppressed spermatogenesis in the rat, dog, and monkey, presumably by not suppressing gonadotropins. Heller, Moore, and Paulsen initiated studies in 1958 to determine the effectiveness of three of these compounds as oral contraceptive agents in normal adult male volunteers. The most potent was N,N¹-bis(dichloroacetyl)-1,8 octanediamine (WIN 18,446). In doses of 125 mg twice daily, WIN 18,446 was demonstrated to be effective in producing severe oligospermia ranging from 0.1 to 2 million per cc in a small number of men. Minor adverse reactions such as bloating and hyperperistalsis were noted by these volunteers.

More importantly, though, it was observed accidentally that men taking either of these analogs could not consume any alcohol. The reason for this was that these bis (dichloroacetyl) diamines interfered with the oxidation of ingested alcohol and resulted in increased blood levels of acetaldehyde. This produced such cardiovascular reactions as arrhythmia and tachycardia. (W. O. Nelson and J. MacLeod examined these drugs independently and drew the same conclusions as Heller and co-workers.) Later, Heller administered disulfiram (Antabuse) to normal adult male volunteers and found that this compound did not have any effect on spermatogenesis. This lent support to the idea that it should be possible to divorce the antispermatogenic property of the bis (dichloroacetyl) diamines from the antioxidative properties. Sterling-Winthrop Research Laboratories have synthesized a variety of analogs but to date have been unsuccessful in effecting such a separation of activities.

Agents That Interfere with Sperm Maturation
Spermatozoa released from the germinal epithelium do not have the ability to fertilize ova but acquire this capability during their passage through the epididymis. Efforts to interfere with this process have focused on studies using the compound α-chlorohydrin (3-chloropropane-1,2-diol). This agent is capable of inducing temporary sterility in rats, guinea pigs, and monkeys. Unfortunately, α-chlorohydrin exerts toxic effects on the bone marrow and kidney. An analog, d-1-amino, 3-chloro-2-propanol hydrochloride, was also effective in producing sterility by interfering with epididymal function. Originally it was claimed to be free of toxic effects, but later studies failed to substantiate these early

findings. Therefore the future in this line of endeavor remains uncertain.

Agents That Directly Disrupt Spermatogenesis
Since colchicine has the ability to inhibit dividing cells in metaphase and since isolated case reports showed it to induce temporary azoospermia when administered to patients with gout, it was thought that colchicine might prove useful as a male contraceptive agent. This was not the case, however, as no alteration in spermatogenesis occurred when colchicine was administered in adequate doses to normal adult males.

A recent observation with another compound, 5-thio-D-glucose, suggests another approach to the problem. Investigators have administered this compound to rats and observed a disruption of spermatogenesis. Used in doses ranging from 10 to 100 mg/kg body weight, 5-thio-D-glucose appears to be safe and effective. Currently, studies are under way in monkeys.

Summary
The short-term approach to male contraceptive development involves the use of nonestrogenic steroids that inhibit gonadotropin secretion. It should be possible by this means to achieve 90 to 100 percent effectiveness. New compounds or, alternatively, new methods of drug delivery are needed to ensure economic use and acceptability. If inhibin can be structurally identified and synthesized, this preparation would be ideal. Since it is already present in body fluids, it should be nontoxic and effective in suppressing FSH secretion, which is necessary for normal spermatogenesis. All this should be accomplished without altering the LH-testosterone axis, and thus libido and sexual potentia would not be affected.

Additional approaches await new information in terms of the basic mechanisms involved in the production, maturation, and delivery of "fertile" sperm. The future is promising, since the nucleus of trained basic science and clinical investigators has increased and the lines of research are becoming more diverse.

38.2 Male Infertility

The ability of the physician to improve testicular function when decreased spermatogenesis exists or, alternatively, to produce a state of temporary infertility when reversible male contraception is desired, represent important contemporary challenges in reproductive medicine. The pressures on the infertile male have increased for several reasons. One is that treatment is limited in effectiveness, because of our present level of understanding of the pathogenic mechanisms involved. Another is the fact that one of the former op-tions to solving the "childless" marriage problem has almost diassappeared due to the lack of available infants for adoption. Furthermore, improved methods for diagnosis have shown that the basis for at least 50 percent of infertile marriages is a defect in the male reproductive system. Although absolute data in terms of prevalence are not available, experience indicates that at least 30 men per 1,000 under age 45 have significant gonadal disorders. Unfortunately, these negative factors have not been offset by improved methods for treatment, though notable exceptions do exist.

It is important to understand the current concepts of testicular physiology in order to identify, categorize, and appropriately manage the infertile male. As previously implied, our knowledge is still limited, but significant advances have occurred in the past decade. For example, we now know that the hypothalamus sends stimulatory and inhibitory signals to the anterior pituitary that are necessary for the proper synthesis and secretion of various glycoprotein hormones. In the case of the reproductive system, the hypothalamus secretes a decapeptide hormone (LHRH). LHRH exerts a stimulatory effect on the pituitary gland to secrete LH and to a lesser extent FSH. These two gonadotropic hormones then act on the testis. LH acts primarily on the interstitial cells of the testis (Leydig cells). FSH exerts its action on the Sertoli cells. Specific biochemical processes are set into motion by these two glycoprotein hormones via the adenyl cyclase and cAMP pathway. LH stimulates the interstitial cells to produce testosterone, which in turn acts on various organs and tissues of the body to initiate pubertal development at the appropriate time and thereafter to maintain normal male sexual characteristics. In many organs of the body, testosterone behaves as a prohormone. This means that before the organ responds positively, testosterone has to be transformed intracellularly into another androgen—dihydrotestosterone (DHT)—by the enzyme system 5α-reductase. In other organs or tissues, testosterone acts directly. An example of an organ in which DHT is the active androgen is the prostate gland, while muscle and bone respond directly to testosterone.

Apart from its action on more distant cells, another important function of testosterone and DHT is to support normal spermatogenesis. This requires a high concentration of androgen within the testes (100 times that of the peripheral circulation). In lower animal species this requirement is facilitated by a protein secreted by the Sertoli cell, ABP. ABP possesses a high affinity for testosterone. This helps maintain high androgen levels within the seminiferous tubules as well as within the ductal system, particularly the head of the epididymis where spermatozoa achieve maturation.

FSH plays another essential role in overall testicular physiology: the secretion of inhibin by the seminiferous tubular compartment of the testis. Presumably the source for inhibin within this compartment is the Sertoli cell. Although the presence of this hormone was postulated some 30 years ago, not until recently was the evidence for its existence sufficiently strong to be acceptable. Inhibin has been shown to be water-soluble, nonandrogenic, nonestrogenic, and peptide in nature. With modern techniques it has been found in aqueous testicular extracts, rete testis fluid, and seminal fluid in several species, including rams, bulls, and men. Furthermore, data demonstrate that inhibin acts primarily to control FSH secretion, with uncertain action on LH. Thus its role in the feedback control of hypothalamic-pituitary function becomes apparent. Future studies should provide the necessary definition of this interaction.

With respect to the principles of feedback control, the hypothalamic-pituitary-testicular axis operates on a negative feedback mechanism common to most endocrine organs. For example, each target organ for a stimulatory hormone produces its own hormone, which acts upon the original organ system that sent out the stimulatory signal. Thus the hormone levels produced by the various target organs, such as the testis, regulate their own metabolic activity by controlling the secretion of their trophic or stimulatory hormone. This means that if the interstitial cells make less than normal amounts of testosterone because of some disorder, the pituitary-hypothalamic system "recognizes" this fact and attempts to overcome the deficiency by increasing the secretion of LHRH and LH. If the interstitial cells are not permanently damaged or absent, they respond to this extra stimulation, and testosterone levels then return to normal. Present information indicates that this feedback hormonal relationship remains abnormal. Thus elevated LH levels are required to maintain normal testosterone levels.

Based on available data, the same situation should hold true in general terms for the feedback relation between the seminiferous tubular compartment and the hypothalamic-pituitary system; that is, under normal circumstances the level of inhibin produced by the Sertoli cells should regulate FSH secretion. If the seminiferous tubules become involved in a pathological process at some point, the damage would be severe enough to impair Sertoli cell function. This would eventually lead to decreased inhibin levels, and FSH secretion would then increase to abnormally high levels.

Using the feedback premise, testicular disorders may be divided into three broad categories: (1) severe diseases of the hypothalamic-pituitary network with impaired secretion (hypogonadotropic syndromes); (2)

primary gonadal disorders with *intact* sites for control mechanisms (eugonadotropic syndromes); and (3) more severe primary gonadal disorders with impairment of one or both sites for control mechanisms (hypergonadotropic syndromes). Table 38.1 lists examples of each of these syndromes.

The majority of males complaining of infertility exhibit so-called adult seminiferous tubule failure with intact feedback control mechanisms. Serum FSH, LH, and testosterone levels are normal; hence they fall into the category of eugonadotropic syndromes. This situation should not be considered static, since these patients may have progressive testicular disease. This means that as the disorder progresses, there is increasing reduplication and biochemical alteration of the membranes that surround the seminiferous tubules (basement membranes and tunica propria). Depending on the extent of the pathology, varying degrees of fibrosis and end-stage hyalinization can be observed when a testicular biopsy specimen is observed microscopically. In some conditions the membrane systems within the interstitial spaces are also involved. Unless severe, this involvement can only be seen by electron microscopy.

As the disease progresses, at some point in time the control mechanisms become impaired. The first one involved is usually the FSH-controlling system. When this occurs, serum FSH increases. With continued damage the interstitium may become involved and testosterone levels can fall below normal adult levels. Then serum LH levels increase. One of the few exceptions to this sequence of events is the Sertoli-cell-only syndrome. Patients with this syndrome lack germinal epithelium, but the Sertoli cells remain as sole occupants of the seminiferous tubules. Usually the interstitium and the interstitial cells are normal; thus plasma testosterone and serum LH levels are normal. Despite the absence of membrane disease and the presence of morphologically normal Sertoli cells, serum FSH levels are pathologically elevated. As stated previously, this implies disturbed Sertoli cell function with presumed lowering of inhibin levels.

Diagnostic Procedures

The reader who is interested in an extensive discussion of the various laboratory procedures that are available should consult specialized journals and textbooks. A few practical comments are included here.

Serum FSH titers Improved radioimmunoassay techniques permit specific measurement of FSH. A "positive" titer should be detected in each adult male, provided adequate methods are used. If serum FSH cannot be detected, steps should be taken to identify the presence of a hypothalamic or pituitary lesion.

Normal FSH levels are frequently encountered in the infertile male with oligospermia; however, if FSH levels are normal in the presence of azoospermia, then posttesticular ductal obstruction must be considered.

Although elevated FSH titers are an indication of serious testicular damage, it is still possible to reverse the disorder with appropriate treatment.

Serum LH titers In the male under 45 years of age, the presence of elevated LH titers is invariably associated with elevated FSH levels. These findings indicate that the disorder is severe, widespread, and essentially irreversible. Moreover, the elevated LH levels reflect markedly impaired androgen production by the interstitial cells, and therefore testosterone replacement therapy should be considered.

Serum testosterone For practical purposes, serum testosterone determinations are rarely indicated, particularly if the pubertal process was normal. In certain

Table 38.1 Male Hypogonadism

Eugonadotropic syndromes

Adult seminiferous tubule failure

Hypergonadotropic syndromes

Klinefelter's syndrome
Classic form
Variant forms

"XYY" syndrome

Sertoli-cell-only syndrome

Reifenstein's syndrome

Functional prepuberal castrate syndrome

"Male" Turner's syndrome

Adult seminiferous tubule failure

Orchitis
Epidemic parotitis
Gonorrhea
Leprosy

Irradiation

Myotonia dystrophica

Adult Leydig cell failure

Hypogonadotropic syndromes

Hypogonadotropic eunuchoidism
Classic form
Variant forms

Delayed puberty

Prepuberal panhypopituitarism (Pituitary dwarfism)

Postpuberal pituitary failure
Selective pituitary failure
Panhypopituitarism

Source: From (10), p. 335.

specific conditions these determinations can be useful —for example, in the full evaluation of the patient with Klinefelter's syndrome, either the classic form or one of the variant forms associated with sex-chromosomal mosaicism.

Seminal fluid examination Impaired fertility in the male must be determined by indirect means. The reason for this is that there are no methods to assess the fertilizing capacity of human sperm.

The best alternative is to examine the seminal fluid and determine the sperm concentration. Since infertile males normally ejaculate sufficient seminal fluid, the conventional means of recording sperm production is to list the number of sperm per ml seminal fluid. Fertility is a relative phenomenon that depends on three known factors (sperm motility, morphology, and numbers) and an indeterminate number of unknown factors.

Proper evaluation of the infertile male dictates examination of at least four to six seminal fluid specimens, since there is considerable variation within an individual. If the sperm morphology and motility are normal, a male should not be considered to have a testicular problem unless the sperm concentration is consistently below 20 million/ml.

Two additional points involving seminal fluid examinations require attention. These are collection and sperm morphology. The only satisfactory way to obtain seminal fluid is to have the patient masturbate into a clean glass container and then submit the fresh specimen for examination within an hour. Condom sheaths should not be used, since sperm motility decreases markedly upon contact with most types of condoms. Interrupted coitus as a means of collecting the seminal fluid is also unsatisfactory, since the initial portion of the ejaculate, which contains the highest density of sperm, may be lost.

The importance of assessing sperm morphology should not be overlooked—for example, the relationship between an increase in tapered forms and a varicocele that exists in some infertile men. Briefly, the seminal fluid smear is prepared similarly to a blood smear. After the slide is air-dried, the smear is stained with a combination of Bryan's sperm stain and Leishman's stain. For normal males, the percentage distribution of the various sperm shapes is as follows: oval = 73, large = 2.7, small = 8.6, taper = 6.1, amorphous = 8.6, duplicate = 1.0, and immature < 0.5. These values are based on the classification of MacLeod. In addition, it is necessary to differentiate the immature germ cells from any white blood cells that may be present in the seminal fluid. If the latter are present, an unsuspected infection of the genital tract may exist and require treatment.

Testicular Disorders

Two examples of testicular disorders are varicocele and nonsymptomatic genitourinary tract infections. Of all types of male infertility the proper management of varicocele leads to the best therapeutic results. In the case of nonsymptomatic infections, the clinician has to be alert because of the low frequency of and the confusion about this condition. Furthermore, patients are not usually checked for this possibility.

Varicocele Varicocele afflicts approximately 10 percent of the male population. Not all of these men are infertile, but in a population of infertile males the incidence of varicocele may be as high as 40 percent. The reason why some men with varicocele have abnormal spermatogenesis and decreased sperm production and others do not is not clear, although many hypotheses have been suggested. The presence of a varicocele permits both testes to be exposed to venous blood that is flowing in a retrograde fashion; in an undetermined manner this disrupts the later stages of spermatogenesis in certain men.

Several years ago MacLeod characterized the abnormal seminal fluid findings in patients with varicocele. Its abnormal characteristics include an increase in tapered and amorphous spermatozoa. Furthermore, greater numbers of immature germ cell forms such as spermatocytes and spermatids are in the ejaculate. Usually these men have oligospermia, and their sperm motility is impaired. Following ligation of the abnormal spermatic and cremasteric veins there is improvement in the seminal fluid findings in approximately 50 to 80 percent of the men. Achievement of normal fertility occurs in approximately 45 percent. It has not been possible to determine in advance which patients will respond to this surgical procedure.

In our experience over the past several years, the patients referred to the Division of Endocrinology for evaluation of varicocele and infertility had been infertile for an average of 42 months. Following surgery, conception occurred with 47 percent of the patients, and the time interval for impregnation to occur ranged from 5 to 15 months after ligation. In monitoring the postsurgical period we found that at least one and usually more than one of the seminal fluid abnormalities had to improve before the chances of achieving fertility became good.

There are many questions with respect to varicocele that require answers. For example, what are the specific biochemical or physicochemical abnormalities present in the spermatozoa in these patients? We know that the number of normal oval-shaped spermatozoa may be only slightly decreased, and "wet-drop" examination of the seminal fluid may reveal fairly good progressive motility, yet these spermatozoa do not penetrate midovulatory cervical mucus (as assessed by the in vitro Kremer test). We have speculated that there may be some alteration in surface properties of the sperm (e.g., in the electrical charge) that prevents normal penetration of female genital tract fluids. Clearly, more investigation is required.

Genitourinary tract infections The relation between genitourinary tract infections and infertility is poorly understood and commonly overlooked. In some countries where venereal diseases are neglected in the early stages or where tuberculosis is still prevalent, genitourinary tract infections are responsible for a large proportion of infertility. Elsewhere the emphasis should be placed on the role of nonsymptomatic infections and the individual impact of the various organisms that might be involved; for example, T. mycoplasma, herpesvirus hominis, cytomegalovirus, and various gram negative organisms have been considered as likely etiologic agents. In an attempt to clarify the issue we compared seminal fluid findings in 22 fertile men whose wives were pregnant in the first trimester with the seminal fluid findings in 21 infertile men whose wives were not pregnant. These studies were performed in collaboration with King Holmes and Ross Alexander. None of the men in either group was symptomatic in terms of genitourinary tract infection. All urine, semen, and expressed prostatic secretion (EPS) samples from each of the men were quantitatively cultured for aerobic bacteria. Additional microbiological studies included cultures of the semen and EPS for mycoplasma hominis, T. mycoplasma, chlamydia trachomatis, cytomegalovirus, and herpesvirus hominis. Also, the seminal fluid specimens from both groups were examined for volume, sperm concentration, motility, agglutination, morphology, and leukocytes. Improved staining techniques were developed to differentiate the white blood cells from the immature germ cells present in the ejaculate (11).

T. mycoplasma was recovered from the EPS or semen of 12 fertile and 7 infertile men. Treatments of these men and their sexual partners with doxycycline was followed by eradication of the mycoplasma infection in each individual, but no improvement in the seminal fluid findings occurred in the infertile men, nor was the seminal fluid leukocyte count reduced in either group. Furthermore, the seminal fluid findings of the fertile men were entirely normal before treatment. Cytomegalovirus was recovered from four men in the fertile group and one in the infertile group. These findings are of interest due to the opinion of some investigators that these organisms have a serious impact on human reproductive function.

In contrast to the above observations, significant bacterial infection was found in three infertile men. Treatments cleared the infection in two, and the semi-nal fluid findings improved markedly. For example, in one patient *S. epidermidis* was present in a concentration of 105 colonies per ml seminal fluid. Cephalaxine treatment reduced the colony count to insignificant levels, and the sperm concentration rose from 7.8×10^6/ml to 37×10^6/ml. Moreover, the number of immature germ cells decreased from 24 percent to 7 percent. In another patient, *E. coli* (4×10^3/ml) was recovered from the seminal fluid and the postprostatic massage urine specimens. Before treatment, the seminal sperm concentration was 0.8×10^6/ml with 80 percent of the sperm agglutinated. Also, 33 percent immature forms were found. Following treatment, sperm agglutination disappeared, and the sperm concentration increased to 22×10^6/ml, while the immature forms dropped to 9 percent.

These examples emphasize the importance of detecting and treating the small number of patients with such infections. One of the intriguing aspects of this problem is the finding of immature germ cells in ejaculate without evidence of orchitis. This indicates an unknown relationship between the accessory glands (e.g., prostate and seminal vesicles) and the germinal epithelium of the testis.

Reviews

Diczfalusy, E., ed. Immunoassay of gonadotrophins. Acta Endocrinol. 63(Suppl.):142, 1969.

Lipsett, M. B., and R. Sherins. The testis. In *Duncan's diseases of metabolism*, 7th ed., eds. P. K. Bondy and L. Rosenberg. Philadelphia: W. B. Saunders, 1974.

Lipsett, M. B., H. Wilson, et al. Studies on Leydig cell pathology: Secretion and metabolism of testosterone. Recent Prog. Horm. Res. 22:245, 1961.

Midgley, A. R., Jr. Radioimmunoassay: A method for human chorionic gonadotropin and human luteinizing hormone. Endocrinology 79:10, 1966.

Midgley, A. R., Jr. Radioimmunoassay for human follicle stimulating hormone. J. Clin. Endocrinol. Metab. 27:295, 1967.

Nieschlag, E., and D. L. Loriaux. Radioimmunoassay for plasma testosterone. Z. Klin. Chem. Klin. Biochem. 4:164, 1972.

Paulsen, C. A., and J. M. Leonard. Clinical trials in reversible male contraception. I. Combination of danazol plus testosterone. In *Regulatory mechanisms of male reproductive physiology*, eds. C. H. Spilman, T. J. Lobl, and K. T. Kitron, p. 197. New York: American Elsevier, 1976.

Santen, R. J., J. M. Leonard, et al. Short- and long-term effects of clomiphene citrate on the male pituitary-testicular axis. J. Clin. Endocrinol. Metab. 33:970, 1971.

References

1. Train, P., J. R. Hendricks, and W. A. Archer. Medical uses of plants by Indian tribes of Nevada. Washington, D.C.: U.S. Department of Agriculture, Bureau of Plant Industry, Division of Plant Exploration and Introduction, part 2, p. 102, December 1941.

2. Cranston, E. M. The effect of *Lithospermum ruderale* on the estrous cycle of mice. J. Pharmacol. 83:130, 1945.

3. Paulsen, C. A., R. B. Leach, J. Lanman, N. Goldston, W. O. Maddock, and C. G. Heller. Inherent estrogenicity of norethindrone and norethynodrel: Comparison with other synthetic progestins and progesterone. J. Clin. Endocrinol. 22:1033, 1962.

4. Sherins, R. J., H. M. Gandy, T. W. Thorslund, and C. A. Paulsen. Pituitary and testicular function studies. I. Experience with a new gonadal inhibitor, 17-a-pregn-4-en-20-yno (2,3-d) isoxazol-17-ol (Danazol). J. Clin. Endocrinol. 32:522, 1973.

5. Skoglund, R. D., and C. A. Paulsen. Danazol-testosterone combination: A potentially effective means for reversible male contraception. A preliminary report. Contraception 7: 357, 1973.

6. Surrey, A. R., and J. R. Mayer. New amebicides. VI. The preparation of some N,N' disubstituted-N,N'-bis (haloacyl)-polymethylenediamines. J. Med. Pharm. Chem. 3:409, 1961.

7. Surrey, A. R., and J. R. Mayer. The preparation and biological activity of some N,N'-bis (haloacyl)-polymethylene-diamines. J. Med. Pharm. Chem. 3:419, 1961.

8. Coulston, F., A. L. Beyler, and H. P. Drobeck. The biologic actions of a new series of bis(dichloroacetyl) diamines. Toxicol. Appl. Pharmacol. 2:715, 1960.

9. Heller, C. G., D. J. Moore, and C. A. Paulsen. Suppression of spermatogenesis and chronic toxicity in men by a new series of bis-(dichloroacetyl) diamines. Toxicol. Appl. Pharmacol. 3:1, 1961.

10. Paulsen, C. A. The testes. In *Endocrinology*, 5th ed., ed. R. H. Williams. Philadelphia: W. B. Saunders, 1974.

11. Couture, M., M. Ulstein, J. M. Leonard, and C. A. Paulsen. Improved staining methods for differentiating immature germ cells from white blood cells in human seminal fluid. Andrologia 8:61, 1976.

39 Assessment of Clinical Testing Methodology

Aníbal Faúndes and Ellen Hardy

Clinical trials are the last link in a long chain of efforts aimed at the development of new therapeutic or prophylactic methods. They constitute a critical assessment of efficacy and safety in humans. Incompetent or inadequate clinical trials may result in unwarranted exposure of the public to toxic effects and to inadequate protection, especially in instances where suitable alternative regimens are already available. Conversely, they can result in rejection of superior methods that could yield a much higher level of safety and effectiveness.

Those who conduct clinical trials have a responsibility to society to conduct the most meaningful tests possible of effectiveness and risks of new therapies. At the same time they have a responsibility to the individual patient not to expose him or her to hazards inconsistent with potential benefits. The clinical testing of contraceptive methods bears a special burden, because any given pregnancy usually represents only a minimum threat to the life and well-being of the mother. At the same time effective contraceptive methods are of the highest importance to the general well-being of mankind. Because of these considerations, efforts to improve the quality of the methodology used in clinical trials of contraceptive methods are of prime importance.

Some investigators and institutions have attempted to meet this challenge to improve and unify procedures—for example, in research design (5, 51, 53, 54, 55, 69, 121, 161, 162) and data analysis (6, 113, 114, 165, 166, 169)—but continued need for improved methods and for greater standardization of methodology is abundantly apparent.

39.1 Evaluation of Data Analysis Procedures

Estimation of Event Rates
Present status Early trials of new contraceptives reported results simply in terms of the percentage of users who became pregnant during the period of study, without considering the number of months each women was exposed to the risk of pregnancy. The next step in sophistication was to calculate the Pearl Index rate, in which the total number of accidental pregnancies is divided by the total number of months of contraceptive use and multiplied by 1,200 (or, in some instances,

1,300) to give the number of pregnancies per 100 woman-years of exposure.

As early as 1960 the importance of the length of the observation period as a factor affecting pregnancy rates was recognized (112). It is a common observation that the Pearl Index pregnancy rate becomes lower the longer a group of contraceptors is followed. This is because the women of higher fecundity and higher incidence of exposure are especially likely to become pregnant and thus be eliminated from the study in the earlier months, leaving behind a group of women with lower fecundity. To overcome this problem, the use of the life tables was proposed (113, 114, 165, 166). In this method, the pregnancy rate is calculated for each ordinal month of use. Cumulative rates can be calculated from monthly rates for any desired interval of experience. Life tables were first used in clinical trials of contraceptives for estimation of pregnancy rates, but they can obviously be used equally well to determine the rate of occurrence of any other event being observed in the trial. Because life tables were first used to analyze the results of clinical trials of intrauterine devices and because Tietze's paper (166) on their application to IUD trials received such wide dissemination, many investigators mistakenly concluded that this approach was appropriate only for IUD studies. An incomplete review of recent publications of clinical studies of new contraceptives revealed that 33 of 53 IUD studies utilized life tables, but only 7 of 100 clinical studies of other contraceptive methods did so.
Recommendations Life tables should be used to analyze data from clinical studies of all new fertility control methods, and they should be applied to all estimates of rates of occurrence of discrete events in such trials.

Criteria for Classification of Events
Considerable ambiguity in interpreting the results of clinical trials of contraceptives arises from the different definitions of events used by different investigators. This serious problem is often further compounded by the failure of investigators to specify the definitions they have employed.
Nonreturnees: Present status Some studies do not include as part of the study population women who make an initial visit to the clinic with the intention of

initiating a method, but who fail to return. Some of these women begin using the method and then later discontinue its use but never return to the clinic to report this fact. Others never initiate use because of some characteristic of the contraceptive. For instance, a neighbor may have told the prospective user that the method produces cancer or thromboembolism, or she may have lost or misplaced the dosage form. All such reasons are related to the characteristics of a method and hence should be accounted for in the study's data collection and analysis procedures. These problems arise less in studies of methods initiated by the physician, such as IUDs, injectables, and implants.

Recommendations When continuation of use of a method is being evaluated, all subjects who accept and are provided with the method should be included in the study. This includes even those who never return to the clinic or ultimately fail to initiate use for whatever reason.

Categories of terminations: Present status The literature indicates general agreement that terminations be classified into the following categories: pregnancies, terminations for medical reasons, terminations for personal reasons, terminations at the investigator's choice, release from study, and subjects lost to follow-up. Subcategories are sometimes introduced. In the case of IUDs, there is the additional category of expulsions. The problems lie with the varying and frequently unnoted definition of the categories (2, 11, 29, 37, 45, 94, 181). The definition of *personal* and *medical* reasons for terminations is an example. Many physicians classify the reason for termination as *personal* if the symptom or side effect, in their judgment, is not attributable to the contraceptive. Other physicians might judge that the same symptom could have been caused by the method and so classify it as a medical reason for discontinuing use.

Problems also arise when additional, nonexclusive categories are added to those noted above. The category "change of method" is sometimes added, but it fails to take into account the important question of why the method was changed (144). Answering this question will place the subject in one of the standard classes of terminators.

The practice of excluding from rate calculations women who discontinue for nonrelevant reasons—as recommended by Tietze (166, 167)—is generally accepted with few exceptions (60). Problems are minimized if the exclusions are limited to the categories of terminations resulting from the investigator's choice and release from the study, as recommended and defined by Tietze (166, 167).

In the analysis, the mode of handling subjects who have been lost to follow-up represents a difficult problem in that the logical procedure varies with the contraceptive method being tested. This category is used for subjects who do not return within a specified time after a scheduled visit and whose reaction to the method therefore remains unknown. In the instance of methods such as long-acting injectables or implants that cannot be discontinued at the will of the subject, it is logical to treat subjects who are lost to follow-up as nonrelevant terminations until the end of the estimated period of effectiveness and relevant from that time on. At the other extreme, in the instance of contraceptives that require a new supply or prescription at each visit, it is logical to assume that the subject discontinued use on the day the prescription or supply ran out (178). Since the women chose not to return for a new supply at the time of loss of protection, the case must be considered a relevant discontinuation. Judgement is harder to make when the contraceptive is commercially available and when the socioeconomic level of the study population is such that they can replenish their supplies themselves.

Such methods as the IUD require the physician's intervention either for discontinuation or for continued use. In such instances, it is logical to wait three or even six months before making an assessment. One is then left with possibilities ranging from all patients having continued uneventful use to all patients having discontinued after pregnancy or for other relevant reasons. It is then logical to reach the compromise of assuming the intermediate possibilities recommended by Tietze, that is, to treat subjects lost to follow-up as nonrelevant discontinuations.

Recommendations The classification of terminations should be restricted to the following categories: pregnancies, termination for medical reasons, termination for personal reasons, termination at the investigator's choice, release from the study, and subjects lost to follow-up. Subcategories within these classifications should be exclusive of the standard categories and should be fully defined.

Medical reasons for termination should include all terminations resulting from health or physical complaints by the wife or husband attributed to the methods, whether or not considered relevant by the investigator.

"Change to another method" should not be listed as a reason for closure; rather, the reasons for the change should be stated and classified under one of the accepted categories.

Exclusion of women who discontinue for nonrelevant reasons should be confined to "terminations at the investigator's choice" and "release from study."

If continuation of a contraceptive requires a new supply or prescription at each visit, terminations prior to return for a new supply should be treated as a relevant discontinuation. In the case of methods that require a physician's intervention to discontinue, subjects lost to follow-up should be treated as nonrelevant discontinuations until the end of the estimated period of effectiveness and relevant from that date on. In the instance of methods that can be either continued or discontinued by the subject without the physician's intervention, it is better to perform a double computation using the alternatives of treating subjects lost to follow-up as relevant and nonrelevant discontinuations (114).

Patient failure and method failure: Present status
Since improper use of a method—such as the omission of a pill or the application of foam too far in advance of coitus—obviously affects a method's performance level adversely, there is a strong temptation to eliminate from calculations events associated with such lapses. The legitimacy of doing so depends upon whether one is trying to assess the potential biological effectiveness of the method or the effectiveness under conditions of actual use. The effectiveness under conditions of actual use will properly include failures related to the sociocultural environment and the psychological behavior of the users. Separation of patient failures from method failures will be subject to quite different criteria in the hands of different investigators. Some will attribute the failures to the subject at the slightest suspicion of deviation from instructions, while others will classify all pregnancies as method failures unless the user had grossly and demonstrably misused the method.

Recommendations Investigators should always report total pregnancy rates. Such rates may be further classified into patient and method failures if a full description of the criteria used for such a classification is presented.

Time Units of Observation
Present status A partial review of the literature showed that nearly 60 percent of the papers reviewed used calendar months as the time unit of analysis. Almost 40 percent used the menstrual cycle as the time unit. Lunar months (28 days) and 30-day months were infrequently used as well. The use of the menstrual cycle as the time unit has biological support, since there is one risk of pregnancy for each individual cycle. In the case of the pill, the use of the cycle is further reinforced by the fact that the treatment itself produces cycles and the number of cycles coincides exactly with the number of prescription units or packages provided to the woman. But when such hormonal contraceptives as long-acting injectables, minipills, or subdermal implants have been tested, cyclic menstrual regularity

is lost; bleeding becomes erratic and the definition of the cycle is left to the criteria of the physician or to the woman herself. Cycle length varies from 15 to 45 or more days. As a result, the tenth ordinal cycle may be the sixth month of use for a subject with polymenorrhea and the thirteenth month for a woman experiencing oligomenorrhea. The use of the calendar month as the unit of time makes analysis feasible in such instances, and the comparison of cases along a time scale will be in error by only a few days.

Recommendation The use of the menstrual cycles as a time unit should be strongly discouraged. Calendar months should be employed as the time unit for analyses of data in the evaluation of all types of contraceptive methods.

Confidence Limits
Present status In order to make the most meaningful comparisons between the performance of methods in different populations or the performance of different methods in the same population, it is necessary that the variability of measurement be known. This is best expressed by indicating upper and lower confidence limits. A partial survey of the literature indicated that in roughly one-tenth of all studies reviewed, the data was analyzed in such a way that the confidence limits could be established and the statistical significance of differences between groups could be evaluated (19, 36, 40, 50, 55, 77, 107, 116, 134, 137, 147, 159, 168). An additional one-fifth of the studies calculated averages and reported ranges. The great majority gave only absolute numbers and percentages of pregnancies and other events. It is noteworthy that some authors provide measurements of statistical significance for their basic research data but do not do the same for their clinical data.

Recommendation Clinical studies should report confidence limits in all possible instances.

Definition of Study Populations
Present status Comparable studies of contraceptive methods generally give very different results in different investigations (185) because the populations studied are of different ages and parity, have different exposure to coitus, or differ in more subtle ways, such as nutritional status (8, 34, 66, 78, 104, 108, 109, 128, 130, 133, 149, 150, 171, 179, 183, 192).

Recommendations If studies are to be easily compared and interpreted, it is essential that the demographic characteristics of the population be described. At a minimum, this should include the age and parity distribution.

39.2 Evaluation of the Role of Research Design

Protocols for Clinical Studies

Present status Many clinical trials have begun without adequate examination of objectives and without sufficient attention to the design necessary to meet the objectives. Inadequate consideration has been given to the number of subjects that will be required to answer the principal questions of the study with acceptable confidence and to the factors that may confuse interpretation of the results.

Typically, research design has been limited to a decision about which data will be registered and evaluated, how frequently women will be examined, the day(s) of the menstrual period on which the method must be initiated, the dosage and schedule of treatment when applicable, sometimes the minimum number of women to enter the study, and the length of the observation period. But even this minimal design is not fully followed in many instances. In some published studies, drugs, devices, dosages, and schedules are mixed and evaluated as a unit without a previous demonstration that those changes do not significantly affect performance (71, 82, 84). Criteria to enter the study such as age, previous fertility, previous use of contraceptives, time postpartum or postabortion, and present lactation are very seldom stated (131, 145, 152, 174, 189).

Recommendations Before clinical studies are begun, the objectives should be carefully set forth and assigned priorities. The design should be reviewed with statisticians, who can advise on design and on factors necessary to meet the minimum objectives, as well as with medical peers, who can aid in identifying the pertinent medical factors that should be studied to provide adequate data on safety and side effects and a correct interpretation of the findings.

Selection of Subjects

Present status Frequently women of unproved fertility, women with little or no sexual contact, and women over 45 are included in clinical tests of contraceptives and given the same weight as other subjects (63, 85, 106). Even if such extremes are avoided, supposedly equivalent groups may vary greatly in identifiable factors that dispose to pregnancy or side effects. One evident solution to this problem is to break the total group into more homogeneous subgroups in the final analysis of the data. As one method of facilitating comparison between studies, Reinke and Baker (122) have proposed a *multisort technique*. This technique adjusts for the distortion deriving from the fact that certain subgroups defined by age, parity, marital status, or socioeconomic level have higher or lower rates of pregnancy or other events. The method gives appropriate weights for each group in accordance with the percentage of that group in the study population (60, 122).

Recommendations Research protocols should carefully define the criteria used for accepting subjects into the study in light of the objectives of the study. Subjects should be described in terms of age, parity, marital status, socioeconomic level, and other factors bearing on performance, and the final data analysis should define changes in event rates associated with these variables.

Comparisons between Methods

Present status An ultimate objective of most studies is to determine whether a given method performs better or worse than alternative methods and in what respect. Seldom is there reason to ask whether a contraceptive method gives greater protection against pregnancy than would no method at all. There are, however, frequent questions as to how many of the side effects would be observed even if placebos were given. Much as one would wish to know the answer to these questions, there is seldom ethical justification in administering placebos to patients desiring protection against pregnancy. Comparisons between methods of similar appearance can, however, frequently be conducted on a randomized, double-blind assignment basis (50, 53, 54). This obviously allows much more meaningful comparisons than do comparisons with studies on other methods conducted at other sites or at other times at the same site.

Sometimes, of course, the differences between methods are so obvious that a randomized double-blind study is impossible. This is the case for comparison of a mechanical device with a drug or sometimes even for comparisons between different mechanical devices or for comparisons between materials given on widely different dosage schedules (62, 92, 101, 111, 127, 176, 177).

The comparison of the performance of groups studied at different times is particularly questionable (44). Changes in general knowledge, in attitudes toward contraception, and in the availability of alternative methods are occurring so rapidly that a comparison of two studies conducted a few years apart can be quite misleading.

As discussed above, collaborative studies in which the experience at several different sites is summed together provide measures of effectiveness and side effects over a wider range of patient characteristics and of investigator bias than does any single study. Such studies therefore give a better picture of what is to be expected in general use than does a study at a single site.

Recommendations Wherever possible, randomized double-blind studies should be used as a basis for comparing contraceptive methods. Where this is not possible, every effort should be made to run comparisons under circumstances as parallel as possible. Comparisons between groups studied several years apart should be viewed with skepticism. Multi-investigator, multisite collaborative studies are especially useful in predicting performance under conditions of actual use.

Comparison between Physicians versus Paramedical Prescription of Methods or Insertion of IUDs
Present status There is clear need for transferring a larger proportion of family planning responsibilities from physicians to paramedical personnel. Several publications describe comparative studies of the prescription of pills or insertion of IUDs by physicians versus paramedical personnel (110, 132). Nevertheless, at least in some cases, the comparison may be seriously biased, because the more difficult or complicated cases and borderline indications are referred to the physicians.

Recommendations The continuation of use and side effects observed in women using contraceptives prescribed or inserted by auxiliary personnel should be compared with similar groups of users under physicians' care. Attention should be given, in such studies, to avoiding introduction of bias by reason of referral of difficult or complicated cases from paramedics to physicians.

Follow-Up of Subjects
Present status The loss of large numbers of subjects who fail to return for follow-up visits renders the interpretation of any study uncertain (170). Even the number and percentage of such patients is rarely mentioned.

Recommendations Telephone, mail, mass media, or even home visits should be utilized to try to keep the number of those lost to follow-up under 10 percent of the patients entering the study (one-year duration), and the percentage of such lost patients should always be mentioned.

39.3 Some Specific Problems in Contraceptive Method Evaluation

Evaluation of Subjective Side Effects
Present status The evaluation of side effects that can be objectively measured gives rise to the relatively simple problems of assuring standard procedures and measurements (105). Subjective side effects are very much more difficult to evaluate quantitatively, and, accordingly, they give rise to more complex problems. One alternative is to present the woman with a detailed questionnaire in which she is asked if she has had any of the listed complaints; another is simply to record the side effects reported spontaneously by the subject. There is no doubt that the checklist approach yields a higher incidence of side effects than results from spontaneous reporting (1, 38, 51, 59). The difficulty is that the significance of side effects listed on the checksheet becomes most difficult to evaluate. In one study of side effects associated with placebos (121), placebo pills "caused" a 30 percent decrease in libido and a 16 percent incidence of headaches. It is, of course, also true that without a checksheet women are likely to forget the less impressive problems they had some days, weeks, or months before.

The second problem is the change of frequency of some side effects with time of use. It is often reported that a complaint is found in a high proportion of users in the first month but that it decreases in frequency as time passes (42, 68). This may represent a real decrease in frequency, or it may represent patient selection, with a disproportionate share of those who experienced the symptoms discontinuing.

A third problem is evaluation of side effects of low frequency but extreme seriousness such as carcinoma or thromboembolic disease. The difficulty is further compounded by the fact that some conditions, such as carcinoma, develop only at long intervals after the initial exposure (142).

Recommendations The need for better means of evaluating and interpreting subjective side effects is evident, and research on such methodology should be encouraged. In the meantime it seems best to record subjective side effects only if spontaneously reported by the subject, except in special studies where a suitable placebo group can be included. When side effects appear to change in frequency with time of use, the data should be further analyzed to determine whether they represent a real change in incidence among continuing users or an apparent change resulting from a more rapid dropout rate among the subjects who experience the side effects. Continuing research on indicators of serious complications that occur only with low frequency is to be encouraged, as well as planning, support, and conduct of long-range, prospective epidemiological studies in connection with all methods that obtain widespread use.

Recovery of Fertility after Discontinuation
Present status Women or couples choose the use of reversible methods with the goal of planning their families at will. This includes the possibility of having a baby if desired by simply discontinuing the use of contraceptive methods. Nevertheless, no sufficient studies have been done to demonstrate that reproductive capacity is fully recovered after short-term or long-

term use of contraceptives, including some that are currently widely prescribed (52, 65, 67, 87, 89, 96, 115, 135, 140, 156, 193).

Recommendations There is a need for more comprehensive studies of recovery of fertility after various periods of use of the different contraceptives. These studies should give attention not only to conception but to the outcome of the pregnancy and the characteristics of the newborn.

Measurement of Effects on Bleeding Patterns

Present status Newer fertility control agents such as depo injections or continuous low-dose oral administration of progestins greatly modify bleeding patterns and yield complete distortion of menstrual cycle in a large proportion of cases (3, 4, 22, 28, 31, 36, 43, 47, 64, 81, 95, 139, 141, 172, 180). In spite of this, most investigators continue to analyze bleeding patterns within the framework of a cyclic phenomenon (10, 12, 14, 24, 82, 117). In spite of recognition of this problem (20, 32, 49, 58, 97, 172, 188), only recently have there been attempts to find more objective procedures for analysis of bleeding data (21, 98, 129, 136, 148).

Recommendations Continued research on better methods of analyzing bleeding patterns is needed. In the meantime it is suggested that a time-reference period rather than cycles be used as the basis for computation and comparison.

Evaluation of Acceptability

Present status Although the evaluation of acceptability is listed as an objective in many clinical trials (70, 144, 163), the methodology for such evaluation is still in a primitive state. Demographically, however, acceptance of a method is usually more important than its relative contraceptive effectiveness in determining its effects on population growth. Reports of acceptability are usually confined to the investigator's impression that it is "well accepted," "very well accepted," and the like (23, 37, 57, 74, 91, 93, 95, 99, 103, 116, 123, 137).

Besides being nonquantitative, such interpretations are frequently confined to impressions of primary acceptability. *Primary acceptability* can be defined as the patient's initial choice of a contraceptive after having been informed about the different methods available, but without having had personal experience with each method. This choice will be influenced by the information the patient has received and will therefore reflect in varying degrees the bias of the clinic personnel.

Secondary acceptability represents choice or continuing use by the patient after personal experience

with the method (36, 81, 186, 191). In this instance, the clinical characteristics of the contraceptives and quality of care in the clinic will be factors influencing secondary acceptance. Secondary acceptance in such an instance will, of course, also be a relative matter and will depend upon the alternative methods available. In very carefully controlled comparative studies, continuation rates can serve as indicators of secondary acceptability. Continuation of use is indeed the prime measure of interest from the point of view of the demographic effectiveness of a given contraceptive method (184). Nonetheless, continuation rates are frequently not estimated or reported in clinical trials of contraceptives.

Recommendations There is urgent need for the development of suitable methodology for measurement of both primary and secondary acceptability. Continuation rates should be determined in all clinical trials of contraceptives.

Communication of Results of Clinical Studies

Present status There is a general prejudice against publication of negative results. It is indeed true that negative findings often permit only the most tentative conclusions, because studies that give such negative results will usually be aborted early and the number of subjects and the period of observation will accordingly be relatively small. Notwithstanding these attitudes and factors, early publication of results of clinical studies, whether positive or negative, does serve a very useful purpose. Positive results will stimulate other investigators to initiate trials of their own, thus speeding the evaluation of contraceptive candidates (27, 30, 35, 95, 120, 190). More importantly, however, early publication of negative findings will alert investigators to proceed with care (164). In some instances, failure to publish negative findings results in the repetition of the same research by different investigators, with each believing he is attempting the approach the first time. In such cases, even if each of the individual papers must be regarded as preliminary and the conclusions as highly tentative, the combined evidence from several such investigations may assume sufficient weight to permit relatively firm conclusions. Ethical responsibility to patients requires early communication of high pregnancy rates or undesirable side effects so that the exposure of other subjects to such risks can be minimized.

Recommendations Preliminary clinical findings, especially findings concerning potential health hazards, should be routinely published. Such publications should, of course, be appropriately qualified as to the preliminary and tentative nature of their findings.

39.4 Discussion

Throughout this paper recommendations have been made calling for greater standardization of clinical testing procedures. This is by no means meant to discourage the development of new methodology in clinical testing, in data analyses, or in research design. The need for new methodology is abundantly evident and has been emphasized. The plea for standardization is meant only to urge adoption of common definitions and common procedures until better procedures become evident from studies directed specifically toward methodological improvement.

Some attempts have been made to assess the role of different agencies in improving the quality and efficacy of clinical trials. A review of the literature in the past six years showed that 35 percent of the clinical studies reported were supported by pharmaceutical companies, and only a little over 25 percent were supported by private agencies such as the Ford Foundation, the Population Council, the Rockefeller Foundation, the Pathfinder Fund, and IPPF.[1] Most of the studies sponsored by pharmaceutical companies were done by research groups also supported in part by private agencies. Over half the studies received direct or indirect support from private agencies of international scope. Thirty-five percent were supported by local universities or hospitals and a few by governmental agencies.

Considering the use or nonuse of life tables as an indicator of the quality of the clinical study, it was found that 60 percent of the studies supported by international private agencies but only 10 percent of those supported by the pharmaceutical companies used life-table analyses. These ratios are misleading, however, as the use of life tables for the analysis of results does not by itself guarantee a careful, methodologically correct clinical trial. If more indicators of the quality of the study are added, the ratios become even more unfavorable.

The main conclusion that can be derived from this critical review of the present status of clinical trial design and methodology in contraception is that a much greater effort needs to be applied to improving the situation. It seems that supportive agencies have not placed enough emphasis on providing technical advice or assistance, even to their own grantees, to bring the quality of clinical research up to the standards usually found in biological and social investigations of reproduction.

1. The study included articles published in the *American Journal of Obstetrics and Gynecology*, *Fertility and Sterility*, *Acta Obstetrica et Gynecologica Scandinavica*, and some Latin American journals. The journal *Studies in Family Planning* was intentionally excluded to avoid bias in favor of Population Council–sponsored clinical trials.

Most training programs on reproduction and family planning include research methodology in their curricula, but clinical investigations are usually not mentioned at all. Many clinicians involved in contraceptive research are aware of their need for technical assistance, consultation, or advice, but there are not enough resources available to them for these purposes.

The several critical aspects described here should be the subject of discussion in every forum attended by clinical investigators on contraception. Journal editors and reviewers also have the important role of giving advice to authors when reviewing the drafts of clinical studies submitted to them and of encouraging the publication of papers on clinical research methodology.

Donor agencies should implement mechanisms for assistance at the time of grant application when a project does not fulfill minimum methodological requirements. At the international level, resident advisors and people responsible for international programs at universities and other institutions should be more cautious about encouraging clinical research without providing adequate consultation and training for the investigators involved.

If these needs are not satisfactorily fulfilled, great efforts and resources will continue to be spent to produce results often of doubtful validity and impossible to compare with parallel experience in the same field.

References

1. Andeleman, M. B., J. Zackler, N. L. Slutsky, and M. M. Jacobson. Family planning and public health. Int. J. Fertil. 13:405, 1968.

2. Andeleman, M. B. Fertility control with 15-8-5. Fertil. Steril. 21:314, 1970.

3. Apelo, R., and I. Veloso. Clinical experience with microdose d-Norgestrel as an oral contraceptive. Fertil. Steril. 24:191, 1973.

4. Aznar-Ramos, R., J. Giner-Velázquez, and J. Martínez-Manautou. Contraceptive efficacy of single and divided doses of chlormadinone acetate. Contraception 4:37, 1971.

5. Aznar-Ramos, R., J. Giner-Velázquez, R. Lara-Ricalde, and J. Martínez-Manautou. Incidence of side-effects with contraceptive placebo. Am. J. Obstet. Gynecol. 105:1144, 1969.

6. Balakrishnan, T. R., J. D. Allingham, and J. F. Kantner. Analysis of oral contraceptive use through multiple decrement life table techniques. Demography 7:459, 1970.

7. Balin, H., L. S. Wan, and R. Rajan. Sequential approach to oral contraceptive therapy. Int. J. Fertil. 14:300, 1969.

8. Banaharnsupawat, L., and A. Rosenfield. Immediate post-partum IUD insertion. Obstet. Gynecol. 38:276, 1971.

9. Boria, M. C., M. Gordon, and M. L. Stone. Some observations on the use of "M" intrauterine contraceptive devices. Contraception 4:193, 1971.

10. Bergsjo, P., and O. Keller. Low-dose chlormadinone acetate for contraception. Int. J. Fertil. 17:35, 1972.

11. Bernstein, G. S. Clinical effectiveness of an aerosol contraceptive foam. Contraception 3:37, 1971.

12. Bernstein, G. S., and P. Seward. Daily chlormadinone acetate as an oral contraceptive. Contraception 5:369, 1972.

13. Bernstein, G. S., R. Israel, P. Seward, and D. R. Mishell. Clinical experience with the Cu-7 intrauterine device. Contraception. 6:99, 1972.

14. Board, J. A. Continuous norethindrone, 0.5mg, as an oral contraceptive agent. Am. J. Obstet. Gynecol. 109:531, 1971.

15. Bollinger, C. C., T. C. Carrier, and W. L. Ledger. Intrauterine contraception in Indians of the American Southwest. Am. J. Obstet. Gynecol. 106:669, 1970.

16. Bolognese, R. J., S. L. Corson, M. S. Piver, and M. S. Nemser. The intrauterine device: Three years of clinical experience. Fertil Steril. 19:294, 1968.

17. Bolognese, R. J., S. L. Corson, and M. S. Piver. The Saf-T-Coil, an IUD. Fertil. Steril. 19:957, 1968.

18. Bourman, J. A. Experience with oral contraceptives in the immediate puerperium: Effect on breast engorgement and menstrual flow. Fertil. Steril. 21:39, 1970.

19. Buchman, M. I. A study of the intrauterine contraceptive device, with and without an extracervical appendage or tail. Fertil. Steril. 21:348, 1970.

20. Burch, T. K., J. J. Macisco, and M. P. Parker. Some methodological problems in the analysis of menstrual data. Int. J. Fertil. 12:67, 1967.

21. Bye, P. G. T. The assessment of menstruation. Report of the WHO Task Force on Acceptability of Fertility Regulating Methods, April 1–3, 1974.

22. Casavilla, F., J. Stubrin, C. Maruffo, B. van Nynatten, and V. Perez. Daily megestrol acetate for fertility control: A clinical study. Contraception 6:361, 1972.

23. Cittadini, E., P. Quartaro, and F. Romano. Our experience with sequential estrogen-progestin treatments to inhibit ovulation. Int. J. Fertil. 14:180, 1969.

24. Clarman, A. D. A trial of a one dose a month oral contraceptive. Am. J. Obstet. Gynecol. 107:461, 1970.

25. Corson, S. L., R. J. Bolognese, and S. Nemser. The shell loop—a new IUD. Contraception 3:115, 1971.

26. Corson, S. L., R. J. Bolognese, S. Nemser, and G. Boose. The silicone shell IUD. Contraception 6:127, 1972.

27. Coutinho, E. M., C. E. R. Mattos, A. R. S. Sant'Anna, J. Adeodato Filho, M. C. Silva, and H. J. Tatum. Long-term contraception by subcutaneous silastic capsules containing megestrol acetate. Contraception 2:313, 1970.

28. Coutinho, E. M., C. E. R. Mattos, A. R. S. Sant'Anna, J. Adeodato Filho, M. C. Silva, and H. J. Tatum. Further studies on long-term contraception by subcutaneous silastic capsules containing megestrol acetate. Contraception 5:389, 1972.

29. Creasy, M. R. K., J. E. Hillig, and J. A. Morris. Physiologic control of conception with an intramuscular progestogen-estrogen: Clinical experience. Contraception 1:271, 1970.

30. Croxatto, H., S. Díaz, S. Vera, M. Echart, and P. Atria. Fertility control in women with a progestogen released in microquantities from subcutaneous capsules. Am. J. Obstet. Gynecol. 105:1135, 1969.

31. Croxatto, H. B., S. Díaz, P. Atria, S. Cheviakoff, S. Rosatti, and H. Oddo. Contraceptive action of megestrol acetate implants in women. Contraception 4:155, 1971.

32. Chizzae, L., F. T. Brayer, J. J. Macisco, and M. P. Parker. The length and variability of the human menstrual cycle. JAMA 203:89, 1968.

33. Diddle, A. W., W. H. Gardner, and P. J. Williamson. Oral contraceptive medication and headache. Am. J. Obstet. Gynecol. 105:507, 1969.

34. DiSaia, P. J., C. D. Davis, and B. Z. Taber. Continuous tablet therapy for oral contraception. Obstet. Gynecol. 31:119, 1968.

35. El-Mahgoub, S., and M. Karim. Depot estrogen as a monthly contraceptive in nulliparous women with mild uterine hypoplasia. Am. J. Obstet. Gynecol. 112:575, 1972.

36. El-Mahgoub, S., and M. Karim. The long-term use of injectable norethisterone enanthate as a contraceptive. Contraception 5:21, 1972.

37. El-Mahgoub, S., M. Karim, and R. Ammar. Long-term use of depot medroxyprogesterone acetate as a contraceptive. Acta Obstet. Gynecol. Scand. 51:251, 1972.

38. El-Tawil, N. Z., A. H. Shabaan, A. Ibrahim, and C. R. García. Effect of a new low-dosage oral contraceptive pill on blood electrolytes. A combined clinical and laboratory evaluation. Fertil. Steril. 20:405, 1969.

39. Esquivel, A., and L. E. Laufe. Conception control by single monthly injection. Obstet. Gynecol. 31:634, 1968.

40. Faúndes, A., G. Rodríguez, G. Mora, and S. Letelier. Post-abortion insertion of the copper T-200 and Lippes loop. A comparative study. Contraception 8:583, 1973.

41. Feldman, J. G., and J. Lippes. A four-year comparison between the utilization and use-effectiveness of sequential and combined oral contraceptives. Contraception 3:93, 1971.

42. Ferrari, A., J. C. Meyselles, J. M. Sartoretto, and A. Soares Filho. The menstrual cycle in women treated with d-Norgestrel 37.5 micrograms in continuous administration. Int. J. Fertil. 18:133, 1973.

43. Foley, M., B. Law, J. Davies, and K. Fotherby. Clinical trial and laboratory investigation of a low-dose progestogen-only contraceptive. Int. J. Fertil. 18:246, 1973.

44. Fortier, L., Y. Lefebvre, M. Larose, and R. Lanctot. Canadian experience with a copper-covered intrauterine contraceptive device. Am. J. Obstet. Gynecol. 115:291, 1973.

45. Franck, R., W. M. Alpern, and D. E. Echbangh. Oral contraception started early in the puerperium. Am. J. Obstet. Gynecol. 103:112, 1969.

46. Fuchs, F., and A. Risk. The Antigon-F, an improved intrauterine contraceptive device. Contraception 5:119, 1972.

47. Furuhjelm, M., and K. Carlstrom. Amenorrhea following use of continued oral contraceptives. Acta Obstet. Gynecol. Scand. 52:373, 1973.

48. Gambrell, R. D. Immediate post-partum oral contraception. Obstet. Gynecol. 36:101, 1970.

49. Geist, S. H. The variability of menstrual rhythm and character. Am. J. Obstet. Gynecol. 20:320, 1930.

50. Goldsmith, A., R. Goldberg, H. Eyzaguirre, and N. Lizana. Immediate post-abortal intrauterine contraceptive device insertion: A double blind study. Am. J. Obstet. Gynecol. 112:957, 1972.

51. Goldzieher, J. W. The incidence of side-effects with oral or intrauterine contraceptive. Am. J. Obstet. Gynecol. 102: 91, 1968.

52. Goldzieher, J. W., and D. C. Hines. Seven years of clinical experience with a sequential oral contraceptive. Int. J. Fertil. 13:399, 1968.

53. Goldzieher, J. W., L. E. Moses, E. Averkin, C. Scheel, and B. Z. Taber. Nervousness and depression attributed to oral contraceptives. A double-blind, placebo-controlled study. Am. J. Obstet. Gynecol. 111:1013, 1971.

54. Goldzieher, J. W., L. E. Moses, M. A. Averkin, C. Scheel, and B. Z. Taber. A placebo-controlled double-blind crossover investigation of the side-effects attributed to oral contraceptives. Fertil. Steril. 22:609, 1971.

55. Greaney, M. O., B. Z. Taber, and S. A. Bessler. Methodology in oral contraceptive research. Fertil. Steril. 19:339, 1968.

56. Guiloff, E., J. Zañartu, C. Toscanini, and G. Ogaz. Estudio clínico del anillo de nylon intrauterino usado para el control de la fertilidad humana. Rev. Méd. de Chile 94:686, 1966.

57. Guiloff, E., E. Berman, A. Montiglio, R. Osorio, and Ch. Lloyd. Clinical study of a once-a-month oral contraceptive: Quinestrol-quingestanol. Fertil. Steril. 21:110, 1970.

58. Gunn, D. L., P. M. Jenkin, and A. C. Gunn. Menstrual periodicity: Statistical observations on a large sample of normal cases. J. Obstet. Gynecol. Br. Commonw. 44:829, 1937.

59. Guttorm, E. Menstrual bleeding with intrauterine contraceptive device. Acta Obstet. Gynecol. Scand. 9:16, 1971.

60. Hall, M. F., and W. A. Reinke. Factors influencing contraception continuation rates: The oral and the intrauterine methods. Demography 6:335, 1969.

61. Hall, R. E. A four-year report on Loop D. Int. J. Fertil. 13:309, 1968.

62. Hall, R. E. Continuation and pregnancy rates with four contraceptive methods. Am. J. Obstet. Gynecol. 116:671, 1973.

63. Harris, J. W., H. G. McQuarrie, A. E. Anderson, H. S. Ellsworth, and R. A. Stone. The T-Cu-300 IUD. A preliminary report.

64. Heinen, G., W. Rindt, J. Yeboa, and H. Umla. Hormonal contraception with 0.5 mg chlormadinone acetate by continuous administration. Contraception 3:45, 1971.

65. Hernandez-Torres, A., and A. P. Satterthwaite. Norgestrel ethinyl estradiol. An oral contraceptive. Am. J. Obstet. Gynecol. 108:183, 1970.

66. Herzog, G. W., and S. Sanle. Control of fertility by monthly injection of estrogen-progesterone. Obstet. Gynecol. 32:111, 1968.

67. Hill, A. M. Contraception with the Gräfenberg ring. A review of 33 years' experience. Am. J. Obstet. Gynecol. 103: 200, 1969.

68. Hines, D. C., and J. W. Goldzieher. Large-scale study of an oral contraceptive. Fertil. Steril. 19:841, 1968.

69. Hines, D. C., and J. W. Goldzieher. Clinical investigation: A guide to its evaluation. Am. J. Obstet. Gynecol. 105: 450, 1969.

70. Homemann, B., and M. Osler. Medroxyprogesterone acetate as a contraceptive. Int. J. Fertil. 17:210, 1972.

71. Horne, H. W., and J. M. Scott. Intrauterine contraceptive devices in women with proven fertility: A five-year follow-up study. Fertil. Steril. 20:400, 1969.

72. Horowitz, A. J. A study of contraceptive effectiveness and incidence of side-effects with the use of the Mäjzlin spring. Contraception 4:23, 1971.

73. Horowitz, A. J. A study of contraceptive effectiveness and incidence of side-effects with the use of the Dalkon shield. Contraception 7:1, 1973.

74. Ingemanson, C. A. Experiences with Lippes silicone-shell loop. Contraception 4:305, 1971.

75. Ishihama, A., and T. Inove. Clinical field test of a new contraceptive vaginal foam tablet. Contraception 6:401, 1972.

76. Jaramillo, M. G., and J. B. Londono. Rhythm: A hazardous contraceptive method. Demography 5:433, 1968.

77. Jepson, S., and S. Kullander. Experience with chlormadinone acetate in continuous low-dose as an oral contraceptive. Fertil. Steril. 21:307, 1970.

78. Jorgensen, V. One year contraceptive follow-up of adolescent patients. Am. J. Obstet. Gynecol. 115:184, 1973.

79. Kaltreider, D. F. Clinical evaluation of ethinylestrenol and mestranol as a contraceptive. Fertil. Steril. 19:589, 1968.

80. Karrer, M. C., and E. R. Smith. Two thousand woman-years' experience with a sequential contraceptive. Am. J. Obstet. Gynecol. 102:1029, 1968.

81. Kesserü, E., E. Larrañaga, H. Hurtado, and G. Benavides. Fertility control by continuous administration of d-Norgestrel, 0.03 mg. Int. J. Fertil. 17:17, 1972.

82. Kesserü, E., E. Larrañaga, and J. Parada. Post-coital contraception with d-Norgestrel. Contraception 7:367, 1973.

83. Kullander, S. Experiences with an IUCD (Margulis coil). Obstet. Gynecol. 21:482, 1970.

84. Kushner, D. H., W. J. Jaffurs, C. E. Tounsend, and M. A. Thomas. Surgical and obstetrical complications of intrauterine devices in a specialty hospital. Int. J. Fertil. 14:48, 1969.

85. Landesman, R., R. E. Kaye, and K. H. Wilson. Experience with the copper "T" intrauterine device. Contraception 7:477, 1973.

86. Larrañaga, A., and E. Berman. Clinical study of a once-a-month oral contraceptive: Quinestrol-quingestanol. Contraception 1:137, 1970.

87. Larsson-Cohn, V. The length of the first three menstrual cycles after combined oral contraceptive treatment. Acta Obstet. Gynecol. Scand. 48:416, 1969.

88. Laufe, L. E., P. B. Brickner, P. E. Ryser, and J. L. Ammer. An evaluation of the use-effectiveness of the Saf-T-Coil in private practice. Contraception 9:23, 1974.

89. Lee, R. A. Contraceptive and endometrial effects of medroxiprogesterone acetate. Am. J. Gynecol. 104:130, 1969.

90. Leiman, G. Depo-medroxiprogesterone acetate as a contraceptive agent: Its effect on weight and blood pressure. Am. J. Obstet. Gynecol. 114:97, 1972.

91. Lippes, J., and S. S. Ogra. The loop, age seven. Int. J. Fertil. 13:444, 1968.

92. Lippes, J., and J. G. Feldman. A five-year comparison of the continuation rates between women using loop D and oral contraceptives. Contraception 3:313, 1971.

93. Maqueo-Topete, M., E. Berman, J. Soberon, and J. J. Calderon. A pill-a-month contraceptive. Fertil. Steril. 20:884, 1969.

94. Maqueo, M., T. W. Mischler, and E. Berman. The evaluation of quingestanol acetate as a low-dose oral contraceptive. Contraception 6:117, 1972.

95. Martínez-Manautou, J., V. Cortéz, J. Giner, R. Aznar, J. Casasola, and H. W. Rudel. Low-doses of progestogen as an approach to fertility control. Fertil. Steril. 11:49, 1966.

96. Matsumato, S., T. Ito, T. Shiozaki, Y. Iijima, and T. Tamada. Influence of long-term use of intrauterine devices on reproductive organs. Int. J. Fertil. 18:326, 1968.

97. Matsumoto, S., Y. Nogami, and S. Ohkuri. Statistical studies of menstruation: A criticism of the definition of normal menstruation. Gunma J. Med. Sci. 11:294, 1962.

98. Mayes, D. G. The analysis of bleeding patterns. Report of the WHO Task Force on Acceptability of Fertility Regulating Methods, April 1–3, 1974.

99. McDaniel, E. G. Trial of a long-acting injectable contraceptive as a substitute for the IUCD and the pill in a remote region in Thailand. Demography 5:699, 1968.

100. McDaniel, E. G., and T. Pardthaisong. Depo-medroxiprogesterone acetate as a contraceptive agent: Return of fertility after discontinuation of use. Contraception 8:401, 1973.

101. Melton, R. J., and J. D. Shelton. Pill versus IUD: Continuation rates of oral contraceptive and Dalkon shield users in Maryland clinics. Contraception 4:319, 1971.

102. Miller, G. H., and L. R. Hughes. Lactation and genital involution effects of a new low-dose oral contraceptive on breast-feeding mothers and their infants. Obstet. Gynecol. 35:44, 1970.

103. Mishell, D. R., and N. D. Freid. Life-table analysis of a clinical study of a once-a-month oral steroid contraceptive. Contraception 8:37, 1973.

104. Mishell, D. R., R. Israel, and N. Freid. A study of the copper T intrauterine contraceptive device (TCU 200) in nulliparous women. Am. J. Obstet. Gynecol. 116:1092, 1973.

105. Morris, N. M., and J. R. Udry. Depression of physical activity by contraceptive pills. Am. J. Obstet. Gynecol. 104:1012, 1969.

106. Moses, L. E., J. W. Goldzieher, and I. G. Moses. Evaluation of a new combination oral contraceptive: Lynestrenol-mestranol (Lyndiol). Fertil. Steril. 20:715, 1969.

107. Neisuler, R. F., and D. R. Mishell. Clinical trial of a new IUD: The silicone-shell loop. Contraception 2:99, 1970.

108. Ostergard, D. R., and E. M. Broen. The Dalkon shield: A clinical evaluation. Contraception 4:313, 1971.

109. Ostergard, D. R. Intrauterine contraception in nulliparas with the Dalkon shield. Am. J. Obstet. Gynecol. 116:1088, 1973.

110. Ostergard, D. R., and E. M. Broer. The insertion of intrauterine devices by physicians and paramedical personnel. Obstet. Gynecol. 41:257, 1973.

111. Portnuff, J. C., S. C. Ballon, and A. Langer. The intrauterine contraceptive device: A prospective five year clinical study. Am. J. Obstet. Gynecol. 114:934, 1972.

112. Potter, R. G. Length of the observation period as a factor affecting the contraceptive failure rate. Milbank Mem. Fund Quart. 38:140, 1960.

113. Potter, R. G. Additional measures of use effectiveness of contraception. Milbank Mem. Fund Quart. 41:400, 1963.

114. Potter, R. G. Application of life table techniques to measurement of contraceptive effectiveness. Demography 3:297, 1966.

115. Powell, L. C., and R. J. Seymour. Effects of depo-medroxiprogesterone acetate as a contraceptive agent. Am. J. Obstet. Gynecol. 110:36, 1971.

116. Preston, S. N. A report of a collaborative dose-response clinical study using decreasing doses as combination oral contraceptives. Contraception 6:17, 1972.

117. Prsic, J., and P. M. Kićović. Low-dose lynestrenol as a contraceptive method. Contraception 8:315, 1973.

118. Ragas, M. I., and M. B. Sammour. Sociomedical studies of 60,000 applicants for family planning. Am. J. Obstet. Gynecol. 105:156, 1969.

119. Ramírez, C. Estudio sobre planificación familiar con diapositivos intrauterinos en un área rural. Rev. Chil. Obstet. Ginecol. 35:11, 1970.

120. Rashbaum, W. K., and R. C. Wallach. Immediate postpartum insertion of a new intrauterine contraceptive device. Am. J. Obstet. Gynecol. 109:1003, 1971.

121. Reidenberg, M. M., and D. T. Lowenthal. Adverse nondrug reactions. New Engl. J. Med. 279:678, 1968.

122. Reinke, W. A., and T. D. Baker. Measuring effects of demographic variables on health service utilization. Health Serv. Res. (Chicago) Spring:61, 1967.

123. Rice-Wray, E., A. Peña, and M. Maqueo. Ovanon: A new sequential oral contraceptive. Int. J. Fertil. 13:453, 1968.

124. Rice-Wray, E., S. A. deFerrer, I. Pérez-Huerta, and J. Gorodovsky. Clinical evaluation of a new combined oral contraceptive. Contraception 1:389, 1970.

125. Rice-Wray, E., I. I. Beristain, and A. Cerbantes. Clinical study of a continuous daily micro-dose progestogen contraceptive d-Norgestrel. Contraception 5:279, 1972.

126. Rice-Wray, E., J. Gorodovsky, and A. Peña. A modified sequential contraceptive. Contraception 5:457, 1972.

127. Rifai, S. F. A new contraceptive device with reduced expulsion rate. Am. J. Obstet. Gynecol. 104:1113, 1969.

128. Rodriguez, A., A. Pérez, P. Vela, J. Espinoza, and C. Lonnberg. Experiencia con el método del ritmo en el período de postparto. Rev. Chil. Obstet. Ginecol. 29:193, 1964.

129. Rodríguez, G., A. Faúndes, and L. Atkinson. An approach to the analysis of menstrual patterns in the clinical evaluation of contraceptives. Stud. Fam. Plann., 7:42, 1976.

130. Roland, M., M. Friedman, and R. J. Hessekiel. Norgestrel, a low dose, oral progestogen for fertility control. Obstet. Gynecol. 31:637, 1968.

131. Roland, M., D. Leisten, and L. J. Caruso. A regimen for fertility control with a cyclic progestogen. Obstet. Gynecol. 41:595, 1973.

132. Rosenfield, A. G., and C. Limcharden. Auxiliary midwife prescription of oral contraceptives. Am. J. Obstet. Gynecol. 114:942, 1972.

133. Rubio, B., and E. Berman. Once-a-month oral contraceptive: Quinestrol-quingestanol. Obstet. Gynecol. 35:933, 1970.

134. Rubio, B., E. Berman, M. Plains, A. Larrañaga, and E. Guiloff. A new postcoital oral contraceptive. Contraception 1:303, 1970.

135. Rubio, B., T. W. Mischler, and E. Berman. Further experience with a once-a-month oral contraceptive: Quinestrol-quingestanol. Fertil. Steril. 23:734, 1972.

136. Rubio, B., T. W. Mischler, and E. Berman. Contraception with a daily low-dose progestogen: Quingestanol acetate. Fertil. Steril. 23:668, 1972.

137. Sajadi, H. E., G. Borazjani, and M. S. Ardekany. Medroxiprogesterone acetate (MPA) for contraception. Int. J. Fertil. 17:217, 1972.

138. Schwallie, P. C., and J. R. Assenzo. Contraceptive use-efficacy study utilizing depo-provera administered as an injection once every six months. Contraception 6:315, 1972.

139. Schwallie, P. C., and J. R. Assenzo. Contraceptive use-effectiveness study utilizing medroxyprogesterone acetate administered as an intramuscular injection once every 90 days. Fertil. Steril. 24:331, 1973.

140. Scommega, A., A. W. Lee, and S. Barushek. Evaluation of an injectable progestin-estrogen as contraceptive. Am. J. Obstet. Gynecol. 107:1147, 1970.

141. Scutchfield, F. D., W. Newton-Long, B. Corey, and C. W. Tyler. Medroxyprogesterone acetate as an injectable female contraceptive. Contraception 3:21, 1971.

142. Seigel, D., and P. Corfman. Epidemiological problems associated with studies of the safety of oral contraceptives. JAMA 203:950, 1968.

143. Seymour, R. J., and L. C. Powell. Depo-medroxiprogesterone acetate as a contraceptive. Obstet. Gynecol. 36:589, 1970.

144. Shah, P. N. Acceptability and clinical effectivity of the oral progestagens for fertility control in Indian women. Fertil. Steril. 19:286, 1968.

145. Shah, P. N. Evaluation of oral progestagens for contraception in Indian women. Am. J. Obstet. Gynecol. 105:512, 1969.

146. Silvermann, E., M. L. Stone, and E. B. Connell. The "M," a new intrauterine contraceptive device. Am. J. Obstet. Gynecol.

147. Snowden, R., and M. Williams. The use effectiveness of the Dalkon shield in the United Kingdom. Contraception 7:91, 1973.

148. Snowden, R. Report on a planning meeting of the WHO Task Force on Acceptability of Fertility Regulating Methods, Geneva, Appendix D:23, March 1973.

149. Sobrero, A. J., and D. Pierotti. Mäjzlin intrauterine contraceptive spring. Obstet. Gynecol. 36:911, 1970.

150. Soichet, S. Depo-provera (medroxiprogesterone acetate) as a female contraceptive agent. Int. J. Fertil. 14:33, 1969.

151. Soichet, S. Ypsilon: A new silicone-covered stainless steel intrauterine contraceptive device. Am. J. Obstet. Gynecol. 114:938, 1972.

152. Solish, G. I., G. K. Schuyler, and G. Majzlin. Effectiveness of the Majzlin spring intrauterine contraceptive device. Am. J. Obstet. Gynecol. 114:106, 1972.

153. Sölvell, L., and L. Nilsson. A clinical study on a sequential oral contraceptive—Orisec. Acta Obstet. Gynecol. Scand. (Suppl. 6):1, 1968.

154. Sölvell, L., L. Nilsson, and H. Westholm. Amount of menstrual blood loss during sequential oral contraceptive therapy—Orisec. Acta Obstet. Gynecol. Scand. 47(Suppl. 6):27, 1968.

155. deSouza, J. C., and E. M. Coutinho. Control of fertility by monthly injections of a mixture of norgestrel and a long-acting estrogen. Contraception 5:395, 1972.

156. Spain, W. T. Systemic effect of a sequential regimen. Int. J. Fertil. 13:431, 1968.

157. Stany, J. A comparison between the efficacy and side effects of oral contraception using closely related combined and sequential preparations. Acta Obstet. Gynecol. Scand. 48 (Suppl. 3):26, 1969.

158. Stenström, B. Oral contraception using a sequential method. Acta Obstet. Gynecol. Scand. 47:443, 1968.

159. Sturtevant, F. M., and R. B. Wait. High-dose estrogen sequential oral contraception. Contraception 3:187, 1970.

160. Swartz, D. P., I. S. Cho, and H. T. Felton. General observations from five years of use of antifertility agents in a public hospital. Int. J. Fertil. 13:332, 1968.

161. Swyer, G. I. M. Collection and evaluation of data on contraception. Int. J. Fertil. 13:366, 1968.

162. Taber, B. Z. Proving new drugs. A guide to clinical trials. Los Altos, Calif.: Geron-X, Inc., 1969.

163. Tatum, H. J., E. M. Coutinho, J. Adeodata Filho, and A. R. Sant'Anna. Acceptability of a long-term contraceptive steroid administration in humans by subcutaneous silastic capsules. Am. J. Obstet. Gynecol. 105:1139, 1969.

164. Tejuja, S. Use of subcutaneous silastic capsules for long-term steroid contraception. Am. J. Obstet. Gynecol.

165. Tietze, C., and S. Lewit. Recommended procedures for the study of use effectiveness of contraceptive methods. In *IPPF Medical Handbook*. London: IPPF, 1964.

166. Tietze, C. Intrauterine contraception. Recommended procedures for data analysis. Stud. Fam. Plann. 18 (Suppl.):1, 1967.

167. Tietze, C. Intrauterine contraception: Research report (Seventh Progress Report). Stud. Fam. Plann. 18:20, 1967.

168. Tietze, C. Experience with new IUDs. Contraception 1:73, 1970.

169. Tietze, C., and S. Lewit. Statistical evaluation of contraceptive methods. Obstet. Gynecol., 1974.

170. Timonen, H., and T. Luukkainen. The use effectiveness of the copper-T-200 in a simulated field trial. Contraception 9:1, 1974.

171. Tompkins, M.G. SC 11800 sequential papel. Fertil. Steril. 21:77, 1970.

172. Treloar, A.E., R.E. Boynto, B.G. Behn, and B.W. Brown. Variation of the human menstrual cycle through reproductive life. Int. J. Fertil. 12:77, 1967.

173. Tyler, E.T. Studies of "mini-micro" contraceptive doses of a new progestagen. Int. J. Fertil. 13:460, 1968.

174. Tyler, E.T., E.M. Matsner, and M. Gotlis. Modified sequential oral contraception employing mestranol and chlormadinone. Obstet. Gynecol. 34:820, 1969.

175. Tyler, E.T., S.L. Cole, M. Levin, and J. Elliot. A clinical evaluation of long term continuous use of norethynodrel-mestranol for contraception. Fertil. Steril. 20:871, 1969.

176. Tyler, E.T., M. Levin, J. Elliot, and H. Dolman. Present status of injectable contraceptives: Results of seven years of study. Fertil. Steril. 21:469, 1970.

177. Tyson, J.E.A., and H.H. Washburn. Canadian country-sponsored family planning. Obstet. Gynecol. 35:377, 1970.

178. Vessey, M., and P. Wiggins. Use-effectiveness of the diaphragm in a selected family planning clinic population in the United Kingdom. Contraception 9:15, 1974.

179. Viel, B., and S. Lucero. An analysis of three years' experience with intrauterine devices among women in the western area of the city of Santiago, July 1, 1964, to June 30, 1967. Am. J. Obstet. Gynecol. 106:765, 1970.

180. Vollmann, R.F. Degree of variability of the length of the menstrual cycle in correlation with age of women. Gynaecologia 142:310, 1956.

181. Wallach, E., and C.R. Garcia. Contraception with an intra-muscular estrogen-progestogen preparation administered monthly. Contraception 1:185, 1970.

182. Wamsteker, E.F. Clinical and laboratory experience with a modified low dosage sequential oral contraceptive. Int. J. Fertil. 13:436, 1968.

183. Weinberg, G., and C. Bailin. Postpartum insertion of the safety filament bow. Obstet. Gynecol. 41:925, 1973.

184. Westoff, Ch.F., and N.B. Ryder. Duration of use of oral contraception in the United States, 1960–1965. Public Health Rep. 83:277, 1968.

185. WHO. Advances in methods of fertility regulation. WHO Tech. Rep. No. 527, 1973.

186. Willson, J.R., and W.J. Ledger. Complications associated with the use of intrauterine contraceptive devices in women of middle and upper socio-economic class. Am. J. Obstet. Gynecol. 100:649, 1968.

187. Winkel, C.A., D.L. Barelay, and L. Dayle. A clinical study of the Inhiband. Obstet. Gynecol. 39:917, 1972.

188. Ylostalo, P., and S. Vuopala. Contraceptive treatment with low doses of gestagen in cases with medical history of hepatosis of pregnancy. Acta Obstet. Gynecol. Scand. 52:221, 1973.

189. Zañartu, J., M. Gajardo, J. Garrido, C. Millan, C. Navarro, M. Pupkin, G. Rodríquez-Moore, S. Stone, J. Lolas, C. Toscanini, G. Ogaz, C. González, S. Milesi, E. Morales, and C. Pozo. Tratamiento secuencial con estrógenos y progestagenos en el control de la fertilidad humana. Rev. Med. Chil. 94:696, 1966.

190. Zañartu, J., E. Rice-Wray, and J.W. Goldzieher. Fertility control with long-acting injectable steroid. Obstet. Gynecol. 28:513, 1966.

191. Zañartu, J., M. Gajardo, J. Garrido, E. Guiloff, C. Millan, C. Navarro, M. Pupkin, G. Rodríquez-Moore, S. Stone, R. Wild, C. Toscanini, G. Ogaz, C. González, S. Milesi, E. Morales, and C. Pozo. Control de la fertilidad humana con una combinacion de estrógenos y progestagenos. Experiencia de 3 anos en 3.300 mujeres. Rev. Med. Chil. 94:675, 1966.

192. Zañartu, J., and C. Navarro. Fertility inhibition by an injectable progestogen acting for three months. Obstet. Gynecol. 31:627, 1968.

193. Zañartu, J. Long term contraceptive effect of injectable progestogens: Inhibition and reestablishment of fertility. Int. J. Fertil. 13:415, 1968.

40 Historical Charts

On the following pages will be found a set of eighteen historical charts tracing the development of the major areas of research on the female and male reproductive systems. Each chart is divided into three major sections: biological processes, methodological advances, and contraceptive methods. Each section is further broken down into three subsections: period before 1960, period 1960–1974, and major gaps, methodological needs, or contraceptive possibilities. (Missing subsections may be taken to indicate no major advances during the period.) In several of the tables, it was found convenient to include additional subheads to outline the process of advance in major subareas; for example, the gonadotropin hormone table is divided into three parts: LH, FSH, and hCG. (In such cases, the methodolgical advance and contraceptive methods sections refer to all subareas.)

The charts included and the individuals most responsible for assembling them are as follows:

Hypothalamus
Frederick Naftolin and James Brauer

Releasing Factors
I. LH and FSH Releasing Factors
II. Prolactin Releasing and Inhibiting Factors (PRF and PIF)
Madhwa Raj

Gonadotropin Hormones
I. Luteinizing Hormone (LH)
II. Follicle Stimulating Hormone (FSH)
III. Human Chorionic Gonadotropin (hCG)
William Moyle

Prolactin
William Moyle

Ovary
I. Gonadotropin Binding
IIa. Follicular Phase: Follicular Growth
IIb. Follicular Phase: Steroidogenesis
III. Luteal Phase
IV. Steroidogenic Pathways
Anastasia Makris

The Menstrual Cycle
Irwin Thompson and Philip Darney

Oogenesis and Ovum Maturation
John Biggers

Oviduct, Oviducal Fluid, and Ovum Transport
John Biggers and Philip Darney

Uterotubal Junction
Philip Darney

Uterus
Philip Darney

Cervix and Vagina
Philip Darney

Testis
I. Leydig Cells
II. Sertoli Cells
III. Blood-Testis Barrier
IV. Hormonal Control of Spermatogenesis
V. Spermatogenesis
Martin Dym

Epididymis
David Hamilton

Mammalian Male Accessory Sex Glands
Lauro Cavazos and Peter Ofner

Spermatozoon
Everett Anderson

Capacitation and Fertilization
Everett Anderson

Preimplantation and Implantation
I. Blastocyst Formation
II. Metabolism of the Preimplantation Stage
III. Implantation
John Biggers and Koji Yoshinaga

Placental Proteins
Philip Darney

Biological Processes: Significant Discoveries

Period before 1960

Environmental factors influence reproduction.

1904 Marshall. *Z. J. Microsc. Sci.* (n. s.) 48:323.

1905 Heape. *Proc. R. Soc. Lond. (Biol.)* 76:260.

Ovulation induction via electrical transcranial stimulation.

1933 Hinsey and Markey. *Proc. Soc. Exp. Biol. Med.* 31:270.

1936 Marshall and Verney. *J. Physiol.* (Lond.) 86:327.

1937 Harris. *Proc. R. Soc. Lond. (Biol.)* 122:374.

1937 Haterius and Derbyshire. *Am. J. Physiol.* 119:324.

Vascular link: description of the hypothalamo–hypophyseal–portal system.

1930 Popa and Fielding. *J. Anat.* 65:88.

1933 Popa and Fielding. *J. Anat.* 67:227.

1936 Wislocki and King. *Am. J. Anat.* 58:421.

1949 Green and Harris. *J. Physiol.* (Lond.) 108:359.

Development of concept of neurosecretion.

1940 Scharrer and Scharrer. *Res. Publ. Assoc. Res. Nerv. Ment. Dis.* 20:170.

Portal system is a constant feature of vertebrates from cyclostomes to man.

1951 Green. *Am. J. Anat.* 88:225.

Permanent interruption of portal system abolishes pituitary function.

1950 Harris. *J. Physiol.* (Lond.) 111:347.

1952 Harris and Jacobsohn. *Proc. R. Soc. Lond. (Biol.)* 139:263.

Interruption of portal system abolishes castration cell formation.

1952 Harris and Jacobsohn. *Proc. R. Soc. Lond. (Biol.)* 139:263.

Exchanging pituitaries between sexes allows normal sexual development and function.

1936 Greep. *Proc. Soc. Exp. Biol. Med.* 34:754.

Description of role of testis in sexual differentiation of hypothamic–pituitary axis.

1936 Pfeiffer. *Am. J. Anat.* 58:195.

Reciprocal relationship between gonads and brain on pituitary function proposed.

1932 Holweg and Junkmann. *Klin. Wochenschr.* 11:321.

1932 Moore and Price. *Am. J. Anat.* 50:13.

Effect of stimulation or ablation of specific hypothalamic regions on reproductive function.

1943 Dey. *Anat. Rec.* 87:85.

1956 Sawyer and Robinson. *J. Clin. Endocrinol. Metab.* 16:914.

1957 Critchlow. *Anat. Rec.* 127:283.

1957 Saul and Sawyer. *Fed. Proc.* 16:112.

Description of "critical period" of LH release in cycling female rat.

1949 Everett, Sawyer, and Markee. *Endocrinology* 44:234.

Active amine control of gonadotropins.

1948 Markee, Sawyer, and Hollinshead. *Recent Prog. Horm. Res.* 2:117.

1952 Markee, Everett, and Sawyer. *Recent Prog. Horm. Res.* 7:139.

Anatomical considerations: demonstration of neuronal projections from medial basal hypothalamus to median eminence.

1951 Spatz. *Acta Neuroveget.* 3:1.

1954 Horstmann. *Z. Zellforsch. Mikrosk. Anat.* 39:588.

Posterior pituitary secretion as prototype for anterior pituitary control. Short feedback (pituitary to hypothalamus).

1959 Sawyer and Kawakami. *Endocrinology* 65:622.

CLINICAL CONSIDERATIONS

Precocious puberty related to hypothalamic lesions and tumors.

1955 Jolly. *Sexual Precocity.* Springfield, Ill.: Thomas.

Hypothalamic amenorrhea.

1946 Reifenstein. *Med. Clin. North Am.* 30:1103.

Pseudocyesis.

1951 Fried et al. *JAMA* 145:1329.

Anorexia nervosa.

1950 Nemiah. *Medicine* 29:225.

Period 1960–1974

Extrahypothalamic influences.

1970 Harris and Naftolin. *Br. Med. Bull.* 26:3 (review).

Role of posterior hypothalamus on estrous behavior.

1958 Law and Meagher. *Science* 128:1626.

Anterior hypothalamus and preoptic area: functional effects of anterior deafferentation and identification of preoptic area as initiator of sexual cycling in rodents.

1961 Everett. In: *Control of Ovulation.* Ed. Villee. New York: Pergamon Press, p. 101.

1969 Halász. In: *Frontiers in Neuroendocrinology.* Eds. Ganong and Martini. New York: Oxford University Press, p. 307.

1970 Gorski. *Am. J. Anat.* 129:219.

1970 Kalra and Sawyer. *Endocrinology* 87:1124.

1970 Koves and Halasz. *Neuroendocrinology* 6:180.

Cycling in female rhesus with deafferented medial basal hypothalamus.

1974 Knobil. *Recent Prog. Horm. Res.* 30.1.

Use of dimorphosis and plasticity in localizing hypothalamic structures controlling sexual differentiation and cycling sexual dimorphism in the preoptic area.

1961 Barraclough and Gorski. *Endocrinology* 68:68.

1973 Raisman and Field. *Brain Res.* 54.1.

Failure of neonatally administered ring A reduced androgens to cause anovulatory sterility.

1971 Brown-Grant, Naftolin, and Sherwood. *Horm. Behav.* 2:173.

Pretreatment with antiestrogen blocks androgen-induced sterility.

1972 McDonald and Doughty. *J. Endocrinol.* 55:455.

Production of estrogen from androgen precursors by hypothalamus from newborn rats.

1974 Reddy, Naftolin, and Ryan. *Endocrinology* 94:117.

Difference in brain differentiation between primates and rodents.

1973 Karsch, Dierschke, and Knobil. *Science* 179:484.

1973 Stearns, Winter, and Faiman. *J. Clin. Endocrinol. Metab.* 37:635.

1974 Knobil. *Recent Prog. Horm. Res.* 30:1.

Testosterone implants: androgen sterilization as a result of testosterone implants in the arcuate nucleus.

1972 Nadler. *Neuroendocrinology* 9:349.

1974 Short. *INSERM* 32:121.

MEDIAN EMINENCE

Neurohemal organ structure: electron-microscopic observations on nerve endings surrounding the primary capillary plexus of the portal system.

1961 Barry and Cotte. *Z. Zellforsch. Mikrosk. Anat.* 53:417.

1961 Kobayashi, Bern, Nishioka, and Hyodo. *Gen. Comp. Endocrinol.* 1:545.

1963 Kobayashi, Yamamoto, and Inatomi. *Endocrinol. Jap.* 10:69.

1967 Wittkowski. *Z. Zellforsch. Mikrosk. Anat.* 81:344.

1969 Bergland and Torach. *Z. Zellforsch. Mikrosk. Anat.* 99:1.

Median eminence — transport capacity.

1971 Knigge and Silverman. In: *Median Eminence: Structure and Function.* Eds. Knigge, Scott, and Weindel. Basel:Karger, p. 350.

Tanycyte structure: specialized ependymal cells linking the third ventricle with the portal system.

1965 Leveque, Stutinsky, Stoeckel, and Porte. *C. R. Acad. Sci. [D]* (Paris) 260:4621.

Capacity of tanycytes to transport a variety of substances from the third ventricle through the median eminence.

1972 Ondo, Mical, and Porter. *Endocrinology* 91:1239.

Sexual dimorphism of tanycytes.

1968 Kumar. *Z. Zellforsch. Mikrosk. Anat.* 90:28.

Sexual cyclicity of tanycytes.

1969 Knowles and Kumar. *Philos. Trans. R. Soc. Lond. (Biol.)* 256:357.

Periventricular glandular structures.

1972 Weindl and Joynt. In: *Median Eminence: Structure and Function.* Eds. Knigge, Scott, and Weindl. Basel:Karger, p. 290.

Localization of LRF decapeptide in median eminence and other diencephalic areas.

Tanycytes (median eminence):

1974 Zimmerman, Hsu, Ferin, and Kozlowski. *Endocrinology* 95:1.

Nerve endings (median eminence):

1974 Pelletier, Labrie, and Puviani. *Endocrinology* 95:314.

Specific hypothalmic nuclei:

1974 Palkovits, Arimura, Brownstein, Schally, and Saavedra. *Endocrinology* 96:5.

In contrast to LRF localization, TRF is generalized.

1974 Winokur and Utiger. *Science* 185:265.

NEUROTRANSMITTERS

Granules.

1965 Fuxe, Hökfelt, and Nilsson. *Am. J. Anat.* 117:33.

1972 Hökfelt and Fuxe. In: *Median Eminence: Structure and Function.* Eds. Knigge, Scott, and Weindl. Basel:Karger, p. 181.

Physiologic correlates.

1972 Hökfelt and Fuxe. In: *Median Eminence: Structure and Function,* p. 181.

Specific role of catecholamines in gonadotropic dynamics.

1971 Kamberi, Mical, and Porter. *Endocrinology* 89:1042.

1972 McCann et al. In: *Median Eminence: Structure and Function.*

Lack of measurable catecholamine in portal blood.

1971 Ruf, Dreifuss, and Carr. *J. Neurovisc. Relat.,* Suppl. X, 65.

Pharmacologic blockade of ovulation.

1971 Kordon. *Neuroendocrinology* 7:202.

1971 Kalnins and Ruf. *Schweiz. Med. Wochenschr.* 101:1124.

Catecholamines in hypothalamic developmental mechanisms.

1971 Weiner and Ganong. *Neuroendocrinology* 8:125.

1972 Weiner and Ganong. *Neuroendocrinology* 9:65.

Influence of catecholamines on sexual behavior.

1974 Everitt et al. *Eur. J. Pharmacol.* 29:187.

Influence of catecholamines on eating behavior.

1973 Simpson and Dicara. *Pharmacol. Biochem. Behav.* 1:413.

Anatomy of fluorescent pathways.

1971 Ungerstedt. *Acta Physiol. Scand.* (Suppl. 367): 1.

Catecholamine fluctuations during ovarian cycle.

1971 Ahren et al. *Endocrinology* 88:1415.

Microanatomic localization and measurement of active amines and their enzymes.

1974 Saavedra et al. *Nature* 248 (5450): 695.

Measurements and manipulations by catecholamines on ovarian steroids.

1973 Gunaga and Menon. *Biochem. Biophys. Res. Commun.* 54:440.

Effect of steroid antimetabolites on active amine enzymes.

1973 Parvez and Parvez. *J. Neurochem.* 20:1011.

Hypothalamic formation of catechol-estrogen.

1973 Fishman. *Endocrinol. Soc. Proc.* (Abstr.) 39:A-68.

Effect of gonadal steroids on hypothalamic indoleamines.

1973 Giulian, Pohorecky, and McEwen. *Endocrinology* 93:1329.

Effect of antimetabolites on hypothalamic indoleamine enzymes.

1974 Victor, Baumgarten, and Lovenberg. *J. Neurochem.* 22:541.

Effect of sex steroids on catecholamine enzymes.

1972 Beattie, Rodgers, and Soyka. *Endocrinology* 91:276.

Localization of releasing factors by bioassay: evidence for separate LRF and FSH-RF.

1968 Watanabe and McCann. *Endocrinology* 82:664.

Role of prostaglandins in gonadotropin control.

1974 Behrman and Caldwell. In: *Reproductive Physiology.* Ed. Greep. London: MTP International Review of Science.

GENERAL HYPOTHALAMIC METABOLISM

Effects of steroids on hypothalamic active amine enzymes.

1973 Beattie and Soyka. *Endocrinology* 93:1453.

1973 Parvez and Parvez. *J. Neurochem.* 20:1011.

1973 Simpson and Dicara. *Pharmacol. Biochem. Behav.* 1:413.

Hypothalamic isoenzyme activity.

1972 Morishita, Nagamachi, Kawamoto, Yoshida, Ozasa, and Adachi. *Acta Endocrinol.* (Kbh.) 71:226.

Alterations in hypothalamic cyclic AMP.

1973 Gunaga and Menon. *Biochem. Biophys. Res. Commun.* 54:440.

Aromatization of androgens by hypothalamus.

1974 Naftolin, Ryan, Davies, Reddy, Flores, Petro, Kuhn, White, Takaoski, and Wolin. *Recent Prog. Horm. Res.* 31:295.

Ring A reduction of progesterone by hypothalamus.

1973 Cheng and Karavolas. *Endocrinology* 93:1157.

Corticoid metabolism by hypothalamus.

1965 Sholiton, Werk, and McGee. *Cortisol and Cortisone Metabolism* 14:1122.

Ring A reduction of androgens by hypothalamus.

1969 Jaffe. *Steroids* 14:483.

In vitro aromatization of androgens localized to anterior hypothalamus.

1972 Naftolin, Ryan, and Petro. *Endocrinology* 90:295.

Estrogen metabolism by hypothalamus.

1975 Fishman and Norton. *Endocrinology* 96(4):1054.

Oxidative activity in the hypothalamus.

1971 Schiaffini and Marin. *Neuroendocrinology* 7:302.

Specific binding of estrogen.

1965 Eisenfeld and Axelrod. *J. Pharmacol. Exp. Ther.* 150:469.

1970 Kato. *Excerpta. Med. Found. Int. Cong. Ser.* 219:764.

Reports of specific binding of androgens by the hypothalamus.

1973 Kato and Onouchi. *Endocrinol. Jap.* 20(4):432.

Inhibition of hypothalamic estrogen binding by antiestrogen.

1968 Kato, Kobayashi, and Villee. *Endocrinology* 82:1049.

Failure of DHT to inhibit nuclear uptake of radioactivity after administration of tritiated testosterone.

1974 Sheridan, Sar, and Stumpf. *Endocrinology* 95:1749.

Rentention of estradiol by cell nuclei in hypothalamus.

1970 Zigmond and McEwen. *J. Neurochem.* 17:889.

Evidence that androgens affect estrogen binding kinetics in hypothalamus.

1974 Korach and Muldoon. *Endocrinology* 94:785.

FINAL COMMON PATHWAY—ARCUATE NUCLEUS

Estradiol implants into arcuate nucleus and subsequent gonadal atrophy.

1963 Lisk and Newton. *Science* 139:223.

Karyometric measurement in arcuate nucleus during reproductive manipulation.

1964 Ifft. *Anat. Rec.* 148:599.

Tritiated amino acid incorporation in specific hypothalamic nuclei in various reproductive states.

1973 Litteria. *Brain Res.* 55:234.

Cytological changes in arcuate nucleus following castration.

1971 Brauer. *J. Comp. Neurol.* 143:411.

Estradiol-induced lesion of arcuate nucleus and subsequent pituitary tumorigenesis.

1975 Brawer and Sonnenschein. *Anat. Rec.* 181:524.

Cytological changes in arcuate nucleus during sexual cycling.

1974 King. *Cell Tissue Res.* 153:497.

Hypothalamic uptake of tritiated estradiol.

1968 Pfaff. *Science* 161:1355.

1971 Stumpf. *Am. Zoologist* 11:725.

Immunohistochemical localization of LRF. Immunofluorescent localization of LRF to preoptic area and scattered cells in anterior hypothalamus.

1973 Barry, Bubois, and Poulain. *Z. Zellforsch. Mikrosk. Anat.* 146:351.

Localization of LRF immunoreactivity to arcuate neurones and tanycytes.

1974 Zimmerman et al. *Endocrinology* 95:1.

Single-unit localization of cells projecting to median eminence.

1971 Harris, Makara, and Spyer. *J. Physiol.* (Lond.) 218:86P.

1973 Sawaki and Yagi. *J. Physiol.* (Lond.) 230:75.

Stimulus-secretion coupling.

1973 Poisner. In: *Frontiers in Neuroendocrinology.* Eds. Ganong and Martini. New York: Oxford University Press.

Lesions of arcuate nucleus with subsequent degeneration in median eminence.

1970 Rethelyi and Halász. *Exp. Brain Res.* 11:145.

1972 Raisman. In: *Median Eminence: Structure and Function.* Eds. Knigge, Scott, and Weindl. Basel:Karger, p. 109.

Major Gaps in Our Knowledge

Structure of releasing factor in portal blood.

Structure of releasing factor bound to pituitary cell.

Function of tanycyte in gonadotropin control.

Detailed analysis of median eminence connections.

Cellular structure of final common hypophysiotrophic pathway.

Rationalization of extrahypothalamic influences (anatomic and physiologic).

Site of difference between rodents and primates in brain differentiation. Cellular mechanism involved in hypothalamic differentiation induced by presence of testes in developing rodents and sheep.

Methodological Advances

Period 1960–1974

Falck-Hillarp methods (induced catecholamine fluorescence).

1962 Falck et al. *J. Histochem. Cytochem.* 10:348.

Perfusion fixation for electron microscopy.

1962 Palay et al. *J. Cell Biol.* 12:385.

Single-unit recording.

1971 Harris, Makara, and Sawyer. *J. Physiol.* (Lond.) 218:86P.

1973 Sawaki and Yagi. *J. Physiol.* (Lond.) 230:75.

1973 Cross. *J. Reprod. Fertil.* (Suppl.) 20:97.

Microelectrophoresis.

1969 Steiner, Ruf, and Albert. *Brain Res.* 12:74.

Induced axon degeneration as a marker for identifying hypothalamic projections at the electron-microscopic level.

1972 Raisman. In: *Median Eminence: Structure and Function.* Basel:Karger, p. 109.

Deafferentation: isolation of medical basal hypothalamus from the CNS in vivo by means of the Halász knife.

1969 Halász. In: *Frontiers in Neuroendocrinology.* Eds. Ganong and Martini. New York: Oxford University Press, p. 307.

Hypothalamo-hypophysiotropic area.

1962 Halász, Pupp, and Uhlarik. *J. Endocrinol.* 25:147.

Diffusion-free autoradiographic steroid uptake studies.

1968 Stumpf. *Science* 162:1001.

1968 Pfaff. *Endocrinology* 82:1149.

Portal bleeding.

1966 Worthington. *Nature* 210:710.

1967 Porter and Smith. *Endocrinology* 81:1182.

1968 Wyss et al. *J. Clin. Endocrinol. Metab.* 28:1824.

Isolated removal of individual hypothalamic nuclei.

1973   Palkovits. *Brain Res.* 59:444.

In vivo perfusion of isolated brain.

1971   White. In: *Fourth Karolinska Symposium*, p. 200.

Methodological Needs

Satisfactory immunohistochemistry specific techniques for studying tanycytes. Fiber optics for direct observation of intraventricular processes.

Contraceptive Possibilities

Inhibition of the release by the hypothalamus of gonadotropin releasing hormone.

Blocking the midcycle surge of hypothalamic luteinizing hormone releasing hormone.

Possible role for prostaglandin inhibitors in ovulation control.

I. LH and FSH Releasing Factors

Biological Processes: Significant Discoveries

Period before 1960

Recognition of environmental influence and interaction with brain to modulate sexual rhythms and cyclicity.

1936 Marshall. *Philos. Trans. R. Soc. Lond. (Biol.)* 226:423.

1942 Marshall. *Biol. Rev.* 17:68.

Induction of ovulation and pseudopregnancy in rats and rabbits through electrical stimulation of the head.

1936 Harris. *J. Physiol.* (Lond.) 88:361.

1936 Marshall and Verney. *J. Physiol.* (Lond.) 86:327.

Recognition of the involvement of the hypothalamic area in the induction of ovulation.

1937 Haterius and Derbyshyre. *Am. J. Physiol.* 119:324.

1937 Harris. *Proc. R. Soc. Lond. (Biol.)* 122:374.

Discovery of hypophysio-hypothalamic portal system.

1930 Popa and Fielding. *J. Anat.* 65:88.

1936 Wislocki and King. *Am. J. Anat.* 58:421.

Confirmation that the direction of blood flow is from hypothalamic to hypophyseal end in the portal system. This gave impetus to the possibility of humoral transmitters regulating hypophyseal function.

1947 Green and Harris. *J. Endocrinol.* 5:136.

1951 Barnett and Greep. *Science* 113:185.

1953 McConnell. *Anat. Rec.* 115:175.

1955 Worthington. *Bull. Johns Hopkins Hosp.* 97:347.

Stereotaxically inflicted lesions in precise areas in infundibulum of rats cause testicular and ovarian atrophy and cessation of estrous cycle.

1936 Cahane and Cahane. *Rev. Fr. Endocrinol.* 14:472.

Dissociation of centers controlling tonic and ovulatory surge of LH in guinea pig by stereotaxic lesions.

1942 Dey, Leninger, and Ranson. *Endocrinology* 30:323.

1953 Bogdanove and Halmi. *Endocrinology* 53:247. (rats)

The pituitary requires blood supply from the hypothalamic portal system for normal gonadotropic function. If it receives supply from systemic sources, as in pituitary grafts, only prolactin activity is seen.

1949 Harris. *Nature* 163:70.

1954 Everett. *Endocrinology* 54:685.

1958 Eckles, Ehni, and Kirschbaum. *Anat. Rec.* 130:295.

Development of concept of neurosecretion.

1940 Scharrer and Scharrer. *Res. Publ. Assoc. Res. Nerv. Ment. Dis.* 20:170.

Concept of neuroendocrines secreted into the portal system.

1947 Green and Harris. *J. Endocrinol.* 5:136.

1948 Harris. *J. Physiol.* 107:418.

Period 1960–1974

Demonstration of a luteinizing hormone releasing factor (LRF) in extracts of hypothalamic tissue that could stimulate the pituitary to release LH.

1960 McCann, Taleisnik, and Friedman. *Proc. Soc. Exp. Biol. Med.* 104:432.

1961 Harris. In: *Control of Ovulation*. Ed. Villee. New York: Pergamon Press, p. 56.

First demonstration of FSH releasing activity in rat hypothalamic extracts in vivo and in vitro.

1964 Igarashi and McCann. *Endocrinology* 74:440.

1966 Mittler and Meites. *Endocrinology* 78:500.

Purification of FSH releasing activity from hypothalamus using sephadex gel filtration, phenol extraction, and CMC chromatography.

1966 Schally et al. *Endocrinology* 79:1087.

1967 Schally et al. *Endocrinology* 81:822.

Development of assay systems for FSH releasing activity based on depletion of pituitary FSH activity in female and male rats.

1966 Schally et al. *Endocrinology* 79:1084.

Belief that FSH-RF and LRF activities are due to two different substances.

1960 McCann et al. *Proc. Soc. Exp. Biol. Med.* 104:432.

1963 Guillemin et al. *C. R. Acad. Sci.* [*D*] (Paris) 256:504.

1968 Schally et al. *Recent Prog. Horm. Res.* 24:497.

Questioning of the earlier belief that FSH-RF and LRF are different.

1970 White. In: *Mammalian Reproduction*. Eds. Gibian and Plotz. New York: Springer-Verlag, p. 84.

CHEMICAL STUDIES WITH RELEASING FACTORS

Initial extraction of LRF from ovine and bovine hypothalami and its partial purification using sephadex gel filtration and CMC column chromatography.

1964 Guillemin, Jutiz, and Sakiz. *C. R. Acad. Sci.* [*D*] (Paris) 256:504.

1964 Schally and Bowers. *Endocrinology* 75:312.

Further purification by rechromatography and column electrophoresis, ultrafiltration, and partition chromatography.

1967 Schally et al. *Endocrinology* 81:77.

1971 Amos et al. In: *Gonadotropins*. Eds. Saxena, Beling, and Gandy. New York: Wiley-Interscience, p. 26.

1971 Arimura, Kastin, and Schally. In: *Gonadotropins*, p. 32.

Because highly purified LRF is ninhydrin negative, yields high amino acid content upon hydrolysis, and is destroyed by proteolytic enzymes, it is a polypeptide.

1964 Guillemin. *Recent Prog. Horm. Res.* 20:89.

1964 Schally and Bowers. *Endocrinology* 75:608.

1965 McCann et al. *Excerpta Med. Found. Int. Cong. Ser.* 87:292.

Highly purified ovine LRF was obtained and described as a small peptide with p-Glu residue at -NH₂ terminus.

1970 Amos et al. *Proc. Endocrine Soc.*, June 1970, p. 61.

Isolation of a nonapeptide with LRF activity from porcine and ovine hypothalamus.

1971 Amos et al. *Biochem. Biophys. Res. Commun.* 44:205.

1971 Schally et al. *Biochem. Biophys. Res. Commun.* 43:393.

Discovery that porcine LRF is a decapeptide and determination of its amino acid sequence. Synthesis of a biologically active decapeptide.

1971 Matsuo et al. *Biochem. Biophys. Res. Commun.* 43:1334.

1971 Matsuo et al. *Biochem. Biophys. Res. Commun.* 45:922.

Discovery that ovine LRF is a decapeptide, identical to the porcine LRF.

1971 Burgus et al. *C. R. Acad. Sci. [D]* (Paris) 273:1611.

1972 Burgus et al. *Proc. Natl. Acad. Sci. USA* 69:278.

Synthesis of the decapeptide with full biological activity.

1971 Guillemin et al. *C. R. Acad. Sci. [D]* (Paris) 273:508.

It was proposed that LRF and FSH-RF activities are due to the same molecule, since the synthetic decapeptide stimulated release of both FSH and LH and inactivation of LRF is accompanied by loss of FSH-RF activity.

Microgram amounts of LRF cause discharge of LH and FSH in various species.

1971 Arimura et al. *Science* 174:511.

1972 Reeves et al. *J. Anim. Sci.* 35:84. (laboratory animals)

1972 Kastin et al. *J. Clin. Endocrinol. Metab.* 34:753. (humans)

1972 Yen et al. *J. Clin. Endocrinol. Metab.* 34:1108.

1972 Abe et al. *Endocrinol. Jap.* 19:77. (humans)

1973 Knobil et al. In: *Hypothalamic Hypophysiotropic Hormones: Clinical and Physiological Studies.* Eds. Gual and Rosemberg. Amsterdam: Excerpta Medica. (subhuman primates)

Synthesis of analogues which are up to fifty times more potent than natural LRF.

1973 Monahan et al. *Proc. Endocrine Soc.* June 1973.

1974 Fujino et al. *Biochem. Biophys. Res. Commun.* 57:1248.

Synthesis of analogues of LRF which act as partial agonists and as true competitive antagonists of LRF.

1972 Vale et al. *Science* 176:933.

Preparation and potency estimation of various analogues of LRF: structure-activity studies.

1974 Grant and Vale. *Curr. Top. Exp. Endocrinol.* 2:37.

BIOLOGICAL AND CLINICAL STUDIES

Development of a sensitive bioassay for LRF and its use to study LRF levels in human subjects.

1972 Malacara, Seyler, and Reichlin. *J. Clin. Endocrinol. Metab.* 34:271.

1973 Seyler and Reichlin. *J. Clin. Endocrinol. Metab.* 37:197.

1973 Seyler and Reichlin. *Endocrinology* 92:295.

Presence of LRF activity in human median eminence.

1964 Croxatto, Arrau, and Croxatto. *Nature* 204:584.

1967 Schally et al. *J. Clin. Endocrinol. Metab.* 27:755.

1970 Schally et al. *J. Clin. Endocrinol. Metab.* 31:291.

LRF from various sources stimulates LH release in humans.

1970 McCann et al. *Nature* 221:570.

1971 Kastin et al. *J. Clin. Endocrinol. Metab.* 32:287.

Normal women, postmenopausal women, women with secondary amenorrhea, and normal adult men respond to LRF.

1970 Kastin et al. *Am. J. Obstet. Gynecol.* 108:177.

1970 Kastin et al. *J. Clin. Endocrinol. Metab.* 31:689.

Ovine LRF increases plasma LH levels in men.

1971 Naftolin, Harris, and Bobrow. *Nature* 232:496.

Stimulation of spermatogenesis in humans by LRF.

1973 Schally et al. *Science* 179:341.

Induction of ovulation in humans with LRF.

1971 Kastin et al. *J. Clin. Endocrinol. Metab.* 33:980.

1972 Zarate et al. *Fertil. Steril.* 23:672.

Comprehensive review of effects of LRF in human subjects.

1972 Kastin, Gual, and Schally. *Recent Prog. Horm. Res.* 28:201.

1973 *Japanese Conference on LH/FSH Releasing Hormones, Tokyo.* Eds. Yamamura, Kurachi, and Kumahara. Tokyo: Daiichi Seiyaku Co.

Localization of LRF in hypothalamus and median eminence using immunofluorescent, immunoperoxidase techniques.

1974 Barry et al. *Endocrinology* 95:1416.

1974 Pelletier et al. *Endocrinology* 95:314.

1974 Zimmerman et al. *Endocrinology* 95:1.

Demonstration of a midcycle elevation in LRF in plasma of women, using radioimmunoassay.

1974 Arimura et al. *J. Clin. Endocrinol. Metab.* 38:510.

Rhesus monkeys are relatively insensitive to LRF given under various conditions.

1972 Ehara, Ryan, and Yen. *Contraception* 6:465.

Rhesus monkeys respond to LRF if given around midcycle, are less sensitive at other times. No clear dose-response relation could be established.

1972 McCormack and Spies. *Proc. Soc. Exp. Biol. Med.* 141:263.

1974 Ferrin et al. *J. Clin. Endocrinol. Metab.* 38:231.

Testicular atrophy in rabbits upon active immunization with LRF and blockade of ovulation by anti-LRF serum in rats.

1973 Schally et al. *J. Reprod. Fertil.* (Suppl.) 20:119.

1973 Fraser and Gunn. *Nature* 244:160.

1974 Arimura et al. *Endocrinology* 95:323.

Half-life, metabolism, and excretion of LRF.

1973 Redding et al. *J. Clin. Endocrinol. Metab.* 37:626.

Oral and intranasal administration of LRF raises serum LH.

1972 Amos et al. *J. Clin. Endocrinol. Metab.* 35:175.

1973 London et al. *J. Clin. Endocrinol. Metab.* 37:829.

Analysis of interaction of gonadal hormones with hypothalamic areas to modify pituitary function.

1971 Knobil et al. In: *Gonadotropins.* Eds. Saxena, Beling, and Gandy. New York: Wiley-Interscience, p. 72. (subhuman primates)

1973 Barraclough et al. *J. Reprod. Fertil.* (Suppl.) 20:161. (laboratory animals)

1974 Knobil. *Recent Prog. Horm. Res.* 30:1. (subhuman primates)

Mode of action of LRF involves binding of LRF to the pituitary (involves Ca^+) and activation of adenyl cyclase system.

1971 Justis et al. In: *Gonadotropins.* Eds. Saxena, Beling, and Gandy. New York: Wiley-Interscience, p. 64.

1973 Grant, Vale, and River. *Biochem. Biophys. Res. Commun.* 50:771.

LRF stimulates release of preformed gonadotropins; this is not inhibited by inhibitors of mRNA or protein synthesis.

1972 Baulieu. In: *Endocrinology.* Ed. Scow. Amsterdam: Excerpta Medica, p. 30.

Involvement of prostaglandins in LRF stimulation of LH secretion.

1971   Amos et al. *Proc. Int. Union Physiol. Sci.* 9:17.

1974   Ratner et al. *Prostaglandins* 5:165.

Release of LRF is under catecholaminergic control, and the evidence indicates a stimulatory role for norepinephrine and dopamine.

1974   McCann et al. *Adv. Neurol.* 5:435.

Role of catecholamines in hypothalamic function.

1971   Wurtman and Anton-Tay. In: *Frontiers in Neuroendocrinology.* Eds. Martini and Ganong. New York: Oxford University Press, p. 45.

Puberty: The LH response to LRF in the prepubertal child is much less than in the adult. However, the FSH response functions as in normal adult subjects.

1972   Roth et al. *J. Clin. Endocrinol. Metab.* 35:926.

1974   Franchimont et al. *Clin. Endocrinol.* 3:27.

Adults: Under comparable circumstances, the pattern of LH and FSH release in response to LRF in males is the same as in females.

1974   Besser and Mortimer. *J. Clin. Pathol.* 27:173.

Pregnancy: During and following pregnancy, the LRF response is severely curtailed.

1973   Zarate et al. *Am. J. Obstet. Gynecol.* 116:1211.

1974   LeMaire et al. *J. Clin. Endocrinol. Metab.* 38:916.

Steroids: Evidence that changes in pituitary sensitivity to LRF are dependent on the steroid milieu has been obtained using eugonadal, agonadal, and steroid treated subjects. Generally, castration and hypo- or agonadism are associated with augmented responses to LRF. However, response to FSH is disproportionately augmented.

Estrogen treatment of hypo- or agonadal subjects diminishes response to LRF and reverses the ratio to LH predominance. Initial response to LRF increases after estrogen treatment, followed by a decrease that is dose- and time-dependent.

1970   Central Actions of Estrogenic Hormones. In: *Advances in the Biosciences,* vol. 14. Ed. Raspe. New York: Pergamon Press.

1973   *Japanese Conference on LH/FSH Releasing Hormones.* Eds. Yamamura, Kurachi, and Kumahara. Tokyo: Daiichi Seiyaku Co.

In normally cycling women, the effects of estrogens are always positive. In men of any gonadal state the effect of estrogen is suppressive.

Progesterone has little effect on LRF response, or appears to augment estrogen effect.

Testosterone administration diminishes release of radioimmunoassayable FSH in response to LRF in men. The response of LH under these circumstances is variable and apparently dose-related.

Estrogen-progestin combinations may suppress the LRF response during chronic administration (contraception). During acute administration of chlormadinone-estradiol combination, augmentation of LRF response was noted. Medroxyprogesterone acetate, a long-acting progesterone analogue, does not suppress the LH response to LRF, but appeared to suppress the rise of FSH in women.

1973   *Hypothalamic Hypophysiotropic Hormones: Clinical and Physiological Studies.* Eds. Gual and Rosemberg. Amsterdam: Excerpta Medica.

1973   *Japanese Conference on LH/FSH Releasing Hormones.* Eds. Yamamura, Kurachi, and Kumahara. Tokyo: Daiichi Seiyaku Co.

Major Gaps in Our Knowledge

Radioimmunoassay for LRF is based on antibodies to the decapeptide and the results obtained are in conflict with biologic data. This methodology requires further refinement.

Ever since the development of the concept of releasing factors and isolation of FSH/LH-RF, the question of a separate FSH-RF has not been resolved. More work needs to be done in this area.

Though extensive studies have been conducted on the structure-activity relation of LRF, an effective analogue that can inhibit LRF activity and be clinically used is yet to be synthesized.

Study of the mechanism of action of releasing factors is in its infancy.

The role of gonadal hormones and other factors influencing various brain centers to effect optimal release of the releasing factor and the right combination of FSH and LH needs to be studied more extensively. In this regard, the pioneering work of Knobil and coworkers on the monkey, and Yen et al. on the human, has significantly added to our understanding of the interactions of steroids with the primate hypothalamus. Metabolism of steroids in these areas of the brain has been studied by:

1975   Naftolin et al. *Recent Prog. Horm. Res.* 31:295.

The possibility of using LRF chronically needs further exploration.

Modification or exhaustion of the pituitary gonadotropins by releasing hormone needs to be explored.

1973   Greep. *Reprod. Fertil.* (Suppl.) 18:1.

Preliminary investigations on the effects of LRF on spermatogenesis and induction of ovulation are under way. Detailed investigations in this area are necessary prior to clinical application of LRF for these purposes.

While progress has been made recently in the localization of LRF using immunofluorescent and immunoperoxidase techniques, opinion is still not unanimous in this area, and further investigations are needed.

Though a midcycle elevation in plasma LRF has been reported, thorough and extensive studies are still necessary. Possible enzymatic degradation of LRF in plasma needs to be investigated in detail.

There is a suggestion of episodic release of LRF in rats. More work is needed to confirm this in rats and in other species.

1974   Blake and Sawyer. *Endocrinology* 94:730.

The mode of action of brain monoamines in bringing about release of FSH/LH-RF needs to be investigated in greater detail.

II. Prolactin Releasing and Inhibiting Factors (PRF and PIF)

Biological Processes: Significant Discoveries

Period before 1960

Autografts of anterior pituitary to renal capsule secrete prolactin in increased quantities, suggesting removal from an inhibitory effect of hypothalamus.

1950 Desclin. *Ann. Endocrinol.* (Paris) 11:656.

1954 Everett. *Endocrinology* 54:685.

1956 Everett. *Endocrinology* 58:786.

1958 Nikitovitch-Weiner and Everett. *Endocrinology* 62:522.

The above observations are paralleled by observations that stalk transection in women with breast cancer leads to persistent lactation.

1958 Eckles, Ehni, and Kirschbaum. *Anat. Rec.* 130:295.

Galactorrhea follows treatment with tranquilizers in humans and animals.

1956 Kehl et al. *C. R. Soc. Biol.* (Paris) 150:981.

1956 Polishuk and Kulcsar. *J. Clin. Endocrinol. Metab.* 16:292. (humans)

Period 1960–1974

Evidence that secretion of prolactin is chronically inhibited by the hypothalamus (in vivo experiments using hypothalamic lesions, stalk section, pituitary transplantation, and CNS depressant drugs; in vitro experiments using pituitary-hypothalamus coincubation).

1963 Everett and Nikitovitch-Weiner. In: *Advances in Neuroendocrinology*. Ed. Nalbandov. Urbana, Ill.: University of Illinois Press, p. 289.

1963 Meites, Nicoll, and Talwalkar. In: *Advances in Neuroendocrinology*, p. 238.

1964 Bogdanove. *Vitam. Horm.* 20:205.

1966 Meites and Nicoll. *Ann. Rev. Physiol.* 28:57.

Inhibition of prolactin secretion is mediated by a neurohumoral agent.

1963 Talwalkar et al. *Am. J. Physiol.* 205:213.

Discovery of PIF in rat hypothalamic extracts.

1963 Danon et al. *Proc. Soc. Exp. Biol. Med.* 114:366.

1964 Gala and Reele. *Proc. Soc. Exp. Biol. Med.* 115:1030.

Confirmation of the presence of PIF in hypothalamic extracts of domestic animals.

1965 Schally et al. *Proc. Soc. Exp. Biol. Med.* 118:350.

In vivo inhibition of prolactin secretion by PIF.

1966 Kuroshima et al. *Endocrinology* 78:216.

1967 Arimura et al. *Endocrinology* 80:972.

Purification and separation of PIF by sephadex and CMC column chromatography and countercurrent distribution.

1968 Schally et al. *Recent Prog. Horm. Res.* 24:497.

1971 Schally et al. *J. Biol. Chem.* 246:7230.

1974 Schally et al. *Fed. Proc.* 33:237.

Concentration of PIF changes during estrous cycle.

1967 Sar and Meites. *Proc. Soc. Exp. Biol. Med.* 125:1018.

1970 Danon and Sulman. *Neuroendocrinology* 6:295.

PIF lowers plasma prolactin concentrations.

1970 Amenomori and Meites. *Proc. Soc. Exp. Biol. Med.* 143:492.

1970 Voogt and Meites. *Neuroendocrinology* 6:220.

1972 Arimura et al. *Endocrinology* 90:378.

Dopamine also reduces prolactin level in human plasma.

1971 Kleinberg et al. *J. Clin. Endocrinol. Metab.* 33:873.

Intraventricular infusion of dopamine reduces plasma prolactin levels in rats.

1971 Kamberi et al. *Endocrinology* 89:1042.

1974 Takahara et al. *Endocrinology* 95:462.

Presence of a PRF in the hypothalami of birds and mammals.

1968 Chen et al. *J. Gen. Comp. Endocrinol.* 11:489.

1970 Nicoll et al. In: *Hypophysiotropic Hormones of the Hypothalamus: Assay and Chemistry*. Ed. Meites. Baltimore: Williams & Wilkins, p. 115.

1973 Schally et al. *Science* 179:341.

Synthetic TRF is capable of releasing prolactin in rats, humans, and sheep.

1971 Bowers et al. *Biochem. Biophys. Res. Commun.* 45:1033.

1971 Jacobs et al. *J. Clin. Endocrinol. Metab.* 33:996. (humans)

1971 Tashjian et al. *Biochem. Biophys. Res. Commun.* 43:516.

1973 Convey et al. *Endocrinology* 92:421.

Orally administered TRF also stimulates prolactin release in men.

1974 Rabello, Snyder, and Utiger. *J. Clin. Endocrinol. Metab.* 39:571.

Ergot alkaloids inhibit prolactin release.

1971 Lu, Koch, and Meites. *Endocrinology* 89:229.

1971 Wuttke, Cassel, and Meites. *Endocrinology* 88:737.

Ergot derivatives such as ergocornine, 2-bromo-ergocryptine (CB-154), and compound 83636 are effective in suppressing prolactin secretion.

1971 Welsch et al. *Am. J. Physiol.* 221:1714. (animals)

1971 Lutterbeck, Pryor, Varga, and Venner. *Br. Med. J.* 3:228. (humans)

1971 Pasteels, Danguy, Frerotte, and Ectors. *Ann. Endocrinol.* (Paris) 32:188. (humans)

1974 Lemberger et al. *J. Clin. Endocrinol. Metab.* 39:579. (humans)

Suggestion that PIF is probably a small polypeptide.

1973 Schally, Arimura, and Kastin. *Science* 179:341.

Prolactin release inhibiting activity of hypothalamus can be totally accounted for by the endogenous catecholamines in the hypothalamus.

1974 Shaar and Clemens. *Endocrinology* 95:1202.

Major Gaps in Our Knowledge

Investigations on PRF and PIF are still in their infancy. Purification and elucidation of structure, mechanism of action, and control of their release need to be pursued.

While TRF has been shown to release prolactin, its physiological significance and possible use to modify prolactin release in health, disease, and various reproductive states need to be investigated.

Releasing Factors (continued)

Methodological Advances

Period before 1960

Development of remote-control method of electrical stimulation of the nervous system.

1934 Chaffe and Light. *Yale J. Biol. Med.* 7:83.

Application of the technique of stimulating hypothalamus through permanently implanted electrodes to study the effects on hormone secretion.

1947 Harris. *Philos. Trans. R. Soc. Lond. (Biol.)* 232:385.

Publication of a comprehensive map of hypothalamic areas controlling the secretion of the hormones of the anterior pituitary gland.

1955 Harris. *Bull. Johns Hopkins Hosp.* 97:358.

Development of techniques for isolation and purification of proteins and polypeptides, ion exchange chromatography, sephadex column chromatography, electrophoresis, amino acid analysis, Edman degradation of peptides, solid phase synthesis of peptides. Development of techniques of hypophysectomy, bioassays for FSH and LH, electron microscopy.

Period 1960–1974

Preparation of antisera to LRF and development of a radioimmunoassay to LRF.

1972 Schally, Justis, and Kerdelhue. In: *Hypothalamic Hypophysiotropic Hormones: Clinical and Physiological Studies.* Eds. Gual and Rosemberg. Amsterdam: Excerpta Medica.

1973 Arimura et al. *Endocrinology* 93:1092.

1973 Jeffacote et al. *J. Endocrinol.* 57:189.

Contraceptive Possibilities

Disruption of normal menstrual cycle is possible by administration of LRF during early follicular phase.

Induction of ovulation using exogenously administered LRF by a suitable, simple delivery means (intranasal) at or around midcycle would make the rhythm method safer and more reliable.

Inhibition of LRF activity during follicular, ovulatory, or luteal phase using structural analogues may be useful in controlling fertility in the human female.

Antibodies to LRF may prove to be useful in control of fertility in animals, if not in humans. The effects of such antibodies on libido, secondary sexual characters, and work potential of domestic animals should be carefully considered.

Gonadotropin Hormones

I. Luteinizing Hormone (LH)

Biological Processes: Significant Discoveries

Period before 1960

LH isolated from pituitary glands and shown to be a glycoprotein.

1940 Li et al. *Science* 92:355.

1940 Shedlovsky et al. *Science* 92:178.

1959 Squire and Li. *J. Biol. Chem.* 234:520.

1959 Ward et al. *Biochim. Biophys. Acta* 32:305.

LH required for androgen production and maintenance of normal Leydig cells.

1927 Smith and Engle. *Am. J. Anat.* 40:159.

1927 Zondek and Aschheim. *Arch. Gynaekol.* 130:1.

1930 Smith. *Am. J. Anat.* 45:205.

1936 Greep et al. *Anat. Rec.* 65:261.

1940 Fraenkel-Conrat et al. *Endocrinology* 27:809.

Indirectly (via androgen production) LH maintains partial spermatogenesis, secondary sex characteristics.

1937 Greep and Fevold. *Endocrinology* 21:611.

Androgen administration inhibits LH production (measured by effects on pituitary morphology).

1952 Nelson. *CIBA Found. Colloq. Endocrinol.* 4:271.

LH required for estrogen and progestin production as well as for maintenance of the ovarian interstitial cells.

1942 Greep et al. *Endocrinology* 30:635.

1942 Simpson et al. *Endocrinology* 30:969.

LH causes ovulation and induces the follicle to lutenize.

1942 Greep et al. *Endocrinology* 30:635.

1947 Hisaw. *Physiol. Rev.* 27:95.

LH secretion is periodic with peak in middle of cycle near point of ovulation.

1958 McArthur et al. *J. Clin. Endocrinol. Metab.* 18:460.

Estrogen inhibits (high dose) and stimulates (low dose) LH secretion.

1934 Hohlweg. *Klin. Wochenschr.* 13:92.

1940 Hellbaum and Greep. *Am. J. Anat.* 67:287.

1951 Funnell et al. *J. Clin. Endocrinol. Metab.* 11:98.

Secretion of LH inferred from pituitary content. For a discussion of validity of this procedure:

1961 Greep. In: *Sex and Internal Secretions.* Ed. Young. Baltimore: Williams & Wilkins, 3rd ed., ch. 4.

Cell types responsible for gonadotropin secretion distinguished from those secreting other hormones at light-microscopic level:

1954 Dawson. *Anat. Rec.* 120:810. (subhuman primates)

1956 Herlant. *Arch. Biol.* (Liege) 67:539.

and at electron-microscopic level by size and staining of intracellular granules:

1955 Farquhar and Rinehart. *Anat. Rec.* 121:394.

However, the cell types responsible specifically for LH secretion (as opposed to FSH secretion) are not clearly defined.

Gonadotropins are released in response to neural stimuli. (see table on Releasing Factors).

Developmental biology of anterior pituitary described.

1953 Pearse. *J. Pathol. Bacteriol.* 65:355.

1956 Jost and Tavernier. *C. R. Acad. Sci.* [D] (Paris) 243:1353.

Period 1960–1974

LH was highly purified from several sources, shown to be composed of two subunits (α and β), which were separable after mild treatments, and its amino acid sequence was determined. The α subunit is common to all glycoproteins (LH, FSH, TSH, hCG) sequenced to date. The β subunit confers the hormone-specific biological and immunological properties to the reconstituted molecule. Neither subunit alone is biologically active. The carbohydrate residues and the terminal amino acids of LH were shown to be heterogeneous, and as a result, most "pure" LH preparations are probably not a single species. Sheep LH served as the model hormone for these discoveries.

Preliminary investigation of the 3-dimensional structure showed that the shape of the intact molecule is different from the sum of the shapes of the subunits.

1972 Bewley et al. *Biochemistry* 11:932.

1973 Moudgal et al. *Recent Prog. Horm. Res.* 30:47.

1974 Ward. *Recent Prog. Horm. Res.* 29:333.

Sheep:

1971 Papkoff et al. *J. Am. Chem. Soc.* 93:1531.

1972 Lin et al. *J. Biol. Chem.* 247:4351.
Humans:

1969 Reichert et al. *J. Biol. Chem.* 244:5110.

1971 Pierce et al. *Recent Prog. Horm. Res.* 27:165.

1972 Sairam et al. *Biochem. Biophys. Res. Commun.* 48:530. (α chain)

1973 Shome and Parlow. *J. Clin. Endocrinol. Metab.* 36:618. (β chain)

Plasma levels of LH measured throughout the life cycles of several species, including humans. Levels of LH, FSH, estrogen, progestin, and androgen are correlated Midcycle peak of LH identified immunologically. Direct measurement showed that estradiol was both stimulatory and inhibitory to LH release. Estradiol is required for midcycle LH surge; antiestradiol blocks surge. Pituitary LH release occurs in a pulselike manner.

Humans:

1966 Midgley. *Endocrinology* 79:10.

1967 Faiman and Ryan. *J. Clin. Endocrinol. Metab.* 27:1711.

1967 Rosselin and Dolais. *Pierse Med.* 75:2027.

1968 Midgley and Jaffe. *J. Clin. Endocrinol. Metab.* 28:1699.

Subhuman Primates:

1971 Hotchkiss, Atkinson, and Knobil. *Endocrinology* 89:177.

1974 Knobil. *Recent Prog. Horm. Res.* 30:1.

Laboratory Animals:

1974 Neill and Smith. In: *Current Topics in Experimental Endocrinology.* Eds. James and Martini. New York: Academic Press, vol. 2, p. 73.

Kinetics of LH secretion established: LH levels are a direct reflection of LH secretion from the anterior pituitary as the metabolic clearance rate of LH is independent of the reproductive state of animal. Half-life of LH is about 20 minutes (human) and may be biphasic with a component of 200 minutes.

1968 Gay and Bogdanove. *Endocrinology* 82:359.

1968 Kohler et al. *J. Clin. Invest.* 47:38.

1969 Gay et al. *Proc. Soc. Exp. Biol. Med.* 130:1344.

1973 Rebar et al. *J. Clin. Endocrinol. Metab.* 37:917. (humans)

Gonadotropin Hormones (continued)

Episodic release of LH.

Ovariectomized Monkeys:

1970 Dierschke et al. *Endocrinology* 87:850.

Humans:

1972 Yen et al. *J. Clin. Endocrinol. Metab.* 34:671.

Electron-microscopic anatomy of pituitary correlated with granules. Isolated size of granules measured and hormone content demonstrated by assay. FSH and LH shown to exist in separate cells and in the same cell when measured by immunohistologic procedures but may be present in separate cells when the pituitary cells are cloned in vitro. It is assumed that synthesis of hormones and release follows pattern of enzyme synthesis in pancreatic tissue.

1964 Midgley. *Exp. Cell. Res.* 32:606. (humans)

1969 Costoff and McShan. *J. Cell. Biol.* 43:564.

1970 Nakane. *J. Histochem. Cytochem.* 18:9.

1971 Farquhar. *Mem. Soc. Endocrinol.* 19:79.

1973 Steinberger et al. *Endocrinology* 92:18.

1973 Schally et al. *Endocrinology* 93:893.

Role of LH in males and females evaluated in detail using antiserum to LH. LH is required for steroid synthesis (estrogen, progesterone, testosterone) during most phases of the reproductive life span; for ovulation; and for growth of testes and full follicle development. It is also required for pregnancy maintenance in the rat between days 8 and 12.

1963 Bourndel and Li. *Acta Endocrinol.* (Kbh.) 42:473.

1963 Hayashida. *J. Endocrinol.* 26:75.

1974 Moudgal et al. *Recent Prog. Horm. Res.* 30:47.

Mechanism of action of LH: earlier studies indicated that LH binds to gonadal cells and as a consequence promotes cyclic AMP formation by activating adenyl cyclase. The elevated cyclic AMP levels are thought to activate protein kinases by causing the dissociation of a regulatory subunit from a catalytic subunit. The activated protein kinases promote the phosphorylation and activation or inactivation of enzymes or proteins responsible for increased steroidogenesis, ovulation, or lutenization. Prostaglandins may play a role in this process. Recent studies indicate that only a very small fraction of the total receptors need to be occupied for maximal stimulation of steroidogenesis, but a much larger fraction must be filled before any cyclic AMP accumulation can be measured. It is not clear why there are so many "spare receptors," nor is it certain that cyclic AMP is the mediator of the LH effect. Since ovulation requires much larger concentrations of LH than steroidogenesis, presumably more receptors need to be filled for this effect to occur. Ovulation and lutenization require elevated levels of LH for only 2 hours. The LH (hCG) receptor has been isolated.

1966 Marsh et al. *J. Biol. Chem.* 241:543.

1966 Marsh and Savard. *Steroids* 8:133.

1970 Kuehl et al. *Biol. Reprod.* 2:154.

1971 Dufau et al. *Biochim. Biophys. Acta* 252:574.

1971 Lee and Ryan. *Endocrinology* 89:1515.

1972 Catt et al. *Nature* 239:280.

1973 Dufau et al. *J. Biol. Chem.* 248:6973.

1973 Gospodarowicz. *J. Biol. Chem.* 248:5042.

1973 Moudgal et al. *Recent Prog. Horm. Res.* 30:47.

1973 Moyle and Ramachandran. *Endocrinology* 93:127.

Major Gaps in Our Knowledge

Although the primary amino acid sequence of the LH molecule from several species is known, little is known about the 3-dimensional structure of the molecule. The disulfide bonds must be established, and the tertiary, quaternary, and carbohydrate structures must be identified to determine how the molecule interacts with its target organ receptors. Evidence suggests that the carbohydrate residues of hCG are not important for biological function; they are important for stabilization of the hormone in circulation. Similar studies must be carried out with LH.

1971 Dufau et al. *Biochem. Biophys. Res. Commun.* 44:1022.

1975 Moyle et al. *J. Biochem.* 250:9163.

Because LH is a heterogeneous glycoprotein and because the structure of the molecules in circulation has not been elucidated, there is a great need to confirm the plasma levels of LH as measured by radioimmunoassay, by bioassay using newly devised, highly sensitive assays. There is also a need to examine critically the most sensitive bioassays, including the "redox" assay. Further along this line, there is a requirement for a standardized universally accepted radioimmunoassay system for LH. This would necessitate distribution of a common well-characterized antiserum along with highly purified species-specific LH. Inasmuch as our understanding of reproductive function is increasingly dependent on reliable quantitative estimates of circulating hormone levels, the need to improve the assay systems is urgent.

1972 Chayen et al. *Clin. Endocrinol.* 1:219.

Although the kinetics of LH clearance rates have been studied, knowledge of how the hormone is metabolized is scanty. Inasmuch as circulating levels of LH are dependent on the addition and removal of hormones from the blood, knowledge of hormone metabolism is as important as determining secretion rates. It is also not clear that the circulating form(s) of LH are identical to that (those) in the pituitary. Some evidence is available suggesting that the circulating glycoprotein (FSH) may be different from that in the pituitary. Are similar differences found with LH? Are differences related to partial degradation products (i.e., hormones missing various carbohydrate or protein residues), or are the differences related to hormone function (i.e., hormones versus prohormones)?

Although it is well documented that FSH and LH are stored in granules in the anterior pituitary, the mechanisms of synthesis, storage, and release are not understood because the cell biology of the gonadotrophs has not been studied extensively. This is critically in need of development.

What are the roles of cyclic AMP, calcium, prostaglandins, protein kinases, and LRF in this process? Is there more than one gonadotropin releasing factor? How do steroids (estrogen) modulate LH and FSH secretion in response to LRF? It is not clear how FSH and LH are secreted at different rates throughout the estrous or menstrual cycle. At one time it was postulated that identification of the cell types responsible for LH and FSH storage would clarify this problem. As it appears that this question of differential release cannot be answered by further work in this area, new approaches must be taken to solve the perplexing dilemma of differential release. Better procedures are necessary for the study of LH and FSH secretion from pituitary cells in vitro.

Recent studies suggest that the nocturnal release of LH during sleep may play a key role in the development of puberty. This very ill-defined area should be studied further.

1947 Rubin et al. *Life Sci.* 14:1041.

The mechanism of action of LH in stimulating steroidogenesis and causing ovulation is still far from understood. Quantitative measurements of cellular processes must be made under physiological conditions. For example, cyclic AMP is postulated to mediate the LH stimulation of steroidogenesis. Nonetheless, LH can stimulate steroidogenesis without stimulating cyclic AMP accumulation if physiological levels of LH are added to Leydig cells. Much higher levels of LH must be used to stimulate cyclic AMP synthesis. The relationship between gonadotropin stimulation and prostaglandin synthesis is also unclear. Although a large number of studies have described binding of LH to its receptor and the receptor has even been "isolated," it is not known how the hormone-receptor complex mediates hormone action. Why are only 1% of the receptors filled for complete stimulation of steroidogenesis? Even less is known about the manner in which LH stimulates ovulation.

1973 Moyle and Ramachandran. *Endodocrinology* 93:127.

II. Follicle Stimulating Hormone (FSH)

Biological Processes: Significant Discoveries

Period before 1960

Fractionation of pituitary extracts led to the two-hormone concept of gonadal stimulation.

1931 Fevold, Hisaw, and Leonard. *Am. J. Physiol.* 97:291.

FSH was isolated and characterized first in 1942 and shown to be a glycoprotein in 1949.

1942 Chow et al. *Endocrinology* 30:650.

1949 Li et al. *Science* 109:445.

1956 Steelman et al. *Endocrinology* 59:256.

Basic physiology of FSH:

Female: Maturation of egg-bearing follicles.

1943 Casida et al. *Am. J. Vet. Res.* 4:76.

Female: Early onset of ovarian maturation.

1953 Simpson and Van Wagenen. *Anat. Rec.* 115:370.

Male: Testis growth by actions on the seminiferous tubles.

1937 Greep and Fevold. *Endocrinology* 21:611.

Male: FSH has no effect on Leydig cells.

1937 Greep and Fevold. *Endocrinology* 21:611.

Male: FSH may be responsible for multiplication of spermatogonia and spermatocytes. Androgens influence final stages of spermatogenesis.

1952 Nelson. *CIBA Found. Colloq. Endocrinol.* 4:271.

Female and Male: FSH does not increase estrogen or androgen production on its own, but is synergistic with LH.

1939 Fevold. *Anat. Rec.* (Suppl. 2) 73:19.

Estrogen inhibits FSH synthesis and secretion.

1937 Meyer and Hertz. *Am. J. Physiol.* 120:232. (males)

1940 Biddulph et al. *Endocrinology* 26:280. (females)

The concept of "inhibin," a substance from the seminiferous tubles that suppresses FSH.

1932 McCullagh. *Science* 76:1920.

1940 McCullagh and Schneider. *Endocrinology* 27:899.

Period 1960–1974

FSH was highly purified, shown to be composed of two subunits (α and β) that were separable by mild treatments, and its preliminary amino acid sequence determined. The α subunit was shown to be common to FSH, LH, TSH, and hCG. The β subunit was shown to confer the hormone-specific biological and immunological properties to the reconstituted molecule. Neither subunit alone has significant biological activity.

1974 Shome and Parlow. *J. Clin. Endocrinol. Metab.* 39:199. (human α chain)

1974 Shome and Parlow. *J. Clin. Endocrinol. Metab.* 39:203. (human β chain)

Plasma levels of FSH have been measured throughout the life cycles of several species, including humans. Correlations of LH, FSH, and steroid levels have been made. FSH shows a midcycle peak in the estrous and menstrual cycles corresponding to that of LH. The follicular levels are higher than luteal levels.

1967 Faiman and Ryan. *J. Clin. Endocrinol. Metab.* 27:1711. (humans)

1970 Ross et al. *Recent Prog. Horm. Res.* 26:1. (humans)

Kinetics of FSH secretion established; plasma FSH levels are a reflection of secretion from the pituitary. Half-life of FSH is longer than that of LH (up to 2 hours), possibly due to the fact that the FSH β chain had more carbohydrate than LH β chain.

1970 Gay et al. *Fed. Proc.* 29:1880.

Pulsatile FSH secretion.

1972 Yen et al. *J. Clin. Endocrinol. Metab.* 34:671.

Pattern of FSH storage and secretion (see LH section of this table)

Role of FSH in male and female reevaluated using antiserum to FSH: Anti-FSH has little effect on spermatogenesis and/or fertility.

1971 Monastinsky et al. *Fertil. Steril.* 22:318.

Anti-FSH reduces fertility in rabbits and in some rats, although effects are nowhere near as dramatic as those of anti-LH.

1969 Talcat and Laurence. *Endocrinology* 84:185.

Use of antiserum to FSH does not have the same dramatic effects as antiserum to LH (this observation was unexpected based on early data).

Mechanism of FSH action: recent evidence indicates that FSH binds to gonadal cells at different receptors than LH. After binding, FSH initiates the synthesis of cyclic AMP and activation of protein kinases similarly to LH. The biological activity of FSH is thought to depend on the phosphorylation of specific enzymes and proteins. In the ovary, FSH has been shown to increase LH (hCG) receptors. In the testis, FSH also induces the synthesis of androgen binding proteins. This protein, secreted by the Sertoli cells, helps to concentrate testosterone needed for sperm development.

1972 Dorrington et al. *Biochem. Biophys. Res. Commun.* 46:1523.

1973 Hansson et al. *Nature (New Biol.)* 246:56.

1974 Channing and Kammerman. *Biol. Reprod.* 10:179.

1974 Means et al. *J. Biol. Chem.* 249:1231.

1974 Zeleznik et al. *Endocrinology* 95:818.

Major Gaps in Our Knowledge

Although the preliminary structure of human FSH has been determined, it needs to be confirmed. The structure of other FSH molecules needs to be determined. The 3-dimensional structure needs to be established.

The reasoning in the similar subsection of the LH section of this table applies even more to FSH. Historically, the FSH radioimmunoassays have not been as reliable as the LH radioimmunoassays.

Although FSH clearance has been studied, we have no idea how the molecule is metabolized. Recently, differences between pituitary FSH and circulating FSH have been detected. Are these related to the metabolism of the hormone or are they related to the functional form of the molecule?

1973 Peckam et al. *Endocrinology* 90:1660.

1974 Bogdanove et al. *Endocrinol. Res. Commun.* 1:87.

Are there regulatory mechanisms of FSH production/secretion distinct from those in common with LH?

The failure of anti-FSH to disrupt fertility in females as does anti-LH is enigmatic. As FSH seems to be required to initiate follicular development, one would expect anti-FSH effects in the female to be very dramatic. The reasons for this failure need to explored. In addition, the role of FSH in the male is still controversial, even after the discovery of the fact that it binds specifically to Sertoli cells, promotes cyclic AMP synthesis, and stimulates androgen binding protein secretion. Although FSH can do these things, is FSH required for male fertility?

Although a start has been made on the mechanism of FSH action, the solution to this problem is very distant. Unlike the case with LH, there is no good way of attempting to correlate changes in function with changes in cellular metabolites. This is primarily because there is no easily quantified response to FSH available. Perhaps the solution to this problem will lie with measurements of androgen binding protein synthesis by Sertoli cells in vitro.

Are there specific FSH effects which are necessary for normal spermatogenesis?

The interest in "inhibin," postulated decades ago to suppress FSH levels in males, has been renewed. Preparations with "inhibin" activity have been isolated from rete testis:

1975 Setchell and Jacks. *J. Endocrinol.* 62(3):675.

From semen:

1975 Franchimont. *J. Steroid Biochem.* 6(6):1037.

From bull testis extracts:

1975 de Kretser et al. *Biol. Reprod.* 12:317.

More information is needed on the control mechanism of FSH levels.

III. Human Chorionic Gonadotropin (hCG)

Biological Processes: Significant Discoveries

Period before 1960

hCG was discovered in the urine of pregnant women but was not fully purified until 1960.

1913 Ashner. *Arch. Gynaekol.* 99:534.

1927 Aschheim and Zondek. *Klin. Wochenschr.* 6:1321.

The hCG content of blood, urine, and the placenta was measured throughout pregnancy. hCG levels were found to rise after 4 weeks, reach a peak between 8 and 12 weeks, and decline thereafter.

1928 Aschheim and Zondek. *Klin. Wochenschr.* 7:1453.

1952 Haskins and Sherman. *J. Clin. Endocrinol. Metab.* 12:385.

1953 Diczfalusy. *Acta Endocrinol.* (Kbh.) (Suppl.) 12:9.

1953 Loraine and Matthew. *J. Obstet. Gynecol.* 60:640.

hCG was also found to prolong the life of the primate corpus luteum.

1938 Browne and Venning. *Am. J. Physiol.* 123:26.

1944 Itisaw. *Yale J. Biol. Med.* 17:119.

hCG was thought to be secreted from the placenta; this was confirmed using placental cells in culture.

1938 Gey et al. *Science* 88:306.

Reports that hCG was secreted by the Langhans cells in the cytotrophoblast proved later to be incorrect.

Aside from the knowledge that hCG was mainly "LH-like" in character, little was known about its mode of action prior to 1960.

1939 Newton. In: *Sex and Internal Secretions.* Ed. Young. Baltimore: Williams & Wilkins, 2nd ed., p. 720.

1961 Zarrow. In: *Sex and Internal Secretions.* Ed. Young. Baltimore: Williams & Wilkins, 3rd ed., p. 892.

Period 1960–1974

Human chorionic gonadotropin was highly purified from pregnancy urine, trophoblastic tumors, or chorionic tissue and was shown to consist of two nonidentical subunits. The sequences of the carbohydrate residues and the amino acids in both subunits have been determined. The α subunit (MW = 14,000) is similar to that of LH, FSH, and TSH. The β subunit (MW = 24,000) confers the hormone-specific biological and immunological properties to the reconstituted molecule. hCGβ is similar but not identical to LHβ; it has four more carbohydrate chains and a C-terminal fragment of 30 more amino acids than LHβ. Neither subunit of hCG alone is active. In addition, the tertiary structure of the molecule cannot be explained by the tertiary structure of the subunits. "Pure" preparations of hCG have an activity of 10,000–20,000 IU/mg. This range is large, due primarily to small differences in the carbohydrate structures of various preparations; no preparation is likely to be a single species.

Purification.

1960 Got and Bourillon. *Biochim. Biophys. Acta* 42:502.

1960 Reisfeld and Hertz. *Biochim. Biophys. Acta* 43:540.

1970 Ashitaka. *Acta Obstet. Gynecol. Jap.* 17:124.

1971 Canfield et al. *Recent Prog. Horm. Res.* 27:121.

Structure (amino acid sequences).

1969 Bahl. *J. Biol. Chem.* 244:575.

1970 Swaminathan and Bahl. *Biochem. Biophys. Res. Commun.* 40:422.

1972 Bahl et al. *Biochem. Biophys. Res. Commun.* 48:416.

1973 Morgan et al. *Mol. Cell Biochem.* 2:97.

1974 Hilgenfeldt et al. *Hoppe Seylers Z. Physiol. Chem.* 355:1051.

Desialylation results in shortened half-life and reduced activity in vivo but no reduction in vitro.

1971 Van Hall et al. *Endocrinology* 88:456.

The apparent primary physiological role of hCG is to rescue the corpus luteum and thus maintain progesterone and estrogen secretion at sufficient levels to prevent menstruation. Administration of hCG to monkeys in the latter half of the luteal phase temporarily enchances progesterone secretion and prolongs the life of the luteal cells. hCG also stimulates estrogen secretion for longer times.

1972 Neill and Knobil. *Endocrinology* 90:34.

Antisera to hCG shorten the menstrual cycle.

1969 Schumberger and Anderer. *Acta Endocrinol.* (Kbh.) 60:861.

1971 Moudgal et al. *J. Clin. Endocrinol. Metab.* 32:579.

Further, an elevation of plasma chorionic gonadotropin levels shortly after implantation has been observed, and some evidence is available that the preimplanting blastocyst is synthesizing gonadotropins.

1973 Braustein et al. *Am. J. Obstet. Gynecol.* 115:447.

1973 Knobil. *Biol. Reprod.* 8:246.

1974 Haour and Saxena. *Science* 185:444.

hCG also inhibits the immune response and may be necessary to suppress lymphocyte function during and after implantation.

1973 Adcock et al. *Science* 181:845.

1973 Marz et al. *Biochem. Biophys. Res. Commun.* 55:717.

hCG may have some TSH-like activity.

1974 Nisula et al. *Biochem. Biophys. Res. Commun.* 59:86.

Unlike the pituitary gonadotropins, hCG is not stored in granules but is apparently secreted from cells in the synctiotrophoblast as it is synthesized.

1962 Midgley and Pierce. *J. Exp. Med.* 115:289.

1970 Dreskin et al. *J. Histochem. Cytochem.* 18:862.

Also unlike LH, hCG has a very long half-life in plasma.

1969 Yoshimi et al. *J. Clin. Endocrinol. Metab.* 29:225.

Some evidence exists that the secreted (plasma) form of hCG may be different from the placental form.

1969 Koide. *Proc. Soc. Exp. Biol. Med.* 132:1137.

Clones of cells from choriocarcinoma have been isolated which secrete hCG with differing immunological to biological potencies.

1971 Kohler et al. *Acta Endocrinol.* (Kbh.) 5153:137.

The binding of iodinated hCG to ovarian and testicular cells was found to have a very high affinity (10^{10} M^{-1}) due to the slow rate of dissociation of hCG from the receptor (hCG dissociates approximately 100 times slower than LH). Bound hCG remains intact. Once-bound hCG stimulates steroidogenesis and cyclic AMP accumulation similar to LH. The carbohydrate portions of hCG are necessary for the full biological potency: removal of these residues yields a molecule which binds well but fails to stimulate adenylate cyclase and inhibits the stimulatory effects of the intact molecule. Because hCG is stable to iodination, it has been used to characterize the LH receptor. Less than 1% of the cellular receptors need to be filled before maximal response to hCG is observed.

Binding.

1967 Lunenfeld and Eshkol. *Vitam. Horm.* 25:137.

1969 DeKretser et al. *Endocrinology* 88:332.

1971 Lee and Ryan. *Endocrinology* 89:1515.

1972 Catt et al. *Biochim. Biophys. Acta* 279:194.

Solubilized receptors.

1973 Dufau et al. *J. Biol. Chem.* 248:6973.

1973 Gospodarowicz. *J. Biol. Chem.* 248:5042.

1974 Charreau et al. *J. Biol. Chem.* 249:4189.

Carbohydrates.

1975 Moyle et al. *J. Biol. Chem.* 250:9163.

Steroidogenesis and cyclic AMP.

1971 Dufau et al. *Biochim. Biophys. Acta* 252:574.

1975 Moyle et al. *J. Biol. Chem.* 250:9163.

Spare receptors.

1972 Catt et al. *Nature* 239:280.

Major Gaps in Our Knowledge

The primary structure of hCG has been nearly completed; however, the chemistry of similar gonadotropins in nonhumans is not yet complete. Knowledge of this structure will be important for the development of animals models. Also, as in the case of the other gonadotropins, little is known about the 3-dimensional structure of hCG. The search for hCG inhibitors will proceed rationally only when the tertiary structure of the molecule is known relative to the biologically active site(s) on the molecule.

Even though evidence exists to show that hCG can "rescue" the corpus luteum, more work needs to be carried out to make this convincing for the human. In addition, the effects of hCG on the immunological system need clarification as to their physiological relevance. To utilize effectively the potential of anti-hCG in controlling fertility, we must better understand the physiological role of hCG.

We need to understand the significance of the TSH-like activity in hCG for reproductive biology.

The factors controlling hCG secretion are unknown. If a method were known which prevented the synthesis and/or secretion of hCG, which is apparently necessary for pregnancy, then a method for the prevention of pregnancy might become available.

Even though the mechanism of action of hCG has been actively pursued, it has remained mysterious. Efforts should be directed to determine what happens after hCG binds to its receptor. The roles of cyclic AMP and protein kinases in this process need clarification. The effects of hCG analogues need to be tested, in the hope of finding inactive materials which have the same affinity for the receptors. Any nonfunctional analogue which can bind to the cells with similar affinity as hCG will be a very useful specific antagonist likely to block fertility.

Gonadotropin Hormones (continued)

Methodological Advances

Period before 1960

Development of techniques used in isolation, purification, and characterization of proteins.

Sephadex:

1959 Porath and Flodin. *Nature* 183:1657.

Ion exchange chromatography:

1956 Peterson and Sober. *J. Am. Chem. Soc.* 78:751.

Alcohol precipitation:

1946 Cohn et al. *J. Am. Chem. Soc.* 68:459.

Hydroxylapatite chromatography:

1951 Swingle and Tiselius. *Biochem. J.* 48:171.

Electrophoresis (paper):

1951 Kunkel and Tiselius. *J. Gen. Physiol.* 35:89.

Centrifugation:

1937 Tiselius et al. *Nature* 140:848.

Sequencing procedures:

1945 Sanger. *Biochem. J.* 39:507.

1950 Edman. *Acta Chem. Scand.* 4:283.

Kaolin procedure for purifying human urinary gonadotropins from urine:

1955 Albert. *Proc. Staff Meet. Mayo Clin.* 30:552.

Development of procedures for hypophysectomy.

1927 Smith. *JAMA* 88:158.

Development of procedures for histological examination of anterior pituitary.

1956 Herlant. *Arch. Biol.* (Liege) 67:89.

Development of electron-microscopic techniques.

1952 Palade. *Anat. Rec.* 114:427.

1954 Farquhar and Rinehart. *Endocrinology* 54:516.

Designation of the first international gonadotropin standard.

1958 Albert et al. *J. Clin. Endocrinol. Metab.* 18:1117.

Development of procedures for bioassaying LH.

1941 Greep et al. *Proc. Soc. Exp. Biol. Med.* 46:644.

1942 Simpson et al. *Endocrinology* 30:969.

Development of procedures for extracting LH.

1940 Li et al. *Science* 92:355.

1940 Shedlovsky et al. *Science* 92:178.

Development of bioassays for FSH.

1953 Steelman and Pohley. *Endocrinology* 53:604.

Bioassay for hCG—used for detection of pregnancies at early stages.

1928 Aschheim and Zondek. *Klin. Wochenschr.* 7:1453. (mice)

1931 Friedman and Lapham. *Am. J. Obstet. Gynecol.* 21:405. (rabbits)

1934 Shapiro and Zwarenstein. *Nature* 133:762. (amphibians)

Ovarian weight augmentation in immature females in presence of hCG.

1955 Brown. *J. Endocrinol.* 13:59. ·

Period 1960–1974

Improvement of protein sequencing procedures.

1967 Edman and Begg. *Eur. J. Bioch.* 1:80.

Use of CNBR for peptide cleavage.

1962 Gross and Witkip. *J. Biol. Chem.* 237:1856.

Preparation of cell suspensions for anterior pituitary and methods for culturing cells improved.

1971 Sayers et al. *Acta Endocrinol.* (Kbh.) *Suppl.* 153:11.

LH

Development of procedures to purify LH in quantities sufficient to do amino acid sequencing.

1962 Squire et al. *Biochemistry* 1:412.

1963 Reichert and Parlow. *Endocrinology* 73:285. (humans)

Procedures for dissociating LH and isolation of subunits.

1964 Li and Starman. *Nature* 202:291.

1967 Papkoff and Samy. *Biochim. Biophys. Acta* 147:175.

Improvements in LH bioassays.

1961 Parlow. In: *Human Pituitary Gonadotropins.* Ed. Albert. Springfield: Thomas, p. 300.

1972 Catt et al. *J. Clin. Endocrinol. Metab.* 34:123.

1972 Dufau et al. *Endocrinology* 90:1032.

Development of procedures for labeling proteins and thereafter LH radioimmunoassays.

1963 Greenwood et al. *Biochem. J.* 89:114.

1966 Midgley. *Endocrinology* 79:10.

Development of procedures for immunization of rabbits with LH.

1971 Vaitukaitis et al. *J. Clin. Endocrinol. Metab.* 33:988.

1974 Moudgal et al. *Recent Prog. Horm. Res.* 30:47.

Procedures for isolating LH by affinity chromatography.

1972 Gospodarowicz. *J. Biol. Chem.* 247:6491.

Electrophoresis in polyacrylamide gels.

1964 Ornstein. *Ann. N.Y. Acad. Sci.* 121:321.

Distribution of NIH-LH for general study (1959).

1968 Rosemberg. In: *Gonadotropins.* Ed. Rosemberg. Los Altos: Geron-X, p. 383.

FSH

Development of procedures to purify FSH.

1970 Papkoff and Ekblad. *Biochem. Biophys. Res. Commun.* 40:614.

1974 Parlow and Shome. *J. Clin. Endocrinol. Metab.* 39:195. (humans)

Separation of FSH subunits.

1970 Papkoff and Ekblad. *Biochem. Biophys. Res. Commun.* 40:614.

Development of FSH radioimmunoassay.

1967 Faiman and Ryan. *J. Clin. Endocrinol. Metab.* 27:1711.

1970 Gay et al. *Fed. Proc.* 29:1880.

hCG

Radioimmunoassay for hCG.

1962 Brody and Carlstrom. *J. Clin. Endocrinol. Metab.* 22:564.

Use of the β subunit for preparation of antisera to improve radioimmunoassay specificity and avoid LH cross-reaction.

1972 Rayford et al. *Endocrinology* 91:144.

Improvements in hCG iodination for radioimmunoassay.

1966 Midgley. *Endocrinology* 79:10.

Radioligand receptor assay.

1972 Catt et al. *J. Clin. Endocrinol. Metab.* 34:123.

Bioassay of hCG in cell suspensions.

1972 Dufau et al. *Endocrinology* 90:1032.

Development of procedures for characterization and removal of the sugar residues from hCG.

1969 Bahl. *J. Biol. Chem.* 244:575.

Development of procedures for cloning choriocarcinoma cells in vitro.

1971 Kohler et al. *Acta Endocrinol.* (Kbh.) 5153:137.

Methodological Needs

Isolated cell suspensions have proven to be a powerful tool for studying endocrine cell biology. The full value of this procedure cannot be realized until methods are developed for separation of the pituitary cells according to their functions (i.e., hormone content).

In addition to separating cells according to function, methods should be developed to allow analysis of single cells. It is unlikely that all cells in a related population are identical. For example, some cells may have more LRF receptors than others and would be more likely to respond to stimulation. Other cells may contain hormone granules but may not be able to respond to LRF. If we know why potentially active cells are responsive or unresponsive, we would have a very useful tool for developing new contraceptives.

Procedures for radiolabeling LH and LRF to very high specific activity without altering their biological activities would be extremely useful. It is not clear how individual cells and/or individual clusters of receptors bind the hormones. Current measurements allow only an average value to be determined. In addition, the present labeling procedures for LH give specific activity as an average value (i.e., one mole of iodine per mole of hormone). It is almost certain that the label is not evenly distributed 1:1 with each individual molecule. Procedures are required to remove nonlabeled material from labeled material.

New methods for bioassaying hormones should be developed and tested. The redox assay shows potential here.

1972 Chayen. *Clin. Endocrinol.* (Oxford) 1:219.

Since the glycoprotein hormones are quite heterogeneous — due principally to differences in carbohydrate content — better methods should be developed to purify and analyze them. This is true for all glycoprotein molecules, and any new techniques for dealing with this difficult class of compounds would be welcomed.

FSH

Procedures are needed for measuring FSH effects on end-product synthesis in vitro.

Structural and biological methods are needed which can be used to determine the active site in the FSH molecule.

Analytical procedures are needed for studying biochemical effects of FSH in the germinal epithelium (e.g., culture techniques, enzyme assays, protein analysis).

Polypeptide synthesis techniques suitable for large peptides or small proteins are needed.

hCG

We need improved methods for studying luteal function related to implantation in primates, so that the role of hCG (MCG) can be defined precisely. To do this, we need to purify and characterize nonhuman chorionic gonadotropins to the same degree as hCG. Then we will be able to prepare specific antisera (using the β subunit) so that we can measure the precise time of chorionic gonadotropin secretion; study the biochemistry of chorionic gonadotropin secretion in vitro at a time when the placenta is just beginning to develop rather than after implantation has already occurred; and determine the best time to terminate pregnancy.

To facilitate purification of chorionic gonadotropins, procedures of affinity chromatography need to be improved.

Contraceptive Methods
Period before 1960

Inhibition of spermatogenesis by androgen administration (due to LH).

1940 Heckel. *J. Urol.* 43:286.

1941 Selye and Friedman. *Endocrinology* 28:129.

Period 1960–1974

Inhibition of the midcycle LH surge: early birth control pills and estrogens. Reviews:

1965 Pincus. In: *The Control of Fertility.* New York: Academic Press, p. 59.

1972 Haller. In: *Hormonal Contraception.* Los Altos, Calif.: Geron-X, ch. 2.

Possibilities for the Future
LH

One of the most satisfactory methods of contraception developed to date relies on altering the levels of circulating gonadotropins. It seems reasonable to follow in this direction by utilizing other approaches:

1. A chemical derivative of LRF may act only on the pituitary gonadotropin to block LH release required for ovulation.

2. Knowledge of how individual cells secrete or fail to secrete LH in response to LRF may enable us to develop procedures for converting responsive cells into nonresponsive cells.

3. At the other end of the picture, it is likely that derivatives of LH will be found which inhibit the effect of the hormone on cell function. To date, this process looks promising, in that chemically modified hCG molecules are inhibitors of the effects of hCG on cyclic AMP accumulation (Moyle and Bahl, unpublished observations). Inasmuch as more LH binding must be required for ovulation to occur than for steroidogenesis (only 1% of the receptors are used in the latter process), development of inactive LH derivatives which remained bound to 90% of the specific target cell receptors would inhibit ovulation but probably not alter normal steroidogenesis.

4. It is becoming clear that the carbohydrate residues on LH play a role in transport of the hormone to the cell. If a procedure could be developed in which the sugar residues were not attached to the hormone, then sufficient hormone might not get to the ovary to promote ovulation.

FSH

The following possibilities should be investigated:

Blocking of FSH binding to Sertoli cells or other sites that are currently unknown.

Specific inhibition of secretion of FSH, without change in LH secretion.

Inhibition of the FSH active site within the molecule by using peptide or protein analogues or inhibitors. However, generation or administration of anti-FSH antibody to prevent its action is not a feasible approach in the human for fertility control because of compensatory FSH secretion by the pituitary and the large amounts of antibody necessary to neutralize FSH activity.

Interference with intracellular processes of the Sertoli cell or germ cell, which represent specific actions of FSH that are necessary for normal sperm production.

Administration of specific inhibitor of FSH secretion, such as "inhibin."

Blocking of FSH cellular site of action by a peptide or protein analogue.

Blocking of specific cellular effects of FSH critical for normal sperm production and/or function.

hCG

Although the relationship between the production of hCG and rescue of the corpus luteum is not completely proven, it is certainly suggested. Thus, any method of interfering with hCG secretion during or shortly after implantation will effectively terminate pregnancy. One approach to this end is by active hCG immunization. With all the conceivable pitfalls of this procedure, however, other approaches should be undertaken. These will be clear only after we learn what signals and controls hCG synthesis and its consequent secretion.

Antibodies to hCGβ are being developed as an approach to fertility control.

1974   Talwar. *Karolinska Symp*. 7:370.

Prolactin

Biological Processes: Significant Discoveries

Period before 1960

Hormone discovered (later named prolactin) that induces milk secretion in rabbits.

1928 Stricker and Grueter. *C. R. Soc. Biol. [D]* (Paris) 99:1978.

Prolactin partially purified and crystallized; not found in the human pituitary.

1937 White et al. *Science* 86:82.

Prolactin maintains corpus luteum function and early pregnancy in the rat but probably not in the monkey or human; role in male unclear.

1941 Astwood. *Endocrinology* 28:309.

1944 Hisaw. *Yale J. Biol. Med.* 17:119.

1949 Holstrom and Jones. *Am. J. Obstet. Gynecol.* 58:308. (humans)

Lactation stimulates prolactin secretion as measured in urine.

1933 Lyons and Page. *Proc. Soc. Exp. Biol. Med.* 31:303.

Cell types producing prolactin identified in the anterior pituitary as acidophiles, containing secretory granules 600 μ or larger in diameter; prolactin-secreting cell different from cells producing the other pituitary hormones.

1933 Wolfe and Cleveland. *Anat. Rec.* 55:233.

1957 Hedinger and Farquhar. *Schweiz. Z. Allg. Pathol.* 20:766.

Relationship of prolactin secretion to hypothalamic control recognized, and the connection of the pituitary to the median eminence inhibits prolactin secretion.

1954 Everett. *Endocrinology* 54:685.

Grafted pituitary disrupts normal estrous cycles in mice; prolactin induces pseudopregnancy and delays cycles.

1954 Mulbach and Boot. *Cancer Res.* 19:492.

Period 1960–1974

Human prolactin identified and partially sequenced. Ovine prolactin sequenced. Large degree of homology with human placental lactogen and human growth hormone.

1969 Li et al. *Nature* 224:695.

1970 Li et al. *Arch. Biochem. Biophys.* 141:705.

1971 Guyda and Friesen. *Biochem. Biophys. Res. Commun.* 42:1068.

1973 Niall et al. *Recent Prog. Horm. Res.* 29:387.

Prolactin levels measured in several species, including humans. Average level in mature females is slightly higher than in mature males and immature animals. Secretion is pulsatile at 30 minute intervals. Plasma levels show diurnal fluctuation with a maximum 6–8 hours after onset of sleep. Prolactin levels remain elevated for about 3 months postpartum only in women who breast feed. Prolactin surge is simultaneous with LH and FSH surge at ovulation.

1972 Frantz et al. *Recent Prog. Horm. Res.* 28:527.

1972 Meites et al. *Recent Prog. Horm. Res.* 28:471.

1973 Friesen and Hwang. *Annu. Rev. Med.* 24:251.

1974 Neill and Smith. In: *Current Topics in Experimental Endocrinology.* Eds. James and Martini. New York: Academic Press, vol. 2, p. 73.

Secretory kinetics: half-life of prolactin about 15–20 minutes. Estradiol increases prolactin secretion. TRH increases prolactin secretion at same time it increases THS secretion. PIF (not yet isolated) decreases prolactin secretion.

1970 Neill. *Endocrinology* 87:1192.

1971 Bowers et al. *Biochem. Biophys. Res. Commun.* 45:1033.

1971 Tashjian et al. *Biochem. Biophys. Res. Commun.* 43:516.

1972 Freeman and Neill. *Endocrinology* 90:292.

1972 L'Hermite et al. In: *4th Tenovus Workshop on Prolactin and Carcinogenesis,* Cardiff, Wales. Eds. Griffiths and Boyns, p. 81. (Humans)

Prolactin secreting cells identified unequivocally in man by staining, electron microscopy, and immunofluorescent procedures.

1967 Herlant and Pasteels. *Methods Achiev. Exp. Pathol.* 3:250.

1970 Herbert and Hayashida. *Science* 169:378.

1972 Pasteels et al. *J. Clin. Endocrinol. Metab.* 34:959.

Biological role of prolactin reinvestigated: it is found to be luteotropic, as well as luteolytic, depending on time of administration.

1966 Malven and Sawyer. *Endocrinology* 78:1259.

1966 Malven and Sawyer. *Endocrinology* 79:268.

Ergot alkaloids (ergocornine, ergocryptine) found to inhibit prolactin secretion and, as a consequence, terminate early pregnancy in the rat.

1968 Kisch and Shelesnyak. *J. Reprod. Fertil.* 15:401.

1971 Lu et al. *Endocrinology* 89:229.

Mechanism of prolactin action: prolactin receptors found in several tissues — receptor concentration influenced by hormonal state of animal. Subsequent steps in action are unknown but prolactin thought to modify action of other hormones.

1973 Turkington. *Recent Prog. Horm. Res.* 29:417.

1974 Kelly et al. *Endocrinology* 95:532.

1974 Posner et al. *Endocrinology* 95:521.

1974 Posner et al. *Proc. Natl. Acad. Sci. USA* 71:2407.

Major Gaps in Our Knowledge

Although structural studies on human prolactin have begun, the amino acid sequence of the molecule has not been completed. This needs to be done. In addition, the tertiary structure of the molecule needs to be investigated. It would also be desirable to find short fragments of the molecule having biological activity. The importance of other forms of prolactin needs clarification.

The measurements of prolactin have been made with the RIA. This gives a picture of the immunological activity corresponding to circulating prolactin levels. The radioligand receptor assay should be applied to many of these studies to confirm the levels from the point of view of bioassay.

Biological effects of prolactin upon spermatogenesis and prostate are unknown.

Biological role of prolactin in any androgen responsive tissue remains to be elucidated.

Although estradiol and TRF have been shown to stimulate prolactin release, the relative contributions of these compounds to the physiologically important release of prolactin need further study (especially with TRF). Prolactin inhibitory factor (PIF) needs identification.

Although the cell types responsible for prolactin secretion have been identified, virtually nothing is known about their cell biology. This needs to be studied further in purified cell suspensions in vitro.

After decades of study, the biological role of prolactin in the reproductive process (exclusive of lactation) is very unclear. Under what conditions is prolactin luteotropic or luteolytic in humans? Why are prolactin antisera so ineffective in blocking fertility even in the rat? Are the ergot alkaloids altering pituitary release or biological function of other hormones? What antigonadotropic role does prolactin play? The answer to this last question may provide the basis for a new contraceptive.

Prolactin (continued)

Although prolactin binding sites have been found, practically nothing is known about the mechanism of action. This area needs careful exploration. It is also important to determine the physiological relevance of the binding sites to the mechanism of action. Just because a tissue binds a hormone, this does not mean that it responds to the hormone.

Methodological Advances

Period before 1960

Bioassays for prolactin:

Crop sac:

1933   Riddle et al. *Am J. Physiol.* 105:191.

Appearance of deciduoma:

1953   Astwood. *Endocrinology* 5:74.

Maintenance of early gestation:

1941   Cutuly. *Proc. Soc. Exp. Biol. Med.* 48:315.

For other assays and protein chemistry advances, see the table on Gonadotropin Hormones.

Period 1960–1974

Development of affinity chromatography.

1968   Cuatrecasas et al. *Proc. Natl. Acad. Sci. USA* 61:636.

Application of affinity chromatography to purify human prolactin from amniotic fluid.

1971   Greyda and Friesen. *Biochem. Biophys. Res. Commun.* 42:1068.

Development of the ''sequenator'' for determining amino acid sequences.

1967   Edman and Begg. *Eur. J. Biochem.* 1:80.

Development of prolactin RIA.

1971   Bryant et al. *Hormones* 2:129.

1971   Hwang et al. *Proc. Natl. Acad. Sci. USA* 68:1902.

Development of prolactin radioligand assay.

1973   Shiu et al. *Science* 180:968.

Development of sensitive prolactin bioassays.

1971   Kleinberg and Frantz. *J. Clin. Invest.* 50:1557.

In vitro culturing procedures for mammary tissue.

1967   Turkington and Topper. *Endocrinology* 80:329.

Methodological Needs

Development of more sensitive prolactin bioassays.

Better methods for blocking prolactin secretion so that the effects of prolactin on the reproductive process can be studied.

Procedures for isolating the prolactin secreting pituitary cells.

Techniques for studying the action of prolactin upon Leydig cells, tubular cells (Sertoli and germinal epithelium), prostate, and male breast.

Contraceptive Possibilities

Some evidence indicates that prolactin may play an antigonadotropic role in humans. In males, high levels of prolactin are correlated with decreased testosterone levels and loss of libido. In females, the short period of high prolactin levels associated with breast feeding are correlated with amenorrhea.

Inhibition of secretion: PIF (not yet identified or available) would be valuable in fertility control if a critical role of prolactin could be demonstrated.

Chronic stimulation of high levels of prolactin, as by TRF, might be valuable if it shows an inhibitory effect on spermatogenesis, sperm maturation, or sperm transport without inhibition of factors critical for sexual function and if chronic hyperprolactinemia is without detrimental effects upon breast and prostate. Similarly, the chronic administration of prolactin may have the advantage of being unassociated with any CNS effects of chronic TRH administration.

I. Gonadotropin Binding

Biological Processes: Significant Discoveries

Period before 1960

Proposition that protein hormone (insulin) localized on cell membrane initiates the regulation of its metabolic effects.

1949 Levine et al. *J. Biol. Chem.* 179:985.

First evidence that hormone binding to hormonesensitive tissues leads to specific metabolic effects (insulin on various insulin-sensitive tissues).

1949 Stadie et al. *Am. J. Med. Sci.* 218:265.

1952 Haugaard and Marsh. *J. Biol. Chem.* 194:33.

1952 Hills and Stadie. *J. Biol. Chem.* 194:25.

Period 1960–1974

Evidence that specific protein hormone (insulin) receptors are located on the cell surface: enzymes used to destroy insulin responsiveness of cells.

1966 Kuo et al. *Life Sci.* 5:2257.

1969 Fain et al. *J. Biol.* 244.

1969 Kono. *J. Biol. Chem.* 244:1772.

1969 Kono. *J. Biol. Chem.* 244:5777.

Localization of gonodotropin receptors on cell surface (testes). Solubilization of receptors with retention of hormonal specificity and high binding affinity; affinity constants determined.

1972 Dufau et al. *Proc. Natl. Acad. Sci. USA* 69:2414.

1972 Lerdenberger and Rochect. *Endocrinology* 91:901.

1973 Catt et al. *J. Clin. Endocrinol. Metab.* 36:73.

1973 Dufau and Catt. *Nature (New Biol.)* 242:246.

Ovary shown to concentrate ^{125}I-labeled hCG and LH, inferring that binding sites for the hormones exist at target organs such as the ovary.

1966 Eshkol. *Recent Research on Gonadotropic*

Hormones. Edinburgh: Livingstone, Ltd., p. 202.

1968 Espland et al. In: *Gonadotropins.* Ed. Rosemberg. Los Altos: Geron-X, p. 177. (rats)

1968 Naftolin et al. In: *Gonadotropins,* p. 373. (human LH RIA)

Characteristics of gonadotropins bound to gonadal tissue found to vary with age and functional and maturational state of gonadal tissue.

1971 Lee and Ryan. *Endocrinology* 89:1515.

1972 Figarova et al. *Endocrinol. Exp.* (Bratisl.) 6:85.

1972 Presl et al. *J. Endocrinol.* 52:585.

1972 Schombert and Tyney. *Biol. Reprod.* 7:127.

1973 Channing and Kammerman. *Endocrinology* 92:531.

1973 Channing and Kammerman. *Endocrinology* 93:1035.

1973 Lee et al. *J. Clin. Endocrinol. Metab.* 36:148.

1973 Midgley. In: *Receptors for Reproductive Hormones.* Eds. O'Malley and Means. New York: Plenum, p. 365.

The number of receptors for LH and hCG appears to increase as the follicle increases in size. The number of receptors is thought to be a function of a priming or maturational effect of FSH on the growing follicle, not all sites on the cells from the largest follicles being occupied (porcine).

1973 Channing. *Excerpta Medica Int. Cong. Ser.* 273:915.

1974 Channing and Kammerman. *Biol. Reprod.* 10:179.

FSH appears to be a factor in integrating the development of the binding sites in ovarian cells to LH (hCG). FSH induced hCG binding localized in the theca and granulosa cells.

1972 Figarova et al. *Endocrinol. Exp.* (Bratisl.) 6:85.

1973 Zeleznik and Midgley. *Program 55th Annual Meeting Endocrine Soc,* Chicago, Ill. (Abstr. 41).

1974 Zeleznick, Midgley, and Reichert. *Endocrinology* 95:818.

In vivo and in vitro studies of LH (hCG) binding in ovarian tissue have shown that binding of these hormones is extensive in luteal tissue and probably localized at the cell membrane. The binding is specific with high affinity for LH and hCG. Binding affinity shown to be a saturable process dependent on time, pH, and salt concentration. Binding requires native gonadotropin and neither binding nor competition for binding occurs with subunits of LH or hCG (rat, monkey, human).

1971 Lee and Ryan. *Endocrinology* 89:1515.

1972 Lee and Ryan. *Proc. Natl. Acad. Sci. USA* 69:3520.

1973 Ashitaka et al. *Proc. Soc. Exp. Biol. Med.* 142:395.

1973 Lee and Ryan. *J. Clin. Endocrinol. Metab.* 36:148.

1973 Rajaniemi and Vanha-Pertulla. *Hormones* 103:1.

Thecal and granulosa cell binding occurred if there was FSH pretreatment.

1972 Figarova et al. *Endocrinol. Exp.* (Bratisl.) 6:85.

The receptor for the gonadotropins is part protein and part lipid in nature.

1973 Lee and Ryan. In: *Receptors for Reproductive Hormones.* Eds. O'Malley and Means. New York: Plenum, p. 419.

1973 Lee and Ryan. *Program, 55th Annual Meeting Endocrine Soc.,* Chicago, Ill. (Abstr.).

Adenyl cyclase is also part of the receptor complex or at least closely associated with it.

1973 Danzo. *Biochem. Biophys. ACTA* 304:560.

^{125}I-hCG shows binding to corpora lutea in pregnancy, but not to term corpora lutea, and low persistent binding to interstitial tissue at all times. Surface-binding autoradiographic studies: binding to corpora lutea of pregnancy appeared to increase with time and has been related to the increase in progesterone production during pregnancy.

1973 Midgley. In: *Receptors for Reproductive Hormones.* Eds. O'Malley and Means. New York: Plenum, p. 363.

1973 Pepe and Rothchild. *Endocrinology* 92:1200.

1974 Midgley et al. In: *Gonadotropins and Gonadal Function.* Ed. Mougdal. New York: Academic Press, pp. 416.

^{125}I-FSH has been found to bind predominantly to granulosa cells of developing follicles. Receptors for FSH appear to be present from Stage 1 (Pederson et al. 1968) through Stage 7 of follicular maturation. The number of receptors appears to increase through Stage 5, and thereafter both the number of receptors and affinity remain constant. The plateauing of receptor number and affinity occurs prior to theca differentiation and cavitation (Stage 6).

1972 Cons. Thesis, University of California at San Francisco.

1972 Rajaniemi and Vanha-Pertulla. *Endocrinology* 90:1.

1974 Presl et al. *Endocrinol. Exp.* (Bratisl.) 8:1.

1976 Nimrod et al. *Endocrinology* 98:56.

Prolactin appears to bind largely to luteal tissue, with a small degree of binding seen on follicular granulosa cells. Binding with the luteal tissue scattered with no real localization (rat).

1972 Carlsson et al. *Acta Obstet. Gynecol. Scand.* 51:175.

1973 Midgley. In: *Receptors for Reproductive Hormones*. Eds. O'Malley and Means. New York: Plenum, p. 363.

Major Gaps in Our Knowledge

LH is measured in the plasma at all phases of the cycle. Before and after the midcycle surge (humans), the levels of LH are low "tonic" levels, for which there is high specificity for LH binding. At midcycle, there is an LH surge, with LH reaching plasma concentrations 10 times tonic levels. This surge induces luteinization, ovulation, corpus luteum formation, and rapid growth. Further research is needed to determine whether the binding sites for LH are different at this time, and if so, how they differ from the binding sites for LH ascribed to luteal tissue.

An intriguing question concerns the function of the ovarian stroma in the reproductive cycle. It is capable of secreting steroids, mainly androgens, but there is some evidence that it may be a major source of progesterone, especially in the preovulatory phase. Studies of binding affinity of ovarian tissues for gonadotropins have thus far failed to show significant binding to stromal or interstitial itssue. If future studies show this compartment to be significantly steroidogenic at different parts of the cycle, not only the significance, but also the control mechanisms (if not gonadotropic) involved must be questioned.

LH and hCG have been shown to have almost interchangeable properties, including structure, immunologic cross-reactivity, and biologic actions. Unresolved is whether they share the same tissue receptor. There are conflicting studies, most of which suggest a common receptor. However, recent studies have inferred possible separate receptors. Immature rats pretreated with FSH do not bind hCG. Rats treated with FSH, then LH, subsequently exhibited a significant increase in hCG uptake, indicating that LH was needed to uncover the hCG receptor.

1972 Kammerman et al. *Endocrinology* 91:65.

1972 Lee and Ryan. *Proc. Natl. Acad. Sci. USA* 69:3520.

1972 Liedenberger and Reichert. *Endocrinology* 91:901.

1974 Midgley et al. In: *Gonadotropins and Gonadal Function*. Ed. Mougdal. New York: Academic Press, p. 416.

1974 Wardlaw et al. *Program 55th Annual Meeting, Endocrine Soc.*, Chicago, Ill. (Abstr. 463).

Most studies on gonadotropin binding have confirmed that specific binding is localized on the plasma membrane. In comparable studies, other researchers have shown that the bulk of radiolabeled hormone has been found in subcellular fractions that are clearly distinguishable from the plasma membrane fraction and unspecifically fixed. There may have to be a reevaluation of the concept of gonadotropins being unable to enter the cell and its possible physiological significance.

1972 Coulson et al. In: *Gonadotropins*. Eds. Saxena et al. New York: Wiley-Interscience, p. 227.

1972 Rajaniemi and Vanha-Pertulla. *Endocrinology* 90:1.

1973 Rao and Saxena. *Biochim. Biophys. Acta* 313:312.

The mechanism of spontaneous luteolysis may be associated with a decline in the luteal tissue receptor of LH (hCG). The control of availability of these receptors is not known.

1974 Midgley et al. In: *Gonadotropins and Gonadal Function*. Ed. Mougdal. New York: Academic Press, p. 416.

Solubilization of the receptors will help to characterize them and to determine the mechanisms involved in translating receptor-gonadotropin interaction with the rest of the cell. Attempts at solubilizing receptors have been initiated by investigators, but the data obtained have been fragmentary and fraught with technical difficulties.

1974 Lee and Ryan. In: *Gonadotropins and Gonadal Function*. Ed. Mougdal. New York: Academic Press, p. 444.

Most of the binding studies, especially those of FSH, have been done using radioautography. This approach has served to localize binding within ovarian tissue, but has not given information as to specificity of the binding sites, affinity, and number of receptors per cell. In addition, there is not yet enough information to correlate binding characteristics and biological activity of the gonadotropins. In vitro competitive binding experiments using purer and more biologically active gonadotropins will yield more accurate information about the binding of gonadotropins to cells and the subsequent biological effects.

One of the current beliefs is that FSH-induced maturation of the follicle leads to development or integration of the LH receptor, presumably on the granulosa cell. The mechanisms are unknown. Some investigators have theorized that FSH may induce estrogen synthesis, which then acts to stimulate formation of LH receptors. However, recent evidence has not substantiated this theory.

1974 Midgley et al. In: *Gonadotropins and Gonadal Function*. Ed. Mougdal. New York: Academic Press, p. 416.

IIa. Follicular Phase: Follicular Growth

Biological Processes: Significant Discoveries

Period before 1960

Hypophysectomy is shown to inhibit gonadal development (dogs), and later the anterior pituitary is shown to contain gonadotropic factors.

1910 Crowe et al. *Bull. Johns Hopkins Hosp.* 21:127.

1912 Aschner. *Pfluegers Arch.* 65:341.

1930 Smith. *Am. J. Anat.* 45:205.

1933 Hill and Parks. *Proc. R. Soc. Lond. (Biol.)* 113:530.

1933 White. *Proc. R. Soc. Lond. (Biol.)* 114:64.

1935 McPhail. *Proc. R. Soc. Lond. (Biol.)* 117:45.

Successful pituitary transplant studies show that gonadal function is dependent on anterior hypophyseal secretion.

1926 Aschheim. *Z. Geburtshilfe Gynaekol.* 90:387.

1926 Zondek. *Z. Geburtschilfe Gynaekol.* 90:372.

1927 Smith and Engle. *Am. J. Anat.* 40:159.

FSH is shown to produce follicular development in 21–25-day-old immature rats.

1931 Fevold et al. *Am. J. Physiol.* 97:291.

1933 Fevold et al. *Am. J. Physiol.* 104:710.

1934 Fevold et al. *Am. J. Physiol.* 109:655.

1934 Wallen and Laurence. *J. Pharmacol. Exp. Ther.* 51:263.

1936 Evans et al. *Univ. Calif. Put. Anatomy* 1:255.

Basic anatomy of the developing follicles defined. Follicular development shown to be independent of pituitary control in preantral stages, dependent in later stages.

1926 McKenzie. *Univ. Missouri Agric. Exp. Sta. Bull.* 86.

1930 Smith. *Am. J. Anat.* 45:205.

1930 Swezy and Evans. *Science* 71:46.

1935 Lane and Greep. *Anat. Rec.* 63:139.

1937 Dempsey. *Am. J. Physiol.* 120:126.

1949 Paesi. *Acta Endocrinol. (Kbh.)* 3:84.

1949 Paesi. *Acta Endocrinol. (Kbh.)* 3:173.

1952 Mandl and Zuckerman. *J. Endocrinol.* 8:126.

1956 von Burki and Kellner. *Acta Anat. (Basel)* 27:309.

Follicles destined to ovulate shown to undergo a preovulatory swelling in the hours preceding ovulation. Only well-matured follicles shown to be sensitive to gonadotropic stimulation resulting in the initiation of swelling.

1934 Grant. *Proc. R. Soc. Edinburgh (Biol.)* 58:1.

1936 Myers et al. *Anat. Rec.* 65:381.

1941 Hammond and Wodzicki. *Proc. R. Soc. Lond. (Biol.)* 130:1.

1947 Hisaw. *Physiol. Rev.* 27:95.

1951 Talbert et al. *Endocrinology* 59:687.

FSH initiates follicular growth.

1942 Greep et al. *Endocrinology* 30:635.

LH initiates estrogen secretion.

1942 Greep et al. *Endocrinology* 30:635.

In monkey (hypophysectomized), subcutaneous injections of LH/FSH induce follicular growth but not luteinization. Subcutaneous protocol followed by intravenous injections of LH/FSH induce luteinization, suggesting a different surge effect of LH/FSH vs. ''tonic'' levels.

1928 Allen. *Anat. Rec.* 39:315.

1932 Hisaw et al. *Proc. Soc. Exp. Biol. Med.* 30:39.

Removal of one ovary from a cyclic rat resulted several weeks later in compensatory increase in the weight of the in situ ovary.

1920 Acai. *Am. J. Anat.* 28:59.

Demonstration that human pituitary gonadotropin (hPG) could be used to stimulate ovarian function in women with amenorrhea. Normal pregnancies followed hPG-induced ovulation.

1958 Gemzell et al. *J. Clin. Endocrinol. Metab.* 18:1333.

Pattern of follicular growth documented in humans: Two periods of folliculogenesis distinguished during one reproductive cycle.

1951 Block. *Acta Endocrinol. (Kbh.)* 8:33.

Period 1960–1974

Classification of the different stages of follicle development in the mouse according to the number of granulosa cells, stage of proliferation, atresia or maturation, and luteinization, using parameters such as follicle size, number of granulosa cells present, and antral formation as the characteristics defining the stages.

1970 Pederson. *Acta Endocrinol. (Kbh.)* 62:117.

Movement of the follicle from nonproliferative to proliferative pools independent of pituitary. Possible influence of larger atretic follicles that reduce growth initiation.

1972 Biggers and Scheutz, Eds. *Oogenesis.* Baltimore: University Park Press.

1973 Anderson et al. *Anat. Rec.* 125:264.

1973 Peters et al. In: *The Development and Maturation of the Ovary and Its Function.* Ed. Peters. Excerpta Med. Found. Int. Cong. Ser. 267.

1974 Schwartz et al. *Biol. Reprod.* 10:236.

THECA

Morphological studies showing changes and developments of thecal compartment of follicle. Undifferentiated concentric layer of avascular stroma has little organelle development and no apparent enzymatic steroidogenic activity in preantral follicle. Antral follicle contains vascularized hypertrophied, luteinized, apparently steroid-secreting, organelle-rich internal stroma layer of stroma (theca interna). Development and timing of differentiation of theca interna is species-dependent and may be dependent on degree of LH receptors present.

1962 Jacoby. In: *The Ovary.* Ed. Zuckerman. New York: Academic Press, vol. I, p. 189.

1963 Parlow. *Endocrinology* 73:509.

1966 Adams et al. *Am. J. Anat.* 119:303.

1968 Varma and Guraya. *Experientia* 24:398.

1969 Byskov. *Z. Zellforsch. Mikrosk. Anat.* 100:285.

1969 Christensen and Gilliam. In: *The Gonads.* Ed. McKerns. New York: Appelton-Century-Crofts, p. 415.

1969 Fawcett et al. *Recent Prog. Horm. Res.* 30:367.

1971 Guraya. *Physiol. Rev.* 51:78.

1974 Greenwald. In: *Gonadotropins and Gonadal Function.* Ed. Mougdal. New York: Academic Press, p.205.

Differentiated theca in antral follicle shown to contain active Δ^5, 3α-hydroxy steroid dehydrogenase and 17α-HSD, and also some enzymes involved in NADPH production.

1966 Baille et al. *Developments in Steroid Histochemistry.* New York: Academic Press.

1970 Brandau. In: *Gonadotropins and Ovarian Development.* Eds. Butt, Cooke, and Ryle. London: Livingston, p. 307.

1971 Guraya. *Physiol. Rev.* 51:785.

1972 Guraya. *Acta Anat. (Basel)* 82:284.

1972 Guraya. *Acta Endocrinol. (Kbh.)* 69:109.

GRANULOSA CELLS

Generally, granulosa cells increase in number in the developing follicle but do not contain organelles to the same degree as theca. Histochemical, morphological, and enzymatic studies have shown them to be protein rather than general steroid producing cells. The avascular granulosa cell compartment becomes vascularized after ovulation.

1960 Arvy. *Z. Zellforsch. Mikrosk. Anat.* 51:406.

1961 McKay et al. *Obstet. Gynecol.* 18:13.

1961 Novikoff et al. *J. Histochem. Cytochem.* 51:406.

1962 Belt. *Anat. Rec. (Abstr.)* 142:214.

1962 Bjorkman. *Acta Anat. (Basel)* 51:125.

1970 Brandau. In: *Gonadotropins and Ovarian Development.* Eds. Butt, Cooke, and Ryle. London: Livingston, p. 307.

1971 Guraya. *Physiol. Rev.* 51:785.

1972 Nicosia. *Fertil. Steril.* 23:802.

Changes that follicle cells undergo during follicular maturation shown by electron-microscopic studies to be aimed directly at providing oocyte with the isolated environment needed for its maturation and the substances necessary for metabolism. Quiescent follicle shown only partially to protect egg from environment.

1972   Anderson. In: *Oogenesis.* Eds. Biggers and Scheutz. Baltimore: University Park Press, p. 87.

1974   Zamboni. *Biol. Reprod.* 10:125.

Both FSH and LH are required to effect maturation of follicles at an early stage of their maturation, and long before they become steroidogenic. Early antral formation requires gonadotropins.

1969   Ryle. *J. Reprod. Fertil.* 20:307.

1970   Eskol et al. In: *Gonadotropins and Ovarian Development.* Eds. Butt, Cooke, and Ryle. London: Livingston, p. 249.

1973   Ross et al. *Excerpta Med. Found. Int. Cong. Ser.* 273:903.

1974   Moore and Greenwald. *Am. J. Anat.* 139:37.

Pituitary control of maturation and ovulation shown to be separable phenomena.

1972   Balin and Glasser. In: *Reproductive Biology.* Amsterdam: Excerpta Medica.

1972   Saxena et al. *Gonadotropins.* New York: Wiley-Interscience.

1972   Schwartz and Hoffman. In: *Reproductive Biology.* Eds. Balin and Glasser. Amsterdam: Excerpta Medica, p. 438.

The storage of cholesterol-containing lipid droplets shown to be conditioned by gonadotropins in all phases of the cycle. Prolactin believed to favor cholesterol storage, while LH induces cleavage of cholesterol esters so that both gonadotropins act synergistically to regulate synthesis and storage of cholesterol, controlling its supply for steroidogenesis. Prolactin action is similar in interstitial and luteal compartments.

1968   Armstrong. *Recent Prog. Horm. Res.* 24:255.

1969   Armstrong et al. *Endocrinology* 85:393.

1969   Behrman and Armstrong. *Endocrinology* 85:474.

1969   Hilliard et al. In: *The Gonads.* Ed. McKerns. New York: Appleton-Century-Crofts, p. 55.

1969   Zarrow and Clark. *Endocrinology* 84:340.

1970   Armstrong et al. *Endocrinology* 86:634.

1970   Behrman et al. *Endocrinology* 87:1251.

1973   Flint et al. *Biochem. J.* 132:313.

1973   Flint and Armstrong. *Biochem. J.* 132:301.

1973   Guraya. *Acta Endocrinol. (Kbh.)* (Suppl. 171) 72:1

Anatomical changes described by electron microscopy of the preovulatory follicle during swelling. Changes in theca interna, hyperemia, decreased G-6-P dehydrogenase activity, intracellular space, and nuclear changes in the granulosa cells. LH treatment advances these changes earlier than the spontaneous LH surge.

1970   Hori et al. *Endocrinol. Jap.* 17:489.

Final stages of follicular growth initiated by a rise in secretion of LH and FSH, with the selective transport of FSH into the follicular fluid of a number of developing follicles. Estradiol concentration then begins to rise in the follicular fluid.

1974   McNatty et al. *J. Endocrinol.* 64:555. (humans)

FSH blockage at proestrus by antisera will not effect ovulation or estrogen synthesis, but it will affect the growth and follicular development of subsequent cycles.

1973   Schwartz et al. *Endocrinology* 92:1165.

1974   Rao et al. In: *Gonadotropins and Gonadal Function.* Ed. Mougdal. New York: Academic Press, p. 213.

FOLLICULOGENESIS DURING PREGNANCY AND NONPREGNANCY

LH deprivation (neutralization by antisera, or hypophysectomy) leads to disappearance of Graafian follicles ordinarily present during pregnancy. FSH promotes follicular growth up to the preantral stage.

1966   Lostroh and Johnson. *Endocrinology* 79:991.

1974   Rao et al. In: *Gonadotropins and Gonadal Function.* Ed. Mougdal. New York: Academic Press, p. 213.

Atretic granulosa cells from larger antral follicles shown to distintegrate and disappear, with the hypertrophied theca forming conspicuous patches of interstitial glands in ovarian stroma. Glands morphologically and histochemically shown to be steroid producing, believed to be capable of producing androgens, estrogens, and progesterone to variable degree in various species (humans, laboratory animals). Reversion of interstitial glands in some species back to stromal tissue. Maintenance, development, and accumulation of interstitial glands in other species.

1956   Knigge and Leathem. *Anat. Rec.* 124:697.

1971   Guraya. *Physiol. Rev.* 51:785.

1973   Guraya. *Acta Endocrinol. (Kbh.)* (Suppl. 72) 171:1.

1974   Resko, Brenner, and West. *Endocrinology* 95(4):1094.

Major Gaps in Our Knowledge

Early work suggested that the granulosa (stimulated possibly by estrogen) produces an inductor substance that elicits theca interna formation in the late stages of follicular development. The controlling factors in the development of specific follicular compartments have not been elucidated, including intercompartmental relationships, if any.

1943   Bullough. *J. Endocrinol.* 3:235.

1947   Hisaw. *Physiol. Rev.* 27:95.

1950   Dubreuil. *Obstet. Gynecol.* 49:282.

Does estrogen have a role in follicle cell development and germ cell proliferation? Evidence compiled by early workers indicates that exogenous estrogen stimulates mitotic activity in germinal epithelium. There was also evidence suggesting that new oogenic cycles were initiated by follicular fluid estrogen. More recent work suggests that labeled estradiol enters the nuclei of granulosa cells of the large follicle. More work needs to be done in this area.

1961   Young. In: *Sex and Internal Secretions.* Baltimore: Williams & Wilkins, 3rd. ed. p. 459.

1972   Berger et al. *Fertil. Steril.* 23:783.

1973   Tjalve and Applegren. *Experientia* 29:1143.

Preovulatory estrogen surge seems to require the low tonic levels of LH and is coupled to folliculogenesis, but the relationship between the two phenomena has not been established.

1969   Chatterton et al. *Endocrinology* 84:252.

1972   Schwartz. *Annu. Rev. Physiol.* 34:425.

The mechanisms that determine which and how many follicles reach full maturation are unknown. The factors that determine the receptivity of the follicles to further gonadotropin action remain unknown. There is some evidence in primates that intraovarian steroids may be determinants in follicular growth (monkeys).

1970   Hoffman et al. *Geburtshilfe Frauenheilkd.* 30:347.

The physiological significance of ovarian androgens elaborated by the ovaries, other than as intermediates in estrogen synthesis, is not known. There was a suggestion in the early 1950s that androgens elaborated by the estrous interstitium might have an effect in regulating follicular growth (monkeys).

1936   Hill and Gardner. *Proc. Soc. Exp. Biol. Med.* 34:78.

1937 Parkes. *Nature* 139:965.

1938 Deansley. *Proc. R. Soc. Lond.* B126:122.

1938 Hill. *Anat. Rec.* (Suppl. 3) 70:37.

1958 Payne et al. *Endocrinology* 59:306.

Restoration of gonadal function in hypophysectomized animals with gonadotropin treatment is less effective the longer the hypophysectomized state. This suggests that mature follicles which form corpora lutea may feedback and control early primordial follicle development. No recent work.

1936 Foster. *Anat. Rec.* 67:48.

1937 Fevold et al. *Endocrinology* 21:343.

1937 Foster et al. *Endocrinology* 21:249.

The role of the granulosa cells in oocyte maturation is unknown. The granulosa cells comprising the cumulus and corona radiata may be different from the other granulosa cells of the preovulatory follicle, undergoing unknown changes. The maturation of oocytes has been attributed to the effect of progestins and gonadotropins.

1969 Foote and Thibault. *Ann. Biol. Anim. Biochem. Biophys.* 9:393.

1972 Nicosia. *Fertil. Steril.* 23:791.

1972 Norman and Greenwald. *Anat. Rec.* 173:95.

Follicular atresia occurs at all stages of follicular development. The causes of atresia are not known, although early investigators suggested that factors in atresia of relatively mature follicles were related and possibly identical to those factors stimulating ovulation, with gonadotropins implicated as the principal factors.

1938 Harman and Kirgis. *Am. J. Anat.* 63:79.

1951 Dawson and McCabe. *J. Morphol.* 88:543.

Another suggestion was that atresia is due to defective differentiation of theca interna with resulting loss of estrogen necessary for maturation of the granulosa cells.

1947 Hisaw. *Endocrinology* 64:276.

Although follicular atresia occurs at all stages of follicular development, the granulosa cells of primordial, primary, and small secondary follicles are relatively more resistant to atresia. The larger atretic follicles have been shown to undergo some degree of luteinization and have slight steroid-synthesizing enzymatic activities. These activities and the relationship to atresia are unknown.

1962 Deane et al. *Am. J. Obstet. Gynecol.* 83:281.

1963 Rubin et al. *Endocrinology* 73:748.

1966 Baille et al. *Developments in Steroid Histochemistry.* New York: Academic Press.

1968 Guraya. *Proc. 6th Cong. Int. Reprod. Animal Insem. Artif.,* Paris, vol. I, p. 141.

1971 Borzynski et al. *Comp. Biochem. Physiol.* 40:595.

1972 Delforge et al. *Fertil. Steril.* 23:1.

The gonadotropic environment may be implicated in rescuing follicles from atresia. Massive doses of PMS to hamsters result in superovulation. The critical time during the cycle at which developing follicles are recruited for eventual ovulation or rescued from atresia is unknown.

1961 Greenwald. *J. Reprod. Fertil.* 2:351.

The mechanisms governing follicular atresia and the rescue of follicles from atresia may be answered by utilizing in part the phenomenon of ovarian hypertrophy after excision or irradition of the contralateral ovary. Accompanying hypertrophy is superovulation of the remaining functional gonad, which implies that normally atretic follicles have been rescued. Part of the mechanism of hypertrophy may involve increased FSH secretion.

1974 Greenwald. In: *Gonadotropins and Gonadal Function.* Ed. Mougdal. New York: Academic Press.

The significance of follicular atresia is not known. The atretic follicles are thought to contribute to interstitial gland development which is steroid secreting. The significance of these glands in cyclic ovarian activity in the female is unknown.

1969 Koering. *Am. J. Anat.* 126:73.

1971 Speroff and Vande Wiele. *Am. J. Obstet. Gynecol.* 109:234.

Recent morphologic evdence has documented the presence of "nexus" or "gap" junctions between granulosa cells of antral follicles. These gap junctions appear to exclude the diffusion of substances from the areas where follicle cell contact is mediated by these junctions. The function of these gap junctions is unknown, but their presence enables direct intercellular contact and may also ensure the isolation and stability of the follicular environment during critical phases of oocyte maturation.

1941 Merk. *Proc. 29th Annu. Mtg. Electr. Microsc. Soc. Am.* Ed. Anceneau. Clactons Pat. Div., p. 554.

1969 Brightman and Reese. *J. Cell. Biol.* 40:648.

1970 McNutt and Weinstein. *J. Cell Biol.* 47:666.

1972 Espey and Stubbs. *Biol. Reprod.* 6:168.

1973 Merk et al. *Anat. Rec.* 175:107.

1974 Zamboni. *Biol. Reprod.* 10:129.

Origin of granulosa cells unknown. Recent evidence indicates that their possible origin may be from undifferentiated stromal cells.

1971 Stenger and Onken. *Cytobiologie* 3:240.

1974 Guraya et al. *Z. Zellforsch. Mikrosk. Anat.*

FSH was shown to increase the uptake of ^{14}C-thymidine and DNA synthesis into cultured mouse ovaries and to increase in vivo protein synthesis and subsequently to increase the proportion of follicles containing five or more layers of granulosa cells. These studies also suggested that the continued presence of FSH was necessary in order for continued stimulation to occur.

1968 Crooke and Ryle. In: *Gonadotropins.* Ed. Rosemberg. Los Altos: Geron-X, p. 193.

FSH remains at low tonic levels throughout the nonfertile estrous or menstrual cycle, except for a preovulatory surge coincident with the LH surge. Whether the FSH surge or the tonic FSH is responsible for transition of follicles into the proliferative pool is not known.

1974 Neill and Smith. In: *Current Topics in Exp. Endocrinol.* Eds. James and Martin. New York: Academic Press, vol. 2, p. 73.

1974 Schwartz. *Biol. Reprod.* 10:236.

Studies have shown that in short-cycling animals, follicles due to reach full maturation and ovulation probably move into the proliferative pool before the cycle in which they ovulate. When follicle growth starts for a given set of follicles is not known. The problem has not been studied in animals with longer cycles.

1966 Peters and Levy. *J. Reprod. Fertil.* 11:227.

1968 Lunenfield and Eskol. In: *Gonadotropins.* Ed. Rosemberg. Los Altos: Geron-X, p. 197.

There is some evidence that luteal progesterone may inhibit follicular growth except when high levels of FSH are present. The physiological significance of this observation, seen in hypophysectomized hamsters which had not experienced a preovulatory FSH surge, is not yet known.

1974 Greenwald. In: *Gonadotropins and Gonadal Function.* Ed. Mougdal. New York: Academic Press, p. 205.

IIb. Follicular Phase: Steroidogenesis

Biological Processes: Significant Discoveries

Period before 1960

Transplantation of ovary demonstrated the endocrine function of ovary.

1900 Halban. *Monatschr. Geburtsch. Gynaekol.* 12:496. (guinea pigs)

1900 Knauer. *Arch. Gynaekol.* 60:322. (rabbits)

Extracts of ovaries and placenta shown to produce hypertrophy of uterus.

1912 Schickele. *Biochem. Z.* 38:191.

1913 Aschner. *Arch. Gynaekol.* 99:534.

1913 Tillner. *Arch. Gynaekol.* 100:641.

1914 Okintschitz. *Arch. Gynaekol.* 102:333.

1915 Hennau. *Monatschr. Geburtsch. Gynaekol.* 41:1.

Description of changes of nature of follicular fluid as ovulation approached.

1918 Robinson. *Proc. R. Soc. Edinburgh (Biol.)* 52:302.

Development of theca interna described in late follicular growth.

1937 Mossman. *Am. J. Anat.* 61:289.

Follicle shown to be source of estrus-producing hormone.

1917 Stockard and Papanicolau. *Am. J. Anat.* 22:225.

1922 Allen. *Am. J. Anat.* 30:297. (mice)

1922 Long and Evans. *Mem. Univ. Calif.* 6:1 (rats)

1923 Allen and Doisy. *JAMA* 81:819.

Follicular hormone (estrogen) shown to induce vaginal cornification (rats).

1923 Allen and Doisy. *JAMA* 81:819.

Isolation and purification of pure estrogens.

1929 Doisy et al. *Am. J. Physiol.* 90:329. (humans)

1929 Butenandt. *Dtsch. Med. Wochenschr.* 55:2171.

Extraction of estrogenic hormone (estrone) from follicular fluid and human placenta.

1925 Laqueur et al. *Versl. Akad. Wetensb. Amsterdam* 38:890.

1925 Zondek and Brahn. *Klin. Wochenschr.* 4:2445.

1926 Ralls et al. *J. Biol. Chem.* 69:357.

1927 Laqueur. *Klin. Wochenschr.* 6:1859.

Extraction of estrone from human (female) urine.

1927 Aschheim and Zondek. *Klin. Wochenschr.* 6:1322.

Structure and molecular weight of the estrogens elucidated.

1932 Adam et al. *J. Soc. Chem. Ind.* 51:259.

1932 Bernal. *J. Soc. Chem. Ind.* 51:259.

1932 Marrian. *J. Soc. Chem. Ind.* 49:515.

1932 Marrian and Haselwood. *J. Soc. Chem. Ind.* 51:277.

1933 MacCorquodale et al. *J. Biol. Chem.* 101:753.

1934 Butenandt, Haworth, and Shedrick. *J. Chem. Soc.* 864:1934.

1934 Cohen and Marrian. *Biochem. J.* 28:1603.

1935 Cohen et al. *Biochem. J.* 29:1577.

Properties and potency of estrogenic compounds elucidated. Summarized by:

1939 Doisy. In: *Sex and Internal Secretions.* Ed. Allen. Baltimore: Williams & Wilkins.

Estradiol identified as the major follicular fluid estrogen.

1935 MacCorquodale et al. *Proc. Soc. Exp. Biol. Med.* 32:1182.

Theca interna, theca lutein, and interstitial tissue shown to secrete estrogens and androgens.

1938 Corner. *Physiol. Rev.* 18:154.

1938 Deansly. *Proc. R. Soc. Lond. (Biol.)* 126:122.

1948 Johnson. *Endocrinology* 62:340.

Histochemical studies showed that the various compartments of the ovary are all capable of steroidogenesis, but to different degrees. Progesterone, estrogens, and androgens appeared to be synthesized by the ovary.

1943 Dempsey and Bassett. *Endocrinology* 33:3.

1947 Claesson and Hillarp. *Acta Physiol. Scand.* 13:115.

1948 Claesson et al. *Acta Physiol. Scand.* 16:183.

1948 Dempsey. *Recent Prog. Horm. Res.* 3:127.

1950 Shippel. *J. Obstet. Gynaecol. Br. Empire* 57:362.

Estrogen synthesized by follicular tissue. Maximum synthesis requires both theca and granulosa cells.

1959 Falck. *Acta Physiol. Scand.* (Suppl.) 47:163.

Ascorbic acid depletion in ovary (rats) shown after gonadotropin administration: an index of the initiation of steroidogenesis.

1947 Everett. *Endocrinology* 41:364.

1948 Levin and Jarly. *Endocrinology* 43:154.

1948 Miller and Everett. *Endocrinology* 42:421.

Chorionic gonadotropins found to induce ovulation.

1933 Cole and Miller. *Am. J. Physiol.* 104:165.

1944 Folley and Malpress. *Proc. R. Soc. Lond.* B132:164.

1949 Folley et al. *J. Endocrinol.* 6:121.

Numerous early studies initiated the use of enzymatic biochemistry as an approach (and an alternative to gross and fine morphology studies) to elucidate the enzymatic profile of the steroid-producing tissues.

1951 Samuels et al. *Science* 113:490.

1954 Huseby et al. *Proc. Soc. Exp. Biol. Med.* 86:580.

1956 Beyer and Samuels. *J. Biol. Chem.* 219:69.

1956 Samuels and Helmreich. *Endocrinology* 58:435.

1956 Slaunwhite and Samuels. *J. Biol. Chem.* 220:341.

Experimental ovulation in nonhuman primates: FSH, then intravenous LH/FSH protocol required.

1935 Hisaw et al. *Anat. Rec.* (Suppl.) 64:34.

Granulosa cells of the follicle shown to contain and secrete progesterone.

1954 Nishizuka. *Univ. Kioto* 31:215.

Progesterone found in the follicular fluid.

1942 Duyvene. *Arch. Gynaekol.* 172:455.

1951 Bryans. *Endocrinology* 48:733.

1954 Zander. *Nature (New Biol.)* 174:406.

Physiological evidence that progesterone is produced by the unruptured preovulatory follicle (nonprimate).

1939 Astwood. *Am. J. Physiol.* 126:162.

1941 Hammond and Wodzicki. *Proc. R. Soc. Lond.* B130:1.

1944 Winsatt. *Am. J. Anat.* 74:129.

Development of synthetic estrogens and gestagens.

1945 Solmsen. *Chem. Rev.* 37:481.

1955 Dodds. *Br. Med. Bull.* 11:131.

1956 Rock et al. *Recent Prog. Horm. Res.* 13:323.

1958 St. Whitlock. *Ann. N.Y. Acad. Sci.* 71:479.

Demonstration that ovulation in mature rabbits is induced by pregnancy urine or anterior pituitary extracts or FSH/LH fraction with both hormones required for ovulation.

1929 Bellerly. *J. Physiol. (Lond.)* 67:22.

1929 Friedman. *Am. J. Physiol.* 90:617.

1930 Jones. *Anat. Rec.* 145:264.

1931 Leonard. *Am. J. Physiol.* 198:406.

1935 Foster et al. *Anat. Rec.* 62:75.

1935 Foster et al. *Anat. Rec.* (Suppl.) 64:8.

1937 Foster et al. *Endocrinology* 21:249.

Period 1960–1974

ESTROGEN SYNTHESIS

Estradiol-17β is the predominant estrogen secreted by the human ovary throughout the menstrual cycle. Estrogen peaks at two points through the cycle: midcycle just before ovulation and around day 22 during the luteal phase.

1970 Abraham and Klaiber. *Am. J. Obstet. Gynecol.* 108:528.

1970 Mikhail et al. *Steroids* 15:333.

Estrogen during the follicular phase is synthesized mainly by the follicles and not by the stroma (humans).

1969 Somma et al. *J. Clin. Endocrinol. Metab.* 29:457.

Estradiol secretion is greatest from the ovary containing the preovulatory follicle. In vivo measurement of estrogen in the ovarian vein (humans).

1972 Baird. *Proc. 4th Int. Cong. Endocrinol.*, Washington, D.C. June 1972, p. 851.

Maximum estrogen synthesis from ovary requires theca and granulosa cells.

1968 Ryan et al. *J. Clin. Endocrinol. Metab.* 28:355.

1975 Makris and Ryan. *Endocrinology* 96:598.

Granulosa cells shown to aromatize androgens more efficiently than does theca.

1965 Ryan and Short. *Endocrinology* 76:108. (horses)

Estrogen synthesis from progesterone and pregnenolone requires the whole sliced rabbit follicle.

1973 YoungLai. *Acta Endocrinol.* (Kbh.) 74:775.

Estrogen synthesis in mare mainly through Δ^4-pathway.

1970 YoungLai and Short. *J. Endocrinol.* 47:321.

Preovulatory surge of estrogen precedes the preovulatory surge of LH and falls after the surge.

1968 Burger et al. *J. Clin. Endocrinol. Metab.* 28:1508.

1968 Hori et al. *Endocrinol. Jap.* 15:215.

1969 Uchida et al. *Endocrinol. Jap.* 16:239.

1971 Barraclough et al. *Endocrinology* 88:1437.

1971 Hotchkiss et al. *Endocrinology* 89:177.

Synthesis of estrogen by the ovary is greatest in the proestrous ovary and minimal in the diestrous ovary. LH inhibits formation of estradiol-17β in the proestrous ovary (rats).

1969 Chatterton et al. *Endocrinology* 84:252.

PROGESTERONE SYNTHESIS

Marked increase in the secretion of progesterone occurring within hours after the peak concentration of LH and just before ovulation.

1970 Yussman and Taymor. *J. Clin. Endocrinol. Metab.* 30:396.

Plasma progesterone increases after the LH surge has occurred (preovulatory phase) (monkeys).

1970 Kirton et al. *J. Clin. Endocrinol. Metab.* 30:105.

Preovulatory ovary of the rat responds with increased progesterone secretion when injected with LH.

1967 Yoshinaga et al. *J. Endocrinol.* 38:423. (rats)

1969 Uchida et al. *Endocrinol. Jap.* 16:239. (rats)

Preovulatory progesterone is at least partially follicular. The early signs of luteinization of the parietal granulosa cells coincide with preovulatory progesterone secretion.

1967 Flerko et al. *Acta Morphol. Acad. Sci. Hung.* 15:163.

Final stage of follicular growth initiated by the rise of LH and FSH at the end of the luteal phase. There is a selective transport of FSH into the follicular fluid, which is then followed by a rise in follicular fluid estradiol-17β.

1974 McNatty et al. *J. Endocrinol.* 64:555.

Dissociation between LH effect on steroidogenesis and ovulation. Inhibition of LH-induced PGF formation inhibited ovulation but not steroidogenesis.

1972 Grinwich et al. *Prostaglandins* 1:97.

1972 O'Grady et al. *Prostaglandins* 1:97.

1973 Armstrong et al. *Adv. Biosci.* 9:90.

Cyclic AMP shown to rise in follicles approaching ovulation after LH exposure. The levels of cAMP found to decrease to almost zero after an hour (rabbits).

1973 LeMaire et al. *Prostaglandins* 3:367.

1973 Marsh et al. *Biochim. Biophys. Acta* 304:197.

Stroma or interstitial glands of the ovary source of androgens.

1968 Rice and Savard. *J. Clin. Endocrinol. Metab.* 26:593.

Major Gaps in Our Knowledge

FSH has been shown to stimulate follicular morphogenesis. Whether the follicle also becomes steroidogenic due to FSH alone is not known. There is evidence that FSH is only morphogenic and stimulates follicular growth to the stage where LH receptors develop. Other workers have demonstrated that high doses of human FSH induce estrogen synthesis in the rat.

1945 Greep et al. *Endocrinology* 30:635.

1967 Eshkol and Lunefeld. *Acta Endocrinol.* (Kbh.) 54:91.

1968 Rosenberg and Joshi. In: *Gonadotropins*. Ed. Rosemberg. Los Altos, Calif.: Geron-X, p. 91.

1970 Petnuez et al. *Acta Endocrinol.* (Kbh.) 63:454.

1971 Jewelwicz et al. *J. Clin. Endocrinol. Metab.* 32:688.

The role of cAMP in the preovulatory follicle appears to be variable. Reports of induction of oocyte maturation and luteinization by cAMP have been contradicted by other workers who have interpreted a suppressive role for cAMP.

1972 Keyes et al. *Endocrinology* 91:197.

1972 Tsafriri et al. *J. Reprod. Fertil.* 31:39.

1973 LeMaire et al. *Prostaglandins* 3:367.

Plasma levels of 17-OH progesterone rose in the follicular phase and reached an initial peak on the day of, or the day preceding, the LH peak. After 2 to 4 days, levels of this hormone subsequently decreased about 50% and then increased again during the luteal phase. These fluctuations parallel the change in estradiol, and the suggestion has been made that they may reflect estrogen synthesis. On the other hand, one could postulate that 17-OH progesterone levels represent physiologically important preovulatory biosynthesis in progestogens.

1969 Strott et al. *J. Clin. Endocrinol. Metab.* 29:1157.

Ovary (continued)

Studies, particularly cytological and histological, have determined that the steroid-synthesizing enzymes reside in the follicular theca. Other studies have given evidence, however, that the preovulatory granulosa cells have considerable aromatizing capacity and, after the preovulatory LH surge, are capable of significant progesterone synthesis. Some demonstrable steroid dehydrogenase activity in normal bovine granulosa has been reported, but no NADPH-producing enzymes have thus far been found. The parietal cells but not the cells of the cumulus oophorus show signs of luteinization before ovulation, coincident with the onset of preovulatory progesterone secretion. The differences in these observations, in addition to the observed theca-granulosa synergism in estrogen production, leave open the questions of whether the granulosa cells are steroid-producing and of the physiological significance of preovulatory steroid production by the follicular compartments.

1962 Bjorkman. *Acta Anat.* 51:125.

1963 Rubin et al. *Endocrinology* 73:748.

1967 Flerko et al. *Acta Morphol. Acad. Sci. Hung.* 15:163.

1968 Label and Levy. *Acta Endocrinol.* (Suppl.) (Kbh.) 59:1.

Androgens are known to be elaborated by the ovarian interstitium. A possible role for elevated testosterone levels has recently been proposed. Increased testosterone secretion on diestrus-2 and proestrus may facilitate the prolonged FSH secretion at proestrus and estrus.

1973 Dupon and Kim. *J. Endocrinol.* 59:653.

1974 Gay. *Science* 184:75.

The physiological significance of the observed synergism between follicular compartments with respect to estrogen synthesis remains to be elucidated.

Verification that in vitro techniques reflect metabolic physiological processes is needed.

There is an abrupt rise and fall of progesterone and estrogen in the follicular fluid of the preovulatory follicle. The concentrations decline just before ovulation. The factors governing this decline and the physiological significance are not known.

1971 Moore et al. *J. Reprod. Fertil.* 27:484.

1972 Knobil. In: *The Use of Non-human Primates in Research on Human Reproduction.* Eds. Diczfalusy and Standley. Stockholm: Karolinska Institutet, p. 137.

1972 YoungLai. *J. Reprod. Fertil.* 30:157.

Resolution of the roles played by, and the interaction between, cell types is important to the understanding of the mechanisms whereby the ovary secretes steroid A into the circulation at one time, and steroid B at another time, which may be the precursor of A.

Progesterone synthesis and secretion during the preovulatory phase of the cycle may have the interstitium as a major source. Measurement of progesterone secretion in hamsters after irradiation had destroyed the follicles indicated that the progesterone secretion was not inhibited. Rabbit interstitium has also been designated as a probable site for progesterone secretion. In the monkey, there is evidence that preovulatory progesterone is secreted in large quantities by both ovaries, independent of the presence of the preovulatory follicle. This is in contrast to the source of progesterone during the luteal phase. The rise in preovulatory progesterone secretion can be correlated with an increased development of the interstitial glands in both ovaries.

1963 Hilliard et al. *Endocrinology* 72:59.

1971 Norman and Greenwald. *Endocrinology* 89:598.

1975 Resko et al. *J. Clin. Endocrinol. Metab.* 41(1):120.

There is no direct evidence that the gonadotropins have a direct effect on the synthesis of estrogen. It remains to be determined whether the gonadotropins have a general effect on the promotion of general follicular growth, of which one manifestation may be autoprogramming of the follicle to produce estrogen at a given phase of its maturation.

Morphological studies suggest estradiol-17β production is decreased when theca interna cell metabolism is inhibited by high levels of LH (humans).

1972 Delforge et al. *Fertil. Steril.* 23:1.

Treatment of cycling rats on the day before proestrus with LH antiserum blocks estrogen secretion, whereas treatment with FSH antiserum is not effective.

1969 Schwartz. *Recent Prog. Horm. Res.* 25:1.

Active immunization of the endogenous LH reduces ovarian size and vaginal cyclicity in the mature ovary. The follicles are small and atretic. Estrogen secretion is reduced after an acute dose of anti-LH at diestrus.

1974 Schwartz. *Biol. Reprod.* 10:236.

It is suggested that FSH and LH have a dual role in estrogen secretion at proestrus. Initially there is promotion of estrogen secretion by the gonadotropins and then inhibition (rats).

1968 Hori et al. *Endocrinol. Jap.* 15:215.

III. Luteal Phase

Biological Processes: Significant Discoveries

Period before 1960

First description of corpus luteum. Recognition of association of corpus luteum with fetus in vitro. Recognized as an organ of internal secretion.

1872 Graaf. *Mulierum Organis Gen. Lugduni Batavonum ex off. Hackeana.*

1898 Prenant. *Rev. Gen. Sci.* 9:646.

1903 Bonn. *Arch. Gynaekol.* 67:438.

1910 Frankel. *Arch. Gynaekol.* 91:705.

Embryo and functional state of endometrial lining shown to be dependent on the integrity of the corpus luteum.

1910 Bouin and Ancel. *J. Physiol. Path. Gen.* 12:1.

1910 Frankel. *Arch. Gynaekol.* 91:705.

1928 Corner. *Am. J. Physiol.* 86:74.

Demonstration that corpus luteum inhibits estrus in guinea pegs, and excision of corpora lutea shortens cycle and induces ovulation.

1911 Lark. *Dtsch. Med. Wochenschr.* 37:17.

1917 Hark and Hesselberg. *J. Exp. Med.* 25:285.

1920 Papanicolaou and Stockard. *Proc. Soc. Exp. Biol. Med.* 17:143.

1937 Dempsey. *Am. J. Physiol.* 116:201.

Ovarian extracts shown to produce uterine hypertrophy.

1912 Adler. *Arch. Gynaekol.* 95:349.

Demonstration that a lipoid fraction (progesterone) of luteal extract inhibits estrus and ovulation in the guinea pig.

1926 Papanicolaou. *JAMA* 86:1422.

1927 Loewe and Lange. *Arch. Exp. Path. Pharmakol.* 120:48.

1927 Parkes and Bellerby. *J. Physiol.* 64:233.

1928 Payne et al. *Am. J. Physiol.* 86:243.

1936 Lahr and Riddle. *Proc. Soc. Exp. Biol. Med.* 34:280.

1936 Selye et al. *Proc. Soc. Exp. Biol. Med.* 34:472.

The histological dating of the human corpus luteum of menstruation. Identification of thecal and granulosa cells and the histological identification of the theca as the major estrogen-producing site.

1938 Corner. *Physiol. Rev.* 18:154.

1956 Corner. *Am. J. Anat.* 98:377.

Histochemical studies show that theca interna and interstitial cells synthesize estrogen and androgen.

1938 Corner. *Physiol. Rev.* 18:154.

1938 Deanesley. *Proc. Zool. Soc. Lond.* A108:31.

1942 Pfeiffer and Hooker. *Anat. Rec.* 83:543.

1943 Hernandez. *Am. J. Anat.* 93:127.

1947 Claesson and Hillarp. *Acta Anat.* (Basel) 3:109.

Histochemical studies show that the follicular and luteal granulosa cells secrete progesterone.

1954 Nishizuka. *Acta Sch. Med. Univ. Kioto* 31:215.

1955 Green. *Endocrinology* 56:621.

Persistence of corpora lutea and nonestrous state during lactation. Luteal life tied to litter size; lactation reflex due to suckling young.

1922 Long and Evans. *Mem. Univ. Calif.* 6:1.

1925 Hammond. In: *Reproduction in Rabbits*. Edinburgh: Oliver & Boyd.

1926 Parkes. *Proc. R. Soc. London* B100:51.

Description of luteal function, development, and control by luteolytic and luteotropic factors. Invasion of vascular network into granulosa from theca interna after rupture of the follicle.

1943 Basset. *Am. J. Anat.* 73:251.

Description of length of luteal function and rate of involution in various species throughout the estrous, menstrual, pregnant, and lactating states.

1942 Brewer. *Am. J. Obstet. Gynecol.* 44:1048.

1944 Hisaw. *Yale J. Biol. Med.* 17:119.

1948 Harrison. *Biol. Rev.* 23:296.

1949 Bergman. *Acta Obstet. Gynecol. Scand.* (Suppl.) 29:4.

1950 Meyer and McShan. In: *Menstruation and Its Disorders*. Ed. Engle. Springfield: Thomas. p. 62.

1956 Corner. *Am. J. Anat.* 98:377.

1957 Dickie et al. *Anat. Rec.* 127:187.

Hypophysectomy found to have a species-dependent effect on luteal function.

1930 Smith. *Am. J. Anat.* 56:205. (rats)

1931 Smith and White. *JAMA* 97:1861. (rabbits)

1933 Selye et al. *Endocrinology* 17:494.

1934 Pencharz and Lyons. *Proc. Soc. Exp. Biol. Med.* 31:1131.

1935 McPhail. *Proc. R. Soc. London* B117:45.

1936 Bunde and Greep. *Proc. Soc. Exp. Biol. Med.* 35:235. (rats)

Estrogen shown to maintain structure and function of the corpora lutea.

Rabbit (directly):

1937 Robson. *J. Physiol.* 90:435.

1951 Hammond and Robson. *Endocrinology* 49:384.

Rat (via pituitary):

1937 Reece and Turner. *P. Soc. Exp. Biol. Med.* 36:283.

Discovery that anterior pituitary lobe extracts were luteotropic (rats), with inhibition of estrus resulting and inducing decidual formation.

1922 Long and Evans. *Mem. Univ. Calif.* 6:1.

1926 Till. *Am. J. Physiol.* 79:170.

1928 Brauha. *Liege Med.* 21:1211.

Ovaries of monkeys shown to be responsive to anterior pituitary implants and extracts to induce both ovulation and luteinization.

1928 Allen. *Am. J. Anat.* 42:467.

1929 Courrier et al. *C. R. Soc. Biol.* (Paris) 101:1093.

1930 Hartman. *Proc. Soc. Exp. Biol. Med.* 27:338.

Formulation of the concept of a luteotropic hormone from the pituitary gland.

1941 Astwood. *Endocrinology* 28:309.

1941 Evans et al. *Endocrinology* 28:433.

Initial work on luteotropic and luteolytic agents. Prolactin is luteotropic in rats and mice.

1949 Desclin. *C. R. Soc. Biol.* (Paris) 143:1004.

1955 Moore and Nalbandov. *J. Endocrinol.* 13:18.

1956 Everett. *Endocrinology* 58:786.

Prolactin found to enhance the movement of cholesterol into the corpus luteum to be stored (rats).

1947 Everett. *Endocrinology* 41:364.

Uterus shown to have a luteolytic effect in some species.

1923 Loeb. *Proc. Soc. Exp. Biol. Med.* 20:441.

1939 Robson. *J. Physiol.* (Lond.) 95:83.

1950 Bradbury et al. *Recent Prog. Horm. Res.* 5:151.

1953 Verlardo et al. *Endocrinology* 53:216.

Uterus shown not to have a luteolytic effect in women after hysterectomy.

1958 Whitelaw. *J. Obstet. Gynaecol. Br. Commonw.* 65:917.

Period 1960–1974

PROGESTERONE SYNTHESIS AND LUTEINIZATION

The steroidogenic ability of the corpus luteum was found to be species-dependent. Enzymes that synthesized progesterone and 20β-hydroxy-4-pregnen-3-one are found in the bovine through the primate. They possess the additional enzymes to produce E_1 and E_2. Most other species shown to present an intermediate enzymatic profile. Δ-5 pathway thought to be insignificant in luteal tissue. No correlation has been found between complexity of enzymatic profile and functional length of corpus luteum.

1962 Huang and Pearlman. *J. Biol. Chem.* 237:1060. (humans)

1962 Mason et al. *J. Biol. Chem.* 237:1801. (cattle)

1963 Mikhail et al. *J. Clin. Endocrinol. Metab.* 23:1267. (humans)

1963 Ryan. *Acta Endocrinol.* (Kbh.) 44:81. (humans)

1966 Telegdy and Savard. *Steroids* 8:149. (rabbits)

1967 Cook et al. *Endocrinology* 81:573. (sows)

1967 Kaltenbach et al. *Endocrinology* 81:1407. (sheep)

Production of progesterone by corpus luteum. Demonstration of the formation of progesterone by porcine luteal tissue in vitro.

1960 Duncan, Bowerman, and Hearn. *Proc. Soc. Exp. Biol. Metab.* 104:17.

INITIATION OF LUTEINIZATION

The ability of granulosa cells to luteinize in culture spontaneously and to respond to either LH or FSH in culture with increased steroidogenesis was determined to be a function of the size of the follicle source for the cells. Smaller antral follicle granulosa cells did not spontaneously luteinize and required a combination of gonadotropins to increase steroidogenesis, establishing the concept that events prior to ovulation influence the metabolism of the lutein granulosa cells.

1970 Channing. *Recent Prog. Horm. Res.* 26:589.

LH given to PMS-primed immature rats prior to ovulation resulted in a significant increase in progesterone secretion after ovulation.

1969 Hashimoto and Wiest. *Endocrinology* 84:885.

Direct effect of LH initiating luteinization shown in the rabbit. Transplanted follicles luteinized when exposed to endogenous or exogenous gonadotropin.

1969 Keyes. *Science* 164:846.

1969 Keyes and Armstrong. *Endocrinology* 85:423.

MAINTENANCE OF LUTEAL FUNCTION (LH AND FSH)

There are three basic pituitary–corpus luteum relationships, based on current information: LH-luteotropic (humans, cattle, sheep), no direct pituitary dependence (rabbits), combination of LH, FSH, and prolactin (hamsters).

1968 Greenwald and Rothchild. *J. Anim. Sci.* 27 (Suppl. 1): 139.

Hypothesis based on experiments in the pig that after ovulation the development and steroidogenic capacity of the corpus luteum was independent of the pituitary in a nonpregnant animal. The intact pituitary was necessary only before ovulation. The feedback inhibition of steroids on the pituitary was demonstrated by the fact that pharmacological doses of progesterone inhibited preovulatory or pregnant pig pituitary secretion, and therefore normal luteal development and function.

1964 Brinkley, Norton, and Nalbandov. *Endocrinology* 74:9.

1964 Brinkley, Norton, and Nalbandov. *Endocrinology* 74:14.

Corpus luteum of the cycle in sheep is never independent of pituitary gonadotropins.

1968 Kaltenbach et al. *Endocrinology* 82:753.

In primates, the pituitary appears to be necessary for maintenance of the corpus luteum throughout the postovulatory period. LH is the principal luteotropic factor in humans. It has been suggested that the length of the human luteal phase is dependent on residual tonic LH following the ovulatory LH surge. Direct correlation has been shown between the level of tonic LH throughout the luteal phase and the length of that phase.

1965 Savard et al. *Recent Prog. Horm. Res.* 21:285.

1970 Vande Wiele et al. *Recent Prog. Horm. Res.* 26:63.

1971 Mougdal et al. *J. Clin. Endocrinol. Metab.* 32:579.

1972 Macdonald and Greep. *Fertil. Steril.* 23:466.

1972 Mougdal et al. *J. Clin Endocrinol. Metab.* 35:113.

1972 Vaudckerchove and Dhont. *Ann. Endocrinol.* (Paris) 33:205.

Hysterectomy in monkey had no effect on ovarian cycle.

1969 Neill, Johansson, and Knobil. *Endocrinology* 84:464.

Injection of LH antibodies into pregnant rats before day 12 of gestation induced fetal abortion or resorption. Progesterone, but not prolactin, maintained gestation in the face of antibodies. Strong evidence that LH and not prolactin was the luteotropic factor, with respect to maintaining progesterone synthesis.

1968 Raj, Sairam, and Mougdal. *J. Reprod. Fertil.* 17:335.

1970 Raj and Moudgal. *Endocrinology* 86:874.

LH shown to increase conversion of cholesterol to progesterone, probably by increased activity of cholesterol esterase activity.

1968 Armstrong. *J. Anim. Sci.* 27 (Suppl. 1):181.

1969 Behrman and Armstrong. *Endocrinology* 85:474.

Demonstration that LH or preparations with LH activity were specific in supporting or stimulating the synthesis of progestins in vitro in corpora lutea.

1962 Mason. *J. Biol. Chem.* 237:1801.

1964 Mason and Savard. *Endocrinology* 74:664.

Cyclic AMP implicated in the mechanism of the luteotropic action of LH. Rapid formation of cAMP after luteal tissue exposed to LH, and the ability of cAMP to increase steroidogenesis taken as evidence.

1966 Marsh et al. *J. Biol. Chem.* 241:5436.

1966 Marsh and Savard. *J. Reprod. Fertil.* (Suppl.) 1:113.

1971 LeMaire et al. *Steroids* 17:65.

1972 Kolena and Channing. *Endocrinology* 90:1543.

Prostaglandin implicated as a mediator in the action of LH on the activation of adenyl cyclase in luteal tissue.

1970 Kuehl et al. *Science* 169:883.

1970 Speroff and Ramwell. *J. Clin. Endocrinol. Metab.* 30:345.

1971 Marsh. *Ann. N.Y. Acad. Sci.* 180:416.

LH shown to stimulate biosynthesis of prostaglandin-type material from radioactive precursors.

1972 Chaslow and Pharriss. *Prostaglandins* 1:107.

Prostaglandins (PGEs, PGAs, and PGFs) found to mimic to some degree the steroidogenic effect of LH in minced ovaries of pseudopregnant rats, bovine corpora lutea.

1968 Pharriss and Wyngarden. In: *Gonadotropins*. Ed. Rosemberg. Los Altos: Geron-X, p. 122.

1970 Sellner and Wickersham. *J. Anim. Sci.* 31:230.

1970 Speroff and Ramwell. *J. Clin. Endocrinol. Metab.* 30:345.

PROLACTIN

Prolactin has been shown to have a luteotropic effect in both ovine and rat corpora lutea. Use of antiprolactin antibodies in the ewe led to a fall in progesterone secretion. Removal of the uterus before hypophysectomy allowed restoration of complete luteal function with a combined LH-prolactin treatment.

1973 Denamur, Martinet, and Short. *J. Reprod. Fertil.* 91:1329.

1973 Goding et al. *Excerpta Medica Found. Int. Cong. Ser.* 273:927.

Prolactin found to maintain cholesterol esterase and synthetase activity in rat luteal tissue.

1970 Behrman. *Endocrinology* 96:251.

Prolactin luteotropic effect in rat inhibited by PGF_2.

1973 Behrman. *Excerpta Medica Found. Int. Cong. Ser.* 273:927.

LUTEOLYTIC AGENTS (UTERUS AND PROSTAGLANDINS)

Isolation from bovine endometria of a substance or complex which reduced luteal weights and steroidogenesis in hamsters.

1970 Lukaszewaska and Hansel. *Endocrinology* 86:261.

Prostaglandin ($F_{2\alpha}$) in pharmacological doses shown to be luteolytic in several species. Significant decreases in progesterone secretion and profound degeneration of the corpus luteum.

1969 Pharriss and Wyngarden. *Proc. Soc. Exp. Biol. Med.* 130:92. (rats)

1970 Karmin and Filscie. *Lancet* 1:57. (humans)

1970 Kirton et al. *Proc. Soc. Exp. Biol. Med.* 133:314. (monkeys)

A uterine luteolytic factor does not appear to be operative in primates. This is in contrast to other species where the uterine luteolysin is identified as prostaglandin $F_{2\alpha}$.

1972 Henzl. *Res. Prostaglandins.* 1:1.

1973 Hansel et al. *Biol. Reprod.* 8:222.

Existence of a hormonal luteolysin produced by the uterus substantiated in the cow, but believed unlikely to be the mechanism in controlling the human corpus luteum.

1966 Hansel. *J. Reprod. Fertil.* (Suppl.) 1:33.

Basically, the effects of prostaglandins given in vivo are luteolytic, in sharp contrast to effects seen in vitro, where there appears to be a steroidogenic effect in luteal tissue. The key to the problem may be the mechanism of luteal support, which is seen to vary from species to species. The role of prostaglandins in these various mechanisms is unknown, and until there is adequate correlation between the two, the role of prostaglandin in luteal function will remain unclear.

The mechanism of action of prostaglandins as uterine luteolysins is not known. Recent evidence indicates interactions of the luteolysins with the hypophyseal or follicular luteotropins at the luteal level.

1972 Pharriss et al. *Recent Prog. Horm. Res.* 28:51.

LH deprival at critical stages (which are species-dependent) induces luteolysis. Induction of luteolysis by either LH deprivation or PGF_2 administration induces similar and profound structural changes (with hamsters and rats) in both thecal and granulosa cells, leucocytic infiltration, and decreased vascularity. The process of luteolysis and controlling factors will be further explained once there is enough information to correlate ultrastructural changes associated with processes of intracellular steroid synthesis and metabolism.

1967 Greenwald. *Arch. Anat. Microsc. Morphol. Exp.* (Suppl. 3–4) 56:281.

1972 Channing. *Prostaglandins* 2:327.

1972 Okamura et al. *Fertil. Steril.* 23:475.

1973 Leavitt et al. *Am. J. Anat.* 136:235.

Some evidence indicates a compromising of the vascular network such that the engorged ovary leads to a cessation of luteal function or a localized shunting of blood away from the corpus luteum.

1970 Pharriss et al. *J. Reprod. Fertil.* (Suppl.) 10:97.

1972 Novey. *Proc. Soc. Stud. Reprod.* A17:24.

In vitro evidence suggests a direct effect on steroidogenesis, with a possible inhibition of prolactin maintenance (through regulation of cholesterol ester formation), of progesterone synthesis.

1971 Behrman et al. *Lipids* 6:791.

1972 Demers et al. *Adv. Biosci.* 9:701.

It appears that the luteolytic effect of PGF (and to a lesser degree of PGE) is dependent on the stage of gestation in the rat, and may be related in part to the LH surge at midgestation. The ovary appears to be most sensitive to the PGF at this time, antagonizing the effect of LH.

1974 Fuchs et al. *Acta Endocrinol.* (Kbh.) 76:583.

The mechanisms regulating uterine luteolysis (PG) are not known. It has been proposed that a rise in luteal estrogens triggers uterine PG production. If this hypothesis is correct, the regulation of luteal phase estradiol and the suppression of this luteolytic complex by pregnancy is unknown.

1970 Karsch et al. *Endocrinology* 87:1228.

1972 Caldwell et al. *Prostaglandins* 1:217.

Pregnancy inhibits uterine luteolysin with the young embryo the source of the antiluteolysin. The embryonic antiluteolysin is not known.

1964 Moor and Rowson. *Nature (New Biol.)* 201:522.

1965 Pickles et al. *J. Obstet. Gynaecol. Br. Commonw.* 72:185.

The mechanism of uterine luteolysin transport to ovary is unknown. There have been observations that in sheep, uterine luteolysin is transported by a local rather than a systemic route. Neural, humoral transport via the oviduct and the lymphatic system has not been evident, but there is some evidence for uterine vein transport of luteolysin to the ovary.

1966 Innskeep and Butcher. *J. Anim. Sci.* 25:1164.

1971 Baird and Land. *J. Reprod. Fertil.* 26:133.

1971 McCracken et al. *Recent Prog. Horm. Res.* 27:133.

Irradiation of the ovaries during the luteal phase, with destruction of all the follicles, will apparently prolong the functional life of the corpus luteum. This observation implies a luteolysin in some follicles which remains to be defined.

1969 Rivera and Sherman. *Am. J. Obstet. Gynecol.* 103:986.

In human and some nonprimate species, there is no evident uterine luteolysin. However, there are some data, still conflicting, that PGF_2 may cause luteolysis in humans. Recent work indicates that the time of the menstrual cycle may be important in demonstrating a luteolytic effect. The presence of prostaglandin receptors in human tissue argues for a role in human luteal function.

1971 Karim. *Contraception* 3:173.

1972 Hiller et al. *Br. Med. J.* 4:333.

1972 Lehman et al. *Prostaglandins* 1:269.

1973 Wentz and Jones. *Obstet. Gynecol.* 4:172.

1974 Powell et al. *Lancet* 1:1120.

ESTROGENS IN THE CORPUS LUTEUM

Homogenates of whole luteal ovaries shown to convert ^{19}C steroids to estrogens. Radioactive estrogens formed in corpora lutea of bovine ovaries perfused with radioactive acetate.

1966 Romanoff. *J. Reprod. Fertil.* (Suppl.) 1:89.

1968 Patawardhan and Romanoff. *J. Endocrinol.* 41:461.

Estrogen found formed from ^{14}C-acetate in human corpus luteum.

1964 Hammerstein, Rice, and Savard. *J. Clin. Endocrinol. Metab.* 24:597.

Isolated corpora lutea or luteal stromal tissues not capable of forming estrogens from acetate, progesterone, or androstenedione (nonprimate).

1965 Savard, Marsh, and Rice. *Recent Prog. Horm. Res.* 21:285.

1965 Savard and Telegdy. *Steroids* 6 (Suppl. 2):205.

1968 Patawardhan and Romanoff. *J. Endocrinol.* 41:46.

Luteinized theca synthesized estrogens from radioactive precursors, whereas luteinized granulosa cells did not. No synergism seen in the luteinized cells as in the human nonluteinized follicle cells.

1969 Channing. *J. Endocrinol.* 45:297.

Estrogen essential for the normal function of rabbit corpora lutea. Maintenance of the corpus luteum in rabbit found to be independent of pituitary, except indirectly. LH thought to induce estrogen synthesis by the follicles, which then maintain corpus luteum.

1967 Keyes and Nalbandov. *Endocrinology* 80:938.

1968 Spies, Hilliard, and Sawyer. *Endocrinology* 83:354.

Estrogen in other species appears to require the pituitary for its luteotropic effect. Mediation via the pituitary assumed (sheep).

1963 Gardner, First, and Casida. *J. Anim. Sci.* 22:132.

Estrogen as a luteolysin implicated in primates. The source of estrogen appears to be luteal. Luteal synthesis of estrogen increases as progesterone decreases. Estrone the predominant estrogen.

1974 Butler, Hotchkiss, and Knobil. *J. Steroid Biochemistry* (Abstr.)5:376.

Some correlation between prostaglandin and estrogen in the late luteal phase is evidenced by a rise in plasma PGF levels. Estrogen treatment results in progesterone falling and in some cases a rise in PGF.

1972 Auletta et al. *Contraception* 6:411.

Estrogen in humans found to be consistently luteolytic when given to subjects within a week after ovulation.

1971 Johannson and Gemzell. *Acta Endocrinol.* (Kbh.) 68:551.

1973 Gore et al. *J. Clin. Endocrinol. Metab.* 36:615.

Estrogen luteolytic in cows.

1965 Niswender et al. *J. Anim. Sci.* 24:986.

The possible effect on estrogen synthesis in the corpus luteum, and subsequent luteolysis, by PGF has been indicated in the hamster. PGF treatment increased ovarian estradiol output by pregnant hamsters with a concomitant decrease in progesterone secretion.

1974 Labhsetwar. *Fed. Proc.* 33:61.

Major Gaps in Our Knowledge

Is there a "luteostatic factor" in the ovum which inhibits the luteinization process as indicated by the work of Nalbandov? Removal of the ova results in luteinization of the follicular granulosa cells and formation of corpora lutea in the rabbit, accompanied by increased secretion of progesterone by the ovectomized ovary. LH injected into the ovectomized follicle results in the luteinization process, initiated by ovectomy, continuing until a corpus luteum is formed.

1970 El-Fouly et al. *Endocrinology* 87:288.

1970 Cropper et al. *52nd Endocrine Soc. Meeting,* St. Louis, Mo., p. 80 (Abstr.).

1971 Nekola et al. *Anat. Rec.* (Abstr.) 169:387.

Other workers have demonstrated that cells have luteinized in a follicle which still had the egg contained in it because ovulation had been inhibited.

1972 O'Grady et al. *Prostalgandins* 1:97.

1973 Armstrong et al. *Adv. Biosci.* 9:90.

Recent work has indicated that a substance in follicular fluid may inhibit the follicle cell luteinization. Fluid from small follicles inhibited the luteinization in vitro of granulosa cells. The nature of this inhibiting factor remains to be determined.

1975 Channing and Tsafriri *Endocrinology* 96:922.

Intrafollicular injections of cAMP prevents the luteinization of follicles normally caused by the intrafollicular injection of LH. Since cAMP is generally supposed to be an intracellular mediator of LH, the significance and validity of this observation are not clear.

1972 LeMaire et al. *Biol. Reprod.* 6:109.

What is the role of FSH in luteal function? There is evidence in the rhesus monkey that one of the actions of FSH is to stimulate the production of new LH receptors on the granulosa cells, and this may be important for subsequent luteinization.

1974 Channing and Kammerman. *Biol. Reprod.* 10:179.

MAINTENANCE OF LUTEAL FUNCTION (LH AND FSH)

Although FSH in the rat and other species has not been implicated in the maintenance of the corpus luteum, work in the hamster has shown that FSH and prolactin are the minimum luteotropic complex. Whether this is a species-specific phenomenon or whether further work will implicate FSH in luteal function in other species remains to be seen.

1967 Greenwald. *Endocrinology* 80:118.

1973 Greenwald. *Endocrinology* 92:235.

The interaction between the LH-cAMP activation system is unknown. Adenylate cyclase is located in the plasma membrane fraction and possibly in proximity to the LH receptor. A receptor–adenylate cyclase complex may exist which might undergo conformational changes secondary to gonadotropin-receptor interactions and thereby activate the catalytic properties of the adenylate cyclase. The nature of this complex, if it exists, is unknown; nor has the mechanism of the activation of the adenylate cyclase been clarified. Ca^{++} may be an essential factor in these membrane-located processes, in analogy to a postulated role in the adrenals.

1969 Dorrington and Baggett. *Endocrinology* 84:989.

1971 Stansfield et al. *Biochim. Biophys. Acta* 227:413.

The mechanism of action by which the LH-cAMP system stimulates steroidogenesis in luteal tissue is not known. Recent work in adrenal tissue has led to the theory that ACTH-cAMP stimulates the synthesis of a short-lived protein which is nonenzymatic and which stimulates the side chain cleavage of cholesterol. An analogous mechanism might exist in ovarian tissue.

1972 Gill. *Metabolism* 21:559.

1973 Joachanicz and Armstrong. *Endocrinology* 83:769.

1973 Savard. *Biol. Reprod.* 8:183.

Cyclohexamide and puromycin inhibit the stimulatory action of LH and cAMP, thus indicating that the protein formation involved in these regulatory processes does not precede cAMP stimulation, but is a consequence of it. A cAMP dependent protein kinase detected in the ovary might be involved.

1966   Marsh et al. *J. Biol. Chem.* 241:5436.

1970   Kuo et al. *Biochim. Biophys. Acta* 212:79.

1971   Hermier et al. *Biochim. Biophys. Acta* 244:625.

On the other hand, cAMP has been shown in adrenal tissue to inhibit the conversion of pregnenolone to progesterone both in the adrenal and the corpus luteum. The physiological role (if any) of cAMP enhancing a step in the steroidogenic pathway while inhibiting another step remains to be elucidated.

1968   Koritz et al. *Endocrinology* 82:620.

1969   Sulimovice and Boyd. *Eur. J. Biochem.* 7:549.

1971   Berger and Jones. *Endocrinology* 89:722.

PGE has been suggested as an intermediate in LH-stimulated cAMP levels in ovarian tissue. PGF possibly enhances cAMP formation in the ovary. Kuehl has suggested a "dual regulatory system," where PGF is a mediator in regulatory processes antagonistic to those processes in which PGE is a mediator. The evidence supporting this theory is not complete and is not substantiated by all the data.

1973   Goldberg et al. *Pharmacology and the Future of Man: Proc. 5th Int. Congr. Pharmacology,* Basel:Karger, p. 140.

1973   Kuehl et al. *Adv. Biosci.* 9:155.

cGMP may prove to be another physiologically important cellular factor in ovarian cellular function. It is present in very small amounts in the cell, and only recently has methodology been developed to measure it with any accuracy. While there is no established effect on ovarian tissue by cGMP, future work may show cellular responses to cGMP. Recently, it has been shown that adrenal cells exposed to ACTH will react by a rise in cGMP at low ACTH levels which do not produce a rise in cAMP. Although there is no detectable rise in cAMP, corticosterone production was shown to increase as cGMP rose. Higher doses of ACTH were required to generate cAMP.

1974   Sharma et al. *FEBS Letters* 45:107.

Even though the placenta becomes dominant in pregnancy after 6–8 weeks, the corpus luteum continues to function and exist throughout pregnancy — although total luteal steroidogenesis is significantly decreased. The gonadotropic environment of pregnancy extends the two-week life span of the cyclic corpus luteum to 8–10 weeks. The reason the luteal function wanes after this, in spite of increased hCG levels, remains to be elucidated, as does the functional role of hCG after the first trimester.

1972   Csapo et al. *Am. J. Obstet. Gynecol.* 112:1061.

PROLACTIN

LH appears to be directly or indirectly the principal luteotropic factor. The role of prolactin as a luteotropin has not been clearly established in any species. In some species, it appears to act synergistically with LH, and may be physiologically important in maintaining or rescuing the corpus luteum of pseudopregnancy or pregnancy (e.g., rats, cattle, hamsters), whereas LH may function in the initiation and maintenance of the corpus luteum.

1967   Ucida et al. *Endocrinol. Jap.* 16:227.

1971   Yoshinaga et al. *Endocrinology* 88:1126.

1972   Behrman et al. *J. Endocrinol.* 52:419.

1972   Mougdal et al. *J. Endocrinol.* 52:413.

1974   Raj et al. In: *Gonadotropins and Gonadal Function.* Ed. Mougdal. New York: Academic Press, p. 271.

1975   Smith et al. *Endocrinology* 96:219.

Prolactin's main function may be to maintain cholesterol stores, so that the ovary can rapidly respond to LH.

1968   Hillard et al. *Endocrinology* 82:122.

1969   Armstrong et al. *Endocrinology* 86:634.

Prolactin in the primate has thus far not been shown to be physiologically necessary in corpus luteum function. Recent work, however, has shown that human granulosa cells in tissue culture require prolactin for normal progesterone secretion, although supraphysiological levels of the hormone are inhibitory. This again raises the possibility of prolactin's function in the primate corpus luteum.

1974   McNatty et al. *Nature* 250:653.

The cellular source of luteal estrogen is not known. A suggestion has been offered of synergism between luteal stromal tissue and luteal theca to effect estrogen synthesis in those species, such as the human, which secrete estrogen during the luteal phase. The smaller antral follicles have also been suggested as the source of luteal phase estrogen.

1968   Patawardhan and Romanoff. *J. Endocrinol.* 41:46.

LUTEOLYSIN

The triggering mechanism leading to luteolysis in the infertile human menstrual cycle is unknown. In the pregnant primate, hCG is probably the factor preventing luteolysis during pregnancy. There may be an inherent life span of the nonfertile primate corpus luteum, or an intraovarian involvement. Estradiol and testosterone have been shown to shorten the life span of the corpus luteum. Estrogen, injected immediately after ovulation, will prevent nidation. A direct effect on the corpus luteum was inferred, since plasma progesterone falls without a fall in LH. The physiological control of luteal function by steroid has not been determined.

1960   Hoffman. *Geburtshilfe Frauenheilkd.* 20:1153.

1973   Gore et al. *J. Clin. Endocrinol. Metab.* 36:615.

1973   Knobil. *Biol. Reprod.* 8:246.

The relationship recently noted between PGF and estrogen in subhuman primates remains to be further defined. This is of importance if there is a physiological effect of these compounds in luteolysis. Since the human corpus luteum also synthesizes estrogen, the possible role of this steroid as a luteolytic agent has important implications in fertility control. The observed luteolytic effect of estrogen cannot yet be explained by a direct effect on progesterone synthesis. Conversion of acetate to progesterone in the presence of estradiol was unaffected, compared to control-incubated corpus luteum (monkey).

1974   Archer. *J. Steroid Biochem.* (Abstr.) 5:312.

OTHER GAPS

In some species, the production rate of 20α-dihydroprogesterone has been suggested as an index of luteal regression. Early signs of corpus luteum regression have been associated with a shift from high levels of progesterone to the dihydroprogesterone. The physiological significance and the mechanisms involved in the shift are not known.

1967   Lindner and Shelesnyak. *Acta Endocrinol.* (Kbh.) 56:27.

1967   Zmigrod. *Acta Endocrinol.* (Kbh.) 56:16.

1973   Little et al. *Excerpta Med. Found. Int. Cong. Ser.* 273:864.

In the human, the corpus luteum preserves its capacity to produce hormones throughout pregnancy. However, its contribution to the plasma hormonal patterns after 6–8 weeks of gestation is overshadowed by placental and other sources. 17-hydroxy-progesterone, which is considered to reflect corpus luteum activity during pregnancy, shows a significant increase in plasma levels in the 33rd week of gestation. The significance of this and the possible function of the corpus luteum late in pregnancy are unknown.

1969   Yoshimi et al. *J. Clin. Endocrinol. Metab.* 29:225.

1971   LeMaire et al. *Steroids* 17:65.

1972   Tulchinsky et al. *Am. J. Obstet. Gynecol.* 112:1095.

1974   Hodgen and Tullner. *56th Meeting Endocrine Soc.*, Abstr. A-248.

The contribution of the preimplantation blastocyst to luteal maintenance is basically unknown. Recent evidence has indicated that it exerts a luteotropic effect. The rise in plasma progesterone occurred sooner in pregnant rabbits than in pseudopregnancy. In the ewe, it has been shown that the blastocyst luteotropic factor overcomes the luteolytic action of PGF, which LH is incapable of doing. Not only is the importance of elucidating the nature of this factor and its relationship to luteal function obvious, but it also raises the question of whether the pseudopregnant animal is an analogous model to the pregnant animal.

1972   Wilson et al. *Proc. 5th Annu. Meeting Soc. Study Reproduction,* June 1972 (Abstr.) 15.

1974   Beling et al. *J. Steroid Biochem.* 5:363.

1974   Fuchs and Beling. *Endocrinology* 95:1056.

IV. Steroidogenic Pathways

Biological Processes: Significant Discoveries

Period before 1960

Demonstration, using an isotopically labeled substrate, of conversion to pregnanediol in a pregnant female. First use of isotopically labeled material to describe steroidogenesis.

1945   Bloch. *J. Biol. Chem.* 157:661.

Cholesterol synthesis from acetate demonstrated in theca and granulosa cells surrounding the growing ovum of laying hens.

1954   Popjak. *Arch. Biochem. Biophys.* 48:102.

Radioactive cholesterol converted to estrone in a pregnant woman.

1957   Werbin et al. *J. Am. Chem. Soc.* 79:1012.

Pregnenolone identified as the steroidal component resulting from cholesterol side chain cleavage in the adrenal.

1954   Saba et al. *J. Am Chem. Soc.* 76:3862.

1956   Staple et al. *J. Biol. Chem.* 219:845.

Pregnenolone shown to be biochemical precursor for steroid biosynthesis in adrenal, placental, testicular, and ovarian tissue.

1952   Nissim and Robson. *J. Endocrinol.* 8:329.

1954   Pearlman et al. *J. Biol. Chem.* 208:231.

1956   Hayano et al. *Recent Prog. Horm. Res.* 12:79.

1965   Savard et al. *Recent Prog. Horm. Res.* 21:281.

1969   Tamaoki et al. In: *The Gonads.* Ed. McKerns. New York: Appleton-Century-Croft, p. 547.

Identification of the conversion of pregnenolone to progesterone by the enzyme complex 5, 3α-hydroxysteroid dehydrogenase.

1951   Samuels et al. *Science* 113:490.

1954   Pearlman, Cerceo, and Thomas. *J. Biol. Chem.* 208:231.

Isolation of labeled estrone from the urine of a pregnant mare that had received a large dose of ^{14}C-acetate.

1954   Heard et al. *Recent Prog. Horm. Res.* 9:383.

Demonstration in ovarian tissue of estrone and estradiol-17α synthesis from ^{14}C-testosterone.

1956   Baggett et al. *J. Biol. Chem.* 221:931.

The isolation of 19α hydroxyandrostenedione as an intermediate in the aromatization of androgens (perfusion through beef adrenal glands).

1955   Meyer. *Experientia* 11:99.

Conversion of ^{21}C steroids, pregnenolone, and progesterone to androgens by 17-hydroxylation and side chain cleavage.

1956   Solomon et al. *J. Am Chem. Soc.* 78:5453. (adrenal)

1956   Slaunwhite and Samuels. *J. Biol. Chem.* 220:341.

Aromatization of androgens to estrogens by tracer techniques in the whole ovary.

1956   Baggett et al. *J. Biol. Chem.* 221:931.

1956   Wotiz et al. *J. Biol. Chem.* 222:482.

Evidence for placental aromatization of androgens as the major pathway in the synthesis of estrogens.

1958   Ryan. *Biochim. Biophys. Acta* 27:658.

Period 1960–1974

Squalene, mevalonate, and lanosterol identified as intermediates in cholesterol biosynthesis in the corpus luteum.

1966   Helig and Savard. *Biochemistry* 5:2944.

Radioactive cholesterol shown to be converted to isocaproic acid and progesterone in homogenates of bovine corpus luteum.

1961   Tamaoki and Pincus. *Endocrinology* 69:527.

Description of the cholesterol side chain cleavage enzymes in the mitochondrial fraction of bovine corpus luteum.

1963   Ichii et al. *Steroids* 2:631.

Purification and properties of the enzymes involved in pregnenolone conversion to progesterone. Localization in microsomes of the corpora lutea.

1966   Cheatum and Warren. *Biochim. Biophys. Acta* 122:1.

Theca favors the Δ-5 pathway, and granulosa apparently predominates in the Δ-4 pathway.

1965   Ryan and Smith. *J. Biol. Chem.* 236:705.

1966   Ryan and Petro. *J. Clin. Endocrinol. Metab.* 26:46.

Elucidation of estrogenic pathways in the ovary using radioactive precursors. Isolation of intermediates showing that estrogens share with neutral hormones a common biogenic pathway from acetate.

1961   Ryan and Smith. *J. Biol. Chem.* 236:705.

1961   Ryan and Smith. *J. Biol. Chem.* 236:710.

1961   Ryan and Smith *J. Biol. Chem.* 236:2204.

1961   Smith and Ryan. *Endocrinology* 69:869.

1961   Smith and Ryan. *Endocrinology* 69:970.

Enzymes in steroidogenic pathways found in the elements of the endoplasmic reticulum of the microsomal and soluble fractions of tissue homogenates (testes).

1967   Inano et al. *Biochim. Biophys. Acta* 137:540.

1968   Samuels. In: *Metabolic Pathways,* 3rd ed. New York: Academic Press, vol. II.

Description of 17α-hydroxylation of pregnenolone and progesterone in the human ovary.

1961   Warren and Salhanick. *J. Clin. Endocrinol. Metab.* 21:1218.

Stroma in the human ovary found to be the most active part of the ovary in converting ^{21}C steroids to ^{10}C steroids (androgens).

1968   Sauaro. In: *The Ovary*. Ed. Mack. Springfield: Thomas, p. 10.

Major Gaps in Our Knowledge

The steroidogenic enzymes have been extensively investigated in testes but not at all in ovarian tissue. The controlling factors in the ovarian tissue enzymes may be different than in the testes, and need to be studied.

Although the general pathways of steroidogenesis are known, little is known about the factors that determine the choice of pathway at a branch point and how these factors vary during the cyclic processes characteristic of the female reproductive tract. The gonadotropins are one of the classes of agents of extraovarian origin most likely to have a role.

Few of the enzymes involved in steroidogenesis have been isolated in pure form, studied kinetically, or studied in the conventional enzyme approach.

The three major compartments of the ovary possess the full array of enzymes required for steroidogenesis. Yet each compartment has, in general, its own distinctive hormonal product. The factors controlling the biochemical profile of each ovarian compartment are not known and require further study.

The events that occur after LH-stimulated activation of the adenyl cyclase and that result in increased steroidogenesis are not known. Presumably the LH effect in steroidogenesis parallels the ACTH stimulation of the cholesterol side chain cleavage step in the adrenal, which is also mediated by cyclic AMP. The mechanism of action of ACTH also is not known, but a nonenzymatic protein has been implicated in the process of side chain cleavage. This protein has been termed a "carrier protein," but its function has not been established.

1972   Ungar et al. *Excerpta Med. Found. Int. Cong. Ser.* 256:26.

Elucidation of the steps in the mechanism of aromatization remains. This has an important implication in developing methods of external interference that would have a specific rather than a generalized effect on fertility control.

Methodological Advances

Period before 1960

Use of lipoid solvents for extraction of tissue hormones.

1912   Iscovesco. *C. R. Soc. Biol.* (Paris) 73:104.

X-ray used selectively to destroy fistollicles without destroying permanent ovarian function.

1926   Parkes. *Proc. R. Soc. Lond.* (Biol.) 100:72.

1927   Bramhill et al. *Proc. R. Soc. Lond.* (Biol.) 101:29.

1927   Parkes. *Proc. R. Soc. Lond.* (Biol.) 101:71.

1927   Parkes. *Proc. R. Soc. Lond.* (Biol.) 101:421.

1927   Parkes. *Proc. R. Soc. Lond.* (Biol.) 102:51.

1927   Zondek. *Klin. Wochenschr.* 6:248.

Methodology developed for the isolation and separation of the ovarian steroids, especially progesterone and estrogens.

1933   Allen and Meyer. *Am. J. Physiol.* 106:55.

Methods for obtaining ovarian vein blood first devised.

1950   Paschkis and Rakoff. *Proc. Soc. Exp. Biol. Med.* 68:485.

1954   Neher and Zarrow. *J. Endocrinol.* 11:323.

1958   Edgar and Ronaldson. *J. Endocrinol.* 16:378.

The collection of follicles and corpora lutea timed more accurately with respect to the moment of ovulation.

1952   Deane. *Am. J. Anat.* 91:363.

Paper chromatography developed, permitting sufficient purification and isolation of steroids in microgram quantities.

1955   Brown. *Biochem. J.* 60:185.

1960   Smith. *Endocrinology* 67:698.

1960   Svendsen. *Acta Endocrinol.* (Kbh.) 35:161.

Development of radioimmunoassay for insulin, based on the principle of antigen-antibody interactions and using radioactively labeled hormones.

1956   Berson et al. *J. Clin. Invest.* 35:170.

1959   Berson and Yalow. *J. Clin. Invest.* 38:1996.

1959   Berson and Yalow. *J. Clin Invest.* 38:2017.

1960   Yalow and Berson. *J. Clin. Invest.* 39:1157.

Labeling of protein hormones with iodine by substitution of the iodine into tyrosine groups.

1957   Hughes. *Ann. N.Y. Acad. Sci.* 70(1):3.

1958   McFarlane. *Nature* 182:53.

Application of electron microscope to studies of reproductive tissue.

1959   Lever. *Anat. Rec.* 124:111.

FOLLICULAR PHASE: STEROIDOGENESIS

Assay of estrogens: production of hypertrophy and hyperplasia of the uterus in castrate or immature rabbit.

1912   Iscovesco. *C. R. Soc. Biol.* (Paris) 73:16.

1920   Herrmann. *Wien. Klin. Wochenschr.* 26.

Vaginal cornification in ovariectomized animals developed as unit of measurment of estrogen.

1923   Allen and Doisy. *JAMA* 81:819.

1928   Kahnt and Doisy. *Endocrinology* 12:760.

1936   Lyons and Templeton. *Proc. Soc. Exp. Biol. Med.* 33:587.

Identification of high levels of estrogenic material in urine of pregnant women allowed for the isolation of greater amounts of estrogen in order to study its physical, chemical, and biological properties.

1927   Aschheim and Zondek. *Klin. Wochenschr.* 6:1322.

Color reaction developed for quantitative measure of estrogen in urine.

1931 Kober. *Biochem. Z.* 239:209.

Isolation and purification methods developed for estrogenic substances.

1928 Thayer et al. *J. Biol. Chem.* 79:53.

1928 Zondek. *Klin. Wochenschr.* 7:485.

1929 Doisy et al. *Am. J. Physiol.* 90:329.

1930 Butenandt. *Z. Physiol. Chem.* 191:127.

1930 Veler et al. *J. Biol. Chem.* 87:357.

First synthetic estrus-producing compound synthesized (1 keto-1, 2, 3, 4, tetrahydrophenanthrene).

1933 Cook et al. *Nature* 131:56.

LUTEAL PHASE

Basis of bioassay for progesterone established by observation that uteri of sterile mated rabbits undergo marked progestational proliferation changes as corpora lutea develop.

1910 Ancel and Bouin. *J. Physiol. Path. Gen.* 12:1.

1912 Adler. *Arch. Gynaekol.* 95:349.

Bioassay of progesterone using lipoid extracts of luteum index of progestation proliferation of the endometrium.

1929 Corner and Allen. *Am. J. Physiol.* 88:326.

1930 Allen. *Am. J. Physiol.* 92:174.

1930 Clauberg. *Zentralbl. Gynaekol.* 54:2757.

Assay for progesterone developed, based on the induction of sexual receptivity in oophorectomized guinea pigs.

1936 Demsey, Hertz, and Young. *Am. J. Physiol.* 116:201.

1939 Hertz et al. *Endocrinology* 21:533.

Assay of progesterone as pregnanediol in urine. Basis of clinical assay of progesterone.

1938 Vinning and Braun. *Am. J. Physiol.* 123:209.

Spectrophotometric methods developed in assay for progesterone.

1942 Reynolds and Ginshing. *Endocrinology* 31:147.

1954 Zander and Simmer. *Klin. Wochenschr.* 32:529.

1958 Short. *J. Endocrinol.* 16:415.

1958 Sommerville and Deghpaude. *J. Clin. Endocrinol. Metab.* 18:1223.

Isolation of pure crystalline progesterone preparations from corpus luteum and determination of its physical and chemical properties and structure.

1929 Corner and Allen. *Am. J. Physiol.* 88:326.

1930 Corner and Allen. *Proc. Soc. Exp. Biol. Med.* 27:403.

1931 Fils and Slotta. *Klin. Wochenschr.* 10:1639.

1932 Allen. *J. Biol. Chem.* 98:591.

1932 Fevold and Hisaw. *Proc. Soc. Exp. Biol. Med.* 29:620.

1934 Budenandt and Wiln. *Klin. Wochenschr.* 47:936.

1934 Slotta et al. *Ber. Chem. Ges.* 67:1947.

1934 Allen and Wintersteine. *Science* 80:190.

1934 Hartman and Wiltsteiner. *Helv. Chim. Acta* 17:878.

1934 Butenandt and Schmidt. *Ber. Chem. Ges.* 67:1901.

Prolongation of corpus luteum shown under conditions of sterile mating (pseudopregnancy) with changes similar to early changes in pregnancy.

1910 Ancel and Bouin. *J. Physiol. Path. Gen.* 12:1.

1914 Hammond and Marshall. *Proc. R. Soc. Lond. (Biol.)* 87:422.

1930 Hammond and Marshall. *Proc. R. Soc. Lond. (Biol.)* 105:607.

1935 Foster and Hisaw. *Anat. Rec.* 62:75.

Progesterone-albumin conjugates synthesized which were antigenic in rabbits.

1959 Erlanger et al. *J. Biol. Chem.* 234:1090.

Esterification of progestogen alcohol shown to form an injectable drug with a long duration of action.

1954 Junkmann. *Naunyn Schmiedebergs Arch. Pharmakol.* 223:244.

Progestogen esters, including norethindrone enanthate, synthesized.

1958 Junkmann and Witzel. *Z. Vitam. Horm. Fermentforsch.* 9:97.

Medroxyprogesterone acetate synthesized.

1958 Babcock et al. *J. Am. Chem. Soc.* 80:2902.

Period 1960–1974

The use of radiation to study selectively in the ovary the effect of destruction of ovarian structures on variables such as growth and steroidogenic capacity after irradiation.

1962 Lacassagne et al. In: *The Ovary.* Ed. Zuckerman. London: Academic Press, vol. 2, p. 463.

Development of a technique to collect ovarian vein blood allowed for a more direct and accurate measure of patterns of steroid secretion from the ovary.

1962 Eto et al. *Jap J. Anim. Reprod.* 8:34.

Gas-liquid chromatography

1963 Horning et al. In: *Methods of Biochemical Analysis* Ed.Glick. New York: Wileu Interscience, vol. II, p. 69.

Principle of radioimmunoassay first applied to steroids.

1963 Murphy et al. *J. Clin. Endocrinol. Metab.* 23:293.

Constant infusion techniques that allow the in vivo determination of production rate of a hormone.

1964 Tait and Burstein. *Hormones* 5:441.

Perfusion of the dog ovary in vivo, allowing determination of the control of steroid secretion.

1964 Aakvaag et al. *Biochim. Biophys. Acta* 86:380.

1964 Aakvaag and Eik-Nes. *Biochim. Biophys. Acta* 86:380.

Transplantation of the ovary to the neck, a more accessible site for the study of ovarian steroid secretion in vivo.

1968 Baird et al. *J. Endocrinol.* 42:283.

Development of anti-LH serum which allows in vivo inhibition of LH and the subsequent effect on steroid synthesis and secretion as a result of the inhibition.

1969 Loewit et al. *Endocrinology* 84:224.

GONADOTROPIN BINDING

Development of improved techniques for labeling protein hormones with significant retention of biologic activity.

1969 Monroe and Midgley. *Proc. Soc. Exp. Biol. Med.* 130:151.

1970 Castro et al. *Proc. Soc. Exp. Biol. Med.* 133:582.

1972 Miyachi et al. *J. Clin. Endocrinol. Metab.* 34:23.

Development of enzymatic (lactoperoxidase) method to iodinate protein hormone, which allows for significantly greater retention of biological activity.

1972 Miyachi et al. *J. Clin. Endocrinol. Metab.* 34:23.

Labeling with ^{125}I of protein hormones with high specific activity, without the inhibition of the biological and immunological activity of the hormone.

1963 Greenwood et al. *Biochem. J.* 89:114.

Development of techniques and criteria to measure directly the binding of hormones to specific receptors and to characterize these receptors.

1974 Cuatrecasus. *Annu. Rev. Biochem.* 43:169.

Use of insulin covalently linked to large polymers, which prevents entry of the hormone into the cell.

1969 Cautrecasus. *Proc. Natl. Acad. Sci. USA* 63:450.

1970 Turkington. *Biochem. Biophys. Res. Commun.* 41:1362.

1971 Blatt and Kim. *J. Biol. Chem.* 246:4895.

Human sex hormone binding globulin shown to be present in circulating plasma.

1974 Anderson. *Clin. Endocrinol.* 3:69.

FOLLICULAR PHASE: STEROIDOGENESIS

Histochemical and cytochemical methods for identification of enzymatic systems within the steroid-producing tissues and the hormonal target organs, permitting a more conclusive functional interpretation of morphological findings.

Characterized antisera used in biochemical experiments such as elucidation of the biosynthesis of gonadotropins, location of tissue bound to gonadotropins by tagged or labeled antibody technique, i.e., studies of mechanism of LH and FSH stimulation of steroidogenesis using tissue slices and single-cell suspensions.

1960 Wakabayashi and Tasnaoki. *Endocrinology* 79:477.

1962 Midgley. *J. Exp. Med.* 115:289.

1963 Midgley. *Exp. Cell Res.* 32:606.

1971 Mougdal et al. *J. Biol. Chem.* 246:4983.

1971 Moyle et al. *J. Biol. Chem.* 246:4978.

1972 Behrman et al. *J. Endocrinol.* 52:419.

Antibodies obtained from conjugates of E$_2$-hemisuccinate coupled to bovine serum albumin, which inhibited the biological effects of E$_2$.

1968 Ferin et al. *Endocrinology* 83:565.

1969 Abraham. *51st June Meeting Endocrine Soc.*

Radioimmunoassay for estrogens using a digitoxin conjugate.

1968 Oliver et al. *J. Clin. Invest.* 47:1035.

Development of the protein-binding method based on the experiments in the uterus that demonstrated the presence of a specific estrogen-binding protein (rats).

1962 Jensen and Jacobsen. *Recent Prog. Horm. Res.* 18:387.

1964 Talwar et al. *Proc. Natl. Acad. Sci. USA* 52:1059.

1968 Korenman. *J. Clin Endocrinol. Metab.* 28:127.

1969 Corker and Exley. *J. Endocrinol.* 43:777.

Estrone-albumin conjugates made which generated antisera in rabbits that had some degree of specificity for estrone and estradiol.

1968 Sehon et al. *Abstr. 133rd Am. Chem. Soc. Meeting*, San Francisco, p. 19.

Development of synthetic, high purity prostaglandins with reasonable stability and shelf life. Discovery that acetylenic fatty acids and nonsteroidal anti-inflammatory agents are potent inhibitors of PG synthetase. Prostaglandin inhibitors provided an important tool for the study of the physiological role of prostaglandins in reproduction.

1971 Fried. *Ann. N.Y. Acad. Sci.* 180:38.

1971 Smith and Willis. *Nature (New Biol.)*.

1971 Vane. *Nature (New Biol.)* 231:235.

Development of PG radioimmunoassay.

1971 Jaffee et al. *Science* 171:494.

1971 Caldwell et al. *J. Clin. Endocrinol. Metab.* 33:171.

LUTEAL PHASE

First CBG assays for progesterone and 17α-hydroxyprogesterone using dog CPG as the assay protein.

1967 Murphy. *J. Clin. Endocrinol. Metab.* 27:973.

1967 Niel et al. *J. Clin. Endocrinol. Metab.* 27:1167.

Preparation of a single generation of functional corpora lutea in immature rats by inducing ovulation with PMS and mechanical stimulation of the cervix.

1964 Guillet and Rennels. *Tex. Rep. Biol. Med.* 22:78.

The use of tissue culture of granulosa and thecal cells as a method of studying the mechanism of luteinization.

1966 Channing. *Nature* 210:5042.

1966 Bergman, Bjersing, and Nilsson. *Acta Pathol. Microbiol. Scand.* [A] 68:461.

1969 Channing. *J. Endocrinol.* 43:381.

Antisera to 11α-hemisuccinyl progesterone generated with a high degree of specificity.

1972 Thorneycroft and Stone. *Contraception* 5:129.

1970 Niswender and Midgley. In: *Immunologic Methods in Steroid Determination*. Eds. Peron and Caldwell. New York: Appleton-Century-Crofts.

Gondadal function shown modified by injected LH antisera (female and male rats).

1963 Bourdel and Li. *Acta Endocrinol.* (Kbh.) 42:473.

1963 Hayashida. *J. Endocrinol.* 26:75.

1968 Laurence et al. *Endocrinology* 82:1190.

1971 Talaat and Laurence. *Fertil. Steril.* 22:18.

Methodological Needs

A method for isolating pure thecal cells in order to study the biochemistry of this tissue.

A sensitive steroid assay, so that the steroidogenic capacity of individual cells can be studied. This may be of importance in determining, within a population of cells, whether all or part of the cells have a similar or dissimilar biochemical profile.

A method to time ovulation in primates more closely. This is necessary in order to obtain more meaningful data in a species where it is not practical to use a large number of animals.

Development of rapid analytical techniques to replace the slower analysis of products of enzymatic reactions by isotope dilution technqiues. This is necessary to speed information that would contribute to the elucidation of the mechanisms involved in the steroidogenic pathway.

Contraceptive Methods

Period 1960–1974

Evaluation of luteolytic agents as contraceptives suggested.

1968 Pincus. *Harvey Lect.* 62:165.

Certain anabolic steroids have been shown to shorten luteal phase, presumably by inhibiting the release of pituitary gonadotropins (but not hCG) on the ovary. Possible applications as a morning-after pill.

1971 Nagvi and Warren. *Steroids* 18:731. (rat)

1973 Bolch and Warren. *Am. J. Obstet. Gynecol.* 117:122. (humans)

Aminoglutethimide shown to depress rapidly plasma progesterone levels in rats and to lead to abortion.

1972 Glasser. *Endocrinology* 90:1363.

Suppression of luteal phase progesterone levels by oral progesterone, in order to provoke menses whether or not fertilization has occurred, shown to have high failure rate.

1972 Nygren et al. *Contraception* 5:445.

Possibilities for the Future

Use of exogenously administered ovarian steroid binding proteins to interfere with ovulation, implantation, or ovarian-endometrial synchrony.

LUTEAL PHASE

Evidence that the blastocyst contributes a factor that increases luteal progesterone before the cycle progesterone would increase opens the possibility that, once the luteotropic agent is identified, an antibody or other inhibitor to the agent could be developed as a contraceptive. An extremely early method of detection of fertilization would, however, be necessary.

Estrogens have been found to interfere with early pregnancy. While the evidence is not complete, the most likely point of interference is luteal. These studies demonstrate significant reduction of progesterone.

1973 Gore et al. *J. Clin. Endocrinol. Metab.* 36:615.

If gestation requires a functional corpus luteum, at least in early pregnancy (as in humans), a chemical inhibition of luteal function is a possibility in preventing term pregnancy. Interference with the steroidogenic capacity of the luteal cells or vascular interference is feasible. Androstane derivatives have demonstrated an ability stoichiometrically to inhibit 3β-hydroxysteroid dehydrogenase. Certain asymmetrical estrogens have been found to localize in the corpus luteum and to interfere with estrogen production.

Various synthetic progestogens have been shown to suppress postovulatory plasma progesterone levels.

1971 Johansson. *Acta Endocrinol.* (Kbh.) 68:779.

Amine-exidase inhibitors with phenylhydrazine structure have been found to suppress progesterone synthesis in the rat, probably by inhibiting the release of LH — perhaps by interfering with the hypothalamic neurotransmitter that stimulates the synthesis of LRF.

1966 Robson. *Br. Med.* (Abstr.) 6:489.

FOLLICULAR PHASE: STEROIDOGENESIS

The development of immunization techniques through hormones of low molecular weight which are not normally antigenic make possible an approach to fertility control, although the field is only in its early stage of development. The difficulties of assessing the possible long-term effects of active immunization of naturally occurring hormones must be overcome. It may be possible in the short term — by passive immunization or by synthetic inhibitors or competitive antagonists — to neutralize the effects of endogenous hormone.

If ovulation can be inhibited, but near normal steroidogenesis (luteal phase) is retained, there might be minimal disruption of normal nonfertile-cycle processes.

STEROIDOGENIC PATHWAYS

There are several types of synthetic steroids which have been shown selectively to inhibit steroidogenic enzymes in the ovary (but not adrenal) of rats. Studies of long-term system effects of such inhibition and possible use of these synthetics as possible contraceptives are of interest.

1973 Goldman et al. *Acta Endocrinol.* (Kbh.) 73:146.

Oxymetholone has been identified as a potent inhibitor of 3β-ol steroid dehydrogenase and steroid isomerase (rats, cattle, bacterial systems), human placenta, and corpus luteum of pregnancy. In a recent work where humans were treated with the drug, it was found to inhibit the length of the luteal phase if given within a few days after ovulation. Further work needs to be done to determine whether the in vivo effect was directly on the ovary.

1963 Ferrari and Arnol. *Biochim. Biophys. Acta* 77:349.

1968 Goldman. *J. Clin. Endocrinol. Metab.* 18:1539.

1968 Neville and Engel. *J. Clin. Endocrinol. Metab.* 28:49.

1973 Klacher et al. *J. Clin. Endocrinol. Metab.* 36:142.

Inhibition of cholesterol conversion to pregnenolone by interference with the cytochrome P-450 oxidase system, e.g., amphenone, glutethemide, metyrapone, and imidazoles. In rats, depression of progesterone leads to abortion or resorption of fetus in 72 hours. Clinical trials have not yet led to optimal conditions or an agent whereby the inhibition of luteal progesterone synthesis will lead to effective pregnancy termination and minimal side effects.

1972 Salhanick. In: *Proc. 4th Int. Cong. Endocrinol.,* Washington, D.C. Ed. Scrow. Amsterdam: Excerpta Medica.

1973 Salhanick et al. In: *The Regulation of Mammalian Reproduction.* Eds. Segal, Crozier, Corfman, Condliffe. Springfield: Thomas, p. 520.

In humans, aminogluthemide at 2 g/day for 5 days will depress progesterone levels by 50%, but levels must be reduced 80–90% for several days to induce abortion of 2-month gestations.

1972 Salhanick. In: *Proc. 4th Int. Cong. Endocrinol.,* Washington, D.C. Ed. Scrow. Amsterdam: Excerpta Medica.

The Menstrual Cycle

Biological Processes: Significant Discoveries

Period before 1960

Early concepts of cyclic endometrial responses to ovarian hormonal stimulation.

1928 Corner. *Am. J. Physiol.* 86:74.

Increasing potency of pituitary after castration.

1929 Engle. *Am. J. Physiol.* 88:101.

1929 Evans and Simpson. *Am. J. Physiol.* 89:371.

Negative feedback by estrogen on gonadotropin demonstrated in rats.

1930 Meyer et al. *Proc. Soc. Exp. Biol. Med.* 27:202.

Development of "push-pull" theory of interaction between hypophyseal and gonadal hormone production.

1930 Moore and Price. *Proc. Soc. Exp. Biol. Med.* 28:38.

1932 Moore and Price. *Am. J. Anat.* 50:13.

Influence of estrogen on stimulation of follicular development by causing increased LH secretion from the pituitary.

1934 Hohlweg. *Klin. Wochenschr.* 13:92.

1935 Lane. *Anat. Rec.* 61:141.

Inhibition of ovulation by progesterone in rabbits.

1937 Makepeace et al. *Am. J. Physiol.* 119:512.

Hypothesis and demonstration of the role of FSH and LH in follicular development.

1939 Fevold and Fiske. *Endocrinology* 24:823.

1942 Greep, Van Dyke, and Chow. *Endocrinology* 39:635.

Demonstration of a "critical period" for LH release on the afternoon of proestrus in the 4-day rat.

1949 Everett et al. *Endocrinology* 44:234.

1953 Everett and Sawyer. *Endocrinology* 52:83.

Possible facilitatory role of progesterone in induction of LH release.

1940 Everett. *Endocrinology* 27:681.

1944 Everett. *Endocrinology* 34:136.

Ovulation.

1950 Pfeiffer. *Proc. Soc. Exp. Biol. Med.* 45:455.

Demonstration of urinary peak of gonadotropins prior to ovulation and conception by bioassay.

1948 Farris. *Am. J. Obstet. Gynecol.* 56:347.

1949 Lloyd et al. *J. Clin. Endocrinol. Metab.* 9:636.

1959 McArthur. In: *Recent Progress in Endocrinology of Reproduction.* Ed. Lloyd. New York: Academic Press.

Investigation of cyclic variation in circulating estrogens during the menstrual cycle by bioassay and demonstration of midcycle peak.

1944 Markee and Berg. *Stanford Med. Bull.* 2:55.

1947 Littrell and Tom. *Endocrinology* 40:292.

Demonstration by chemical assay of daily changes in urinary estrogen levels during the menstrual cycle with midcycle peak.

1955 Brown. *Lancet* 1:320.

Measurement of circulating plasma progestins during the menstrual cycle.

1950 Forbes. *Am. J. Obstet. Gynecol.* 60:180.

Period 1960–1974

Urinary excretion patterns of FSH and LH established in human menstrual cycle, and hormonal interrelationships described.

1966 Bell et al. *Acta Endocrinol.* (Kbh.) 51:578.

Plasma levels of LH measured with demonstration of midcycle LH "ovulatory" surge.

1966 Midgley and Jaffe. *J. Clin. Endocrinol. Metab.* 26:1375.

1967 Odell, Ross, and Rayford. *J. Clin. Invest.* 46:248.

Plasma levels of FSH measured with demonstration of early FSH rise and low midcycle rise. Higher levels in early cycle 10–15 mIU/ml.

1967 Faiman and Ryan. *J. Clin. Endocrinol. Metab.* 27:1711.

Initial measurements of circulating gonadal steroids by newer methods of increased sensitivity including competitive protein binding and double isotope derivative methods.

Progesterone:

1967 Neill et al. *J. Clin. Endocrinol. Metab.* 27:1167.

1968 Yoshimi and Lipsett. *Steroids* 11:527.

17-hydroxyprogesterone:

1968 Strott and Lipsett. *J. Clin. Endocrinol. Metab.* 28:1426.

Estrogens:

1969 Baird and Guevara. *J. Clin. Endocrinol. Metab.* 29:149.

Administration of 2.5 mg norethynodrel and 0.1 mg mestranol abolished midcycle LH and FSH peaks as measured by radioimmunoassay.

1969 Swerdloff and Odell. *J. Clin. Endocrinol. Metab.* 29:157.

Small daily doses of progestins disrupt the LH secretion pattern but do not invariably abolish the LH peak.

1970 Larsson-Cohn et al. *Acta Endocrinol.* (Kbh.) 63:216.

Contraceptive effect of injectable progestogen medroxyprogesterone acetate is shown to depend primarily on the suppression of ovulation.

1967 Mishell. *Am. J. Obstet. Gynecol.* 99:86.

1970 Goldzieher et al. *Contraception* 2:225.

1972 El Mahgoub et al. *J. Reprod. Med.* 8:288.

Some 60% of women receiving low-dose chlormadinone ovulate during treatment.

1966 Martínez-Mantanou et al. *Fertil. Steril.* 17:49.

1967 Martínez-Mantanou et al. *Br. Med. J.* 2:730.

Demonstration of rise in circulating progesterone at the time of LH surge and prior to ovulation.

1970 Yussman and Taymor. *J. Clin. Endocrinol. Metab.* 30:396.

Simultaneous immunoassay of FSH, LH, progesterone, 17-hydroxyprogesterone, and estradiol-17β during the menstrual cycle.

1971 Mishell et al. *Am. J. Obstet. Gynecol.* 111:60.

1972 Abraham et al. *J. Clin. Endocrinol. Metab.* 34:312.

Demonstration of episodic secretion of LH and FSH by secretory bursts at 60–90 minute intervals.

1971 Midgley and Jaffe. *J. Clin. Endocrinol. Metab.* 33:962.

1972 Yen et al. *J. Clin. Endocrinol. Metab.* 34:671.

Circulating steriod levels in menstrual cycle established.

Realization of importance of circulating estrogen in regulation of menstrual cycle by positive stimulation of LH secretion.

1970 Vande Wiele et al. *Recent Prog. Horm. Res.* 26:104.

1972 Monroe, Jaffe, and Midgley. *J. Clin. Endocrinol. Metab.* 34:342.

1974 Thompson et al. *Am. J. Obstet. Gynecol.* 118:788.

Possible feedback effect of gonadal steroids at the pituitary level shown by modulation of pituitary responses to exogenous LRH.

1973 Thompson et al. *J. Clin. Endocrinol. Metab.* 37:152.

1974 Jaffe and Keye. *J. Clin. Endocrinol. Metab.* 39:850.

Elucidation by radioimmunoassay of circulating levels of LH, FSH, estrogen, and progesterone in the normal cycle; resemblance to human menstrual cycle, but relatively low levels of estradiol and progesterone in the luteal phase.

1970 Monroe et al. *Endocrinology* 86:1012.

1971 Hotchkiss, Atkinson, and Knobil. *Endocrinology* 89:177.

1974 Knobil. *Recent Prog. Horm. Res.* 30:1.

Hourly pulsatile ("circhoral") secretion of gonadotropins demonstrated in ovariectomized monkeys, but not intact animals.

1970 Dierschke et al. *Endocrinology* 87:850.

Demonstration of positive estrogen stimulus for LH release with need for sustained stimulus of 30–40 hours' duration.

1973 Karsch et al. *Endocrinology* 92:798.

Elaboration of concept that increasing estrogen (E2) stimulates release of gonadotropins.

1969 Schwartz. *Recent Prog. Horm. Res.* 25:1.

Measurement of increasing peripheral E2 levels and LH surge.

1970 Yoshinaga et al. *Endocrinology* 87:693.

1972 Naftolin et al. *J. Endocrinol.* 53:17.

Possible role of progestins (progesterone and 20α-dihydroxyprogesterone) in the regulation of LH release.

1969 Goldman et al. *Endocrinology* 85:1137.

1971 Barraclough et al. *Endocrinology* 88:1437.

Temporal relationships of circulating levels of E2, P, and LH in 4-day estrous cycle (rats): E2 peaks at 1200 hours on diestrus I and proestrus at 0800 hours; P peaks at 2300 hours on diestrus I and proestrus at 2300 hours; LH peaks in proestrus at 1800 hours.

1974 Kalra and Kalra. *Endocrinology* 95:1711.

Major Gaps in Our Knowledge

HORMONAL ENVIRONMENT

Unanswered questions pertaining to gonadotropin releasing factors include: the putative existence of an FSH-releasing factor; mechanisms controlling LRF synthesis and release; the role of LRF in regulation of gonadotropin ovulatory surge, possibly by increased LRF release at midcycle.

1972 Malacara, Seyler, and Reichlin. *J. Clin. Endocrinol. Metab.* 34:271.

1974 Arimara et al. *J. Clin. Endocrinol. Metab.* 38:510.

Continuing problems pertaining to gonadotropins (GTs) include: factors regulating GT synthesis and release in the pituitary; physiologic significance of incremental changes in GT release; possible polymorphism of circulating GTs.

1970 Spiro. *Annu. Rev. Biochem.* 39:599.

1973 Peckham et al. *Endocrinology* 92:1660.

The role of estrogen in triggering the LH ovulatory surge.

Mechanisms inhibiting LH release after mono-ovulation in the human.

Lack of information about ovarian function includes the following significant areas: the selection process of the follicle that will ovulate; factors controlling maturation of the oocyte; factors influencing the life span of the human corpus luteum; the physiologic role of metabolites of progesterone.

OVULATION INHIBITION

What are long-term effects of oral-contraceptive-induced hypertension?

What effect does ovarian steroid administration during pregnancy have on the fetus?

Do oral contraceptives protect against development of breast cancer?

What is the relationship of oral contraceptive use to cervical dysplasia?

What oral contraceptive estrogen dose achieves the best balance between safety, efficacy, and acceptability?

What is the clinical significance of oral-contraceptive-induced changes in carbohydrate and lipid metabolism?

Should nursing mothers use oral contraceptives?

Methodological Advances

Period before 1960

Initial bioassays for estrogens.

1924 Allen and Doisy. *Am. J. Physiol.* 69:577.

1934 Fluhmann. *Endocrinology* 18:705.

1945 Hartman and Littrell. *Science* 102:178.

Development of procedures for bioassay of urinary gonadotropins.

"Total" gonadotropins:

1943 Klinefelter et al. *J. Clin. Endocrinol. Metab.* 3:529.

LH:

1941 Greep et al. *Proc. Soc. Exp. Biol. Med.* 46:644.

FSH:

1953 Steelman and Pohley. *Endocrinology* 53:604.

1955 Brown. *J. Endocrinol.* 13:59.

Initial iodination of insulin and quantitation by radioimmunoassay techniques.

1958 Berson and Yalow. *Adv. Biol. Med. Phys.* 6:349.

1959 Berson and Yalow. *J. Clin. Invest.* 38:1996.

Demonstrated antigenicity of steroid molecules linked to haptens.

1959 Erlanger et al. *J. Biol. Chem.* 234:1090.

1959 Lieberman et al. *Recent Prog. Horm. Res.* 15:165.

Development of long-acting steroid analogues.

1957 Junkmann. *Recent Prog. Horm. Res.* 13:389.

Period 1960–1974

Improvements in bioassays for urinary excretion of FSH and LH.

1961 Parlow. In: *Human Pituitary Gonadotropins.* Ed. Albert. Springfield: Thomas.

1963 Loraine and Bell. *Lancet* 1:1340.

Iodination of polypeptide hormones for labeling.

1963 Greenwood et al. *Biochem. J.* 89:114.

Development of radioimmunoassays for glycoproteins.

FSH:

1967 Faiman and Ryan. *J. Clin. Endocrinol. Metab.* 27:444.

LH:

1966 Midgley. *Endocrinology* 79:10.

1967 Aono et al. *Am. J. Obstet. Gynecol.* 98:996.

Early development of steroid assay by competitive protein-binding procedures.

1964 Murphy. *Nature* 201:679.

1967 Murphy. *J. Clin. Endocrinol. Metab.* 27:973.

Development of steroid-hapten antibodies and subsequent development of radioimmunoassay for steroids.

1969 Abraham. *J. Clin. Endocrinol. Metab.* 29:866.

1970 Caldwell et al. In: *Immunologic Methods in Steroid Determination.* Eds. Peron and Caldwell. New York: Appleton.

Passive immunization by antibodies to hormones as an experimental technique to block ovulation.

Antigonadotropins:

1963 Young et al. *Nature* 197:1117.

1974 Moudgal et al. *Recent Prog. Horm. Res.* 30:47.

Antiestrogen:

1969 Ferin et al. *Endocrinology* 85:1070.

Methodological Needs

Procedures for rapid assay of gonadotropins in peripheral plasma.

Improved methods for evaluation of follicular maturation.

Improved assay methods for LRF.

Satisfactory methods for prediction or detection of ovulation.

Bioassay in relation to peripheral plasma gonadotropins.

Contraceptive Methods

Period before 1960

Concept of use of "safe period" for fertility control.

1932 Ogino. *Zentralbl. Gynaekol.* 56:721.

1962 Hartman. *Science and the Safe Period.* Baltimore: Williams & Wilkins.

Synthesis of norethyndrone.

1951 Djerassi et al. *J. Am. Chem. Soc.* 73:1523.

Demonstration of inhibition of ovulation by orally active progestins in rabbits.

1953 Pincus and Chang. *Acta Physiol. Lat. Am.* 3:177.

Inhibition of ovulation by modification of gonadotropin release and the loss of LH surge through the use of oral contraceptives (humans).

1956 Pincus et al. *Endocrinology* 59:695.

1957 Rock, Garcia, and Pincus. *Recent Prog. Horm. Res.* 13:323.

1958 Pincus et al. *Am. J. Obstet. Gynecol.* 75:1333.

Extensive field trials of oral contraceptives demonstrate their effectiveness.

1958 Pincus et al. *Am. J. Obstet. Gynecol.* 75:1333.

Period 1960–1974

Probable luteolytic function of estrogen administered as postcoital contraceptive.

1966 Morris and van Wagenen. *Am. J. Obstet. Gynecol.* 96:804.

1973 Gore et al. *J. Clin. Endocrinol. Metab.* 36:615.

IUD as delivery system for intrauterine progesterone for contraception.

1970 Scommegna et al. *Fertil. Steril.* 21:201.

Norethindrone acetate demonstrated to be an effective contraceptive, although less so than medroxyprogesterone acetate when both are injected at 3-month intervals.

1973 Chinnatamby. *Aust. N.Z. J. Obstet. Gynecol.* 11:223.

1973 Kessern et al. *Acta Eur. Fertil.* 4:203.

Low-dose progestins may have a contraceptive effect through alteration of cervical mucus, interference with progesterone synthesis and metabolism, or inhibition of ovulation while allowing luteinization.

1968 Diczfalusy. *Am. J. Obstet. Gynecol.* 100:136.

1968 Zanartu et al. *Br. Med. J.* 2:263.

Oral contraceptives (OCs) having lower (10–20 μg) estrogen content shown to have somewhat increased pregnancy and intermenstrual bleeding rates.

1972 Preston. *Contraception* 6:17.

Medroxyprogesterone acetate demonstrated to be a highly effective contraceptive when injected intermuscularly at either 3- or 6-month intervals.

1971 Bloch. *S. Afr. Med. J.* 45:777.

1972 Schwallie and Assenzo. *Contraception* 6:315.

1972 Zanartu and Onelto. *Aust. N.Z. J. Obstet. Gynecol.* 10:65.

1973 Schwallie and Assenzo. *Fertil. Steril.* 24:331.

1974 McDaniel and Pardthaisong. *Am. J. Obstet. Gynecol.* 119:175.

OC use causes changes in carbohydrate and lipid metabolism; these are of unknown significance.

1966 Wynn et al. *Lancet* 11:720.

1969 Beck. In: *Metabolic Effects of Gonadal Hormones and Contraceptive Steroids.* Eds. Salhanick et al. New York: Plenum, p. 97.

1969 Spellacy. *Am. J. Obstet. Gynecol.* 104:448.

1970 Doar and Wynn. *Br. Med. J.* 1:149.

1971 Stokes and Wynn. *Lancet* 11:677.

1971 Spellacy et al. *Fertil. Steril.* 22:217.

1973 Spellacy et al. *Fertil. Steril.* 24:419.

OCs observed in a prospective study to be highly effective and generally safe for most women; risk of developing serious illness is small and mortality of a low order of magnitude, much lower than that associated with pregnancy.

1974 Royal College of General Practitioners. *Oral Contraceptives and Health: An Interim Report from the Oral Contraception Study for the Royal College of General Practitioners.* New York: Pitman Medical.

Liver and gallbladder dysfunction associated with OC use.

1968 Gershberg et al. *Obstet. Gynecol.* 31:186.

1973 Boston Collaborative Drug Surveillance Program. *Lancet* 1:1399.

1974 Editorials. *Br. Med. J.* 3:3; 4:430.

1974 Royal College of General Practitioners. *Oral Contraceptives: An Interim Report.* New York: Pitman Medical.

No evidence of association of OC use with breast, endometrial, or cervical cancers.

1972 Erb and Kallenber. *Acta Endocrinol.* (Kbh.) 30:143.

1972 Vessey et al. *Br. Med. J.* 3:719.

1973 Boston Collaborative Drug Surveillance Program. *Lancet* 1:1399.

1974 Royal College of General Practitioners. *Oral Contraceptives: An Interim Report.* New York: Pitman Medical.

OC use during lactation may lower the volume and nutrient content of milk, but the lower the dose and the later after onset of lactation OC use is initiated, the less the effect.

1971 Borglin and Sandlholm. *Fertil. Steril.* 22:39.

1972 Koetsawang et al. *Fertil. Steril.* 23:24.

1973 Barsivala and Virkar. *Contraception* 7:307.

Continuation and use-effectiveness rates of OCs found to be lower than expected.

1967 Jones and Maudlin. *Stud. Fam. Plann.* 24:1.

1968 Westoff and Ryder. *Public Health Rep.* 83:277.

OC use associated with increased mortality due to thromboembolic disease of less than 3 per 100,000.

1967 Royal College of General Practitioners. *J. R. Coll. Gen. Pract.* 13:267.

1968 Vessey and Doll. *Br. Med. J.* 2:199.

1969 Sartwell et al. *Am. J. Epidemiol.* 90:365.

1970 Inman and Vessey. *Br. Med. J.* 2:203.

1974 Badaracco and Vessey. *Br. Med. J.* 1:215.

OCs cause slight hypertension and aggravate preexisting hypertension.

1971 Laragh. *Am. J. Obstet. Gynecol.* 109:210.

1974 Spellacy and Burk. *Fertil. Steril.* 25:467.

1974 Royal College of General Practitioners. *Oral Contraceptives: An Interim Report.* New York: Pitman Medical.

Slight delay in return to fertility after OC use; appears unrelated to duration of use.

1974 Royal College of General Practitioners. *Oral Contraceptives: An Interim Report.* New York: Pitman Medical.

Nonphysician distribution of OCs proposed.

1974 Atkinson et al. *Stud. Fam. Plann.* 5:242.

1974 Smith et al. *Br. Med. J.* 4:161.

1975 Huber and Huber. *Stud. Fam. Plann.* 6:49.

Possibilities for the Future

Modification of gonadotropin release by manipulation of LRF production or release. Possible use of analogues of LRF as competitive antagonists.

Possible disruption of progesterone secretion by interference with corpus luteum function, i.e., use of "luteolytic" factors.

Interference with implantation by use of competitive progesterone antagonists.

Alterations in ovum transport.

Biological Processes: Significant Discoveries

Period before 1960

Demonstration that primordial germ cells are rich in alkaline phosphatase in humans and mice. The finding was exploited to establish the continuity of the germ cell line from the primordial germ cell to the primary oocyte at diplotene.

1953 McKay et al. *Anat. Rec.* 117:201.

1957 Mintz. *J. Embryol. Exp. Morphol.* 5:396.

Demonstration that rabbit and human oocytes will spontaneously complete meiosis in vitro without the addition of hormones.

1935 Pincus and Enzmann. *J. Exp. Med.* 62:665.

1939 Pincus and Saunders. *Anat. Rec.* 75:537.

Meiotic prophase is completed in all oocytes about the time of birth, although there is considerable variation among species.

1959 Jones and Krohn. *Nature* 185:1115.

Period 1960–1974

Demonstration of the high ameboid activity of mouse primordial germ cells in vitro, supporting the view that these cells actively migrate from the yolk sac to the gonadal ridge.

1963 Blandau, White, and Rumery. *Fertil. Steril.* 14:482.

DNA synthesis in preparation for meiosis occurs in the preleptotene stage.

1959 Sirlin and Edwards. *Exp. Cell. Res.* 18:190.

1962 Rudkin and Griech. *J. Cell Biol.* 12:169.

In humans and monkeys, structures similar to lamp-brush chromosomes exist in the diplotene stage of the meiotic prophase.

1967 Baker and Franchi. *Chromosoma* 22:358.

Chromosomes at diplotene stage incorporate radioactive precursors of RNA and protein in a similar fashion to amphibian oocytes.

1969 Baker, Beaumont, and Franchi. *J. Cell Sci.* 4:655.

In mice, spontaneous meiotic maturation occurs when oocytes are placed in vitro in a simple, chemically defined medium; pyruvate is an important component of the medium in the absence of cumulus cells. If cumulus cells are present, glucose will support maturation, indicating that the cumulus cells can feed the oocyte.

1967 Biggers, Whittingham, and Donahue. *Proc. Natl. Acad. Sci. USA* 58:560.

1968 Donahue. *J. Exp. Zool.* 169:237.

Oocytes derived from immature mice (<15 days old) do not mature spontaneously in vitro, suggesting that some maturational factor is involved.

1972 Szybek. *J. Endocrinol.* 54:527.

Spontaneous meiotic maturation of rhesus monkey oocytes is depressed in the nonbreeding season, suggesting a trophic gonadotropic effect necessary for maturation.

1974 Smith and Conaway. *Proc. Soc. Study Reprod.* Ottawa, Canada.

LH acts on the follicle cells.

1970 Channing. *Recent Prog. Horm. Res.* 26:589.

1974 Ericsson, Challis, and Ryan. *Dev. Biol.* 40:208.

Demonstration using the Cartesian diver technique that LH, but not FSH, directly stimulates respiration of granulosa cells.

1968 Hamberger. *Acta Physiol. Scand.* 76:410.

In rats, spontaneous meiotic maturation does not occur in organ cultures of follicles, unless the follicles are explanted shortly after the proestrous rise of LH, FSH, and prolactin.

1970 Lindner. In: *The Regulation of Mammalian Reproduction.* Eds. Segal, Crozier, Corfman, and Condliffe. Springfield: Thomas.

In rats, meiotic maturation can be stimulated in follicle organ cultures by the addition to the system of LH, FSH, cAMP, and prostaglandin E_2.

1973 Lindner et al. *Recent Prog. Horm. Res.* 29:79.

Meiotic maturation is not directly stimulated by cAMP since in mice, dibutyryl cAMP and theophylline inhibit spontaneous maturation.

1974 Wan Kyoo Cho, Stern, and Biggers. *J. Exp. Zool.* 187:383.

Oocytes from adult mice synthesize protein during spontaneous meiotic maturation.

1972 Stern, Rayyis, and Kennedy. *Biol. Reprod.* 7:341.

Although dibutyryl cAMP arrests spontaneous nuclear maturation in vitro in mice, it does not block protein synthesis, suggesting that independent cytoplasmic maturation also occurs.

1974 Stern and Wassarman. *J. Exp. Zool.* 189:275.

A lysine-rich protein, synthesized in adult mouse oocytes undergoing spontaneous maturation in vitro, comigrates with lysine-rich histone (f1).

1974 Wassarman and Sorensen. *Fed. Proc.* 33:1413.

Detailed description of the fine structure of the mammalian oocyte.

1960 Chiquoine. *Am. J. Anat.* 106:149.

1960 Anderson and Beams. *J. Ultrastruct. Res.* 3:432.

1960 Odor. *J. Biophys. Biochem. Cytol.* 7:567.

1964 Adams and Hertig. *J. Cell Biol.* 21:387.

1967 Baker and Franchi. *J. Cell Sci.* 2:213.

Immature mammalian oocytes are connected by intracellular bodies.

1967 Zamboni and Gondos. *J. Cell Biol.* 35:192.

1967 Weakley. *J. Anat.* 101:435.

1969 Ruby, Dyer, and Skalko. *J. Morphol.* 127:307.

Description of the development of cortical granules.

1967 Szollosi. *Anat. Rec.* 159:431.

1968 Anderson. *J. Cell Biol.* 37:514.

Major Gaps in Our Knowledge

Although we know that LH acts on the follicle cells, we do not know how it controls meiotic maturation. Does it involve removal of an inhibitory influence, or is an active intermediate molecule involved (e.g., 1-methyl adenine) as in echinoderms? The organ culture of follicles and the culture of denuded ova do not seem able to provide the answers.

We need to learn more about the types of protein synthesis involved in meiotic maturation and how they participate.

We need to determine whether cytoplasmic maturation is involved in maturation of the oocyte, as is the case in amphibia.

Oogenesis and Ovum Maturation (continued)

Methodological Advances

Period before 1960

Development of simple chemically defined media for the culture of preimplantation mouse embryos.

1956 Whitten. *Nature* 177:96.

Advancements in techniques of fixation, microtomy, and microscopy to learn more about the submicroscopic organization of cells.

1952 Palade. *J. Exp. Med.* 95:285.

1953 Fernandez-Moran. *Exp. Cell Res.* 5:255.

1953 Porter and Blum. *Anat. Rec.* 117:685.

1955 Matson. *J. Biophys. Biochem. Cytol.* 1:183.

Contraceptive Possibilities

Shedding of the zona pellucida following sperm penetration might offer an approach to immunological fertility control.

1972 Shivers et al. *Science* 178:1211.

Biological Processes: Significant Discoveries

Period before 1960

Physical characteristics of human oviducal fluid described.

1898 Bond. *J. Physiol.* (Lond.) 22:296.

The oviduct does not depend on influx from the peritoneal cavity for its fluid volume.

1891 Workressensky. *Zentralbl. Gynaekol.* 15:849.

1956 Bishop. *Am. J. Physiol.* 187:347.

Exogenous estrogen shown to accelerate the passage of ova through the oviduct.

1937 Burdick and Whitney. *Endocrinology* 21:637.

Estrogen is responsible for stimulating regeneration of the oviducal epithelium.

1928 Allen. *Morphol.* 46:479.

1928 Allen. *Am. J. Anat.* 42:467.

Oviducal ciliated cells increase during the follicular phase and decrease during the luteal phase.

1932 Westmann. *Acta Obstet. Gynecol. Scand.* 12:282.

1934 Westmann. *Acta Obstet. Gynecol. Scand.* 13:263.

1935 Joachimovits. *Biol. Generalis* 11:281

Progesterone probably provides the normal stimulation to atrophy and deciliation of oviducal epithelium.

1951 Andrew. *Am. J. Obstet. Gynecol.* 62:28.

1968 Good and Moyer. *Fertil. Steril.* 19:37.

Ovarian estrogen and progesterone affect the height and ultrastructure of oviducal epithelium, amount and structure of the different types of secretory granules, ciliogenesis, deciliation, and the rate of cilia beat.

1951 Andrews. *Am. J. Obstet. Gynecol.* 62:28.

1954 Flerko. *Mikroscop. Anat. Forsch.* 61:99.

1956 Borell et al. *Acta Obstet. Gynecol. Scand.* 35:36.

1959 Hashimoto et al. *J. Jap. Obstet. Gynecol. Soc.* 6:384.

Various enzymes are found in the cytoplasm of oviducal cells, and these may vary in activity with changes in secretions of ovarian steroids.

1953 Foraker et al. *Obstet. Gynecol.* 2:500.

1955 Augustin and Moser. *Arch. Gynaekol.* 185:759.

1959 Levy et al. *Endocrinology* 65:932.

Patterns of oviducal motility are associated with changes in glycogen content of oviducal musculature which varies with the reproductive cycle — low postmenses, higher postovulation, and highest in pregnancy — as does glycogen content of myometrium.

1939 Joel. *J. Obstet. Gynaecol. Br. Commonw.* 46:721.

1940 Joel. *Mschr. Gebrurtsh. Gynaekol.* 110:252.

1959 Fredricsson. *Acta Morphol. Neerl. Scand.* 38:109

Demonstration in the rabbit that ova pass from the fimbria into the ostium of the ampulla even if a ligature is placed between the ampulla and fimbria, thus ruling out the "vacuum hypothesis" in egg transport.

1958 Clewe and Mastroianni. *Fertil. Steril.* 9:13.

Demonstration in the rabbit that segmental movements occur in the oviduct and that they play a major role in the transport of ova.

1958 Black and Asdell. *Am. J. Physiol.* 192:63.

1961 Harper. *J. Reprod. Fertil.* 2:522.

As eggs pass through the oviduct, a mucin layer is deposited around them. Estrogen is responsible for the synthesis and storage of mucin in the oviducal epithelium, and progesterone is needed for its discharge. Embryonic degeneration may result if the mucin layer becomes too thin as a result of exogenous estrogen administration.

1954 Bassich and Hamilton. *J. Embryol. Exp. Morphol.* 2:81.

1957 Greenwald. *J. Exp. Zool.* 135:461.

1958 Greenwald. *Anat. Rec.* 130:477.

The density, cytological characteristics, and ultrastructure of the oviducal epithelium vary with species, segments of the oviduct, hormonal conditions, and reproductive phases, but cyclic changes are more profound in species with longer reproductive cycles.

1942 Alden. *Anat. Rec.* 34137:170.

1966 Horstmann and Stegner. In: *Handbuch der microscopischenanatomie des menschen.* Heidelberg: Springer, p. 35.

Oviducal activity is altered by prostaglandins.

1937 Euler. *J. Physiol.* (Lond.) 88:213.

1963 Eliasson. *Biochem. Pharmacol.* 12:405.

Period 1960–1974

OVIDUCAL FLUID

Oviduct fluid appears to form partly as a transudate of blood plasma and partly by active secretion. Recent physiological evidence for the latter is provided by demonstration of proteins in oviduct fluid not found in blood plasma, and demonstration by the short-circuit technique of Ussing and Zerahn of the active transport of Cl.

1971 Brunton and Brinster. *Am. J. Physiol.* 221:658.

1971 Shapiro, Jenrsch, and Yard. *J. Reprod. Fertil.* 24:403.

1972 Feigelson and Kay. *Biol. Reprod.* 6:244.

Flow of oviducal fluid through the isthmus is very low except for 3–6 days after estrus — the time when the egg passes into the uterus.

1968 Bellve and McDonald. *J. Reprod. Fertil.* 15:357.

Progesterone suppresses the amount of fluid in the oviducts and counteracts the stimulatory effect of estrogens.

1968 Hamner and Fox. *J. Reprod. Fertil.* 16:121.

Estrogen stimulates the production of fluid by the oviduct, with highest production at estrus.

1961 Mastroianni and Wallach. *Am. J. Physiol.* 200:815.

1970 McDonald and Bellve. *J. Reprod. Fertil.* 20:51.

Estrogens decrease the osmolarity of oviducal fluid but have no effect on its specific gravity or viscosity.

1969 Stambaugh et al. *J. Reprod. Fertil.* 18:51.

Electrolytic and enzymatic constituents of oviducal fluid quantitated for several animals.

1957 Olds and VanDenmark. *Fertil. Steril.* 8:345.

1963 Gregoire and Rakoff. *J. Reprod. Fertil.* 6:467.

1965 Hamner. *Fertil. Steril.* 19:137.

1965 Holmdahl and Mastroianni. *Fertil. Steril.* 16:587.

1966 Perkins and Goode. *J. Anim. Sci.* 25:465.

Fluids obtained from different segments of the oviduct have different compositions.

1969 David et al. *J. Reprod. Fertil.* 19:285.

Concentrations of pyruvate and lactate are raised considerably during the first 4–6 days after ovulation in the rabbit, whereas the rise in concentration of glucose is only marginally significant.

1956 Holmdahl and Mastroianni. *Fertil. Steril.* 16:587.

The pO_2 in the ampullary region of the oviduct, in situ in unanesthetised rabbits, shown by means of a platinum electrode to be 60 mm Hg.

1965 Mastroianni and Jones. *J. Reprod. Fertil.* 9:99.

Recommended reviews:

1969 Hafez and Blandau, eds. *The Mammalian Oviduct.* Chicago: University of Chicago Press.

1974 Johnson and Foley, eds. *The Oviduct and Its Functions.* New York: Academic Press.

OVUM TRANSPORT

In rabbits, cilia play a major role in the transport of ova, possibly by creating a flow of fluid toward the ostium; also, the presence of the cumulus cells is essential for the cilia to move the ova.

1969 Blandau. In: *The Mammalian Oviduct.* Eds. Hafez and Blandau. Chicago: University of Chicago Press.

In monkeys, the cilia of the fimbria are replaced during each ovarian cycle, and their regeneration is associated with the secretion of estrogen.

1969 Brenner. In: *The Mammalian Oviduct.* Eds. Hafez and Blandau. Chicago: University of Chicago Press.

There are no cyclic changes in the ciliated cells of the human oviduct.

1963 Shimoyama. *J. Jap. Obstet. Gynecol. Soc.* 15:1237.

1964 Hashimoto. *J. Jap. Obstet. Gynecol. Soc.* 11:92.

1966 Clyman. *Fertil. Steril.* 17:281.

In rabbits, the rate of movement of ova through the oviduct is not uniform; it is rapid through the ampulla and slow through the isthmus.

1961 Harper. *J. Reprod. Fertil.* 2:522.

Proposal that the ova are held at the junction between the ampulla and the isthmus by means of a "physiological sphincter."

1961 Greenwald. *Fertil. Steril.* 12:80.

1964 Brundin. *Acta Physiol. Scand.* 60:295.

1964 Brundin. *Acta Physiol. Scand.* 61:219.

1970 El-Banna and Hafez. *Anat. Rec.* 166:469.

Muscular contractions of the oviduct are complex, stimulated by the mesosalpinx and mesotubarium, and vary in frequency and amplitude with the reproductive cycle in response to ovarian steroids.

1961 Harper. *J. Reprod. Fertil.* 2:522.

1961 Greenwald. *Fertil. Steril.* 12:80.

1963 Greenwald. *Fertil. Steril.* 14:666.

1965 Harper. *J. Endocrinol.* 77:114.

1965 Harper. *J. Endocrinol.* 31:217.

1966 Chang. *Endocrinology* 79:939.

1967 Greenwald. *Anat. Rec.* 157:163.

Proposal that the orderly movements of the oviduct at the time of ovulation are related to the increased secretion of progesterone and a fall in the level of estrogens.

1971 Boling and Blandau. *Biol. Reprod.* 4:174.

In rabbits, the degree of adrenergic innervation increases from the ovarian to the uterine end of the oviduct (based on the content of norepinephrine in different regions of the oviduct).

1964 Brundin. *Acta Physiol. Scand.* 62:156.

In rabbits, the functional adrenergic innervation of the oviduct is modified by the endocrine state.

1968 Longley, Black, and Currie. *J. Reprod. Fertil.* 17:579.

1973 Polidoro, Howe, and Black. *J. Reprod. Fertil.* 35:331.

The response of the oviduct to stimulation of its α and β receptors varies with the reproductive cycle, although it has no cholinergic nerve supply. The isthmus and ampulla have different innervation and response.

1960 Sandburg et al. *Acta Obstet. Gynecol. Scand.* 39:506.

1964 Brundin. *Acta Physiol. Scand.* 60:295.

1965 Brundin. *Acta Physiol. Scand.* (Suppl.) 259:1.

In the oviducal isthmus, but not the ampulla, there is a rich adrenergic plexus and circular muscle fiber.

1964 Brundin and Wirsen. *Acta Physiol. Scand.* 61:505.

1967 Owman et al. *Obstet. Gynecol.* 30:763.

PGE_1 relaxes the isthmic circular muscle but contracts the longitudinal muscle.

1963 Sandberg et al. *Acta Obstet. Gynecol. Scand.* 42:269.

Prostaglandins affect differently the proximal and distal segments of the oviduct.

1965 Horton et al. *J. Physiol.* (Lond.) 180:514.

PGE_1 and PGE_2 suppress, while $PGF_{1\alpha}$ and $PGF_{2\alpha}$ increase, oviduct contractions. The sensitivity of the oviduct to $PGF_{2\alpha}$ is increased at the time of expected ovulation.

1974 Spilman. Unpulished presentation from colloquium: Prostaglandins and reproductive physiology. Detroit, Mich. April 4, 1974.

Prostaglandin $F_{2\alpha}$ levels are higher in oviducal fluids than in circulating serum and vary with the menstrual cycle.

1974 Swtantarta et al. *Fertil. Steril.* 25:250.

SPERM TRANSPORT

IUDs interfere with sperm transport through the oviducts of sheep but not of primates.

1965 Hawk. *Reprod. Fertil.* 10:267.

1973 Hafez. In: *Handbook of Physiology.* Eds. Astwood and Greep. Baltimore: Williams & Wilkins, sec. 7, vol. 2, pt. 2, p. 112.

Glucose utilization and lactate accumulation by sperm are stimulated by oviducal fluids.

1966 Restall and Wales. *Aust. J. Biol. Sci.* 19:883.

Factors necessary for capacitation of rabbit sperm are present in the oviduct.

1962 Adams and Chang. *J. Exp. Zool.* 151:159.

1967 Hamner and Sojka. *Proc. Soc. Exp. Biol. Med.* 124:689.

No significant quantity of antibody has been found in oviducal fluid.

1967 Ackerman. *Nature* 213:253.

In semen-immunized rabbits, slightly fewer sperm reach the fibriated end of the oviduct than in unimmunized animals.

1969 Behrman. In: *The Mammalian Oviduct.* Eds. Hafez and Blandau. Chicago: University of Chicago Press, p. 364.

Eggs collected from unimmunized and semen-immunized rabbits implanted at the same rates in unimmunized recipient rabbits, but implanted at lower rates in semen-immunized recipients.

1969 Behrman. In: *The Mammalian Oviduct.* Eds. Hafez and Blandau. Chicago: Univeristy of Chicago Press, p. 367.

Major Gaps in Our Knowledge

There is an extensive literature on the composition of oviducal fluid from several species (rabbits, sheep, cattle, monkeys, and humans) in several reproductive states, collected by cannulation over relatively long periods. The literature begins in 1960 with the work of Clewe and Mastroianni, (*J. Reprod. Fertil.* 1:146). The following reviews provide comprehensive coverage:

1966 Restall. *Adv. Reprod. Fertil.* 2:181.

1974 Brackett and Mastroianni. In: *The Oviduct and Its Functions*. Eds. Johnson and Foley. New York: Academic Press, p. 133.

There are now sufficient indications in the literature to suggest that the local environment in the oviduct may vary from place to place. If this is so, the physiological meaning of much of the analytical work will be obscure. The study of the microenvironment of the preimplantation embryos as they pass along the oviduct is therefore of high priority. This includes both ionic and organic components.

Studies are needed to demonstrate the role of directional flows of oviduct fluid in controlling the microenvironment of the embryos.

There is evidence that the microenvironment in the oviduct is high in K^+ in comparison to plasma. Studies are required to determine how this high level of K^+ is produced and regulated.

Combined manometric and electrophysiological studies have shown that the movements of the oviduct of the rabbit are very complex. The nature of these movements needs to be analyzed in greater detail. The implications of possible frequency gradients need to be thoroughly explored and their patterns related to the endocrine status of the animal.

1974 Talo. *Biol. Reprod.* 11:3351.

There is ample evidence of a relation between the endocrine status of the animal and the functional state of the adrenergic innervation. This relationship needs to be elucidated in more detail.

A quantitative evaluation of the density of adrenergic nerve fibers in various portions of the oviduct is needed.

What is the pattern of cyclic changes in the muscle contractions of the oviducal isthmus?

What are the causes of ectopic pregnancy? Why are there species differences in the incidence of the condition?

What is the molecular basis for species differences in the hormone dependence of oviducal ciliated cells?

Does estrogen merely initiate ciliogenesis in the oviducal epithelium, or is its presence necessary for completion of the process?

By what mechanism does progesterone antagonize estrogen and inhibit oviducal ciliogenesis?

What is the significance for fertility of a shortened segment of oviduct?

Does the contraction of muscle within the folds regulate possible functions of gamete transport?

What is the mechanism of egg transport through the oviducal isthmus?

What is the mechanism of the physiologic stricture of the ampullary-isthmic junction?

What effect do hormones have on the muscular contraction of the ampulla and isthmus and the stricture of the ampullary-isthmic junction?

Is the opening of the ampullary-isthmic junction controlled by hormonal or pharmacologic factors?

Are hormones concentrated differently in the different regions of the oviduct?

Which immunoglobulins are transferred into the oviducal fluid?

Do the mucosal folds have an important role in gamete transport?

What are the roles of muscle and cilia in egg transport through the oviducal ampulla?

How are the ciliated cells arranged on the folds? Does this arrangement affect sperm transport?

What effect do hormones have on the biochemical and biophysical properties of the oviduct?

What is the significance of species differences in the presence of oviducal bursae?

Methodological Advances

Period before 1960

"Laparoscopy" using a cystoscope first described in humans.

1910 Jacobaeus. Cited in Steptoe. *Laparoscopy in Gynecology*. London: Livingston, 1967.

Introduction of the oviducal insufflation test of tubal patency in women.

1920 Rubin. *JAMA* 75:661.

Abdominal window technique.

1926 Westman. *Munch. Med. Wochenschr.* 73:1293.

Use of silver stains to define nerve networks.

1929 Harting. *Z. Zellforsch. Mikrosk. Anat.* 9:544.

Short-circuit method for the measurement of active ion transport.

1951 Ussing and Zerahn. *Acta Physiol. Scand.* 23:40.

Demonstration of the feasibility of collecting oviduct fluid in the rabbit by cannulation of the fimbriated end; demonstration that oviduct fluid can be secreted against a considerable hydrostatic pressure.

1956 Bishop. *Am. J. Physiol.* 187:347.

Period 1960–1974

Development of methods for continuous collection of oviducal fluid.

1961 Mastroianni et al. *Fertil. Steril.* 12:417.

1963 Hamner and Williams. *J. Reprod. Fertil.* 5:143.

Use of formaldehyde-induced fluorescence for the demonstration of biogenic amines.

1965 Flock and Owman. *Acta Univ. Lund.* (Sect. II) 7:1.

Maintenance of oviducts in organ and tissue culture preparations.

1969 Rumery. In: *The Mammalian Oviduct*. Eds. Hafez and Blandau. Chicago: University of Chicago Press, p. 445.

Development of techniques allowing in vivo observation of exteriorized oviducts.

1971 Blandau. In: *Methods in Mammalian Embryology*. Ed. Daniel. San Francisco: Freeman, p. 1.

Development of a nonsurgical technique to obtain unimplanted eggs from the human uterus in situ.

1972 Croxatto et al. *Am. J. Obstet. Gynecol.* 112:662.

Use of a strain gauge transducer to measure ampullary muscle contractions.

1974 Garcia et al. *Fertil. Steril.* 25:301.

Methodological Needs

The adaptation of micropuncture and ultramicrochemical techniques for the analysis of small samples of oviducal fluid collected from the neighborhood of the embryos as they move along the oviduct.

The adaptation of ion-sensitive and other electrodes to measure the concentration of various constituents of the oviduct in situ.

Instrumentation for measurement of oviducal ciliary activity.

Improved instrumentation for measuring oviducal muscle contractions.

Tissue and organ culture techniques that support the cytosol estrogen receptor system.

Methods for separating the thin oviducal muscle layers from mucosa so that biochemical studies of the muscle may be done.

A model for ectopic pregnancy in humans.

Contraceptive Methods

Period before 1960

Various methods of tubal ligation at laparotomy described.

1919   Madlener. *Zentralbl. Gynaekol.* 43:380.

1925   Irving. *Am. J. Obstet. Gynecol.* 8:353.

1930   Bishop and Nelms. *N.Y. State J. Med.* 30:214.

1934   Aldridge. *Am. J. Obstet. Gynecol.* 27:471.

1961   Uchida. *Proc. 3rd World Conf. Obstet. Gynecol.* 1:26.

Colpotomy used to expose the tubes for ligation.

1928   Babcock. *Am. J. Obstet. Gynecol.* 17:573.

1949   Boysen and McRae. *Am. J. Obstet. Gynecol.* 58:488.

1953   Evans. *Am. J. Obstet. Gynecol.* 66:393.

Culdoscopy first described and suggested as sterilization procedure.

1944   Decker and Cherry. *Am. J. Surg.* 64:40.

Period 1960–1974

Electrocoagulation and cutting of the Fallopian tubes through the laparoscope introduced and evaluated.

1970   Steptoe. *Br. Med. Bull.* 26:60.

Laparoscopic electrocoagulation without cutting suggested and evaluated.

1970   Liston et al. *Lancet,* February: 382.

Laparoscopic electrocoagulation through a device permitting a single wound technique suggested and evaluated.

1973   Wheeless and Thompson. *Obstet. Gynecol.* 42(5):751.

Cryosurgery to occlude tubes found unsatisfactory.

1972   Martens. In: *Human Sterilization.* Springfield: Thomas, p. 305.

Culdoscopy used for tubal ligation and occlusion with clips.

1963   Clymna. *Obstet. Gynecol.* 21:343.

1964   Hyanshi and Nishio. In: *Proc. 7th Intl. Conf. Planned Parenthood Fed.,* Singapore, Feb. 1963. Eds. Cadburg et al. Amsterdam: Excerpta Medica, p. 623.

Postcoital estrogens probably do not work by altering the rate of ovum passage through the oviduct.

1972   Croxatto et al. *Fertil. Steril.* 23:447.

Tantalum clips applied laparoscopically found to have high failure rate.

1972   Davidson and Donald. *Scott. Med. J.* 17(6):210.

1972   Palmer. Presentation at Int. Conf. Contraception, Sterilization and Abortion, May 1972, Paris, France.

1974   Wheeless. *Obstet. Gynecol.* 44:752.

Spring-loaded clips applied through laparoscope evaluated.

1972   Hulka and Omran. *Fertil. Steril.* 23(9):633.

1973   Hulka et al. *Am. J. Obstet. Gynecol.* 116:715.

Silastic rubber bands applied to tubes through the laparoscope.

1974   Yoon, Wheeless, and King. *Am. J. Obstet. Gynecol.* 120(1):132.

Very small suprapubic incisions under local anesthesia used for tubal ligation of the Pomeroy type.

1971   Saunders and Munsick. *Obstet. Gynecol.* 78:273.

1974   Osathanondh. *Contraception* 10:251.

Possibilities for the Future

Premature opening of the ampullary-isthmic junction might have a contraceptive effect.

Alteration of the direction or rate of oviducal ciliary beat by chemical or pharmacologic means in order to interfere with gamete transport.

Pharmacologic or immunologic alteration of the sperm capacitors present in the oviduct to interfere with the process of capacitation.

Drug-induced changes in oviducal fluid volume might exert a contraceptive effect if the dilution of an essential constituent or the concentration of an inhibitor of egg cleavage resulted.

Use of pharmacologic agents to control oviduct secretions or embryonal development. Alteration of the secretory products of the oviduct so as to affect gamete transport or embryonal development.

Use of immune mechanisms to produce antibodies to sperm or egg antigens, so that the antibodies could pass with the transudate into the oviducal fluid.

Since oviducal fluid is partially a transudate, specific drugs might be delivered to gametes via transudation to alter physiologic events.

Use of pharmacologic agents to alter tubal motility and thereby interfere with gamete transport and/or ovulatory-endometrial synchrony.

Uterotubal Junction

Biological Processes: Significant Discoveries

Period before 1960

Mammals differ markedly in the morphology and anatomy of the uterotubal junction.

1942   Alden. *Anat. Rec.* 84:134.

1952   Novak and Rubin. *Ciba Found. Clin. Symp.* 4(6):179.

1954   Lisa et al. *Surg. Gynecol. Obstet.* 99:159.

1959   Vasen. *Int. J. Fertil.* 4:309.

Pressures required to open the uterotubal junction vary with the menstrual cycle, but these variations are not understood.

1925   Rubin. *JAMA* 84:661.

1940   Bernstein and Feresten. *Endocrinology* 26:946.

The number of sperm passing the uterotubal junction varies with the reproductive cycle, but the number entering the oviduct is always far smaller than the number in the uterus.

1949   Blandau and Odor. *Anat. Rec.* 103:93.

Depending on the species, ovarian steroids do or do not speed egg transport through the oviduct and the uterotubal junction.

1959   Balck and Asdell. *Am. J. Physiol.* 197:1275.

1959   Noyes et al. *J. Endocrinol.* 18:108.

Occlusion of the uterotubal junction may be affected by contraction of the uterine muscle girdling the intramural portion of the oviduct.

1959   Vasen. *Int. J. Fertil.* 4:309.

Period 1960–1974

Nonmotile sperm and inert particles, as well as normal sperm, pass the uterotubal junction.

1961   Egli and Newton. *Fertil. Steril.* 12:5.

The area of the uterotubal junction serves as a sperm reservoir for up to 48 hours after coitus. Sperm from the reservoir probably pass continually into the oviducts.

1965   Rigby and Glover. *J. Anat.* 99:416.

1966   Rigby. *J. Reprod. Fertil.* 11:153.

Lowered fertility, observed after progestogen treatment of sheep and cattle, may be accounted for by a decrease in sperm transport through the uterotubal junction.

1962   Hancock. *Anim. Breeding Abstr.* 30:285.

1969   Quinlivan and Robinson. *J. Reprod. Fertil.* 19:73.

Surgical removal of the uterotubal junction, followed by uterotubal reanastomosis, reduced by half the rate of implantation, indicating that sperm migration, fertilization, and egg transport can occur in the absence of the junction.

1969   David et al. *Fertil. Steril.* 20:250.

The uterotubal junction is probably not the major barrier to egg transport through the oviduct.

1961   Greenwald. *Fertil. Steril.* 12:80.

1970   El-Banna and Hafez. *Anat. Rec.* 166:469.

Major Gaps in Our Knowledge

What mechanisms are involved in the transport of sperm and eggs through the uterotubal junction?

What are the effects of reproductive cycle changes, changes in ovarian function, and exogenous hormones on the patency of the uterotubal junction?

What is the relative importance of the uterotubal junction as compared to other portions of the oviduct in controlling entry of eggs into the uterus? as compared to the cervix in controlling entry of sperm into the oviduct?

What are the histological and histochemical changes in the uterotubal junction following changes in levels of ovarian steroids, copulation, and at the time of egg transport to the uterus?

Methodological Advances

Period before 1960

Development of equipment to measure the pressure required to open the uterotubal junction.

1928   Anderson. *Am. J. Anat.* 42:255.

1958   Stavorski and Hartmann. *Obstet. Gynecol.* 11:622.

Methodological Needs

Device for improved visualization of the uterotubal junction.

See also the Oviduct and Uterus tables.

Contraceptive Methods

Period before 1960

Administration of carbolic acid and tincture of iodine into the uterus to produce sterility from endometrial and tubal scarring.

1941   Salgado. *An. Bras. Cien.* 503.

Period 1960–1974

Quinacrine introduced transcervically into the uterine fundus shown to be unreliable in producing tubal occlusion.

1970   Zipper et al. *Fertil. Steril.* 21:581.

1973   Davidson and Wilkins. *Contraception* 7:333.

1974   Alvarado et al. In: *Hysteroscopic Sterilization.* New York: Symposia Specialists, p. 85.

Silver nitrate paste introduced transcervically shown to be unsatisfactory for tubal occlusion with high complication rate.

1973   Ringrose. *Obstet. Gynecol.* 42:151.

Use of cyanoacrylate tissue adhesives for tubal occlusion.

1965   Corfman et al. *Science* 148:1348.

1970   Omran and Hulka. *Int. J. Fertil.* 15:226.

1972   Richart et al. In: *Human Sterilization.* Springfield: Thomas, p. 360.

Methyl 2-cyanoacrylate shown to require two applications to occlude tubes.

1972   Stevenson and Taylor. *J. Obstet. Gynecol.* 79:1028.

Solid intratubal devices of dacron or teflon inserted transcervically shown to adhere poorly to tubal tissue.

1970   Omran and Hulka. *Int. J. Fertil.* 15:226.

1973   Richart and Neuwirth. Unpublished report of current studies of intratubal devices sponsored by WHO, Geneva.

Silicone rubber introduced transcervically shown to occlude tubes unreliably, although some compounds were better than others.

1967   Hefnawi et al. *Am. J. Obstet. Gynecol.* 99:421.

1970   Racshit. *J. Obstet. Gynecol. Ind.* 20:618.

1974   Erb et al. *Contemp. Obstet. Gynecol.* (February 19):82.

Hysteroscopy used for transcervical occlusion at the uterotubal junction with relatively high complication and failure rates.

1973   Semm. *Endoscopy* 5:218.

Possibilities for the Future

Devices or materials to close the uterotubal junction temporarily or permanently.

Pharmacologic agents to close the junction.

Biological Processes: Significant Discoveries

Period before 1960

Ovarian and, specifically, follicular extracts shown to induce estrus.

1905 Marshall and Jolly. *Philos. Trans. R. Soc. Lond. (Biol.)* 198:99.

1912 Adler. *Arch. Gynaekol.* 95:349.

1923 Allen and Doisy. *JAMA* 81:819.

1924 Allen and Doisy. *Am. J. Physiol.* 69:577.

Hysterectomy in guinea pigs is followed by ovulation and formation of a corpus luteum.

1922 Loeb. *Proc. Soc. Exp. Biol. Med.* 20:441.

1927 Loeb. *Am. J. Physiol.* 83:202.

Involution of the uterus following delivery is due to a decrease in the size of individual myometrial cells.

1921 Kurimitsu and Loeb. *Am. J. Physiol.* 55:422.

Estrogen isolated from the urine of pregnant women.

1929 Doisy et al. *Am. J. Physiol.* 90:329.

Progesterone demonstrated necessary for the maintenance of pregnancy.

1930 Allen and Corner. *Proc. Soc. Exp. Biol. Med.* 27:403.

1935 Allen et al. *Science* 82:153.

Progesterone is isolated.

1932 Allen. *J. Biol. Chem.* 98:591.

Hypophysectomy or oophorectomy near term results in prolonged gestation.

1933 Selye et al. *Proc. Soc. Exp. Biol. Med.* 30:589.

1935 McPhail. *Proc. R. Soc. London* B117:34.

1938 Boe. *Acta Pathol. Microbiol. Scand.* (Suppl.) 26:1.

In some mammals (rats, mice, rabbits), exogenous progesterone delays parturition.

1938 Boe. *Acta Pathol. Microbiol. Scand.* (Suppl.) 26:1.

1938 Heckel and Allen. *Am. J. Obstet. Gynecol.* 35:131.

1959 Kroc et al. *Ann. N.Y. Acad. Sci.* 75:942.

Following hypophysectomy or oophorectomy, unrestrained uterine activity, which can be controlled by high doses of progesterone, results in termination of intrauterine pregnancy.

1933 Pencharz and Long. *Am. J. Anat.* 53:117.

1933 Selye et al. *Proc. Soc. Exp. Biol. Med.* 30:589.

1938 Heckel and Allen. *Am. J. Obstet. Gynecol.* 35:131.

1941 Courrier. *Soc. Biol.* 135:820.

Removal of fetuses or fetal death *in utero* was observed not to disturb the course of pregnancy.

1938 Newton. *Physiol. Rev.* 18:419.

1943 Van Wagenen and Newton. *Surg. Gynecol. Obstet.* 77:539.

Hysterectomy prolongs the luteal phase in some species with its effect depending on the timing of hysterectomy in relation to luteal regression.

1941 Greep. *Anat. Rec.* 80:465.

1942 Heckel. *Surg. Gynecol. Obstet.* 75:379.

1946 Chu et al. *J. Endocrinol.* 4:392.

Hysterectomy does not affect the reproductive cycle in some other species, including humans.

1907 Carmichael and Marshall. *Proc. R. Soc. London* B79:387.

1919 Drips. *Am. J. Anat.* 25:117.

1925 Hartman. *Am. J. Anat.* 35:25.

1934 Cheval. *Proc. R. Soc. Med.* 27:1395.

1936 Burford and Diddle. *Surg. Gynecol. Obstet.* 62:701.

1941 Jones and TeLinde. *Am. J. Obstet. Gynecol.* 41:682.

1960 TeLinde and Wharton. *Am. J. Obstet. Gynecol.* 80:844.

Classification of animals into those that do and those that do not abort after oophorectomy during pregnancy suggested a role for the ovary in pregnancy maintenance in the former group and a role for the placenta in the latter.

1962 Amoroso and Finn. In: *The Ovary.* Ed. Zuckerman. New York: Academic Press, vol. 1.

Progesterone increases uterine weight — although not as much as does estradiol — but does not increase rate of mitosis in uterine cells.

1950 Noyes et al. *Fertil. Steril.* 1:3.

Estrogens cause a marked increase in uterine anabolic activity and biosynthesis.

1956 Herranean and Meuller. *J. Biol. Chem.* 223:369.

1957 Herranean and Meuller. *Biochim. Biophys. Acta* 24:223.

Rapid uterine growth induced by estradiol is associated with early stimulation of various metabolic pathways.

1958 Meuller et al. *Recent Prog. Horm. Res.* 14:95.

Glycogen content of myometrium is lowest postmenses, higher postovulation, and highest during pregnancy.

1958 Brody. *Acta Endocrinol. (Kbh.)* 27:377.

Blood levels of catecholamines are not elevated during pregnancy.

1959 Israel et al. *Obstet. Gynecol.* 14:68.

Failure to demonstrate concentration of radioactive progesterone in the uteri of rats.

1950 Riegel et al. *Endocrinology* 47:311.

Estradiol 17-β, estrone, and estriol shown to promote rat uterine growth to different degrees — estradiol 17-β most and estriol least; the latter inhibits the effect of the other two.

1954 Hisaw et al. *J. Clin. Endocrinol. Metab.* 14:1134.

Certain estrogens ("impeded estrogens") have the capacity to promote uterine growth in rats only to a limited extent and to inhibit the growth induced by estrone.

1955 Huggins and Jensen. *J. Exp. Med.* 102:335.

The uterine sugar transport system has many characteristics of other tissues but is also responsive to estrogen.

1953 Szego and Roberts. *Recent Prog. Horm. Res.* 8:419.

1966 Barker and Warren. *Endocrinology* 78:1205.

1967 Roskoski and Steiner. *Biochim. Biophys. Acta* 135:717.

Myometrium is spontaneously contractile, but is restrained during pregnancy.

1956 Csapo. *Recent Prog. Horm. Res.* 12:405.

Semen found to have a stimulatory effect on the uterus both in vivo and in vitro.

1930 Kurzrok and Lieb. *Proc. Soc. Exp. Biol. Med.* 28:268.

Identification of prostaglandins.

1936 von Euler. *J. Physiol. (Lond.)* 88:213.

Period 1960–1974

OVARIAN STEROIDS: EFFECTS ON THE MYOMETRIUM

Progesterone inhibits both spontaneous and oxytocin-induced activity of myometrial strips, apparently by altering the muscle's capacity to propagate an action potential.

1961 Kuriyama and Csapo. *Am. J. Obstet. Gynecol.* 82:592.

1962 Marshall. *Physiol. Rev.* 42:213.

Progesterone is probably important in myometrial hypertrophy of pregnancy. Declining progesterone levels after delivery facilitate postpartum involution.

1962 Woessner. *Biochem. J.* 83:304.

1965 Csapo et al. *Nature* 207:1378.

1969 Csapo and Wiest. *Endocrinology* 85:735.

1969 Rao et al. *Endocrinology* 85:1057.

Placental progesterone is critical in "non-corpus-luteum-dependent" species to pregnancy maintenance but seems not to be a dynamic factor in parturition.

1964 Hendricks. *Obstet. Gynecol.* 24:357.

1971 Hobson. *Adv. Reprod. Physiol.* 5:67.

1972 Davies and Ryan. *Vitam. Horm.* 30:239.

In other mammals (guinea pigs, humans), exogenous progesterone has no delaying effect on parturition.

1962 Brenner and Hendricks. *Am. J. Obstet. Gynecol.* 83:1094.

1964 Schofield. *J. Endocrinol.* 30:347.

The placenta has a local restraining effect, mediated by progesterone, on myometrial activity.

1960 Zarrow et al. *Fertil. Steril.* 11:370.

1965 Kumar and Barnes. *Am. J. Obstet. Gynecol.* 97:717.

1968 Porter. *J. Reprod. Fertil.* 15:437.

1969 Csapo and Wiest. *Endocrinology* 85:735.

Maintenance of pregnancy correlates more closely with uterine than with plasma progesterone levels.

1969 Csapo and Wiest. *Endocrinology* 85:735.

Concentration of endogenous progesterone is higher in the uterus than in plasma.

1970 Wiest. *Endocrinology* 87:43.

Progesterone found unlikely to have inhibitory effect on myometrium in some species.

1970 Porter. *J. Endocrinol.* 46:425.

There is no decline in progesterone in humans prior to labor; a decline does occur during labor and after parturition.

1968 Llauro et al. *Am. J. Obstet. Gynecol.* 101:867.

1968 Yannone et al. *Am. J. Obstet. Gynecol.* 101:1058.

The pattern of myometrial contractility is primarily under the influence of progesterone.

1968 Csapo and Wood. In: *Recent Advances in Endocrinology.* Ed. James. Boston: Little, Brown, p. 207.

Estriol infused into the uterine cavity increases myometrial activity.

1969 Klopper et al. *Brit. J. Med.* 2:786.

Optimal hormone replacement to maintain pregnancy requires a combination of estrogen and progesterone.

1962 Amoroso and Finn. In: *The Ovary.* Ed. Zuckerman. New York: Academic Press, vol. I, p. 451.

OVARIAN STEROIDS: EFFECTS ON UTERINE METABOLISM

Estrogenic compounds demonstrated to induce specific enzymatic changes.

1960 Marks and Banks. *Proc. Natl. Acad. Sci. USA* 46:447.

1963 Levy. *J. Biol. Chem.* 238:775.

1963 McKearns. *Biochim. Biophys. Acta* 73:507.

1964 Yielding et al. *Can. J. Biochem.* 42:727.

1965 Tompkins et al. *J. Biol. Chem.* 240:3793.

Maximum growth and maturation of the endometrium depends on the cyclical pattern and an optimal quantitative ratio of estrogen to progesterone.

1968 Good and Moye. *Fertil. Steril.* 19:371.

Estradiol 17β, but not estradiol 17α, stimulates an increase in uterine cyclic AMP within 15 sec. This effect is blocked by propanalol, a β-adrenergic blocker, but not by other blocking agents.

1967 Szego and Davis. *Proc. Natl. Acad. Sci. USA* 58:1711.

1969 Szego and Davis. *Mol. Pharmacol.* 5:470.

Progesterone increases the activity of uterine glucose-6-phosphate dehydrogenase, NADP + isocitric dehydrogenase, NADP + malic dehydrogenase, succinic dehydrogenase, total uterine RNA and DNA, and uterine glycogen storage.

1966 Lerner et al. *Endocrinology* 78:111.

1969 Hughes et al. *Am. J. Obstet. Gynecol.* 105:707.

1969 Murdoch and White. *J. Endocrinol.* 43:167.

Estrogen inhibits the capacity of progesterone to increase uterine acid and alkaline phosphatase and succinic dehydrogenase activity.

1966 Murdoch and White. *J. Endocrinol.* 42:187.

1969 Murdoch and White. *J. Endocrinol.* 43:167.

Progesterone and estrogen often have antagonistic effects on enzyme activity.

1967 Singhal and Valadares. *J. Biol. Chem.* 242:2593.

1970 Aldeen. *J. Endocrinol.* 46:405.

1970 Singhal and Valadares. *Am. J. Physiol.* 218:312.

Estradiol directly induces the uterus to synthesize a protein (IP); the amount of IP synthesized is directly proportional to the amount of estradiol bound to nuclear receptors, and synthesis is blocked by actinomycin D.

1972 Katzenellenbogen and Gorski. *J. Biol. Chem.* 247:1299.

Medroxyprogesterone acetate makes the endometrium atrophic throughout the period of its use.

1970 Mishell et al. In: *Proc. 6th World Congress Fertil. Steril.,* Tel Aviv, p. 7.

1972 El Maghoub et al. *Acta Obstet. Gynecol. Scand.* 51:251.

Norethindrone enanthate does not invariably affect an atrophic endometrium.

1957 Davis and Weid. *Geburtshilfe Frauenheilkd.* 17:916.

OVARIAN STEROIDS: MECHANISM OF UTERINE ACTION

Estradiol is localized, concentrated, and persistent in the female accessory organs.

1962 Jensen and Jacobsen. *Recent Prog. Horm. Res.* 18:387.

Anabolic activity and biosynthesis in the uterus are prevented if enzyme synthesis is blocked.

1961 Mueller et al. *Proc. Natl. Acad. Sci. USA* 47:164.

1963 Ui and Mueller. *Proc. Natl. Acad. Sci. USA* 50:256.

A protein receptor for estradiol in uterine tissues participates in its intranuclear transfer.

1966 Toft and Gorski. *Proc. Natl. Acad. Sci. USA* 55:1574.

1968 Jensen et al. *Proc. Natl. Acad. Sci. USA* 59:632.

RNA synthesis is a significant and early event in the control of uterine metabolism by estrogen.

1963 Hamilton. *Proc. Natl. Acad. Sci. USA* 49:373.

1963 Noteboom and Gorski. *Proc. Natl. Acad. Sci. USA* 50:250.

1966 Means and Hamilton. *Proc. Natl. Acad. Sci. USA* 56:1594.

After estrogen administration ribosomal, messenger, and transfer RNA all increase in the uterus; RNA is a common pathway for the response of the uterus to estrogen.

1963 Billing et al. *Biochem. J.* 112:563.

1965 Segal et al. *Proc. Natl. Acad. Sci. USA* 54:782.

1967 Barker and Warren. *Endocrinology* 80:536.

1968 Hamilton et al. *Proc. Natl. Acad. Sci. USA* 59:1265.

1968 Hamilton et al. *J. Biochem.* 243:408.

Actinomycin D fails to inhibit all uterine metabolic responses to estrogen; these unaffected responses must be independent of RNA synthesis.

1966 Nicolette and Mueller. *Endocrinology* 79:1162.

Cyclic AMP increases protein and RNA synthesis and lipid and glycogen metabolism in uterine tissue.

1967 Hechter et al. *Arch. Biochem. Biophys.* 122:449.

1970 Sharma and Talwar. *J. Biol. Chem.* 245:1513.

The increase in glucose utilization of the uterus stimulated by estradiol represents a secondary response resulting from biological amplification via a genomic mechanism rather than a primary response of the uterus to estradiol.

1965 Aaronson et al. *Proc. Soc. Exp. Biol. Med.* 120:9.

1966 Barker et al. *Endocrinology* 78:1005.

1966 Eckstein and Villee. *Endocinology* 78:409.

1967 Singhal et al. *Metabolism* 16:271.

The persistent effects of the affinity-labeling compounds (4 mercuri-17α- and 17β-estradiols) are compatible with the existence of a macromolecular estrogen receptor.

1968 Chin and Warren. *J. Biol. Chem.* 243:5056.

1969 Muldoon and Warren. *J. Biol. Chem.* 244:5430.

1971 Ellis and Warren. *Steroids* 17:331.

Progesterone uptake by the uterus demonstrated and presence of a specific uterine cytoplasmic progesterone receptor substantiated.

1963 Wiest. *J. Biol. Chem.* 238:94.

1967 Wichman. *Acta Endocrinol.* (Kbh.) (Suppl.) 116:1.

1967 O'Malley et al. *Recent Prog. Horm. Res.* 25:105.

1970 Milgrom and Baulieu. *Endocrinology* 87:276.

1970 O'Malley et al. *Proc. Natl. Acad. Sci. USA* 67:501.

1972 Davies and Ryan. *Endocrinology* 90:507.

Both the placenta (except in humans) and the uterus metabolize progesterone to less active substances; the biological activity of progesterone appears limited mostly to the progesterone molecule itself.

1967 Wichman. *Acta Endocrinol.* (Kbh.) (Suppl.) 116:1.

1969 Wiest. *Ciba Found. Study Group* 35:56.

1972 Davies and Ryan. *Endocrinology* 90:507.

1973 Wiest. *Endocrinology* 73:310.

NEURAL AND OTHER ENDOCRINE CONTROL OF THE UTERUS

Adrenalin inhibits (via β receptors) and noradrenalin stimulates myometrium.

1968 Shabanah et al. *Am. J. Obstet. Gynecol.* 100:974.

Uterine transplantation experiments in several species indicate that major nervous pathways to the uterus are *not* necessary for uterine luteolytic action, that the luteolytic effect is mediated by local and systemic pathways, and that only endometrium is essential for uterine luteolytic action.

1962 Butcher et al. *Endocrinology* 70:442.

1963 Anderson et al. *Nature* 198:311.

1963 Zhordania and Gotsiridze. *Int. J. Fertil.* 8:849.

1964 Melampy et al. *Endocrinology* 74:501.

1966 DuMesnil Du Buisson. *J. Reprod. Fertil.* 12:413.

1967 Caldwell et al. *Endocrinology* 80:477.

1968 Caldwell et al. *J. Reprod. Fertil.* 17:567.

1968 Harrison et al. *J. Endocrinol.* 39:xiii.

1970 Niswender et al. *J. Anim. Sci.* 30:935.

The fetal pituitary and adrenal cortex influence the initiation of parturition.

1964 Binns et al. *Ann. N.Y. Acad. Sci.* 111:571.

1969 Liggins. *J. Endocrinol.* 42:323 and 45:515.

1969 Milic and Adamsons. *J. Obstet. Gynaecol. Br. Commonw.* 76:102.

1971 Anderson et al. *J. Obstet. Gynaecol. Br. Commonw.* 78:481.

Pregnancy is prolonged in the absence of fetal pituitary or adrenal glands unless exogenous adrenocorticotropic hormone is administered.

1967 Liggins et al. *Am. J. Obstet. Gynecol.* 98:1080.

PROSTAGLANDINS AND THE UTERUS

Laboratory synthesis of prostaglandins.

1964 Bergstrom et al. *Biochim. Biophys. Acta* 90:207.

1964 Dorp. *Biochim. Biophys. Acta* 90:204.

1965 Wallach. *Life Sci.* 4:361.

Prostaglandins found in amniotic fluid during labor.

1968 Karmin. *J. Obstet. Gynaecol. Br. Commonw.* 73:903.

Induction of labor with $PGF_{2\alpha}$ and demonstration of correlation between $PGF_{2\alpha}$ blood levels and uterine contractions.

1968 Karim. *Br. Med. J.* 4:621.

Increase in fetal cortisol leads to increase in fetoplacental estrogen and increase in synthesis and release of maternoplacental prostaglandin $F_{2\alpha}$.

1971 Liggins et al. *Nature* 232:629.

1972 Challis et al. *J. Reprod. Fertil.* 30:485.

1973 Currie et al. *Mem. Soc. Endocrinol.* 20:95.

Increase in $PGF_{2\alpha}$ in uterine vein correlated with increase in production of estrone and estradiol 17β and precedes labor by 12–24 hours.

1972 Challis et al. *J. Reprod. Fertil.* 30:485.

1973 Currie et al. *Mem. Soc. Endocrinol.* 20:95.

Elevated levels of $PGF_{2\alpha}$ found in venous blood of women in labor.

1973 Sharma. *Br. Med. J.* (5855):709.

1974 Challis et al. *Prostaglandins* 6(4):281.

Concentrations of $PGF_{2\alpha}$ in the umbilical cord plasma is higher in patients in active labor than in patients at cesarean section.

1974 Challis et al. *Prostaglandins* 6(4):281.

In the process of uterine activation, the prostaglandin step cannot be bypassed by oxytocin.

1974 Csapo and Csapo. *Life Sci.* 14:719.

Estrogen induces $PGF_{2\alpha}$ production in the myometrium and maternal cotyledons and thereby increases the sensitivity of the myometrium to oxytocin.

1973 Liggins. *Recent Prog. Horm. Res.* 29:111.

Regulation of intracellular calcium through pathways involving adenyl cyclase and cyclic AMP may be the basis for the effects of prostaglandins on the myometrium.

1972 Carsten. *J. Reprod. Med.* 9(6):277.

1974 Carsten. *Prostaglandins* 5(1):33.

Prostaglandins increase in vitro adenyl cyclase activity of the myometrium — more in the luteal than the follicular phase.

1973 Beatty et al. Paper read at the 6th Annual Meeting Soc. Stud. Reprod., August 1973, Oregon.

Elevated levels of $PGF_{2\alpha}$ are found in the uterine vein before onset of uterine activity.

1973 Currie. *Mem. Soc. Endocrinol.* 20:95.

Intra-aortic infusion of $PGF_{2\alpha}$ causes uterine contractions like those at normal term.

1971 Liggins. *Nature* 232:629.

1973 Liggins. *Recent Prog. Horm. Res.* 29:111.

Estrogens, both endogenous and exogenous, act directly on the sheep uterus to release $PGF_{2\alpha}$.

1973 Barcikowski et al. Paper read at the 6th Annual Meeting Soc. Stud. Reprod., August 1973, Oregon.

$PGF_{2\alpha}$ is the luteolytic factor in sheep.

1972 McCracken et al. *Nature (New Biol.)* 238:129.

Exogenous cortisol and $PGF_{2\alpha}$ initiate parturition in the rabbit; the latter depresses plasma progesterone more rapidly than does the former.

1973 Abel et al. *Prostaglandins* 4:431.

$PGF_{2\alpha}$ caused luteolysis but did not cause uterine contractions in cows and goats.

1973 Currie and Thorbun. *Prostaglandins* 4:201.

1973 Lamond et al. *Prostaglandins* 4:269.

Acetylenic fatty acids and nonsteroidal anti-inflamatory agents are potent inhibitors of prostaglandin synthetase.

1971 Collier and Flower. *Lancet* 2:852.

Intra-amniotic concentrations of $PGF_{2\alpha}$ are higher in spontaneous than in induced labor, suggesting that the release of $PGF_{2\alpha}$ is a cause and not a result of uterine contraction.

1974 Hillier et al. *Obstet. Gynaecol. Br. Commonw.* 81:257.

Myometrium contains specific binding proteins for both $PGF_{2\alpha}$ and PGE_1 located in both the cytosol and microsomal fractions. Binding capacity is influenced by the reproductive cycle and by exogenous progesterone and estradiol.

1974 Kimball. Unpublished paper read at the colloquium on Prostaglandins and Reproductive Physiology, April 4, 1974, Detroit, Michigan.

IUDs AND THE UTERUS

A leukocytic infiltration of the endometrium results after IUD insertion.

1963 Jessen et al. *Am. J. Obstet. Gynecol.* 85:1023.

1965 Greenwald. *J. Reprod. Fertil.* 9:9.

1965 Hawk et al. In: *Intrauterine Contraception.* Eds. Segal et al. Excerpta Med. Int. Cong. Ser. 86:189.

1965 Moyer and Mishell. In: *Intrauterine Contraception,* p. 159.

1966 Ginther et al. *J. Anim. Sci.* 25:472.

The antifertility effect of the IUD is directly correlated with the intensity of the leukocytic response it evokes in the endometrium.

1965 Mastroianni and Rosseau. *Am. J. Obstet. Gynecol.* 93:416.

1967 Parr et al. *J. Exp. Med.* 126:523.

1969 Marston and Kelly. *J. Endocrinol.* 43:95.

1971 El-Sahwi and Moyer. *Fertil. Steril.* 22:398.

Lytic enzymes from polymorphs or degenerating cells of the endometrium may be responsible for the antifertility effect of the IUD in some species but not in others.

1964 Doyle and Margolis. *Fertil. Steril.* 15:597.

1969 Parr et al. *Biol. Reprod.* 1:1.

1970 Joshi and Kraemer. *Contraception* 2:339.

Luteal regression in some species is caused by a local luteolytic effect from the stimulated part of the uterus; denervating the uterine segment containing the IUD suppresses the effect.

1966 Bland and Donovan. *J. Physiol.* (Lond.) 186:503.

IUDs, in some species, interfere with development and maintenance of the corpus luteum, as evidenced by shortened estrous cycles, but in others, including humans, cycles remain unaffected.

1968 Corfman and Segal. *Am. J. Obstet. Gynecol.* 100:448.

1968 Hawk. *J. Anim. Sci.* 27 (Suppl. 1):119.

1969 Anderson et al. *Recent Prog. Horm. Res.* 25:57.

Presence of the IUD alters the timing of LH release from the pituitary, but ovulation is not disturbed.

1966 Ginther et al. *J. Anim. Sci.* 25:1262.

1968 Corfman and Segal. *Am. J. Obstet. Gynecol.* 100:448.

1968 Jankiraman and Casida. *J. Reprod. Fertil.* 15:395.

Presence of an IUD results in myometrial hypertrophy and changes in myometrial activity.

1962 Man. In: *Intraduterine Contraceptive Devices.* Eds. Tietze and Lewit. Excerpta Med. Int. Cong. Ser. 54:91.

1966 Israel and Davis. *JAMA* 195:764.

1966 Johnson et al. *Obstet. Gynecol.* 28:526.

1968 Behrman and Burchfield. *Am. J. Obstet. Gynecol.* 100:194.

1969 Parr and Segal. *Fertil. Steril.* 17:174.

Changes in uterine motility do not alter sperm transport or result in premature uterine explusion of ova.

1964 Malkani and Sujan. *Am. J. Obstet. Gynecol.* 88:963.

1965 Moyer and Mishell. In: *Intrauterine Contraception.* Eds. Segal et al. Excerpta Med. Int. Cong. Ser. 86:159.

Movement of ova through the oviducts of naturally ovulating rabbits, monkeys, and humans is not altered by the presence of IUDs.

1966 Ishihama et al. *Yokohama Med. Bull.* 17:45.

1967 Kar. *Proc. 8th Int. Conf. Int. Planned Parenthood Fed.,* April 1967, Santiago, Chile, p. 393.

1967 Kelly and Marston. *Nature* 214:735.

1967 Mastroianni et al. *Am. J. Obstet. Gynecol.* 96:649.

The effectiveness of IUDs in preventing pregnancy is correlated with size and, to some extent, shape of the device.

1970 Tietze and Lewit. *Stud. Fam. Plann.* 55:1.

Oxygen uptake is increased and the ovulatory increase in nonphospholipid-to-phospholipid ratio is retarded after IUD insertion.

1967 Glasser. *Fed. Proc.* 56:536.

1968 Corfman and Segal. *Am. J. Obstet. Gynecol.* 100:448.

There are no changes in endometrial levels of alkaline phosphatase, glycogen, nucleic acids, or other substances as a result of IUD insertion.

1965 Hall et al. *Am. J. Obstet. Gynecol.* 93:1031.

1965 Kar and Kamboj. *Indian J. Exp. Biol.* 3:141.

1968 Corfman and Segal. *Am. J. Obstet. Gynecol.* 100:448.

Relationship between IUD surface area in contact with endometrium and contraceptive effectiveness postulated.

1965   Davis and Israel. In: *Intrauterine Contraception.* Eds. Segal et al. Exerpta Med. Int. Cong. Ser. 86:135.

1969   Zipper et al. *Am. J. Obstet. Gynecol.* 105:1274.

Endometrial maturation accelerated and growth stimulated in presence of IUD.

1969   Joshi and Sujan-Tejuja. *Fertil. Steril.* 20:98.

IUDs cause early, asynchronous development of the endometrium and may, thereby, interfere with implantation.

1967   Tamada et al. *Am. J. Obstet. Gynecol.* 98:811.

1969   Wynn and Sawaragi. *J. Reprod. Fertil.* (Suppl.) 8:45.

Abnormal myometrial activity in the presence of IUDs may be caused by prostaglandin release.

1971   Chaudhari. *Lancet* 1:480.

The use of IUDs for up to 3 years does not influence subsequent fertility experience.

1968   Tietze. *Proc. 6th World Conf. Fertil. Steril.*, Tel Aviv.

1974   Tatum et al. *Proc. 3rd Int. Conf. Intrauterine Contraception,* Cairo, p. 13.

Major Gaps in Our Knowledge

What inhibits the human myometrium during pregnancy and thereby prevents premature expulsion of the fetus?

By what mechanism does the primate fetus influence the timing of parturition?

Does the conceptus produce substances which inhibit or stimulate the myometrium?

To what extent can the extensive information regarding the rodent uterus be extrapolated to the human?

What factors might alter progesterone's effectiveness in sensitizing the myometrium? Among the possibilities are (1) uterine volume, (2) rate of change of uterine volume, (3) oxytocin, (4) nervous stimuli, (5) catecholamines, and (6) estrogens.

Of what importance is myometrial activity during gamete transport and implantation?

What part does relaxin play as a physiological regulator of uterine activity?

What part does the relationship between cyclic AMP and prostaglandin play in myometrial contraction?

Does a decline in the ratio of progesterone to estrogen account for the increasing sensitivity of the myometrium to oxytocin as pregnancy progresses?

What is the importance of progesterone (and its ratio to estrogen) in maintaining pregnancy in various species?

How are changes in fetal adrenocortical activity translated into the increased myometrial activity of labor? Do glucocorticoids interfere with progesterone synthesis in the placenta?

Do IUDs have a spermatodepressive and/or spermatocidal mechanism of action?

Do copper-bearing IUDs initiate destruction of unfertilized eggs within the oviduct?

What is the mechanism of increased menstrual bleeding associated with IUDs?

What is the relationship of IUDs to pelvic inflammatory disease?

What are the precise and primary molecular mechanisms involved in estrogen's action on the uterus?

Of what importance is endometrial lysosomal activity in the human menstrual cycle?

1972   Henzl et al. *J. Clin. Endocrinol. Metab.* 34:860.

Does ethyl alcohol reduce myometrial activity by adrenalin release and/or by inhibition of prostaglandin release or synthesis?

Are prostaglandins the "intrinsic myometrial stimulant" whose activity is modified by progesterone?

What are the immediate and long-range effects on infants whose mothers have been treated with prostaglandins or prostaglandin synthetase inhibitors? Are these compounds teratogenic?

What is the mechanism of action of postcoital estrogens?

Methodological Advances

Period before 1960

Development and refinement of methods of enzymatic assay.

1953   Glock and McLean. *Biochem. J.* 55:400.

1955   Kornberg. In: *Methods of Enzymology.* Eds. Colowick and Kaplan. Vol. 1, p. 441.

1955   Ochoa. In: *Methods of Enzymology,* p. 739.

Progesterone assayed on the basis of its effect on uterine carbonic anhydrase.

1957   Pincus et al. *Endocrinology* 61:528.

Development of nylon and polypropylene materials suitable for use as intrauterine devices.

Period 1960–1974

Chromatography applied to the measurement of ovarian steroids.

1961   Bush. *The Chromatography of Steroids.* Oxford: Pergamon Press.

Multiple decrement life tables applied to the evaluation of IUD effectiveness.

1966   Potter. *Demography* 3:297.

1973   Tietze and Lewit. *Stud. Fam. Plann.* 4:35.

Enzyme affinity labeling used to identify enzyme active sites for estrogen binding.

1962   Wolfsy et. al. *Biochemistry* 1:1031.

1964   Baker. *J. Pharm. Sci.* 53:347.

1966   Holkin et al. *Proc. Natl. Acad. Sci. USA* 55:797.

Commercial processes for prostaglandin synthesis devised.

1970   Pike. *Fortschr. Chem. Org. Naturst.* 28:313.

1971   Corey. *Ann. N.Y. Acad. Sci.* 18:24.

Autoradiography used to observe the cellular distribution of estradiol and progesterone.

1968   Stumpf. *Endocrinology* 83:777.

Uterus (continued)

Radioimmunoassay of endogenous estradiol and progesterone.

1973 Wiest. *Endocinology* (Suppl.) 92:65.

Radioimmunoassay of prostaglandins.

1974 Cornette et al. *Prostaglandins* 5(2):155.

Gas chromatography–mass spectrometry assay for prostaglandins.

1972 Axen et al. In: *The Prostaglandins: Clinical Applications in Human Reproduction.* Ed. Southern. Mt. Kisco: Futura Publ.

Platelets and traumatized tissue secrete prostaglandins; therefore, assays must be performed in presence of indomethacin and with anticoagulated plasma.

1972 Silver et al. *Prostaglandins* 2(2):75.

1973 Smith. *J. Clin. Invest.* 52(4):965.

Methodological Needs

Improved methods of recording and interpreting myometrial activity in humans.

Steroid-specific antibodies that can interfere with hormone function without disturbing placental nutritive and transfer activities, so that the role of estrogen and progesterone on the maintenance of pregnancy can be evaluated.

A complete analysis of the enzymes responsible for progesterone-influenced glycogen accumulations.

Devices for more precise measurement of uterine size.

Polymers for prescribed release of drugs in the uterine cavity.

Methods of separation of myometrium from endometrium and for separation of the three major cells types of the endometrium.

A sensitive and promptly interpretable pregnancy test.

A sensitive and specific self-administered pregnancy test.

Assay method for the measurement of the progesterone receptor in human endometrium.

Protocols for treating various side effects associated with IUD use.

Polymers that will release intrauterine hormones at constant rates for periods longer than 1 year.

An IUD with low puerperal expulsion rate.

Better methods of comparing IUD effectiveness, incorporating blind studies and standardizations.

1975 Jain. *Contraception* 11:243.

Polymers that will release prostaglandins subcutaneously at desired rate.

Contraceptive Methods
Period before 1960

Intrauterine devices (IUDs) of natural materials and metals.

1929 Grafenburg. As cited in: *Proc. Conf. Intrauterine Contraceptive Devices.* Eds. Tietze and Lewit. Excerpta Med. Int. Cong. Ser. 54 (1962).

1934 Ota. *Jap. J. Obstet. Gynecol.* 17:210.

1959 Ishihama. *Yokohama Med. Bull.* 10:89.

1959 Oppenheimer. *Am. J. Obstet. Gynecol.* 78:445.

Use of hypertonic solutions (saline, urea, or glucose) injected intra-amniotically to induce abortion.

1934 Abruel. Reprinted in: *Textbook of Contraceptive Practice.* Eds. Peel and Potts. London: Cambridge Univ. Press (1969).

1971 Craft and Musa. *Lancet* 2:1058.

Transcervical injection of pastes to provoke abortion.

1944 Weilerstein. *JAMA* 125:205.

1947 Barns. *Lancet* 2:825.

Hysterotomy or hysterectomy to remove products of conception.

1973 Potts and Diggory. As cited in: *Human Reproduction: Conception and Contraception.* Eds. Hafez and Evans. New York: Harper & Row, p. 415.

Dilation and curettage to remove products of conception.

1973 Beric. As cited in: *Human Reproduction,* p. 412.

Vacuum aspiration to remove products of conception.

1958 T'sai. *Chinese J. Obstet. Gynecol.* 6:445.

1958 Wu and Wu. *Chinese J. Obstet. Gynecol.* 6:447.

Period 1960–1974

IUDs of nylon or plastic in various shapes underwent clinical trial and had widespread use.

1962 Tietze and Lewit, eds. *Proc. Conf. Intrauterine Contraceptive Devices,* April 30–May 11, New York. Excerpta Med. Int. Cong. Ser. 54.

IUDs with elemental copper underwent clinical trial and had initial use.

1969 Zipper. *Am. J. Obstet. Gynecol.* 101:979.

1969 Zipper et al. *Am. J. Obstet. Gynecol.* 105:1274.

1972 Tatum. *Contraception* 6(3):179.

IUDs medicated with progestogens undergo clinical trial.

1970 Scommegna et al. *Fertil. Steril.* 21:201.

Estrogens used postcoitally to prevent implantation.

1966 Morris and Van Wagenen. *Am. J. Obstet. Gynecol.* 96:804.

1970 Morris. *Ann. Intern. Med.* 73:656.

Vacuum aspiration with flexible plastic cannula and without cervical dilatation to remove products of conception early in gestation.

1971 Goldsmith and Margolis. *Am. J. Obstet. Gynecol.* 110:580.

1972 Beric et al. *Am. J. Obstet. Gynecol.* 114(2):273.

Laminaria tents used to dilate cervix sufficiently to permit extraction of products of conception.

1971 Manabe. *Am. J. Obstet. Gynecol.* 110:743.

1972 Eaton et al. *Obstet. Gynecol.* 39(4):533.

Cytotoxic drugs not believed promising as abortifacients in humans.

1970 Van Wagenen et al. *Am. J. Obstet. Gynecol.* 108:272.

Expulsion, pregnancy, or infection rates not increased when IUDs inserted immediately after abortion.

1972 Tatum. *Am. J. Obstet. Gynecol.* 112:1000.

1973 Nygren and Johansson. *Contraception* 7:299.

1974 Timonen and Luukkainen. *Contraception* 9:153.

PGE$_2$ and PGF$_{2\alpha}$ can induce labor or abortion when administered by intravenous, intravaginal, intra-amniotic, oral (or extraovular) routes.

1972 Karim. *J. Reprod. Fertil.* (Suppl.) 16:105.

1973 Karim et al. *Res. Prostaglandins* 2(6):1.

1973 Naftolin. In: *Prostaglandins and Cyclic AMP*. New York: Academic Press, p. 157.

Insertion of IUDs immediately postpartum demonstrated; expulsion rates higher.

1966 Liss and Andros. *Am. J. Obstet. Gynecol.* 94:1068.

1967 Zatuchni. *Stud. Fam. Plann.* 1:1.

1974 Rosenfield and Castadot. *Am. J. Obstet. Gynecol.* 118:1104.

Progestin-releasing IUD reported to increase retention rate, produce a secretory endometrium, and have a local effect to prevent implantation.

1968 Doyle and Clewe. *Am. J. Obstet. Gynecol.* 101:564.

1972 Tatum. *Am. J. Obstet. Gynecol.* 112:1000.

Contraceptive effectiveness of IUD releasing 65 mcg/day of progestin equal to that of oral contraceptives but bleeding incidence greater:

1974 Manautou et al. *Proc. 3rd Int. Conf. Intrauterine Contraception*, Cairo.

Possibilities for the Future

Can the monthly period of endometrial receptivity to implantation be pharmacologically suppressed?

Can zygote-endometrial synchrony be pharmacologically altered?

Can "impeded estrogens" be used to block or inhibit estrogen action on the uterus?

Can myometrial activity be pharmacologically influenced in order to prevent or disrupt implantation?

Cervix and Vagina

Biological Processes: Significant Discoveries

Period before 1960

The uterine cervix plays a distinct role in the process of sperm migration.

1866   Sims. *Uterine Surgery.* New York: Woods.

1930   Cary. *N.Y. State J. Med.* 30:131.

1942   MacLeod et al. *J. Urol.* 48:225.

Cervical stimulation creates pseudopregnancy in rats.

1922   Long and Evans. *Mem. Univ. Calif.* 6:82.

Cervical stimulation can result in "reflex ovulation" in some species.

1930   Fee and Parkes. *J. Physiol. (Lond.)* 70:385.

1936   Marshall and Verney. *J. Physiol.* (Lond.) 86:327.

Vaginal mucosa responds to ovarian hormones by proliferation, differentiation, and desquamation of its cells.

1933   Papanicolaou. *Am. J. Anat.* (Suppl.) 52:519.

Height and secretion of endocervical cells vary cyclically with ovarian hormone stimulation.

1949   Hamilton. *Contrib. Embryol.* 33:81.

Cervical mucus is a heterogeneous secretion with the rheological properties of viscosity, elasticity, spinnbarkeit, thixotrophy, and tack.

1941   Blair et al. *Nature* 147:453.

Sperm are unable to penetrate progestational mucus which is scanty, viscous, and cellular.

1946   Pommerenke. *Am. J. Obstet. Gynecol.* 52:1023.

1952   Cohen et al. *Fertil. Steril.* 3:201.

Period 1960–1974

One-third of women tested had sterile cervical mucus; the others commonly grew the lactobacilli, diphtheroids, coagulase negative staphylococci, nonhemolytic streptococci, *E. coli,* and yeasts. Treatment of chronic cervicitis caused by these and other organisms increased subsequent probability of conception.

1962   Sobrero. *Ann. N.Y. Acad. Sci.* 97:591.

Cervical mucus has bacteriostatic and bacteriocidal activity against certain strains. This activity is present during all phases of the menstrual cycle but is least pronounced at ovulation.

1962   Rozansky et al. *Proc. Soc. Exp. Biol. Med.* 110:876.

1970   Enhorning et al. *Am. J. Obstet. Gynecol.* 106:532.

Cervical mucus contains inorganic salts and organic compounds including carbohydrates, lipids, enzymes, amino acids, and proteins — IgG, IgA, and secretory IgA — which may be of immunologic importance.

1962   Moghissi et al. *Am. J. Obstet. Gynecol.* 83:149.

1970   Schumacher. *Fertil. Steril.* 21:697.

Nerve fibers of the cervix are in intimate contact with the glandular epithelium and may transmit impulses through the sympathetic nerve system to the pituitary gland to influence its secretory activity.

1964   Giro. *Les Fonctions du Col Uterin.* Paris: Masson, p. 114.

Possible relationship of cervical dilation at midcycle to rapid chondroitin sulfate synthesis.

1966   Stevens et al. *Am. J. Obstet. Gynecol.* 95:959.

Cervical mucus is more copious and has decreased viscosity at ovulation.

1968   Vickery et al. *Physiol. Rev.* 48:135.

Cervix secretes mucoid substances of epithelial origin composed of glycoproteins, mostly sialomucins.

1970   Davajan et al. *Obstet. Gynecol. Survey* 25:1.

Endocervical secretions are generally alkaline, most so at midcycle in women; optimum pH for sperm penetration is 7–9.

1964   Giro. *Les Fonctions du Col Uterin.* Paris: Masson, p. 114.

1970   MacDonald et al. *Obstet. Gynecol.* 35:202.

Major Gaps in Our Knowledge

Are sperm retained in cervical mucus for long periods capable of ascending the uterus and tubes and fertilizing the ovum?

What is the importance, if any, of pheromones in human reproduction?

Are there properties of the vagina or cervix other than cervical mucus viscosity which might permit self-detection of the time of ovulation?

What is the true structure of cervical mucus?

To what extent does the antitrypsin of cervical mucus counteract the proteolytic enzymes of sperm and seminal fluid?

Of what significance is the cervically or vaginally initiated neurohumoral reflex resulting in neurohypophyseal release of oxytocin?

How effective is the vaginal route of prostaglandin administration to induce abortion?

Of what importance to future fertility is cervical trauma during abortion?

Of what importance is cervical dilation as an adjunct to midtrimester abortion with prostaglandins?

Methodological Advances

Period before 1960

Vulcanization of rubber by Goodyear and Hancock in 1844–1845.

Liquid latex manufacturing processes developed 1930–1935. See:

1963   Himes. *Medical History of Contraception.* New York: Gamut Press, pp. 201–202.

Chemical vehicles developed in the early 1950s which, when warmed, adhere to the vaginal mucosa and spread. See:

1973   Langmyhr. In: *Human Reproduction: Conception and Contraception.* Eds. Hafez and Evans. New York: Harper & Row, p. 286.

Aerosol vehicles in glass or metal containers using sreon gas under pressure developed in the early 1950s.

Methodological Needs

A process for fixation of cervical mucus that will avoid artifacts that conceal the true ultrastructure.

Radioimmunoassays for oxytocins to elucidate cervically or vaginally neurohumoral reflexes resulting in release of oxytocin.

Polymers that will release drugs into the vagina at prescribed rates.

A device for precise measurement of cervical mucus viscosity.

Contraceptive Methods

Period before 1960

Rubber cervical cap first described in 1838 and widely used until largely displaced by the vaginal diaphragm.

1838   Widde. *Das weibliche Gebar unvermogen. Eine medicinisch-juridische Abhandlung zum Gebrauch fur practische Geburtshelfer*. Berlin: Aerzte und Jeristen, p.16.

Vaginal diaphragm described in 1891.

1891   Mensinga. *Ein Beitrag zum Mechanismus der Conception*. Leipzig, p. 8.

Vaginal sponge containing a spermicide suggested for contraception.

1879   Besant. *The Law of Population: Its Consequences, and Its Bearing upon Human Conduct and Morals*. London (pamphlet), p. 32.

Vaginal suppositories containing a spermicide in a dispersant vehicle first manufactured.

1895   Chunn. *State Med. J.* 32:340.

Vaginal tablets containing spermicidal agents, and in some varieties producing CO_2 when moistened, evaluated.

1952   Tietze. In: *Proc. 3rd Int. Conf. Planned Parenthood*. Bombay.

1966   Tietze et al. *J. Fam. Welfare* 13:2.

Spermicides incorporated into vaginal creams and jellies designed to be used alone undergo trials of contraceptive effectiveness.

1952   Tietze. In: *Proc. 3rd. Int. Conf. Planned Parenthood*. Bombay.

1956   Wulff and Jonas. *Am. J. Obstet. Gynecol.* 72:549.

1961   MacLeod et al. *JAMA* 176:427.

1964   Rovinsky. *Obstet. Gynecol.* 23:125.

Period 1960–1974

Contraceptive foam comprised of a dispersant cream, a spermicide (usually nonylphenoxy-polyethoxethanol), and freon under pressure field tested and then widely used.

1961   Paniagua et al. *JAMA* 177:125.

1965   Kleppinger. *Pa. Med.* 68:31.

1967   Tietze and Lewitt. *J. Sex. Res.* 3:295.

Oral administration of small doses of progesterone may produce cervical mucus hostile to sperm.

1965   Rudel et al. *Fertil. Steril.* 16:158.

1971   Segal and Tietze. *Rep. Popul. Family Plann.* New York.

Contraceptive effect of the progestogen norethindrone enanthate shown to result primarily from alteration of cervical mucus.

1967   Bedoga-Hevia et al. In: *Proc. 5th World Congr. Gynecol. Obstet.*, Sydney. Eds. Wood and Walters. New York: Appleton–Century, p. 340.

1968   Kesseru and Larranaga. *Ginecol. Obstet.* (Lima) 14:339.

1969   Archari. *J. Obstet. Gynecol. India* 19:731.

1972   El Mahgoub and Karim. *Contraception* 5:21.

Possibilities for the Future

What is the reliability and utility of predicting ovulation from cervical mucus composition?

What are the possibilities of stimulating production of a cervical mucus hostile to sperm?

What is the significance of heavy metal ions in cervical mucus for sperm penetrability and viability?

What is the safety, efficacy, and acceptability of vaginal pessaries used to administer contraceptive steroids?

What are the possibilities for stimulating production of antisperm antibodies in the cervical mucus?

I. Leydig Cells

Biological Processes: Significant Discoveries

Period before 1960

Observation of clusters of epithelial cells.

1850 Leydig. *Z. Wiss. Zool.* 2:1.

Interpretation of epithelial cells (Leydig cells) as an interstitial gland of the testis; its secretions prophetically described as important for the development of the secondary sexual characteristics of the male.

1903 Bovin and Ancël. *Arch. Zool. Exp. Genet.* 1:437.

Demonstration that Δ^5-3β-hydroxysteroid dehydrogenase is an essential enzyme in the production of steroids.

1951 Samuels et al. *Science* 113:490.

Period 1960–1974

Confirmation that Leydig cells convert precursors to testosterone much more efficiently than the seminiferous tubules and, therefore, that they are the principal source of androgens.

1965 Christensen and Mason. *Endocrinology* 76:646.

1973 Van der Molen et al. In: *The Endocrine Function of the Human Testis.* New York: Academic Press, vol. 1, p. 533.

Description of the fine structure of Leydig cells and correlation of structure and function. Demonstration that Leydig cells contain abundant smooth endoplasmic reticulum. Suggestion that this organelle is important in steroid synthesis.

1961 Christensen and Fawcett. *J. Biophys. Biochem. Cytol.* 9:653.

Demonstration that Leydig cells can synthesize cholesterol from acetate. Enzymes for this conversion are located in the microsomal fraction.

1965 Gaylor et al. *Biochemistry* 4:1144.

Confirmation that Leydig cell lipid granules store esterified cholesterol in preparation for androgen synthesis. Decrease in lipid granules correlated with a decrease in the amount of cholesterol esters and an increase in plasma testosterone levels. Hydrolysis of the cholesterol ester appears to be LH-dependent.

1970 Aoki. *Protoplasma* 71:209.

1971 Bartke. *J. Endocrinol.* 49:317.

1973 Moyle, Jungas, and Greep. *Biochem. J.* 134:407.

1973 Neaves. *Biol. Reprod.* 8:451.

In the ram, the testosterone levels in testicular lymphatics are about two-thirds that in blood from the internal spermatic vein (i.e., much higher than the concentration in arterial blood). This suggests that the seminiferous tubules are bathed in fluid containing high androgen levels.

Demonstration that there are very high levels of testosterone within the rete testis fluid.

1963 Lindner. *J. Endocrinol.* 25:483.

1974 Harris and Bartke. *Endocrinology* 95:701.

With ^{3}H fucose and electron-microscopic radioautography, the Leydig cells were shown to produce glycoproteins for export.

1974 Lalli. *Ann. Meet. Soc. Stud. Reprod.*, Ottawa, Canada, p. 38.

Definitive demonstration of a well-defined system of lymphatic channels in the intertubular region of the mammalian testis.

1969 Fawcett, Heidger, and Leak. *J. Reprod. Fertil.* 19:109.

1973 Fawcett, Neaves, and Flores. *Biol. Reprod.* 9:500.

Demonstration that plasma testosterone levels fluctuate markedly in rats and mice.

1973 Bartke et al. *Endocrinology* 92:1223.

Specific receptor for estradiol-17β demonstrated in Leydig cells.

1973 Mulder et al. *FEBS Lett.* 31:131.

Cholesterol side-chain cleavage enzymes found in the inner mitochondrial membrane. This is an important rate-limiting step in steroid synthesis and it is LH-dependent.

1964 Toren et al. *Steroids* 3:381.

1973 Moyle, Jungas, and Greep. *Biochem. J.* 134:415.

Demonstration that all the enzymes required to convert pregnenolone to testosterone are located in the microsomal fraction.

1973 Tamaoki. *J. Steroid Biochem.* 4:89.

LH binds specifically to Leydig cells. Receptor(s) isolated and partially purified.

1971 DeKretser, Catt, and Paulsen. *Endocrinology* 80:332.

1971 Moudgal, Moyle, and Greep. *J. Biol. Chem.* 246:4983.

1973 Dufau, Charreau, and Catt. *J. Biol. Chem.* 248:6973.

The binding of LH to Leydig cells leads to an activation of adenyl cyclase and cAMP formation. Cyclic AMP stimulates steroidogenesis. FSH does not result in these events.

1971 Robison, Butcher, and Sutherland. In: *Cyclic AMP.* New York: Academic Press.

1972 Cooke et al. *FEBS Lett.* 25:83.

1974 Dorrington and Fritz. *Endocrinology* 94:395.

Major Gaps in Our Knowledge

The identity of the glycoproteins produced by the Leydig cells remains unknown. Is this secretion under LH control?

Little is known concerning the mechanism by which the LH-receptor unit interacts with adenyl cyclase. The sequence of events by which cyclic AMP stimulates testosterone production has not been clarified. Protein kinases are likely involved.

There is evidence that damage to the germinal epithelium leads to Leydig cell hyperplasia. In addition to a systemic feedback to the Leydig cells, the possibility exists that there is a direct feedback link between the seminiferous epithelium and the neighboring Leydig cells. This remains to be clarified.

Do prolactin or other hormones have a role in Leydig cell function?

Recent evidence suggest that there may be several different LH receptors on the surface of the Leydig cell. This remains to be fully clarified. Morphological detection of the LH receptors, using ultrastructural techniques, should be carried out.

The role of high-affinity steroid receptors for other steroids remains a mystery.

The mechanism by which testosterone is released from the Leydig cells is unclear. Is there a pulse release?

Characterization of Leydig cell 17-ketoreductase.

II. Sertoli Cells

Biological Processes: Significant Discoveries

Period before 1960

Discovery of high-branched supporting cells, later named Sertoli cells.

1865   Sertoli. *Morgagni* 7:31.

Syncytial nature of Sertoli cells postulated.

1871   von Ebner. In: *Untersuchungen über den Bau der Samenkanalchen.* Leipzig.

1940   Rolshoven. *Z. Zellforsch. Mikrosk. Anat.* 31:156.

1945   Rolshoven. *Z. Zellforsch. Mikrosk. Anat.* 33:439.

The definitive demonstration, by electron microscopy, that the Sertoli cells are individual and not syncytial.

1955   Burgos and Fawcett. *J. Biophys. Biochem. Cytol.* 1:287.

Period 1960–1974

Fine structure of Sertoli cells studied with the electron microscope.

1963   Brokelman. *Z. Zellforsch. Mikrosk. Anat.* 59:820.

1966   Nagano. *Z. Zellforsch. Mikrosk. Anat.* 73:89.

1973   Dym. *Anat. Rec.* 175:639.

Discovery of a factor in the fetal testis that inhibits the Müllerian duct and the accumulation of evidence for its production by the Sertoli cells.

1969   Jost. *Philos. Trans. R. Soc. Lond. (Biol.)* 259:119.

1973   Josso. *Endocrinology* 93:829.

Description of the complex active role of the Sertoli cell in sperm release and residual body retention.

1969   Fawcett and Phillips. *J. Reprod. Fertil.* (Suppl.) 6:405.

Identification of occluding junctions between seminiferous epithelium.

1967   Flickenger and Fawcett. *Anat. Rec.* 158:207.

1967   Nicander. *Z. Zellforsch.* 83:375.

Identification of the occluding junctional complexes between Sertoli cells as the structural basis of the blood-testis permeability barrier.

1970   Dym and Fawcett. *Biol. Reprod.* 3:308.

1970   Fawcett, Leak, and Heidger. *J. Reprod. Fertil.* (Suppl.) 10:105.

Sertoli cells phagocytize degenerating germ cells and residual bodies during normal spermatogenesis.

1969   Sapsford, Rae, and Cleland. *Aust. J. Zool.* 17:729.

1973   Dym. *Anat. Rec.* 175:639.

The Sertoli cells secrete fluid into the lumen of the seminiferous tubules against a pressure gradient.

1967   Setchell. *J. Reprod. Fertil.* 14:347.

It appears well established that the seminiferous tubules are capable of converting pregnenolone and progesterone to testosterone. This is most likely carried out by the Sertoli cells.

1965   Christensen and Mason. *Endocrinology* 76:646.

1969   Hall, Irby, and DeKretser. *Endocrinology* 84:48.

1973   Lacy. *The Endocrine Function of the Human Testis.* New York: Academic Press, vol. 1, p. 493.

1974   Harris and Bartke. *Ann. Meet. Soc. Stud. Reprod.,* Ottawa, Canada, p. 145.

The tight junctions between Sertoli cells divide the seminiferous epithelium into two compartments: (1) a basal compartment, containing the mitotically active spermatogonia, and (2) an adluminal compartment, containing the meiotically active spermatocytes and spermatids.

1970   Dym. and Fawcett. *Biol. Reprod.* 3:308.

1973   Dym. *Anat. Rec.* 175:639. (subhuman primates)

Identification of an androgen binding protein (ABP) and demonstration that it is produced by the Sertoli cells in response to FSH stimulation.

1973   French and Ritzen. *J. Reprod. Fertil.* 32:479.

Demonstration that FSH is bound to the plasma membrane of Sertoli cells. FSH increases cyclic AMP levels in Sertoli cells; LH does not. The Sertoli cell is the primary target for FSH.

1970   Castro, Seiguer, and Mancini. *Proc. Soc. Exp. Biol. Med.* 133:582.

1972   Chowdhury and Steinberger. *J. Reprod. Fertil.* 29:173.

1974   Dorrington and Fritz. *Endocrinology* 94:395.

1974   Means. *Life Sci.* 15:371.

1974   Thanki and Steinberger. *Proc. Meeting Endocrine Soc.*

Success in isolating and culturing pure populations of Sertoli cells from immature rats. Addition of FSH to culture medium results in (1) increased cyclic AMP levels; (2) increased protein synthesis; (3) increased synthesis of androgen binding protein.

1974   Tung et al. *Meet. Am. Soc. Cell Biol.*

Discovery that high levels of androgen in rete testis fluid can be maintained in hypophysectomized rats by administration of C_{21} steroids. This can be best explained by conversion of these compounds to testosterone and dihydrotestosterone in the seminiferous tubules, probably by the Sertoli cells.

1974   Harris and Bartke. *Ann. Meet. Soc. Stud. Reprod.,* Ottawa, Canada.

Major Gaps in Our Knowledge

De novo steroid synthesis by the Sertoli cells remains to be demonstrated. There is evidence that cholesterol does not freely permeate into the seminiferous epithelium. This may partially explain why incubation of seminiferous tubules with cholesterol fails to result in androgen production. This type of study should be repeated using cultured Sertoli cells.

The occluding junctions between Sertoli cells near the base of the seminiferous tubules constitute a tight permeability barrier that isolates meiotic and postmeiotic germ cells from the general circulation. Further studies are needed to discover the mechanism controlling the opening and closing of this barrier and to determine whether the barrier is indeed essential for fluid secretion and germ cell differentiation.

There is evidence for production by the seminiferous tubules of a factor ("inhibin") that exerts a negative feedback on FSH release by the pituitary. Other evidence suggest a local feedback from the tubules to the Leydig cells. Further research is needed to determine whether these factors originate in the germ cells or in the Sertoli cells. Efforts are necessary to isolate and characterize these factors.

The role and, indeed, the importance of androgen binding protein (ABP) remain to be clarified.

Gap junctions have been implicated in electrical communication between adjoining cells. The role of the gap junctions separating Sertoli cells remains to be worked out.

Data at the biochemical level are accumulating concerning the response of the Sertoli cells to FSH. Concomitant morphological studies at the ultrastructural level should be carried out in an attempt to correlate the structure and function of the cell.

More data are required concerning the need for a compartmentalization of the seminiferous epithelium. One function of the occluding junctions between Sertoli cells may be to prevent sperm antigens from leaking into the systemic circulation and eliciting an autoantigenic response.

The importance of the fluid secreted by the Sertoli cells into the lumen of the seminiferous tubules remains to be clarified.

The role of tubular fluid secretion in sperm release and spermiogenesis must be determined.

The full control of germ cell differentiation is likely mediated by the Sertoli cells, although we still do not know what they contribute to the germ cells. More information is required, on both the morphological and biochemical levels, concerning the response of the Sertoli cells to hormone withdrawal, antifertility agents, antiandrogens, etc.

III. Blood-Testis Barrier

Biological Processes: Significant Discoveries

Period before 1960

Certain dyes, when injected into the bloodstream, stained most tissues of the body but not the testis.

1906   Bouffard. *Ann. Inst. Pasteur Lille* 20:539.

Period 1960–1974

Demonstration that dyes do not pass readily into seminiferous tubules of adults.

1967   Kormano. *Histochemie* 9:327.

Analysis of the composition of rete testis fluid and comparison with testicular lymph and blood plasma. Demonstration that many substances normally found in lymph and plasma are present in very low concentrations in rete testis fluid. The amount of proteins, for example, is only 3 to 10% of that found in peripheral plasma.

1969   Setchell, Voglmayr, and Waites. *J. Physiol.* (Lond.) 200:73.

Demonstration that testosterone is present in high concentrations in rete testis fluid: rete testis fluid, 45 ng/ml; circulating arterial plasma, 1.7 ng/ml; internal spermatic vein, 135 ng/ml.

1974   Harris and Bartke. *Endocrinology* 96:701.

Use of the electron microscope and electron-opaque intercellular tracers to localize the main morphological site of the barrier to tight junctions between Sertoli cells.

1970   Dym and Fawcett. *Biol. Reprod.* 3:308.

1970   Fawcett, Leak, and Heidger. *J. Reprod. Fertil.* (Suppl.) 10:105.

Demonstration that there is a blood-testis barrier in primates with ultrastructural tracer techniques. Analysis of total proteins in rete testis fluid of monkeys confirmed this. Suggestion that gonadotropins may not have ready access to the spermatocytes and spermatids beyond the barrier.

1973   Dym. *Anat. Rec.* 175:639.

Studies on the penetration of vascularly introduced substances into rete testis fluid: (1) antifertility agents (esters of methanesulphonic acid) passed readily into rete testis fluid; (2) ^{125}I-labeled albumin did not penetrate into the rete testis; (3) testosterone freely entered RTF, but cholesterol did not.

1972   Waites et al. *Schering Workshop on Contraception: The Masculine Gender*. Ed. Raspe. New York: Pergamon Press, p. 101.

Demonstration that RTF contains most plasma proteins but in much lower concentrations than in blood.

1973   Koskimies. *J. Reprod. Fertil.* 34:433.

Major Gaps in Our Knowledge

There is evidence indicating that the rete testis epithelium may be more permeable than the seminiferous tubules. The significance of this remains unclear.

The full functional significance of the barrier remains unclear. Is it necessary for meiosis and speriogenesis to proceed? What controls the development of the barrier? Can the barrier be broken down in the adult?

What is the function of the specific proteins within the rete testis fluid? Apart from androgen binding protein, Setchell suggested that one of these proteins may be inhibin.

Is the blood-testis barrier important in the penetration of antifertility agents into the seminiferous epithelium?

What is the role of the barrier in the immunological isolation of the spermatids and spermatocytes from the general circulation?

IV. Hormonal Control of Spermatogenesis

Biological Processes: Significant Discoveries

Period before 1960

Extracts of testis shown to promote growth of comb on capons.

1928   McGee et al. *Am. J. Physiol.* 87:406.

Castration effects (prostate and seminal vesicle atrophy, testological regression) reversed by injection of testis extracts.

1928   Moore and McGee. *Am. J. Physiol.* 87:436.

1930   Moore et al. *Am. J. Anat.* 45:109.

Principle of negative feedback control of the release of gonadotropins in the male (rat) with gonadal androgen.

1932   Moore and Price. *Am. J. Anat.* 50:13.

Demonstration that testosterone is capable of maintaining spermatogenesis in the hypophysectomized rat.

1934   Walsh, Cuyler, and McCullagh. *Am. J. Physiol.* 107:508.

First crystallization of androgen from urine and testis extracts.

1931   Butenandt. *Z. Klin. Chem.* 44:925.

Synthesis of diandrosterone.

1935   Ruzicka and Wettstein. *Helv. Chim. Acta* 18:1264.

Synthesis of testosterone.

1935   Butenandt and Hanisch. *Z. Physiol. Chem.* 237:89.

Concept developed of dual control of male gonad: FSH controls spermatogenesis, LH controls Leydig cells.

1936   Greep, Fevold, and Hisaw. *Anat. Rec.* 65:261.

Suggestion that androgens produced by Leydig cells may control spermatogenesis.

1937   Nelson. *Proc. Soc. Exp. Biol. Med.* 34:825.

Administration of testosterone to normal men produces atrophy of germinal epithelium.

1950   Heller et al. *Fertil. Steril.* 1:45.

Period 1960–1974

After hypophysectomy, LH or testosterone is capable of maintaining near normal spermatogenesis, qualitatively. Role of FSH remained unclear.

1967   Clermont and Harvey. *Ciba Found. Study Colloq. Endocrinol.* 16:173.

Studies on hypophysectomized men revealed that Pergonal (HMG) or hCG can maintain spermatogenesis. Difficult to separate LH and FSH actions of above hormones.

1964   Macleod, Pazlanos, and Ray. *Lancet* 1:1196.

1968   Mancini et al. *Am. J. Anat.* 112:203.

Using organ culture, it has been shown that spermatogenesis may proceed through prophase of the meiotic divisions, but no further, in the absence of hormones.

1966   Steinberger and Steinberger. *Exp. Cell Res.* 44:249.

There is a marked increase of protein, RNA, and DNA synthesis in testes of 20-day-old rats injected with FSH or PMS. LH had no effect. Protein synthesis did not increase in the adult.

1967   Means and Hall. *Endocrinology* 81:1151.

Demonstration that membranes isolated from seminiferous epithelium were able to bind FSH. Membranes from the interstitial area did not bind any FSH.

1972   Means and Vaitukaitis. *Endocrinology* 90:39.

Testis tissue can produce dihydrotestosterone from testosterone. It is possible that DHT is the active androgen in the seminiferous tubules as it is in other tissues.

1972   Folman, Haltmeyer, and Eik-Nes. *Am. J. Physiol.* 222:653.

Evidence is accumulating that the Sertoli cells and/or the spermatogonia may release a factor (inhibin) which regulates the release of FSH by the pituitary.

1972   Van Thiel et al. *J. Clin. Invest.* 51:1009.

1974   Krueger, Hodgen, and Sherins. *Endocrinology* 95:955.

1974   Setchell. *J. Reprod. Fertil.* 37:165.

1974   Lee. *Int. Res. Commun. Med. Sci.* 2:1406.

In humans, it appears established that both FSH and LH are required for initiation, maintenance, and recovery of spermatogenesis.

1974   Vilar. In: *The Endocrine Function of the Human Testis*. New York: Academic Press, vol. 2.

Demonstration that the testis secretes estradiol.

1974   Loriaux et al. *J. Clin. Endocrinol. Metab.* 39:627.

Damage to the seminiferous tubules results in higher levels of circulating FSH. LH levels are not affected, provided there is no lesion of the Leydig cells. Testosterone levels also remain normal.

1973   Franchimont. In: *The Endocrine Function of the Human Testis*. New York: Academic Press, vol. 1.

Demonstration that FSH stimulates the secretion of androgen binding protein by the Sertoli cells.

1973   French and Ritzen. *J. Reprod. Fertil.* 32:479.

Demonstration that FSH is probably required for late spermatid maturation.

1967   Steinberger and Duckett. *J. Reprod. Fertil.* (Suppl.) 2:75.

Hormones regulate the survival of the germ cells, not the rate of their maturation.

1967   Clermont and Harvey. *Ciba Found. Study Colloq. Endocrinol.* 16:173.

Major Gaps in Our Knowledge

The role of FSH in spermatogenesis is not clear. It may be necessary for completion of spermiogenesis. Testosterone is essential for normal completion of meiosis.

Little information is available concerning the changes in the metabolism of proteins, lipids, or carbohydrates following hormonal alterations.

Early studies pointed out that there are differences in the responses of rodent and human testes to hypophysectomy. This suggests that more work is required on the response of the primate testis to hormonal depletion.

More detailed analysis of the respective roles of FSH and LH on the testis is needed. Use of specific and potent antisera to the specific hormones may provide additional data.

After FSH interacts with the Sertoli cell membranes, several events occur resulting in an increase in cyclic AMP-dependent protein kinase. Subsequent events leading to transcription and translation are not known.

Classical studies on the hormonal control of the seminiferous epithelium show that it involves pituitary ablation. It is not known whether the other pituitary hormones affect the testis. Use of antisera to the specific gonadotropins may provide information on this topic.

Evidence is accumulating that there is a transfer of testosterone from testicular venous blood directly to the testicular artery. The significance of this remains to be clarified.

Little is known concerning the transport of testosterone into the seminiferous tubules; the cell type(s) that testosterone acts upon; the conversion of testosterone to metabolites within the seminiferous epithelium; and the role of estrogens in tubular function.

The role of prolactin in spermatogenesis must be ascertained.

Characteristics of androgen receptors in the germinal epithelium must be determined, including the site of action of androgens (testosterone, DHT) and the differences between general epithelium androgen receptors and those in other androgen responsive tissues (e.g., epididymis, prostate, and hypothalamus). Direct effects of estrogens and other steroids upon the germinal epithelium, especially those that may not affect gonadotropin secretion, must also be found.

The quantitative relationship between sperm production and intratesticular testosterone production must be worked out.

V. Spermatogenesis

Biological Processes: Significant Discoveries

Period before 1960

Classification of spermatogenesis into well-defined cellular associations using the development of the acrosome as revealed by the PAS staining technique.

1952 Leblond and Clermont. *Am. J. Anat.* 90:167.

Demonstration that the wall of the seminiferous tubules contains contractile cells.

1958 Clermont. *Exp. Cell Res.* 15:438.

Temperature sensitivity of spermatogenesis determined.

1924 Moore et al. *Am. J. Anat.* 34:337.

1926 Moore et al. *Am. J. Anat.* 37:351.

Groups of germ cells (spermatocytes, spermatids) are joined together because of incomplete cytokinesis.

1959 Burgos and Fawcett. *J. Biophys. Biochem. Cytol.* 1:287.

Period 1960–1974

Classification of human and monkey spermatogenesis into a specific number of cellular associations.

1963 Clermont. *Am. J. Anat.* 112:35.

1969 Clermont. *Am. J. Anat.* 126:57.

Calculation of the duration of the spermatogenic process in rodents, monkeys, and humans.

1963 Heller and Clermont. *Science* 140:184.

1965 Clermont and Harvey. *Endocrinology* 76:80.

1973 Clermont and Antar. *Am. J. Anat.* 136:153.

Reserve stem cell and renewing stem cell concept described in rodents, monkeys, and humans.

1968 Clermont and Bustos-Obregón. *Am. J. Anat.* 122:237.

1972 Clermont. *Physiol. Rev.* 52:198.

Reserve stem cell theory challenged. Evidence suggested that all spermatogonial stem cells divide to produce more differentiated germ cells, except for the early stem cells (A_s). When the A_s divide, half of them yield other A_s and half yield differentiated spermatogonia.

1971 Huckins. *Cell Tissue Kinet.* 4:139.

1971 Huckins. *Anat. Rec.* 169:533.

Demonstration that large numbers of germ cells (spermatogonia) are joined by cytoplasmic bridges.

1971 Dym and Fawcett. *Biol. Reprod.* 4:195.

Demonstration that during the normal spermatogenic process, large numbers of germ cells degenerate.

1956 Oakberg. *Am. J. Anat.* 99:391.

1962 Clermont. *Am. J. Anat.* 111:111.

A description of the differentiation of the mammalian spermatid using the electron microscope.

1975 Fawcett and Bloom. *Textbook of Histology.* Philadelphia: Saunders.

Use of the electron microscope to examine human seminiferous epithelium. A knowledge of the normal morphology is essential for future studies.

1970 Vilar, Paulsen, and Moore. In: *The Human Testis.* Eds. Rosemberg and Paulsen. New York: Plenum Press.

1971 Rowley, Berlin, and Heller. *Z. Zellforsch. Mikrosk. Anat.* 112:139.

Demonstration that a lactate dehydrogenase (LDH-x) is a unique isoenzyme found only in testis. It is probably synthesized in the spermatocytes during early meiotic prophase.

1970 Blackshaw and Elkington. *Biol. Reprod.* 2:268.

Adenyl cyclase is present in the seminiferous epithelium, in germ cells and Sertoli cells. Demonstration of a unique type of cyclic nucleotide phosphodiesterase "f," which appears in testis at 40 days of age; this appears to be associated with the formation of early spermatids. Phospho-diesterase may be important in regulating FSH action in the testis.

1970 Hollinger. *Life Sci.* 9:533.

1972 Monn, Desautel, and Christensen. *Endocrinology* 91:716.

1974 Dorrington and Fritz. *Endocrinology* 94:395.

1974 Means. *Life Sci.* 15:371.

Demonstration in the trout that late spermatids synthesize protamines and that these replace histones previously present. Specific enzymes are involved.

1969 Marushige and Dixon. *Dev. Biol.* 19:397.

Somatic-type histones are present in pachytene spermatocytes and early spermatids. These are displaced from the chromatin during sperm condensation and are sequestered in the residual body. These histones are replaced by an arginine-cysteine rich sperm chromosomal protein.

1974 Bellve and Romrell. *Meet. Am. Soc. Cell Biol.*

Successful isolation and characterization of mammalian sperm basic chromosomal proteins; these appear to be species-specific.

1969 Coelingh et al. *Biochim. Biophys. Acta* 188:353.

1973 Kistler et al. *J. Biol. Chem.* 248:4532.

Determination of primary structure of bull sperm basic chromosomal protein.

1972 Coelingh. *Biochim. Biophys. Acta* 285:1.

A number of enzymes have been localized in the seminiferous epithelium. Most of these studies are still in the cataloguing stage since little information is available on the function of the individual enzymes.

1970 Blackshaw. In: *The Testis.* Eds. Johnson, Gomes, and Van Denmark. New York: Academic Press, vol. 2, p. 73.

Confirmation that blood glucose is an important source of energy for the seminiferous epithelium. In some species, the spermatogonia and the Sertoli cells store glycogen. This may provide a source of substrate as well.

1969 Free and Van Denmark. *Comp. Biochem. Physiol.* (B) 30:323.

The seminiferous tubules contain abundant fatty acids and other lipids. Metabolism of lipid by the testis is still poorly understood. A consistent observation is that when the seminiferous tubules are damaged in any way, there is a sudden and remarkable increase in the total amount of lipid. Another consistent change is that in impaired spermatogenesis there is a drop in the amount of fatty acid.

1970 Johnson. In: *The Testis.* Eds. Johnson, Gomes, and Van Denmark. New York: Academic Press.

Demonstration that there is abundant protein and RNA synthesis during spermatogenesis. Pachytene spermatocytes take up labeled uridine and amino acids avidly. Arginine is taken up by spermatids during their condensation.

1965 Monesi. *Exp. Cell Res.* 39:197.

1974 Kierzenbaum and Tres. *J. Cell Biol.* 60:39.

Major Gaps in Our Knowledge

The proliferative behavior of the spermatogonial population in humans is largely unknown. How many divisions do the different spermatogonial types undergo? Which is the stem cell?

The factors that determine stem cell renewal and/or differentiation remain unknown. The factors initiating meiosis are unknown.

Germ cell bridges are probably important for the synchronous development of a particular segment of a seminiferous tubule. However, the factors controlling the synchrony among adjacent lengths of tubules are unknown.

The importance of germ cell degeneration in normal testis is unknown. Are the dying germ cells defective in some way?

It appears that there are specific meiotic proteins in mammals. More work is required to identify and characterize them.

It is well known that advanced spermatogenic cells (and sperm) are antigenically foreign and can induce an autoantigenic response in the individual. This rarely occurs under normal conditions since the foreign antigens are anatomically isolated from the circulation. Efforts are required to identify and isolate the specific antigens.

The role of histones in nuclear condensation remains unknown. The mechanism by which the histones are removed and replaced by "protamines" is not known.

Data are required concerning the role of the various testicular enzymes.

Mechanisms by which spermatogenesis is inhibited in naturally occurring human and primate male infertility remain to be explored.

A complete biochemistry of mammalian meiosis should be worked out, with specific reference to processes unique to meiosis and distinct from those in mitosis.

Are there any naturally occurring inhibitors of meiosis?

Specific biochemical sites of hormonal requirements and control in spermatogenesis remain to be determined.

The reversibility of long-term suppression of spermatogenesis by androgens needs to be studied.

Gene regulation during meiosis and spermiogenesis must be explored.

Methodological Advances

Period before 1960

HORMONAL CONTROL OF SPERMATOGENESIS

Injection of steroids (estrogens, progestogens, androgens) interferes with gonadotropin release and results in spermatogenic disruption.

1950 Heller et al. *Fertil. Steril.* 1:415.

1959 Heller et al. *Fed. Proc.* 18:1057.

Period 1960–1974

LEYDIG CELLS

Use of Leydig cell tumors to study steroid secretion.

1970 Moyle and Armstrong. *Steroids* 15:681.

Use of dispersed Leydig cells as a bioassay system to measure LH and hCG activity in vitro.

1974 Mendelson, Dufau, and Catt. *Meet. Endocrine Soc.*

Separation of interstitial tissue from the tubules.

1965 Christensen and Mason. *Endocrinology* 76:646.

Separation of cell types of blood or bone marrow.

1969 Miller and Phillips. *J. Cell Physiol.* 78:191.

Separation techniques applied to testis.

1970 Lam, Furrer, and Bruce. *Proc. Natl. Acad. Sci. USA* 65:192.

1972 Meistrich. *J. Cell Physiol.* 80:299.

SERTOLI CELLS

Separation of the rodent testis into tubule and interstitial tissue fractions for separate biochemical analysis.

1965 Christensen and Mason. *Endocrinology* 76:646.

Introduction of peroxidase and lanthanum as electron-opaque probes of extracellular spaces.

1966 Graham and Karnovsky. *J. Histochem. Cytochem.* 14:291.

1967 Revel and Karnovsky. *J. Cell Biol.* 33:7.

Techniques developed to culture Sertoli cells.

1974 Tung et al. *Meet. Am. Soc. Cell Biol.*

Freeze fracture technique.

1963 Moor and Mühlethaler. *J. Cell Biol.* 17:609.

1966 Branton. *Proc. Natl. Acad. Sci. USA* 55:5.

Cultures of myoid and Sertoli cells.

1975 Steinberger et al. *Endocrine Res. Commun.* 2:261.

BLOOD-TESTIS BARRIER

Development of methods for cannulation of rete testis and seminiferous tubules permits study of the composition of the tubular fluid.

1966 Voglmayr, Waites, and Setchell. *Nature* 210:861.

1969 Tuck et al. *Aust. J. Exp. Biol. Med. Sci.* 47:32.

HORMONAL CONTROL OF SPERMATOGENESIS

Use of an organ culture system of seminiferous tubules to study hormonal control of spermatogenesis.

1965 Steinberger and Steinberger. *J. Reprod. Fertil.* 9:243.

Development of a procedure to prepare radioactively labeled FSH.

1971 Vaitukaitis. *Endocrinology* 89:1356.

SPERMATOGENESIS

Use of whole mounts of seminiferous tubules for histological analysis. Radioautography of the whole mounted tubules.

1968 Clermont and Bustos-Obregón. *Am. J. Anat.* 122:237.

1968 Dym. *Anat. Rec.* 160:342.

Demonstration that cells of different sizes from mouse spleen could be separated according to their different sedimentation velocities ("staput" technique).

1969 Miller and Phillips. *J. Cell Physiol.* 73:191.

The use of the "staput" technique to separate relatively pure populations of germ cells. Electron-microscopic studies of the isolated germ cells.

1970 Lam, Furrer, and Bruce. *Proc. Natl. Acad. Sci. USA* 65:192.

1972 Meistrich. *J. Cell Physiol.* 80:299.

1974 Bellve and Romrell. *Meet. Am. Soc. Cell Biol.*

Methodological Needs

Development and improvements in the sensitivity of the radioimmunoassay technique.

The electron-microscopic radioautographic localization of steroids within cells remains a problem. New techniques must be developed.

LEYDIG CELLS

Techniques for isolating single Leydig cells and studying the mechanism by which LH stimulates steroidogenesis in the individual cell.

Inhibitors of 17-ketoreductase.

SERTOLI CELL

Improvements in the methods for the isolation of pure populations of Sertoli cells for biochemical and morphological analyses.

Preparation of a potent antisera to FSH.

Characterization of the FSH receptor.

Inhibitors of FSH binding.

Culture techniques for Sertoli cell tumors or normal Sertoli cells.

Definition of biochemical activities specific to Sertoli cells, other than androgen binding protein synthesis.

In vivo techniques for studying tubular fluid formation.

BLOOD-TESTIS BARRIER

Techniques for studying appearance in testicular fluid of systematically administered substances in humans.

In vivo techniques for studying the integrity of blood-testis barrier.

HORMONAL CONTROL OF SPERMATOGENESIS

Preparation of a potent and highly specific antiserum to purified FSH for biological neutralization experiments.

Isolation techniques for characterization of steroid receptors in Sertoli cells or germ cells.

Noncompetitive blockers of gonadotropin receptors.

Improved techniques for preparing radioactive gonadotropin tracers.

SPERMATOGENESIS

Further improvements in the technique for isolating and culturing individual populations of germ cells.

Methods for isolating and culturing mitotically spermatogonial cells.

Animal models to study factors determining the quantity of sperm produced.

Assays of specific parameters of sperm function required for fertility (e.g., protamine content, structural proteins and enzymes required for motility).

Identification of cellular constituents unique to individual stages of spermatogenesis.

Microtechniques to permit protein and enzyme analysis upon testicular biopsy specimens in humans and animals.

Contraceptive Methods

Period before 1960

HORMONAL CONTROL OF SPERMATOGENESIS

Administration of testosterone propionate daily or testosterone enanthate weekly resulted in infertility without suppression of libido or potentia.

1950 Heller et al. *Fertil. Steril.* 1:415.

1965 MacLeod. In: *Agents Affecting Fertility.* Eds. Austin and Perry. Boston: Little, Brown, p. 92.

1973 Reddy and Rao. *Contraception* 5:295.

SPERMATOGENESIS

Nitrofurens and theophenes inhibit spermatogenesis in man, but with undesirable side effects.

1957 Nelson and Bunge. *J. Urol.* 77:275.

Period 1960–1974

HORMONAL CONTROL OF SPERMATOGENESIS

Antisera to testosterone and antiandrogens have been used in attempts to block male fertility. Results are not clear but libido is probably affected.

1964 Neri et al. *Endocrinology* 74:593.

1970 Prasad et al. *Contraception* 2:165.

Danazol acts directly on Leydig cells to suppress spermatogenesis. This results in decreased sperm count.

1971 Sherins et al. *J. Clin. Endocrinol. Metab.* 32:522.

Demonstration that some compounds, such as methallibure, will inhibit pituitary function and ultimately the testis.

1973 Labhsetwar and Walpole. *J. Reprod. Fertil.* 31:147.

Implants containing testosterone, and others containing synthetic progestogens, inhibited spermatogenesis for months without depressing libido and potentia.

1973   Coutinho and Melo. *Contraception* 8:207.

1973   Frick and Bartsch. In: *Physiology and Genetics of Reproduction, Part A*. Eds. Coutinho and Fuchs. New York: Plenum Press, p. 259.

1973   Johansson and Nygren. *Contraception* 8:219.

SPERMATOGENESIS

Exposure of the testis to temperatures of 37° to 40°C leads to aspermatogenesis.

Drugs, such as nitrogen mustards, ethyleneamene derivatives, and mono- and diesters of methene sulphonic acid, in low doses, interrupt spermatogenesis by destroying spermatogonia or arresting their division.

1959   Jackson. *Pharmacol. Rev.* 11:135.

1970   Jackson. *Br. Med. Bull.* 26:79.

Dinitropyrolles (or F1616) inhibit spermatogenesis effectively in rats, but cause toxic effects in dogs.

1964   Patanelli and Nelson. In: *Recent Progress in Hormone Research*. Ed. Pincus. New York: Academic Press, vol. 20, p. 491.

Diamines have antispermatogenic activity in rats, monkeys, and dogs, but WIN 18,446 is incompatible with alcohol in humans.

1961   Beyler et al. *Endocrinology* 69:819.

1962   Drobeck and Coulston. *Exp. Mol. Pathol.* 1:201.

1963   Heller et al. *Exp. Mol. Pathol.* (Suppl.) 2:107.

1965   Nelson and Patanelli. In: *Agents Affecting Fertility*. Eds. Austin and Perry. Boston: Little, Brown, p. 78.

Possibilities for the Future

Binding of FSH to its receptor.

Binding of testosterone to the cellular site of action in the germinal epithelum, if the receptor is shown to have different specificity than that in other androgen-responsive tissues.

Androgen-produced suppression of spermatogenesis.

LEYDIG CELLS

Quantitative reduction of intratesticular testosterone production sufficient to inhibit spermatogenesis while maintaing secondary sexual characteristics.

A combination of 17-ketoreductase inhibition with enough androgen to maintain sexual function and to prevent compensatory LH rise.

Administration of inhibitors of steroid biosynthesis, e.g., aminoglutethimide.

Inhibition of LH action to Leydig cell.

SERTOLI CELLS

Androgen binding protein (ABP) appears to be under FSH control. If ABP is indeed required for normal male fertility, then a specific antiserum to FSH may selectively interfere with ABP production. The reduction of plasma FSH using antisera should be specific and should not interfere with LH and testosterone levels.

FSH binding.

Tubular fluid production.

BLOOD-TESTIS BARRIER

Breakdown of blood-testis barrier may facilitate transport of peptide or protein inhibitors of specific processes essential to normal spermatogenesis.

Breakdown of barrier may inhibit the initiation of meiosis.

SPERMATOGENESIS

Midpachytene spermatocytes are very vulnerable to heat treatment.

Meiosis and, in particular, the two maturation divisions may be especially sensitive to certain drugs and other noxious treatments. See:

1970   Jackson. *Br. Med. Bull.* 26:79.

Hormonally dependent stages of spermatogenesis, particularly meiosis and spermiogenesis, may be vulnerable to inteference, as is any metabolic step unique to and essential for meiosis.

Specific protein synthesis occurs within the spermatids; perhaps methods could be devised to interfere selectively with the synthetic processes, especially protamine synthesis.

Low doses of colchicine may depress sperm counts in man.

1972   Merlin. *Fertil. Steril.* 23:180.

Cadmium results in spermatogenic disruption, due to a specific effect on the vasculature of the testis.

1963   Gunn, Gould, and Anderson. *Am. J. Pathol.* 42:685.

Epididymis

Biological Processes: Significant Discoveries

Period before 1960

Discovery that the capacity for sperm motility increases along the epididymis.

1897 Hammar. *Arch. Anat. Entwickelungsgesch.* (Suppl.), p. 1.

1911 Tournade and Regaud. *C. R. Assoc. Anat.*, p. 252.

1913 Tournade. *C. R. Soc. Biol.* (Paris) 74:738.

1924 Redenz. *Arch. Mikrosk. Anat.* 103:595.

1926 Benoit. *Arch. Anat. Histol. Embryol.* (Strasbourg) 5:173.

1928 Moore. *J. Exp. Zool.* 50:455.

1929 Hammond and Asdell. *Br. J. Exp. Biol.* 4:155.

1930 Yochem. *Physiol. Zool.* 3:309.

1935 Munro. *Proc. Soc. Exp. Biol. Med.* 33:255.

1944 Collery. *Proc. R. Ir. Acad.* 49B:213.

1949 Mukherjee and Bhattacharya. *Proc. Zool. Soc.* (Bengal) 2:149.

1952 Nishikawa and Waide. *Bull. Natl. Inst. Agric. Sci.* (Tokyo) G3:68.

Evidence that sperm maturation depends upon the epididymis and its secretions.

1888 Von Ebner. *Arch. Mikrosk. Anat.* 31:236.

1893 Van der Strict. *C. R. Soc. Biol.* (Paris) 45:799.

1897 Hammar. *Arch. Anat. Entwidklungsgesch.* (Suppl.), p. 1.

1897 Myers-Ward. *J. Anat. Physiol.* 32:135.

1900 Henry. *Arch. Anat. Microsc. Morphol. Exp.* 3:229.

1901 Regaud. *C. R. Soc. Biol.* [D] (Paris) 53:616.

1924 Redenz. *Arch. Mikrosk. Anat.* 103:595.

1926 Benoit. *Arch. Anat. Histol. Embryol.* (Strasbourg) 5:173.

1928 Wagenseil. *Z. Zellforsch. Mikrosk. Anat.* 7:141.

Dissenting view that the epididymis plays no role in sperm maturation.

1931 Young. *J. Exp. Biol.* 8:151.

Clarification of hormonal control of the epididymis.

1926 Benoit. *Arch. Anat. Histol. Embryol.* (Strasbourg) 5:173.

1928 Moore. *J. Exp. Zool.* 50:455.

1949 Wislocki. *Endocrinology* 44:167.

1957 Allen and Slater. *Anat. Rec.* 129:255.

1958 Allen and Slater. *Anat. Rec.* 130:731.

1958 Cavazos. *Anat. Rec.* 132:209.

1959 Allen and Slater. *Am. J. Anat.* 105:117.

Descriptive studies on epididymal morphology.

1857 Becker. *Naturg. Mensch. Thiere* 2:71.

1901 Regaud. *Arch. Anat. Microsc.* 4:101, 231.

1926 Benoit. *Arch. Anat. Microsc.* 5:173.

1957 Nicander. *Acta Morphol. Neerl. Scand.* 1:99.

1957 Nicander. *Acta Morphol. Neerl. Scand.* 1:337.

1957 Reid and Cleland. *Aust. J. Zool.* 5:223.

1958 Reid. *Q. J. Microsc. Sci.* 99:295.

Discovery of the absorptive function of the epididymis.

1920 von Möllendorff. *Ergeb. Physiol.* 18:141.

1928 Wagenseil. *Z. Zellforsch. Mikrosk. Anat.* 7:141.

1933 Young. *Z. Zellforsch. Mikrosk. Anat.* 17:729.

1952 Mason and Shaver. *Ann. N. Y. Acad. Sci.* 55:585.

1954 Shaver. *Anat. Rec.* 119:177.

Discovery of the secretion of glycerylphosphorylcholine (GPC) by the epididymis.

1957 Dawson, Mann, and White. *Biochem. J.* 65:627.

1959 Dawson and Rowlands. *Q. J. Exp. Physiol.* 44:26.

Period 1960–1974

Clarification of parameters of sperm maturation.

General reviews:

1967 Orgebin-Crist. *Ann. Biol. Anim. Biochim. Biophys.* 7:373.

1969 Orgebin-Crist. *Biol. Reprod.* (Suppl.) 1:155.

1975 Orgebin-Crist, Danzo and Davis. In: *Handbook of Physiology* (*Endocrinology*). Eds. Astwood and Greep. Baltimore: Williams & Wilkins.

Morphological changes:

1963 Fawcett and Hollenberg. *Z. Zellforsch. Mikrosk. Anat.* 60:276.

1965 Bedford. *J. Anat.* 99:891.

1969 Fawcett and Phillips. *J. Reprod. Fertil.* (Suppl.) 6:405.

1971 Bedford and Nicander. *J. Anat.* 108:527.

Increased susceptibility to cold shock along the duct:

1967 Quinn and White. *Aust. J. Biol. Sci.* 20:1205.

Increased permeability to dyes:

1953 Ortavant. *C. R. Soc. Biol.* [D] (Paris) 147:1552.

1960 Glover. *J. Reprod. Fertil.* 1:121.

1962 Glover. *Int. J. Fertil.* 7:1.

Changes in electrophoretic mobility:

1963 Bedford. *Nature* 200:1128.

Changes in the pattern of motility:

1964 Blandau and Rumery. *Fertil. Steril.* 15:571.

1967 Voglmayr et al. *J. Reprod. Fertil.* 14:87.

1969 Gaddum. *Anat. Rec.* 161:471.

Lipid changes:

1964 Dawson and Scott. *Nature* 202:292.

1967 Scott, Voglmayr, and Setchell. *Biochem. J.* 102:456.

1973 Poulos, Voglmayr, and White. *J. Reprod. Fertil.* 32:309.

Protein changes:

1971 Lavon, Volcani, and Danon. *J. Reprod. Fertil.* 24:219.

Increase in -S-S- bonds:

1973 Bedford, Bent, and Calvin. *J. Reprod. Fertil.* 33:19.

1973 Bedford, Calvin, and Cooper. *J. Reprod. Fertil.* (Suppl.) 18:199.

1974 Bedford and Calvin. *J. Exp. Zool.* 187:181.

Changes in metabolic patterns:

1970 O'Shea and Voglmayr. *Biol. Reprod.* 2:326.

1973 Scott. *J. Reprod. Fertil.* (Suppl.) 18:65.

1973 Frankel, Peterson, and Freund. *Proc. Soc. Exp. Biol. Med.* 143:1231.

Role of carnitine in sperm maturation and maintenance:

1965 Marquis and Fritz. In: *Recent Research on Carnitine.* Ed. Wolf. Cambridge: MIT Press, p. 27.

1965 Marquis and Fritz. *J. Biol. Chem.* 240:2193.

1965 Marquis and Fritz. *J. Biol. Chem.* 240:2197.

1972 Casillas. *Biochim. Biophys. Acta* 280:545.

1973 Casillas. *J. Biol. Chem.* 248:8227.

1973 Brooks, Hamilton, and Mallek. *Biochem. Biophys. Res. Commun.* 52:1354.

1974 Brooks, Hamilton, and Mallek. *J. Reprod. Fertil.* 36:141.

Discovery of androgen binding protein.

1973 French and Ritzen. *J. Reprod. Fertil.* 32:479.

1973 Hansson et al. *Steroids* 22:19.

Discovery of steroid synthetic capacity of epididymis.

Biochemical studies:

1968 Hamilton, Jones, and Fawcett. *J. Reprod. Fertil.* 18:156 (Abstr).

1969 Inano, Machino, and Tamaoki. *Endocrinology* 84:997.

1970 Frankel and Eik-Nes. *J. Reprod. Fertil.* 23:441.

1970 Frankel and Eik-Nes. *Endocrinology* 87:646.

1970 Hamilton and Fawcett. *Proc. Soc. Exp. Biol. Med.* 133:693.

Histochemical studies:

1966 McGadey, Baillie, and Ferguson. *Histochemie* 7:211.

Elucidation of uptake metabolism, and, metabolic effects of steroid hormones on epididymis.

1969 Tveter and Aakvaag. *Endocrinology* 85:683.

1969 Gloyna and Wilson. *J. Clin. Endocrinol. Metab.* 29:970.

1969 Inano, Machino, and Tamaoki. *Endocrinology* 84:997.

1971 Blaquier. *Biochem. Biophys. Res. Commun.* 45:1076.

1973 Blaquier and Calandra. *Endocrinology* 93:51.

1973 Danzo, Orgebin-Crist, and Toft. *Endocrinology* 92:310.

1973 Djøseland, Hansson, and Haugen. *Steroids* 21:773.

1973 Ofner et al. *Symp. Southwest Found. Research Education*, March 1–3, 1973, San Antonio, Texas (1975).

1974 Ofner, Leav, and Cavazos. In: *Structure and Function of Male Sex Accessory Organs*. Ed. Brandes. New York: Academic Press, chap. 11.

1975 Hansson et al. In: *Handbook of Physiology (Endocrinology)*. Eds. Astwood and Greep. Baltimore: Williams & Wilkins.

Clarification of the role of the epididymis in absorption of electrolytes and particulate material from the lumen.

1951 Clubb. Thesis, University of Rochester.

1964 Burgos. *Anat. Rec.* 148:517.

1965 Crabo. *Acta Vet. Scand.* (Suppl.) 6(5):1.

1965 Nicander. *Z. Zellforsch. Mikrosk. Anat.* 66:829.

1965 Nicander, Paulsson, and Selander. *4th Scand. Congr. Cell Res.* p. 51.

1966 Sedar. *J. Cell Biol.* 31:102A.

1967 Friend and Farquhar. *J. Cell Biol.* 35:357.

1969 Friend. *J. Cell Biol.* 41:269.

1969 Waites and Setchell. In: *Advances in Reproductive Physiology*. Ed. McLaren. London: Logos Press Ltd., vol. 4, p. 1.

Study of the electrolyte composition along the length of the duct.

1965 Crabo. *Acta Vet. Scand.* (Suppl.) 6(5):1.

1971 Levine and Marsh. *J. Physiol.* (Lond.) 213:557.

Proof that the epididymis synthesizes glycerylphosphorylcholine (GPC) from ^{32}P-orthophosphate.

1963 Scott, Baggett, and Rowlands. *Biochem. J.* 87:507.

1963 Scott, Baggett, and White. *Aust. J. Exp. Biol. Med. Sci.* 41:363.

1963 Scott, Wales, Wallace, and White. *J. Reprod. Fertil.* 6:49.

1966 Wallace, Wales, and White. *Aust. J. Biol. Sci.* 19:849.

1968 Scott and Dawson. *Biochem. J.* 108:457.

Elucidation of the fine structure of the epididymal epithelium.

1968 Hamilton, Jones, and Fawcett. *J. Reprod. Fertil.* 18:156 (Abstr.).

1969 Holstein. *Zwanglose. Abhandl. Gebiet. Norm. Pathol. Anat.* 20:1.

1971 Glover and Nicander. *J. Reprod. Fertil.* (Suppl.) 13:39.

1972 Hamilton. In: *Reproductive Biology*. Eds. Balin and Glasser. Amsterdam: Excerpta Medica, p. 268.

1973 Hoffer, Hamilton, and Fawcett. *Anat. Rec.* 175:169.

1975 Hamilton. In: *Handbook of Physiology (Endocrinology)*. Eds. Astwood and Greep. Baltimore: Williams & Wilkins.

Evidence of complex carbohydrate synthesis in the epididymis.

1966 Bose, Kar, and Das Gupta. *Curr. Sci.* 35:336.

1966 Fournier. *C. R. Soc. Biol.* [D] (Paris) 160:1087.

1966 Peyre and Laporte. *C. R. Soc. Acad. Sci.* [D] (Paris) 263:1872.

1966 Neutra and Leblond. *J. Cell Biol.* 30:137.

1968 Rajalaksmi and Prasad. *J. Endocrinol.* 41:471.

1969 Fleischer, Fleischer, and Ozawa. *J. Cell Biol.* 43:59.

Possibility that some seminal antigens are formed in the epididymis.

1969 Barker and Amann. *J. Reprod. Fertil.* 18:155.

1970 Johnson and Hunter. *Proc. Soc. Study Reprod. USA* (Abstr.) 3:8.

1975 Crabo and Hunter. In: *Control of Male Fertility*. Eds. Sciarra, Markland, and Speidel. New York: Harper & Row, p. 2.

Possible role of prostaglandins in the epididymis.

1972 Hunt and Nicholson. *Fertil. Steril.* 23:763.

1974 Hafs, Lewis, and Stenerud. *Proc. Soc. Exp. Biol. Med.* 145:1120.

1974 Bartke and Koerner. *Endocrinology* 95(6):1739.

Major Gaps in Our Knowledge

Real understanding of the role of androgen binding protein in the epididymis.

Understanding of the role of steroids in sperm maturation. That is, do steroids that are formed or transported by the epididymis interact with sperm and do they control the metabolic activity of sperm?

Specificity of the role of the epididymis in the maturation process of spermatozoa.

Role of the initial segment in sperm maturation.

Function of the lymphocyte-like cells, especially with respect to immunological consequences of vasectomy.

A detailed knowledge of the mechanisms of transport and accumulation of small-molecular-weight substances by the epididymis.

An understanding of the dynamic aspects (i.e., secretion and absorption) of control of the luminal environment by the epididymal epithelium.

Understanding of the interactions between epididymal sperm from various segments and their environment under physiological conditions.

Role of gonadotropic hormones and other hormones (thyroid, etc.) in the control of epididymal function.

Biochemical and physiological processes involved in sperm transport in the human male ducts.

Role of sperm antigens in fertility.

Electron-microscopic autoradiography of epididymal secretion.

Understanding of the blood-epididymal barrier.

Effect of epididymis on sperm motility patterns.

Role of intraluminal and systemic androgens in control of epididymal function.

Role of epididymis in sperm removal.

Epididymis (continued)

Methodological Advances

Period 1960–1974

Flushing of the epidymis to analyze the luminal contents.

1965   Crabo. *Acta Vet. Scand.* (Suppl.) 6:5.

1966   Gustafsson. *Acta Vet. Scand.* (Suppl.) 17:1.

1974   Brooks, Hamilton, and Mallek. *J. Reprod. Fertil.* 36:141.

Methodological Needs

Microassays enabling investigators to work on a small number of cells.

Micropuncture and microflow techniques to allow studies of fluid movement, molecular absorption and secretion, and sperm transport.

Contraceptive Methods

Period 1960–1974

Vasectomy.

1975   Sciarra, Markland, and Speidel, eds. *Control of Male Fertility.* New York: Harper & Row.

Use of α-chlorhydrin and related compounds.

1970   Ericsson and Baker. *J. Reprod. Fertil.* 21:5.

1970   Ericsson and Youngdale. *J. Reprod. Fertil.* 21:263.

1974   Coppola and Saldarini. *Contraception* 9:459.

Possibilities for the Future

The role of the human epididymis in sperm maturation is not yet defined and may offer possibilities for contraception.

Transport mechanisms that might be interrupted: sperm along duct; electrolytes in and out of duct; small-molecular-weight compounds such as carnitine.

Hormonal regulatory mechanisms should be explored.

Methods of mechanical obstruction need further study.

Biological Processes: Significant Discoveries

Period before 1960

Embryology of seminal vesicle, prostate, and coagulating gland.

1910 Walker. *Bull. Johns Hopkins Hosp.* 21:182.

1934 Wiesner. *J. Obstet. Gynaecol. Br. Emp.* 41:867.

1936 Price. *Am. J. Anat.* 60:79.

Heterogeneous nature of developing prostate gland established.

1912 Lowsley. *Am. J. Anat.* 13:299.

Establishment of endocrine role of testis in maintenance of accessory sex gland function, castration, hormone replacement.

1930 Moore, Price, and Gallagher. *Am. J. Anat.* 45:71.

1930 Moore, Hughes, and Gallagher. *Am. J Anat.* 45:109.

Establishment of endocrine role of testis in hormonal control of prostatic cancer.

1956 Huggins. *Cancer Res.* 825:30.

Antiandrogenic measures with patients with adenocarcinoma of prostate. Lobes of human prostate differ in responsiveness to sex hormones. Adenocarcinoma originates in the androgen-sensitive zone.

1948 Huggins and Webster. *J. Urol.* 59:258.

Histochemical and cytometric analysis of castration effects and hormone replacement.

1950 Leblond. *Am. J. Anat.* 86:1.

1953 Melampy and Cavazos. *Endocrinology* 52:173.

1954 Cavazos and Melampy. *Endocrinology* 54:640.

Physiological response of zinc to hormones and high level of zinc in prostate established.

1951 Mawson and Fischer. *Nature* 167:859.

1956 Gunn and Gould. *Proc. Soc. Exp. Biol. Med.* 92:17.

Acid phosphatase from prostate, present in semen, becomes a useful index for circulating androgen levels.

1935 Krutscher and Wolbergs. *Z. Physiol. Chem.* 236:237.

Abnormally high levels of acid phosphatase indicate osteoblastic metastases of carcinoma of the prostate.

1936 Gutman, Sproul, and Gutman. *Am. J. Cancer* 28:485.

Identification of acid phosphatase in prostate and prostatic secretion.

1940 Gutman and Gutman. *J. Biol. Chem.* 136:201.

1949 Stafford, Rubinstein, and Meyer. *Proc. Soc. Exp. Biol. Med.* 71:353.

1954 Mann. *The Biochemistry of Semen.* New York: Wiley-Interscience.

Prostaglandins first identified and purified from secretions of male accessory glands.

1936 von Euler. *J. Physiol.* 88:213.

1949 Bergstrom. *Nord. Med.* 42:1465.

Fructose, produced in seminal vesicles, found to be principal natural energy source of ejaculation of spermatozoa.

1946 Mann. *Biochem. J.* 40:481.

Seminal fructose quantities strictly controlled by testicular hormones.

1950 Mann and Parsons. *Biochem. J.* 46:440.

Fructose levels the basis for assessing endogenous androgen production.

1951 Landau and Loughead. *J. Clin. Endocrinol. Metab.* 11:1411.

Period 1960–1974

Fine-structural analysis of endoplasmic reticulum, effects of castration, hormone replacement.

1960 Deane and Porter. *Proc. First Int. Congr. Endocrinol.* Copenhagen, p. 971.

1964 Cavazos et al. *Z. Zellforsch. Mikrosk. Anat.* 63:179.

1965 Szirmai and Van der Linde. *J. Ultrastruct. Res.* 12:380.

1965 Deane and Wurzelmann. *Am. J. Anat.* 117:91.

Correlation of histochemical results with fine-structural observations.

1961 Feagans, Cavazos, and Ewald. *Am. J. Anat.* 108:31.

Loss of ribosomes following castration-lysosomes.

1963 Harkin. *NCI Monograph* 12.

1966 Brandes. *Int. Rev. Cytol.* 20:207.

Glycocalyx definition.

1963 Bennett. *J. Histochem. Cytochem.* 11:14.

1965 Ito. *J. Cell Biol.* 27:475.

Chemical analysis of prostatic secretion.

1964 Mann. In: *The Biochemistry of Semen and of the Male Reproductive Tract.* New York: Wiley.

Identification of 5α-dihydrotestosterone.

1963 Farnsworth and Brown. *JAMA* 183:436. (in vitro)

1970 Morfin et al. *Proc. 3rd Int. Congr. Hormonal Steroids* Hamburg. (in vivo)

Identification of 5α-androstanediol epimers.

1966 Chamberlain et al. *Biochem. J.* 99:610. (in vitro)

1970 Ofner et al. *Proc. 3rd Tenovus Workshop,* Cardiff, Wales. (in vitro)

1970 Morfin et al. *Proc. 3rd Int. Cong. Hormonal Steroids,* Hamburg. (in vivo)

Prostatic and epididymal 6- and 7-hydroxylation.

1974 Ofner, Vena, and Morfin. *Steroids* 24:261.

Fine-structural analysis of effects of estrogen on canine prostate and [19]C-steroid metabolism.

1971 Leav et al. *Endocrinology* 89:465.

Selective enhancement of prostatic RNA by androgen.

1966 Liao, Lin, and Barton. *J. Biol. Chem.* 241:3869.

1967 Liao and Lin. *Proc. Natl. Acad. Sci. USA* 57:379.

Action of 5α-dihydrotestosterone receptors.

1968 Anderson and Liao. *Nature* 219:277.

1968 Bruchovsky and Wilson. *J. Biol. Chem.* 243:2012.

Effects of male sex hormone mediated by intracellular metabolites of circulating androgens.

1971 Robel, Lasnitzki, and Baulieu. *Biochimie* 53:81.

Aspects of androgen-dependent events studied by antiandrogens and cyproterone acetate action.

1970 Neumann et al. *Recent Prog. Horm. Res.* 26:337.

Autoradiographic cellular and subcellular localization of sexual steroids.

1970 Sar, Liao, and Stumpf. *Endocrinology* 86:1008.

1971 Stumpf, Baerwaldt, and Sar. In: *Basic Actions of Sex Steroids on Target Organs.* Basel:Karger, p. 3.

Mechanisms and regulation of polyamine and putrescine biosynthesis in male genital glands.

1969 Williams-Ashman, Pegg, and Lockwood. *Adv. Enzyme Regul.* 7:291.

Effects of castration and hormones in zinc content of human prostate.

1962 MacKenzie, Hall, and Whitmore. *Nature* 193:72.

1964 Schrodt, Hall, and Whitmore. *Cancer* 17:1555.

Relation between zinc content and histologic effects of dithizone.

1962 MacKenzie, Hall, and Whitmore. *J. Urol.* 87:923.

Establishment of a human epithelial cell line MA 160 from prostate with benign hyperplasia.

1970   Fraley, Ecker, and Vincent. *Science* 170:540.

Maintenance of human prostate with benign hyperplasia in organ culture.

1973   Harbitz. *Scand. J. Urol. Nephrol.* 7:6.

Structure and pathology of the human prostate (central and peripheral zones).

1975   McNeal. In: *Normal and Abnormal Growth of the Prostate.* Ed. Goland. Springfield: Charles C Thomas, p. 517.

Bulbourethral gland histochemistry and fine structure.

1961   Feagans, Cavazos, and Ewald. *Am. J. Anat.* 108:31.

1963   Feagans, Belt, and Sheridan. *Acta Anat.* (Basel) 52:273.

Analysis of bulbourethral gland secretions.

1962   Hartree. *Nature* 196:483.

1964   Hart and Greenstein. *Am. Zool.* 4:260 (Abstr.).

Reviews.

1968   Ofner. *Vitam. Horm.* 26:237.

1969   Liao and Fang. *Vitam. Horm.* 27:18.

1970   Wilson and Gloyna. *Recent Prog. Horm. Res.* 26:309.

1971   Williams-Ashman and Reddi. *Annu. Rev. Physiol.* 33:31.

1975   Ofner, Leav, and Cavazos. In: *Normal and Abnormal Growth of the Prostate.* Ed. Goland. Springfield: Charles C Thomas, p. 111.

Recent Source Books.

1974   Brandes. *Male Accessory Sex Organs. Structure and Function in Mammals.* New York: Academic Press.

1975   Goland. In: *Normal and Abnormal Growth of the Prostate.* Springfield: Charles C Thomas.

1975   Thomas and Singhal, eds. *Molecular Mechanisms of Gonadal Hormone Action. Advances in Sex Hormone Research.* Baltimore: University Park Press, vol. 1.

Control of canine prostatic secretion by the autonomic nervous system.

1975   Hamilton and Greep. *Male Reproductive System. Handbook of Physiology,* Sect. V: *Endocrinology.* Baltimore: Williams & Wilkins.

Major Gaps in Our Knowledge

Additional information on the direct role of the accessory sex glands in the fertilization process. What is the major function of the prostate in this regard: to provide diluent and correct nutrients for epididymal spermatozoa?

Role of zinc in physiology of accessory sex glands; function of high zinc content in human prostatic tissue, secretion, and seminal plasma.

Role of polyamines in androgen action on accessory sex glands and male reproduction; role of high polyamine content in prostatic secretion.

Possibility of blocking enzymes responsible for metabolic transformation of testosterone: search for specific inhibitors of accessory-sex-gland 4-en-3-oxosteroid 5α-reductase.

Need to understand fully role of each metabolite of testosterone (and other circulating androgens) in accessory sex gland function.

Androgen metabolism and inhibition of 5α-androstanediol formation: Is there a particular metabolite that is responsible for secretion?

Androgen metabolism in relation to termination of response.

Characterization of cytoplasmic binding proteins for androgen, specifically 5α-dihydrotestosterone, in human accessory sex glands; identification of endogenous compounds and search for agents that are competitive for the cytoplasmic receptor of testosterone/5α-dihydrotestosterone.

Differential effects of estrogens on the accessory sex glands; squamous metaplasia in the prostate; atrophy of epithelium of seminal vesicles and bulbourethral gland.

Comparative effects of estrogen and steroidal and nonsteroidal antiandrogens on accessory sex glands.

Limited information is available on the role of apical plasma membrane and glycocalyx of accessory sex glands; function of glycocalyx in fertility and sterility; possibility to induce infertility by obliterating the mucopoly-saccharide layer with a chemical agent.

Role of connective tissue, basal cells, and smooth muscle of accessory sex glands.

Role of prolactin in synergizing androgen action on accessory reproductive organs.

Endogenous factors, other than androgen, that influence/stimulate accessory sex gland secretions.

Methodological Advances

Period before 1960

Rat-ventral-prostate bioassay of androgens.

Extensive analyses of chemical constituents of accessory glandular secretions and seminal plasma.

1946   Mann. *Biochem. J.* 39:451; 39:458.

1949   Mann et al. *J. Endocrinol.* 6:75.

1954   Koefoed-Johnson and Mann. *Biochem. J.* 57:406.

1954   Williams-Ashman. *Endocrinology* 54:121.

1954   Williams-Ashman and Banks. *J. Biol. Chem.* 208:337.

Prostatic secretion and preparation of fistula for gathering and analyzing prostatic secretion.

1947   Huggins. *Harvey Lect.* 42:148.

Surgical procedures, developed for the dog, first permit collection of prostatic fluid; help relate secretory activity of the gland to endocrine status of the animal.

1953   Huggins and Sommer. *J. Exp. Med.* 97:663.

Maintenance of rodent prostate glands in organ culture; study of androgen effects in organ culture.

1955   Lasnitzki. *J. Endocrinol.* 12:236.

Period 1960–1974

Use of electron microscopy and correlation with histochemistry and membrane studies.

Biochemical methods for in vivo and in vitro studies of target-tissue ^{19}C-steroid metabolism. In vivo: intra-arterial infusion. In vitro: perfusion; superfusion; organ culture; cell culture.

Dry-mount autoradiography of steroids.

Radioimmunoassay of plasma steroids.

Determination of free and bound plasma sex steroids.

Characterization of cytoplasmic and nuclear 5α-dihydrotestosterone receptor in rat accessory sex organs.

Methodological Needs

Techniques for studies on plasma membranes and glycocalyx.

Further development of explant techniques and long-term maintenance of accessory sex glands in organ culture for testing hormones and antifertility compounds.

Further refinement of steroid autoradiography, and development of techniques suitable for electron microscopy.

Establishment of normal culture cell lines of epithelium.

Tissue fractionation techniques for isolation of connective tissue, smooth muscle, epithelium, and basal cells for chemical analysis.

Study of transplanted human prostate tissue in nude mice.

Radioimmunoassay of 5α-dihydrotestosterone receptor.

Characterization of binding proteins for the 5α-androstanediol epimers.

Administration of agents through silastic tubing into the vas deferens.

Contraceptive Possibilities

The following processes are considered vulnerable to contraception:

1. ^{19}C-steroid metabolism in accessory sex glands, e.g., 5-reductase.

2. Binding of 5α-dihydrotestosterone to cytosol receptors.

3. Prostatic secretion: e.g., interference with nerve-induced (acetylcholinergic) secretion, antiandrogen, inhibition of 5α-androstanediol formation, if metabolite (3α) can be shown to act at the level of secretion.

4. Termination of androgenic response.

5. Membrane permeability.

6. Zinc content and transport.

7. Polyamine biosynthesis.

Biological Processes: Significant Discoveries

Period before 1960

Demonstration that removal of animalcules from semen prevented fertilization; spermatogonia identified.

1780 Spallazani. *Dissertazioni di fisica animale e vegetale. Modena.*

Tracing of spermatozoon origin to testis.

1841 von Kolliker. *Beitrage zur Kenntnis der Geschlechtwerhattnisse etc.* Berlin.

Demonstrations that spermatozoa were highly specialized animal cells, including nucleus and cytoplasm.

1865 La Vallette. *Arch. Mikrosk. Anat.* 1:403.

Tracing sequence of changes in germ cells during spermatogenesis in seminiferous tubules.

1865 La Vallette. *Arch. Mikrosk. Anat.* 1:403.

1888 von Ebner. *Arch. Mikrosk. Anat.* 31:236.

1898 Benda. *Verh. Anat. Gesell. (Jena)* 12:264.

1899 Meves. *Arch. Mikrosk. Anat.* 54:329.

Principal morphogenetic events of spermiogenesis:

1. Outgrowth of flagellum.

1897 Meves. *Anat. Anz.* (Jena) 14:168.

2. Acrosomal cap.

1899 Meves. *Mitth. Ver. Sahlesw-Holst.* F:7:43.

1919 Gatenby. *Q. J. Microsc. Sc.* (Lond.) 63:445.

1920 Bowen. *Biol. Bull.* XXIX.

3. Investment of base of flagellum by sheath of mitochrondria.

1897 Benda. *Arch. Physiol. Leipz.* I + II:385; 393.

1898 Meves. *Verhandl. Anat. Gesellsch.* 12:91.

Precise staging of the spermatogenic cycle of the seminiferous epithelium.

1952 Leblond and Clermont. *Ann. N.Y. Acad. Sci.* 55:548.

Detailed description of the submicroscopic features of the spermatozoon that were unachievable with the optics of the light microscope.

1953 Welkins and Randall. *Biochim. Biophys. Acta* 10:192.

1955 Burgos and Fawcett. *J. Biophys. Biochem. Cytol.* 1:287.

1958 Austin and Bishop. *Proc. R. Soc. Lond.* B149:241.

1965 Fawcett. *Z. Zellforsch. Mikrosk. Anat.* 67:279.

The demonstration that spermiogenesis involved complex morphogenetic changes that were out of the range of the light microscope.

1958 Fawcett. *Int. Rev. Cytol.* 7:195.

1959 Afzelius. *J. Biophys. Biochem. Cytol.* 5:269.

Period 1960–1974

Localization of Y chromosome in head of male determining sperm with fluorescent quinacrin dyes.

1970 Barlow and Vosa. *Nature* 226:961.

1970 Pearson and Bobrow. *J. Reprod. Fertil.* 22:177.

Clarification of the origin and structural relationship of the acrosomal cap.

1962 Nicander and Bane. *Z. Zellforsch. Mikrosk. Anat.* 57:390.

1970 Fawcett. *Biol. Reprod.* (Suppl.) 2:90.

1974 Pedersen. *Costers Botrykkeir.* Copenhagen.

1974 Friend and Fawcett. *J. Cell Biol.* 63:641.

Description of cytological changes taking place during the acrosome reaction.

1956 Dan. *Int. Rev. Cytol.* 5:365. (subhuman primates)

1961 Colwin and Colwin. *J. Biophys. Biochem. Cytol.* 10:211.

1970 Yanigamachi and Noda. *J. Ultrastruct. Res.* 31:465.

1971 Bedford. *Am. J. Anat.* 133:213.

Other components of the acrosome:

1. Carbohydrates.

1955 Clermont, Glegg, and Leblond. *Exp. Cell. Biol.* 8(3):453.

2. Enzymes.

1948 Austin. *Nature* 162:63.

1963 Hartree and Srivatava. *J. Reprod. Fertil.* 5:225.

1971 Teichman and Bernstein. *J. Reprod. Fertil.* 27:243.

1973 Zaneveld. *J. Biol. Chem.* 248:564.

Identification of proteolytic enzyme of the acrosome (acrosin).

1965 Srivastava et al. *J. Reprod. Fertil.* 10:61.

1969 Stambaugh and Buckley. *J. Reprod. Fertil.* 19:423.

1969 Stambaugh and Buckley. *Fertil. Steril.* 23:348.

1974 Brown and Hartree. *J. Reprod. Fertil.* 36:195.

Successful in vitro fertilization of mammalian eggs.

1969 Edwards, Bavister, and Steptoe. *Nature* 221:592. (subhuman primates)

1973 Gould, Kline, and Williams. *Fertil. Steril.* 24:260.

1973 Steptoe. *J. Reprod. Med.* 10:211.

Demonstration of selective recognition of egg by postacrosomal membrane and its fusion with the oolemma.

1968 Barros and Franklin. *J. Cell Biol.* 37:C13.

1969 Stefanini, Oura, and Zambioni. *J. Submicrosc. Cytol.* 1:1.

1970 Yanagimachi and Noda. *Am. J. Anat.* 128:429.

Discovery of universal occurrence of a 9 + 2 pattern of microtubules in the oxoneme of cilia and flagella (sperm tails) in plant and animal kingdoms.

1961 Fawcett. In: *The Cell.* Eds. Brachet and Mirsky. New York: Academic Press, p. 217.

Description of outer dense fibers and 9 + 9 + 2 pattern of flagellar structure as typical of mammals.

1965 Fawcett. *Z. Zellforsch. Mikrosk. Anat.* 67:279.

1970 Pedersen. *J. Ultrastruct. Res.* 33:457.

Demonstration of a sliding mechanism in generation of sperm tail movements.

1968 Satir. *J. Cell Biol.* 39:77.

1971 Summers and Gibbons. *Proc. Natl. Acad. Sci. USA* 68:3092.

Isolation and characterization of tubulin.

1970 Stephens. *J. Mol. Biol.* 47:353.

1973 Olmsted and Borisy. *Annu. Rev. Biochem.* 42:507.

1973 Wilson and Meza. *J. Cell Biol.* 58:709.

Development of a method employing colchicine for isolation of tubulin.

1967 Shelanski and Taylor. *J. Cell Biol.* 34:549.

1967 Wilson and Friedkin. *Biochemistry* 6:3126.

Isolation of dynein, a protein with ATPase activity, and its localization in the arms of the doublets.

1965 Gibbons. *Arch. Biol.* (Liege) 76:317.

1965 Gibbons and Rowe. *Science* 149:424.

Isolation of linkage protein nexin.

1970 Stephens. *Biol. Bull.* 139:438.

Isolation and partial chemical characterization of outer fibers of sperm flagellum.

1973 Price. *J. Cell Biol.* 59:272.

1973 Baccetti et al. *J. Submicrosc. Cytol.* 5:237.

The proposal of a fluid mosaic model of the plasma membrane.

1972 Singer and Nicolson. *Science* 175:720.

Demonstration of regional differences in sperm membrane by binding of colloidal iron and lectins.

1971 Cooper and Bedford. *Anat. Rec.* 169:300.

1971 Flechon. *J. Microscopie* 11:53.

1972 Yanagimachi et al. *Am. J. Anat.* 135:497.

Demonstration of continued morphological and biochemical differentiation of spermatozoa in the epididymis.

1963 Fawcett and Hollenberg. *Z. Zellforsch. Mikrosk. Anat.* 60:276.

1969 Fawcett and Phillips. *J. Reprod. Fertil.* (Suppl.) 6:406.

1973 Bedford et al. *J. Reprod. Fertil.* (Suppl.) 18:199.

Demonstration of the immunological properties of spermatozoa.

1957 Metz. In: *Beginnings of Embryonic Development.* Eds. Tyler et al. Washington, D.C.: Am. Assoc. Adv. Sci., p. 23.

1963 Tyler and Bishop. In: *Mechanisms Concerned with Conception.* Ed. Hartman. New York: Macmillan, p. 397.

Major Gaps in Our Knowledge

The biochemical mechanisms of chromatin condensation, its biological significance, and its rapid reversal to form the male pronucleus.

The factors that normally trigger the acrosome reaction when sperm reaches the vicinity of the ovulated egg.

Although there is some indication that the enzyme bound to the inner acrosomal membrane permits the sperm to gain access to the egg, the relative importance of zona lysis in mechanical penetration by a motile sperm needs further investigation.

It is known that substances within the cortical granules prevent polyspermy; however, the mechanism by which they block polyspermy is not know.

It has been found that the acrosomal hydrolases are chemically distinct from the equivalent ones of the lysosomes; this suggests the need for further characterization of the antigenic properties of these enzymes to determine the feasibility of specific immunosuppresion of their activity without undesirable consequences outside of the reproductive tract.

The ultrastructure of the postacrosomal region of the sperm is well known. Still largely unknown is the chemical basis for the specificity of this segment of the sperm surface and the molecular mechanisms involved in gamete attachment and fusion.

In some animals, the detachment of sperm heads from sperm tails is a genetic defect and can be induced in vitro by brief exposure to endopeptidase. Since this region is a vulnerable site in the structural integrity of the spermatozoon, we need to know the nature of this linkage.

Much is known about dynein, the protein mainly involved in transduction of chemical energy to mechanical work in motility. We now need to characterize the nexin links, radial spokes, and other minor components of the axoneme, as well as the chemical fractionation of the doublets, to identify the basis for specific binding of dynein and spoke protein to particular protofilaments in the wall of the doublets.

Information is needed concerning the chemical nature and function of those fibrous components that are peculiar to spermatozoa.

It is quite clear that membranes play a central role in capacitation, in the acrosome reaction, and in the recognition and attachment of the gametes. We need to know: (i) the significance of the unique patterns revealed by freeze-cleaving within the lipid bilayer in different regions of the sperm membrane; (ii) how the membrane intercalated particles are related to those oligosaccharides on the outer surface that appear to be the basis for the regional specificity of the sperm membrane; and (iii) the nature of the internal organization of the membrane during different stages of maturation and in the different environments encountered in the male and female reproductive tracts.

Physiological significance of cyclic nucleotide stimulation of sperm motility.

Specific energy requirements necessary to maintain sperm motility.

Biochemical mechanism(s) by which sperm motility is maintained in cervical mucus.

Characterization of sperm cyclase, its specificity, and its activators.

Elucidation of biochemical processes with chemical or physiological characteristics which are unique to the spermatozoon (e.g., enzyme activators or inhibitors, membrane stability).

Specific abnormalities in sperm function which are associated with naturally occurring male infertility; knowledge of these abnormalities will provide a basis for interfering with those processes essential for the capacity for fertilization.

Methodological Advances
Period before 1960

Advancements in techniques of microtomy and microscopy to learn more about the submicroscopic organization of cells.

1952 Pallade. *J. Exp. Med.* 95:285.

1953 Porter and Blum. *Anat. Rec.* 117:685.

1953 Fernandez-Moran. *Exp. Cell Res.* 5:255.

1955 Watson. *J. Biophys. Biochem. Cytol.* 1:183.

Period 1960–1974

Introduction of aldehyde fixation for electron microscopy.

1963 Sabatini, Bemsch, and Barnett. *J. Cell Biol.* 17:19.

Development of freeze-fracture technique for the study of membranes.

1963 Moor and Mühlethaler. *J. Cell Biol.* 17:609.

1966 Branton. *Proc. Natl. Acad. Sci. USA* 55:5.

Availability of high-speed cinematographic equipment for analysis of germ cell and sperm tail movements.

1963 Blandau, White, and Rumery. *Fertil. Steril.* 14:482.

1972 Phillips. *J. Cell Biol.* 53:561.

Availability of molecular probes for the study of spermatozoon structures.

1971 Edelman and Millette. *Proc. Natl. Acad. Sci. USA* 68:2436.

1973 Mercado and Rosado. *Biochim. Biophys. Acta* 298:639.

1973 Pihlaja and Roth. *J. Ultrastruct. Res.* 44:293.

1974 Mercado et al. *Biochem. Biophys. Res. Commun.* 56:185.

Methodological Needs

Methods for the immunological or biochemical interference with sperm mobility.

Assay to detect the antigenic properties of acrosomal enzymes.

Spermatozoon (continued)

More sophisticated methods for the molecular dissection of the mature spermatozoon.

In vitro techniques to assay human sperm biochemical processes necessary for fertility (e.g., steps involved in chromatin decondensation, pronucleus formation, maintenance of motility).

Techniques for immunological and physiochemical characterization of specific structural proteins or enzymes present in spermatozoa from a single subject.

In vitro models for study of zona pellucida penetration and pronucleus formation, using human spermatozoa.

Contraceptive Possibilities

Cyclic AMP formation in mature spermatozoa may be vulnerable to contraception, if a specific spermatozoal cyclase can be demonstrated and if sperm motility is dependent upon it.

Introduction of noncompetitive inhibitors of enzymatic processes unique to spermatozoa that abolish motility.

Interference with cervical mucus factors that maintain sperm motility.

Inhibition of cervical mucus formation.

Drugs to induce premature release of acrosomal enzymes in female tract.

Administration of inhibitors of sperm function required for fertilization.

Capacitation and Fertilization

Biological Processes: Significant Discoveries

Period before 1960

Observation that spermatozoa enter the egg.

1843 Barry. *Philos. Trans. R. Soc. Lond. (Biol.)* 128.

Demonstration that fertilization involves union of sperm nucleus with that of the ovum.

1875 Hertwig. *Morphol. Jahrbuch* (Liepzig) 1:347.

Male and female nuclei which unite in fertilized ovum contain half as many chromosomes as the somatic cells.

1883 van Beueden. *Bull. Acad. R. Belg.* 11.

Discovery that there is a physiological change occurring in the female genital tract that prepares the spermatozoon for fertilization: capacitation.

1951 Austin. *Aust. J. Sci. Res.* B4:581.

1951 Chang. *Nature* 168:687.

1952 Austin. *Nature* 170:326.

Successful in vitro fertilization of mammalian eggs.

1951 Chang. *Nature* 184:466.

1960 Thibault and Dauzier. *C.R. Acad. Sci.* [D] (Paris) 250:1358.

Discovery that capacitated sperm can be decapacitated by brief incubation in seminal plasma.

1957 Chang. *Nature* 179:258.

Description of cortical granules in the mammalian egg.

1956 Austin. *Exp. Cell Res.* 10:533.

Fine-structural description of the developing mammalian oocyte.

1959 Sotelo and Porter. *J. Biophys. Biochem. Cytol.* 5:327.

1960 Anderson and Beams. *J. Ultrastruct. Res.* 3:432.

1960 Chiquoine. *Am. J. Anat.* 106:149.

Discovery of the presence of hyaluronidase in the acrosome.

1958 Austin and Bishop. *Proc. R. Soc. Lond. (Biol.)* 149:241.

Further clarification of the presence of proteolytic activity in human semen.

1958 Thorsteinsson. *Am. J. Physiol.* 194:341.

Detailed description of the submicroscopic features of spermatozoa that had been beyond the reach of the light microscope.

1953 Wilkins and Randall. *Biochim. Biophys. Acta* 10:192.

1955 Burgos and Fawcett. *J. Biophys. Biochem. Cytol.* 1:287.

1958 Austin and Bishop. *Proc. R. Soc. Lond.* B149:241.

1965 Fawcett. *Z. Zellforsch. Mikrosk. Anat.* 67:279.

Period 1960–1974

Finding that decapacitation factor (DF) is a definite substance.

1962 Bedford and Chang. *Am. J. Physiol.* 202:179.

Discovery of a corona-penetrating enzyme in the acrosome.

1968 Zaneveld, McRori, and Williams. *Fed. Proc.* 27:567.

Isolation of the lytic enzyme acrozonase (acrosin) from the acrosome.

1968 Stambaugh and Buckley. *Science* 161:158.

1971 Stambaugh and Buckley. *Biol. Reprod.* 3:275.

Recognition that acrozonase (acrosin) can be inhibited by plant and animal polypeptide inhibitors and also by seminal plasma trypsin inhibitor.

1968 Stambaugh and Buckley. *Science* 161:585.

1970 Zaneveld, Srivastava, and Williams. *J. Reprod. Fertil.* 20:377.

Finding that, upon ejaculation, an acrozonase inhibitor from seminal plasma is added to acrozonase, and during capacitation in the uterus it is removed.

1970 Zaneveld, Srivastava, and Williams. *J. Reprod. Fertil.* 20:377.

Subcellular localization of hyaluronidase and acrozonase.

1969 Stambaugh and Buckley. *J. Reprod. Fertil.* 19:423.

Description of the origin of cortical granules.

1967 Szollosi. *Anat. Rec.* 158:431.

1968 Anderson. *J. Cell Biol.* 37:514.

Further clarification of the fine structure of oocytes.

1964 Beams. In: *Cellular Membranes in Development*. Ed. Locke. New York: Academic Press, p. 175.

1967 Baca and Zamboni. *J. Ultrastruct. Res.* 19:354.

1967 Hertig and Adams. *J. Cell Biol.* 34:647.

1974 Anderson. *J. Cell Biol.* 47:711.

Discovery that mammalian sperm undergo capacitation and the acrosome reaction in vitro.

1969 Banister. *J. Reprod. Fertil.* 18:544.

1969 Yanagimachi. *J. Reprod. Fertil.* 18:275.

Proposal of a fluid mosaic model for the plasma membrane.

1972 Singer and Nicolson. *Science* 175:720.

Demonstration of regional differences in sperm membrane by binding of colloidal iron and lectins.

1971 Flechon. *J. Microscopie* 11:53.

1972 Yanagimachi et al. *Am. J. Anat.* 135:497.

Description of cytological changes taking place during the acrosomal reaction.

1961 Colwin and Colwin. *J. Biophys. Biochem. Cytol.* 10:211.

1970 Yanagimachi and Noda. *J. Ultrastruct. Res.* 31:465.

1971 Bedford. *Am. J. Anat.* 133:213.

Demonstration of selective recognition of egg by postacrosomal membrane and its fusion with the oolemma.

1968 Barros and Franklin. *J. Cell Biol.* 37:C13.

1969 Stefanini, Oura, and Zamboni. *J. Submicrosc. Cytol.* 1:1.

1970 Yanagimachi and Noda. *Am. J. Anat.* 128:429.

Successful in vitro fertilization of mammalian eggs.

1954 Dauzier, Thibault, and Wintenberger. *C.R. Acad. Sci.* [D] (Paris) 238:844.

1959 Chang. *Nature* 184:466.

1964 Yanagimachi and Chang. *J. Exp. Zool.* 186:361.

1969 Edwards, Bavister, and Steptoe. *Nature* 221:632.

1973 Gould, Kline, and Williams. *Fertil. Steril.* 24:260.

Discovery of a neuraminidase-like factor (NLF) in the acrosome which renders the bound sialic acids active.

1970 Srivastava, Zaneveld, and Williams. *Biochem. Biophys. Res. Commun.* 39:575.

Recognition that cervical mucus presents a physical barrier that sperm must penetrate to reach the uterine cavity and the possible influence of proteolytic enzymes of semen on sperm migration.

1970 Moghissi and Syner. *Int. J. Fertil.* 15:43.

1970 Moghissi and Syner. *Fertil. Steril.* 21:234.

1971 Syner and Moghissi. *Biochem. J.* 126:1135.

Capacitation and Fertilization (continued)

Major Gaps in Our Knowledge

Although much information has been obtained concerning capacitation with the existing methodology, we still need information concerning the precise timing of sperm incubation, control of the numbers of sperm incubated to avoid overloading the capacitating ability of a particular site, and the use of adequate statistical methods for anlyzing the significance of differences observed when the effects of various treatments are compared.

Information concerning the hormonal control of capacitation is controversial, and therefore careful study should be made to determine in a precise manner whether or not endocrine factors are necessary for capacitation.

The current theory of capacitation requires the removal of a sperm-coating substance; however, nothing is known about the biochemical mechanism involved in the removal of this substance.

There is some suggestion that the neuraminidase (NLF) located in the sperm acrosome is different from other neuraminidases, and this suggests the need for further characterization of the antigenic properties of these enzymes to determine the feasibility of specific immunosuppression of their activity without undersirable consequences outside the reproductive tract.

It is postulated that acrozonase is involved in sperm passage through the zona pellucida; however, nothing is known concerning the role of other acrosomal enzymes in the fertilization process.

Some investigators have achieved certain success in the subcellular localization of acrosomal enzymes. There is, nevertheless, a need to develop cytobiochemical techniques to demonstrate the exact location of the enzymes.

Investigations are needed to explain the biochemical mechanisms of chromatin condensation, its biological significance, and its rapid reversal to form the male pronucleus.

There is a need to know about the factors that normally trigger the acrosome reaction when sperm reach the vicinity of the ovulated egg.

Continued efforts should be devoted to the biochemical understanding of the initial events of fertilization.

While some progress has been made in isolating a decapacitation factor, efforts should be made to isolate specific substances active in capacitation from the female reproductive tract.

While the need for capacitation has been well defined in a few mammals, further study is needed in a variety of mammals (and other species) to determine how widespread this phenomenon is.

Although some investigators have suggested that capacitation is a membrane-related phenomenon, there is no direct morphological evidence that changes occur in the sperm plasma membrane during capacitation. Therefore, investigators should continue to probe the sperm plasma membrane with a wide variety of techniques employed by anatomists.

There is some evidence that there is a change in spermial oxygen consumption as a result of their exposure to secretions of the female tract. However, the relation that this apparent increase bears to the phenomenon of capacitation should be investigated.

While it is well known that sperm gain access to the egg by passing through the zona pellucida, further study should be made concerning the identification of the sperm head zona lysin.

Evidence indicates that the equatorial segment fuses with the oolemma and enters the egg unchanged. Wee need to know the functional significance of the equatorial region of the acrosome.

Although experimental evidence suggests that cortical granules are involved in blocking polyspermy, further study is needed to unravel the biochemical processes by which this is achieved.

A suggestion is made that the zona pellucida in some animals is involved in blocking polyspermy; however, much work is needed to clarify its origin and chemical composition.

It is known that the sperm initiates meiotic cleavage; however, nothing is known about the biochemistry of this important event.

Methodological Advances

Period before 1960

Advancements in techniques of microtomy and microscopy to learn more about the submicroscopic organization of cells.

1952 Palade. *J. Exp. Med.* 95:285.

1953 Porter and Blum. *Anat. Rec.* 117:685.

1953 Fernández-Moran. *Exp. Cell Res.* 5:255.

1955 Watson. *J. Biophys. Biochem. Cytol.* 1:183.

Development of zone electrophoresis in starch gels.

1955 Smithies. *Biochem. J.* 61:629.

Period 1960–1974

Introduction of aldehyde fixation for electron microscopy.

1963 Sabatini, Bensch, and Barnett. *J. Cell Biol.* 17:19.

Development of freeze-fracture technique for the study of membranes.

1963 Moor and Mühlethaler. *J. Cell Biol.* 17:609.

1966 Branton. *Proc. Natl. Acad. Sci. USA* 55:5.

Discovery of the liquefaction of primate semen coagulata with tryspin permits is use for in vitro studies.

1967 Roussell and Austin. *Int. J. Fertil.* 12:288.

Development of a radioimmunoassay to follow the progress of the capacitation process.

1973 Oliphant and Brackett. *Biol. Reprod.* 9:404.

Development of an in vivo capacitation system.

1958 Chang. *Endocrinology* 63:619.

1958 Noyes et al. *Nature* 181:1209.

1967 Bedford and Shalkovsky. *J. Reprod. Fertil.* 13:361.

Development of a chemically defined medium for culturing mouse oocytes.

1967 Biggers, Whittingham, and Donahue. *Proc. Natl. Acad. Sci. USA* 58:560.

Species specificity of sperm capacitation in the rabbit.

1967 Bedford and Shalkovsky. *J. Reprod. Fertil.* 13:361.

1970 Bedford. *Biol. Reprod.* (Suppl.) 2:128.

1970 Seitz et al. *Fertil. Steril.* 21:325.

Development of an in vitro capacitation system.

1965 Kirton and Hofs. *Science* 150:168.

1967 Ericcson. *J. Reprod. Fertil.* (Suppl.) 2:65.

1969 Yanagimachi. *J. Exp. Zool.* 170:269.

1969 Yanagimachi. *J. Reprod. Fertil.* 18:275.

In vitro fertilization of the mammalian egg.

1960 Thibault and Dauzier. *C.R. Acad. Sci. [D]* (Paris) 250:1358.

1964 Yanagimachi and Chang. *J. Exp. Zool.* 156:361.

1968 Whittingham. *Nature* 220:592.

1969 Edwards, Barrister, and Steptoe. *Nature* 221:632.

1970 Brackett. *Fertil. Steril.* 21:169.

Methodological Needs

Methods for the immunological or biochemical interference with sperm motility.

Methods for microbiochemical analysis of cortical granules.

Assay to detect the antigenic properties of acrosomal enzymes.

More sophisticated biochemical methods for the molecular dissection of the mature spermatozoon, egg, and early events of fertilization.

Cytobiochemical techniques for the precise detection of acrosomal enzymes.

Contraceptive Possibilities

The reversible inhibition of capacitation by substances in the epididymal and seminal plasma shows the necessity for further investigation of these substances. Such identification might lead to the development of antifertility agents that would maintain spermatozoa in the decapacitated state.

Study of acrosomal hyaluronidase antibodies.

1973   Metz. *Fed. Proc.* 32:2057.

Study of the protease acrosin and the feasibility of immunological inhibition of its activity to prevent sperm penetration of the zona pellucida.

1973   Zaneveld et al. *Biol. Reprod.* 9:219.

Investigation of sperm specific isoenzyme lactic dehydrogenase.

1972   Goldbert and Lerum. *J. Biol. Chem.* 247:2044.

Attempts to render the zona pellucida impenetrable through treatment with trypsin-like enzymes.

1970   Gwatkin et al. *Nature* 227:182.

Experiments with nonenzymatic agents such as plant lectins and the zona substance in vitro.

1973   Oikawa et al. *Nature* 241:246.

Preimplantation and Implantation

I. Blastocyst Formation

Biological Processes: Significant Discoveries

Period 1960–1974

Description of the growth in volume and cell number of the rabbit blastocyst.

1964 Daniel. *Am. Nat.* 98:85.

Accumulation of evidence that two distinct cell populations areise in the mouse by the blastocyst stage: outer cells, which form the trophoblast, and inner cells, which form the inner cell mass. The evidence is based on:

1. Differences in the rate of cell multiplication.

1972 Barlow, Owen, and Graham. *J. Embryol. Exp. Morphol.* 27:431.

2. Differences in the cell junctions between adjacent inner and outer cells.

1967 Schlafke and Enders. *J. Anat.* 102:13.

1969 Calarco and Brown. *J. Exp. Zool.* 171:253.

3. Differences in the ability of groups of outside and inside cells to seal and form liquid-filled vesicles; outside cells form vesicles whereas inside ones cannot.

1971 Gardner. *Adv. Biosci.* 6:279.

4. Differences in the ability to induce a decidual reaction in a pseudopregnant uterus; outside cells can induce this reaction whereas inside ones cannot.

1972 Gardner. *J. Embryol. Exp. Morphol.* 28:279.

Recognition that the formation of junctional complexes between adjacent outer cells is a necessary prerequisite for the formation of the blastocyst.

1971 Enders. In: *The Biology of the Blastocyst.* Ed. Blandau. Chicago: University of Chicago Press.

Demonstration by means of the lanthanum technique and freeze fracture that the junctional complexes are associated with compaction of the morula and consist of tight and gap junctions.

1974 Ducibella et al. *Proc. Soc. Am. Cell Biol.,* San Diego.

Collection of data suggesting that the inner cell mass only differentiates after the creation of an inner microenvironment by the intimately apposed trophoblast cells.

1967 Tarkowski and Wroblewska. *J. Embryol. Exp. Morphol.* 18:155.

1972 Hillman, Sherman, and Graham. *J. Embryol. Exp. Morphol.* 28:263.

Discovery that the preimplantation rabbit blastocoele fluid is rich in potassium and low in chloride in comparison with blood plasma.

1960 Lutwak-Mann. *J. Reprod. Fertil.* 1:3176.

1970 Smith. *Experientia* 26:736.

Demonstration that the trophoblast forms an epithelium-like outer membrane capable of the active transport of ions.

1969 Cross and Brinster. *Exp. Cell Res.* 58:125.

1970 Cross and Brinster. *Exp. Cell Res.* 62:303.

1970 Gamow and Daniel. *Wilhelm Roux Arch.* 169:261.

Demonstration that the rabbit blastocyst can heal itself and reexpand after removal of a portion of the trophoblast.

1968 Gardner and Edwards. *Nature* 218:346.

Demonstration that cytochalasin β causes collapse (loss of fluid) from the mouse blastocyst and that on removal of the drug, blastocoele fluid reforms; the formation of the fluid seems to depend on ouabain-sensitive sites on the blastocyst.

1974 Borland. Thesis, University of Delaware.

1974 Dizio and Tasca. *Proc. Soc. Am. Cell Biol.,* San Diego.

Recommended Reviews.

1972 Biggers. In: *The Water Metabolism of the Fetus.* Eds. Barnes and Seeds. Springfield: Charles C Thomas, ch. I.

1974 Herbert and Graham. In: *Current Topics in Developmental Biology.* Eds. Moscona and Monroy. New York: Academic Press, vol. 8, ch. 5.

Major Gaps in Our Knowledge

A critical stage in the development of the morula is the establishment of an outer epithelial layer of cells which creates a special internal microenvironment. This epithelial membrane is established by the formation of junctional complexes. We need to determine what causes the formation of this membrane and the physiological role of the tight and gap junctions.

The transport properties of this trophoblastic membrane need to be determined. There is evidence that Na and Cl are actively transported (Cross, *Biol. Reprod.* 8:566 [1970]). However, these facts do not explain why blastocoele fluid is rich in K and poor in Cl. Studies are also needed on the transport of other substances, such as glucose, amino acids, and proteins such as uteroglobin (blastokinin).

A major question is how water is accumulated in the blastocoele, for this substance must play a major role in the swelling of the blastocyst. By estimating the chemical potential of water inside and outside the blastocyst, Tuft and Boving (*J. Exp. Zool.* 174:165) concluded that water is actively transported.

The active transport of water is not generally accepted as a normal physiological process, and the question therefore needs critical study. The application of methods of irreversible thermodynamics could help determine whether the movement of water, coupled to active ion transport, is sufficient to account for the observed blastocyst expansion.

The role of the internal microenvironment, caused by the transport properties of the trophoblast, in the differentiation of the inner cell mass needs to be determined.

II. Metabolism of the Preimplantation Stage

Biological Processes: Significant Discoveries

Period 1960–1974

The development of the late 2-cell mouse embryo requires an exogenous source of carbon, and the number of compounds that can be utilized to support development is restricted: pyruvate, lactate, oxaloacetate, and phosphoenolpyruvate.

1963 Brinster. *Exp. Cell. Res.* 32:205.

1965 Brinster. *J. Exp. Zool.* 158:59.

The carbon sources that can support development of the preimplantation mouse embryo change with development, being restricted to pyruvate and oxaloacetate at the 1-cell stage, and increasing to several others by the 8-cell stage (glucose, malate, citrate, and α-oxoglutarate).

1966 Brinster and Thomason. *Exp. Cell Res.* 43:303.

1967 Biggers, Whittingham, and Donahue. *Proc. Natl. Acad. Sci. USA* 58:560.

Hexokinase and phosphofructokinase is present in all mouse preimplantation stages of development.

1968 Brinster. *Enzyme* 34:306.

1971 Brinster. *Arch. Roux-Ocefa* 166:300.

Lactate can be produced from glucose in small amounts by the fertilized ovum and 2-cell stage of the mouse, indicating that the glycolytic pathway is intact but held in an inhibited state.

1969 Wales. *Aust. J. Biol. Sci.* 22:701.

The ratio of ATP to ADP in the unfertilized and fertilized ovum and 2-cell stage of the mouse is very high and falls with development.

1971 Quinn and Wales. *J. Reprod. Fertil.* 25:133.

1973 Quinn and Wales. *J. Reprod. Fertil.* 32:231.

1973 Ginsberg and Hillman. *J. Embryol. Exp. Morphol.* 30:267.

Demonstration by the use of enzyme recycling methods that there is high citrate in 2-cell mouse embryos which, acting in concert with the high levels of ATP, could severely inhibit phosphofructokinase activity. This phenomenon could largely explain the inability of glucose to support early development.

1974 Barbehenn, Wales, and Lowry. *Proc. Natl. Acad. Sci. USA* 71:1056.

Application of biometrical methods for the systematic determination of the nutritional requirements of mouse embryos in chemically defined media.

1965 Biggers and Brinster. *J. Exp. Zool.* 158:39.

1965 Brinster. *J. Reprod. Fertil.* 10:227.

Development of the principle of enzymatic cycling for the measurement of metabolites in histological sections or single cells.

1966 Lowry et al. *J. Biol. Chem.* 236:2746.

Demonstration of the feasibility of measuring enzyme activity (LDH) in small batches of mouse embryos, including the study of enzymes.

1965 Brinster. *Biochim. Biophys. Acta* 110:439.

1967 Auerbach and Brinster. *Exp. Cell Res.* 46:89.

1967 Rapola and Kaskimies. *Science* 157:1311.

A marked change in the morphology of mitochondria occurs in the mouse between the 2- and 8-cell stages of development, and the correlation of this observation with changes in the ability of the embryo to use malate, citrate, and oxoglutarate.

1968 Wales and Biggers. *J. Reprod. Fertil.* 15:103.

1971 Kramen and Biggers. *Proc. Natl. Acad. Sci. USA* 68:2556.

1971 Stern, Biggers, and Anderson. *J. Exp. Zool.* 176:179.

CO_2 is fixed by all mouse preimplantation stages and is incorporated into nucleic acids, protein, and lipid. This finding is consistent with the view that pyruvate is not only required for energy but also to supply anapleurotic pathways.

1967 Biggers, Whittingham, and Donahue. *Proc. Natl. Acad. Sci. USA* 58:560.

1969 Wales, Quinn, and Murdoch. *J. Reprod. Fertil.* 20:561.

1970 Graves and Biggers. *Science* 167:1506.

Bicarbonate is an essential component of the medium for the culture of preimplantation mouse embryos, and adequate synthesis of macromolecules does not occur in its absence.

1973 Quinn and Wales. *J. Reprod. Fertil.* 3:289.

Preimplantation mouse embryos accumulate leucine and methionine by specific, chemically mediated active transport systems.

1974 Borland and Tasca. *Dev. Biol.* 30:169.

The pathways of energy metaolism may be different in the rabbit and mouse.

1961 Fridhandler. *Exp. Cell Res.* 22:303.

1969 Brinster. *Exp. Cell Res.* 54:205.

Protein synthesis is detectable in the early cleavage stages of the mouse and rabbit.

1964 Mintz. *J. Exp. Zool.* 157:85.

1967 Monesi and Salfi. *Exp. Cell Res.* 46:632.

1969 Manes and Daniel. *Exp. Cell Res.* 55:261.

Synthesis of RNA occurs very early in the cleavage in the mouse and rabbit.

1964 Mintz. *J. Exp. Zool.* 157:85.

1967 Monesi and Salfi. *Exp. Cell Res.* 46:632.

1969 Woodland and Graham. *Nature* 221:327.

1969 Manes. *J. Exp. Zool.* 172:303.

Two-cell mouse embryos are very sensitive to actinomycin D, raising the possibility that genetic activation is required throughout cleavage.

1964 Mintz. *J. Exp. Zool.* 157:85.

1966 Thomson and Biggers. *Exp. Cell Res.* 41:411.

Studies on glucose phosphate isomerase reveal that the paternal genome may be activated much earlier than had been demonstrated in fish, amphibia, and birds.

1971 Chapman, Whitten, and Ruddle. *Dev. Biol.* 26:153.

1973 Brinster. *Biochem. Genet.* 9:187.

When the giant cell transformation of the trophoblast occurs in the mouse, the nuclei of the cells acquire 500–1000 times the haploid DNA content.

1972 Chapman, Ansell, and McLaren. *Dev. Biol.* 29:48.

1972 Sherman, McLaren, and Walker. *Nature* 238:175.

Major Gaps in Our Knowledge

Comparative studies on other species comparable to those on the mouse are required urgently.

A systematic study of the energy charge in unfertilized ova and preimplantation cleavage stages of several species to determine what feedback systems may control metabolism during early development.

Further studies on the nature of specific macromolecules synthesized in the preimplantation embryo. At present there is no information on lipids, although it is known that in some species there is an abundance of lipid droplets.

A much more thorough study of ion metabolism in preimplantation stages, particularly with respect to the role of K^+ in the regulation of metabolism.

At present we know relatively little about the role of membranes and permeability changes in early mammalian development. Some progress could be made by the joint application of electrophysiological and tracer techniques.

III. Implantation

Biological Processes: Significant Discoveries

Period before 1960

Lactation causes a delay in implantation in some rodents.

1891 Lataste. *C. R. Soc. Biol.* (Paris) 43:21.

Corpus luteum is necessary for establishment and maintenance of pregnancy.

1928 Corner. *Am. J. Physiol.* 86:74.

Lactational delay in implantation in the rat is due to low estrogen secretion.

1941 Krehbiel. *Anat. Rec.* 81:381.

1942 Weichert. *Anat. Rec.* 83:1.

Hormonal requirements for epithelial plaque formation and decidualization of the endometrium in the rhesus monkey established.

1935 Hisaw. *Anat. Rec.* 64:54.

1936 Hisaw and Greep. *Proc. Soc. Exp. Biol. Med.* 35:29.

1937 Hisaw, Greep, and Fevold. *Am. J. Anat.* 61:483.

Blastocyst attaches to the uterine wall on the 9th day in the rhesus monkey.

1938 Wislocki and Streeter. *Contrib. Embryol. Carnegie Instit. Wash.* 27:1.

Implantation of human ova takes place between 5th and 6th days of age.

1945 Hertig and Rock. *Contrib. Embryol. Carnegie Inst. Wash.* 31:67.

1954 Hertig et al. *Contrib. Embryol. Carnegie Inst. Wash.* 35:199.

Progesterone alone cannot induce implantation in ovariectomized rats; hormonal requirement varies depending on time of ovariectomy.

1956 Canivenc, Laffargue, and Mayer. *C. R. Soc. Biol.* 150:2208.

1957 Cochrane and Meyer. *Proc. Soc. Exp. Biol.* 96:155.

Importance of synchronous development of the uterus and embryo for successful implantation established.

1950 Chang. *J. Exp. Zool.* 114:197.

1951 Beatty. *Nature* 168:995.

1952 Noyes. *Fertil. Steril.* 3:1.

1956 McLaren and Michie. *J. Exp. Biol.* 33:394. (mice)

1960 Noyes and Dickman. *J. Reprod. Fertil.* 1:186. (rats)

Period 1960–1974

Preimplantation surge of estrogen in the rat proposed.

1960 Shelesnyak. *Endeavour* 19:81.

Surge demonstrated directly by measurement of estrogen by bioassay.

1969 Yoshinaga et al. *Endocrinology* 85:103.

Surge demonstrated by radioimmunoassay.

1969 Shaikh and Ahluwalia. *Biol. Reprod.* 1:378.

Clarification of the steroidal control of the uterine receptivity and refractoriness in the rat.

1963 Psychoyos. *C.R. Soc. Biol.* (Paris) 257:1153.

1970 Meyers. *J. Endocrinol.* 46:341.

1974 Yoshinaga and Greep. In: *Progress in Reproduction Research and Population Control.* Eds. Husain and Guttmacher. Quebec: Publications International, p. 137.

Prolactin is essential for progesterone secretion, which in turn is necessary for ovum implantation. Ergocornine injection interrupts prolactin secretion and inhibits implantation.

1963 Shelesnyak and Barnea. *Acta Endocrinol.* (Kbh.) 43:469.

LH is required for ovarian hormone secretion, which in turn is necessary for implantation in the rat.

1968 Raj et al. *J. Reprod. Fertil.* 17:335.

FSH is required for estrogen secretion prior to implantation in lactating rats.

1974 Raud. *Biol. Reprod.* 10:327.

The decidual reaction is preceded by early modification of the capillary permeability of the uterus.

1960 Psychoyos. *C.R. Soc. Biol.* [*D*] (Paris) 154:1384.

The induction of deciduomata in the rat.

1963 Finn and Kemp. *J. Embryol. Exp. Morphol.* 11:673.

Structural differentiation of luminal membranes in the rat uterus during normal and experimental implantations.

1966 Nilsson. *Z. Anat. Entwicklungsgesch.* 125:152.

A morphological analysis of the early implantation stages in the rat.

1967 Enders and Schlafke. *Am. J. Anat.* 120:185.

A study of the early stages of implantation in mice.

1967 Finn and McLaren. *J. Reprod. Fertil.* 13:259.

Hormonal interplay controlling egg implantation in the rat.

1967 Psychoyos. *Adv. Reprod. Physiol.* 2:257.

Patterns of cell division in the mouse uterus during early pregnancy.

1967 Finn and Martin. *J. Endocrinol.* 39:593.

DNA synthesis and cell proliferation during formation of deciduomata in mice.

1967 Zhinkin and Samoshkina. *J. Embryol. Exp. Morphol.* 17:593.

Changes in protein patterns of the uterus during maintenance of the blastocyst in rabbits.

1967 Beier. *Verh. Dtsch. Zool. Ges.* 31:139.

"Blastokinin," inducer and regulator of blastocyst development in the rabbit uterus.

1967 Krishnan and Daniel. *Science* 158:490.

"Uteroglobin," a hormone-sensitive endometrial protein involved in blastocyst development.

1968 Beier. *Biochim. Biophys. Acta* 160:289.

Influence of estrogen and progesterone on the incorporation of ^{35}S-methionine by blastocysts in ovariectomized mice.

1968 Weitlauf and Greenwald. *J. Exp. Zool.* 169:463.

Temporal changes in protein synthesis by mouse blastocysts transferred to ovariectomized recipients.

1969 Weitlauf. *J. Exp. Zool.* 171:481.

Uptake and incorporation of amino acids by cultured mouse embryos: estrogen stimulation.

1971 Smith and Smith. *Biol. Reprod.* 4:66.

Implantation and development of mouse eggs transferred to the uteri of nonprogestational mice.

1969 Cowell. *J. Reprod. Fertil.* 19:239.

Resumption of development by quiescent blastocysts transferred to primed ovariectomized recipients in the marsupial, *Macropus eugenii.*

1970 Tyndale-Biscoe. *J. Reprod. Fertil.* 23:25.

Studies on the development of the implantation reaction in the mouse uterus: influence of actinomycin D.

1973 Finn and Bredl. *J. Reprod. Fertil.* 34:247.

Differential effects of estrogen on the uptake of nucleic acid precursors by mouse blastocysts in vitro.

1973 Harper and Lee. *J. Reprod. Fertil.* 33:327.

The effect of progesterone and estradiol on blastocysts cultured within the lumina of immature mouse uteri.

1973   Grant. *J. Embryol. Exp. Morphol.* 29:617.

Steroid hormone production by pig blastocyst.

1973   Perry, Heap, and Amoroso. *Nature* 245:45.

Influence of the trophoblast upon differentiation of the uterine epithelium during implantation in the mouse.

1974   Pollard and Finn. *J. Endocrinol.* 62:669.

Evidence for a preimplantation rise in estradiol-17β level on day 4 of pregnancy in the mouse.

1974   McCormack and Greenwald. *J. Reprod. Fertil.* 41:297.

Binding of estradiol to rabbit blastocysts and its possible role in implantation.

1974   Bhatt and Bullock. *J. Reprod. Fertil.* 39:65.

Steroidogenesis in the preimplantation rat embryo and its possible influence on morula-blastocyst transformation and implantation.

1974   Dickmann and Dey. *J. Reprod. Fertil.* 37:91.

Steroidogenesis in rabbit preimplantation embryos.

1975   Dickmann, Dey, and Gupta. *Proc. Natl. Acad. Sci. USA* 72:298.

Major Gaps in Our Knowledge

Uterine receptivity for blastocysts; mechanism by which hormones control the receptivity.

Cause of ectopic pregnancy.

Physiological significance of uteroglobin and blastokinin.

Basic elements of implantation in humans remain unknown.

Nature of stimulus from embryos that initiates implantation.

Extent to which there is a uterine control of embryonic development.

Function of decidua.

Growth of vascular system.

Mode of action of estrogens in implantation.

Reason for high incidence of implantation in oviduct of human.

Reason why the conceptus is not rejected by the maternal organism.

Role of ovarian steroid binding proteins in human endometrial function in general and in implantation in particular.

Methodological Advances

Period before 1960

BLASTOCYST FORMATION

Short-circuit method for the measurement of active ion transport.

1951   Ussing and Zerahn. *Acta Physiol. Scand.* 23:40.

Development of methods for the in vitro culture and the efficient transfer to uterine foster mothers of preimplantation mouse embryos.

1950   Chang. *J. Exp. Zool.* 114:197.

1956   Whitten. *Nature* 177:96.

1957   Whitten. *Nature* 179:1081.

1958   McLaren and Biggers. *Nature* 182:877.

METABOLISM OF PREIMPLANTATION STAGES

Demonstration that preimplantation mouse embryos could be partially cultivated to the blastocyst stage in vitro in simple chemically defined media.

1956   Whitten. *Nature* 177:96.

1957   Whitten. *Nature* 179:1081.

Development of methods of superovulation with gonadotropins in mice for the production of synchronous batches of mouse preimplantation stages.

1956   Gates. *Nature* 177:754.

1959   Edwards and Gates. *J. Endocrinol.* 18:292.

Development of very sensitive fluorometric pyridine nucleotide methods for measuring metabolites.

1956   Greengard. *Nature* 178:632.

IMPLANTATION

Deciduoma formation after traumatization of the endometrium of the guinea pig.

1907   Loeb. *Proc. Soc. Exp. Biol. Med.* 4:93.

1908   Loeb. *Proc. Soc. Exp. Biol. Med.* 5:102.

Induction of pseudopregnancy in the rat by means of electrical stimulation.

1931   Shelesnyak. *Anat. Rec.* 49:179.

Transfer of blastocysts into extrauterine sites.

1947   Fawcett et al. *Am. J. Anat.* 81:413.

1950   Fawcett. *Anat. Rec.* 108:71.

Direct observation of rabbit blastocyst implantation within a uterine segment using a plastic chamber in vivo.

1952   Boving. *Science* 116:211.

Period 1960–1974

BLASTOCYST FORMATION

Use of culture methods and transfer of embryos to uterine foster mothers to produce chimeras.

1961   Tarkwoski. *Nature* 190:857.

1962   Mintz. *Am. Zool.* 2:432.

Introduction of lanthanum as electron-opaque probes for the detection of tight junctions.

1964   Karnowsky. *J. Cell Biol.* 27:137A.

Introduction of the freeze-fracture technique for the study of membranes.

1963   Moor and Mühlethaler. *J. Cell Biol.* 17:609.

IMPLANTATION

Visualization of early implantation sites by systemic injection of blue dye (blue reaction).

1960   Psychoyos. *C.R. Acad. Sci.* [D] (Paris) 251:3072.

Method for local injection to induce implantation.

1961   Yoshinaga. *J. Reprod. Fertil.* 2:35.

Induction of deciduomata in hamsters and rats by injection of air.

1963   Orsini. *J. Endocrinol.* 28:119.

In vitro development of the explanted embryonic shields from rabbit blastocyst.

1967 Waddington and Waterman. *Am. J. Anat.* 53(67):355.

Hormone secretion during early pregnancy in the mouse.

1969 Finn and Martin. *J. Endocrinol.* 45:57.

Methodological Needs

BLASTOCYST FORMATION

Adaptation of micropuncture and ultramicrochemical techniques for the analysis of blastocoele fluid under various experimental conditions.

METABOLISM OF PREIMPLANTATION STAGES

The development of defined media for the culture in vitro of the preimplantation stages of several other species, particularly rats and a subhuman primate.

The development of ultrasensitive techniques for many more metabolites to use in the analysis of single embryos or batches of a few embryos. These techniques include enzymatic cycling, electron probe, mass spectrometer, ion- and substrate-sensitive electrodes.

The development of electron-probe techniques for the analysis of ions in single embryos.

Contraceptive Methods
Period 1960–1974

Ergocornine shown to prevent implantation in rats, probably by suppression of progesterone production, but only at doses likely to be toxic in humans.

1963 Shelesnyak and Barnea. *Acta Endocrinol.* (Kbh.) 43:469.

High doses of estrogen (25 mg DES) administered within 72 hours of coitus prevent pregnancy.

1971 Kuchera. *JAMA* 4:562.

1973 Blye. *Am. J. Obstet. Gynecol.* 115:1044.

1974 Kuchera. *Contraception* 10:47.

Postcoital estrogens may prevent implantation by inhibiting postovulatory progesterone production, resulting in an endometrium unable to support nidation.

1972 Nilsson and Nygren. *Ups. J. Med. Sci.* 77:3.

High doses of estrogen administered over long periods of time in abnormal pregnancies associated with vaginal malignancy.

1974 Herbst et al. *Am. J. Obstet. Gynecol.* 119:713.

Antiestrogenic compound ICI 46474 prevents implantation.

1967 Harpar and Walpole. *J. Endocrinol.* 37:83.

Treatment of pregnant rats with tranquilizers causes delayed implantation.

1958 Chambon. *Bull. Acad. Natl. Med.* 192:243.

1965 Mayer. In: *Biol. Counc. Symp. Agents Affecting Fertility.* Eds. Austin and Perry. London: Churchill.

Reserpine causes delayed implantation.

1960 Mayer et al. *Ann. Endocrinol.* 21:1.

Antiserum to LH prevents implantation.

1968 Raj et al. *J. Reprod. Fertil.* 17:335.

Antiserum to estrogen prevents implantation.

1969 Ferin, Zimmering, and Vande Wiele. *Endocrinology* 84:893.

Possibilities for the Future

Interference with the immunologic mechanism by which the maternal tissues fail to reject the conceptus may provide a basis for contraception.

Substances to block plasma, cytoplasmic, or nuclear ovarian steroid receptors to interfere with their effect on endometrium and/or implantation may be contraceptive.

Active immunization against the nonhormonal protein uteroglobin (blastokinin) specific to the pregnant uterus of the rabbit might prevent implantation.

Placental Proteins

Biological Processes: Significant Discoveries

Period before 1960

Disruption of pregnancy by antisera to placental antigens demonstrated.

1903   Dobrowski. *Bull. Int. Cracovie.* 5:226.

1940   Cohen and Nedzel. *Proc. Soc. Exp. Biol. Med.* 43:249.

1949   Loeb et al. *J. Exp. Med.* 89:287.

Period 1960–1974

Active immunization with placental extracts resulted in fetal death and kidney damage to the mother in rats and rabbits.

1966   Okunda and Grollman. *Arch. Pathol.* 32:246.

1968   Menge. *Proc. Soc. Exp. Biol. Med.* 127:1271.

Antiserum to whole placentas found not only to induce abortion but also to cause kidney and liver damage in mice and rats.

1949   Loeb et al. *J. Exp. Med.* 89:287.

1968   Koren et al. *Am. J. Obstet. Gynecol.* 102:340.

When rabbit anti–rat placenta serum was absorbed with rat lymphocytes, the toxicity of the antisera disappeared but abortifacient activity was retained.

1972   Beer et al. *J. Exp. Med.* 135:1177.

Injection of antiserum to rhesus monkey placental extracts causes abortion in the species.

1972   Behrman and Amano. *Contraception* 5:357.

1974   Behrman et al. *Am. J. Obstet. Gynecol.* 118:616.

Active immunization with human placental lactogen shown to disrupt fertility in rats and rabbits.

1970   El Tomi et al. *Endocrinology* 87:1811.

1971   El Tomi et al. *Am. J. Obstet. Gynecol.* 109:74.

Both active and passive immunization of the baboon with human placental lactogen results in abortion during early pregnancy.

1971   Stevens et al. *Abstr. 4th Mtg. Soc. Stud. Reprod.* Boston, June 1971.

1971   Stevens et al. *Biol. Reprod.* 5:97.

Rats receiving anti–human placental lactogen serum, returned to normal estrous cycles after abortion but failed to conceive upon repeated mating for 11 months postimmunization.

1972   Gusdon. *Am. J. Obstet. Gynecol.* 112:472.

Injections of hCG alone found not to have an antifertility effect in rabbits.

1967   Glass and Mroueh. *Am. J. Obstet. Gynecol.* 97:1082.

1970   Goldzeiher et al. *Contraception* 2:323.

Antisera to hCG shown capable of interfering with reproduction in nonhuman species.

1969   Schlumberger and Anderer. *Acta Endocrinol.* (Kbh.) 60:681.

1971   Mougdal et al. *J. Clin. Endocrinol. Metab.* 32:579.

Antibodies that inactivate hCG demonstrated in women actively immunized with complex hCG antigen.

1973   Stevens. *Obstet. Gynecol.* 42:485.

Active immunization with hapten-coupled hCG shown to lower levels of LH for 1–2 months in postmenopausal women and longer in premenopausal women.

1973   Steven and Crystle. *Obstet. Gynecol.* 42:485.

1974   Stevens. In: *Immunological Approaches to Fertility Control.* Ed. Diczfalusy. Stockholm: Karolinska Institute, p. 365.

Antibodies produced to the β subunit of hCG have cross-reactivity with human LH, but not baboon LH.

1974   Stevens. In: *Immunological Approaches to Fertility Control.* Ed. Diczfalusy. Stockholm: Karolinska Institute, p. 368.

Uteroglobin, a nonhormonal protein specific to the pregnant rabbit, identified.

1968   Beier. *Biochim. Biophys. Acta* 160:289.

Placenta-specific proteins (SP₁ and PP₅) isolated from term human placentas.

1972   Bohn. *Arch. Gynaekol.* 212:165.

Purified gonadotropin preparations are not homogeneously pure antigens.

1972   Laurence and Hassouna. In: *Handbook of Physiology (Endocrinology)*. Eds. Astwood and Greep. Baltimore: Williams & Wilkins, vol. 2, pt. 2, p. 339.

Major Gaps in Our Knowledge

What are the effects of antibodies specific for placental lactogen in primates?

Methodological Needs

An animal model for the development of immunogens to induce the formation of specific antibodies against reproductively active substances.

Synthetic, pure, and hormonally active gonadotropins for homogeneously pure antigen development.

An antigen that will elicit antibodies specific for hCG and not react with human LH.

Contraceptive Methods

Period 1960–1974

> Antibodies to hCG β as an approach to fertility control.

1974 Talwar. *Karolinska Symp.* 7:370.

Possibilities for the Future

Highly specific constituents of the placenta (and sperm) appear to offer the best opportunity for immunological control of fertility, especially if it becomes possible to induce local immunity restricted to a limited portion of the reproductive tract.

1974 Diczfalusy. In: *Immunological Approaches to Fertility Control.* Ed. Diczfalusy. Stockholm: Karolinska Institute, p. 26.

An antigen specific for hCG which does not react with LH might control ovulation without interfering with ovarian steroidogenesis.

Name Index

Aakvaag, A., 419
Acevedo, H. F., 272
Acone, A. B., 274
Adam, D. E., 379
Afzelius, B. A., 452, 454
Agrawal, K. M. L., 14, 16
Aiken, J. W., 227
Ajika, K., 97
Albagli, L., 390
Albert, A., 265
Alexander, R., 464
Alford, F. P., 265, 266
Allen, E., 137, 146
Allen, J. M., 415, 416, 418
Allison, V. F., 403
Aloj, S. M., 13
Alumot, E., 416
Alvarado, A., 181
Amann, R. P., 388, 412
Amos, B., 452
Amoss, M., 90
Anderson, D., 273
Anderson, E., 95
Anderson, K. M., 407
Anderson, R. G. W., 137, 138
Anderson, T. J., 192
Anderson, W. A., 381
Anika, J., 384
Annison, E. F., 415
Ansell, J., 162
Aoki, A., 327
Aonuma, S., 389, 391, 438
Appelgren, L. E., 417
Archer, W. A., 458
Aref, I., 225
Arimura, A., 66, 71, 72
Armstrong, D. T., 230, 407
Aron, C., 97
Artzt, K., 159, 163
Aschkenasy, A., 269
Ashitaka, T., 16
Ashitaka, Y., 11, 12, 16
Atkinson, L. E., 62, 71
Auletta, F. J., 207, 222
Austin, C. R., 140, 383, 385,
  395, 434–451

Bacetti, B., 455
Bagshawe, K. D., 11, 265
Bahl, O. P., 2, 11–24, 259
Bahr, J. M., 40–43
Baird, D. T., 44–48, 274–275
Baillie, A., 403
Baker, H. W. G., 267
Baker, T. D., 469
Baker, V., 419
Banerjee, B. N., 419
Bardin, C. W., 97, 251, 255, 256,
  265, 266, 275, 276
Barker, K. L., 239
Barker, L. D. S., 412
Barlow, P. W., 161

Barraclough, C. A., 63, 64, 67,
  68, 96
Barros, C., 389, 390, 439, 445,
  446
Bartke, A., 280
Bastians, L. A., 137
Batchley, F. R., 222, 224
Baulieu, E. E., 91, 239, 246, 247,
  248, 249, 251, 254, 276, 402
Bavister, B. D., 140, 388, 389,
  390, 437, 439, 442, 444
Beach, F. A., 98
Beattie, C. W., 66
Beatty, R. A., 431
Beck, J. W., 63, 65
Bedford, J. M., 383, 386, 387,
  388, 390, 394, 411, 412, 413,
  434–451
Behrman, H. R., 220, 223, 230
Bell, C., 133, 134
Bell, J. J., 11, 12
Bellerby, C. W., 171, 203
Bellisario, R., 12, 14, 16, 17, 18
Behrman, S. J., 430, 432
Belt, W. D., 403
Bengtsson, L. P., 197, 228
Bennett, D., 159, 160, 163, 431
Bennett, H. S., 408
Benoit, M. J., 417, 418
Bergström, S., 428
Berliner, D. L., 276
Bermant, G., 97, 98, 99
Bernstein, M. H., 383
Berson, S. A., 265
Berthold, A. A., 270
Bertrand, J., 269
Bewley, T. A., 13
Bey, E., 412
Beyer, C., 96, 99, 254
Bhalla, R. C., 228
Bhalla, V. K., 281
Bhargava, P. M., 382
Bhattacharya, A. N., 66
Bidlack, W. R., 381
Biggers, J. D., 140, 159
Biglieri, E. G., 275
Birge, C. A., 106
Bishop, D. W., 139, 140, 381,
  412
Bishop, M. W. H., 412
Black, D. L., 133
Blackshaw, A. E., 416
Blackshaw, A. W., 381
Bland, K. P., 225
Blandau, R. J., 132–145, 214,
  380, 383, 411, 412
Blaquier, J., 254, 255, 420
Bliss, E. L., 269
Blivaiss, B. B., 269
Bloch, E., 272
Bloom, G., 411
Blum, J. J., 379, 454

Bodenheimer, S., 269
Bodke, R. R., 134
Boettcher, B., 430
Bogdanove, E. M., 68, 76, 265
Bøhmer, T., 417
Bohnet, H. G., 30
Boling, J. L., 132–145
Bolognese, R. J., 167, 222
Bolt, D. J., 63, 67
Bonner, J., 236
Bonnevie, K., 160
Bonney, W. A., 229
Boon, D. A., 265
Borgen, M. L., 62
Bosu, W. T. K., 71
Bourillon, R., 11, 12
Bowers, C. Y., 91
Boyar, R., 63, 70, 265, 268
Boyse, E. A., 431
Brachet, A., 157
Bradbury, J., 61
Brady, R. O., 270
Braendle, W., 16
Brandes, D., 402, 405, 406
Braunstein, G. D., 13, 20
Bredderman, P. J., 391
Breed, W. G., 229
Brenner, R. M., 132–145, 167,
  250
Brenth, B. J., 280
Bresciana, F., 246
Breuer, H., 417
Brinster, R. L., 140, 159
Broderson, S. H., 132–145
Brokaw, C. J., 453, 454
Brooks, D. E., 379, 381, 417
Brossmer, R. M., 12, 18
Brown, C. R., 384, 385, 393
Brown, E. H., 159
Brown, P. D. C., 393
Brown-Grant, K., 63, 78, 97
Brownie, A., 273
Brown-Woodman, P. D. C.,
  393
Bruchovsky, N., 254, 276, 407
Brummer, H. C., 227
Brundin, J., 132, 134, 135
Brunton, W. J., 139
Brusilow, S., 139
Bryan, J. H. D., 383, 388
Buckley, J., 384, 385, 393
Buehr, M., 162
Burgos, M. H., 388, 414
Burgus, R., 90
Burnes, R. K., 402
Burnstock, G., 134
Busby, W. F., 382
Butenandt, A., 253, 270
Butler, W. J., 392
Butler, W. R., 62

Bygdeman, M., 167, 226, 229,
  230
Byrnes, W. W., 268

Cable, Y. D., 266
Calandra, R. S., 420
Calarco, P. G., 159
Caldwell, B. V., 63, 225, 227,
  230
Caligaris, L., 63, 64, 67, 70
Calvin, H. C., 413
Calvin, H. I., 387, 390, 394
Camacho, A., 273, 275
Campbell, H. T., 90
Canales, E. S., 72
Canfield, R. E., 2, 11, 12, 13, 16
Cargille, C. M., 72
Carlson, J. C., 219
Carlson, R. B., 12, 14, 16, 18
Carmen, L. B., 13
Carpen, E., 65
Carr, D. H., 162
Carsten, M. E., 227
Casillas, E. R., 380, 413, 417, 421
Castellano, M. A., 381
Castro, A. E., 281
Catt, K. J., 13, 16, 19, 245–263,
  267, 277
Cavazos, L. F., 402–410, 418
Cerini, M. E. D., 223
Chaikoff, I. L., 270, 325
Challis, J. R. G., 227
Chamberlain, B., 172
Chamberlain, E., 420
Chamley, W. A., 71, 72, 219
Chang, C. C., 189, 190, 192, 199
Chang, M. C., 140, 171, 225,
  226, 383, 385, 388, 389, 390,
  392, 418, 434–451
Chang, T. S. K., 391
Chang, Y., 11
Channing, C. P., 16, 220, 221
Channing, C. R., 256, 258, 260
Chapman, V. M., 159, 162
Chari, S., 267
Charreau, E. H., 17
Charters, A. C., 66
Chasalow, F. I., 220
Chatterjee, A., 219, 223
Chaudhuri, G., 228
Cheng, P., 392
Chester, R., 227
Chowdhury, A. K., 280
Chowdhury, M., 267
Christensen, A. K., 272, 321,
  323, 324, 325
Christiansen, R. O., 282
Christie, M., 219
Church, R. B., 239
Church, R. L., 97
Clark, J. H., 248, 249, 250, 251,
  260

Clemens, J. A., 31, 107
Clemens, L., 99
Clermont, Y., 279, 293–301, 322, 338
Clewe, T. H., 139, 193
Clifton, D. K., 63, 64
Closset, J., 15
Clubb, R. W., 414
Cole, F. E., 16
Collier, J. G., 229
Comfort, A., 98
Cook, M. J., 224
Cooper, G. W., 412, 445, 447
Cooper, R. L., 192
Coppings, R. J., 63
Cordes, E. H., 394, 395
Corfman, P. A., 180, 185
Corner, G. W., 146
Corson, S. L., 167, 222
Cottle, M. K., 134
Coudert, S. P., 224
Coulston, F., 460
Coutinho, E. M., 137, 212, 225, 226
Cox, R. F., 239
Crabo, B., 412, 413, 414, 416, 417, 428
Cramer, O., 93
Cranston, F. M., 458
Cronin, T. J., 71
Cross, B. A., 97, 416
Croxatto, H. B., 193, 195
Crystal, C. D., 71
Csapo, A., 71, 146, 226, 227, 228, 230
Cuadros, A., 190, 195
Cumming, I. A., 69
Curtis, G. C., 64

Dahl, E., 405
Dailey, R. A., 65
Damjanov, I., 163
Dan, J. C., 445
Dandekar, P. V., 442
Daniel, J. C., Jr., 140
Danielsson, H., 270
Danzo, B. J., 16, 420
Darabi, K. F., 178–187
Darin-Bennett, A., 380, 392
Daughaday, W. H., 269
Dauzier, L., 443
David, K., 270
Davidson, J. M., 68, 90–102
Davidson, O. W., 181
Davies, D. V., 269
Davis, B. K., 389, 391, 438
Davis, H. J., 193, 194
Davis, R. H., 179, 180
Davis, S. L., 62
Dawson, R. M. C., 413, 415
Deane, H., 403, 404
Debeljuk, L., 70
DeFeo, V. J., 269
DeKretser, D. M., 256, 258, 267, 327
Dempsey, E., 403
Desautel, M., 282
DeSombre, E. R., 249, 250
Dever, N. Y., 267
Devlin, J., 227
Diamond, J., 414
Diaz-Infante, A., 220
Dickson, G. H., 237

Diczfaluzy, E., 420
Diekman, N. A., 62, 65, 70
Dierschke, D. J., 55–89
Dingle, J. T., 411
Dirscherl, W., 417
Djøseland, O., 419
Döcke, F., 68
Dodge, A. H., 272
Domanski, E., 68
Domm, L. V., 321
Donini, S., 14
Donovan, B. T., 225
Dorfman, R. I., 203, 276
Dörner, G., 68
Dorrington, J. H., 275, 281
Dott, H. M., 392, 411
Doty, P., 236
Dougherty, T. F., 276
Downie, J., 225
Doyle, L. L., 193
Drori, D., 97
Dubois, M. P., 383
Duby, R. T., 228
Ducker, M. J., 65
Duckett, G. E., 265, 267
Dufau, M. L., 16, 17, 18, 256, 258, 259, 260, 261
Du Mesnil du Buisson, F., 443
Dunn, L. C., 159, 160
Dunn, M. V., 227
Dym, M., 311, 347
Dyrenfurth, I., 63
Dziuk, P. J., 443

Eagling, E. M., 227
Eaton, G. J., 159, 160
Ebner, V. von, 302
Edwards, R. G., 441, 442
Eglington, G., 225
Eik-Nes, K. B., 270, 274, 275, 276, 326, 330, 417, 418, 419
Eisenfeld, A., 68, 246, 248, 253, 254
Eleftheriou, B. E., 96, 97
Eliasson, R., 226, 229
Elkington, J. S. H., 282
Ellicott, A. R., 66
Ellinger, J. V., 225
Elliot, P. R., 416
Ellory, J. C., 381
El Sahwi, S., 190, 195, 228
Engle, E. T., 50
Erb, R. A., 182
Erdos, T., 246, 247
Erickson, B. J., 380
Ericsson, J. L. E., 405
Ericsson, R. J., 419, 420, 440
Eskes, T. K. A. B., 156
Evans, J. I., 267
Everett, J. W., 63, 64, 65, 66, 78, 269
Ewing, L. L., 266, 275, 277

Faiman, C., 70, 71, 265, 267, 268, 269
Falck, B., 134
Farquhar, M. G., 414, 415
Faúndes, A., 466–477
Fawcett, D. W., 297, 302–320, 323, 324, 338, 347, 353–378, 411, 417, 455
Feagans, W. M., 403, 406, 408
Feder, H. H., 64

Feigelson, M., 139
Ferin, M., 63, 64, 68, 69
Fernstrom, J. D., 269
Ficher, M., 272, 273, 277
Field, P. M., 96, 219, 230
Fielding, U., 108
Filshie, G. M., 167
Finkelstein, M., 273
Finn, C. A., 146–156
Fischer, E., 405
Fiske, V. M., 269
Fléchon, J.-E., 370, 383
Fleischer, B., 415
Flerko, B., 68, 95, 96
Flickinger, C. J., 418
Flipse, R. J., 380
Flower, R. J., 229
Folman, Y., 97
Foote, R. H., 391
Forchielli, E., 270, 271, 276, 277
Ford, J. J., 71, 72
Foster, D. L., 62, 63, 66, 70, 72
Fox, B., 97
Fox, C. A., 97
Franchimont, P., 62, 267
Frankel, A. I., 417, 418
Franklin, L. E., 384
Frantz, A. G., 105, 106
Fraser, L. R., 442
Frasier, S. D., 269, 274, 275
Freisen, H. G., 25–32
French, F. S., 254, 255, 282
Frenkel, G., 413
Freund, M., 216, 380, 381
Frick, J., 332
Friedman, S., 280
Friend, D., 264, 369, 371, 414, 415
Friesen, H., 105, 257, 258
Fritz, G. R., 65
Fritz, H., 385, 386, 388, 393
Fritz, I. B., 275, 282, 416, 417, 418, 428
Fuchs, A. R., 223
Fugita, M., 403
Fujino, M., 91
Fulka, J., 411
Furst, A., 189
Futoran, J. M., 194
Fuxe, K., 93, 94, 96

Gaddum, P., 383, 388, 412
Gaddum-Rosse, P., 132, 133, 137, 138
Gallagher, T. F., 282
Ganong, W. F., 96, 97
Garbers, D. L., 382, 390, 413, 455
Garcia, C.-R., 136, 178
Gardner, R. L., 161, 162
Garner, D. L., 383
Gaur, R. D., 390
Gay, V. L., 62, 63, 64, 70, 72, 76, 267
Gaylor, J., 325
Gemzell, C., 49–54
Gerson, T., 270, 325
Gessa, G. L., 99
Gibbons, I. R., 381, 452–457
Gibbons, R., 380
Gillespie, A., 227
Gillim, S. W., 272
Gilman, J. P. W., 189

Gilmore, R. S., 237
Gilula, N. B., 312, 313
Ginther, O. J., 229
Gladstone, L., 236
Glascock, R. F., 245
Glass, L. E., 140
Glasser, S. R., 239, 249
Gledhill, B. L., 387
Glover, T. D., 388, 411, 412, 415, 417, 421, 428
Gloyna, R. E., 407, 417
Gluecksohn-Schoenheimer, S., 160
Gluecksohn-Waelsch, S., 159, 160
Goding, J. R., 63, 65, 71
Goldberg, E., 130, 430, 447
Goldberg, V. J., 219–235
Goldenberg, R. L., 16, 61
Goldzieher, J. M., 266
Gomez-Mont, F., 269
Gordon, M., 384, 388, 389
Gorski, J., 239, 240, 245–263
Gorski, R. A., 96, 98
Gospodarowicz, D., 2, 3, 13, 14, 259
Got, R., 11, 12, 14
Gould, K. G., 385, 389, 441
Gould, T., 405
Goverde, B. C., 12
Goy, R. W., 67, 98
Graesslin, D., 11, 12
Graham, C. F., 159, 161
Graham, E. F., 392
Grant, L. J., 97
Grant, P. S., 159
Graves, C. N., 140
Green, J. D., 109, 265
Green, M. M., 159, 160
Greenstein, J. S., 406
Greenwald, G. S., 135, 203, 228
Greep, R. O., 70, 265, 278, 327
Grieves, S. A., 225, 227
Griffiths, 256
Grimek, H. J., 12
Grinwich, D. L., 220, 221
Grogan, D. E., 413
Groth, D., 402, 405
Grumbach, M. M., 70, 268
Grüneburg, H., 159
Gual, C., 69
Guevara, A., 269
Guiliana, G., 97
Guillemin, R., 90–102
Gulyas, B. J., 393
Gunn, R. M. C., 412
Gunn, S., 405
Gurpide, M., 33–39, 246
Gustafsson, B., 415, 428
Gutierrez-Najar, A. J., 179
Gutknecht, G. D., 224
Guyon, J. C., 188
Gwatkin, R. B. L., 159, 385, 389, 437, 446, 448

Hafiez, A. A., 265, 266
Hafs, H. D., 389, 440
Hagino, N., 65, 66
Halász, B., 68, 95, 96
Halkerston, I. D., 270, 276
Hall, M. N., 188, 205
Hall, P. F., 270, 271, 275, 276, 281, 325, 327
Haltmeyer, G. C., 276
Hamberg, M., 229

Hamberger, L. A., 327
Hamburg, D. A., 274
Hamburger, C., 50
Hamilton, D. W., 411–426
Hamilton, T. H., 238, 239, 240
Hammerstein, J., 195
Hammond, J., Jr., 157
Hammonds, J., 71, 72
Hamner, C., 132–145, 390, 393, 437
Han, S. S., 16
Hanada, A., 385
Hancock, J. L., 431, 443
Hanisch, G., 270
Hansel, W., 221, 224, 225
Hansen, D., 172
Hansson, V., 273, 282, 420
Haour, F., 17, 20
Harkin, J. C., 405
Harkness, R. A., 97
Harms, P. G., 95, 443
Haro, R. T., 189
Harper, M. J. K., 134, 135, 225
Harris, G. W., 108, 265
Harris, M., 280, 419
Harrison, F. A., 224
Harrison, R. A. P., 379–401
Hart, B. L., 98
Harting, K., 134
Hartman, C. G., 412
Hartmann, J. F., 385
Hartree, E. F., 385, 390, 393, 406, 417
Harvey, S. C., 279, 322
Haspels, A. A., 205
Hathaway, R. R., 420
Haugen, C. M., 98
Hauger, R. L., 62
Hawk, H. W., 228
Haymaker, W., 95
Haynes, N. B., 97
Hefnawi, F., 182, 190, 196, 197
Heindel, J. J., 282
Hellbaum, A. A., 265
Heller, C. G., 267, 269, 322, 460
Heller, R. E., 406
Helminen, H. J., 405
Helmreich, H., 277
Hendrickx, A. G., 71
Henle, G., 413
Henricks, J. R., 167, 458
Henzl, M. R., 226
Hertz, R., 11
Hervonen, A., 134, 135
Hicks, J. J., 390, 413
Higgs, G. W., 134
Hilgenfeldt, V., 12, 13
Hilliard, J., 136, 224
Hillman, N., 159, 160, 161
Hirsch, J. G., 190
Hochereau-de Reviers, M. T., 387
Hodgen, G. D., 14, 71
Hoekstra, W. G., 245
Hoffer, A. P., 414, 417
Hoffman, J. C., 71
Hökfelt, T., 93, 94, 96, 97
Holland, T. R., 13, 18, 19
Holmberg, N. G., 269
Holmdahl, T. H., 139
Holmes, K., 464
Holstein, A. F., 421
Hooker, C. W., 274
Hooley, R. D., 69

Horan, A. H., 411
Hori, T., 63
Horton, E. W., 224, 225, 230
Horton, R., 264–292
Hoskins, D. D., 380, 382, 387, 413, 428
Howard, R. P., 267
Howland, B. E., 63
Hsu, Y., 159
Huang, H. F. S., 416
Huang, R. C., 241
Huang-Yang, Y. H. J., 388
Huckins, C., 338
Hudson, B., 273, 417, 419
Huggins, C., 269, 405
Hulka, J. F., 179, 180, 183, 217
Hum, G. V., 18
Hunt, D. M., 225
Hunt, W. I., 229
Hunter, A. G., 389, 390, 412, 416
Hunter, G. I., 71
Hunter, J., 402
Hunter, R. H. F., 388, 434, 451
Hutchison, C. F., 385

Ichihara, I., 324
Ichii, S., 272
Ichijo, S., 268
Ingelman-Sundberg, A., 137
Inskeep, E. K., 230
Iritani, A., 390
Ismail, A. A. A., 97
Israel, R., 190, 193, 196
Ito, S., 408
Ito, T., 274
Iwamatsu, T., 140, 390, 444

Jackson, G. I., 64
Jackson, H., 394, 421
Jacobson, H. I., 246, 259
Jaffe, R. B., 62, 69, 71
Janowsky, D. S., 99
Jeffrey, J., 405, 408
Jenson, E. V., 245–263
Jewelewiez, R., 222
Job, J. C., 268
Johansson, E. D. B., 191, 207
Johnsen, S. G., 267
Johnson, A. D., 412, 416, 421
Johnson, B. H., 266, 277
Johnson, M. H., 161, 162
Johnson, W. L., 383, 388, 389, 390, 391
Johnston, P., 99
Jonas, H. A., 63, 65
Jones, A. R., 394
Jones, G. S., 222
Jones, I. C., 265
Jones, R., 381
Jones, T. M., 277
Jonsson, G., 134
Joshi, S. G., 195
Jost, A., 274
Jouan, 254
Judd, H. L., 267
Jung, R., 227
Jungblut, P. W., 246, 248, 250, 251

Kaley, G., 228
Kalra, S. P., 94, 97
Kamberi, I. A., 28
Kammerman, S., 256, 258, 260

Kammerman, W., 13, 16
Kanerva, L., 134
Kapen, S., 64
Kaplan, S. L., 25, 268
Karim, S. M. M., 167, 226, 227, 230
Karlson, W., 226
Karsch, F. J., 62, 63, 64, 67, 70, 72, 79, 222, 223
Kastin, A. J., 275
Kato, J., 246
Kaye, G. I., 414
Kelch, R. P., 268, 274, 275
Kelly, W. A., 228
Kenny, F. T., 240
Kent, J. R., 274
Kesserü, E., 206
Keverne, E. B., 65
Keye, W. R., Jr., 69
Keyhani, E., 380, 381
Keys, A., 269
Kille, J. W., 139, 140
Killian, G. L., 388
King, R. J. B., 246, 247, 248, 251
Kinouchi, T., 274
Kirchner, M. A., 275, 276
Kirkham, W. B., 160
Kirkpatrick, J. F., 229
Kirsh, R. E., 171
Kirton, K. T., 222, 223, 224, 225, 389, 440
Kitrilakis, S., 194
Klein, J., 159
Kloeck, F. K., 227
Klug, A., 452
Knigge, K. M., 96
Knight, J., 26
Knobil, E., 56, 63, 64, 72, 96, 207, 222
Knowler, J. T., 239
Knuchel, W., 417
Kocen, B. C., 404
Koefoed-Johnson, H. H., 411
Koehler, K., 445
Koering, M. J., 222, 223
Kohler, P. O., 266
Kolata, G. B., 228
Kolena, J., 221
Kolodny, R. C., 99
Komarek, R. J., 413
Komisaruk, B., 98
Kordon, C., 97
Koreman, S. G., 264, 274, 275
Koritz, S. B., 276
Kormano, M., 338
Kovacs, J., 403
Koves, K., 68, 96
Kraft, L. A., 416
Kreuz, L. E., 269
Krey, L. C., 63, 64, 68, 69, 72
Krieger, D., 108–127, 265
Kroener, W. F., 178
Kuchera, L. K., 205
Kuehl, F. A., 221, 281, 282
Kulin, H. E., 67
Kwok, R., 172

Labhsetwar, A. P., 219, 222, 223, 224, 225, 230
Lacy, D., 272, 281
Land, R. B., 70
Landefeld, T. D., 12
Lansing, E., 99

Lardner, T. J., 214–218
Lardy, H. A., 382, 412, 413, 428
Larks, S. D., 136
Larsen, J. W., 227
Larsson, K., 99
Laschet, U., 99
Lasnitzki, I., 407
Lau, I. F., 225, 226
Lauersen, 167
Laurence, K. A., 128–131
Lavon, R., 413
Lawson, G. M., 12
Lawton, E. E., 64
Leach, R. B., 459
Leathem, J. H., 269, 280, 416
Leav, I., 402, 405, 407
Leavitt, 248, 251
Lebech, P., 194
Leblond, C. P., 403, 415
Lee, C. Y., 13, 16, 17, 256, 258
Leeson, C., 418
Leeson, T., 418
Legan, S. J., 64, 79
Lehfeldt, H., 205
Lehman, F., 222
Leidenberger, F., 16
Lein, A., 108–127
LeMaire, W. J., 220, 222, 230
Leonard, J. M., 267
Leroy, F., 156
Lerum, J., 447
Levak-Svajger, B., 163
Levine, S., 97, 99
Lewis, P. E., 71
Lewitt, S., 188, 197, 199
Leydig, F. von, 270
Leyendecker, G. S., 63, 64, 72
Leymarie, P., 266
Li, C. H., 1, 2, 3, 11, 13, 18, 26
Liao, S., 239, 240, 248, 249, 253, 254, 255, 256
Liao, T.-H., 3
Libertun, C., 69
Libertun, D., 95
Licht, P., 13
Lieberman, S., 33–39
Liedholm, P., 196
Liefer, R. W., 70
Liggins, G. C., 227
Lin, T. P., 161
Linck, R. W., 362
Lincoln, G. A., 418
Lindemann, C. B., 381, 456
Lindholmer, C., 391
Lindner, H. R., 219, 221, 225, 230, 254, 258, 274
Lingrel, J. B., 241
Linkie, D. N., 71
Lippes, J., 188, 192
Lipsett, M., 33–39, 272, 274, 275, 276
Lisk, R. D., 68, 99, 251
Lissak, K., 97
Liston, W. A., 179
Lloret, A. P., 272
Lockard, A. R., 241
Loeb, P. M., 239
Loewit, K., 190
Loir, M., 387
Loisel, G., 270

Longcope, C., 267, 274
Longo, F. L., 445, 447
Loriaux, D. L., 267
Lostroh, A. J., 61, 278, 279
Louis, T. M., 230
Lowsley, O. S., 404
Lubicz-Nawrocki, C. M., 418
Lubliner, J., 454
Lucas, W. M., 270
Lunaas, T., 416
Lunde, D. T., 274
Lutwak-Mann, C., 391, 392, 393, 402, 404, 406
Luukkainen, T., 191, 251
Lyman, C., 402

McCann, S. M., 62, 63, 90–102, 268
McCarthy, B. W., 239
McClintock, K. M., 98
McCormack, C. E., 55–89
McCracken, J., 224, 230
McCullagh, D. R., 267
McCullagh, E. P., 420
McDaniel, E. P., 211
Macdonald, G. J., 71
McDonald, M. J., 16
MacDonald, P. C., 274
McGadey, J., 417
McGee, L. C., 270
McGuire, J. S., Jr., 276
McGuire, W. L., 239, 247, 248, 251
McLaren, A., 157–166
McLaren, D. S., 269
McLean, B. K., 69
MacLeod, J., 460, 463
MacLeod, R. M., 106
McNeal, J. E., 404
McRorie, R. A., 381, 383, 384, 385
McShan, W. H., 12
Maddock, W. O., 269, 459
Magee, K., 65
Mahi, C. A., 388, 390
Mahler, H. R., 394, 395
Maia, H. S., 225, 226
Mainwaring, W. I. P., 253, 254, 255, 256
Malacara, J. M., 69
Malkani, P. K., 228
Malven, P. V., 62, 63, 65, 70
Mancini, R. E., 256, 258, 281, 383, 430
Mandl, J. P., 225
Maneely, R. B., 418
Manes, C., 159
Mann, D., 64
Mann, T., 379, 381, 391, 392, 393, 402, 404, 405, 406, 412, 415, 417, 427–433
Markert, C. L., 381
Marley, B. P., 223
Marquis, N. R., 416, 417, 418, 428
Marrian, G. F., 269
Marsh, J., 221
Marshall, F. H. A., 434
Marshall, J. C., 266
Marshall, J. M., 133
Marston, J. H., 228
Martens, F. W., 179
Martin, J. E., 69

Martinez Manautou, J., 193
Martini, L., 63, 93, 95, 96, 97
Marushige, K., 237, 387
Marushige, Y., 387
März, L., 12, 13, 16, 19
Masaki, J., 392
Mason, H. F., 271
Mason, K. E., 269, 414
Mason, N. R., 272, 321, 325
Masson, G., 280
Masters, C. J., 382
Mastroianni, L., 132–145, 379
Matsuo, H., 90
Matta, K. L., 16
Mattner, P. E., 443
Mayer, J. R., 460
Mayes, D., 273
Means, A. R., 238, 240, 241, 257, 258, 260, 281, 282
Mears, E., 203
Meeker, C., 183
Meier, A. H., 31
Meites, J., 31, 269
Meizel, S., 387, 388, 393
Melampy, R. M., 71, 72, 402, 403, 404, 406
Menge, A. C., 430
Menkin, M. F., 441
Mercado, E., 445
Merz, W. E., 11, 12, 13
Mess, B., 93, 95
Metz, C. B., 381, 384, 389, 395, 430, 431, 444, 445, 447
Meyer, R. K., 70, 268
Meyerson, B. J., 99
Michael, R. F., 65, 98
Michael, R. P., 274
Middleton, A., 344
Midgley, A. R., Jr., 16, 62, 258, 265, 273
Migeon, C. J., 269, 273, 275
Milgrom, E., 251
Millette, C. F., 455
Mills, J. A., 139
Mills, S. C., 380, 382
Millward, J. T., 140
Minassian, E. S., 382
Mintz, B., 161
Mishell, D. R., Jr., 190, 192, 209–213, 228
Miyamoto, H., 389, 444, 446
Moawad, A. H., 228
Mohla, S., 239, 249
Mohri, H., 393
Mok, E., 223
Mollendorff, W. von, 414
Monahan, M., 90, 91
Monden, Y., 97
Money, J., 99
Monie, I. W., 161
Monroe, S. E., 63, 72, 265
Mont, F. G., 269
Moore, C. R., 265, 402, 404, 418
Moore, D. J., 460
Moore, N. W., 161
Morgan, F. J., 12, 13, 14
Morgenstern, L. L., 228
Morgentaler, H., 279
Mori, K. F., 11, 13, 18, 19
Morishige, W. K., 71
Morita, Z., 383, 392
Morris, J. McL., 172, 203–208

Morris, M. D., 270, 325
Morse, H. C., 322
Morton, B., 382–383, 390, 391, 412, 413
Morton, D. B., 384, 389
Moser, G. C., 160
Moss, R. L., 98
Mougdal, N. R., 256
Moulding, T. S., 183
Mounib, M. S., 390
Moyer, D. L., 190, 195, 196, 197, 228
Moyle, W. R., 19, 259, 260, 325, 326
Mueller, G. C., 238, 240, 246, 249, 250
Mukerji, S. K., 388, 393
Mulinos, M. G., 269
Mullen, J. O., 417, 419
Murad, F., 281
Murdoch, R. N., 381, 420
Murota, S., 323
Murphy, B. E. P., 273
Murphy, H. D., 281

Naftolin, F., 65, 108–127, 265, 266, 276
Naftolin, R., 99
Nakano, R., 72
Nalbandov, A. V., 40–43, 71
Naller, R., 63
Nance, D. M., 99
Nankin, H. R., 265
Nauta, W. J. H., 95
Neaves, W. B., 321–337
Neill, A. R., 382
Neill, J. D., 65, 67
Nelson, L., 379, 383
Nelson, W. O., 171, 203, 267, 282, 460
Nequin, L. G., 66
Nett, T. M., 60
Netter, A. A., 63
Neumann, F., 279, 280
Neutra, M., 415
Neuwirth, R. S., 179, 180, 183
Nevo, A. C., 379
Ney, R. L., 269
Niall, H. D., 26
Nicander, L., 411, 412, 414, 417
Nicholson, N., 229
Nicoll, C. S., 31
Nicolson, G. L., 445
Nieschlag, E., 267
Nillius, S. J., 62
Nishikawa, Y., 411
Nisula, B. C., 13
Niswender, G. D., 40, 63, 71, 97, 265
Niwa, K., 444
Noda, Y., 446
Noriega, C., 140
Norman, C., 393
Norman, R. L., 69, 219
Northcutt, R. C., 275
Notides, A. C., 240, 247, 248
Noumura, T., 272, 274
Novy, M. J., 224
Noyes, R. W., 228, 385
Nugent, C. A., 273
Nylander, I., 269

Odell, W. D., 64, 67, 265, 266, 267, 268, 269, 275
O'Donnell, J. M., 381
Odor, D. L., 137
Ofner, P., 402, 405, 407, 419, 421
Ogawa, S., 440
Ogra, S. S., 226
O'Grady, J. P., 220, 227
Oikawa, T., 385, 448
Ojamura, H., 223
Ojeda, S. R., 93
Okumura, E., 346
Oliphant, G., 389, 391, 440, 445
Olson, J. D., 140
O'Malley, B. W., 236–244, 247, 248, 249, 251, 252, 253, 255
Omran, K. F., 179, 180, 183
Oppenheimer, W., 188
O'Rand, M. G., 384
Oregin-Crist, M. C., 386, 388, 411, 412, 418
Oritz, E., 403, 418
Ortavant, R., 412, 443
O'Shea, T., 381, 392
Osler, M., 194
Ostergard, D. R., 62
Overstreet, J. W., 386
Owman, C., 134

Pace, M. M., 392
Paesi, F. J. A., 265
Pallini, V., 455
Palmiter, R. D., 241
Pandian, M. R., 18
Pannabecker, R., 272
Papkoff, H., 1–10, 13, 259
Parkes, A. S., 171, 203, 269
Parlow, A. F., 4, 5, 15, 62, 72
Patek, E., 137
Patterson, D. L., 98, 380
Pauerstein, C. J., 134
Paul, J., 237
Paul, W. E., 265
Paulsen, C. A., 264, 265, 267, 275, 458–465
Pazos, R., Jr., 269
Pearlman, W. H., 253, 275
Pearson, D. J., 416
Peck, E. J., 138
Pedersen, R. A., 159
Pelletier, J., 71
Pepe, G. J., 71
Perloff, W. H., 269
Perry, J. S., 161
Personne, P., 381
Peterson, N. T., Jr., 267
Peterson, R. E., 97
Peterson, R. N., 380, 381
Pettitt, A. J., 272
Pfaff, D., 96, 98, 254
Pharriss, B. B., 220, 221, 222, 230
Phillips, D., 364, 411, 455
Pichles, V. R., 225, 230
Picket, D. W., 413
Pierce, J. G., 2, 3, 13, 14
Pierrepoint, C. G., 418
Pikó, L., 383, 445, 446
Pincus, G., 171, 274
Pitkin, R. M., 182
Pitkjanen, I. G., 443
Polakoski, K. L., 381, 385, 388

Polge, C., 431
Pomerantz, L., 269
Popa, G. T., 108
Porter, D. G., 146–156
Porter, J. C., 93, 95, 403, 404
Posse, N., 226
Potter, R. G., 188
Poulos, A., 380, 388
Poyser, N. L., 224, 226, 229, 230
Prasad, M. R. N., 331, 418, 421
Prelog, V., 280
Premkumar, E., 382
Presl, J., 16
Price, D., 265, 272, 402, 404, 406, 418
Price, J. M., 455
Proudfit, C. M., 66
Przekop, F., 68
Psychoyos, A., 156
Puca, G. A., 246, 248, 250
Purvis, K., 97

Qazi, M. H., 11
Quinn, P. J., 381, 388, 392, 412, 413
Quinones, R., 181

Radford, H. M., 66
Raff, E. C., 379
Raisman, G., 96
Rajaneimi, M., 256, 258
Rajaniemi, H. J., 16
Rakha, A. M., 64, 65, 66
Rakshit, B., 182
Rall, T. W., 281
Rambourg, A., 415
Ramirez, V. D., 62, 70, 268
Ramwell, P. W., 219–235
Randolph, P. W., 279
Rao, Ch. V., 13, 16, 17
Raska, K., 159
Rasmussen, H., 228
Rathnam, P., 12, 13, 15
Ratner, A., 219, 229, 230
Ravenholt, R., 214
Raynaud-Jammet, M., 239
Reddi, A. H., 282, 402, 419
Reddy, K. J., 331
Redenz, E., 411
Reed, J. O., 269
Reeves, J. J., 63, 65, 69, 72
Reichert, L. E., Jr., 12, 16, 256, 257, 258, 281
Reichlin, S., 267
Reid, J. T., 269
Reinius, S., 140
Reinke, W. A., 469
Reisfeld, R. A., 11
Reiter, E. O., 61, 67, 70
Resko, J. A., 67, 72, 98, 253, 274
Restall, B. J., 71, 379, 384
Reyes, A., 389
Reyes, F. I., 71
Richart, R. M., 178–187
Richman, K. A., 220
Riesen, J. W., 65
Rifkind, A. B., 268
Rikmenspoel, R., 379, 454, 455
Rinaldini, L. M., 269
Ringrose, C. A., 181, 182
Riondel, A., 273
Rippel, R. H., 72
Risley, P. L., 418

Ritzen, E. M., 282
Rivarola, M. A., 273
Rizkallah, T., 265
Robel, P., 407
Roberts, I. K., 430
Roberts, T. K., 392
Robertson, G. G., 160
Robertson, H. A., 64, 65, 66
Robinson, T. J., 65
Rocca, D., 265
Roche, J. F., 62, 65
Rochefort, H., 247, 249
Rock, J., 441
Rodgers, C., 68
Rogers, B. J., 390
Root, A., 62, 269
Rosad, E., 445
Rose, R. M., 97
Rosen, S. W., 267
Rosenfield, G. C., 240
Rosen-Runge, E. C., 273
Ross, G. T., 14, 19, 40–43, 260
Roth, J. C., 268
Roth, L. J., 246
Rothchild, I., 71, 72
Rowlans, I. W., 415
Ruben, G., 274
Rubens, R., 267
Rubenstein, L., 93
Rubin, R. T., 265
Rubio, B., 206
Rumery, R. E., 138, 411, 412
Rümke, 430
Russ, R. D., 269
Ruzicka, L., 280
Ryan, R. J., 1–10, 13, 16, 17, 251, 256, 258, 260, 265, 267
Rydberg, E., 50

Sachs, C., 134
Saez, J. M., 269, 275
Saginor, M., 274
Sagiroglu, N., 195
Said, S. A. H., 71
Sairam, M. R., 3, 12, 14, 15
Saito, S., 69, 190
Saksena, S. K., 225, 228
Salamon, S., 431
Salamonsen, L. A., 72
Salgado, C., 180
Salhanick, H., 33–39
Salisbury, G. N., 420
Samisoni, J. I., 416
Samuels, L. T., 253, 272, 277
Samy, T. S. A., 2
Sanborn, B. M., 282
Sandberg, F., 225, 226
Sandler, M., 99
Sanger, M., 434
Santen, R. J., 265, 266
Sasano, N., 268
Satir, P., 362, 454
Sato, T., 219
Satoh, P., 271
Savard, K., 270
Saxena, B. B., 12, 13, 15, 17, 20, 258, 265
Scaramuzzi, R. J., 62, 63
Schaffenburg, C. A., 420
Schalch, D. S., 267
Schally, A. V., 90

Schill, W. B., 388, 393
Schimke, R. T., 241, 249
Schlaff, S., 265
Schlumberger, H. D., 18
Schmidt, F. H., 190, 197, 199
Schneider, H. P. G., 94, 95
Schoenfeld, C., 390
Schrader, W. T., 253
Schriefers, H., 276
Schwartz, N. B., 55–89
Schwartz, R. J., 239
Scott, D. E., 96
Scott, T. W., 380, 382, 413, 415, 416, 420
Seamark, R. F., 420
Sedar, W. W., 414
Sedlakova, E., 416
Segal, S. J., 170–177, 203
Seitz, H. M., 139, 441, 442
Sellner, P. G., 221
Semm, K., 179, 185
Serra, B. G., 272
Sertoli, E., 281
Setchell, B. P., 338–352, 386, 388, 413, 414, 415, 417
Shaar, C. J., 107
Shannon, P., 392
Shapiro, A. G., 222
Sharma, O. K., 159
Shaver, S. L., 414
Shaw, S. T., 197
Shearman, R. P., 206
Sherins, R. J., 267, 459
Sherman, J. K., 432
Sherman, M. I., 161, 162
Sherman, M. R., 252
Sheth, N. A., 62, 70
Shettles, L. B., 441
Shevah, Y., 71
Shikita, M., 327
Shimizu, K., 270, 271
Shirley, B. J., 63
Shivers, C. A., 444, 448
Sholl, S. A., 416
Shome, B., 4, 5, 15
Short, R. V., 44–48, 67, 407
Shulman, S., 430
Siegel, F. L., 381
Signoret, J.-L., 98
Siiteri, P., 248, 274, 276
Silver, I. A., 416
Simeone, F. A., 412
Simpson, M. E., 278, 279
Sizonenko, P. C., 269
Sjöberg, N.-O., 134
Skoglund, R. D., 459
Skreb, N., 163
Slater, J. J., 415, 416, 418
Smellie, R. M. S., 239
Smith, B., 61
Smith, E. R., 97
Smith, K. D., 265, 266
Smith, L. J., 159, 160
Smith, P. E., 1, 55
Snow, M. H. L., 161, 162, 163
Sobotta, J., 157, 158
Soichet, S., 194
Solter, D., 163
Soupart, P., 385, 437, 442
Southren, A. K., 276
Sowell, J. G., 419
Speidel, J., 214
Speroff, L., 167, 221

Spies, H. G., 56, 63, 68, 69, 97, 219
Spilman, C. H., 225
Spilman, E. H., 228
Squire, P. G., 1
Srere, P. A., 270
Srivastava, P. N., 385, 389
Stafford, R. O., 404
Stambaugh, R., 140, 223, 384, 385, 386, 393, 445, 447
Staple, E., 270
Starman, B., 2, 3
Starman, B., 2, 3
Stavnezer, J., 241
Stearns, E. L., 67, 97, 267
Steeno, O., 417, 419
Steinberger, A., 273, 276, 278, 280, 281, 282
Steinberger, E., 264–292, 321
Steiner, R. A., 67, 96
Stephens, R. E., 362
Steptoe, P. C., 159, 179, 184
Stevens, L. C., 160, 163
Stevens, V. C., 19, 130
Stevenson, T. C., 182, 185
Steward, V. W., 327
Stewart, D. L., 431
Stewart-Bentley, M., 267
Stone, S. C., 66, 246
Storey, B. T., 380, 381
Stormshak, F., 229
Story, J. C., 63
Strauss, J. F., 223
Strong, P. A., 442
Strott, C. A., 274
Stryker, J. C., 193
Stumpf, W. E., 93, 96, 97, 138, 246, 248, 254
Stylianou, M., 276
Sugawara, S., 139
Sujan, S., 228
Sujan-Tejuja, S., 195
Sulman, F. G., 106
Summers, K. E., 454, 456
Surrey, A. R., 460
Surve, A. H., 223
Suryanarayana, B. V., 269
Sutherland, E. W., 281
Suzuki, S., 139
Svajger, A., 163, 269
Svoboda, D. J., 331
Swaminathan, N., 12
Swerdloff, R. S., 64, 67, 264–292
Swtantarta, S. O., 137
Symons, A. M., 69
Szentágothai, J., 95
Szirmai, J., 403
Szollosi, D., 447
Szontagh, F. E., 63

Tait, J. F., 273, 275
Takahara, J., 28
Takahashi, M., 61
Takayasu, M., 405
Takeguchi, S., 139
Talbot, P., 384
Taleisnik, S., 72, 97
Talwar, G. P., 19, 130, 246, 390
Tamaoki, B. I., 272, 326
Tang, F. Y., 382
Tappel, A. L., 381
Tarkowski, A. K., 161, 163
Tasca, R. J., 159
Tatum, H. J., 188–201

Taut, J. F., 274
Taylor, D. S., 182, 185
Taylor, H. C., 188
Tchen, T., 270
Tcholakian, R. K., 272, 273, 277
Teng, C., 239
Teichman, R. J., 383
Terner, C., 382
Tervit, H. R., 140
Thibault, C., 65, 71, 380, 443
Thiersch, J. B., 175
Thimonier, J., 71
Thompson, H. E., 183, 185
Thornburn, G. D., 230
Thorndike, J., 160
Thorneycroft, I. H., 63
Thurman, J. C., 64
Tietze, C., 167–169, 188, 197, 198, 466
Timonen, H., 191
Timonen, S., 65
Toft, D., 246
Tolis, G., 71, 72
Tomacari, R. L., 72
Tomkins, G. M., 240, 255, 276
Toner, P., 403
Tormey, J., 414
Toth, S. E., 403
Tourney, G., 99
Tovar, E. S., 388
Toyoda, Y., 390, 440, 444
Train, P., 458
Troen, P., 265
Tsafriri, A., 220
Tsai, C. C., 62, 63, 72
Tsuruhara, T., 19
Tubbs, P. K., 416
Tullner, W. W., 272, 274
Turnbull, A., 156
Turner, P. C., 416
Tveter, K. J., 253, 254, 419
Tyler, E., 432
Tyson, J. E., 29

Ui, H., 238, 240
Ungar, F., 276
Unnithan, R. R., 383
Urquart, J., 276
Usui, N., 388, 389, 390, 391, 447
Utiger, R., 108–127

Vaitukaitis, J. L., 13, 14, 19, 281
Vale, W., 91, 94
Van Aarde, G. L., 71
Vandeberg, J. L., 381
van Deenen, L. L. M., 412
Vandenbergh, J. C., 98
Van Denmark, N. L., 275
van der Linde, P. C., 403
Vanderlinde, R. E., 269
van der Molen, H. J., 321, 327
Vande Weile, R. L., 63, 72, 273
Vane, J. R., 227
Van Hall, E. V., 19
Vanha-Perttula, T., 16
van Hell, H., 11, 12
Vankin, L., 160
Van Thiel, D. H., 267
Van Valen, P., 160
van Wagenen, G., 172, 203, 204, 205
Verhage, H. G., 138
Vermeulen, A., 267, 274, 275

Vernon, R. G., 282
Vickery, B. H., 393
Vilar, O., 281
Visser, H. K. A., 70
Voglmayr, J. K., 381, 412, 413, 414, 429
von Berswordt-Wallrabe, R., 279, 280
von Euler, U. S., 226, 229
von Leeuwenhoek, A., 353

Waddington, C. H., 157
Wagenseil, F., 414
Waide, Y., 411
Waites, G. M. H., 338, 414, 415, 417
Wakasugi, N., 160
Wales, R. G., 140, 381, 392, 415, 416
Walker, G., 402
Walker, J. D., 275
Wallace, A. L. C., 66
Wallace, J. C., 415, 416
Wallach, E. E., 62
Wallach, J. C., 140
Wallach, R. C., 139
Walsh, E. L., 267
Walsh, P. C., 267, 268
Waltman, R., 227
Walton, A., 412
Waltz, P. W., 55–89
Ward, D. N., 1–10, 12
Warner, F. D., 362
Warren, J. C., 239
Watson, M. L., 160
Wayneforth, H. B., 71
Webster, R. C., 420
Webster, W. O., 405
Wei, J., 379
Weick, R. F., 62, 63, 64, 65, 68, 70
Weindl, A., 96
Weiner, R., 96, 228
Weinman, D. E., 438, 445
Weintraub, B. D., 20, 267
Weiss, G., 72
Weiss, S. B., 236
Wentz, A. C., 222
Werner, S. C., 269
West, C. D., 273, 420
Westerfeld, W. W., 269
Westrom, L., 197
Wheeless, C. R., 179, 184
White, I. G., 140, 190, 379, 381, 386, 388, 391, 392, 393, 412, 413, 415, 417, 419, 420, 421, 428
White, W., 90
Whitten, W. K., 18, 98, 140, 159
Whittingham, D. G., 444
Wickersham, E. W., 221
Wide, L., 62, 71
Wiesner, B., 402
Wiest, W. G., 138, 251
Wilde, C. E., 11
Wilkins, C., 181
Wilks, J. W., 220, 225, 227
Williams, K. E., 227
Williams, W., 140
Williams, W. L., 139, 140, 383, 384, 385, 386, 388, 389, 390, 393, 436, 438, 445

Williams-Ashman, H. G., 245–263, 402, 404, 406, 419
Willis, A. L., 229
Wilmut, I., 431
Wilson, J. D., 239, 240, 253, 254, 255, 256, 274, 275, 276, 407, 417, 418, 430
Wilson, L., 225
Wintenberger, S. L., 140
Winter, J. S. D., 70, 265, 268, 269
Wiqvist, N., 167, 230
Wislocki, G. B., 108, 418
Witters, W. L., 381
Wolfe, J. M., 269
Wolstenholme, G. F. W., 26
Wotiz, H. H., 247
Wood, C., 442
Woods, J. E., 321
Woods, M. C., 278, 279
Wroblewska, J., 161, 162, 163
Wu, S. H., 415
Wudl, L., 159
Wurtman, R. J., 65, 103–107, 269
Wurzelmann, S., 403, 404
Wyngarden, L. J., 222

Yago, N., 272
Yalow, R. S., 265
Yamaguchi, Y., 405
Yamaji, T., 57, 62, 63, 67
Yanagimachi, R., 171, 383, 385, 388, 389, 390, 391, 434–451
Yang, N. S. T., 220, 221
Yang, W. H., 13
Yannone, M. E., 71
Yates, F. E., 276
Yates, R., 316
Yen, S. S. C., 62, 63, 69, 72, 108–127
Ying, S.-Y., 70
Yoon, B., 179
Young, D. G., 276
Young, L. G., 379
Young, W. C., 411, 414
Yuthasastrakosol, P., 63

Zacharias, L., 65, 269
Zachmann, M., 275
Zamboni, K., 445, 446, 447
Zanartu, J. J., 206
Zaneveld, L. J. D., 381, 384, 386, 445, 447
Zarate, A., 71
Zeilmaker, G. H., 63, 64, 161
Zeleznik, A. J., 258, 260
Zimmerman, W., 135
Zipper, J. A., 180, 181, 185, 188, 189, 190, 192
Zittle, C. A., 413
Zor, U., 219, 221, 229
Zubay, G., 236
Zubiran, S., 269

Subject Index

AAG. *See* Alpha l-acid glycoprotein
Abcor Corp., 216
Abortifacients, 170
  from natural products, 175
  prostaglandins as, 148–149
Abortion, 167–169
  bioengineering aspects of, 215
  cervical damage during, 155
  disadvantages of, 175
  effect of pheromones on, 98
  hypertonic saline-induced, 149
  illegality of, 168
  IUD insertion after, 191
  prostaglandin-induced, 226
  sequelae of, 168
Abortuses, chromosomal abnormalties of, 163
ABP. *See* Androgen-binding protein
Acepromazine Maleate, and ampullar transport, 136
Acetylcholine, 103
  and release of gonadotropin-releasing factors, 94
  in spermatozoa motility, 383
  and uterine contraction, 227
Acidophilic activation, in hormone-receptor interaction, 248
Acriflavine, in seminiferous tubules, 348
Acromegaly
  response to releasing factors, 126
  therapeutic agents for, 125
Acrosin
  in aging spermatozoa, 393
  conversion of proacrosin to, 387–388
  and DF, 438
  inhibitory role of, 386
  role in egg penetration, 385
Acrosome, of spermatozoon, 354, 356–359, 368, 443, 445
Acrosome phase, of spermiogenesis, 297–298
Acrosome reaction, of spermatozoa, 388–391
  and fertility control, 448
ACTH. *See* Adrenocorticotropic hormone
Actin, and sperm motility, 454
Actinomycin D, stimulation of implantation by, 153, 154
Additional tubular fluid (ATF), ionic composition of, 340
Adenine nucleotides, as energy source for spermatozoa, 379
Adenohypophysis. *See also* Anterior pituitary;

Hypophysectomy; Pituitary gland
  gonadotropin secretion of, 112
  hypothalamic control of, 109
Adenosine diphosphate (ADP), as energy source for spermatozoa, 379
Adenosine triphosphate (ATP)
  as energy source for spermatozoa, 379, 395, 453
  in mammalian semen, 428
  in spermatozoa metabolism, 383
Adhesives, tissue, for tubal occlusion, 182
Adjuvant procedures, 128
Adolescence, testicular hormonal function during, 274. *See also* Puberty
Adrenal cortex
  hormones produced by, 123
  role in parturition of, 149
Adrenal glands, sulfated steroids secreted by, 36
Adrenalin
  and labor, 150
  and uterine relaxation, 151
Adrenal medulla, as neuroendocrine transducer, 104
Adrenal steroids, positive feedback by, 63–64
Adrenocorticotropic hormone (ACTH)
  action of nonadrenal hormones on CNS regulation of, 124
  hypothalamic regulation of, 124
  receptor binding studies for, 257
Adrenocorticotropic hormone (ACTH) secretion
  CNS regulation of, 123
  control of, 123–124
  feedback regulation of, 123–124
Age, and pituitary-gonadal axis, 267–269. *See also* Puberty
Agency for International Development (AID), International Training Project, 184. *See also* Clinical trials; Family planning programs
Aggression, and gonadotropin secretion, 97
Alcohol, and male accessory gland secretions, 429
Alpha estradiol, and epithelium of seminal vesicles, 403
Alpha l-acid glycoprotein (AAG), 118
Amebicides, contraceptive value of, 460
Amenorrhea. *See also* Menstrual cycle
  anovulation associated with, 50
  and elevated prolactin levels, 28

and hPG therapy, 53
  hypothalamic, 112
  microadenomas associated with, 30
  primary, 51
  secondary, 52
American Association of Anatomists, 96
Amino acids. *See also* Proteins; *specific proteins*
  and blood-testis barrier, 343–344
  in embryonic development, 140
  NH₂-terminal, 4
  in RTF, 340
  synthetic, 105
Amino acid sequences
  determinations of, 3–5
  for hCG subunits, 14
  for prolactin, 26
Aminoglutethemide, effect on progesterone levels, 174
Amniocentesis, 163
Amniotic cavity, development of, 157
Amniotic fluid, concentrations of prolactin in, 30
Amphenone, as contragestational agent, 174
Ampulla tubae uterinae. *See also* Fallopian tubes; Uterus
  contractile activities in, 134
  egg transport through, 132
  fluorescent fibers in, 134
  and gamete transport, 133
  smooth muscle in, 135
Ampullar-isthmic junction,
  and egg retention, 132
  and gamete transport, 133
  movement of ovum at, 134
Anatomy, and CNS control of gonadotropin secretion, 95–97
Andrenogenital syndrome, 59
Androgen-binding proteins (ABP), 37, 255
  action of Sertoli cells on, 314
  in epididymal function, 420
  synthesis of, 39
  in testicular tissue, 282
Androgen-protein complex, and spermatogenesis, 282
Androgen-receptor complexes, 254
Androgens, 123
  and accessory sex glands, 406–407
  activity of, 42, 406
  and adult sexual behavior, 98
  and epididymal function, 418
  formation from pregnenolone of, 271
  in hormone-receptor interaction, 253–256
  Leydig cell biosynthesis of, 325

and LH in eugonadal men, 266
  and maintenance of spermatogenesis, 280
  and male infertility, 461
  negative feedback mechanisms of, 57
  neonatal organization of gonadotropin secretion by, 67
  and neural control of gonadotropin secretion, 59
  substitution of exogenous, 331–332
  testicular origin of, 273–277, 321–323
  unbound, 275
Androgen synthesis, 270–272
Androstenediol, and maintenance of spermatogenesis, 280
Androstenedione
  conversion of, 35
  and maintenance of spermatogenesis, 280
  secretion of, 37, 274
Anesthetics, and gonadotropin secretion, 58–59, 112
Anorexia nervosa, and gonadotropin release, 112
Anovulation, treatment of, 50, 54. *See also* Clomiphene; Ovulation
Anterior hypothalamus, and sexual dimorphism, 91. *See also* Hypothalamus
Anterior pituitary, retention of radioactive hormone by, 246. *See also* Adenohypophysis; Pituitary gland
Antibodies. *See also* Immunology
  to estrogen receptors, 130
  for fertility regulation, 129–130
  to sperm, 129
Antiestrogens, 203. *See also* Estrogens
Antifertility. *See also* Contragestational agents
  postcoital, 204
  postovulatory, 204
  in RTF, 345
Antigens, sperm coating, 430–431. *See also* Immunology; *specific antigens*
Antigon F, 194
Antineoplastic agents, contraceptive properties of, 458
Antiprogestational compounds, 173–174
Antrum, follicular, fluid of, 40–41, 42. *See also* Follicle
Aqueous ammonium sulfate fractionation techniques, 1

Arias-Stella reaction, 206
Artificial insemination, 341–342
  deep-frozen semen for, 427
Asialo-hCG, steroidogenic
  activities of, 259
Aspermatogenesis, allergic, 129,
  130. *See also* Spermatogenesis
Association for Voluntary
  Sterlizations (AVS), 184
ATF. *See* Additional tubular fluid
ATP. *See* Adenosine triphosphate
Atresia, of ovarian follicles, 40,
  42, 76. *See also* Follicle
Atropine, and gonadotropin
  releasing factors, 95
Autonomic nervous system, and
  gamete transport, 133–135
Avidin, estrogen action on, 241
Axonemes
  chemical dissection of, 374
  of sperm tail, 362–363, 364

Barbiturates, in RTF, 345. *See
  also* Drugs
Barium sulfate, 183
Battelle Memorial Institute,
  Population Study Center, 167
Battelle Northwest, fertility control
  devices developed by, 215,
  216
Behavior
  aggressive, 97
  hormonal effect on, 98–99
  masculine, 322, 333
  sexual, 92, 97–98
Binding, of hCG, 16–17
Binding sites
  measurement of, 260
  for ovarian follicles, 41
Bioassays, development of, 27,
  265
Biocarbonates, and sperm
  metabolism, 140
Bioengineering, reproductive and
  contraceptive aspects of,
  214–218
Biomaterials, development of,
  216–217
Biopsy, testicular, 277–278
Biosynthetic particle, 34–35
Birth control. *See* Contraception;
  Fertility control
Blastocoele, development of, 157,
  158
Blastocyst, endometrial receptivity
  of, 153
Blastokinin, 153
Blastotoxins, for termination of
  pregnancy, 175
Bleeding
  associated with clinical trials,
  471
  IUD-associated, 196–197
Blood supply
  and follicular growth, 40
  testicular, 345–346
Blood-testis barrier
  amino acids and, 343–344
  carbohydrates and, 343
  disturbances of, 347
  effects on spermatozoa of, 350
  establishment of, 338, 341–342
  localization of, 347

maintenance of, 310–313,
  350–351
  permeability of, 345
  structure of, 345–347
Boar, spermatozoa of, 361. *See
  also* Pig
Brain tissue, and steroid
  metabolism, 117. *See also
  specific brain tissues*
Breastfeeding, prolactin levels
  during, 28, 29. *See also*
  Lactation
Breasts, development of, 42
''Bridge cells,'' 304. *See also*
  Sertoli cells
Buffered ethanolic precipitation
  techniques, 1
Bulbourethral glands, 402
  secretory products of, 406
Bull, spermatozoa of, 366, 415,
  443. *See also* Cow

Cadmium, effect on blood-testis
  barrier, 348
Calcium
  and fertilization process, 140
  in RTF, 340
  in spermatozoa metabolism,
  381–383
  and uterine contraction, 227
cAMP. *See* Cyclic adenosine
  monophosphate
Cancer
  and injectable contraceptives,
  212
  mammary
    and DMPA, 210
    estrogen-receptor content of,
    248
  therapeutic agents for, 106
Cannula, for uterine injection, 185
Capacitation, of spermatozoa,
  388–391, 434–451
  control of, 438–439
  decapacitation, 437–438
  in domestic animals, 443–444
  effects of chemical agents on,
  438
  factors required for, 437
  morphological aspects of,
  435–436
  and oviductal fluids, 139, 141
  physiological aspects of, 435–436
  recapacitation, 437–438
  in vitro, 140, 440–443
Capillaries, testicular, 345–346
Capping, on spermatozoon
  surface, 373
Carbohydrates
  and blood-testis barrier, 343
  in epididymis, 415
  in RTF, 340
Carbolic acid, uterine injection of,
  180. *See also* Contraceptives
Carnitine, in epididymis, 416–418
Carotid body, 104
Castration
  birth control by, 332
  and LH surges, 57
Castration cells, 60
Catecholamines, 103. *See also*
  Dopamine; Epinephrine;
  Norepinephrine

action on human uterus of, 150,
  151
  effects of gonadotropin release
  of, 93–94
  identification of, 108
  in regulation of LRF secretion,
  110
  storage of, 104
  synthesis of, 104
Cats
  oviducts of, 138
  ovulatory pattern of, 109
CBG. *See* Corticosteroid-binding
  globulin
Central nervous system (CNS)
  controlling functions of, 108
  and onset of puberty, 119
Central nervous
  system–hypothalamic complex,
  and gonadotropin secretion, 109
Central nervous system pathways,
  97
Cephalaxine, 464
Cervix, uterine. *See also* Uterus
  during abortion, 155
  bioengineering approaches, 215
  mucus secretion in, 154–155
  perforation of, 197
CG. *See* Chorionic gonadotropin
Chalones, spermatogonial, 294,
  349
Chicken, progesterone receptors
  in, 251–253
Childhood, testicular hormonal
  function during, 274. *See also*
  Adolescence; Puberty
Chimpanzee, chorionic
  gonadotropin of, 14. *See also*
  Primates
Chlorpromazine
  effect on reproductive function,
  103
  and prolactin release, 106
Cholesterol, 36, 270
Cholesterol synthesis, testicular,
  325
Chorionic gonadotropin (CG), 2
  and antiprogestational
  compounds, 173
  chimpanzee (chCG), 14
  gorilla (goCG), 14
  human (hCG)
    amino acid sequences of
    subunits of, 14–16
    antibody production against,
    129
    beta subunit of, 259
    binding of radioiodinated, 6
    biological properties of, 13–14
    chemical composition of, 14
    clinical applications of, 19–20
    function relationships of, 18–19
    immunization against, 46
    immunological properties, 13
    iodination of, 257
    location of receptors for, 258
    microheterogeneity of, 12
    physicochemical properties of,
    12–13
    preparation of subunits of, 12
    purification of, 11–12
    receptor binding studies for, 257
    structure of, 18–19

Chromatography
  affinity, 7, 31
  for isolating hCG, 11
  for purification of estrogen
  receptors, 250
Chromosome structure, hormonal
  regulation of, 236–238
Cilia, oviductal, 132, 136
Ciliary pathways, of oviduct, 133
Circadian periodicity. *See also*
  Diurnal variation
  of ACTH, 123–124
  effect on gonadal steroids of, 124
  of GH, 125
Circular dichroic (CD) spectrum,
  of native hCG, 13
Clinical intervention, possibilities
  for, 44, 45–46
Clinical studies, need for, 43
Clinical trials, 466–477. *See also*
  Fertility control
  comparison between methods,
  469
  public response to, 471
Clips
  electrocoagulation of Fallopian
  tubes by, 179
  oviductal, 216
Clogestone acetate, 206
Clomiphene
  effect of administration of, 119
  and estradiol retention, 246
  failure with, 53
  treatment with, 53–54
Clomiphene citrate, 51
  and LH release, 6
CNS. *See* Central nervous system
Coagulating gland, 402, 406, 407
Colchicine, contraceptive value of,
  460
Cold, and fertilizing ability of
  spermatozoa, 391–392
Colpotomy, tubal ligation
  procedure at, 178, 186
Comparative studies, on steroid
  feedback mechanisms, 55–56.
  See also Clinical trials;
  Methodology
Computer techniques, in hormone
  studies, 38, 80, 81
Conception, confirmation of, 52.
  See also Fertilization
Condom, contraceptive value of,
  355
Congenital defects, etiology of, 164
Contraception
  vs. abortion, 168
  and capacitation of spermatozoa,
  439
  clinical testing of, 466
  condom use, 355
  diaphragm for, 355
  in female tract, 434
  inhibition of ovarian hormones,
  38
  intrauterine, 188–202 (*see also*
  Intrauterine contraceptive
  devices)
  male, 157, 158, 317, 458–460
  Leydig cell function
    suppression, 331–332
  spermatogenic inhibition, 332,
  333

Contraception (continued)
postcoital, 103–108
rhythm method of, 436
and sperm membrane, 395
vaginal, 155
Contraceptives
acceptability of, 471
evaluation of, 470–471
injectable, 209–213
male, 212, 328
and mammary cancer, 210
progestogens as, 205–206
steroidal, 36
Contractions, oxytocin-induced, 227
Contragestational activity, nonsteroidal compounds, 170–171
Contragestational agents
examples of, 204
need for development of, 176
Cooperative Statistical Program (CSP), 188
Copper
spermatodepressive action of, 195
in uterine cavity, 189–190
Copper 7 (IUD), effectiveness of, 199
Copper T (IUD). See also Intrauterine contraceptive devices
effectiveness of, 199
insertion of, 196
long-lasting, 191–192
postabortion insertion of, 191
postpartum insertion of, 191
Corona-penetrating enzyme, 384
Corpus luteum
activity of, 45
human, 45
interference with function of, 46
maintenance of, 221–222
prolongation of function of, 224
Corticosteroid-binding globulin (CBG), 118
Corticosteroids, role in labor of, 149
Cow
gonadotropin-binding studies in, 258
LH of, 14
prolactin levels in, 30
Cryosurgery, of Fallopian tubes, 179–180
Culdoscopy, ligation procedures at, 178, 184, 186
Cumulus oophorus, ovarian, 135–136, 446
Cyanoacrylates, for tubal occlusion, 180
Cycle, ovarian, 49. See also Menstruation; Ovulation
Cyclic adenosine monophosphate (cAMP)
as energy source for spermatozoa, 379
FSH stimulation of, 281–282
in mammalian semen, 428
and protein synthesis in testicular tissue, 282
in spermatozoa metabolism, 382
in sperm maturation, 413

synthesis during capacitation, 435
Cyproterone, in hormone-receptor interaction, 254
Cyproterone acetate, contraceptive value of, 459–460
Cyst formation, and human gonadotropins, 50
Cytomegalovirus, 464
Cytoplasmic body, of spermatid, 298
Cytoplasmic protein receptors, 148
Cytosol, and estrogen-receptor complex, 247

Dalkon shield (IUD), 193–194, 197, 198
Danazol, contraceptive value of, 459
Decapacitation factor (DF), 437–438
Decapeptides, LRF, 91, 110
Decidualization, of uterus, 152. See also Menstruation
Dehydroisoandrosterone, 35
Deoxyribonucleic acid (DNA)
in spermatogenesis, 296
in trophoblast giant cells, 162
Depomedroxyprogesterone acetate (DMPA)
as contraceptive agent, 209–212
side effects of, 210
DF. See Decapacitation factor
DHEA (androgen), and maintenance of spermatogenesis, 280
Diaphragm, contraceptive value of, 355
Diethylstilbestrol. See also Interceptives
and epithelium of seminal vesicles, 403
postovulation administration of, 173
Dieting, and cessation of ovulation, 50. See also Nutrition
Dihydrotestosterone (DHT), 99
and male infertility, 461
in prostatic nuclei, 254
protein synthesis and, 255
synthesis of, 35
Dihydroxyprogesterone acetofenide, contraceptive value of, 209
Diphenylethlene, contragestational effects of, 172
Diplotene stage, in spermatogenesis, 296
Diurnal (circadian) rhythm, and gonadal secretion, 265
Diurnal variation
and ovulation, 59
in plasma TSH concentrations, 121
in prolactin levels, 29, 30
and sexual cyclicity, 58
in steroid regulation, 65
DMPA. See Depomedroxyprogesterone acetate
DNA. See Deoxyribonucleic acid
d-norgestrel, as contraceptive, 206
Dog, absence of seminal vesicles in, 407

Dopamine, 103. See also Catecholamines
concentrations of, 104
effects on gonadotropin release, 93
and prolactin secretion, 27, 106–107
Dopaminergic (DA) systems, 96
Dopamine synthesis, blocking of, 105
Dose-response relationships, 266
Doxycycline, for genitourinary tract infections, 464
Drugs
adrenregic blocking, 94
alterations in reproductive function caused by, 103
barbiturates, 345
and brain monoamine neurotransmitters, 105
development of, 39
effects on gonadal secretion, 66
and male accessory gland secretions, 429
Dynein, 374
in flagellar axoneme, 453
in tail of spermatozoon, 363
Dystocia, in rats, 149

Edema, uterine, 151
Egg
degeneration of, 49
oviduct transportation of, 135–136, 225–226
structural components of, 445–446
transportation of, 132–138
Egg cylinder, formation of, 162–163
Egg envelope, penetration of, 357
Egg transfer, 163–164
Electrocoagulation, of Fallopian tubes, 179–180
Electrophysiological antidromic firing technique, 97
Electrophysiology, of myometrium, 150
Embden-Meyerhof pathway, 416
Embryo
effect of oviductal fluid on, 142
growth regulation of, 162
role of oviduct in survival of, 141–142
steroid production of, 161
Embryogenesis, 157–166
growth and differentiation, 162–164
morphology of, 157–159
and oviductal fluids, 139
trophoblast giant cell transformation, 161–162
in vitro techniques for study of, 159–161
Emotional stress
and cessation of ovulation, 50
influence on reproductive function, 108
Endocrine cells, signal system of, 103
Endocrine glands, enzymatic processes in, 36. See also Enzymes
Endocrinology

behavioral, 98
concept of feedback in, 55
Endoderm, embryonic, 163
Endometrium. See also Uterus
and DMPA therapy, 209, 210
effect of estrogen on, 152, 206
infiltration of leukocytes into, 190
major cell types of, 153
regulation of, 146
reproductive role of, 151–154
Environment
influence on reproductive function, 108
and steroid regulation, 58, 64
Enzymes, acrosomal, 358, 374, 495
of prostate gland, 405
sperm, 380–382
in steroidogenesis, 271–272
Enzyme systems, on biosynthetic particle, 34
Epidemiology, of induced abortion, 167–168
Epididymis
ABP in, 37
absorption process in, 414–415
biochemistry of, 412–413
control of, 418–421
glycolytic activity of, 416
metabolism by, 418–419
morphological features of, 411–412
physiology of, 412–414
secretions of, 415–418
spermatozoa in, 350, 386
sperm maturation in, 411–413
steroid-binding proteins in, 420
Epinephrine, 103. See also Catecholamines
concentrations of, 104
effect on gonadotropin release, 93
Epinephrine synthesis, control of, 104
Epithelium
seminal vesicle, 403
seminiferous, 311
cycle of, 299
organization of, 302–304
standing gradient hypothesis, 315
Ergocornine, and progesterone levels, 174
Ergot alkaloids, for termination of pregnancy, 170
ESMODEL, 74
Estradiol, 104
and androgen synthesis, 277
conversion of, 35
conversion of testosterone to, 256
critical level of, 44
DMPA effect on levels of, 210
effect on FSH, 267
effect on LH response to SRF, 118
and LH inhibition, 267
in LRF secretion, 111
in men, 37
oviductal accumulation of, 138
production and release of, 115
regulation of production of, 38
regulatory function of, 116

Estradiol (continued)
 secretion of, 36-37
 synthesis of, 33
 testicular secretion of, 274
Estradiol enanthate, contraceptive
 value of, 209
Estrogenic compounds,
 contragestational activity of,
 171
Estrogen-receptor complexes,
 246-249
 and RNA synthesis, 249
Estrogen receptors, antibodies to,
 130
Estrogens. See also
 Clomiphene
 and accessory sex glands,
 407-408
 activity of, 42
 carcinogenicity of, 212
 effects on peripheral nervous
 system of, 98
 egg transport and, 136
 and endometrium, 152, 206
 and follicular development, 46
 formation of, 117
 and GH levels, 125
 and gonadotropin secretion, 59
 in hormone receptor interaction,
 245
 as interceptives, 203-205
 during labor, 149, 150
 during luteal phase, 45
 modeling of, 74, 77, 81, 82
 negative feedback mechanisms
 of, 57
 ovulatory surge of LH and, 6
 and ovum transport, 136-137
 positive feedback of, 55, 57,
 63-64
 postcoital administration of,
 170-173, 205
 in postovulatory period, 206-207
 and prolactin levels, 31, 106
 regulatory function of, 118, 210,
 211
 and response to dopamine, 94
 stimulation of implantation by,
 153, 154
 unbound, 275
 uterine effects of, 151
Estrogen secretion, by Sertoli
 cells, 323
Estrone, conversion of estradiol to,
 35
Estrone sulfate, conversion of,
 35
Estrus, and pheromones, 98
Ethamoxytriphetol, and estradiol
 retention, 246
Ethinyl estradiol
 and epithelium of seminal
 vesicles, 403
 as interceptive, 205
Ethyl alcohol, and premature
 labor, 150
Ethynodiol diacetate, as coital
 progestogen, 206
Ethynyl testosterone, contraceptive
 value of analogs of, 459
Eugonadotropic syndromes, 462
Experimental studies. See also
 Clinical trials; Methodology

animal, 55-56 (see also specific
 animals)
 controversy over human
 application of, 146
 human, 43
 in vitro vs. in vivo, 442, 444
Explant techniques, 408
Expulsion, IUD-associated, 196

Fallopian tubes. See also Oviducts
 alteration of, 178
 capacitation of spermatozoa in,
 437-438
 chemical sclerosing agents for
 occlusion of, 180-182
 contraction of, 225
 methods of closure of, 178-183
Family planning programs, 472.
 See also Clinical trials
 sterilizations in, 184
Fatty acids, in mammalian semen,
 428
Feedback
 concept of, 55
 internal, 57, 63
 negative, 57
 positive, 55, 63-64
 steroid, 68-69
Feminization, testicular, 278
Fertility. See also Infertility
 enzyme inhibition for blocking
 of, 394
 immunologic interference with,
 128-131
 recovery after contraceptive use,
 470-471
 regulation of male, 458-465
Fertility control, 448. See also
 Contraception
 bioengineering aspects of, 216,
 217
 devices for, 216, 217
 and endometrial physiology,
 151-154
 immunological approach to,
 448
 Leydig cells and, 330, 333
 life tables for, 466
 types of, 207-208
Fertilization
 bioengineering involvement in,
 215
 electron-microscopic study of,
 374
 enzymes implicated in, 384-385
 human experiments in, 441-443
 inhibition of, 447-448
 morphology of, 444-447
 nature of, 434
 and oviductal fluids, 139, 141
 physiology of, 444-447
 sperm-egg fusion and, 446
 in vitro, 139-143
 in vitro vs. in vivo, 444
Fetoscopy, 163
Fetus
 and hypertonic saline-induced
 abortion, 149
 parturition role of, 149-150
Fimbriectomy, 179
Flagella, of mammalian sperm,
 361, 452. See also
 Spermatozoa

Flutamide, in hormone-receptor
 interaction, 254
Follicle, ovarian. See also Ovaries;
 Oviducts
 cellular compartmentalization in,
 33
 effects of steroids on, 61
 hormonal regulation of, 40-43
 inhibition of development of, 46
 mechanical rupture of, 45
 normal development of, 44-45
 stimulation of development of,
 45-46
Follicle radius, modeling of, 75,
 76, 81
Follicle stimulating hormone
 (FSH), 1
 ABP synthesis stimulated by, 37
 amino acid sequences for
 subunits of, 15
 biological roles of, 6
 concentration of, 44
 control system for, 61
 and diagnosis of male infertility,
 462
 differential feedback of gonadal
 steroids on secretions of, 72
 effects on Leydig cells, 327-328
 human (hFSH), 2, 5
 induction of LH receptors by,
 260-261
 iodination of, 257
 isolation of, 2
 location of receptors for, 258
 modeling of, 82
 negative feedback mechanisms
 of, 57
 ovulation control of, 49
 prepuberal appearance of, 6
 production of, 267
 receptor binding studies for, 257
 regulation of ABP by, 39
 response to LRF stimulation, 115
 role of, 6-7
 role in spermatogenesis,
 278-279
 in testes, 317
 and testicular physiology, 277,
 461
Follicle-stimulating-hormone
 releasing factor (FRF), 91
Follicular fluid, and capacitation of
 spermatozoa, 389
Freeze-cleaving studies, of
 spermatozoon, 369
Freeze-fracturing, method of, 367
Fructolysis, in mammalian semen,
 428-429
Fructose, in seminal vesicles, 403
FSH. See Follicle stimulating
 hormone
Fundus, perforation of, 197-198.
 See also Uterus

Galactin, See Prolactin
Galactorrhea, 52
 and elevated prolactin levels, 28
 microadenomas associated with,
 30
 therapeutic agents for, 106
Gametes, oviductal environment
 of, 139-141, 142
Gamete transport, 132-138

bioengineering involvement in,
 215
Gametogenesis, hormonal
 regulation of, 40. See also
 Ovulation
Gamma amino butyric acid, 103
Gamma globulin, in seminiferous
 tubule, 348
Gelatin resorcinol formalin (GRF),
 180
Genetic defects, in mouse
 embryos, 160-161
Genetics, and embryonic
 development studies, 157-159
Genitalia, male differentiation of,
 313
Genitourinary tract infections, and
 male infertility, 464
Germ cells, relation of Sertoli cells
 to, 303
GH. See Growth hormone
Glands. See also Pituitary gland
 mammalian accessory sex,
 402-410
 steroid-secreting, 33
Glucocorticoids, 123
 and labor, 149, 150
Glucose, in embryonic
 development, 140
Glutethimide, effect on
 progesterone levels, 174
Glycerol, for storage of semen,
 431
Glycerylphosphorylcholine (GPC),
 in epididymis, 415
Glycocalyx, on epithelia of
 accessory sex glands, 408
Glycoprotein hormones, amino
 acid sequences of, 3, 15, 16
Glycoproteins, microheterogeneity
 in, 12
Gonadal steroids, regulatory
 functions of, 108. See also Sex
 steroids
Gonadectomy, effects·of, 405
Gonadotropin-binding studies, 257
 and target cell activation, 260
 in vitro, 258-260
Gonadotropin concentrations, in
 hypogonadal patients, 115
Gonadotropin-controlling centers,
 localization of, 92
Gonadotropin injection, DMPA
 inhibition of, 209, 210
Gonadotropin preparations, for
 induction of ovulation, 50-51
Gonadotropin receptors, 256-261
 location of, 258
 solubilization, 261
Gonadotropin release, 265
 inhibition of, 116
 PGs and, 219-220
Gonadotropin-releasing factors,
 control of, 92-95
Gonadotropin-releasing hormone
 (GnRH), 49, 62
 for induction of ovulation, 50
 isolation of, 265
 and LH release, 60
Gonadotropins
 access to seminiferous tubules of,
 349
 brain centers controlling, 92

Gonadotropins (continued)
cyclic changes in release of, 114–115
development of RIAs for, 5–6
human (hPG), methods of treatment with, 50, 52–54
immunization against, 46
iodinated, 257–258
isolation of, 1–2
mode of action of, 6
normal cyclic secretions of, 60
plasma levels of, 265–267
preparation of labeled, 257
primary action of, 41
subunits of, 2–3
Gonadotropin secretion
behavioral components of, 97
control of, 90–92, 109–119
effect of brain neurotransmitters on, 106
effect of surgical stress on, 66
influence of nonreproductive factors on, 269
pattern of, 112
by pituitary gland, 265–267
regulation of, 266–267
Gorilla, chorionic gonadotropins of, 14
Graafian follicle, growth of, 44
Granulosa cells
luteinization of, 42
mediation of LH action on, 220–221
Gravidity, and copper T use, 190
GRF. See Gelatin resorcinol formalin
Growth hormone (GH)
in primate, 27
release of
hypothalamic regulation of, 125
stimulation of, 122
secretion of
CNS regulation of, 125
control of, 124–126
feedback regulation of, 125
Guinea pig
myometrium of, 147, 151
spermatozoa of, 364, 368, 369
Gynecomastia, 275

Haloperidol, 105
Hamster
capacitation of spermatozoa in, 439
spermatid of, 360
sperm motility in, 455
in vitro fertilization in, 444
hCG. See Chorionic gonadotropin, human
Hexestrol, synthesis of, 245
HHH. See Hormones, hypothalamic hypophysiotropic
Hirsutism, androgen levels in, 276
Histones, sperm, 237, 387–388
Homosexuality, and serum testosterone, 99
Hormone Distribution Program, 26
Hormone-receptor interaction, 245–263
Hormone receptors, steroid, 245–256
Hormones. See also Gonadotropins; Steroids;

specific hormones
classification of, 103
effect of nutrition on, 269
glycoprotein, 5, 15, 16
hypothalamic
hypophysiotropic, 90, 112
synthetic, 113
immunization against, 46
ovarian, 38, 120
reassociated form, 3
role in contraception of, 207
steroid, 134
Horses, gonadotropin-binding studies in, 258
Humans
effect of neurally active drugs on gonadotropin secretion in, 66
effect of surgical stress on gonadotropin secretion in, 66
environmental influences on steroid regulations in, 64
feedback dormancy in
during lactation, 71–72
during pregnancy, 71–72
during puberty, 70
site of action of steroid feedback in, 68–69
steroid feedback mechanisms in, 56–72
Humegon, 51
Hyaluronidase
released by spermatozoa, 384
role in fertilization, 394
Hydrolases, acrosomal, 374, 383. See also Enzymes
Hydroxyprogesterone, testicular secretion of, 274
Hyperbolic LH Production Model, 73
Hypergonadotropic syndromes, 462
Hyperkalemia, and renin secretion, 104
Hyperpolarization, of myometrial cell membranes, 150, 151
Hypogonadism, male, 462
Hypogonadotropic ovarian failure, 51
Hypophysectomy
arrest of spermatogenesis induced by, 279
decline in gonadotropin concentration following, 113
effects on reproductive system of, 1
and estrogen production, 54
and maintenance of spermatogenesis, 280
and prolactin levels, 31
and testicular protein, 282
and testosterone synthesis, 327
Hypopituitarism, 51
Hypothalamic dysfunction, and gonadotropin release, 112
Hypothalamic-hypophyseal-gonadal system, integrated, 118–119
Hypothalamic-hypophseal-ovarian feedback system, 43
Hypothalamic hypophysiotropic hormones (HHH), 90, 112
Hypothalamic neurons, 104
Hypothalamic-pituitary-gonadal

axis, 264–270
Hypothalamic-releasing-factor release, and PGs, 230
Hypothalamus
and anterior pituitary, 108
monoamine neurotransmitters in, 104
nuclei of, 95
turnover of catecholamines in, 94
Hysterectomy
and corpus luteum function, 174
for female sterilization, 183
Hysteroscopy, for sterilization, 184–185

ICGH. See Interstitial-cell-stimulating hormone
IITRI, 215, 216, 217
Imidazoles, effects on progesterone levels, 174
Immunization, against pituitary gonadotropins, 46
Immunoassays, for prolactin, 26
Immunofluorescence techniques, 93
Immunoglobulins, in cervical mucus, 155
Immunology. See also Antibodies
and contragestational activity, 174–175
reproductive, 128–130
Implantation
physiology of, 152–154
preparation for, 151–152
prevention of, 153
progesterone levels during, 174
Implant techniques, 408
Indoleamines, identification of, 108
Indomethacin, uterine effects of, 227
Infection
genitourinary tract, 464
pelvic, IUD-associated, 197
Infertility. See also Fertility
enzyme defects associated with, 278
female, 50, 129
male, 129, 460–464
diagnostic procedures for, 462
and prostaglandins, 229
Inhibin, 460
Inhibition, reciprocal, 55
Inhibitors, safety of, 38
Inositol, in seminal vesicles, 403
Insects, reproductive biology of, 56
"Inside-outside" theory, environmental, 161
Instrumentation, for detection of reproductive events, 216
Insulin secretion, control of, 104
Interception
estrogen, 205
postcoital, 203–208
Interceptives. See also Morning-after pill
examples of, 204
stilbestrol as, 203–204
Intercourse, sexual, prolactin levels during, 106
Interstitial-cell-stimulating

hormone (ICSH), 1
action on androgen biosynthetic pathway, 276
in Leydig cell function, 278
Interstitial tissue
from atretic follicles, 42
of testis, 346
Intratubal devices, for female sterilization, 182–183
Intrauterine contraceptive devices (IUDs). See also specific devices
accidental pregnancy with, 199
advantages and disadvantages of, 199–200
bioengineering work on, 216
biomaterials for, 216, 217
and capacitation of spermatozoa, 440
clinical trials with, 466–467
copper-bearing, 192 (see also Copper T)
design of, 215
early history of, 188
effective life in utero, 191
and elevated cervical mucus copper levels, 155
fluid-filled, 194
hormone-releasing, 193
mechanism of action of, 194–196
medicated, 189–190
postabortion insertion of, 191
postpartum insertion of, 190–191
and prostaglandin synthesis, 228–229
removal of, 198–199
and septic abortions, 194
side effects of, 196–198
size and shape of, 188–189
stainless steel, 197
T-shaped, 188
ypsilon-shaped, 194
Iodine, tincture of, uterine injection of, 180
Isoelectric focusing, 2
Isolation techniques, 2, 3. See also Experimental studies
Isoproterenol, and ampullar transport, 136
Isthmus of oviduct
contractile activities in, 134
egg transport through, 132–133
fluorescent fibers in, 134
and gamete transport, 133
IUD. See Intrauterine contraceptive devices

Joint Program for Study of Abortion (JPSA), 167, 183

Karyopyknotic index, and ovarian response to hPG, 52
Klinefelter's syndrome, 462
androgen biosynthesis in, 278
and chromosomal anomalies, 296
Leydig cell steroidogenesis in, 275
Krebs-cycle pathway, 416

Labor
amplitude of contractions during, 148
oxytocin-induced, 148

575   Subject Index

Labor (continued)
  premature
    control of, 150
    and incompetence of cervix, 155
    progesterone and, 147
    prostaglandin levels during, 227, 230
Lactate, and epididymal spermatozoa, 416
Lactation
  chlorpromazine-induced, 103
  feedback dormancy during, 60, 61, 71-72
  prolactin secretion and, 119
Lactotropes, during pregnancy, 25
Laparoscopy, 178
Laparotomy, 178, 184
Latex Leaf (IUD), 192
L-DOPA, and prolactin levels, 28, 106
Leydig cell function
  biological significance of, 328
  feedback control of, 328
  research in, 334
  suppression of, 331
Leydig cells
  androgens produced by, 272, 313, 325
  biochemistry of, 329
  and biosynthesis of steroids, 314
  and blood-testis barrier, 346
  cytochemistry of, 329
  effects of FSH on, 327-328
  effects of LH on, 326-327
  and fertility control, 321
  in Golgi complex, 324
  gonadotropin control of, 274
  lipid droplets in, 324
  lipofuscin in, 324
  lysosomes in, 324
  microbodies in, 324
  mitochondria of, 324
  morphology of, 323, 329
  normally functioning, preservation of, 331
  origin of testicular androgens, 321-322
  physiology of, 330
  production of, 270
  and seminiferous tubules, 322
  smooth reticulum of, 324
  testosterone secreted by, 37
  testosterone synthesized by, 33
LH. See Luteinizing hormone
LHRF. See Luteinizing-hormone releasing factor
LHRH, and elevated prolactin levels, 29-30
Life tables, 466, 477. See also Clinical trials
Light-dark cycles, and gonadotropin secretion, 58
Lipids
  and aging of spermatozoa, 393
  on spermatozoon surface, 367
Lipofuscin granules, in Leydig cells, 324
Lippes loop (IUD), 188
  copper-bearing, 192
  insertion of, 196
  postabortion insertion of, 191
  postpartum insertion of, 190
  uterine reaction to, 198

Lithospermum ruderale, and testicular function, 458
LRF. See Luteinizing-hormone releasing factor
Luteal phase
  inadequate, 46
  prolactin during, 29
Luteinizing hormone (LH), 1
  action of, 6-7
  amino acid sequences for subunits of, 3, 4, 5, 15
  binding of radioiodinated, 6
  biological roles of, 6
  concentration of, 44
  control system for, 61
  and diagnosis of male infertility, 462
  differential feedback of gonadal steroids on secretions of, 72
  effects on Leydig cells, 326-327
  iodination of, 257
  location of receptors for, 258
  modeling of, 74, 77, 81, 82
  negative feedback mechanisms of, 57
  ovulation control of, 49
  prepuberal appearance of, 6
  production of, 266-267
  pulsatile pattern of release of, 6
  receptor binding studies for, 257
  release of, and PGs, 219
  response to LRF stimulation, 114
  role in spermatogenesis, 278-279
  signal apparatus for, 103
  steroidogenic action of, 327
  subunits of, 3
Luteinizing-hormone releasing factor (LRF or LHRF), 62, 91
  activity of, 60
  availability of, 92
  characterization of, 90
  isolation of, 265
  localization of, 97
  mechanism of pituitary response to, 112-113
  metabolism of, 111-112
  priming effect of, 118
  responses of adult male pituitary to, 113
  routes of administration of, 114
  secretion of
    increased, 116
    regulation of, 110
    release pattern for, 109-110
  synthetic, 113
Luteolysin, uterine, 174
Luteolysis, 45
  mechanism of PG action on, 223
Luteolytic effect, 207
Lymph
  concentrations of various substances in, 342
  from spermatic cord, 338
Lytic agents, in fertilization, 445

Magnesium
  in RTF, 340
  in spermatozoa, 381
Majzlin spring (IUD), 197
Mammals
  accessory sex glands of, 402-410
  fertilization in, 444

inhibition of fertilization in, 444-448
  LH in, 2
  mating behavior of, 274
  spermatogenesis in, 293-299
  spermatozoa of, 354, 358, 379-401, 454-456
Mammotropin. See Prolactins
Marsupials, sperm of, 365
Masculinity
  expression of, 333
  Leydig cells and, 322
Mating, and precipitation of ovulation, 97. See also Intercourse, sexual
Maturation process, 119. See also Puberty
  role of gonads in, 268-269
Meiosis, in spermatogenesis, 295-297
Melatonin, and control of gonadotropin release, 95
Melengestrol, in IUD development, 193
Menarche, of blind girls, 65
Menopause
  atrophy of tissues following, 154
  ovary during, 42
Menstrual cycle
  and DMPA injections, 210, 211
  effect of emotional problems on, 109
  follicular development during, 44
  gonadotropin release during, 114
  and myometrium, 148
  and ovarian secretion of hormones, 36
  steroidal regulation of, 118
  synchronization of, 98
  as time units of observation in clinical trials, 468
Menstrual fluid, PGs in, 225
Menstruation
  and IUD-associated bleeding, 190, 196
  medical control of, 47
  normal, 51
  occurrence of, 49
Metabolites, for sperm motility, 379. See also Enzymes
Methodology, in reproductive science, 408. See also Experimental studies
  clinical testing, 466-477
  data collection, 61
Methotrexate, for termination of pregnancy, 175
Methyl cyanoacrylate, for tubal occlusion, 180
Metyrapone, effect on progesterone levels, 174
Microadenomas, of pituitary gland, 30
Microcirculation, in ovarian arteries, 40
Microheterogeneity, of hCG, 12
Microiontophoretic technique, for mapping hormonal feedback action, 96
Micropinocytosis, in epididymis, 404
Microsomal system, electron transport in, 34

Midbrain, stimulatory projections of, 97
Milk production, effect of prolactin on, 31
Mineralocorticoids, 123
Minilaparotomy, 186
Mitochondrial system, electron transport in, 34
Modeling, 80, 81
  in endocrinology, 56
  heuristic value of, 73
  in reproductive biology, 73
Molecular biology, advances in, 242
Molecular exclusion processes, 2
Monitoring therapy, for induction of ovulation, 52
Monkey
  effect of surgical stress on gonadotropin secretion of, 66
  egg transport in, 136
  environmental influences on steroid regulation of, 64
  for experimentation, 56
  feedback dormancy in, 70, 71-72
  gonadotropin-binding studies in, 258
  internal feedback mechanisms in, 63
  negative feedback mechanisms in, 62
  neonatal exposure to androgens, 67
  oviduct transport in, 132-133, 135-136
  positive feedback mechanisms in, 63-64
  Sertoli-Sertoli cell junctions in, 347
  site of action of steroid feedback in, 68-69
  spermatogonia in, 294
  spermatozoon in, 370
Morning-after pill, 103-108
Mouse
  carbohydrate metabolism in, 159
  egg cylinders of, 163
  genetic defects in embryos of, 160
  sperm motility in, 455
  in vitro fertilization, 444
Mucus
  cervical, 154, 209
  vaginal, 154
Multiple unit method, for mapping sites of hormonal feedback action, 96
Multisleeved model, of copper T IUD, 191
Mutations, and embryogenesis, 159
Myometrial tension, intrauterine pressure recordings of, 148
Myometrium
  action of saline on, 149
  electrophysiology of, 150
  infiltration of leukocytes into, 190
  physiology of, 150-151
  during pregnancy, 146-147
  prostaglandins produced by, 228
  regulation of, 146, 151
  stimulation of, 148-149
Myosin, 454

Nafoxidine, and estradiol retention, 246
National Institutes of Health (NIH), Contraceptive Development Program, 212, 458
Neonates, TSH secretions of, 121
Nerve degeneration techniques, 96
NET. See Norethindrone
Neuraminidase, activity in spermatozoa of, 385. See also Enzymes
Neuroendocrine transducers
  hypothalamic-releasing-factor cells, 103–104
  identification of, 104
  signal systems of, 103
Neuroendocrinology, 103
Neurons, signal systems of, 103
Neurotransmitters
  characteristics of, 103
  in gonadotropin regulation, 125
  identification of, 108
  and secretion of gonadtropin-releasing factors, 92
Nicotinamide-adenine dinucleotide (NAD), in mammalian semen, 428
Noradrenalin, and labor, 150
Noradrenergic fibers, in hypothalamus, 96
Norepinephrine, 103, 134
  concentrations of, 104
  effect on gonadotropin release of, 93
Norethindrone (NET), and luteal-phase progesterone levels, 173
Norethindrone enanthate
  as contraceptive agent, 209, 212
  inhibition of ovulation caused by, 211
Norgestrieone, as coital progestogen contraceptive, 206
Norsteroids, as interceptive agents, 205
"Nurse cells," 317. See also Sertoli cells
Nursing. See Breastfeeding
Nutrition
  effect on spermiogenesis, 299
  and reproductive function, 269

Oligomenorrhea
  anovulation associated with, 50
  hPG therapy in presence of, 53
  secondary, 52
Oligospermia, enzyme defects associated with, 278
Oncolytic agents, for termination of pregnancy, 175
Oocyte
  enlargement of, 40
  role of, 42
Oophorectomy, and prolactin levels, 31
Oral contraception, discontinuation of, 50. See also Contraception
Orchitis, allergic, 331
Orciprenaline, and premature labor, 150

Osteoporosis, premature development of, 212
Ovalbumin, 241
Ovariectomy
  bilateral hormone circulation after, 115
  modeling of, 81
  pulsatile discharge of LH after, 56
Ovaries
  bioengineering involvement in, 215
  cellular compartmentalization in, 33
  cyclical vs. continuous suppression of, 47
  and gonadotropin release, 114–118
  and hypophysis, 41
  polycystic, acyclicity associated with, 119
  secretion of, 38
  steroid hormones secreted by, 36
Oviductal cells, biology of, 137–138
Oviductal clips, 216, 217
Oviducts, 132–142
  deciliation of, 137
  fluid composition in, 139–140
  function of, 139–141
  hot water destruction of, 183
  innervation of, 134–135
  pharmacological influences on, 142
  physiology of, 138–142
  in vitro, 138
Ovulation-inducing hormone (OIH), 41
Ovulation
  coitus-induced, 97
  DNA inhibition of, 209, 210
  drug alteration of, 105
  endogenous PG synthesis in, 220
  and gonadotropin secretion, 97–98
  hormonal control of, 49
  induction of, 49–54
  luteinization during, 37
  modeling of, 82
  pathophysiology of, 50
  peak, 41, 42
  physiology of, 49
  precipitation of, 57
  prediction of, 154
  prevention of, 42
  spurt, 41
  timing mechanism for, 96
Oxygen, for sperm motility, 379
Oxytocin
  response of human uterus to, 148
  role in labor of, 150, 155
  for termination of pregnancy, 170

Parity, and copper T IUD use, 190
Parturition. See also Labor
  fetal role in, 149–150
  effect of PGs on, 227–228
Pasteur effect, in immature spermatozoa, 387
Pathfinder Fund, 472
Patients, selection for induction of ovulation, 51–52

Pearl Index, of pregnancy rate, 466
Pelvic inflammatory disease (PID), IUD-associated, 197
Penetration
  enzymatic assistance for, 445
  in vitro, 443
Pentobarbital
  effect on gonadotropin secretion, 66
  and LH secretion, 56
  and ovulation, 59
Peptides, nonspecific bound radioactivity of, 257–258
Pergonal, 51
Pharmacological intervention. See also Drugs
  and luteal function, 46
  for ovarian follicle, 43
Pharmacology, neurotransmitter, 103
Pheromones, behavioral-social effects on reproduction of, 98
Phospholipid, sperm, 380. See also Spermatozoa
Physiology
  ovarian, 47, 49
  oviductal, 138–142
  TRH, 121–122
PIF. See Prolactin-inhibiting factor
Pig
  capacitation of spermatozoa of, 443
  gonadotropin-binding studies in, 258
  oviducts of, 138
  oviduct transport in, 132
  prolactin of, 26
Pigeon, prolactin levels in, 30
Pigeon cropsac assay, for prolactin, 26
Pimozide, 105, 106
Pineal gland
  LRF concentrations in, 112
  as neuroendocrine transducers, 104
Pituitary gland
  central nervous control of gonadotropic function of, 91–92
  gonadal secretion by, 265–267
  human gonadotropin from (hPG), 50
  ovarian response to, 52
  hypothalamic regulation of, 109
  LRF sensitivity of, 113, 116
  and maturation process, 268
  portal blood of, 106
  prolactin and, 25
  and reproductive system, 1
Pituitary-hypothalamic dysfunction, 51
Pituitary luteotropic stimulus, 45
Pituitary tissue, and steroid metabolism, 117
Pituitary tumor, sign of, 50
Placenta
  estradiol synthesized by, 35
  and hypertonic saline-induced abortion, 149
Placental components, for immunological reactions, 175
Plant extracts, and testicular

function, 458
Plants, abortifacient action of, 175
Plasmalemma, of spermatozoa, 360, 412
Polarization microscopy, 355
Polyacrylamide disc-gel electrophoresis, 2
Polycystic ovary syndrome, 49, 50
Polymers. See also Drugs
  biodegradable, as contraceptive agents, 212
  for release of drugs, 217
Pomeroy technique, of tubal ligation, 178–179, 183, 184
Population control, 434. See also Fertility control
Population Council, 472
  IUD research of, 193
  JPSA of, 167, 183
  research on injectable contraceptives of, 213
  sterilization programs of, 183
Population Information Program (George Washington University Medical Center), 168
Populations, for clinical trials, 468
Postmenopausal women
  extract from urine of (hMG), 50, 51
  gonadotropin levels in, 115, 267
  oviductal ciliation of, 137
Postpartum period
  follicular development during, 44
  prolactin levels during, 29
Postpartum women, prolactin secretion in, 105
Potassium, in RTF, 340
Pregnancy
  accidental IUD-associated, 199
  ectopic
    early detection of, 11, 19
    and morning-after pill, 205
  effect of IUDs on subsequent, 198
  feedback dormancy during, 60, 61, 71–72
  follicular development during, 44
  interruption of, 149 (see also Abortion)
  multiple pregnancies, 50
  myometrium during, 146–148
  normal, early detection of, 11, 19
  pharmacological termination of, 170
  prolactin concentrations during, 25, 120
Pregnancy Termination Study (Carolina Population Center), 167
Pregnant mare serum gonadotropin (PMG), 2
Pregnenolone
  and androgen synthesis, 277
  conversion of cholesterol to, 270–271, 326
  formation of androgens from, 271
  and maintenance of spermatogenesis, 280
Preimplantation, in vitro, 140. See also Implantation
Preleptotene stage, in spermatogenesis, 295

Premarin, 205
Premenopausal women, bilateral ovariectomies in, 115
Preovulatory phase, 49
Preparatory phase, during capacitation of spermatozoa, 390
Prepuberty, feedback dormancy during, 60. *See also* Puberty
PRF. *See* Prolactin-releasing factor
Primates. *See also specific primates*
  capacitation of spermatozoa in, 441
  corpus luteum of, 44
  gonadotropin-binding studies in, 258
  luteolysis in, 222–224
  mating behavior of, 274
  oviduct activity in, 135, 136, 142
  pregnancy of, 170
  Sertoli-Sertoli cell junctions in, 347
  spermatogonia in, 294
  steroid feedback mechanisms in, 56–72
Proestrus, modeling of, 82
Progesterone
  accumulation, of oviductal cells, 138
  action on myometrium, 147–148
  and androgen synthesis, 277
  antiprogestational compounds, 173–174
  conversion of, 35
  and deciliation of oviduct, 137
  discovery of, 146
  effects on endometrium of, 152
  effect on LH response to LRF, 118
  formation from pregnenolone, 271
  and gonadotropin secretion, 59
  and hyperpolarization of myometrial cell membranes, 150, 151
  in hypophysectomized rat, 61
  LH surge elicited by, 56
  in LRF secretion, 111
  during luteal phase, 45
  and myometrium, 151
  negative feedback mechanisms of, 57
  neutralization of, 130
  ovarian, 38
  oviductal accumulation of, 138, 141
  positive feedback mechanism of, 57, 63–64
  in postovulatory period, 207
  preovulatory, contraceptive action of, 207
  production and release, 115
  regulation of production of, 38
  regulatory function of, 116
  role of, 42
  secretion of, 36
  uterine supply of, 147
Progesterone-block theory, of pregnancy maintenance, 147–148
Progesterone receptors
  in chick oviduct, 251–253

in mammalian tissues, 251
purification of, 253
Progestins
  cessation of spermatogenesis caused by, 332
  in hormone-receptor interaction, 251–253
  and implantation, 153
  and ovum transport, 136–137
Progestogens
  as contraceptive agents, 205–206, 212
  definition of, 207
Prolactin-inhibiting factor (PIF), of hypothalamus, 27, 120
  effect of dopamine on, 106
Prolactin release, stimulation of, 122
Prolactin-releasing factor (PRF), 27
Prolactins
  activity of, 31
  assays of, 26–27
  biological effects of, 31
  chemistry of, 26
  effect of dopamine on, 105–106
  effect on males of, 31
  effects on maternal behavior of, 31
  human, 25, 28
  hypothalamic regulation of, 109
  luteotropic role of, 29
  and pituitary, 25–27
Prolactin secretion, 27–30, 120
  alterations in, 120
  control of, 119–120
  direct pituitary modifiers of, 120
  in disease, 120
  in normal individuals, 120
  pharmacological effects on, 120
Prostaglandins (PGs)
  activity of, 45
  effects of, 223
  and egg transport, 137
  and gonadotropin release, 219–220
  in human semen, 225
  immunization against, 46
  for induction of abortion, 167
  and myogenic activity, 148–149
  regulatory activity of, 223
  and release of gonadotropin-releasing factors, 95
  reproduction role of, 219–235
  response of human uterus to, 148
  in seminal plasma, 229
  in seminal vesicles, 404
  uterine contractions caused by, 170, 226
  in veterinary practice, 230
  in vivo effects on pregnant human uterus, 226
Prostaglandin synthesis, and uterine cell stretch, 147
Prostate gland, 402
  cytological characteristics of, 404–405
  effects of gonadectomy on, 405
  secretory function of, 405–406
Proteins
  and blood-testis barrier, 341, 344
  endometrium-secreted, 153

epididymal plasmal, 416
flagellar, 363
in RTF, 340–341
steroid-binding, 118, 420
Protein synthesis, in reproductive tissues, hormonal regulation of, 240–241
Pseudocyesis, 109
  and gonadotropin release, 112
Puberty
  feedback dormancy during, 70
  gonadotropin levels during, 268
  onset of, 119
  and pheromones, 98

R-2323, contraceptive value of, 211
Rabbit
  capacitation of spermatozoa in, 438
  interstitial gland of, 42
  myometrium of, 147, 148
  oviduct of, 132–133, 134, 136
  ovulatory pattern of, 109
  prolactin levels in, 30
  response to PGs in, 149
  RNA synthesis in, 159
  spermatozoa of, 366
  in vitro fertilization of, 139
Radioactive steroids, 408
Radioimmunoassays (RIAs), 265, 273–274
  of ACTH, 124
  development of, 129
  of gonadotropic hormonal levels, 41
  for pregnancy detection, 52
  for prolactin, 27
Radioligand-receptor assay, 257
Radioreceptor assay, for prolactin, 27
Ram. *See also* Sheep
  Sertoli cells in, 305–307, 308
  spermatozoa of, 415
Rat
  androgen metabolism in, 421
  blood-testis permeability barrier in, 313
  coitus-induced ovulation in, 97
  effect of surgical stress on gonadotropin secretion of, 66
  environmental influences on steroid regulations of, 64
  estradiol activity in, 124
  for experimentation, 55–56
  follicle phase of, 56
  gonadotropin-binding studies in, 258
  gonadotropin secretion in, 58
  LH in, 14
  maintenance of spermatogenesis in, 281
  myometrium of, 147
  neonatal exposures to androgens, 67
  ovarian follicles of, 75
  oviduct transport in, 132–133
  ovulatory pattern of, 109
  positive feedback mechanisms in, 63–64
  pregnancy in, 148
  site of action of steroid feedback in, 68–69

spermatogonial population of, 293, 360, 455
steroid feedback mechanisms, 56–72
Receptor binding, prevention of, 242
Receptor masking, phenomenon of, 7
Receptors
  gonadotropin, 7
  induction of, 260
  labeling of LH-hCG, 17–18
  solubilization of LH-hCG, 17
  steroid hormone, 245–256
Reduced triphosphopyridine nucleotide (TPNH), ICSH action on, 277
Reductases, in androgen metabolism, 276. *See also* Enzymes
Relaxin
  in rats, 149
  as regulator of myometrium, 151
Renal juxtaglomerular cells, as neuroendocrine transducers, 104
Replacement therapy, for maintenance of spermatogenesis, 279
Reproductive biology, systems analysis approach to, 73–82
Reproductive duct system, development of, 42
Reproductive tissue function, blocking of, 241
Reproductive tissues
  androgen binding in, 253–256
  estrogen binding in, 245
  hormonal regulation of protein synthesis in, 240
Research design, for clinical studies, 469–470
Resection, wedge, for induction of ovulation, 54
Reserpine
  effect on reproduction function, 103
  and prolactin release, 106
Respiration, in mammalian semen, 428–429
Retardation, as sign of nucleolar abnormality, 159
Rete testis
  ABP in, 37
  and seminiferous tubules, 338–339
  spermatozoa in, 386
Rete testis fluid (RTF)
  concentration of spermatozoa in, 340
  concentration of various substances in, 342
Retroprogestogen, as contraceptive, 206
Rhesus monkeys. *See also* Monkeys; Primates
  inhibitors in seminal plasma of, 386
  vaginal "cocktail" in, 98
RIAs. *See* Radioimmunoassays
Ribonucleic acid (RNA) synthesis
  effect of receptor complex on, 249, 256

Ribonucleic acid (RNA)
  synthesis (continued)
  estrogen stimulation of, 238
  FSH-induced, 281
  hormonal effects on, 140
  in spermatogenesis, 296
Ribonucleoprotein (RNP), 255
Ritodrine, and premature labor, 150
RNA. See Ribonucleic acid
RNP. See Ribonucleoprotein
Rodents. See also Mouse; Rat
  coagulating gland in, 402, 406, 407
  female sexual receptivity in, 99
  spermatozoa of, 365, 436
RTF. See Rete testis fluid

Saf-T-Coil (IUD)
  insertion of, 196
  postpartum insertion of, 190
Salicylates, and male accessory secretions, 429
Salicylic acid, in RTF, 345
Salpingitis, IUD-associated, 197
Seasonal variation
  and ovarian function, 56
  in prolactin levels, 30
Seminal plasma
  active factor in, 437–438
  antigenicity of, 430–431
  decapacitation factor in, 389
  inhibitors in, 386
Seminal vesicles, 402
  biochemical characteristics of, 403
  cytological structure of, 402–403
Seminiferous tubules
  effects of hormones on, 281–282
  inhibition of function of, 38–39
  layers of, 346
  and Leydig cells, 322
  rate of penetration of substances into, 342
  and rete testis, 338–339
  and size of testis, 332
Serotonin, 93, 103
  concentrations of, 104
  and control of gonadotropin release, 95
  and prolactin release, 28
  synthesis of, 105
Sertoli cells, 33
  characteristics of, 302
  cytoplasmic matrix of, 307–309
  cytoplasmic organelles, 305–307
  FSH bound to, 282
  and germ cells, 300
  localization of FSH in, 281
  meiosis-inducing effect of, 249
  nucleus of, 304–305
  phagocytic function of, 310
  response to injury of, 316
  in ruminants, 305–307
  secretory functions of, 313–315
  and spermatogenesis, 281–282
  and sperm release, 309–310
  ultrastructure of, 304–309
Sertoli-Sertoli cell junction, 347
Sex chromosomes, in spermatogenesis, 296
Sex glands, mammalian accessory, 402–410

Sex-hormone-binding globulin (SHBG), 118
Sexual receptivity, and ovulatory phase, 436
Sex steroids
  measurement of, 273
  ovarian, 115–118
  regulatory function of, 108
Sexual behavior
  and gonadotropin secretion, 97–98
  and LRF activity, 92
Sexual dimorphism, in preoptic region of rat brain, 96
SHBG. See Sex-hormone-binding globulin
Sheep
  capacitation of spermatozoa of, 443
  effect of surgical stress on gonadotropin secretion, 66
  environmental influences on steroid regulations of, 64
  for experimentation, 55–56
  gonadotropin-binding studies in, 258
  internal mechanisms in, 63
  LH of, 2, 14
  neonatal exposure to androgens, 67
  prolactin of, 26
  steroid feedback mechanisms of, 56–72
Sialic acid
  in human chorionic gonadotropin, 13
  reproductive role of, 6
Silastic rubber, for tubal occlusion, 179, 182
Silicone
  for IUD design, 192
  for tubal occlusion, 182
Silver nitrate
  for tubal occlusion, 180–182
  uterine injection of, 185
Sleep. See also Circadian periodicity
  and GH regulation, 125
  and gonadotropin release, 112
  LH reaction during, 6, 61
  and prolactin secretion, 29
Smooth muscle cells, uterine, 148
  action of PGs on, 149
  membrane potential of, 150
Sodium morrhuate, for tubal ligation, 182
Somatomedin, 124
Somatostatin (SRIH), and TSH secretion, 121
Sorbitol, in seminal vesicles, 403
Sparteine sulfate, for termination of pregnancy, 170
Sperm
  bioengineering involvement with, 215
  effects of copper on, 155
  migration of, 154
  morphology of, 463
  in oviduct, 133, 141
  survival time of, 205
Spermatogenesis, 293–301
  action of testosterone on, 273
  agents disrupting, 460

and blood-testis barrier, 348–349
  depression of, 212
  effect of androgen on, 255
  estrogen secretion and, 37
  feedback control on Leydig cells of, 328
  hormonal control of, 278–282
  inhibition of, 38
  pharmacological interference with, 331
  research on, 299–300
  role of Leydig cells in, 322, 334
  role of Sertoli cells in, 281–282
  suppression of, 332, 333
  termination of, 386
Spermatogonia
  active proliferation of, 293
  categories of, 293
Spermatozoa
  abnormalities of, 427
  acrosomes of, 356–359
  agents interfering with maturation of, 460
  aging of, 429
  antigenicity of, 430–431
  axoneme of, 362–363, 364
  capacitation of, 388–391, 434–451
  capping, 373
  charge density in, 367
  coating material of, 391
  collection of, 429
  control of metabolism for, 382
  damage to, 391–394
  ejaculated, 392
  enzymes of, 380–382
  in epididymis, 392
  fertilizing ability of, 411
  fibrous sheath of, 365–366
  flagellar movement of, 453–454
  formation of, 293
  free-cleaving preparation of, 370, 371, 372, 373
  heads of, 355–359
  human, 353
  irreversible changes in, 386–394
  location of enzymes in, 383
  mammalian, 454–456
  maturation of, 386–388, 411, 414
  mechanisms of environmental and structural maintenance for, 381–382
  metabolism of, 139–141, 142, 379–401
  mitochondrial sheath of, 365, 371
  motility of, 452–457
  nuclei of, 355–356
  outer dense fibers of, 363–365
  phagocytic attack on, 195
  primitive, 452
  protein composition of, 452, 455
  senescence of, 391–394
  steroid action on, 420
  structure of, 353–358, 445, 452, 455
  surface of, 366–373, 435
  survival in female tract of, 436
  tails of, 359–366
Sperm banks, human, 432
Spermicides, 355
Sperm production, 38. See also Spermatogenesis

Sperm release, Sertoli cell participation in, 309
Sperm transport, 436
Spironolactone, 242
SRIH. See Somatostatin
Starch gel electrophoresis, 2
Stein-Leventhal syndrome, 50, 53. See also Polycystic ovary syndrome
Stem cells, spermatogonial, 294
Stereotaxic knife, 95
Sterility, and chromosomal anomalies, 196
Sterilization
  female, 178–186
  bioengineering involvement in, 215
  delivery systems for, 183–185
  for fertility regulation, 178
  transcervical approaches to, 185
  vaginal approach for, 186
  male, 129, 185, 331
Steroidal sulfates, 36
Steroid feedback, site of action of, 59–60
Steroid-hormone-producing cells, subcellular compartmentalization in, 33–34
Steroid hormones
  and capacitation, 440
  interaction with receptors in target cells, 247
Steroid molecules, antigenic rendering of, 129
Steroidogenesis, 261
  control of, 36
  enzymes involved in, 271
  hormonal control of, 276
  local (ovarian) effects of steroids on, 61
  by Sertoli cells, 314
Steroids
  and blood-testis barrier, 344
  chemistry of, 35–36
  contraceptive properties of, 46, 211–212, 458–460
  control of ovaries, 55
  epididymal, 417
  follicular, 40, 43
  hypothalamic metabolism of, 117
  immunization against, 46
  measurement of, 37–38
  native vs. synthetic, 124
  negative feedback by, 62
  ovarian, 118
  precursors of, 36
  in RTF, 341
  testicular, 270–278
  in vivo secretion of, 330
Steroid-spermatozoa interactions, 419–420
Steroid therapy, for male contraception, 332
Stilbestrol, as interceptive, 203–204, 205
Stress
  and ACTH secretion, 123
  effect on GH secretion, 125
  and gonadotropin secretion, 97
  prolactins during, 106
  surgical, and gonadotropin secretion, 58–59, 66

Stress (continued)
  and TSH secretions, 121
Subjects
  for clinical trials, 469
  follow-up of, 470
Subunits, gonadotropin, 2–3
Suckling, and prolactin secretion, 105
Sulfonamides
  and male accessory secretions, 429
  in RTF, 345
Superovulation, 49
Systems analysis approach
  to reproductive biology, 73–82
  to steroid feedback mechanisms, 56

TBG (beta globulin), 275
Teflon plugs, 183
Temperature
  and blood-testis barrier, 347
  and fertilizing ability of spermatozoa, 391–392
Teratocarcinomas, production of, 163
Testes
  blood-testis barrier in, 311–313
  composition of fluids within, 338–441
  disorders of, 463–464
  steroid biochemistry in, 325
  steroid biosynthetic pathways in, 272
  steroid secretion by, 36, 37, 38, 274–276
Testicular pathology, in vitro biosynthesis techniques for, 277–278
Testosterone
  action of ICSH on, 276
  as contraceptive agent, 212
  conversion of, 35
  conversion to dihydrotestosterone, 255–256
  conversion of pregnenolone to, 271, 326
  and diagnosis of male infertility, 462–463
  effect on FSH, 267
  and epididymis function, 418
  in hormone-receptor interaction, 253
  intratesticular, 273
  and LH inhibition, 267
  and male homosexuality, 99
  and male infertility, 461
  in replacement therapy, 332
  secretion of, 37
  in seminiferous tubules, 338
  in Sertoli cells, 282
  synthesis of, 33
  in vitro, 276
  in vivo, 276
Testosterone-estrogen binding globulin (TEBG), 58
Testosterone production
  estrogen blockage of, 407
  by Leydig cells, 322
Testosterone synthesis, rate-limiting step in, 321
Tetrabenazine, effect on reproduction function, 103

Tetracyclines, and male accessory secretions, 429
Tetraploidy, 162
Thalidomide, and male accessory secretions, 429
Theca cells
  LH inhibition of, 45
  luteinization of, 42
  steroids in, 40
5-thio-D-glucose, and spermatogenesis, 460
Thyroidectomy, and prolactin levels, 31
Thyroid-stimulating hormone (TSH), 1
  amino acid sequences for subunits of, 15
  hypothalamic inhibition of, 121
  regulatory function of, 120, 121, 123
  stimulation of, 122
Thyrotropin-releasing factor (TRF), isolation of, 90
Thyrotropin-releasing hormone (TRH), 28
  pharmacological effects of, 122
  and prolactin secretion, 120
  psychotropic actions of, 122–123
  structure of, 121
Thyrotropin secretion, control of, 120
Tissue adhesives, hysteroscopic application of, 185
Tissue-fractionation techniques, 408
Tissue to plasma (T/P) ratio, after LRF injection, 111–112
Toxicity, specificity of, 39
TPNH. See Reduced triphosphopyridine nucleotide
Tracer methods, 37
Training programs, 472
Transcription, in reproductive tissues, hormonal regulation of, 238
Transducers, design of, 214–215
TRH. See Thyrotropin-releasing hormone
Triploidy, 162
Trophoblast cells
  development of, 157, 158
  giant cell transformation of, 161–162
Trypsin inhibitors, and fertilization, 447
TSH. See Thyroid-stimulating hormone
Tubal ligation. See also Sterilization
  methods of, 178
  reversibility of, 185
Tuberoinfundibular (TIDA) system, 96
Tubuli recti. See Rete testis
Tumors
  GH-secreting, 126
  pituitary, 50
  prolactin-secreting, 31
Turner's syndrome, 55
Tyrosyl residues, in biological activity of hCG, 18

Uterine cavity, infiltration of leukocytes into, 190
Uterine cell stretch, mechanisms of, 147, 148
Uterine flushings, 153
Uterine lumen, measurement of, 215
Uteroglobin (blastokinin), antigenic activity of, 153, 175
Uterotubal junction
  bioengineering involvement with, 215
  and gamete transport, 133
Uterus. See also Endometrium; Myometrium
  bioengineering involvement with, 215
  biology of, 146–156
  capacitation of spermatozoa in, 437–438
  catecholamines in, 151
  contractility of, 226
  decidualization of, 152
  effect of luteolytic substances on, 174
  endogenous PG synthesis by, 224
  perforation of, 197
  PG production in, 224–225
  retention of radioactive hormone by, 246
  vascular dynamics of, 151

Vacuum aspiration, for induced abortion, 167. See also Abortion
Vagina
  mucus secretion in, 154–155
  retention of radioactive hormone by, 246
Vaginitis, and ovarian response to hPG, 52
Varicocele, and infertility, 463
Vasculature, and follicular growth, 40
Vasectomy
  advantages of, 185
  and Leydig cell function, 331
  medical sequelae of, 129
Vasopressin, and uterine contraction, 227
Vesiculase, in coagulating gland, 406
Virilization, androgen levels in, 276
Vitelline membrane, and sperm enzymes, 385

World Health Organization (WHO), 212
  injectable contraceptive research of, 209
  Karolinska Symposia of, 128
  research on induced abortion, 168

Yeast extracts, abortifacient action of, 175
Ypsilon (IUD), development of, 194

Zinc
  antifertility effects of, 192
  intrauterine, 192

Zinc chloride, for tubal occlusion, 180
Zona pellucida, 374
  and fertility control, 448
  and sperm enzymes, 385
Zonulae adherentes, 303
Zonulae occludentes, 311
Zygote, and oviductal function, 142. See also Gametes
Zygotene, in spermatogenesis, 295–296